K.J. Lee's Essential Otolaryngology

Notice

K.J. Lee's Essential Otolaryngology

Head and Neck Surgery

Thirteenth Edition

Edited by

YVONNE CHAN, MD, FRCSC, MSc, FARS
Professor and Vice-Chair Education
Otolaryngologist-in-chief, St. Michael's Hospital
Department of Otolaryngology—Head & Neck Surgery
University of Toronto
Toronto, Ontario, Canada

JOHN C. GODDARD, MD
Otology, Neurotology, and Skull Base Surgery
Department of Otolaryngology—Head and Neck Surgery
Northwest Permanente, PC
Portland, Oregon

DERRICK T. LIN, MD, FACS (Guest Editor)
Daniel Miller Professor and Executive Vice-Chair
Department of Otolaryngology, Head and Neck Surgery
Harvard Medical School
Massachusetts Eye and Ear
Mass General Brigham
Boston, Massachusetts

Mc
Graw
Hill

K.J. Lee's Essential Otolaryngology, Thirteenth Edition

1 2 3 4 5 LBC 30 29 28 27 26

ISBN 978-1-266-09215-2
MHID 1-266-09215-3

This book was set in Minion Pro by KnowledgeWorks Global Ltd.
The editor was Sydney Keen Vitale.
The production supervisor was Catherine Saggese.
The digital production manager was Steve Brown.
Project management was provided by Rishi Arora, KnowledgeWorks Global Ltd.
This book is printed on acid-free paper.

Library of Congress Control Number: 2026940551

Contents

Contributors

Nithin D. Adappa, MD [24]
Professor & Vice Chair of Clinical Operations
Department of Otorhinolaryngology
University of Pennsylvania
Division of Rhinology & Skull Base Surgery
Philadelphia, Pennsylvania

Amr H. A. Ahmed, MD, MMSc. [37]
Research Scientist
Division of Thyroid and Parathyroid Endocrine Surgery
Department of Otolaryngology—Head & Neck Surgery
Harvard Medical School
Boston, Massachusetts

Nasser Almutairi, MD [54]
Pediatric Otolaryngology Fellow
Montreal Children's Hospital
McGill University
Montreal, Quebec, Canada

ENT Consultant
King Saud University
Riyadh, Saudi Arabia

Michael Armstrong, MD [10, 30]
Department of Otolaryngology—Head and Neck Surgery
Virginia Commonwealth University (VCU) School of Medicine
Richmond, Virginia

Jamil Asaria, MD [55]
Clinical Lecturer
Division of Facial Plastic and Reconstructive Surgery
Department of Otolaryngology—Head & Neck Surgery
University of Toronto
Director
FACE Toronto
Toronto, Ontario, Canada

Seilesh C. Babu, MD [15]
President and Senior Partner
Michigan Ear Institute
Farmington Hills, Michigan

Caroline A. Banks, MD [19]
Facial Plastic and Reconstructive Surgery
Clinical Associate
Instructor in Otolaryngology
Otolaryngology/Head and Neck Surgery
Massachusetts Eye and Ear Infirmary
Harvard Medical School
Boston, Massachusetts

Pete S. Batra, MD, FACS, FARS [28]
Stanton A. Friedberg, MD Chair in Otolaryngology
Professor and Chairman
Department of Otorhinolaryngology–Head and Neck Surgery
Rush University Medical Center
Chicago, Illinois

Benjamin S. Bleier, MD, FACS, FARS [32]
Professor
Claire and John Bertucci Chair in OHNS
Director of Translational Research
Director of Endoscopic Skull Base Surgery
Director (Co) of Center for Orbital Surgery
Department of Otolaryngology
Harvard Medical School
Boston, Massachusetts

Ciersten Burks, MD [57]
Facial Plastic and Reconstructive Surgery
Harvard Medical School
Mass General Brigham
Boston, Massachusetts

J. Kenneth Byrd, MD, FACS [9, 35]
Associate Professor
Chief
Division of Head and Neck Surgery
Department of Otolaryngology
Medical College of Georgia at Augusta University
Augusta, Georgia

Claudio Callejas, MD [31]
Department of Otolaryngology Head and Neck Surgery
University of Adelaide and Central Adelaide Health Network
South Australia, Australia

Audrey P. Calzada, MD [21]
Otology & Neurotology
California Head and Neck Specialists
San Diego, California

Matthew L. Carlson, MD [18]
Associate Professor of Otolaryngology
Medical Director Cochlear Implant Program
Department of Otolaryngology, Mayo Clinic
Rochester, Minnesota

Yvonne Chan, MD, FRCSC, MSc, FARS [11, 26]
Otolaryngologist-in-Chief
St. Michael's Hospital
Unity Health
Vice Chair Education
Professor
Department of Otolaryngology—Head & Neck Surgery
Temerty Faculty of Medicine
University of Toronto
Toronto, Ontario, Canada

Rebecca Chiffer, MD [17]
Assistant Professor
Department of Otolaryngology—Head and Neck Surgery
Division of Otology/Neurotology
Thomas Jefferson University Hospital
Philadelphia, Pennsylvania

Jerlon Chiu, MD [25]
Ear, Nose, and Throat Institute of Connecticut
Farmington, Connecticut

Marc A. Cohen, MD, MPH [49]
Associate Attending
Memorial Sloan Kettering Cancer Center
New York, New York

Michelle Coppola, AuD [13]
Department of Otolaryngology
University of Miami Miller School of Medicine
Miami, Florida

Sam J. Daniel, MDCM, FRCSC, CPC(HC) [54]
Chair
Chair, Department of Pediatric Surgery
Surgeon-in-Chief, The Montreal Children's Hospital, McGill University Health Centre
Professor, Departments of Pediatric Surgery and Otolaryngology–Head and Neck Surgery
McGill University
Senior Scientist, Child Health and Human Development Program, Centre for Translational Biology, Research Institute of the McGill University Health Centre (RI-MUHC)
Director, McGill Otolaryngology Sciences Laboratory
Montreal, Quebec, Canada

Lillian Datillo, MD [57]
Resident, Harvard Combined Otolaryngology Program
Department of Otolaryngology—Head and Neck Surgery
Boston, Massachusetts

Joel Davies, MD [40]
Resident, Department of Otolaryngology—Head and Neck Surgery
University of Toronto
Toronto, Ontario, Canada

Nicholas L. Deep, MD [18]
Resident Physician
Department of Otolaryngology, Mayo Clinic Arizona
Phoenix, Arizona

Daniel G. Deschler, MD, FACS [33]
Professor of Otolaryngology—Head and Neck Surgery
Harvard Medical School
Vice Chair
Academic Affairs
Mass Eye and Ear
Mass General Hospital
Boston, Massachusetts

Colin L. W. Driscoll, MD [18]
Professor and Chair
Department of Otolaryngology, Mayo Clinic
Rochester, Minnesota

Glen D'Souza, MD [28]
Fellow
Department of Otorhinolaryngology—Head and Neck Surgery
Rush University Medical Center
Chicago, Illinois

Caoimhe C. Duffy, MD, MSc [4]
Department of Otorhinolaryngology–Head and Neck Surgery
Hospital of the University of Pennsylvania
Perelman School of Medicine, University of Pennsylvania
Philadelphia, Pennsylvania

Charles S. Ebert, Jr, MD, MPH FACS, FARS, FAAOA [10]
Co-Director, NeuroRhinology—Advanced Rhinology and Endoscopic Skull Base Surgery Fellowship
Medical Director of Otolaryngic Allergy Services
Professor
Department of Otolaryngology-Head & Neck Surgery
Chapel Hill, North Carolina

Carole Fakhry, MD, MPH [44]
Professor, Department of Otolaryngolgoy
Johns Hopkins School of Medicine
Baltimore, Maryland

Jessica Feinleib, MD, PhD, FASA, CHSE [4]
Assistant Professor
Department of Anesthesiology
National Faculty Veterans Health Administration
Yale School of Medicine
West Haven, Connecticut

John C. Goddard, MD [12, 16]
Otology, Neurotology, and Skull Base Surgery
Department of Otolaryngology—Head and Neck Surgery
Northwest Permanente, PC
Portland, Oregon

Christopher Griffith, MD, PhD [29]
Staff Physician
Department of Pathology
Cleveland Clinic
Cleveland, Ohio

Paavali A. Hannikainen, MD [58]
Resident Physician
Department of Otolaryngology—Head & Neck Surgery
Northwestern University Feinberg School of Medicine
Chicago, Illinois

Meredith Holcomb, AuD [13]
Director
Hearing Implant Program
Associate Professor
Department of Otolaryngology
University of Miami
Miami, Florida

Amanda Hu, MD, FRCSC [50]
Clinical Associate Professor
Laryngologist, Director of the Pacific Voice Clinic
Division of Otolaryngology, Department of Surgery
University of British Columbia
Vancouver General Hospital
Vancouver, British Columbia, Canada

Jacob B. Hunter, MD [17]
Department of Otolaryngology—Head and Neck Surgery
University of Texas Southwestern Medical Center
Dallas, Texas

Ali Jamshidi, MD [6]
The Ohio State University
Department of Neurological Surgery
Columbus, Ohio

Courtney A. Jatana, DDS [38]
Associate Professor
Division of Oral and Maxillofacial Surgery
Ohio State University College of Dentistry
Columbus, Ohio

Kris R. Jatana, MD [38]
Professor
Department of Otolaryngology—Head and Neck Surgery
Nationwide Children's Hospital and Wexner Medical Center at Ohio State University
Columbus, Ohio

Patricia G. Johnson, MD [58]
Rhinology/Skull Base Surgery
Assistant Professor of Otolaryngology—Head and Neck Surgery
New York Medical College
Westchester Medical Center
Valhalla, New York

Matthew J. Kabalan, MD [29]
Clinical Fellow
Head & Neck Institute
Section of Rhinology
Cleveland Clinic
Cleveland, Ohio

Omar Karadaghy, MD [56]
Assistant Professor, Otolaryngology—Head and Neck Surgery
Associate Director, head and Neck Surgery Fellowship Program
Director, Minimally Invasive Head and Neck Surgery
Kansas University Medical Center

Dennis H. Kraus, MD, FACS [49]
Director, New York Head and Neck Institute
Center for Head and Neck Oncology
NS-LIJ Cancer Institute
Professor of Otolaryngology
Hofstra North Shore-LIJ School of Medicine
Hempstead, New York

Andrew P. Lane, MD [25]
Professor
Department of Otolaryngology—Head and Neck Surgery
Director
Division of Rhinology
Skull Base and Sinus Surgery
Johns Hopkins School of Medicine
Baltimore, Maryland

Andrew R. Larson, MD [33]
Assistant Professor
Kaiser Permanente Los Angeles Medical Center
Los Angeles, California

Daniel J. Lee, MD, FRCSC [24]
Lecturer
Division of Rhinology
Department of Otolaryngology—Head & Neck Surgery
St. Michael's Hospital
Unity Health Toronto
North York General Hospital
University of Toronto
Toronto, Ontario, Canada

K. J. Lee, MD, FACS [1, 7, 12, 15, 52]
Associate Clinical Professor
Yale University School of Medicine
Adjunct Associate Clinical Professor
Hofstra University School of Medicine
Emeritus Chief of Otolaryngology
Hospital of St. Raphael
Chief Medical and Experience Officer
IQ-EQ Systems
Intelligent Cloud and Advisory Group
New Haven, Connecticut

Lauren K. Leeper, MD [53]
Department of Otolaryngology—Head and Neck Surgery
University of North Carolina at Chapel Hill School of Medicine
Chapel Hill, North Carolina

Derrick T. Lin, MD, FACS
Daniel Miller Professor and Executive Vice-Chair
Department of Otolaryngology, Head and Neck Surgery
Harvard Medical School
Massachusetts Eye and Ear
Mass General Brigham
Boston, Massachusetts

R. Jun Lin, MD [51]
Associate Professor
Department of Otolaryngology—Head & Neck Surgery
Temerty Faculty of Medicine
University of Toronto
Unity Health Toronto—St. Michael's Hospital
Toronto, Ontario, Canada

Sallie Long, MD [35]
Assistant Professor
Department of Otolaryngology—Head & Neck Surgery
Medical College of Georgia
Augusta, Georgia

Zhonghui Katie Luo, MD, PhD [8]
Assistant Professor
Harvard Medical School
Massachusetts Eye & Ear Infirmary
Boston, Massachusetts

Jordan McNair, AuD [13]
Department of Otolaryngology
University of Miami Miller School of Medicine
Miami, Florida

Tanya K. Meyer, MD [50]
Professor and Residency Program Director
UW Department of Otolaryngology-HNS
University of Washington Medical Center
Seattle, Washington

Theodore R. McRackan, MD [16, 20]
Professor
Director, Skull Base Center
Medical Director, Cochlear Implant Program
Department of Otolaryngology—Head and Neck Surgery
Medical University of South Carolina
Charleston, South Carolina

Ross Merkin, MD [46]
Instructor of Medicine, Harvard Medical School
Assistant in Medicine, Massachusetts General Hospital
Boston, Massachusetts

David Macias, MD [59]
Department of Otolaryngology—Head and Neck Surgery
Northwest Permanente, P.C.
Kaiser Permanente Northwest
Clackamas, Oregon

Alexander Moise, MD [50]
Resident Physician
Division of Otolaryngology
Department of Surgery
University of British Columbia
Vancouver General Hospital
Vancouver, British Columbia, Canada

Eric Monteiro, MD, MSc, FRCSC [40]
Associate Professor
Department of Otolaryngology–Head & Neck Surgery
Temerty Faculty of Medicine, University of Toronto
Otolaryngologist-in-Chief
Department of Otolaryngology–Head & Neck Surgery, Sinai Health
Toronto, Ontario, Canada

Ethan Moritz, MD [55]
Fellow
Division of Facial Plastic and Reconstructive Surgery
Department of Otolaryngology—Head & Neck Surgery
University of Toronto
FACE Toronto
Toronto, Ontario, Canada

James Netterville, MD [39]
Mark C. Smith Professor of Head and Neck Oncology
Vanderbilt University Medical Center
Nashville, Tennessee

João Flavio Nogueira, Jr., MD [22]
Director Sinus and Oto Centro
Department of Otolaryngology—Head and Neck Surgery
Ceara State University
Fortaleza, Ceara

Sarah C. Nyirjesy, MD [5]
Assistant Professor or Otolaryngology-Head and Neck Surgery
Boston University Chobanian and Avedisian School of Medicine
Boston, Massachusetts
(acknowledge John E. Godwin, MD, past author)

Ostap Orishchak, MD [54]
Pediatric Otolaryngology Fellow
Montreal Children's Hospital
McGill University
Montreal, Quebec, Canada

Thomas J. Ow, MD, FACS [42]
Associate Attending
Memorial Sloan Kettering Cancer Center
Associate Professor
Montefiore Medical Center
Albert Einstein College of Medicine
Department of Otorhinolaryngology—Head and Neck Surgery
and Department of Pathology
Bronx, New York

Jonathan Paly, DO [47]
Instructor in Radiation Oncology
Harvard Medical School
Massachusetts General Brigham
Boston, Massachusetts

Kenny P. Pang, MD [2]
Consultant, Otorhinolaryngology–Head and Neck Surgery
Clinical Director
Asia Sleep Centre
Singapore

Sathish Paramasivan, MBBS, BMedSci (Hons), MPH, PhD, FRACS (ORL-HNS) [32]
Rhinology/Skull Base Fellow
Clinical Lecturer
Department of Otolaryngology, Head and Neck Surgery
Massachusetts Eye and Ear Infirmary
Harvard Medical School
The University of Adelaide
South Australia, Australia

Jong Park, MD [46]
Assistant Professor
Medicine-Hematology and Medical Oncology
Harvard Medical School
Massachusetts General Brigham
Boston, Massachusetts

Justine Philteos, MD [36]
Assistant Professor
University of Toronto Medical Center
Toronto, Ontario, Canada

Daniel M. Prevedello, MD [6]
Department of Neurosurgery
Ohio State University Medical Center
Columbus, Ohio

Natasha Pollak, MD, MS [3]
Professor-Depatment of Oto-HNS
Lewis Katz School of Medicine
Temple University
Philadelphia, Pennsylvania

Alkis J. Psaltis, MD [31]
Professor
Department of Otolaryngology Head and Neck Surgery
University of Adelaide and Central Adelaide Health Network
South Australia, Australia

Madeline Pyle, MD [34]
Resident, University of Miami Miller School of Medicine
Miami, Florida

Gregory W. Randolph, MD, FACS, FACE [37]
Director of the General and Thyroid-Parathyroid
Endocrine Surgical Divisions
Mass Eye and Ear Infirmary
Member Endocrine Surgery Service
Mass General Hospital
Boston, Massachusetts

Sarah L. Rohde, MD, MMHC [39]
Associate Professor of Otolaryngology-Head and Neck Surgery
Vanderbilt University Medical Center
Nashville, Tennessee

Sanjeet Rangarajan MD, M Eng. [26]
Associate Professor
Division of Rhinology and Endoscopic Skull Base Surgery
Vice Chair
Innovation and Community Partnerships
Department of Otolaryngology—Head and Neck Surgery
University Hospitals Cleveland Medical Center
Case Western Reserve University School of Medicine
Memphis, Tennessee

Habib Rizk, MD [14]
Associate Professor
Department of Otolaryngology—Head and Neck Surgery
Medical University of South Carolina
Charleston, South Carolina

Allan Rodrigues, MD [7]
Attending Physician
Pulmonary and Critical Care Medicine
Yale New Haven Hospital—Saint Raphael Campus
New Haven, Connecticut

Clark A. Rosen, MD [51]
UCSF Voice and Swallowing Center
Division of Laryngology, Department of Otolaryngology—Head & Neck Surgery
University of California San Francisco
San Francisco, California

Brian W. Rotenberg, MD [2]
Professor-OtoHNS Surgery
Schulich School of Medicine and Dentistry
Western University
London, Ontario, Canada

Zoukaa Sargi, MD, MPH [34]
Professor and Vice Chair for Quality, Performance Improvement, and Value
Department of Otolaryngology
University of Miami
Miami, Florida

Cecelia E. Schmalbach, MD, MSc, FACS [41]
Professor of Otolaryngology—Head & Neck Surgery
Indiana University School of Medicine
Roudebush VA Medical Center
Fesler Hall
Indianapolis, Indiana

Joseph S. Schwartz, MD, FRCSC [24]
Assistant Professor
Rhinology and Skull Base Surgery
Department of Otolaryngology—Head and Neck Surgery
McGill University
Montreal, Canada

Brent A. Senior, MD, FACS, FARS [30]
Harold C. Pillsbury, III Distinguished Professor
Otolaryngology/Head and Neck Surgery
Chief
Rhinology, Allergy, and Endoscopic Skull Base Surgery
University of North Carolina at Chapel Hill
Chapel Hill, North Carolina

Justin Shapiro, MD, MSc [11]
Resident Physician
Department of Otolaryngology—Head & Neck Surgery
Schulich School of Medicine & Dentistry
Western University
Toronto, Ontario, Canada

Raj Sindwani, MD [29]
Vice Chairman
Head and Neck Institute
Professor of Otolaryngology and Neurological Surgery
Cleveland Clinic Lerner College of Medicine (CCLCM)
Co-Director
Minimally Invasive Cranial Base & Pituitary Surgery Program
Burkhardt Brain Tumor & Neuro-Oncology Center
Cleveland Clinic
Cleveland, Ohio

Miriam Smetak, MD [23]
Department of Otolaryngology—Head and Neck Surgery
Washington University School of Medicine in St. Louis
St. Louis, Missouri

Joshua Smith, MD [45]
Assistant Professor, Department of Otolaryngology—Head & Neck Surgery
VA Pittsburgh Healthcare System
University of Pittsburgh Medical Center
Pittsburgh, Pennsylvania

Nizar Taki, MD [55]
Staff Otolaryngologist
Eastern Maine Medical Center
Bangor, Maine

Kenric Tam, MD [43]
Head and Neck Fellow
Memorial Sloan-Kettering Cancer Center
New York, New York

Elina Toskala-Kennedy, MD, PhD, MBA [58]
Professor
Vice Chair, Faculty Affairs
Director of Allergy
Department of Otolaryngology, Head & Neck Surgery
Thomas Jefferson University Hospital
Philadelphia, Pennsylvania

Danielle Trakimas, MD, MSE [44]
Resident Physician
Department of Otolaryngology—Head and Neck Surgery
Johns Hopkins School of Medicine
Baltimore, Maryland

Courtney C. J. Voelker, MD [21]
Pacific Neuroscience Institute
Providence Saint John's Health Center
Santa Monica, California

Randall S. Weber MD, FACS [42]
Professor of Surgery and Perioperative Care
Department of Surgery
The University of Texas at Austin
Dell Medical School
Austin, Texas

Kevin C. Welch, MD, FACS, FARS [27]
Professor
President, American Rhinologic Society
Rhinology & Skull Base Surgery
Department of Otolaryngology—Head & Neck Surgery
Northwestern University
Feinberg School of Medicine
Chicago, Illinois

Cameron Wick, MD [23]
Otologist/Neurotologist
University Hospitals Cleveland Medical Center
Associate Professor
Department of Otolaryngology—Head and Neck Surgery
Case Western Reserve University School of Medicine
Cleveland, Ohio

Lori Wirth, MD [46]
Professor
Medicine-Hematology and Medical Oncology
Harvard Medical School
Massachusetts General Brigham
Boston, Massachusetts

Richard Wong, MD, FACS [43]
Chief, Head and Neck Service
Memorial Sloan Kettering Cancer Center
New York, New York

Juan Carlos Yanez-Siller, MD [27]
Fellow
Department of Otolaryngology—Head & Neck Surgery
Northwestern University
Feinberg School of Medicine
Chicago, Illinois

Wendell G. Yarbrough, MD, FACS, MMHC [48]
Thomas J. Dark Distinguished Professor and Chair
Department of Otolaryngology/Head and Neck Surgery
UNC School of Medicine
Professor and Chief, Otolaryngology Yale
Co-Director, Molecular Virology Program Yale Cancer Center
Director, Head and Neck Disease Center, Smilow Cancer Hospital
New Haven, Connecticut

Daniel M. Zeitler, MD, FACS [20]
Staff Surgeon
Department of Otolaryngology/Head and Neck Surgery
Virginia Mason Medical Center
Clinical Faculty
Department of Otolaryngology/Head and Neck Surgery
University of Washington
Seattle, Washington

Joseph Zevallos, MD, MPH, FACS [45]
Eugene N. Myers, M.D., Professor and Chair
Department of Otolaryngology-Head and Neck Surgery
Interim Deputy Director, UPMC Hillman Cancer Center
University of Pittsburgh Medical Center
Eye and Ear Institute,
Pittsburgh, Pennsylvania

Preface

I finished my Otolaryngology-Head and Neck Surgery Residency at Massachusetts Eye and Ear Infirmary (MEEI), at Harvard, in 1970. Thereafter, I was drafted by the US Army to serve at the Madigan General Hospital in Fort Lewis, Tacoma, Washington. Madigan was just starting a residency training program in Otolaryngology-Head and Neck Surgery. When I studied for my Otolaryngology Board Exam, I read the most recent 5 years of the Laryngoscope and ORL journals, as well as all the textbooks I could find. My wife, Linda, helped not only by locating these journals and books, but she sped up the process by reading them and made "script notes" for me. When I was President of the American Academy of Otolaryngology-Head and Neck Surgery, in 2002, at the Opening Ceremony podium, I announced that Linda "wrote half the book." That was the birth of *Essential Otolaryngology-Head and Neck Surgery*, now in its 13th edition.

Initially, Linda and I did all of the revisions, with Linda doing the typing and proofreading. Since the 11th edition, Dr. Yvonne Chan and Dr. John Goddard have been coeditors. Dr. Derrick Lin joined the team as an associate editor during this most recent, 13th edition.

K. J. Lee's Essential Otolaryngology has been considered by the publishing industry to be one of the most read texts in its field in all the world. It has been translated into many languages. In some countries, it is the "core text" in Otolaryngology-Head and Neck Surgery for their medical school. The first edition was published when I was 31 years old.

I would like to express my sincere appreciation to Yvonne, John, and Derrick for their outstanding collaboration, scholarly rigor, and unwavering commitment to uphold and advance the longstanding tradition of this text, which has been in continuous circulation for 53 years. Some have called it the "Grant's Anatomy" in ENT.

K. J. Lee, MD, FACS*

*Dr. Lee was born in 1940, in Malaya, of Chinese descent.

Acknowledgments

For this 13th edition, I want to thank our two editors, Dr. Yvonne Chan and Dr. John Goddard, who have done a tremendous job. Particularly, I would like to thank the one person who has been by my side, even before the appearance of the very first edition of this book in 1973—my lovely and devoted wife of 53 years, Linda. Our three sons, Ken, Lloyd and Mark, used to help with editorial assistance, but are now busy with their respective professions, law, private equity and media consultant; Jeannie Grenier, my nurse for over 35 years and editorial associate, worked hard on previous editions. I thank the McGraw-Hill staff for their diligence, great work, and congeniality.

I thank my parents for the gene and nurturing environment that allowed me to develop a passion for hard work, a sense for organization, and an ability to distill complex materials into simple facts. These are the three cornerstones that have shaped this book from the first edition. I am thrilled to see these traits are also inherent in Yvonne and John.

And to those newcomers at the frontiers of medical science who have contributed greatly to this edition, I also extend my thanks for taking the time to share their own expertise and, in doing so, helping to keep this book up-to-date.

We are so proud of Yvonne and John.

—K. J. Lee

I would like to thank the many authors who volunteered their time and expertise to help make this book possible. I am indebted to my talented co-editor Dr. John Goddard for his organizational mastery to keep us on track through the planning and editing process. "I would also like to acknowledge our new Guest Editor, Dr. Derrick Lin, whose expertise and leadership were instrumental in the comprehensive modernization of the Head and Neck Surgery section of this edition." I am so grateful to my mentor Dr. K. J. Lee for his ongoing guidance and support over the years as well as his belief in me to work alongside him on so many projects. It is indeed a great honor to be part of the legacy that is "*K. J. Lee's Essential Otolaryngology*." "I am especially appreciative to my fellowship directors, Drs Fred Kuhn, Peter-John Wormald, and Alkis J. Psaltis, whose mentorship extended far beyond surgical training, teaching me to think critically, embrace new perspectives, and continually challenge myself to grow, and whose enduring impact on my career continues to inspire me." Last but not least, I would like to thank my family, especially my parents, Dexter and Phoebe, without their love and support, I would not be who I am today.

—Yvonne Chan

I continue to be honored and humbled to participate in the editing and writing of '*K. J. Lee's Essential Otolaryngology*,' now in the 13th edition. Working alongside Dr. Yvonne Chan, and more recently Dr. Derrick Lin, has been a true joy and I am thankful for the knowledge, effort, and professionalism they bring to this work. I would also like to thank Dr. K. J. Lee for his tireless commitment to this work, and for the vision he has always shown in making this book such a remarkable source of information for all those seeking to learn more about our great field. Finally, I'd like to acknowledge my sons, Luke and Henry, who continue to inspire me to be the best that I can be.

—John C. Goddard, MD

Part 1
General Otolaryngology

Chapter 1
Syndromes and Eponyms

Syndromes and Diseases

Adult Respiratory Distress Syndrome

Adult respiratory distress syndrome (ARDS) is characterized by a delay in onset (12-24 hours) following injury, shock, and/or successful resuscitative effort. Septic shock, extrathoracic trauma, central nervous system (CNS) pathology, fat embolism, oxygen toxicity, head and facial injuries, and massive blood transfusions can lead to ARDS. It is characterized by hypoxia and pulmonary infiltrates secondary to increased pulmonary vascular permeability, microvascular hemorrhage, or both.

Aide Syndrome

Aide syndrome is characterized by decreased pupillary reaction and deep tendon reflex. The etiology is unknown.

Alagille Syndrome

Alagille syndrome is marked by cardiovascular abnormalities, characteristic facial appearance, chronic cholestasis, growth retardation, hypogonadism, mental retardation, vertebral arch defect, temporal bone anomalies in the cochlear aqueduct, ossicles, semicircular canals (SCCs), and subarcuate fossa. Liver transplantation is a possible treatment.

Albers-Schönberg Disease

Albers-Schönberg disease is a genetic disorder also known as osteopetrosis which results in a progressive increase in the density (but also increase in weakness) of the bones in the skeletal system. Vascular nutrition to affected bones is also decreased by this disease. Broken down into three categories, there is osteopetrosis with precocious manifestations, osteopetrosis with delayed manifestations, and pyknodysostosis. In the mandible, treatments include long-term antibiotic therapy, multiple debridements, sequestrectomies, and resection.

Albright Syndrome

Polyostotic fibrous dysplasia usually manifests early in life as multicentric lesions involving the long bones and bones of the face and skull with scattered skin lesions similar to melanotic café au lait spots and precocious puberty in female patients. Frequently, there is an elevation of serum alkaline phosphatase as well as endocrine abnormalities.

Aldrich Syndrome

Thrombocytopenia, eczema, and recurrent infections occur during the first year of life. It is inherited through a sex-linked recessive gene. The bleeding time is prolonged, the platelet count is decreased, and the bone marrow megakaryocytes are normal in number.

Amalric Syndrome

Granular macular pigment epitheliopathy (foveal dystrophy) is associated with sensorineural hearing loss. Visual acuity is usually normal. It may be a genetic disorder or the result of an intrauterine rubella infection.

Aortic Arch Syndrome

See Takayasu Disease.

Apert Syndrome

Apert syndrome is not to be confused with Pfeiffer syndrome, which has different types of hand malformations.

Ascher Syndrome

Ascher syndrome is a combination of blepharochalasis, double lip, and goiter.

Auriculotemporal Syndrome (Frey Syndrome)

Auriculotemporal syndrome is characterized by localized flushing and sweating of the ear and cheek region in response to eating. It usually occurs after parotidectomy. Parasympathetic fibers of the ninth nerve innervate the sweat glands after parotidectomy.

Avellis Syndrome

Avellis syndrome is unilateral paralysis of the larynx and velum palati, with contralateral loss of pain and temperature sensitivity in the parts below the larynx. The syndrome is caused by involvement of the nucleus ambiguus or the vagus nerve along with the cranial portion of the ninth nerve.

Babinski-Nageotte Syndrome

Babinski-Nageotte syndrome is caused by multiple or scattered lesions, chiefly in the distribution of the vertebral artery. Ipsilateral paralysis of the soft palate, larynx, pharynx, and sometimes tongue occurs. There is also ipsilateral loss of taste on the posterior third of the tongue, loss of pain and temperature sensation around the face, and cerebellar asynergia. Horner syndrome with contralateral spastic hemiplegia and loss of proprioceptive and tactile sensation may also be present.

Baelz Syndrome

Painless papules at the openings of the ducts of the mucous glands of the lips with free exudation of mucus are characteristic of Baelz syndrome. Congenital and familial forms are precancerous. Acquired forms are benign and caused by irritating substances.

Bannwarth Syndrome (Facial Palsy in Lymphocytic Meningoradiculitis)

A relatively benign form of acute unilateral or bilateral facial palsy that is associated with lymphocytic reactions and an increased protein level in the cerebrospinal fluid (CSF) with minimal, if any, meningeal symptoms are known as Bannwarth syndrome. Neuralgic or radicular pain without facial palsy and unilateral or bilateral facial palsy of acute onset are symptoms of this syndrome. A virus has been suggested as a possible etiology. Males are more often affected than females, with the greatest number of cases occurring in the months of August and September.

Barany Syndrome

Barany syndrome is a combination of unilateral headache in the back of the head, periodic ipsilateral deafness (alternating with periods of unaffected hearing), vertigo, and tinnitus. The syndrome complex may be corrected by induced nystagmus.

Barclay-Baron Disease

Vallecular dysphagia is present.

Barre-Lieou Syndrome

Occipital headache, vertigo, tinnitus, vasomotor disorders, and facial spasm due to irritation of the sympathetic plexus around the vertebral artery in rheumatic disorders of the cervical spine are characteristic. It is also known as cervical migraine.

Barrett Syndrome

Barrett syndrome is characterized by esophagitis due to change in the epithelium of the esophagus.

Barsony-Polgar Syndrome

A diffuse esophageal spasm, caused by disruption of the peristaltic waves by an irregular contraction resulting in dysphagia and regurgitation, is evidence of this syndrome. It most commonly affects excitable elderly persons.

Basal Cell Nevoid Syndrome

This familial syndrome, non–sex-linked and autosomal dominant with high penetrance and variable expressivity, manifests early in life. It appears as multiple nevoid basal cell epitheliomas of the skin, cysts of the jaw, abnormal ribs and metacarpal bones, frontal bossing, and dorsal scoliosis. Endocrine abnormalities have been reported, and they have been associated with medulloblastoma. The cysts in the jaw, present only in the maxilla and mandible, are destructive to the bone. The basal cell epitheliomas are excised as necessary, and the cysts in the jaw rarely recur after complete enucleation.

Bayford-Autenrieth Dysphagia (Arkin Disease)

Dysphagia lusoria is said to be secondary to esophageal compression from an aberrant right subclavian artery.

Beckwith Syndrome

This is a congenital disorder characterized by macroglossia, omphalocele, hypoglycemia, pancreatic hyperplasia, noncystic renal hyperplasia, and cytomegaly of the fetal adrenal cortex.

Behçet Syndrome

Of unknown etiology, this disease runs a protracted course with periods of relapse and remission. It manifests as indolent ulcers of the mucous membrane and skin, stomatitis, as well as anogenital ulceration, iritis, and conjunctivitis. No definitive cure is known, though steroids help.

Besnier-Boeck-Schaumann Syndrome

Sarcoidosis is present.

Bloom Syndrome

Bloom syndrome is an autosomal recessive growth disorder associated with chromosomal breaks and rearrangements. It is also associated with an unusually high rate of cancer at an early age. Associated with facial erythema, growth retardation, immunodeficiency, infertility, and sun sensitivity, diagnosis is confirmed by chromosome analysis. Anomalous numbers of digits or teeth, asymmetric legs, heart malformation, hypopigmented spots in blacks, protruding ears, sacral dimple, simian line, and urethral or meatal narrowing are less common characteristics. For head and neck tumor patients, there is an increased chance of secondary and primary tumors.

Bogorad Syndrome

Bogorad syndrome is also known as the syndrome of crocodile tears, characterized by residual facial paralysis with profuse lacrimation during eating. It is caused by a misdirection of regenerating autonomic fibers to the lacrimal gland instead of to the salivary gland.

Bonnet Syndrome

Sudden trigeminal neuralgia accompanied by Horner syndrome and vasomotor disorders in the area supplied by the trigeminal nerve are manifestations of this syndrome.

Bonnier Syndrome

Bonnier syndrome is caused by a lesion of Deiters nucleus and its connection. Its symptoms include ocular disturbances (eg, paralysis of accommodation, nystagmus, diplopia), deafness, nausea, thirst, and anorexia, as well as other symptoms referable to involvement of the vagal centers, cranial nerves VIII, IX, X, and XI, and the lateral vestibular nucleus. It can simulate Ménière disease.

Bourneville Syndrome

Bourneville syndrome is a familial disorder whose symptoms include polyps of the skin, harelip, moles, spina bifida, and microcephaly.

Bowen Disease

Bowen disease is a precancerous dermatosis characterized by the development of pinkish or brownish papules covered with a thickened horny layer. Histologically, it shows hyperchromatic acanthotic cells with multinucleated giant cells. Mitoses are frequently observed.

Branchio-Oto-Renal Syndrome

Branchio-Oto-Renal syndrome is an autosomal dominant disorder characterized by anomalies of the external, middle, and inner ear in association with preauricular tissues, branchial cleft anomalies, and varying degrees of renal dysplasia, including aplasia. Many of the following symptoms (but not necessarily all) are present:

A. Conductive or mixed hearing loss
B. Cup-shaped, anteverted pinnae with bilateral preauricular sinuses
C. Bilateral branchial cleft fistulas or sinuses
D. Renal dysplasia

This syndrome is among a group of syndromes characterized by deformities associated with the first and second branchial complexes. The precise incidence of the disorder is unknown.

Briquet Syndrome

Briquet Syndrome is characterized by a shortness of breath and aphonia due to hysteric paralysis of the diaphragm.

Brissaud-Marie Syndrome

Unilateral spasm of the tongue and lips of a hysteric nature are characteristic.

Brown Syndrome

Brown syndrome is a congenital or acquired abnormality of the superior oblique muscle tendon characterized by vertical diplopia and the inability to elevate the eye above midline or medial gaze. This syndrome is of two types: true and simulated. True Brown syndrome is always congenital. Simulated Brown syndrome is either congenital or acquired. The congenital simulated type may be caused by thickening of an area in the posterior tendon or by the firm attachment of the posterior sheath to the superior oblique tendon. The acquired simulated type may be caused by inflammation extending from the adjacent ethmoid cells to the posterior sheath and tendon, an orbital floor fracture, frontal ethmoidal fracture, crush fracture of nasal bones, sinusitis, frontal sinus surgery, or surgical tucking of the superior oblique tendon.

Brun Syndrome

Vertigo, headache, vomiting, and visual disturbances due to an obstruction of CSF flow during positional changes of the head are seen. The main causes of this syndrome include cysts and cysticercosis of the fourth ventricle as well as tumors of the midline cerebellum and third ventricle.

Burckhardt Dermatitis

Burckhardt dermatitis appears as an eruption of the external ear. It consists of red papules and vesicles that appear after exposure to sunlight. The rash usually resolves spontaneously.

Caffey Disease (Infantile Cortical Hyperostosis)

Of familial tendency, its onset is usually during the first year of life. It is characterized by hyperirritability, fever, and hard, nonpitting edema that overlie the cortical hyperostosis. Pathologically, it involves the loss of periosteum with acute inflammatory involvement of the intratrabecular bone and the overlying soft tissue. Treatment is supportive, consisting of steroids and antibiotics. The prognosis is good. The mandible is the most frequently involved site.

Caisson Disease

This symptom complex occurs in men and women who work in high air pressures and are returned too suddenly to normal atmospheric pressure. Similar symptoms may occur in fliers when they suddenly ascend to high altitudes unprotected by counterpressure. It results from the escape from solution in the body fluids of bubbles (mainly nitrogen) originally absorbed at higher pressure. Symptoms include headache; pain in the epigastrium, sinuses, and tooth sockets; itchy skin; vertigo; dyspnea; coughing; nausea; vomiting; and sometimes paralysis. Peripheral circulatory collapse may be present. Nitrogen bubbles have been found in the white matter of the spinal cord. It can also injure the inner ear through necrosis of the organ of Corti. There is a question of rupture of the round window membrane; hemotympanum and eustachian tube obstruction may occur.

Camptomelic Syndrome

The name is derived from a Greek word meaning *curvature of extremities*. The syndrome is characterized by dwarfism, craniofacial anomalies, and bowing of the tibia and femur, with malformation of other bones. The patient has cutaneous dimpling overlying the tibial bend. Respiratory distress is common, and the patient has an early demise in the first few months of life. In the otolaryngologic area, the patient exhibits a prominent forehead, flat facies with a broad nasal bridge and low-set ears, cleft palate, mandibular hypoplasia, and tracheobronchial malacia that contributes to the respiratory distress and neonatal death. This syndrome is not to be confused with Pierre Robin syndrome, which presents with very similar clinical features.

Cannon Nevus

This is an autosomal dominant disorder characterized by spongy white lesions of the oral and nasal mucosa. The lesions are asymptomatic and may be found from the newborn period with increasing severity until adolescence. The histologic picture is that of keratosis, acanthosis, and parakeratosis.

Carcinoid Syndrome

The symptoms include episodic flushing, diarrhea, and ascites. The tumor secretes serotonin. Treatment is wide excision. The tumor may give a positive dopa reaction.

Carotid Sinus Syndrome (Charcot-Weiss-Barber Syndrome)

When the carotid sinus is abnormally sensitive, slight pressure on it causes a marked fall in blood pressure due to vasodilation and cardiac slowing. Symptoms include syncope, convulsions, and heart block.

Castleman Disease

First described by Castelman et al in 1954. It is a benign lymphoepithelial disease that is most often mistaken for lymphoma. It is also known as localized nodal hyperplasia, angiomatous lymph node hyperplasia, lymphoid hamartoma, and giant lymph nodal hyperplasia. Symptoms include tracheobronchial compression, such as cough, dyspnea, hemoptysis, or dysphagia. Masses in the neck are also not uncommon. There are two histologic types: the hyaline vascular type and the plasma cell type. Follicles in the hyaline vascular type are traversed by radially oriented capillaries with plump endothelial cells and collagenous hyalinization surrounding the vessels. The follicles in the plasma cell type are normal in size without capillary proliferation or hyalinization. Intermediate forms exist but are rare. Treatment entails complete excision of the mass. Etiology is unknown.

Cavernous Sinus Syndrome

The cavernous sinus receives drainage from the upper lip, nose, sinuses, nasopharynx, pharynx, and orbits. It drains into the inferior petrosal sinus, which in turn drains into the internal jugular vein. The cavernous sinus syndrome is caused by thrombosis of the cavernous intracranial sinus, 80% of which is fatal. The symptoms include orbital pain (V_1) with venous congestion of the retina, lids, and conjunctiva. The eyes are proptosed with exophthalmos. The patient has photophobia and involvement of nerves II, III, IV, and V_1. The treatment of choice is anticoagulation and antibiotics. The most common cause of cavernous sinus thrombosis is ethmoiditis. The ophthalmic vein and artery are involved as well. (The nerves and veins are lateral to the cavernous sinus, and the internal carotid artery is medial to it.)

Cestan-Chenais Syndrome

Cestan-Chenais syndrome is caused by occlusion of the vertebral artery below the point of origin of the posteroinferior cerebellar artery. There is paralysis of the soft palate, pharynx, and larynx. Ipsilateral cerebellar asynergia and Horner syndrome are also present. There is contralateral hemiplegia and diminished proprioception and tactile sensation.

Champion-Cregah-Klein Syndrome

This is a familial syndrome consisting of popliteal webbing, cleft lip, cleft palate, lower lip fistula, syndactyly, onychodysplasia, and pes equinovarus.

Chapple Syndrome

This disorder is seen in the newborn with unilateral facial weakness or paralysis in conjunction with comparable weakness or paralysis of the contralateral vocal cord, the muscles of deglutition, or both. The disorder is secondary to lateral flexion of the head in utero, which compresses the thyroid cartilage against the hyoid or cricoid cartilages or both, thereby injuring the recurrent or superior laryngeal nerve, or both.

Charcot-Marie-Tooth Disease

This is a hereditary and degenerative disease that includes the olivopontocerebellar, cerebelloparenchymal, and spinocerebellar disorders and the neuropathies. This disease is characterized by chronic degeneration of the peripheral nerves and roots; and distal muscle atrophy in feet, legs, and hands. Deep tendon reflexes are usually nil. It is also associated with hereditary cerebellar ataxia features, optic atrophy, and other cranial involvement. Some suggest that this disease is linked to auditory dysfunction and that it is also linked to other CNS dysfunctions. This disease can be progressive, and it can also spontaneously arrest.

CHARGE Syndrome

CHARGE syndrome (Coloboma of the eye, Heart defects, Atresia of the choanae, Retardation of growth and development, Genital and/or urinary abnormalities and Ear abnormalities and deafness) is a genetic pattern of birth defects that occurs in one in 10,000 births worldwide, without any family history. It involves heart defects, breathing and swallowing difficulties, hearing loss, vision loss, and balance problems.

Major Features of CHARGE Syndrome (Very Common in CHARGE and Relatively Rare in Other Conditions)

Feature	*Includes*	*Frequency (%)*
Coloboma of the eye	Coloboma (sort of like a cleft) of the iris, retina, choroid, macula, or disc (not the eyelid); microphthalmos (small eye) or anophthalmos (missing eye): *Causes vision loss*	80-90
Choanal atresia or stenosis	They can be stenosed or atretic. It can be unilateral or bilateral, bony, or membranous.	50-60
Cranial nerve abnormality	I—Missing or decreased sense of smell	90-100
	IX/X—Swallowing difficulties, aspiration	70-90
	VII—Facial palsy (one side or both)	40
CHARGE outer ear	Short, wide ear with little or no lobe, "snipped off" helix, prominent antihelix which is discontinuous with tragus, triangular concha, decreased cartilage (floppy), often stick out, usually asymmetric	> 50
CHARGE middle ear	Malformed bones of the ossicles: *Conductive hearing loss*	Common
CHARGE inner ear	Mondini defect; small or absent semicircular canals: *Balance problems and sensorineural loss*	90

Minor Characteristics of CHARGE: Significant, But More Difficult to Diagnose or Less Specific to CHARGE

Feature	*Includes*	*Frequency (%)*
Heart defects	Can be any type, but many are complex, such as tetralogy of Fallot	75
Cleft lip ± cleft palate	Cleft lip with or without cleft palate, cleft palate, submucous cleft palate	20
TE fistula	Esophageal atresia, tracheoesophageal fistula (TEF), H-shaped TEF	15-20
Kidney abnormalities	Small kidney, missing kidney, misplaced kidney, reflux	40
Genital abnormalities	Males: small penis, undescended testes Females: small labia, small or missing uterus Both: lack of puberty without hormone intervention	50 25 90
Growth deficiency	Growth hormone deficiency Other short stature	15 70
Typical CHARGE face	Square face with broad prominent forehead, arched eyebrows, large eyes, occasional ptosis, prominent nasal bridge with square root, thick nostrils, prominent nasal columella, flat midface, small mouth, occasional small chin, larger chin with age. Facial asymmetry even without facial palsy	
Palm crease	Hockey-stick palmar crease	50
CHARGE behavior	Perseverative behavior in younger individuals, obsessive-compulsive behavior (OCD) in older individuals	> 50

Chédiak-Higashi Syndrome

Chédiak-Higashi syndrome is the result of an autosomal recessive trait. It is characterized by albinism, photophobia, nystagmus, hepatosplenomegaly, anomalous cellular granules, and development of lymphoma. These patients usually die during childhood of fulminant infections.

Cleft Lip and Palate and Congenital Lip Fistulas

This syndrome is transmitted in an autosomal dominant manner with 80% penetrance; it occurs in 1 per 100,000 live births. Usually bilateral, symmetrically located depressions are noted on the vermilion portion of the lower lip and communicate with the underlying minor salivary glands. The lip pits may be an isolated finding (33%) or be found with cleft lip palate (67% of cases). Associated anomalies of the extremities may include talipes equinovarus, syndactyly, and popliteal pterygia. Congenital lip pits have also been seen in association with the oral-facial-digital syndrome.

Cockayne Syndrome

Cockayne syndrome is an autosomal recessive, progressive bilateral sensorineural hearing loss associated with dwarfism, facial disharmony, microcephaly, mental deficiency, retinitis pigmentosa, optic atrophy, intracranial calcification, and multiple dental caries. Patients succumb to respiratory or genitourinary infection in their teens or twenties.

Cogan Syndrome

Nonsyphilitic interstitial keratitis and vestibuloauditory symptoms are characteristics of Cogan syndrome. Interstitial keratitis gives rise to rapid visual loss. Symptoms include episodic severe vertigo accompanied by tinnitus, spontaneous nystagmus, ataxia, and progressive sensorineural hearing loss. There are remissions and exacerbations. It is believed to be related to periarteritis nodosa. Eosinophilia has been reported in this entity. Pathologically, it is a degeneration of the vestibular and spiral ganglia with edema of the membranous cochlea, SCCs, and inflammation of the spiral ligament. Treatment with steroids has been advocated.

Cyclophosphamide and azathioprine have been used in addition to prednisone (40 mg daily). This syndrome is not to be confused with Ménière disease despite vertiginous symptoms and fluctuating hearing loss. Vogt-Koyanagi-Harada syndrome is also similar but involves alopecia, poliosis, and exudative uveitis. Syphilis is also confused with this syndrome, but in syphilis, the interstitial keratitis is old and usually does not demonstrate active inflammatory changes. Syphilitic involvement of the cornea is often centrally located. Follow-up treatment of patients must be thorough to detect more extensive involvement, such as systemic vasculitis or aortitis.

Collet-Sicard Syndrome

The 9th, 10th, and 11th nerves are involved with normal sympathetic nerves. The etiology is usually a meningioma or other lesion involving the nerves in the posterior cranial fossa.

Conradi-Hünermann Syndrome

The most common variant of chondrodysplasia punctata; this syndrome is characterized by punctate epiphyseal calcifications. Clinical features include saddle nose deformity, micromelia, rhizomelia, short stature, flexion contractures, and dermatoses. This syndrome is also known as chondrodystrophia epiphysialis punctata, stippled epiphysis disease, dysplasia epiphysialis punctata, chondroangiopathia calcarea punctata, and Conradi disease. Some cases point to sporadic mutations and others to autosomal dominant patterns of inheritance. The clinical features of this syndrome are so varied from case to case that only a complete workup can exclude other versions of this syndrome.

Costen Syndrome

Costen syndrome is a temporomandibular joint (TMJ) abnormality, usually due to impaired bite and characterized by tinnitus, vertigo, and pain in the frontal, parietal, and occipital areas with a blocked feeling and pain in the ear. After a careful workup to rule out other abnormalities, the patient is treated with aspirin, heat, and slow exercise of the joint. An orthodontist may help the patient. The TMJ differs from other joints by the presence of avascular fibrous tissue covering the articulating surfaces with an interposed meniscus dividing the joint into upper and lower compartments. The right and left TMJs act as one functional unit. The condyle is made up of spongy bone with marrow and a growth center. The condyle articulates with the glenoid fossa of the temporal bone (squamosa). The squamotympanic fissure separates the fossa from the tympanic bone. The joint is a ginglymoarthrodial joint with hinge and transverse movements. The key supporting ligament of the TMJ is the temporomandibular ligament. The boundaries of the glenoid fossa are as follows:

Anterior:	Margins of the articular eminence
Posterior:	Squamotympanic fissure
Lateral:	Zygomatic process of the temporal bone
Medial:	Temporal spine

The TMJ derives its nourishment from the synovial membrane, which is richly vascularized and produces a mucinous-like substance. The joint has a gliding motion between the meniscus and the temporal bone (upper compartment). It has a hinge motion between the disk and the condyle (lower compartment). It is innervated by the auriculotemporal nerve, masseter nerve, lateral pterygoid nerve, and temporal nerve. It is supplied by the superficial temporal artery and the anterior tympanic branch of the internal maxillary artery. The lateral pterygoid muscle protracts the jaw, and the masseter, medial pterygoid, and temporalis muscles act as elevators. All these muscles are innervated by V_3. The sphenomandibular and stylomandibular ligaments have no function in TMJ articulation.

Cowden Syndrome

This is a familial syndrome characterized by adenoid facies, hypoplasia of the mandible and maxilla, high-arched palate, hypoplasia of the soft palate and uvula, microstomia, papillomatosis of the lips and pharynx, scrotal tongue, multiple thyroid adenomas, bilateral breast hypertrophy, pectus excavatum, and liver and CNS abnormalities.

Creutzfeldt-Jakob Disease

Creutzfeldt-Jakob disease is a rare spongiform encephalopathy. Constitutional symptoms lead to mental retardation and movement disorder.

Cri du Chat Syndrome

A condition caused by a B group chromosome with a short arm; its symptoms are mental retardation, respiratory stridor, microcephaly, hypertelorism, midline oral clefts, and laryngomalacia with poor approximation of the posterior vocal cords.

Crouzon Disease

See Chapter 15.

Curtius Syndrome

A form of hypertrophy that may involve a single small part of the body or an entire system (ie, muscular, nervous, or skeletal systems). It is also known as congenital hemifacial hypertrophy.

Dandy Syndrome

Oscillopsia or jumbling of the panorama common in patients after bilateral labyrinthectomy is characteristic of this syndrome. These patients are unable to focus while walking or moving.

Darier Disease (Keratosis Follicularis)

Autosomal dominant, this skin disorder of the external auditory canal is characterized by keratotic debris in the canal. Some investigators have advocated the use of vitamin A or steroids.

De'Jean Syndrome

Exophthalmos, diplopia, superior maxillary pain, and numbness along the route of the trigeminal nerve are found with lesions of the orbital floor in this syndrome.

Déjérine Anterior Bulbar Syndrome

This syndrome is evidenced by thrombosis of the anterior spinal artery, resulting in either an alternating hypoglossal hemiplegia or an alternating hypoglossal hemianesthetic hemiplegia.

Demarquay-Richter Syndrome

Demarquay-Richter syndrome is a congenital orofacial disorder characterized by cleft lip, cleft palate, lower lip fistulas, and progeria facies. Defective dentition, heart defects, dwarfism, and finger abnormalities may be seen.

DIDMOAD Syndrome

An autosomal recessive disorder associating **d**iabetes **i**nsipidus, **d**iabetes **m**ellitus, **o**ptic **a**trophy, and **d**eafness. Diabetes mellitus is usually juvenile in onset and insulin dependent. Diabetes insipidus has a varied time of onset and is vasopressin sensitive, indicative of degeneration of the hypothalamic cells or of the supraopticohypophyseal tract. The hearing loss is sensorineural and progressive, and primarily affects the higher tones. Urinary tract abnormalities ranging from atonic bladder to hydronephrosis and hydroureter have been reported with this disorder.

DiGeorge Syndrome

Lischaneri reported three categories of this syndrome:

A. Third and fourth pharyngeal pouch syndrome, characterized by cardiovascular and craniofacial anomalies as well as abdominal visceral abnormalities
B. DiGeorge syndrome (thymus agenesis)
C. Partial DiGeorge syndrome (thymic hypoplasia in which the thymus gland weighs less than 2 g)

The patients have small, malformed pinnae with narrow external auditory canals and abnormal ossicles. The patients also have a shortened cochlea of the Mondini type as well as an absence of hair cells in the hook region, hypertelorism with nasal cleft, shortened philtrum, and micrognathia. Other middle ear anomalies include an absence of stapedial muscle, hypoplastic facial nerve, and absent oval window. Most of the findings are symmetrical.

Down Syndrome

See section on trisomy in Chapter 15.

Dysphagia Lusoria

Dysphagia lusoria is secondary to an abnormal right subclavian artery. The right subclavian arises abnormally from the thoracic aorta by passing behind or in front of the esophagus, thus compressing it.

Eagle Syndrome

The patient has elongation of the styloid process or ossification of the stylohyoid ligament causing irritation of the trigeminal, facial, glossopharyngeal, and vagus nerves. Symptoms include recurrent nonspecific throat discomfort, foreign body sensation, dysphagia, facial pain, and increased salivation. Carotidynia may result from impingement of the styloid process on the carotid artery, producing regional tenderness or headaches. The only effective treatment for Eagle syndrome is surgical shortening of the styloid process.

Ectodermal Dysplasia, Hidrotic

See Chapter 15.

Ectodermal Dysplasia, Hypohidrotic

This syndrome consists of hypodontia, hypotrichosis, and hypohidrosis. Principally, the structures involved are of ectodermal origin. Eyelashes and especially eyebrows are entirely missing. Eczema and asthma are common. Aplasia of the eccrine sweat glands may lead to severe hyperpyrexia. The inheritance is X-linked recessive.

18q Syndrome

This syndrome consists of psychomotor retardation, hypotonia, short stature, microcephaly, hypoplastic midface, epicanthus, ophthalmologic abnormalities, cleft palate, congenital heart disease, abnormalities of the genitalia, tapered fingers, aural atresia, and conductive hearing loss.

Eisenlohr Syndrome

Numbness and weakness in the extremities; paralysis of the lips, tongue, and palate; and dysarthria are evidenced.

Elschnig Syndrome

Extension of the palpebral fissure laterally, displacement of the lateral canthus, ectropion of the lower lid, and lateral canthus are observed. Hypertelorism, cleft palate, and cleft lip are frequently seen.

Empty Sella Syndrome

The patient has an enlarged sella, giving the appearance of a pituitary tumor. The syndrome consists of the abnormal extension into the sella turcica of an arachnoid diverticulum filled with CSF, displacing and compressing the pituitary gland. Four causal theories of this syndrome exist: (1) rupture of an intrasellar or parasellar cyst; (2) infarction of a pituitary adenoma; (3) pituitary hypertrophy and subsequent involution; and (4) the most common theory, the syndrome is due to CSF pressure through a congenitally deficient sella diaphragm leading to the formation of an intrasellar arachnoidocele. A trans-septal or trans-sphenoidal route to the sella is a treatment to consider.

The primary empty sella syndrome is due to congenital absence of the diaphragm sella, with gradual enlargement of the sella secondary to pulsations of the brain. Secondary empty sella syndrome may be due to necrosis of an existing pituitary tumor after surgery, postirradiation directed at the pituitary, or pseudotumor cerebri.

Face-Hand Syndrome

A reflex sympathetic dystrophy that is seen after a stroke or myocardial infarction. There may be edema and erythema of the involved parts along with persistent burning.

Fanconi Anemia Syndrome

Patients have aplastic anemia with skin pigmentation, skeletal deformities, renal anomalies, and mental retardation. Death due to leukemia usually ensues within 2 years. The disorder rarely occurs in adults. (A variant is congenital hypoplastic thrombocytopenia, which is inherited as an autosomal recessive trait.) It is characterized by spontaneous bleeding and other congenital anomalies. The bleeding time is prolonged, the platelet count is decreased, and the bone marrow megakaryocytes vary from decreased to absent.

It is associated with unrepaired chromosome breakage. Congenital anomalies of the inner, middle, and external ear could be causes of the deafness that accompanies this syndrome.

Felty Syndrome

Felty syndrome is a combination of leukopenia, arthritis, and enlarged lymph nodes and spleen.

First Bite Syndrome

First bite syndrome is characterized by facial pain, severe cramping in the parotid region with the first bite of each meal. The pain and spasm diminish with subsequent bites. The etiology is unknown but may be related to deep-lobe parotid or infratemporal fossa lesion or surgery. Treatment included Tegretol (carbamazepine), gabapentinoids (calcium channel blockers), and amitriptyline (tricyclic antidepressants and anticholinergic). But there is no conclusive evidence as to the effects of these treatments.

First and Second Branchial Arch Syndromes (Hemifacial Microsomia, Lateral Facial Dysplasia)

This disorder consists of a spectrum of craniofacial malformations characterized by asymmetric facies with unilateral abnormalities. The mandible is small with hypoplastic or absent ramus and condyle. Aural atresia, hearing impairment, tissue tags from the tragus to the oral commissure, coloboma of the upper eyelid, malar hypoplasia, and cleft palate also may be present. Cardiovascular, renal, and nervous system abnormalities have been noted in association with this disorder.

Fish Odor Syndrome

Clinical symptoms of this peculiar syndrome consist of a fish odor emanating from the mucus, particularly in the morning. A challenge test with either choline bitartrate or trimethylamine is diagnostic of this disease. Eating non–choline-containing foods usually helps. No long-term effects are known.

Fordyce Disease

Fordyce disease is characterized by pseudocolloid of the lips, a condition marked by the presence of numerous, small, yellowish-white granules on the inner surface and vermilion border of the lips. Histologically, the lesions appear as ectopic sebaceous glands.

Foster Kennedy Syndrome

Patients with this disorder show ipsilateral optic atrophy and scotomas and contralateral papilledema occurring with tumors or other lesions of the frontal lobe or sphenoidal meningioma. Anosmia may be seen.

Fothergill Disease

The combination of tic douloureux and anginose scarlatina is characteristic of this disease.

Foville Syndrome

Facial paralysis with ipsilateral paralysis of conjugate gaze and contralateral pyramidal hemiplegia are diagnostic. Tinnitus, deafness, and vertigo may occur with infranuclear involvement. Loss of taste of the anterior two-thirds of the tongue with decreased salivary and lacrimal secretions is seen with involvement of the nervus intermedius.

Frey Syndrome

In the normal person, the sweat glands are innervated by sympathetic nerve fibers. After parotidectomy, the auriculotemporal nerve sends its parasympathetic fibers to innervate the sweat glands instead. Also called preauricular gustatory sweating, parotidectomy is considered the most common etiology.

Friedreich Disease

The disease consists of facial hemihypertrophy involving the eyelids, cheeks, lips, facial bones, tongue, ears, and tonsils. It may be seen alone or in association with generalized hemihypertrophy.

Garcin Syndrome

Paralysis of cranial nerves III through X, usually unilateral or occasionally bilateral, is observed in this syndrome. It may be the result of invasion by neoplasms, granulomas, or infections in the retropharyngeal space.

Gard-Gignoux Syndrome

Gard-Gignoux syndrome involves paralysis of the eleventh nerve and the tenth nerve below the nodose ganglion. The cricothyroid function and sensation are normal. The symptoms include vocal cord paralysis and weakness of the trapezius and sternocleidomastoid muscles.

Gardner Syndrome

Gardner syndrome is an autosomal dominant disease whose symptoms include fibroma, osteoma of the skull, mandible, maxilla, and long bones, with epidermoid inclusion cysts in the skin and polyps in the colon. These colonic polyps have a marked tendency toward malignant degeneration.

Gargoylism (Hurler Syndrome)

See Chapter 17.

Gaucher Disease

As an autosomally recessive inherited disorder of lipid metabolism, this syndrome results in a decrease in the activity of the glucocerebrosidase. This leads to an increased accumulation of glucocerebrosides, particularly in the retroendothelial system. There are three classifications of the disease: (1) the chronic non-neuronopathic form, characterized by joint pain, aseptic necrosis, pathologic fractures, hepatosplenomegaly, thrombocytopenia, anemia, and leukopenia; (2) the acute neuronopathic Gaucher disease (infantile form), causing increased neurologic complications that often end in death before the first 2 years of life; and (3) the juvenile and less severe forms than the infantile form.

Gerlier Disease

With the presence of vertigo and kubisagari, it is observed among cowherds. It is marked by pain in the head and neck with visual disturbances, ptosis, and generalized weakness of the muscles.

Giant Apical Air Cell Syndrome

Giant apical air cell syndrome consists of giant apical air cells, spontaneous CSF rhinorrhea, and recurrent meningitis. It is caused by the constant pounding of the brain against the dura overlying the giant apical air cell, which leads to dural rupture and CSF leak.

Gilles de la Tourette Syndrome

Characterized by chorea, coprolalia, and tics of the face and extremities, it affects children (usually boys 5-10 years old). Repetitive facial grimacing, blepharospasms, and arm and leg contractions may be present. Compulsive grunting noises or hiccupping subsequently become expressions of frank obscenities.

Goldenhar Syndrome

A rare, nonhereditary congenital variant of hemifacial microsomia, Goldenhar syndrome is a congenital syndrome of the first and second arch. It is characterized by underdevelopment of craniofacial structures, vertebral malformations, and cardiac dysfunction. Clinical features of this syndrome are malar and maxillary hypoplasia, poor formation of external auditory canal, supernumerary ear tags and antetragal pits, orbit, enlarged mouths, renal anomalies, and missing growth centers in the condyle, causing delayed eruption of teeth and teeth crowding. Intelligence is usually normal or mildly retarded. Maxillofacial reconstruction in young patients demands consideration of future growth and development. It is also recommended for psychologic reasons as well as reasons involving the proper expansion of the skin that will later aid in further reconstruction. This syndrome is not to be confused with Treacher Collins, Berry, or Franceschetti-Zwahlen-Klein syndromes. These tend to show well-defined genetic patterns (irregular but dominant), whereas Goldenhar syndrome does not.

Goodwin Tumor (Benign Lymphoepithelial Lesion)

This syndrome is characterized by inflammatory cells, lymphocytes, plasma cells, and reticular cells.

Gradenigo Syndrome

Due to an extradural abscess involving the petrous bone (Dorello canal). The symptoms are suppurative otitis, pain in the eye and temporal area, abducens paralysis, and diplopia.

Grisel Syndrome

Also known as nasopharyngeal torticollis, it is the subluxation of the atlantoaxial joint and is usually associated with children. It is associated with pharyngitis, nasopharyngitis, adenotonsillitis, tonsillar abscess, parotitis, cervical abscess, and otitis media. This syndrome has been known to occur after nasal cavity inflammation, tonsillectomy, adenoidectomy, mastoidectomy, choanal atresia repair, and excisions of a parapharyngeal rhabdomyosarcoma. Proposals for etiology include overdistention of the atlantoaxial joint ligaments by effusion, rupture of the transverse ligament, excessive passive rotation during general anesthesia, uncoordinated reflex action of the deep cervical muscles, spasm of the prevertebral muscles, ligamentous relaxation from decalcification of the vertebrae, and weak lateral ligaments. Clinical features include spontaneous torticollis in a child, a flexed and rotated head with limited range of motion, flat face, and Sudeck sign (displacement of the spine of the axis to the same side as the head is turned). Treatment includes skeletal skull traction under fluoroscopic control to realign the odontoid process within the transverse ligament sling, followed by 6 to 12 weeks of immobilization. Timely treatment is usually successful.

Guillain-Barré Syndrome

An infectious polyneuritis of unknown etiology ("perhaps" viral) causing marked paresthesias of the limbs, muscular weakness, or a flaccid paralysis. CSF protein is increased without an increase in cell count.

Hallermann-Streiff Syndrome

Hallermann-Streiff syndrome consists of dyscephaly, parrot nose, mandibular hypoplasia, proportionate nanism; hypotrichosis of scalp, brows, and cilia; and bilateral congenital cataracts. Most patients exhibit nystagmus or strabismus. There is no demonstrable genetic basis.

Hanhart Syndrome

A form of facial dysmorphia characterized by (1) bird-like profile of face caused by micrognathia, (2) opisthodontia, (3) peromelia, (4) small growth, (5) normal intelligence, (6) branchial arch deformity resulting in conductive hearing loss, (7) tongue deformities and often a small jaw, and (8) possibly some limb defects as well. Ear surgery should be carefully considered because of the abnormal course of the facial nerve due to this syndrome.

Heerfordt Syndrome or Disease

Uveoparotid fever develops in Heerfordt syndrome. Heerfordt syndrome is a form of sarcoidosis (see Chapter 12).

Hick Syndrome

A rare condition characterized by a sensory disorder of the lower extremities, resulting in perforating feet and ulcers that are associated with progressive deafness due to atrophy of the cochlear and vestibular ganglia.

Hippel-Lindau Disease

Hippel-Lindau disease consists of angioma of the cerebellum, usually cystic, associated with angioma of the retina and polycystic kidneys.

Hollander Syndrome

Appearance of a goiter during the third decade of life related to a partial defect in the coupling mechanism in thyroxine biosynthesis. Deafness due to cochlear abnormalities is often related.

Homocystinuria

Homocystinuria is a recessive hereditary syndrome secondary to a defect in methionine metabolism with resultant homocystinemia, mental retardation, and sensorineural hearing loss.

Horner Syndrome

The presenting symptoms are ptosis, miosis, anhidrosis, and enophthalmos due to paralysis of the cervical sympathetic nerves.

Horton Neuralgia

Patients have unilateral headaches centered behind or close to the eye accompanied or preceded by ipsilateral nasal congestion, suffusion of the eye, increased lacrimation and facial redness, and swelling.

Hunt Syndrome

A. Cerebellar tumor, an intention tremor that begins in one extremity gradually increasing in intensity and subsequently involving other parts of the body
B. Facial paralysis, otalgia, and aural herpes due to disease of both motor and sensory fibers of the seventh nerve
C. A form of juvenile paralysis agitans associated with primary atrophy of the pallidal system

Hunter Syndrome

A hereditary and sex-linked disorder, this incurable syndrome involves multiple organ systems through mucopolysaccharide infiltration. Death, usually by the second decade of life, is often caused by an infiltrative cardiomyopathy and valvular disease leading to heart failure. Physical characteristics include prominent supraorbital ridges, large, flattened nose with flared nares, low-set ears, progressive corneal opacities, generous jowls, patulous lips and prognathism, short neck, abdominal protuberance, hirsutism, short stature, extensive osteoarthritis (especially in the hips, shoulders, elbows, and hands), TMJ arthritis, pseudopapilledema, and low-pressure hydrocephalus. Chondroitin sulfate B and heparitin in urine, mental retardation, beta-galactoside deficiency, and hepatosplenomegaly are also features of this syndrome. There is cerebral storage of three gangliosides: GM_1, GM_2, and GM_3. Compressive myelopathy may result from vertebral dislocation. High spinal cord injury is a great complication in surgery. Neurologic development is often slowed or never acquired. Abdominal abnormalities, respiratory infections, and cardiovascular troubles plague the patient.

Immotile Cilia Syndrome

This syndrome appears to be a congenital defect in the ultrastructure of cilia that renders them incapable of movement. Both respiratory tract cilia and sperm are involved. The clinical picture includes bronchiectasis, sinusitis, male sterility, situs inversus, and otitis media. Histologically, there is a complete or partial absence of dynein arms, which are believed to be essential for cilia movement and sperm tail movement. Also, no cilia movements were observed in the mucosa of the middle ear and the nasopharynx.

Inversed Jaw-Winking Syndrome

When there are supranuclear lesions of the fifth nerve, touching the cornea may produce a brisk movement of the mandible to the opposite side.

Jackson Syndrome

Cranial nerves X, XI, and XII are affected by nuclear or radicular lesion. There is ipsilateral flaccid paralysis of the soft palate, pharynx, and larynx with weakness and atrophy of the sternocleidomastoid and trapezius muscles and muscles of the tongue.

Jacod Syndrome

Total ophthalmoplegia, optic tract lesions with unilateral amaurosis, and trigeminal neuralgia. It is caused by a middle cranial fossa tumor involving the second through sixth cranial nerves.

Job Syndrome

One of the groups of hyperimmunoglobulin E (hyper-IgE) syndromes that are associated with defective chemotaxis. The clinical picture includes fair skin, red hair, recurrent staphylococcal skin abscesses with concurrent other bacterial infections and skin lesions, as well as chronic purulent pulmonary infections and infected eczematoid skin lesions. This syndrome obtained its name from the Biblical passage referring to Job being smitten with boils. It is of interest to the otolaryngologist because of head and neck infections.

Jugular Foramen Syndrome (Vernet Syndrome)

Cranial nerves IX, X, and XI are paralyzed, whereas XII is spared because of its separate hypoglossal canal. Horner syndrome is not present because the sympathetic chain is below the foramen. This syndrome is most often caused by lymphadenopathy of the nodes of Krause in the foramen. Thrombophlebitis, tumors of the jugular bulb, and basal skull fracture can cause the syndrome. The glomus jugulare usually gives a hazy margin of involvement, whereas neurinoma gives a smooth, sclerotic margin of enlargement. The jugular foramen is bound medially by the occipital bone and laterally by the temporal bone. The foramen is divided into anteromedial (pars nervosa) and posterolateral (pars vascularis) areas by a fibrous or bony septum. The medial area transmits nerves IX, X, and XI as well as the inferior petrosal sinus. The posterior compartment transmits the internal jugular vein and the posterior meningeal artery. The right foramen is usually slightly larger than the left foramen.

Kallmann Syndrome

Kallmann syndrome consists of congenital hypogonadotropic eunuchoidism with anosmia. It is transmitted via a dominant gene with variable penetrance.

Kaposi Sarcoma

Patients have multiple idiopathic, hemorrhagic sarcomatosis particularly of the skin and viscera. Radiotherapy is the treatment of choice.

Kartagener Syndrome

The symptoms are complete situs inversus associated with chronic sinusitis and bronchiectasis. It is also called the Kartagener triad.

Cilia and flagella of a patient lack normal dynein side arms of ciliary A-tubes. Deficient mucociliary transport causes sterility in both sexes.

Keratosis Palmaris et Solaris

This disorder is an unusual inherited malformation. If these people live to 65 years of age, 50% to 75% of them develop carcinoma of the esophagus.

Kimura Disease

Kimura disease is a chronic inflammatory condition occurring in subcutaneous tissues, salivary glands, and lymph nodes. Etiology is unknown. Histologically, there is dense fibrosis, lymphoid infiltration, vascular proliferation, and eosinophils. This is different from angiolymphoid hyperplasia with eosinophilia (ALHE). It is much more prevalent in people of Oriental descent. Laboratory studies show eosinophilia and elevated IgE. Differential diagnosis includes ALHE, eosinophilic granuloma, benign lymphoepithelial lesion, lymphocytoma, pyogenic granuloma, Kaposi sarcoma, hamartoma, and lymphoma. Treatment includes corticosteroids, cryotherapy, radiation, and surgery.

The differences between Kimura disease and ALHE are as follows:

Kimura	Age:	30-60 (ALHE age 20-50)
	Sex:	Male (ALHE female)
	Larger lesions	(ALHE < 1 cm)
	Deep	(ALHE superficial)
	More lymphoid follicles than ALHE	
	Fewer mast cells than ALHE	
	Less vascular hyperplasia than ALHE	
	More fibrosis than ALHE	
	More eosinophilia than ALHE	
	More IgE than ALHE	

Kleinschmidt Syndrome

Symptoms include influenzal infections, resulting in laryngeal stenosis, suppurative pericarditis, pleuropneumonia, and occasionally meningitis.

Klinefelter Syndrome

Klinefelter syndrome is a sex chromosome defect characterized by eunuchoidism, azoospermia, gynecomastia, mental deficiency, small testes with atrophy, and hyalinization of seminiferous tubules. The karyotype is usually XXY.

Klinkert Syndrome

Paralysis of the recurrent and phrenic nerves due to a neoplastic process in the root of the neck or upper mediastinum is evidenced. The sympathetics may be involved. (Left-side involvement is more common than right-side involvement.) It can be a part of Pancoast syndrome.

Lacrimoauriculodentodigital Syndrome

Autosomal dominant, occasional middle ear ossicular anomaly with cup-shaped ears, abnormal or absent thumbs, skeletal forearm deformities, sensorineural hearing loss, and nasolacrimal duct obstruction are the characteristics of lacrimoauriculodentodigital syndrome.

Large Vestibular Aqueduct Syndrome

The large vestibular aqueduct as an isolated anomaly of the temporal bone is associated with sensorineural hearing loss. It is more common in childhood than in adulthood. In this syndrome, the rugose portion of the endolymphatic sac is also enlarged. Endolymphatic sac procedures to improve hearing are not often successful. A vestibular aqueduct is considered enlarged if its anteroposterior diameter on a computed tomography (CT) scan is greater than 1.5 mm.

Larsen Syndrome

Larsen syndrome is characterized by widely spaced eyes, prominent forehead, flat nasal bridge, midline cleft of the secondary palate, bilateral dislocation of the knees and elbows, deformities of the hands and feet, and spatula-type thumbs; sometimes tracheomalacia, stridor, laryngomalacia, and respiratory difficulty are present. Therapy includes maintaining adequate ventilation.

Lemierre Syndrome

First discussed by André LeMierre in 1936, usually caused by anaerobic, nonmotile gram-negative rod, *Fusobacterium necrophorum*, Lemierre syndrome can be found in normal flora of oropharynx, gastrointestinal (GI), and female genital tract; sensitive to clindamycin and metronidazole, penicillin, and chloramphenicol. Usually seen in young adults, the infection first begins in the oropharynx, progresses to neck and parapharyngeal abscess, leading to internal jugular and sigmoid sinus thrombosis which can cause septic embolism leading to septic arthritis, liver and splenic abscess. Sigmoid sinus thrombosis findings include headache, otalgia, vertigo, vomiting, otorrhea and rigors, proptosis, retrobulbar pain, papilledema, and ophthalmoplegia.

Lermoyez Syndrome

Lermoyez syndrome is a variant of Ménière disease. It was first described by Lermoyez in 1921 as deafness and tinnitus followed by a vertiginous attack that relieved the tinnitus and improved the hearing.

Lethal Midline Granuloma Syndrome

Destroying cartilage, soft tissue, and bone, this disease manifests itself by a number of entities, including idiopathic midline destructive disease, Wegener granulomatosis, polymorphic reticulosis, nasal lymphoma, and non-Hodgkin lymphoma (NHL). High-dose local radiation totaling 5000 rad is the treatment of choice for localized cases. Chemotherapy involving an alkylating agent (cyclophosphamide) is recommended for disseminated cases.

Löffler Syndrome

Consists of pneumonitis with eosinophils in the tissues. It is possibly of parasitic etiology.

Loose Wire Syndrome

Occurs in patients with stapedectomy and insertion of a prosthesis that attaches to the long process of the incus by means of a crimped wire. It is a late complication, occurring on an average 15 years after surgery. A triad of symptoms is present that improves temporarily with middle ear inflation: auditory acuity, distortion of sound, and speech discrimination. Treatment in revision surgery involves finding the loose wire attachment at the incus and tightening that wire to allow the incus and prosthesis to move as one.

Louis-Bar Syndrome

This autosomal recessive disease presents as ataxia, oculocutaneous telangiectasia, and sinopulmonary infection. It involves progressive truncal ataxia, slurred speech, fixation nystagmus, mental deficiency, cerebellar atrophy, deficient immunoglobulin, and marked frequency of lymphoreticular malignancies. The patient rarely lives past age 20.

Maffucci Syndrome

Maffucci syndrome is characterized by multiple cutaneous hemangiomas with dyschondroplasia and often enchondroma. The origin is unknown, and it is not hereditary. Signs and symptoms of this syndrome usually appear during infancy. It equally affects both sexes and has no racial preference. The dyschondroplasia may cause sharp bowing or an uneven growth of the extremities as well as give rise to frequent fractures. Five to 10% of Maffucci syndrome patients have head and neck involvement giving rise to cranial nerve dysfunction and hemangiomas in the head and neck area. The hemangiomas in the nasopharynx and larynx could cause airway compromise as well as deglutition problems. Fifteen to 20% of these patients later undergo sarcomatous degeneration in one or more of the enchondromas. The percentage of malignant changes is greater in older patients, with the percentage of malignant degeneration approaching 44% in patients older than 40 years.

This syndrome is not to be confused with Klippel-Trenaunay syndrome, which causes no underdeveloped extremities, Sturge-Weber syndrome, or von Hippel-Lindau syndrome. No treatment is known for this syndrome, although surgical procedures to treat the actual deformities are sometimes necessary.

Mal de Debarquement Syndrome

Mal de Debarquement syndrome (or MDDS) is an imbalance or rocking sensation that occurs after prolonged exposure to motion (most commonly after a sea cruise or a long airplane flight). Travelers often experience this sensation temporarily after disembarking, but in the case of MDDS sufferers, it can persist for 6 to 12 months or even many years in some cases.

The imbalance is generally not associated with any nausea, nor is it alleviated by typical motion sickness drugs such as scopolamine or meclizine. Symptoms are usually most pronounced when the patient is sitting still; in fact, the sensations are usually minimized by actual motion such as walking or driving. Diagnosis of MDDS is generally a process of exclusion. The medical literature describes MDDS as a *self-limiting* condition.

Valium and other derivatives (particularly *Klonopin*) have been known to help alleviate some of the severe symptoms in MDDS patients, but there is always a worry that these are habit forming and may prolong the eventual disappearance of the condition. In general, physical activity is recommended for vestibular rehabilitation.

Marcus Gunn Syndrome (Jaw-Winking Syndrome)

Increase in the width of the eyelids during chewing. Sometimes the patient experiences rhythmic elevation of the upper eyelid when the mouth is open and ptosis when the mouth is closed.

Marie-Strümpell Disease

Marie-Strümpell disease is rheumatoid arthritis of the spine.

Masson Tumor

Masson tumor is intravascular papillary endothelial hyperplasia caused by excessive proliferation of endothelial cells. It is a benign condition. Differential diagnosis includes angiosarcoma, Kaposi sarcoma, and pyogenic granuloma.

Melkersson-Rosenthal Syndrome

(Triad: Recurrent orofacial swelling, one or more episodes of facial paralysis, and lingua plicata.) A congenital disease of unknown etiology, it manifests as recurring attacks of unilateral or bilateral facial paralysis (see Chapter 19), swelling of the lips, and furrowing of the tongue. It is associated with high serum levels of angiotensin-converting enzyme during affliction, and is also known as orofacial granulomatosis, cheilitis granulomatosis, Scheuermann glossitis granulomatosis, and Miescher cheilitis.

Treatment should focus on facial paralysis and edema. Steroids and facial nerve decompression have had limited success.

Meyenburg Syndrome (Familial Myositis Fibrosa Progressiva)

Meyenburg syndrome is a disease in which the striated muscles are replaced by fibrosis. Fibrosarcoma rarely originates from this disease.

Middle Lobe Syndrome

A chronic atelectatic process with fibrosis in one or both segments of the middle lobe. It is usually secondary to obstruction of the middle lobe bronchus by hilar adenopathy. The hilar adenopathy may be transient, but the bronchiectasis that resulted persists. Treatment is surgical resection.

Mikulicz Disease

The symptoms of swelling of the lacrimal and salivary glands occur as complications of some other disease, such as lymphocytosis, leukemia, or uveoparotid fever.

Millard-Gubler Syndrome

Patients present with ipsilateral paralysis of the abducens and facial nerves with contralateral hemiplegia of the extremities due to obstruction of the vascular supply to the pons.

Möbius Syndrome

Möbius syndrome is a nonprogressive congenital facial diplegia (usually bilateral) with unilateral or bilateral loss of the abductors of the eye, anomalies of the extremities, and aplasia of the brachial and thoracic muscles. It frequently involves other cranial nerves. Saito showed evidence that the site of nerve lesions is in the peripheral nerve. The etiology could be CNS hypoplasia, primary peripheral muscle defect with secondary nerve degeneration, or lower motor neuron involvement.

Morgagni-Stewart-Morel Syndrome

Occurs in menopausal women and is characterized by obesity, dizziness, psychologic disturbances, inverted sleep rhythm, and hyperostosis frontalis interna. Treatment is supportive.

Multiple Endocrine Adenomatosis

Multiple Endocrine Adenomatosis Type IIA (Sipple Syndrome) Sipple syndrome is a familial syndrome consisting of medullary carcinoma of the thyroid, hyperparathyroidism, and pheochromocytoma.

Multiple Endocrine Adenomatosis Type IIB This multiple endocrine adenomatosis (MEA) variant consists of multiple mucosal neuromas, pheochromocytoma, medullary carcinoma of the thyroid, and hyperparathyroidism. This syndrome is inherited in an autosomal dominant pattern. Mucosal neuromas principally involve the lips and anterior tongue. Numerous white medullated nerve fibers traverse the cornea to anastomose in the pupillary area.

Munchausen Syndrome

Munchausen syndrome was named after Baron Hieronymus Karl Freidrich von Münchausen (1720-1791) by Asher in 1951. The integral features of this syndrome include the following:

A. A real organic lesion from the past that has left some genuine signs but is causing no organic symptoms.
B. Exorbitant lying with dramatic presentation of nonexistent symptoms.
C. Traveling widely with multiple hospitalizations.
D. Criminal tendencies.
E. Willingness to undergo painful and dangerous treatment.
F. Presenting challenging illnesses for treatment.
G. Unruly behavior during hospital stays and early self-discharge without prior approval.
H. Patients often inflict pain on their own children and forcibly create symptoms to indirectly receive hospital treatment.

The patients usually go from one medical center to another to be admitted with dramatic presentations of nonorganic symptoms related to a real organic lesion in the past medical history.

Nager Syndrome (Acrofacial Dysostosis)

Acrofacial dysostosis patients have facies similar to those seen with Treacher Collins syndrome. They also present with preaxial upper limb defects, microtia, atresia of the external auditory canals, and malformation of the ossicles. Conductive and mixed hearing losses may occur.

Nager de Reynier Syndrome

Hypoplasia of the mandible with abnormal implantation of teeth associated with aural atresia characterizes this syndrome.

Neurofibromatosis (von Recklinghausen Disease)

Salient Features

A. Autosomal dominant.
B. Mental retardation is common in families with neurofibromatosis.
C. Arises from neurilemmal cells or sheath of Schwann and fibroblasts of peripheral nerves.
D. Café au lait spots—giant melanosomes (presence of six or more spots > 1.5 cm is diagnostic of neurofibromatosis, even if the family history is negative).
E. Of all neurofibromatoses, 4% to 5% undergo malignant degeneration with a sudden increase in growth of formerly static nodules. These nodules may become neurofibrosarcomas, and they may metastasize widely.

External Features

A. Café au lait spots
B. Fibromas

Internal Features

A. Pheochromocytoma.
B. Meningioma.
C. Acoustic neuroma: bilateral in type 2 neurofibromatosis.
D. GI bleeding.
E. Intussusception bowel.
F. Hypoglycemia (intraperitoneal fibromas).
G. Fibrous dysplasia.

H. Subperiosteal bone cysts.
I. Optic nerve may be involved, causing blindness and proptosis.
J. May present with macroglossia.
K. May involve the parotid or submaxillary gland.
L. The nodules may be painful.
M. Nodules may enlarge suddenly if bleeding of the tumor occurs or if there is malignant degeneration.

The treatment is only to relieve pressure from expanding masses. It usually does not recur if the tumor is completely removed locally.

Nothnagel Syndrome

The symptoms include dizziness, a staggering and rolling gait with irregular forms of oculomotor paralysis, and nystagmus is often present. This syndrome is seen with tumors of the midbrain.

Oculopharyngeal Syndrome

Characterized by hereditary ptosis and dysphagia, oculopharyngeal syndrome is an autosomal dominant disease having equal incidence in both sexes. It is related to a high incidence of esophageal carcinoma. Age of onset is between 40 and 50 years, and it is particularly common among French Canadians. Marked weakness of the upper esophagus is observed together with an increase in serum creatinine phosphokinase. It is a myopathy and not a neuropathy. Treatment includes dilatation and cricopharyngomyotomy.

Ollier Disease

Ollier disease consists of multiple chondromatosis, 10% of which is associated with chondrosarcoma.

Ondine Curse

Failure of respiratory center automaticity with apnea, especially evident during sleep, is symptomatic. Also known as the alveolar hypoventilation syndrome, it may be associated with increased appetite and transient central diabetes insipidus. Hypothalamic lesions are thought to be the cause of this disorder.

Oral-Facial-Digital Syndrome I

See Chapter 17 for oral-facial-digital syndrome I.

A lethal trait in men, it is inherited as an X-linked dominant trait limited to women. Symptoms include multiple hyperplastic frenula, cleft tongue, dystopia canthorum, hypoplasia of the nasal alar cartilages, median cleft of the upper lip, asymmetrical cleft palate, digital malformation, and mild mental retardation. About 50% of the patients have hamartoma between the lobes of the divided tongue. This mass consists of fibrous connective tissue, salivary gland tissue, few striated muscle fibers, and rarely cartilage. One-third of the patients present with ankyloglossia.

Orbital Apex Syndrome

Orbital apex syndrome involves the nerves and vessels passing through the superior sphenoid fissure and the optic foramen with paresis of cranial nerves III, IV, and VI. External ophthalmoplegia is associated with internal ophthalmoplegia with a dilated pupil that does not react to either light or convergence. Ptosis as well as periorbital edema are due to fourth nerve paresis. Sensory changes are secondary to the lacrimal frontal nasal ciliary nerves as well as the three branches of the ophthalmic nerve. The optic nerve is usually involved.

Ortner Syndrome

Cardiomegaly associated with laryngeal paralysis secondary to compression of the recurrent laryngeal nerve is observed with this syndrome.

Osler-Weber-Rendu Disease (Hereditary Hemorrhagic Telangiectasia)

An autosomal dominant disease in which the heterozygote lives to adult life, whereas the homozygous state is lethal at an early age. The patient has punctate hemangiomas (elevated, dilated capillaries, and venules) in the mucous membrane of the lips, tongue, mouth, GI tract, and so on. Pathologically, they are vascular sinuses of irregular size and shape lined by a thin layer of endothelium. The muscular and elastic coats are absent. Because of their thin walls, these vascular sinuses bleed easily, and because of the lack of muscular coating the bleeding is difficult to control. The patient has normal blood elements and no coagulation defect. The other blood vessels are normal. If a person with this disease marries a normal person, what are the chances that the offspring will have this condition? Because the patient with this disease is an adult, we can assume that he is heterozygous, as the homozygote dies early in life. Therefore, the child will have a 50% chance of having this hereditary disease.

Otopalatodigital Syndrome

Otopalatodigital (OPD) syndrome is characterized by skeletal dysplasia, conductive hearing loss, and cleft palate. Middle ear anomalies are also associated with this syndrome. Although the mode of inheritance is not known, some suggest that X-linked recessive inheritance is possible. Symptoms tend to be less severe in females than in males. The diagnosis of OPD syndrome is sometimes based on characteristic facies and deformities of hands and feet. Physical features include mild dwarfism, mental retardation, broad nasal root, frontal and occipital bossing, hypertelorism, small mandible, stubby, clubbed digits, low-set and small ears, winged scapulae, malar flattening, downward obliquity of the eye, and down-turned mouth. The inner ear has been known to display deformities likened to a mild type of Mondini dysplasia. Surgical attempts to improve hearing loss are not always recommended since certain deformities, such as a missing round window, make such attempts unsuccessful.

Paget Disease (Osteitis Deformans)

See Chapter 17.

This term is also used to characterize a disease of elderly women who have an infiltrated, eczematous lesion surrounding the nipple and areola associated with subjacent intraductal carcinoma of the breast.

Paget Osteitis

This disorder is related to sarcomas.

Pancoast Syndrome

See Chapter 7.

Pelizaeus-Merzbacher Disease

An X-linked recessive sudanophilic leukodystrophy. The CNS myelin forms improperly and never matures, sometimes ending in death by the age of 2 or 3 years. Nystagmoid eye movements are characteristic at age 4 to 6 months, followed by a delay in motor development. Prenatal amniocentesis is not useful in detecting this disease. Neonatal stridor, a specific genealogy combined with a characteristic auditory brain stem response (ABR) wave can lead to early diagnosis. Characteristic waves have been known to be missing rostral waves and normal wave I latency. Males are afflicted, whereas females are unknowing carriers.

Pena-Shokeir Syndrome

Rare autosomal recessive, affects newborns with camptodactyly, multiple ankylosis, pulmonary hypoplasia, and facial anomaly. Generally poor prognosis and die shortly after birth.

Peutz-Jeghers Syndrome

The patient has pigmentation of the lips and oral mucosa and benign polyps of the GI tract. Granulosa theca cell tumors have been reported in female patients with this syndrome.

Pheochromocytoma

Pheochromocytoma is associated with neurofibromatosis, cerebellar hemangioblastoma, ependymoma, astrocytoma, meningioma, spongioblastoma, multiple endocrine adenoma, or medullary carcinoma of the thyroid. Pheochromocytoma with or without the tumors may be inherited as an autosomal dominant trait. Some patients have megacolon, others suffer neurofibromatosis of Auerbach and Meissner plexuses.

Pierre Robin Syndrome

Pierre Robin syndrome consists of glossoptosis, micrognathia, and cleft palate. There is no sex predilection. The etiology is believed to be intrauterine insult at the fourth month of gestation, or it may be hereditary. Two-thirds of the cases are associated with ophthalmologic difficulties (eg, detached retina or glaucoma), and one-third are associated with otologic problems (eg, chronic otitis media and low-set ears). Mental retardation is present occasionally. If the patient lives past 5 years, he or she can lead a fairly normal life (see Chapter 17). The symptoms are choking and aspiration as a result of negative pressure created by excessive inspiratory effort. Passing a nasogastric (NG) tube may alleviate the negative pressure. Aerophagia has to be treated to prevent vomiting, airway compromise, and aspiration. Tracheotomy may not be the answer.

A modification of the Douglas lip–tongue adhesion has helped prevent early separation of the adhesion. One theory explains that the cause may be that the fetus's head is flexed, preventing forward growth of the mandible, forcing the tongue up and backward between the palatal shelves, and producing the triad of micrognathia, glossoptosis, and cleft palate.

Plummer-Vinson Syndrome (Paterson-Kelly Syndrome)

Symptoms include dysphagia due to degeneration of the esophageal muscle, atrophy of the papillae of the tongue, as well as microcytic hypochromic anemia. Achlorhydria, glossitis, pharyngitis, esophagitis, and fissures at the corner of the mouth are also observed. The prevalence of this disease is higher in women than in men, and it usually presents in patients who are in their fourth decade. Treatment consists of iron administration, with esophagoscopy for dilatation and to rule out carcinoma of the esophagus, particularly at the postcricoid region. Pharyngoesophageal webs or stenosis may be noted.

This disease is to be contrasted with pernicious anemia, which is a megaloblastic anemia with diarrhea, nausea and vomiting, neurologic symptoms, enlarged spleen, and achlorhydria. Pernicious anemia is secondary to failure of the gastric fundus to secrete intrinsic factors necessary for vitamin B_{12} absorption. Treatment consists of intramuscular vitamin B_{12} (riboflavin).

Folic acid deficiency also gives rise to megaloblastic anemia, cheilosis, glossitis, ulcerative stomatitis, pharyngitis, esophagitis, dysphagia, and diarrhea. Neurologic symptoms and achlorhydria are not present. Treatment is the administration of folic acid.

Potter Syndrome

One of every 3000 infants is born with Potter syndrome. Most of them die during delivery and the rest die shortly after birth. Potter syndrome is characterized by severely malformed, low-set ears bilaterally, a small lower jaw, and extensive deformities of the external and middle ear (eg, an absence of auditory ossicles, atresia of the oval window, and abnormal course of the facial nerve). The cochlear membranous labyrinth is normal in its upper turn but contains severe hypoplasia in its basal turn, a rare cochlear anomaly.

One cause for this syndrome that has been proposed is fetal compression caused by oligoamnios.

Prader-Willi Syndrome

Prader-Willi syndrome affects 1 in 10,000 to 30,000 people. It is a complex genetic condition that affects many parts of the body. In infancy, this condition is characterized by weak muscle tone (hypotonia), feeding difficulties, poor growth, and delayed development. Beginning in childhood, affected individuals develop an insatiable appetite, which leads to chronic overeating (hyperphagia) and obesity. Some people with Prader-Willi syndrome, particularly those with obesity, also develop type 2 diabetes mellitus (the most common form of diabetes).

People with Prader-Willi syndrome typically have mild to moderate intellectual impairment and learning disabilities. Behavioral problems are common, including temper outbursts, stubbornness, and compulsive behavior such as picking at the skin. Sleep abnormalities can also occur. Additional features of this condition include distinctive facial features such as a narrow forehead, almond-shaped eyes, and a triangular mouth; short stature; and small hands and feet. Some people with Prader-Willi syndrome have unusually fair skin and light-colored hair. Both affected males and affected females have underdeveloped genitals. Puberty is delayed or incomplete, and most affected individuals are unable to have children (infertile).

Prader-Willi syndrome is caused by the loss of function of genes in a particular region of chromosome 15. People normally inherit one copy of this chromosome from each parent. Some genes are turned on (active) only on the copy that is inherited from a person's father (the paternal copy). This parent-specific gene activation is caused by a phenomenon called genomic imprinting.

Pseudotumor Cerebri Syndrome

Now known as idiopathic intracranial hypertension, this condition is characterized by increased intracranial pressure without focal signs of neurologic dysfunction. Obstructive hydrocephalus, mass lesions, chronic meningitis, and hypertensive and pulmonary encephalopathy should be ruled out and not confused with this syndrome. The patient is typically a young, obese female with a history of headaches, blurring of vision, or both. Facial pain and diplopia caused by unilateral or bilateral abducens nerve paralysis are less common symptoms. The CSF opening pressure on a patient lies between 250 and 600 mm of water. CSF composition, electroencephalogram (EEG), and CT scans of the head are typically normal. X-rays of the skull may reveal enlargement of the sella turcica or thinning of the dorsum sellae. This simulates a pituitary tumor, but pituitary function is normal. This syndrome is self-limited, and spontaneous recovery usually will occur within a few months. Auscultation of ear canal, neck, orbits, and periauricular regions should be performed for diagnosis, as well as funduscopic examination to identify papilloma. Complete audiologic evaluations, electronystagmography (ENG), and radiographic examinations should also be made. Occlusion of the ipsilateral jugular vein by light digital pressure should make the hum disappear by cessation of blood flow in this structure.

Purpura-Like Syndrome

Purpura-like syndrome is autoimmune thrombocytopenic purpura, which can be accompanied by systemic lupus erythematosus (LE), chronic lymphocytic leukemia, or lymphoma. There seems to be a strong association between syndromes resembling autoimmune thrombocytopenia and nonhematologic malignancies.

Pyknodysostosis

Pyknodysostosis is a syndrome consisting of dwarfism, osteopetrosis, partial agenesis of the terminal phalanges of the hands and feet, cranial anomalies (persistent fontanelles), frontal and occipital bossing, and hypoplasia of the angle of the mandible. The facial bones are usually underdeveloped with pseudoprognathism. The frontal sinuses are consistently absent, and the other paranasal sinuses are hypoplastic. The mastoid air cells are often pneumatized. Toulouse-Lautrec probably had this disease.

Raeder Syndrome

This relatively benign, self-limiting syndrome consists of ipsilateral ptosis, miosis, and facial pain with intact facial sweating. Pain exists in the distribution of the ophthalmic division of the fifth cranial nerve. It results from postganglionic sympathetic involvement in the area of the internal carotid artery or from a lesion in the anterior portion of the middle cranial fossa.

Reichert Syndrome

Neuralgia of the glossopharyngeal nerve, usually precipitated by movements of the tongue or throat, is present.

Reiter Syndrome

Arthritis, urethritis, and conjunctivitis are evident in Reiter syndrome.

Reye Syndrome

Reye Syndrome is an often fatal disease primarily afflicting young children during winter and spring months. Its cardinal pathologic features are marked encephalopathy and fatty metamorphosis of the liver. Though its etiology is unclear, Reye syndrome has been known to occur after apparent recovery from a viral infection, primarily varicella or an upper respiratory tract infection. In some patients, there is also structural damage in cochlear and vestibular tissues of the membranous labyrinth.

Intracranial pressure monitoring and respiratory support may limit brain edema. Tracheal diversion and pulmonary care may be necessary.

Riedel Struma

This disorder is a form of thyroiditis seen most frequently in middle-aged women manifested by compression of surrounding structures (ie, trachea). There is loss of the normal thyroid lobular architecture and replacement with collagen and lymphocyte infiltration.

Rivalta Disease

An actinomycotic infection characterized by multiple indurated abscesses of the face, neck, chest, and abdomen that discharge through numerous sinus tracts.

Rollet Syndrome (Orbital Apex-Sphenoidal Syndrome)

Rollet syndrome is caused by lesions of the orbital apex that cause paralysis of cranial nerves III, IV, and VI. This syndrome is characterized by ptosis, diplopia, ophthalmoplegia, optic atrophy, hyperesthesia or anesthesia of the forehead, upper eyelid and cornea, and retrobulbar neuralgia. Exophthalmos and papilledema may occur.

Romberg Syndrome

Romberg syndrome is characterized by progressive atrophy of tissues on one side of the face, occasionally extending to other parts of the body that may involve the tongue, gums, soft palate, and cartilages of the ear, nose, and larynx. Pigmentation disorders, trigeminal neuralgia, and ocular complications may be seen.

Rosai-Dorfman Disease

Rosai-Dorfman disease is benign, self-limiting lymphadenopathy, and has no detectable nodal involvement. Histiocytosis, plasma cell proliferation, and lymphophagocytosis may all be present.

Rutherford Syndrome

A familial oculodental syndrome characterized by corneal dystrophy, gingival hyperplasia, and failure of tooth eruption.

Samter Syndrome

Samter Syndrome is a triad of:

A. Allergy to aspirin
B. Nasal polyposis
C. Asthma

Scalenus Anticus Syndrome

The symptoms for scalenus anticus syndrome are identical to those for cervical rib syndrome. In scalenus anticus syndrome, the symptoms are caused by compression of the brachial plexus and subclavian artery against the first thoracic rib, probably as a result of spasms of the scalenus anticus muscle bringing pressure on the brachial plexus and the subclavian artery. Any pressure on the sympathetic nerves may cause vascular spasm resembling Raynaud disease.

Schafer Syndrome

Hereditary mental retardation, sensorineural hearing loss, prolinemia, hematuria, and photogenic epilepsy are characteristics. Schafer syndrome is due to a deficiency of proline oxidase with a resultant buildup of the amino acid proline.

Schaumann Syndrome

Schaumann syndrome is generalized sarcoidosis.

Schmidt Syndrome

Unilateral paralysis of the vocal cord, the velum palati, the trapezius, and the sternocleidomastoid muscles is found. The lesion is located in the caudal portion of the medulla and is usually of vascular origin.

Scimitar Syndrome

This congenital anomaly of the venous system of the right lung gets its name from the typical shadow formed on a thoracic roentgenogram of patients afflicted with it. (The scimitar is a curved Turkish sword that increases in diameter toward its distal end.) The most common clinical features are dyspnea and recurrent infections. The cause of scimitar syndrome is abnormal development of the right lung bed. The syndrome may be the result of vascular anomalies of the venous and arterial system of the right lung, hypoplasia of the right lung, or drainage of part of the right pulmonary venous system into the inferior vena cava, causing the scimitar sign on the thoracic roentgenogram.

This syndrome occurs between the fourth and sixth weeks of fetal life. Clinical features include displacement of heart sounds as well as heart percussion shadow toward the right. When dextroposition of the heart is marked, tomography can also help in diagnosis. Bronchography and angiography also aid in diagnosis and in providing exact information for surgical correction.

Seckel Syndrome

Seckel syndrome is a disorder that consists of dwarfism associated with a bird-like facies, beaked nose, micrognathia, palate abnormalities, low-set lobeless ears, antimongoloid slant of the palpebral fissures, clinodactyly, mental retardation, and bone disorders.

Secretion of Antidiuretic Hormone Syndrome

Secretion of antidiuretic hormone syndrome is also referred to as the syndrome of inappropriate secretion of antidiuretic hormone (SIADH). Antidiuretic hormone helps maintain constant serum osmolality by conserving water and concentrating urine. This syndrome involves low serum osmolality, elevated urinary osmolality less than maximally dilute urine, and hyponatremia. This can lead to lethargy, anorexia, headache, convulsions, coma, or cardiac arrhythmias. Increased CSF and intracranial pressure are possible etiologies. Fluid restriction can help prevent this condition.

Sheehan Syndrome

Ischemic necrosis of the anterior pituitary associated with postpartum hypotension characterizes Sheehan syndrome. It is seen in menopausal women and is associated with rheumatoid arthritis, Raynaud phenomenon, and dental caries. Changes in the lacrimal and salivary glands resemble those of Mikulicz disease. Some physicians attribute this syndrome to vitamin A deficiency. A positive LE preparation, rheumatoid factor, and an abnormal protein can be identified in this disorder.

Shy-Drager Syndrome

Usually presented in late middle age, this is a form of neurogenic orthostatic hypotension that results in failure of the autonomic nervous system and signs of multiple systems atrophy affecting corticospinal and cerebellar pathways and basal ganglia. Symptoms include postural hypotension, impotence, sphincter dysfunction, and anhidrosis with later progression to panautonomic failure. Such autonomic symptoms are usually followed by atypical parkinsonism, cerebellar dysfunction with debilitation, or both, and then death. SDS should always be considered when the patient displays orthostatic hypotension, laryngeal stridor, restriction in range of vocal cord abduction (unilaterally or bilaterally), vocal hoarseness, intermittent diplophonia, and slow speech rate. This syndrome is often compared with Parkinson disease. However, SDS involves the nigrostriatal, olivopontocerebellar, brain stem, and intermediolateral column of the spinal cord. It is a multiple system disorder, whereas Parkinson disease involves only the nigrostriatal neuronal system. The symptoms, such as autonomic failure, pyramidal disease, and cerebellar dysfunction, have been associated with pathology of the pigmented nuclei and the dorsal motor nucleus of the vagus.

Sjögren Syndrome (Sicca Syndrome)

Sjögren syndrome is manifested as keratoconjunctivitis sicca, dryness of the mucous membranes, telangiectasias or purpuric spots on the face, and bilateral parotid enlargement. It is a chronic inflammatory process involving mainly the salivary and lacrimal glands and is associated with hyperactivity of the B lymphocytes and with autoantibody and immune complex production. One of the complications of this syndrome is the development of malignant lymphoma. CT aids in the diagnosis.

Sleep Apnea Syndrome

The definition of apnea is a cessation of airflow of more than 10 seconds in duration. The conditions for sleep apnea syndrome are said to be met when at least 30 episodes of apnea occur within a 7-hour period or when 1% of a patient's sleeping time is spent in apnea. The cause of sleep apnea is unclear. Some people believe it is of central origin; others think that it may be aggravated by hypertrophied and occluding tonsils and adenoids. Some investigators classify sleep apnea into central apnea, upper airway apnea, and mixed apnea. Monitoring of the EEG and other brain stem-evoked response measurements may help identify central apnea.

Sluder Neuralgia

The symptoms are neuralgia of the lower half of the face, nasal congestion, and rhinorrhea associated with lesions of the sphenopalatine ganglion. Ocular hyperemia and increased lacrimation may be seen. It is sometimes referred to as Charlin-Sluder neuralgia or Charlin syndrome or Sluder syndrome. Another manifestation is rhinorrhea accompanied by severe ocular and orbital pain, and paroxysmal congestion of the anterior segment of the eye.

Stevens-Johnson Syndrome

Stevens-Johnson syndrome is a skin disease (erythema multiforme) with involvement of the oral cavity (stomatitis) and the eye (conjunctivitis). Stomatitis may appear as the first symptom. It is most common during the third decade of life. Treatment consists largely of steroids and supportive therapy. It is a self-limiting disease but has a 25% recurrence rate. The differential diagnosis includes herpes simplex, pemphigus, acute fusospirochetal stomatitis, chicken pox, monilial infection, and secondary syphilis.

Still Disease

Rheumatoid arthritis in children is sometimes called Still disease (see a pediatric textbook for more details).

Sturge-Weber Syndrome

Sturge-Weber syndrome is a congenital disorder that affects both sexes equally and is of unknown etiology. It is characterized by venous angioma of the leptomeninges over the cerebral cortex, ipsilateral port wine nevi, and frequent angiomatous involvement of the globe, mouth, and nasal mucosa. The patient may have convulsions, hemiparesis, glaucoma, and intracranial calcifications. There is no specific treatment.

Subclavian Steal Syndrome

Stenosis or occlusion of the subclavian or innominate artery proximal to the origin of the vertebral artery causes the pressure in the vertebral artery to be less than that of the basilar artery, particularly when the upper extremity is in action. Hence, the brain receives less blood and may be ischemic. The symptoms consist of intermittent vertigo, occipital headache, blurred vision, diplopia, dysarthria, and pain in the upper extremity. The diagnosis, made through the patient's medical history, can be confirmed by the difference in blood pressure in the two upper extremities, by a bruit over the supraclavicular fossa, and by angiography.

Superior Semicircular Canal Dehiscence Syndrome

Vertigo, oscillopsia induced by loud noise, changes in middle ear, or intracranial pressure, positive Hennebert sign, and Tullio phenomenon. Dehiscence of bone overlying the superior SCC can lead to vestibular as well as auditory symptoms and signs. The vestibular abnormalities include vertigo (an illusion of motion) and oscillopsia (the apparent motion of objects that are known to be stationary) induced by loud noises and/or by maneuvers that change middle ear or intracranial pressure. Patients with this syndrome can have eye movements in the plane of the superior canal in response to loud noises in the affected ear (Tullio phenomenon). Insufflation of air into the external auditory canal or pressure on the tragus can, in some patients, result in similar abnormalities (Hennebert sign).

The auditory abnormalities include autophony, hypersensitivity to bone-conducted sounds, and pulsatile tinnitus. Patients may complain of seemingly bizarre symptoms as hearing their eye movements in the affected ear. They may also experience an uncomfortable sensation of fullness or pressure in the ear brought about by activities that lead to vibration or motion in the long bones such as running. The Weber tuning fork test (512 Hz) often localizes to the affected ear. The audiogram will frequently show an air–bone gap in the low frequencies, and bone conduction thresholds may be better than 0-dB NHL. The findings on audiometry can resemble those in otosclerosis. Some patients with superior canal dehiscence have undergone stapedectomy, which does not lead to closure of the air–bone gap. Acoustic reflex testing can be beneficial in distinguishing an air–bone gap due to superior canal dehiscence from one due to otosclerosis. Acoustic reflexes will be absent in the affected ear of a patient with otosclerosis, whereas these responses will be present in superior canal dehiscence. Patients with intact acoustic reflex responses and an air–bone gap on audiometry should undergo further investigation for superior canal dehiscence, such as a high-resolution CT scan of the temporal bones, before proceeding with surgical exploration of the middle ear.

Some patients have exclusively vestibular manifestations, others have exclusively auditory manifestations, and still others have both auditory and vestibular abnormalities from superior canal dehiscence. The reasons for these differences are not known. The mechanism underlying both the vestibular and auditory manifestations of this syndrome can be understood based upon the effects of the dehiscence in creation of a "third mobile window" into the inner ear.

Vestibular-evoked myogenic potential (VEMP) responses are short-latency relaxation potentials measured from tonically contracting sternocleidomastoid muscles that relax in response to ipsilateral presentation of loud sounds delivered as either clicks or tone bursts. The VEMP response is typically recorded from the sternocleidomastoid muscle that is ipsilateral to the side of sound presentation. Patients with superior canal dehiscence have a lowered threshold for eliciting a VEMP response in the ear(s) affected by the disorder. The VEMP response can also have a larger-than-normal amplitude in superior canal dehiscence. High-resolution temporal bone CT scans have been used to identify dehiscence of bone overlying the superior canal.

The surgery is typically performed through the middle cranial fossa approach. A recent comparison of surgical outcomes in patients who underwent either canal plugging or resurfacing (without plugging of the canal lumen) revealed that complete resolution of vestibular symptoms and signs is more commonly obtained with canal plugging than with resurfacing alone.

Superior Orbital Fissure Syndrome (Orbital Apex Syndrome, Optic Foramen Syndrome, Sphenoid Fissure Syndrome)

There is involvement of cranial nerves III, IV, V1, and VI, the ophthalmic veins, and the sympathetics of the cavernous sinus. The syndrome can be caused by sphenoid sinusitis or any neoplasia in that region. Symptoms include paralysis of the upper eyelid, orbital pain, photophobia, and paralysis of the above nerves. The optic nerve may be damaged as well.

Superior Vena Cava Syndrome

This syndrome is characterized by obstruction of the superior vena cava or its main tributaries by bronchogenic carcinoma, mediastinal neoplasm, or lymphoma. Rarely, the presence of a substernal goiter causes edema and engorgement of the vessels of the face, neck, and arms, as well as a nonproductive cough and dyspnea.

Takayasu Disease

Also called "pulseless disease" and aortic arch syndrome, this disease involves narrowing of the aortic arch and its branches. Possibly an autoimmune disorder, the etiology is unknown. Symptoms often originate in the head and neck area. Sensorineural hearing loss is often an associated symptom. An association has also been found with B-cell alloantigens DR4 and MB3. Steroid treatment and cyclophosphamide have been known to help, as does surgery, although operating during a relatively inactive phase of the disease is recommended.

Tapia Syndrome

Unilateral paralysis of the larynx and tongue is coupled with atrophy of the tongue; the soft palate and cricothyroid muscle are intact. Tapia syndrome is usually caused by a lesion at the point where the 12th and 10th nerves, together with the internal carotid artery, cross one another.

Trauma is the most common cause of this syndrome. Pressure neuropathy due to inflation of the cuff of an endotracheal tube within the larynx, rather than within the trachea, is associated with the palsy of the laryngeal nerve.

Tay-Sachs Disease

An infantile form of amaurotic familial idiocy with strong familial tendencies, Tay-Sachs disease is of questionably recessive inheritance. It is more commonly found among those of Semitic extraction. Histologically, the nerve cells are distorted and filled with a lipid material. The juvenile form is called Spielmeyer-Vogt disease, and the patient is normal until after 5 to 7 years of age. The juvenile form is seen in children of non-Semitic extraction as well.

Tietze Syndrome

Tietze syndrome is a costal chondritis chondropathia tuberosa of unknown etiology. Its symptoms include pain, tenderness, and swelling of one or more of the upper costal cartilages (usually the second rib). Treatment is symptomatic.

Tolosa-Hunt Syndrome

Tolosa-Hunt syndrome is a cranial polyneuropathy usually presenting as recurrent unilateral painful ophthalmoplegia. Cranial nerves II, III, IV, V1, and VI may be involved. The etiology is unknown, and there is a tendency for spontaneous resolution and for recurrence. An orbital venogram may show occlusion of the superior ophthalmic vein and at least partial obliteration of the cavernous sinus. The clinical course often responds well to systemic steroids.

Erroneous diagnoses include inflammation, tumor, vascular aneurysm, thrombus involving the orbit, superior orbital fissure, anterior cavernous sinus, parasellar area, or posterior fossa. An extension of nasopharyngeal carcinoma, mucocele, or contiguous sinusitis must also be ruled out. Sources of infection in the head and neck region, such as the tonsils, can be treated, relieving the pain of ophthalmoplegia.

Tourette Syndrome

A disorder of the CNS, Tourette syndrome is characterized by the appearance of involuntary tic movements, such as rapid eye blinking, facial twitches, head jerking, or shoulder shrugging. Involuntary sounds, such as repeated throat clearing, "nervous" coughing, or inappropriate use of words, sometimes occur simultaneously. Tourette syndrome, in many cases, responds to medication. It has a higher rate of absorption, or binding at D_2 dopamine receptors on cells in the caudate nucleus. The etiology of this syndrome is unknown.

Toxic Shock Syndrome

Cases of toxic shock syndrome have been found related to nasal packing and to staphylococcal infection of surgical wounds. Although the pathogenesis of the disease is incompletely understood, it is believed that packing left too long can cause bacterial overgrowth, leading to toxic shock syndrome. Symptoms include fever, rash, hypotension, mucosal hyperemia, vomiting, diarrhea, laboratory evidence of multiorgan dysfunction, and desquamation during recovery. It has been found that although antibiotic impregnation into the packing material may reduce bacterial overgrowth, it does not provide absolute protection against toxic shock syndrome.

Single-dose antimicrobial prophylaxis has proven highly effective as a treatment. Additionally, screening for toxic shock syndrome toxin (TSST)-1–producing *Staphylococcus aureus* helps point out high-risk patients for this syndrome.

Treacher Collins Syndrome

See Chapter 17.

Trigeminal Trophic Syndrome

Trigeminal trophic syndrome, also called trigeminal neurotrophic ulceration or trigeminal neuropathy with nasal ulceration, involves ulceration of the face, particularly ala nasi, and histologic features, such as chronic, nonspecific ulceration and crusting, erythema, tendency to bleed easily, and predominant granulation tissue. Whether caused by self-induced trauma, surgery, or any process involved with the trigeminal nerve or its connections, the etiologies of nasal ulceration to be excluded with this syndrome are basal cell carcinoma, blastomycosis, leishmaniasis, leprous trigeminal neuritis, lethal midline granuloma, paracoccidioidomycosis, postsurgical herpetic reactivation, pyoderma gangrenosum, and Wegener granulomatosis. Treatment should focus on prevention of trauma to lesion and prevention of secondary infection.

Trotter Syndrome (Sinus of Morgagni Syndrome)

Neuralgia of the inferior maxillary nerve, conductive hearing loss secondary to eustachian tube blockage, preauricular edema caused by neoplastic invasion of the sinus of Morgagni, ipsilateral akinesia of the soft palate, and trismus are observed in Trotter syndrome.

Tube Feeding Syndrome

See Chapter 53.

Turner Syndrome

See Chapter 17.

Turpin Syndrome

Patients have congenital bronchiectasis, megaesophagus, tracheoesophageal fistula, vertebral deformities, rib malformations, and a heterotopic thoracic duct.

Vail Syndrome

Vail syndrome consists of unilateral, usually nocturnal, vidian neuralgia that may be associated with sinusitis.

VATER Syndrome (VACTERL Syndrome)

VATER syndrome is a nonrandom association of vertebral defects, anal atresia, tracheoesophageal fistula with esophageal atresia, renal defects, and radial limb dysplasia. Vascular anomalies, such as ventricular septal defect and single umbilical artery, have also been associated with this syndrome. Vertebral anomalies consist of hypoplasia of either the vertebral bodies or the pedicles, leading to secondary scoliosis in children. Anal and perineal anomalies consist of hypospadias, persistent urachus, female pseudohermaphroditism, imperforate anus, and genitourinary fistulas. GI anomalies include duodenal atresia, esophageal atresia, and tracheoesophageal fistula. Radial anomalies include supernumerary digiti, hypoplastic radial rays, and preaxial lower extremity anomalies. Renal anomalies include aplasia or hypoplasia of the kidneys with ectopia or fusion as well as congenital hydronephrosis and hydroureter. Hold-Oram syndrome is often confused with this syndrome, but VATER syndrome is random, whereas Hold-Oram is inherited. This syndrome is suggested to be formed prior to the fifth week of fetal life during organogenesis.

Vernet Syndrome

See Jugular Foramen Syndrome (Vernet Syndrome).

Villaret Syndrome

Villaret syndrome is the same as the jugular foramen syndrome except that Horner syndrome is present here, suggesting more extensive involvement in the region of the jugular foramen, the retroparotid area, and the lateral pharyngeal space.

Vogt-Koyanagi-Harada Syndrome

Spastic diplegia with athetosis and pseudobulbar paralysis associated with a lesion of the caudate nucleus and putamen, bilateral uveitis, vitiligo, deafness, alopecia, increased CSF pressure, and retinal detachment are evidenced.

von Hippel-Lindau Disease

Associated with cerebellar, medullary, and spinal hemangioblastoma, retinal angiomata, pheochromocytoma, and renal cell carcinoma. Endolymphatic sac tumors can be present.

Wallenberg Syndrome

Also called syndrome of the posterior–inferior cerebellar artery thrombosis or lateral medullary syndrome, Wallenberg syndrome is due to thrombosis of the posteroinferior cerebellar artery giving rise to ischemia of the brain stem (lateral medullary region). Symptoms include vertigo, nystagmus, nausea, vomiting, Horner syndrome, dysphagia, dysphonia, hypotonia, asthenia, ataxia, falling to the side of the lesion, and loss of pain and temperature sense on the ipsilateral face and contralateral side below the neck.

Weber Syndrome

Weber syndrome is characterized by paralysis of the oculomotor nerve on the side of the lesion and paralysis of the extremities, face, and tongue on the contralateral side. It indicates a lesion in the ventral and internal part of the cerebral peduncle.

Whistling Face Syndrome

Also known as craniocarpotarsal dysplasia, whistling face syndrome is mostly transmitted through autosomal dominant genes (although heterogenic transmission is not unknown).

The main physical features are antimongoloid slant of the palpebral fissures, blepharophimosis, broad nasal bridge, convergent strabismus, enophthalmos, equinovarus with contracted toes, flat midface, H-shaped cutaneous dimpling on the chin, kyphosis–scoliosis, long philtrum, mask-like rigid face, microglossia, microstomia, protruding lips, small nose and nostrils, steeply inclined anterior cranial fossa on roentgenogram, thick skin over flexor surfaces of proximal phalanges, ulnar deviation, and flexion contractures of fingers.

Wildervanck (Cervico-Oculo-Acoustic) Syndrome

Wildervanck syndrome consists of mixed hearing loss, Klippel-Feil anomalad (fused cervical vertebrae), and bilateral abducens palsy with retracted bulb (Duane syndrome). Occurring in more female than male subjects, in almost a 75:1 ratio, it has sex-linked dominance with lethality in the homozygous male subject.

Wilson Disease (Hepatolenticular Degeneration)

There are two chief types of Wilson disease: one rapidly progressive that occurs during late childhood and the other slowly progressive occurring in the third or fourth decades. Familial, its symptoms are cirrhosis with progressive damage to the nervous system and brown pigmentation of the outer margin of the cornea, called Kayser-Fleischer ring. It can present with hearing loss as well.

Winkler Disease (Chondrodermatitis Nodularis Chronica Helicis)

Arteriovenous anastomosis and nerve-ending accumulation at the helical portion of the ear are evident. It presents with pain and is characterized by hard, round nodules involving the skin and cartilage of the helix. Ninety percent of all cases occur in men. The treatment is to excise the nodules or administer steroids.

Xeroderma Pigmentosum (Autosomal Recessive)

This disorder presents as photosensitive skin with multiple basal cell epitheliomas. Squamous cell carcinoma or malignant melanoma can result from it. The condition occurs mainly in children. These children should be kept away from the sun.

Eponyms

Abrikossoff Tumor (Granular Cell Myoblastoma)

Causes pseudoepithelial hyperplasia in the larynx, the site most favored in the larynx being the posterior half of the vocal cord. Three percent of granular cell myoblastoma progress to malignancy. In order of decreasing frequency of involvement, the granular cell myoblastoma occurs in tongue, skin, breast, subcutaneous tissue, and respiratory tract.

Adenoid Facies

Adenoid facies is characterized by crowded teeth, high-arched palate, and underdeveloped nostrils.

Adler Bodies

Deposits of mucopolysaccharide are found in neutrophils of patients with Hurler syndrome.

Antoni Types A and B

See Chapter 53.

Arnold-Chiari Malformation

Type I: Downward protrusion of the long, thin cerebellar tonsils through the foramen magnum

Type II: Protrusion of the inferior cerebellar vermis through the foramen

Type III: Bony occipital defect with descent of the entire cerebellum

Type IV: Cerebellar hypoplasia

Arnold Ganglion

Otic ganglion.

Aschoff Body

Rheumatic nodule is found in rheumatic disease.

Ballet Sign

Ballet sign is characterized by paralysis of voluntary movements of the eyeball with preservation of the automatic movements, and is sometimes present with exophthalmic goiter and hysteria.

Bechterew Syndrome

Bechterew syndrome is characterized by paralysis of facial muscles limited to automatic movements. The power of voluntary movement is retained.

Bednar Aphthae

Bednar aphthae is characterized by symmetrical excoriations of the hard palate in the region of the pterygoid plates due to sucking of the thumb, foreign objects, or scalding.

Bezold Abscess

Bezold abscess is abscess in the sternocleidomastoid muscle secondary to perforation of the tip of the mastoid by infection.

Gland of Blandin

Gland of Blandin is a minor salivary gland situated in the anterior portion of the tongue.

Brooke Tumor (Epithelioma Adenoides Cysticum)

Originates from the hair follicles in the external auditory canal and auricle and of basal cell origin. Treatment is local resection.

Broyle Ligament

Broyle ligament is anterior commissure ligament of the larynx.

Brudzinski Sign

With meningitis, passive flexion of the leg on one side causes a similar movement to occur in the opposite leg. Passive flexion of the neck brings about flexion of the legs as well.

Brunner Abscess

Brunner abscess is abscess of the posterior floor of the mouth.

Bruns Sign

Bruns sign is characterized by intermittent headache, vertigo, and vomiting, especially with sudden movements of the head. It occurs in cases of tumor of the fourth ventricle of the brain.

Bryce Sign

A gurgling is heard in a neck mass. It suggests a laryngocele.

Carhart Notch

Dip at 2000 kHz (bone conduction) seen in patients with otosclerosis.

Charcot-Leyden Crystals

Crystals are in the shape of elongated double pyramids, composed of spermine phosphates, and present in the sputum of asthmatic patients. Synonyms are Charcot-Newman crystals and Charcot-Robin crystals. Also found in fungal infection.

Charcot Triad

The nystagmus, scanning speech, and intention tremor are seen in multiple sclerosis.

Cherubism

Familial, with the age of predilection between 2 and 5 years. It is characterized by giant cell reparative granuloma causing cystic lesions in the posterior rami of the mandible. The lesions are usually symmetrical. It is a self-limiting disease with remissions after puberty. The maxilla may also be involved.

Chvostek Sign

Facial twitch obtained by tapping the distribution of the facial nerve. It is indicative of hypocalcemia and is the most reliable test for hypocalcemia.

Curschmann Spirals

Spirally twisted masses of the mucus present in the sputum of bronchial asthmatic patients.

Dalrymple Sign

Upper lid retraction with upper scleral showing is a clinical manifestation of Graves orbitopathy (exophthalmos).

Demarquay Sign

Demarquay sign is characterized by the absence of elevation of the larynx during deglutition. It is said to indicate syphilitic induration of the trachea.

Di Sant'Agnese Test

Di Sant'Agnese test Measures the elevated sodium and chloride in the sweat of cystic fibrotic children.

Dupre Sign

Meningism.

Gustatory Glands of Ebner

These glands are the minor salivary glands near the circumvallate papillae.

Escherich Sign

In hypoparathyroidism, tapping of the skin at the angle of the mouth causes protrusion of the lips.

Flexner-Wintersteiner Rosettes

True neural rosettes of grades III and IV esthesioneuroblastoma.

Galen Anastomosis

An anastomosis between the superior laryngeal nerve and the recurrent laryngeal nerve.

Goodwin Tumor

Benign lymphoepithelioma.

Griesinger Sign

Edema of the tip of the mastoid in thrombosis of the sigmoid sinus.

Guttman Test

In the normal subject, frontal pressure on the thyroid cartilage lowers the tone of voice produced, whereas lateral pressure produces a higher tone of voice. The opposite is true with paralysis of the cricothyroid muscle.

Guyon Sign

The 12th nerve lies directly upon the external carotid artery, whereby this vessel may be distinguished from the internal carotid artery. (The safer way prior to ligation of the external carotid artery is to identify the first few branches of the external carotid artery.)

Glands of Henle

They are the small glands situated in the areolar tissue between the buccopharyngeal fascia anteriorly and the prevertebral fascia posteriorly. Infection of these glands can lead to retropharyngeal abscess. Because these glands atrophy after age 5, a retropharyngeal abscess is less likely to occur after that age.

Hennebert Sign

See Chapter 17. The presence of a positive fistula test in the absence of an obvious fistula is called Hennebert sign. The patient has a normal-appearing tympanic membrane and external auditory canal. The nystagmus is more marked upon application of negative pressure. This sign is present with congenital syphilis and is believed to be due to an excessively mobile footplate or caused by motion of the saccule mediated by fibrosis between the footplate and the saccule.

Hering-Breuer Reflex

A respiratory reflex from pulmonary stretch receptors. Inflation of the lungs sends an inhibitory impulse to the CNS via the vagus nerve to stop inspiration. Similarly, deflation of the lungs sends an impulse to stop expiration. This action is the Hering-Breuer reflex.

Homer-Wright Rosettes

Pseudorosette pattern seen in grade I esthesioneuroblastoma.

Kernig Sign

When the subject lies on the back with the thigh at a right angle to the trunk, straightening of the leg (extending the leg) elicits pain, supposedly owing to the pull on the inflamed lumbosacral nerve roots. This sign is present with meningitis.

Kiesselbach Plexus

This area is in the anterior septum where the capillaries merge. It is often the site of anterior epistaxis and has also been referred to as Little's area.

Koplik Spot

Pale round spots on the oral mucosa, conjunctiva, and lacrimal caruncle that are seen in the beginning stages of measles.

Krause Nodes

Nodes in the jugular foramen.

Lhermitte Sign

A rare complication of radiation to the head and neck region causing damage to the cervical spinal cord, symptoms of Lhermitte sign consist of lightning-like electrical sensation spreading to both arms, down the dorsal spine, and to both legs upon neck flexion.

Lillie-Crowe Test

Used in the diagnosis of unilateral sinus thrombophlebitis. Digital compression of the opposite internal jugular vein causes the retinal veins to dilate.

Little Area

See Kiesselbach Plexus.

Luschka Pouch

See Thornwaldt Cyst.

Marcus Gunn Phenomenon

Unilateral ptosis of the eyelid with exaggerated opening of the eye during movements of the mandible.

Marjolin Ulcer

A carcinoma that arises at the site of an old burn scar. It is a well-differentiated squamous cell carcinoma that is aggressive and metastasizes rapidly.

Meckel Ganglion

Sphenopalatine ganglion.

Mikulicz Cells

These cells are macrophages in rhinoscleroma. (Russell bodies, which are eosinophilic, round structures associated with plasma cells, are also found with rhinoscleroma.)

Mollaret-Debre Test

Performed for cat scratch fever.

Sinus of Morgagni

A dehiscence of the superior constrictor muscle and the buccopharyngeal fascia where the eustachian tube opens.

Ventricle of Morgagni

Ventricle of Morgagni separates the quadrangular membrane from the conus elasticus in the larynx.

Nikolsky Sign

Detachment of the sheets of superficial epithelial layers when any traction is applied over the surface of the epithelial involvement in pemphigus is characteristic of Nikolsky sign. Pemphigus involves the intraepithelial layer, whereas pemphigoid involves the subepithelial layer. The former is a lethal disease in many instances.

Oliver-Cardarelli Sign

Recession of the larynx and trachea is synchronous with cardiac systole in cases of aneurysm of the arch of the aorta or in cases of a tumor in that region.

Parinaud Sign

Extraocular muscle impairment with decreased upward gaze and ptosis is seen in association with pinealomas and other lesions of the tectum.

Paul-Bunnell Test

Paul-Bunnell test measures the elevated heterophile titer of infectious mononucleosis.

Physaliferous Cells

"Soap bubble" cells of chordoma.

Psammoma Bodies

Found with papillary carcinoma of the thyroid.

Rathke Pouch

See Thornwaldt Cyst.

Reinke Tumor

A "soft" tumor variant of lymphoepithelioma in which the lymphocytes predominate. (With the hard tumor the epithelial cells predominate; it is called Schmincke tumor.)

Romberg Sign

If a patient standing with the feet together "falls" when closing the eyes, the Romberg test is positive. It is indicative of either abnormal proprioception or abnormal vestibular function. It does not necessarily distinguish central from peripheral lesions. Cerebellar function is not evaluated by this test.

Rosenbach Sign

Fine tremor of the closed eyelids seen in hyperthyroidism and hysteria.

Rouvier Node
Lateral retropharyngeal node, Rouvier node is a common target of metastases in nasopharyngeal carcinoma.

Russell Bodies
Eosinophilic, round structures; associated with plasma cells found in rhinoscleroma.

Santorini Cartilage
Corniculate cartilage of the larynx, composed of fibroelastic cartilage.

Santorini Fissures
Fissures in the anterior cartilaginous external auditory canal leading to the parotid region.

Schaumann Bodies
Together with asteroids, they are found in sarcoid granuloma.

Schmincke Tumor
The "hard" variant of lymphoepithelioma in which the epithelial cells predominate (see Reinke Tumor).

Schneiderian Mucosa
Pseudostratified ciliated columnar mucosa of the nose.

Seeligmüller Sign
Contraction of the pupil on the affected side in facial neuralgia.

Semon Law
Semon law states that injury to the recurrent laryngeal nerve results in paralysis of the abductor muscle of the larynx (cricoarytenoid posticus) before paralysis of the adductor muscles. During recovery, the adductor recovers before the abductor.

Straus Sign
With facial paralysis, the lesion is peripheral if injection of pilocarpine is followed by sweating on the affected side later than on the normal side.

Sudeck Sign
Sudeck sign is sometimes associated with Grisel syndrome and is recognized by the displacement of the spine of the axis to the same side as the head is turned.

Sulkowitch Test
Determines an increase in calciuria.

Thornwaldt Cyst
A depression exists in the nasopharyngeal vault that is a remnant of the pouch of Luschka. When this depression becomes infected, Thornwaldt cyst results. In the early embryo, this area has a connection between the notochord and entoderm. Thornwaldt cyst is lined with respiratory epithelium with some squamous metaplasia. Anterior to this pit, the path taken by Rathke pouch

sometimes persists as the craniopharyngeal canal, running from the sella turcica through the body of the sphenoid to an opening on the undersurface of the skull.

Tobey-Ayer-Queckenstedt Test

Tobey-Ayer-Queckenstedt test is used in the diagnosis of unilateral and bilateral sinus thrombophlebitis. In cases where the lateral sinus is obstructed on one side, compression of the jugular vein on the intact side causes a rise in CSF pressure, whereas compression of the obstructed side does not raise the CSF pressure.

Toynbee Law

When CNS complications arise in chronic otitis media, the lateral sinus and cerebellum are involved in mastoiditis, whereas the cerebrum alone is involved in instances of cholesteatoma of the attic.

Trousseau Sign

With hypocalcemia, a tourniquet placed around the arm causes tetany.

Tullio Phenomenon

See Chapter 17. This phenomenon is said to be present when a loud noise precipitates vertigo. It can be present in congenital syphilis, with a SCC fistula, or in a postfenestration patient if the footplate is mobile. The tympanic membrane and ossicular chain must be intact with a mobile footplate.

Wartenberg Sign

Intense pruritus of the tip of the nose and nostril indicates cerebral tumor.

Warthin-Finkeldey Giant Cells

Warthin-Finkeldey giant cells are found in the lymphoid with measles.

Warthin-Starry Stain

Warthin-Starry stain is used to identify cat scratch bacillus.

Weber Glands

Weber Glands are minor salivary glands in the superior pole of the tonsil.

Wrisberg Cartilage

Wrisberg cartilage is the cuneiform cartilage of the larynx, composed of fibroelastic cartilage.

Xeroderma Pigmentosa

Xeroderma pigmentosa is hereditary precancerous condition that begins during early childhood. These patients die at puberty.

Zaufal Sign

Saddle nose.

Zellballen

Nest of cells surrounded by sustentacular cells seen in paragangliomas.

Clinical Entities Presenting With Dysequilibrium

The clinical entities presenting with vertigo or dysequilibrium have been named by their mode of presentation. As more information becomes available about clinical entities, the emphasis is shifting toward finding an etiology for the symptoms. When evaluating a patient with vertigo, one should try to differentiate between vertigo of peripheral origin and that of central origin. The following list of differential diagnoses constitutes the more common etiologies of the dizzy patient:

Acoustic Neuroma (Vestibular Schwannoma)

Acoustic neuroma, a benign, slow-growing tumor, has its origin most commonly in the vestibular division of the eighth cranial nerve. Most patients with acoustic neuromas complain of unsteadiness rather than episodic vertigo. As the enlarging tumor spills over into the cochlear division of the eighth nerve or compromises the artery to the inner ear, hearing symptoms become manifest. These symptoms include unilateral tinnitus, hearing loss, or both. Initially the findings may be indistinguishable from Ménière syndrome. With time, there is a progressive hearing loss, with a disproportionate loss of speech discrimination occurring long before a total hearing loss occurs. Acoustic neuroma accounts for 80% of cerebellar–pontine (CP) angle tumors.

Even though the facial nerve is in close proximity, visible signs of facial nerve (VII) palsy occur only rarely in advanced cases. More commonly, the first modality affected by the pressure on the fifth (trigeminal) nerve is demonstrated by altered corneal sensation. Later, there may be symptoms of numbness in any or all divisions of the trigeminal nerve. On rare occasions, trigeminal neuralgia has been a presenting symptom.

The audiologic evaluation may vary from normal pure tone hearing with poor speech discrimination to a pure tone sensorineural hearing loss and poor or absent speech discrimination. A search for the acoustic stapedial reflexes with the impedance bridge may show reflexes present at normal levels without evidence of decay in about 18% of the tumors. The reflexes are helpful when they are absent or show evidence of decay when the behavioral pure tones are in the normal range. ABR is the most sensitive test in detecting acoustic neuromas, abnormal in 82% of small intracanalicular tumors.

When there is an absent caloric response in the suspect ear with no history of dysequilibrium, the vestibular evaluation heightens one's suspicion.

Magnetic resonance imaging (MRI) with intravenous contrast (gadolinium-DPTA) is a reliable and cost-effective method of identifying tumors and may be selected as the first or only imaging technique. Tumors as small as 2 mm may be enhanced and identified.

Presbystasis (Dysequilibrium of Aging) and Cardiovascular Causes

Age-related decline in peripheral vestibular function, visual acuity, proprioception, and motor control has a cumulative effect upon balance and is the most common cause of dysequilibrium.

Arrhythmias usually produce dysequilibrium. They rarely present to the otologist but are seen in consultation with the cardiologist. However, consideration must be given when seeing a new patient with dysequilibrium.

Benign Paroxysmal Positional Vertigo

The symptoms include sudden attacks of vertigo precipitated by sitting up, lying down, or turning in bed. These attacks have been reported to be prompted by sudden movement of the head to the right or left or by extension of the neck when looking upward. The sensation of vertigo is always of short duration even when the provocative position is maintained. Diagnosis can be confirmed by positional testing (Dix-Hallpike test), which indicates positional nystagmus with latency and fatigability.

Etiologies include degenerative changes, otitis media, labyrinthine concussion, previous ear surgery, and occlusion of the anterior vestibular artery. The cause is thought to involve abnormal sensitivity of the SCC ampulla, especially the posterior, to gravitational forces stimulated by free-floating abnormally dense particles (canaliths). These particles can be repositioned and the symptoms resolved in a high percentage of cases, by canalith repositioning procedure.

To effectively carry out the procedure, one should be able to envision the ongoing orientation of the SCCs while carrying out the head maneuvers.

Internuclear Ophthalmoplegia

Internuclear ophthalmoplegia is a disturbance of the lateral movements of the eyes characterized by a paralysis of the internal rectus on one side and weakness of the external rectus on the other. In testing, the examiner has the patient follow his or her finger, first to one side and then to the other, as when testing for horizontal nystagmus. Internuclear ophthalmoplegia is recognized when the adductive eye (third nerve) is weak and the abducting eye (sixth nerve) moves normally and displays a coarse nystagmus ("perhaps" vestibular nuclei involvement). The pathology is in the medial longitudinal fasciculus (MLF). When the disorder is bilateral, it is pathognomonic of multiple sclerosis. When it is unilateral, one should consider a tumor or vascular process.

Intracranial Tumors

There is a small but definite number of patients that present with dysequilibrium associated with primary or secondary intracranial tumors. The use of CT and MRI scanning, without and with intravenous contrast, in selected patients helps identify these otherwise silent lesions.

Ménière Disease

The symptoms, when complete and classically present, include fluctuating sensorineural hearing loss, fluctuating tinnitus, and fluctuating fullness in the affected ear. In addition, as the tinnitus, fullness, and hearing loss intensify, an attack of episodic vertigo follows, lasting 30 minutes to 2 hours. The process may spontaneously remit, never occur again, and leave no residual or perhaps a mild hearing loss and tinnitus. In 85% of the patients, the disease affects only one ear. However, should the second ear become involved, it usually happens within 36 months. The natural history is final remission occurs in about 60% of the patients.

Cochlear hydrops, vestibular hydrops, or Lermoyez syndrome have aural fullness as the common denominator. *Cochlear hydrops* is characterized by the fluctuating sensorineural hearing loss and tinnitus. *Vestibular hydrops* has episodic vertigo as well as aural fullness. *Lermoyez syndrome* is characterized by increasing tinnitus, hearing loss, and aural fullness that is relieved after an episodic attack of vertigo. Recurrence of this phenomenon can be expected. *Crisis of Tumarkin or drop attack* is another variant of Ménière syndrome in which the patient loses extensor powers and falls to the ground suddenly and severely. There is no loss of consciousness, and complete recovery occurs almost immediately. This occurs late in the disease process with no warning.

Audiometric tests show a fluctuating low-tone sensorineural hearing loss and little to no tone decay. The ENG findings commonly show very little between the initial episodes. During the attack, there may be active spontaneous nystagmus with direction changing components even in the midst of caloric testing.

Because the stage at which a spontaneous remission occurs cannot be predicted, several medical and surgical therapies have evolved to alter the natural history. The medical therapies are aimed at the symptoms and include vestibular suppressants, vasodilators, and diuretics. The surgical therapies are either destructive or preservative of residual hearing. The first includes labyrinthectomy or translabyrinthine eighth nerve section when there is no useful hearing. Procedures when there is useful hearing include selective (middle cranial fossa, retrolabyrinthine, or retrosigmoid) vestibular nerve section, gentamicin or streptomycin application to the inner ear. Conservative procedures include those performed on the endolymphatic sac. They range from sac decompression to endolymphatic–mastoid shunts. The latter appears directed at correcting the resultant mechanical or production–reabsorption changes seen in the histopathology of endolymphatic hydrops in the temporal bone. Cochleosacculotomy is indicated in elderly patients with disabling vertigo, poor hearing, and residual vestibular function under local anesthesia.

Glycerol Test It is speculated that the administration of glycerol in an oral dose of 1.2 mL/kg of body weight with the addition of an equal amount of physiologic saline to a patient with Ménière syndrome may have diagnostic value in clinical management. Within 1 hour of administration, the patient may sense an improvement in the hearing loss, tinnitus, and sensation of fullness in the ear with maximum effects occurring within 2 to 3 hours. After 3 hours, the symptoms slowly return.

Metabolic Vertigo

There are no clinical symptoms that separate the metabolic form from other forms of vertigo. A prerequisite may be an abnormally functioning vestibular system. In this instance, the metabolic factor exaggerates or interferes with the compensatory mechanisms and brings about the symptoms. Dietary modification often results in a striking improvement in symptoms.

Hypothyroidism is an extremely rare but definite cause. Many times, the patients are not otherwise clinically hypothyroid.

Allergic causes are very elusive in the management of the dizzy patient, but the screening IgE assay may give a clue. Radioallergosorbent test (RAST) or skin testing may provide more precise findings about an allergic cause and its treatment. When there is no clear-cut history and in the absence of any other clearly defined cause, an allergic management should be undertaken.

Multiple Sclerosis

Multiple sclerosis is one of the more common neurologic diseases encountered in clinical practice. Vertigo is the presenting symptom of multiple sclerosis in 7% to 10% of patients or eventually appears during the course of disease in as many as one-third of the cases. The patient usually complains of unsteadiness along with vertigo. Vertical nystagmus, bilateral internuclear ophthalmoplegia, and ataxic eye movements are other clues to this disease. *Charcot triad* (nystagmus, scanning speech, and intention tremor) may be present. Electronystagmography may show anything from normal findings to peripheral findings to central findings. Auditory brain stem-evoked potentials may show a delay of central conduction. More likely, there is a significant delay of the visually evoked potentials. Research into an etiology for this disorder is pointing to an autoimmune disorder of the myelin.

Oscillopsia (Jumbling of the Panorama) Dandy Syndrome

Since our heads bob up and down while walking, the otolithic system controls eye movement to maintain a constant horizon when walking. When there is bilateral absent vestibular function as seen with ototoxic drug use, *the loss of otolithic function results in oscillopsia,* which is the inability to maintain the horizon while walking.

Otitis Media

Suppurative or serous otitis media may have associated vestibular symptoms. In serous otitis media, the presence of fluid in the middle ear restricting the round window membrane, serous labyrinthitis, may be responsible for the vestibular symptoms. Removing the serous fluid either medically or surgically gives rise to remission of the dizziness.

In the presence of suppuration there may be reversible serous labyrinthitis or irreversible suppurative labyrinthitis, and the more extensive sequestrum with a dead ear and facial nerve palsy. In this instance, judgment about the disease and its effects determines the proper treatment.

Otosclerosis (Otospongiosis)

There appears to be three areas where otosclerosis may bear relation to dysequilibrium. The first occurs in relation to the fixed footplate. There may be a change in the fluid dynamics of the inner ear, giving rise to vestibular symptoms. In a large number of patients, the symptoms are cleared by stapedectomy.

Sometimes vertigo begins after stapedectomy. It may occur with a perilymph fistula that requires revision and repair. A total, irreversible loss of hearing with vertigo may also occur. A destructive surgical procedure of labyrinthectomy with or without eighth nerve section is indicated if the vestibular suppressants fail to control the dysequilibrium.

The coexistence of otosclerotic foci around the vestibular labyrinth with elevated blood fats or blood glucose abnormalities may give rise to vestibular symptoms. Effective treatment requires fluoride therapy.

There is also evidence that an otosclerotic focus may literally grow through the vestibular nerve. In this instance, a reduced vestibular response (RVR) is found on ENG testing. This clinical presentation may look like vestibular neuronitis in the absence of a hearing loss.

Ototoxic Drugs

Ototoxic drugs, predominantly aminoglycoside antibiotics, are usually used in lifesaving situations where no other antibiotics are judged to be as effective. The main symptom is oscillopsia and results from a lack of otolithic input to allow the eyes to maintain a level horizon. This is found while the head is bobbing up and down as the individual walks.

The use of rotational testing, especially at the higher frequencies, may reveal a function that is not evident on caloric testing. The presence of this rotational function indicates intact responses in other areas of vestibular sensitivity. This intact function may separate the patient who will benefit from vestibular rehabilitation from the patient who will not. This may also explain the difference in the degree of disability between patients.

Sometimes the usual vestibular suppressants aid the patient. In other instances, one is frustrated by an inability to adequately treat this condition.

Perilymph Fistula

In the absence of hearing loss, perilymph fistula is a cause of vertigo. The history should be straightforward for impulsive trauma or barotrauma, and the resultant symptoms clearly follow. However, this is not always the case, as a sneeze or vigorous blowing of the nose may be the inciting event. The resultant vertigo may not occur for some time. The clue in the history is one of an episodic nature, usually related to exertion. Many patients are asymptomatic on awakening in the morning, only to have symptoms appear once they are up and around. A positive fistula sign with or without ENG results is helpful, although a negative sign does not rule out a fistula.

Associated symptoms of ear fullness, tinnitus, and mild or fluctuating hearing loss help localize the problem to the ear. Many patients demonstrate nystagmus with the affected ear down;

however, this finding alone is not a reliable sign to determine the pathologic ear. The definitive diagnosis occurs at surgery, but there are instances where there are equivocal findings at surgery.

Posttraumatic Vertigo

Posttraumatic vertigo comprises a history of head trauma followed by a number of possible symptoms, such as dysequilibrium. If there is a total loss of balance and hearing function, the use of vestibular suppressants may result in a cure that is sustained after cessation of the suppressants. In some instances when there is no cure, a labyrinthectomy or eighth nerve section ameliorates the symptoms. Occasionally, there is a progressive hearing loss.

After trauma, delayed Ménière syndrome may develop. This may be resistant to medical therapy and requires surgery. In this instance, endolymphatic sac surgery can improve the symptoms if there is no fracture displacement through the endolymphatic duct.

The statoconia of the otolithic system may have become dislodged by the trauma. With head movement, they roll toward the ampullated end of the posterior SCC. Their weight deflects the ampullary contents producing a gravity stimulus that stimulates a positional vertigo of a posttraumatic type. The nystagmus is said to occur with the affected ear down. The most effective treatment is with habituation exercises. Vestibular neurectomy is also a recommended therapy.

Syphilis: Congenital and Acquired

The neurotologic findings associated with syphilis usually present with bilateral Ménière syndrome. There is a significant hearing loss and usually bilateral absent caloric function. Another common clinical manifestation is the presence of interstitial keratitis. The patients, as a rule, are in their mid-forties; however, when the onset occurs during childhood, the hearing loss is abrupt, bilaterally symmetrical, and more severe.

These patients usually have a positive Hennebert sign (ie, positive fistula test without any demonstrable fistula along with a normal external auditory canal and tympanic membrane). The positive fistula test indicates an abnormally mobile footplate or an absence or softening of the bony plate covering the lateral SCC. The patient may also demonstrate Tullio phenomenon.

Histopathologically, the soft tissue of the labyrinth may demonstrate mononuclear leukocyte infiltration with obliterative endarteritis, inflammatory fibrosis, and endolymphatic hydrops. Osteolytic lesions are often seen in the otic capsule.

The treatment consists of an intensive course of penicillin therapy for an adequate interval. Patients allergic to penicillin should be desensitized to this drug in the hospital and given 20 million units of penicillin intravenously daily for 10 days. The use of steroids may result in a dramatic improvement in hearing and a reduction of vestibular symptoms. Usually, the steroids must be maintained indefinitely to retain the clinical improvement.

Temporal Bone Fracture and Labyrinthine Concussion

Transverse Fracture Because a transverse fracture destroys the auditory and vestibular function, the patient has no hearing or vestibular response in that ear. Initially, the patient is severely vertiginous and demonstrates a spontaneous nystagmus whose fast component is away from the injured side. The severe vertigo subsides after a week, and the patient may remain mildly unsteady for 3 to 6 months. The patient may also have labyrinthine concussion of the contralateral side, and facial nerve palsy is not uncommon.

Longitudinal Fracture Longitudinal fractures constitute 80% of the temporal bone fracture. With this type of fracture, there is usually bleeding into the middle ear with perforation of the tympanic membrane and disruption of the tympanic ring. Thus, there may be a conductive hearing loss from the middle ear pathology and a sensorineural high-frequency hearing loss from a concomitant labyrinthine concussion. There may also be evidence of peripheral facial nerve palsy. Dizziness may be mild or absent except during positional testing.

Labyrinthine Concussion Labyrinthine concussion is secondary to head injury. The patient complains of mild unsteadiness or light-headedness, particularly with a change of head position. Audiometric testing may reveal a high-frequency hearing loss. The ENG may show a spontaneous or positional nystagmus, an RVR, or both. As the effects of the concussion reverse, the symptoms and objective findings also move toward normal.

Vascular Insufficiency and Its Syndromes

Vascular insufficiency can be a common cause of vertigo among people over the age of 50 as well as patients with diabetes, hypertension, or hyperlipidemia. The following syndromes have been recognized among patients with vascular insufficiency.

Labyrinthine Apoplexy Labyrinthine apoplexy is due to thrombosis of the internal auditory artery or one of its branches. The symptoms include acute vertigo with nausea and vomiting. Hearing loss and tinnitus may also occur.

Wallenberg Syndrome Wallenberg syndrome is also known as the lateral medullary syndrome secondary to infarction of the medulla, which is supplied by the posterior inferior cerebellar artery. This syndrome is believed to be the most common brain stem vascular disorder. The symptoms include the following:

A. Vertigo, nausea, vomiting, nystagmus
B. Ataxia, falling toward the side of the brain
C. Loss of the sense of pain and temperature sensations on the ipsilateral and contralateral body
D. Dysphagia with ipsilateral palate and vocal cord paralysis
E. Ipsilateral Horner syndrome

Subclavian Steal Syndrome

Subclavian steal syndrome is characterized by intermittent vertigo, occipital headache, blurred vision, diplopia, dysarthria, pain in the upper extremity, loud bruit or palpable thrill over the supraclavicular fossa, a difference of 20 mm Hg in systolic blood pressure between the two arms, and a delayed or weakened radial pulse. The blockage can be surgically corrected.

Anterior Vestibular Artery Occlusion This symptom complex includes:

A. A sudden onset of vertigo without deafness
B. A slow recovery followed by months of positional vertigo of the benign paroxysmal type
C. Signs of histologic degeneration of the utricular macula, cristae of the lateral and superior SCCs, and the superior vestibular nerve

Vertebrobasilar Insufficiency

The symptoms of vertebrobasilar insufficiency include vertigo, hemiparesis, visual disturbances, dysarthria, headache, and vomiting. These symptoms are a result of a drop in blood flow to the vestibular nuclei and surrounding structures. The posterior and anterior inferior cerebellar arteries are involved. Tinnitus and deafness are unusual symptoms.

Drop attacks without loss of consciousness and precipitated by neck motion are characteristic of vertebrobasilar insufficiency.

Cervical Vertigo

Cervical vertigo can be caused by cervical spondylosis as well as by other etiologies. Cervical spondylosis can be brought about by degeneration of the intervertebral disk. As the disk space narrows, approximation of the vertebral bodies takes place. With mobility, the bulging of the annulus is increased, causing increased traction on the periosteum to which the annulus is attached and stimulating proliferation of bone along the margins of the vertebral bodies to produce osteophytes.

Barre believed that the symptoms of cervical spondylosis (including vertigo) are due to irritation of the vertebral sympathetic plexus, which is in close proximity to the vertebral artery. It is claimed that spondylosis irritates the periarterial neural plexus in the wall of the vertebral and basilar arteries leading to contraction of the vessels. Temporary ischemia then gives rise to vertigo. Others claimed that the loss of proprioception in the neck can give rise to cervical vertigo. Emotional tension, rotation of the head, and extension of the head can cause the neck muscle (including the scalenus anticus) to be drawn tightly over the thyrocervical trunk and subclavian artery, compressing these vessels against the proximal vertebral artery. In elderly individuals, a change from the supine to the upright position may give rise to postural hypotension, which in turn may cause vertebrobasilar insufficiency. The aortic arch syndrome and subclavian steal syndrome may also cause cervical vertigo.

Symptoms include the following:

A. Headache, vertigo
B. Syncope
C. Tinnitus and loss of hearing (usually low frequencies)
D. Nausea and vomiting (vagal response)
E. Visual symptoms, such as flashing lights (not uncommon), due to ischemia of the occipital lobe, supplied by the posterior cerebral artery, a branch of the basilar artery
F. Supraclavicular bruit seen by physical examination in one-third of the patients

Each of these symptoms usually appears when the head or neck assumes a certain position or change of position.

Proper posture, neck exercises, cervical traction, heat massage, anesthetic infiltration, and immobilization of the neck with a collar temporarily are all good therapeutic measures. If traction is required, it can be given as a few pounds horizontally for several hours at a time. For cervical spondylosis without acute root symptoms, heavy traction (100 lb) for 1 to 2 minutes continuously or 5 to 10 minutes intermittently is considered by some to be more effective.

Vertiginous Epilepsy

Dysequilibrium as a symptom of epilepsy is seen in two forms. The first is the aura of a major Jacksonian seizure. The second is the momentary, almost petit mal seizure whose entire brief moment is experienced as dysequilibrium. The diagnosis of the latter form may require a sleep EEG. These patients respond to usual seizure control therapy.

Cortical vertigo either can be as severe and episodic as Ménière disease or it may manifest itself as a mild unsteadiness. It is usually associated with hallucinations of music or sound. The patient may exhibit daydreaming and purposeful or purposeless repetitive movements. Motor abnormalities such as chewing, lip smacking, and facial grimacing are not uncommon. The patient may experience an unusual sense of familiarity (déjà vu) or a sense of strangeness (*jamais vu*). Should the seizure discharge spread beyond the temporal lobe, grand mal seizures may ensue.

Vertigo due to Whiplash Injury

Patients often complain of dizziness following a whiplash injury. In some cases, there is no physiologic evidence for this complaint. In others, ENG has documented objective findings, such as spontaneous nystagmus. The onset of dizziness often occurs 7 to 10 days following the accident, particularly with head movements toward the side of the neck most involved in the whiplash. The symptoms may last months or years after the accident.

Otologic examination is usually normal. Audiometric studies are normal unless there is an associated labyrinthine concussion. Vestibular examination can reveal spontaneous nystagmus or positional nystagmus with the head turned in the direction of the whiplash. The use of ENG is essential for the evaluation of these patients.

Vertigo With Migraine

Vertebrobasilar migraine is due to impairment of circulation of the brain stem. The symptoms include vertigo, dysarthria, ataxia, paresthesia, diplopia, diffuse scintillating scotomas, or homonymous hemianopsia. The initial vasoconstriction is followed by vasodilatation giving rise to an intense throbbing headache, usually unilateral. A positive family history is obtained in more than 50% of these patients. Treatment of migraine includes butalbital (Fiorinal), ergot derivatives, and methysergide (Sansert). The latter has the tendency to cause retroperitoneal fibrosis.

Vestibular Neuronitis

Occasionally referred to as viral labyrinthitis, vestibular neuronitis begins with a nonspecific viral illness followed in a variable period of up to 6 weeks by a sudden onset of vertigo with nausea, vomiting, and the sensation of blacking out, accompanied by severe unsteadiness. The patient, however, does not lose consciousness. The severe attack can last days to weeks. Cochlear symptoms are absent and without associated neurologic deficits. When seen initially, the patient has spontaneous nystagmus to the contralateral side, and ENG demonstrates a unilaterally reduced caloric response. The remainder of the evaluation is negative for a cause. In most patients, vestibular compensation clears the symptoms in time. The remission may be hastened by the effective use of vestibular suppressant medication for a period of up to 6 weeks. After the acute episode has subsided, which may take weeks, the patient continues to experience a slight sensation of light-headedness for some time, particularly in connection with sudden movements. The acute episode may also be followed by a period of positional vertigo of the benign paroxysmal type.

A small percentage of afflicted patients do not respond to vestibular suppression or to vestibular compensation. In these patients, an evaluation for metabolic, otosclerotic, or autoimmune factors is indicated. If these other factors are identified and the appropriate treatment initiated, the symptoms may disappear. If after an appropriate treatment and observation period, and if incapacitating symptoms persist, a retrolabyrinthine vestibular nerve section is indicated. Abnormal myelination has been found in some of these nerve specimens.

Bibliography

Hennekam R, Krantz I, Allanson J, eds. Gorlin's Syndromes of the Head and Neck. 5th ed. New York, NY: Oxford University Press; 2010.

Questions

1. Which of the following is characterized by hypoplastic malar eminences, down-slanting palpebral fissures, normal IQ, and aural atresia?
   A. Waardenburg syndrome
   B. Goldenhar syndrome
   C. Treacher-Collins syndrome
   D. Apert syndrome

2. Zellballen is best described as
   A. Whorled cellular pattern with psammoma bodies
   B. Cellular nests and sustentacular cells
   C. Keratin pearls
   D. Palisading cells and Verocay bodies

3. Sipple syndrome is a familial syndrome consisting of
   A. Medullary carcinoma of the thyroid
   B. Hyperparathyroidism
   C. Pheochromocytoma
   D. All of the above

4. Nonsyphilitic interstitial keratitis and progressive hearing loss with vestibular symptoms is characteristic of
   A. Meniere disease
   B. Alport syndrome
   C. Cogan syndrome
   D. Behçet disease

5. Which of the following syndromes is characterized by cerebellar, medullary, and spinal hemangioblastoma, pheochromocytoma, and bilateral papillary adenocarcinoma of the temporal bone?
   A. Chediak-Higashi syndrome
   B. von Hippel-Lindau syndrome
   C. Takayasu disease
   D. Costen syndrome

Chapter 2
Obstructive Sleep Apnea

Obstructive sleep apnea (OSA) is a highly prevalent disorder typified by repeated episodes of complete or partial pharyngeal collapse and airway obstruction occurring during sleep. It is estimated by the seminal Wisconsin Sleep Cohort that OSA affects 3% of middle-aged women and 9% of middle-aged men, with incidence increasing in parallel with society's worsening obesity rates. This disorder is among the most common problems presenting to Otolaryngology—Head & Neck surgeons, and a recent *NEJM* Editorial has described OSA as a "perioperative epidemic."

Sleep-Disordered Breathing

The term *sleep-disordered breathing* (SDB) refers to a large number of sleep-related breathing problems, of which OSA is just one, the others being beyond the scope of this chapter. Regarding obstructive diseases specifically, the severity can range from simple snoring to life-threatening obstruction. The more commonly employed terms are stated in the following discussion.

Primary Snoring

Primary snoring is defined as snoring without concomitant arousals or sleep fragmentation. All patients with OSA will snore, but not all snorers have OSA. Although not pathological in and of itself, snoring can be associated with altered sleep habits (because of bed partner dissatisfaction). Additionally, there is emerging evidence that the physical trauma of the snoring vibrations on neck structures can be independently associated with carotid artery stenosis and stroke.

Upper Airway Resistance Syndrome

Upper airway resistance syndrome remains poorly defined in the literature. It is generally accepted to consist of respiratory events during sleep that are not severe enough to qualify as apneas or hypopneas, but still lead to sleep fragmentation and daytime symptoms. These patients are more commonly female who are neither overweight nor obese and typically present with psycho-somatic complaints and orthostatic hypotension, with or without temporomandibular joint disorder and bruxism. The sleep test might demonstrate a normal apnea-hypopnea index (AHI), but an increased Respiratory Disturbance Index (RDI) with high Arousal Index, resulting in recurrent frontal cortical arousals and excessive daytime sleepiness.

Obstructive Sleep Apnea

OSA is formally defined as repetitive episodes of airway obstruction consisting of either hypopneas (partial obstruction associated with hypoxia and brief sleep arousal) or apneas (complete obstruction for minimum of 10 seconds associated with hypoxia and brief arousal). In OSA evidence must also exist of respiratory effort being made in association with the decreased or absent airflow to differentiate this from central sleep apnea (in which no respiratory efforts are made). Respiratory events in OSA are more common during stage 2 or rapid-eye-movement (REM) sleep, which in the adult are the largest proportional sleep stages.

Impact of OSA on Personal Health

- Snoring
- Witnessed choking or gasping
- Frequent body moments
- Disproportionate fatigue
- Nocturia
- Daytime somnolence
- Morning headaches
- Sensation of unrefreshing sleep
- Memory loss
- Poor concentration and focus
- Sexual dysfunction
- Personality changes

Impact of OSA on Society

- Increased odds-ratio of motor vehicle accidents (MVA)
- Loss of economic productivity
- Workplace accidents
- Patients with OSA are known to use more health-care resources

Medical Consequences of Untreated OSA

Hypertension

OSA is an independent risk factor for hypertension (HTN) as shown by the Sleep Heart Health Study. This is thought to be associated with increased sympathetic tone from chronic hypoxia and the frequent cortical arousals. Once an apnea occurs, the cardiac output decreases, triggering increased firing of the sympathetic nervous system and associated increased systemic vascular resistance. This cycle happens repeatedly throughout the apneic sleep time and eventually persists throughout the day too. Successful treatment of OSA is known to decrease HTN severity even in patients resistant to pharmacotherapy.

Cardiovascular Disease

OSA is well known to be associated with increased risk of heart attack, stroke, and death. This has been prominently demonstrated in the Busselton Health Study, showing that untreated OSA was an independent mortality risk factor. OSA can also worsen preexisting congestive heart failure by decreasing cardiac output as well as altering catecholamine levels. Cardiac arrhythmias can also be seen in patients with OSA, with the most common being brady- or tachyarrhythmias.

Cerebrovascular Disease

Like the heart, the brain is also under hypoxic stress during OSA. In the midst of apneic events, there can be increases in the intracranial pressure leading to decreased cerebral perfusion, which correspondingly increases stroke risk. Additionally, the snoring associated with OSA can lead to atherosclerotic changes in the carotid arteries, worsening the chance of an embolic event in the brain. Evolving evidence also suggests a link with neurocognitive disorder development (ie, dementias).

Making the Diagnosis

History

Diagnosis begins with a thorough history. Patients should be questioned about sleep habits and hygiene, typical sleep initiation and wake-up times, and shift work, in addition to asking about the standard symptoms and signs of sleep apnea. History can also be used to distinguish fatigue from OSA versus other type of sleep disorders such as insomnia or simple lack of sleep. Comorbidities of OSA should be pursued. It is very important to question patients about their sleepiness at work or while driving, as in some jurisdictions or for certain occupations, the physician is required by law to notify the transportation authorities or company about excessively drowsy patients who are at risk of driving or operating equipment. If possible, a history should be taken from the bed partner, who can both corroborate and expand on the patient's complaints. It is not surprising to find patients who claim to either be asymptomatic, or downplay their symptoms, as over years of untreated disease a process of normalization occurs. Screening tools can be also used to help quantify disease severity. The most commonly employed is the Epworth Sleepiness Scale, which is a validated measure of daytime somnolence (although not specific to OSA) (Figure 2-1).

EPWORTH SLEEPINESS SCALE

Please answer the following questions based on this scale:

0. Would never fall asleep
1. Slight chance of dozing
2. Moderate chance of dozing
3. High chance of dozing

Situation	Chance of Dozing
Reading	______
Watching TV	______
Sitting in a public place (eg, theater or meeting place)	______
Driving a car, stopped at a traffic light	______
As a passenger in a car for an hour without a break	______
During quiet time after lunch without alcohol	______
Lying down to rest when circumstances permit	______
Total Score:	______

Epworth Score < 8 = Normal

Figure 2-1 The Epworth sleepiness scale.

A score over 10 is considered problematic. The Berlin scale is useful as a screening test for OSA as it is more specific, but is also more complex to employ. Quality-of-life scoring is valuable to assess the impact of disease on personal health. Performance vigilance testing is important as a direct measure of the impact of OSA on wakefulness—these tests are widely available on the Internet.

Physical Findings

All patients suspected of having OSA should undergo a complete head and neck examination to assess for areas of obstruction. The body mass index (BMI) should be calculated as well. Specific areas to examine include:

Nose

- Deviated septum
- Turbinate hypertrophy
- Nasal polyposis
- Concha bullosa

The nasal cavity should be examined both with a speculum and endoscope. If the nose is blocked, this can lead to downstream increases in airflow resistance both directly (by nasal obstruction) and indirectly (by forcing mouth opening, which in turn drops the tongue and pushes the hyoid backward).

Nasopharynx

- Adenoid tissue

Oral Cavity

- Size and position of tongue
- Scalloping of tongue edges
- Mandibular or palatine tori
- Assess occlusive status and jaw position

Scalloping of the tongue can indicate relative macroglossia. Jaw occlusion and position (Angle Classification II, in particular) should be noted as a retrognathic jaw means the tongue will be relatively posteriorly position. Tori of large size can also decrease room inside the oral cavity, which can in turn malposition the malleable tongue.

Oropharynx

- Tonsil size and position
- Soft palate thickness and position
- Uvular size, wrinkles, thickness, and position
- Medialized lateral pharyngeal walls

One of the most important physical assessments in OSA is the relationship between the tonsils, tongue, and palate. This can be graded using the Friedman staging system (Figure 2-2). The tonsils are Friedman graded from 0 to 4 as follows: 0 = no tonsil (prior tonsillectomy); 1 = small, lateral to the pillars; 2 = extend to edge of tonsil pillars; 3 = extend beyond tonsil pillars; and 4 = hypertrophic and midline contact. The Friedman palate position grading differs from the anesthesiology Mallampati classification in that with the Friedman system the tongue is not protruded and remains in a neutral position with mouth open. The Friedman palate grades are: I = posterior pharyngeal wall visible; II = uvula visible; III = soft palate visible; and IV = hard palate visible. The Mallampati system is not correct to use when assessing OSA, as it is not an accurate reflection of the patient's oropharyngeal anatomical relationships during sleep.

Hypopharynx

- Size and position of tongue base relative to epiglottis
- Lingual tonsil hypertrophy

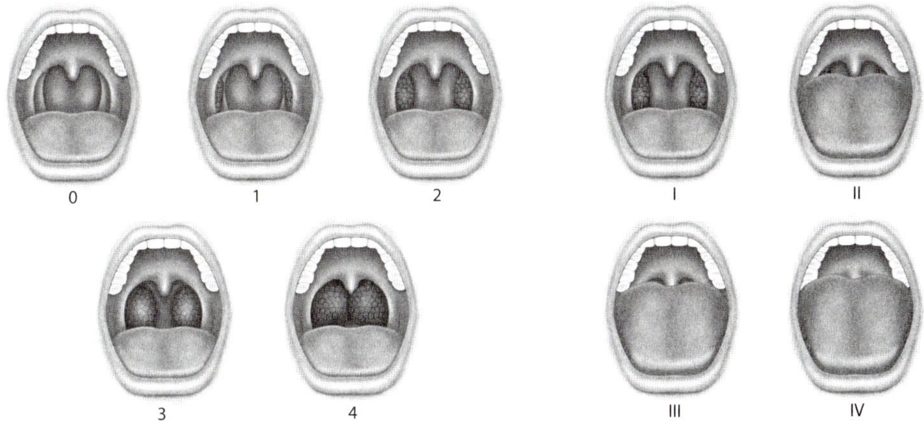

Figure 2-2 Friedman tonsil and palate grading scales.

The hypopharynx should be examined with a flexible fiberoptic endoscope to study both the retropalatal and retrolingual areas. The Mueller maneuver (MM) is a commonly employed test, during which the patient's mouth is closed and nose pinched after which they are asked to inhale, and the examiner can see which areas of the pharynx collapse. This is done with the patient both sitting and lying down. MM is simple to perform and inexpensive but is hampered by poor inter- and intra-rater reliability. Additionally, there is a low correlation with intraoperative findings, and a low positive-predictive value for success at pharyngeal sleep surgery. Another valuable method of endoscopic assessment is to identify areas of obstruction seen in the pharynx at end expiration (which is thought to be the time of the respiration cycle most prone to collapse). This is a more reproducible maneuver and also more valid than the MM.

Supraglottis

- Epiglottis shape
- Epiglottis position relative to posterior pharyngeal wall
- Size and position of tongue base relative to epiglottis

An increasing body of evidence is showing that the larynx may play a more prominent role in OSA than previously thought, especially in cases resistant to standard therapies.

Drug-Induced Sleep Endoscopy

Office-based assessments of the patient are hampered by the fact that anatomical and physiological findings while aware are known to be different from those during sleep. Drug-induced sleep endoscopy (DISE) is a method of examination performed while the patient is asleep, and in recent years has gained considerable traction in the sleep community. Under appropriate anesthetic supervision, sleep is induced via either midazolam or propofol after which the endoscope is inserted and the relevant anatomical subsites examined in a structured fashion. Various protocols, most commonly the VOTE system, allow for valid and reproducible exams to be performed (Figure 2–3). Patients who have very severe OSA or are morbidly obese represent relative contraindications to DISE. There remain open questions regarding the cost-effectiveness of DISE and its predictive value to surgical outcomes. Since it is resource intensive, DISE is not indicated for all patients with OSA but rather is suggested for use in the following situations:

- Where clinical findings do not match sleep study outcomes
- Failure of primary surgery
- Prior to major surgical intervention

Structure	Degree of Obstruction[a]	Configuration[c]		
		A–P	Lateral	Concentric
Velum				
Oropharynx lateral walls[b]				
Tongue Base				
Epiglottis				

For each structure, there should be a classification as to the degree of obstruction and configuration of obstruction. *Open boxes* reflect the potential configuration that can be visualized related to a specific structure. *Shaded boxes* reflect the fact that a specific structure-configuration cannot be seen (for example, oropharynx lateral walls in an anteroposterior direction).

A-P Anteroposterior.

[a]Degree of obstruction has one number for each structure: 0, No obstruction (no vibration); 1, Partial obstruction (vibration); 2, Complete obstruction (collapse); X, Not visualized.

[b]Oropharynx obstruction can be distinguished as related solely to the tonsils or including the lateral walls, with or without a tonsillar component.

[c]Configuration noted for structures with degree of obstruction greater than 0.

Figure 2-3 The VOTE scoring system used during DISE.

Polysomnography

Sleep studies are currently considered the gold standard in making the diagnosis of OSA as well as tracking responses to therapy. The American Academy of Sleep Medicine (AASM) has defined four levels of sleep studies.

Level 1 Polysomnography (PSG) This is the prototypical attended hospital-based overnight study, requiring 6 hours of recording sleep at an efficiency of 70% or better to make an accurate recording. A technician is preset to hook up all recording leads and remains present overnight to adjust or correct as necessary as well as to observe the patients sleep behaviors. Specific recordings made include: EEG, EKG, EOG, nasal airflow, oxygen saturation (SaO_2), thoracic and abdominal movements, leg movements, body position, and snoring sound. From the Level 1 PSG is derived the fundamental diagnostic measure of OSA, that being the apnea-hypopnea index (AHI). Disease severity can be subdivided into mild (AHI < 15), moderate (AHI 15-30), and severe (AHI > 30). Typically blood pressure is at risk when the AHI is greater than 30, but the other cut-offs are less objectively defined. The level 1 PSG is also able to distinguish central from obstructive sleep apnea. Performing this as a split-night study with the addition of continuous positive airway pressure (CPAP) for the second half of the night allows for immediate therapy and titration. Although considered the gold-standard test for OSA, level 1 PSG is also highly resource intensive and expensive, and considered by many practitioners to be overly detailed beyond what is required to initiate and maintain therapy. There are also questions as to the validity of the study, in that patients frequently report that their sleep in the lab was different than that which they have at home.

Level 2 PSG (comprehensive, at home study). This is performed in the patient's home, and includes assessment of PSG, brain activity (EEG), as well as EMG, ECG, EOG, and oxygen levels. This provides similar measures to an in lab study, but is peformed in the home without a technician, thereby reducing the costs.

Level 3 PSG (ambulatory sleep study) This is performed in the patient's home as well but records fewer outcomes, most typically SaO_2, body motion, snoring, and chest movement. Modern devices are far more sensitive than those from the past, and mobile software has also improved accuracy tremendously. In many jurisdictions, ambulatory studies are rapidly overtaking level 1 PSG as the primary test for OSA due to their convenience, decreased cost, and improved accuracy. Patients tend to believe the diagnosis more if the test takes place in their own bed, and this in turn increases therapeutic adherence. As demand increases for sleep diagnostics and technology continues to improve, level 3 ambulatory sleep studies are likely to grow in importance. Practice standards for ambulatory sleep studies have been developed based on American and Canadian Thoracic Society guidelines, and practitioners in sleep medicine and surgery should familiarize themselves with these documents. In general, it is necessary that ambulatory sleep studies when used be part of a comprehensive sleep program, that quality assurance checks exists, and that the result be interpreted by a qualified or experienced sleep expert.

Level 4 PSG This is essentially home oximetry. Although simply to perform, the test is insufficiently detailed for therapeutic planning and can lead to false positive (in patients with mild COPD) and false negatives (in a subgroup of patients with problematic OSA but only mild desaturations). This test is not sufficient for OSA diagnosis.

Nonsurgical Therapy of OSA

Behavioral Modifications

Various conservative measures have been shown to improve both the fundamental indices of OSA as well as symptoms. Patients should be warned against excessive alcohol or sedative consumption as these can disturb respiratory drive. Patients who are feeling sleepy also commonly feel the need to take stimulants (eg, excess caffeine) that can further alter sleep hygiene. Weight reduction is frequently key in OSA, but despite the physician's well-meaning intentions and suggestions, weight loss of the degree needed to alter OSA is frequently unattainable by the patient, and therefore consideration should be given to refer the morbidly obese patient to bariatric surgery. Positional therapy (by retraining the body not to sleep supine) can also be attempted either by commercially available devices or homemade products.

CPAP

CPAP has been considered the gold standard of OSA therapy. It functions as a pneumatic splint to prevent airway collapse. In the past the air pumps were cumbersome and loud but modern devices are both stylish and far quieter. CPAP may be delivered in three main ways, those being via nasal mask, nasal cannula, or full-face mask. When patients are able to tolerate CPAP and wear it frequently, their disease will be effectively treated. Newer machines have built-in compliance monitors as well as self-diagnostics to check for air leak as well as auto-titration of the air pressure. Bilevel positive airway pressure (BiPAP) devices can help deliver higher air pressure than CPAP can by altering the pressure during inspiration versus expiration to more comfortable levels.

The AASM defines adequate therapy as 4 hours per night, 5 nights per week. However, numerous studies indicate that generally only ~50% of patients are still able to use the device at this rate. Although the AHI improvement while on CPAP is almost always robust, generally only the lab-based PSG results are reported, as opposed to long-term results when considered over total sleep time at home, which are likely to be less impressive. It is not sufficient to simply prescribe CPAP as one would a medication; rather, extensive coaching and long-term support should be offered to help maximize therapeutic adherence. Reasons for CPAP nonadherence include:

- Comfort
- Cost
- Claustrophobia
- Convenience
- Side effects (skin rashes, nasal irritation, eye irrigation, and nasal congestion)

Oral Appliance Therapy

Oral-mandibular splints can be utilized to prevent oropharyngeal or hypopharyngeal collapse during sleep. There are numerous marketed devices, but the common theme is to hold the mandible relatively protruded compared to the maxilla, in turn bringing the soft pharyngeal structures forward, thereby opening the airway. Some newer devices can be titrated to patient comfort and also record adherence. Most devices are very effective for snoring, and in some cases, these can also be used as a therapy bridge if CPAP cannot be consistently used. The most common complications of mandibular repositioning devices are temporomandibular joint discomfort, malocclusion, and an overly dry mouth.

Surgical Treatment of OSA

Surgery for OSA is intended to expand the pharyngeal airway, thus restoring patency and improving both AHI and symptomatic outcomes. The modern concept of multilevel surgery suggests that operations should take place at more than one level of the pharynx, the goal being to address the multiple collapsing segments and obtain cure. Multilevel surgery can either be staged or performed simultaneously based on clinician's discretion and patient characteristics. Indications for surgery for OSA include:

- CPAP nonadherence
- Favorable anatomy
- Cardiovascular dysfunction
- Patient preference

Nasal Surgery

Whenever nasal obstruction exists in the setting of OSA, corrective measures should be offered. Options for nasal surgery include:

- Septoplasty (open versus endoscopic)
- Nasal valve surgery (functional septorhinoplasty)
- Turbinate surgery
- Polypectomy
- Endoscopic adenoidectomy
- Removal obstructive concha bullosa

Does Nasal Surgery Affect OSA or Snoring? Nasal surgery is not intended to affect either snoring or the AHI. The nose is not a collapsing segment, and thus altering airflow therein is unlikely to change the patient's OSA. Many patients need to be educated in that regard. Correction of nasal obstruction can, however, improve the perception of sleep quality as well as decrease daytime fatigue.

Does Nasal Surgery Facilitate CPAP Use? Correction of nasal obstruction has been shown to both improve CPAP adherence and potentially decrease the machine's pressure (if nasal CPAP is prescribed). The literature is as yet unable to provide guidance as to the optimal time to resume nasal CPAP use after surgery, so clinicians should use their individual judgement in terms of optimal early resumption versus the effect the mask may have on the healing nose.

Oropharyngeal Surgery

The oropharynx holds some of the most compliant tissues in the upper airway and is frequently cited as the main area of collapse. Numerous surgical options exist, and it is important that the clinicians not have a one-size-fits-all approach, but rather tailor the choice of which procedure to use with the right anatomical characteristics of the patient. The modern options for oropharyngeal surgery include:

- Isolated tonsillectomy
- Uvulopalatopharyngoplasty (UPPP)
- Uvulopalatal flap (UPF)
- Expansion sphincteroplasty (ES)
- Transpalatal advancement pharyngoplasty (TPA)
- Cautery-assisted palate stiffening operation (CAPSO)
- Soft palate implants (SPI)

Isolated Tonsillectomy Extremely hypertrophic tonsils are rare in adults. Both Friedman's original publications and subsequent data suggest that grade 3 or 4 tonsils only occur in 10% to 12% of the population. These patients represent optimal candidates for tonsillectomy, however, and both AHI and symptomatic improvement can be high in this group.

Uvulopalatopharyngoplasty This procedure has long been synonymous with OSA surgery. Introduced by Fujita in 1981, it consists of tonsillectomy simultaneous to trimming of redundant tissue from the soft palate, uvula, and palatoglossus muscles. The posterior pillars are then sutured anteriorly, as is the back of the palate to the front, in order to expand the whole oropharyngeal airway anteriorly. When considering all patients, UPPP has a suboptimal historical success rate of ~50%. However, using the Friedman staging system in a thoughtful manner to perform this procedure on more anatomically favorable patients (ie, those with Friedman tonsil grade 2-4, and palate position I-II), long-term success rates of over 85% can be reliably obtained; this stands in contradistinction to the long-term problematic adherence to CPAP. UPPP is not appropriate as an isolated procedure when tongue base contributions to OSA are strongly suspected. Complications of UPPP include:

- Pain
- Infection
- Bleeding
- Velopharyngeal insufficiency (due to malfunction of levator palatini)
- Nasopharyngeal stenosis (due to over-resection of the levator palatini)

Uvulopalatal Flap UPF is a variant of UPPP introduced by Powell and Riley in which the posterior palate is denuded of mucosa and the resulting defect closed via a rotation flap from the uvula (Figure 2-4). This procedure is advantageous to UPPP because the muscle is left intact, which both decreases pain and minimizes levator dysfunction. Outcomes from surgery are similar to UPPP. UPF is contraindicated if the palate is overly thick as otherwise patients can feel the resulting flap that can lead to problematic gagging.

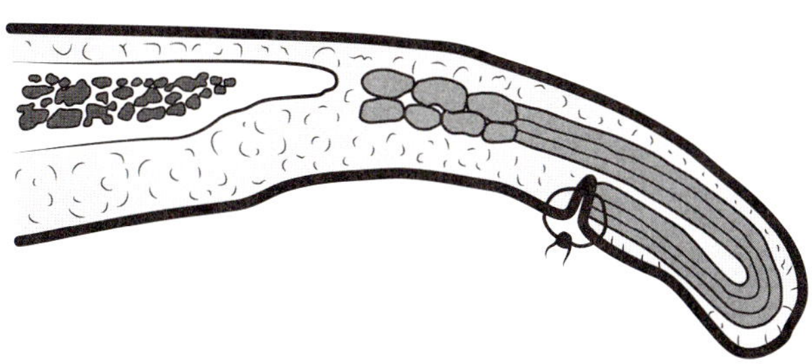

Figure 2-4 Saggital depiction of a completed UPF.

Expansion Sphincter Pharyngoplasty Some patients with OSA have narrowing in the lateral dimension more than the anteroposterior, often caused by excessively thick palatopharyngeus muscles. Pang introduced expansion sphincter pharyngoplasty (ESP) as means of treating this subgroup. The palatopharyngeus muscle is divided two-thirds of the way down its length, and then dissected off the underlying superior constrictor. Two channels are created in the lateral soft palate, and the palatopharyngeal stumps are rotated superolaterally and inset into the palate with a tendon stitch. This has the effect of widely opening the pharynx in the lateral dimension. Randomized level evidence has shown that this procedure is more effective than UPPP for appropriately chosen patients.

Cautery-Assisted Palatal Stiffening Operation and Anterior Palatoplasty This is an office-based surgery in which needle-tip electrocautery is used to remove a diamond-shaped strip of mucosa off the soft palate. This induces scar tissue to form, which stiffens the palate. Although this carries good success for snoring improvement, this procedure is unlikely to be of benefit for OSA. This was further modified to the anterior palatoplasty, introduced by Pang, and had also showed better results for snoring and OSA (Figure 2-5).

Hypopharyngeal and Supraglottic Surgery

The hypopharynx and supraglottis are increasingly being identified as major components of the pathological OSA airway. Surgery on these areas should be contemplated if they are identified as collapsing segments. The options to treat the hypopharynx and supraglottis include:

- Radiofrequency (RF) ablation of the tongue base
- Lingual tonsillectomy
- Hyoid suspension
- Tongue suspension

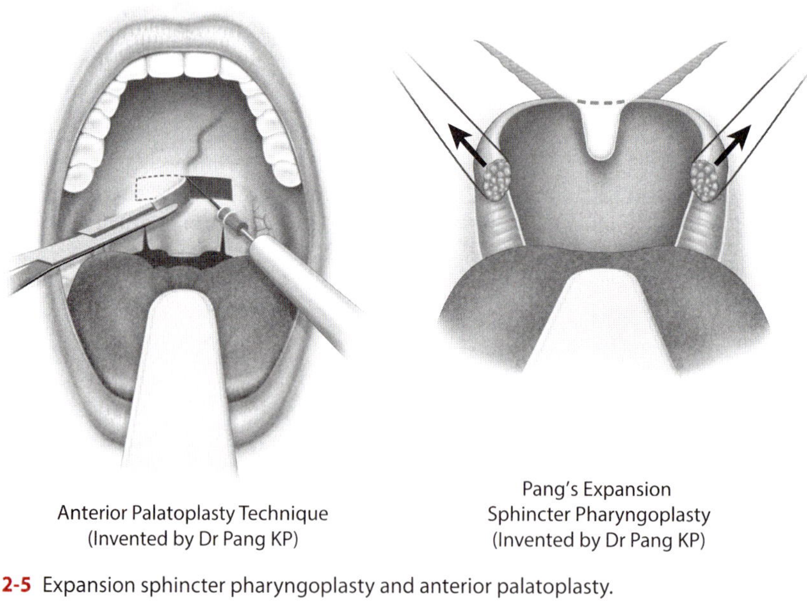

Figure 2-5 Expansion sphincter pharyngoplasty and anterior palatoplasty.

- Midline glossectomy
- Supraglottoplasty

Radiofrequency Ablation of the Tongue Base RF energy is a temperature-controlled method of delivering relatively high power current over a longer period of time, inducing scar tissue via plasma formation but at a lower temperature than seen for typical mono/bipolar cautery. This has significant advantages in terms of reducing pain and swelling after surgery. Numerous published protocols exist, but most involve creating four to six paired lesions at the base of the tongue within the muscle tissue. The resulting scar stiffens the tongue, and also over time reabsorbs, thus volumetrically reducing the tongue size. Potential complications include ulceration, taste change, foreign body sensation, and infection. Tongue base ablation has been shown in several studies to tremendously augment UPPP success rates in higher Friedman stage patients.

Lingual Tonsillectomy The lingual tonsils form part of Waldeyer's lymphatic ring of tissue, and in many patients with OSA, they can be markedly hypertrophic. Multiple methods for reduction exist, most commonly using RF or Coblation technology to shrink them down or ablate at a low temperature. Adequate visualization can be achieved via use of a transoral 70-degree endoscope (Figure 2-6). Potential complications are similar to that of RF ablation of tongue muscle.

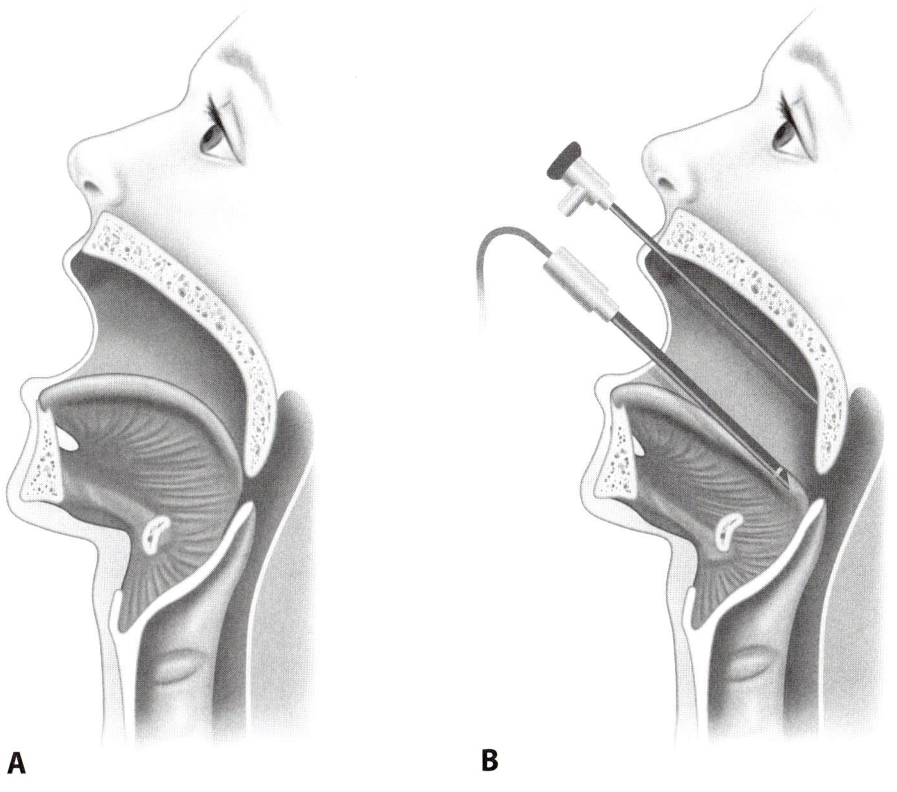

Figure 2-6 (A and B) Before and after views of lingual.

Hyoid Suspension In some patients with OSA, the hyoid bone is thought to be posteriorly positioned, thus dragging the tongue backward too. Suspending the hyoid anteriorly by transecting the strap muscles and affixing it to the thyroid cartilage may open the airway anteriorly. This procedure is not commonly done and is most useful as augmentative as opposed to standalone.

Tongue Suspension The tongue can be suspended from the genial tubercle using a commercially available low-torque screw and suture system (Medtronic). Suspending the tongue is thought to help prevent posterior collapse. Some patients notice the feeling of an altered swallow or foreign body sensation after this surgery.

Midline Glossectomy Resecting tissue from the base of the tongue in the midline may be done transorally using RF or Coblation technology, as well as using the endoscopic microdebrider. Exposure can be improved with the use of endoscopes. The end result is volume reduction at the base of the tongue with an increase in the hypopharyngeal airway. Complications include bleeding from the lingual artery, hypoglossal nerve injury, hematoma, abscess, dysphagia, and taste disturbance.

Supraglottoplasty During DISE or office examination, certain patients are observed to have significant epiglottic collapse either due to configuration of the cartilage or from redundant arytenoid soft tissue. These cases may also be resistant to CPAP because the pneumatic splint can actually augment the epiglottic collapse. Laser or micordebrider trimming of this tissue can markedly open the airway and improve OSA. All standard laryngeal surgery considerations should apply when this type of surgery is contemplated.

Hypoglossal Nerve Stimulation Hypoglossal stimulation has developed into a mainstay of therapy for patients who are not able to tolerate a CPAP and have either failed conventional surgery or have anatomy suitable for this as primary therapy. This technique has been studied extensively and show strong effectiveness to treat cases of primary surgery failure or certain anatomical configurations deemed favorable. The device also shows stronger long-term compliance of use than CPAP. However, the heath economics of the procedure remains a challenge preventing more widespread adoption.

Osseous Surgery for OSA

In addition to soft tissue operations, the other way to consider OSA surgery is by enlarging the bony confines of the pharynx. Options for osseous surgery include:

- Genioglossus advancement
- Maxillomandibular advancement (MMA)

Genioglossus Advancement A rectangular geniotubercle osteotomy is made, the resulting block pulled forward, and then rotated and affixed to the anterior mandible with a screw (after removing the anterior table to prevent cosmetic deformity). This advances the tongue forward, thus opening the posterior airway. Potential complications include dental injury, mental nerve injury, mandible fracture, and hematoma. This procedure, like hyoid suspension, is considered augmentative as opposed to standalone.

Maxillomandibular Advancement Of all surgeries for OSA, this is the single most effective, aside from tracheostomy. By performing a series of osteotomies (LeFort 1 for the maxilla and sagittal split for the mandible), the boney confines of the airway can be moved anteriorly, taking with them the soft-tissue collapsing segments (Figure 2-7). The moved bone is affixed with plates. Typically, orthodontic work may often be required both before and after surgery to optimize healing and occlusion. MMA is most commonly indicated in significantly retrognathic patients who would likely not benefit from traditional soft tissue surgery, although it also has a role as salvage procedure when primary OSA surgery has failed.

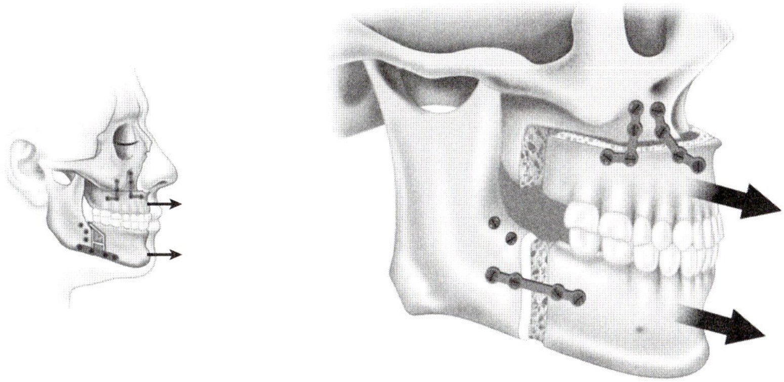

Figure 2-7 Maxillomandibular advancement.

Tracheostomy for OSA Tracheostomy is the only surgery that definitively cures OSA. Via bypass of the obstructive segments, full airway patency is restored. Tracheostomy in this patient population is often challenging due to morbid obesity and perioperative anesthetic and respiratory concerns. This procedure carries significant personal and social implications, and thus it is rarely performed. The indications for tracheostomy for OSA include:

- Failure of conventional therapy (CPAP +/– surgery)
- Not a candidate for traditional pharyngeal expansion procedures
- Significant cardiovascular comorbidities
- Life-threatening OSA

Monitoring After Surgery for Sleep Apnea

A debate has emerged regarding the need for, and the extent of, postoperative SaO_2 monitoring after surgery for OSA. Patients with OSA are theoretically at risk for postoperative respiratory complications because of altered oxygenation physiology, and therefore many hospitals would routinely admit patients for overnight monitoring in high-intensity units. This philosophy has been challenged in recent years because of more modern evidence suggesting that this level of observation is excessive for many patients, that the actual rate of respiratory complications is very low, and that admitted patients do not benefit from observation. Current OSA-specific indications for admission and SaO_2 monitoring after surgery include:

- Severe symptomatic OSA with highly elevated AHI
- Cardiovascular comorbidities
- Major tongue base surgery

Defining Successful Treatment of OSA

Unlike many other disorders of the head and neck, there is a significant disconnect between the symptoms of OSA and the results of PSG testing. Some patients with elevated AHI are relatively asymptomatic, whereas various patients with lower AHI describe disproportionate symptoms. When treating patients with OSA, it is not sufficient to simply aim for a lowered AHI on postoperative PSG, but also to identify improvement in both symptoms and comorbidities.

Broadly speaking, success at surgical therapy should be defined as more than just an AHI improvement and can include such measures as:

- Decrease in AHI to less than 50% of baseline
- Improvement in witnessed apneas (as noted by bed partner) and decrease snoring
- Improvement in daytime symptoms as measured by a valid scale
- Improvement in co-morbidities (eg, HTN)
- Improvement in ancillary measures of OSA (quality of life, performance tests)

Pang-Rotenberg et al introduced the Sleep Goal Index (SGI) to simplify and enable sleep physicians to apply more holistic parameters that better define success outcomes, instead of the unreliable AHI (as we are aware of its inherent inaccuracies ranging from hypopnea definitions, night-to-night variability, different sensors used, and lab-to-lab variability). The SGI is the concise use of main major criteria of the sleep goal:

- P = blood **Pressure**—reduction of either SBP or DBP by 7 mm Hg or both by 5 mm Hg
- G = **Gross** weight/BMI—reduction of GW by 8% or drop in BMI by 2 points
- O = **Oxygenation** (duration of oxygen < 90%)—improvement by 50%
- A = **AHI**—reduction by 50%

Bibliography

1. Young T, Peppard PE, Gottlieb DJ. Epidemiology of obstructive sleep apnea: a population health perspective. *Am J Respir Crit Care Med.* 2002;165(9):1217-1239.
2. Friedman M, Ibraham H, Bass L. Clinical staging for sleep-disordered breathing. *Otolaryngol Head Neck Surg.* 2002;127(1):13-21.
3. George CF. Reduction in motor vehicle collisions following treatment of sleep apnoea with nasal CPAP. *Thorax.* 2001;56(7):508-512.
4. Rotenberg BW, Theriault J, Gottesman S. Redefining the timing of surgery for obstructive sleep apnea in anatomically favorable patients. *Laryngoscope.* 2014. Doi: 101002/lary.24720
5. Pang KP, Baptista PM, Olszewska E, Braverman I, Carrasco-Llatas M, Kishore S, Chandra S, Yang HC, Chan YH, Pang KA, Pang EB, Rotenberg B. SLEEP-GOAL: a multicenter success criteria outcome study on 302 obstructive sleep apnoea (OSA) patients. *Med J Malaysia.* 2020;75(2):117-123.

Questions

1. The definition of an apnea includes:
   A. Cessation of airflow for 10 seconds
   B. Cessation of airflow for 10 seconds with an arousal
   C. Hypoxia after decreased airflow for 10 seconds
   D. Cessation of airflow for 20 seconds with an arousal

2. All of the following are indications for surgery for OSA except:
   A. Nonadherence to CPAP
   B. Patient preference
   C. Favorable anatomy
   D. Small tonsils

3. When performing Friedman staging of a patients oropharynx, which of the following is true?
   A. The tongue is protruded
   B. The patient is instructed to say "ahh"
   C. The patient is asked to swallow
   D. The patient is asked to open mouth without any other action

4. The only curative surgery for OSA is:
   A. UPPP
   B. Tracheostomy
   C. MMA
   D. Lingual tonsillectomy

5. Indications for drug-induced sleep endoscopy include all of the following except:
   A. Mandatory before any surgery takes place
   B. Where clinical findings do not match sleep study outcomes
   C. Failure of primary surgery
   D. Prior to major surgical intervention

Chapter 3
Laser and Radiofrequency Surgery

Lasers in Otolaryngology

History

- *Laser* is an acronym for "light amplification by stimulated emission of radiation."
- In 1917, Albert Einstein described the theoretical basis of lasers in his paper *Zur Quantentheorie der Strahlung.*[1] The first functional laser was constructed in 1957 by Theodore Maiman, a physicist at Hughes Research Laboratories in Malibu, California.

Physics of Lasers

A laser is a resonant cavity flanked by two mirrors and filled with an active medium which can be gas, liquid, or solid. One of the mirrors is 100% reflective and the other is partially reflective (slightly leaky). A laser also has a pump or external energy source. A laser is pumped by passing current through the active medium or by using a flash lamp. When a laser is pumped, energy is absorbed by the atoms of the active medium, raising electrons to higher energy levels. The high-energy electrons then spontaneously decay to their lower-energy "ground state," emitting a photon in a random direction. This process is called *spontaneous emission*. Most of these spontaneously emitted photons are absorbed and decay; however, the photons emitted in the direction of the long axis of the resonant cavity are retained as they bounce between the two mirrors of the laser. When these photons encounter an atom in the excited state, they stimulate the excited electron to decay to its ground state and emit another photon of the same wavelength in the same direction. This process is called *stimulated emission*. When more than half of the atoms in the active medium reach the high-energy state, *population inversion* occurs. This is a necessary condition for a laser to start working. As light is amplified in the active medium through the process of stimulated emission, the partially reflective mirror begins to emanate light which is uniform in wavelength, direction, phase, and polarization. This creates the familiar laser beam (Figure 3-1).

Properties of Laser Light

- Laser light is monochromatic, unidirectional, and uniform in phase and polarization.
- Laser beam widens as it travels, but can be focused with lenses.
- Once laser light exits the main resonance chamber, it is delivered to tissue via one of the two major delivery mechanisms, optical fiber or a waveguide. Light in the visible

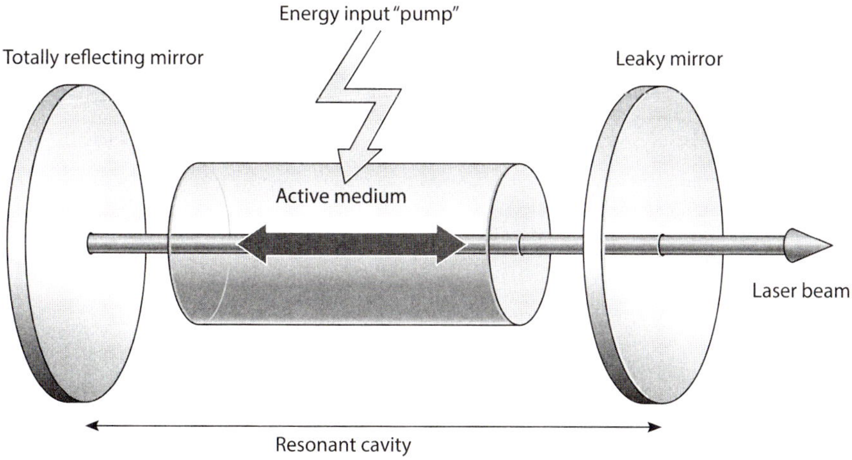

Figure 3-1 Components of a laser include an active medium flanked by two mirrors and a pumping mechanism which delivers energy to the active medium.

spectrum easily travels through an optical fiber and can be delivered directly to target tissues using a handpiece without significant energy loss. Even the near-infrared light of the Nd:YAG laser (1.06 μm) can be delivered through a fiber; however, infrared light of the CO_2 laser (10.6 μm) cannot be delivered via optical fiber, a major shortcoming of this highly popular laser. CO_2 laser light is delivered through waveguides which are essentially a series of articulated hollow tubes lined with mirrors. OmniGuide (Lexington, MA) and Lumenis (Yokneam, Israel) have developed flexible delivery systems for the CO_2 laser, resembling the flexibility of an optical fiber. This allows the surgeon to deliver CO_2 laser light through a handpiece directly to target tissues, though this system can be lossy, especially if bent.

Laser–Tissue Interaction

- Tissue interacts only with laser light that is absorbed, not reflected, transmitted, or scattered.
- In general, lasers with longer wavelengths have deeper tissue penetration. This rule holds for lasers in the visible spectrum, but not for infrared lasers such as CO_2 and Er:YAG. These lasers in the infrared range (3-10 μm) are easily absorbed by water and therefore have shallow tissue penetration.
- Ultraviolet lasers (UV), currently used in ophthalmology, work by tissue heating and photodissociation of molecular bonds. Visible and infrared (IR) lasers, commonly used in otolaryngology, work by heating tissue only. Laser energy is absorbed by tissue and converted to heat.
- *Thermal relaxation time* is the time needed for tissue to dissipate half of its heat.
- A laser characteristically produces a wound with the following layers: tissue vaporization, necrosis, and thermal conductivity and repair (reversible damage) (Figure 3-2).
- High laser energy delivered in short pulses minimizes thermal injury by allowing time for heat to diffuse between pulses.
- Laser parameters under surgeon's control are power, spot size, and exposure time.

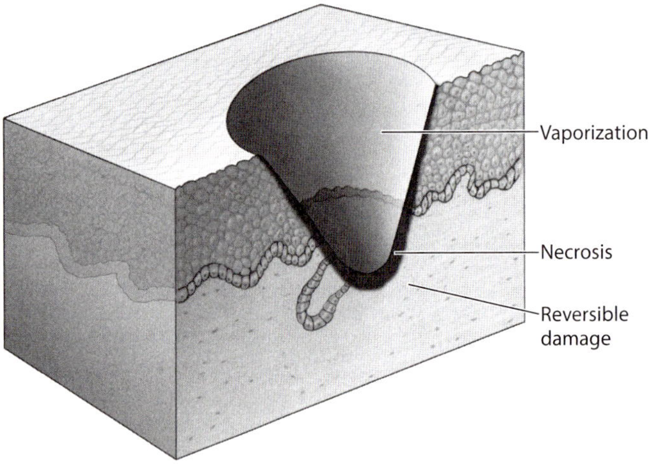

Figure 3-2 Layers of a laser wound.

- Tissue effect depends on the amount of energy deposited into tissue or *fluence*. (J/cm^2).
- The surgeon can change the spot size and energy delivered per unit area by changing the lens strength or simply working in and out of focus.

Chromophores and Their Spectral Characteristics

- *Chromophore*—the target molecule that absorbs laser light. In laser skin resurfacing, the chromophore is **water** contained in the skin. When ablating a vascular lesion, the chromophore is **hemoglobin**. When removing a tattoo, the chromophore is the **dye** contained within the skin. When removing a pigmented skin lesion or dark hair, the chromophore is **melanin**.
- Spectral analysis of hemoglobin shows the highest absorption peak at 405 to 420 nm (*blue*) and two secondary peaks at 538 nm (*green*) and 578 nm (*yellow*). Absorption drops off abruptly at wavelengths longer than 600 nm. Due to shallow tissue penetration of blue light and competitive absorption of blue light by melanin, medical lasers targeting vascular lesions exploit the secondary absorption peaks (530-600 nm) (Figure 3-3). Examples of lasers targeting hemoglobin in vascular lesions are potassium titanyl phosphate (KTP) 532 nm (*green*) and pulsed dye laser (PDL) 595 nm (*yellow-orange*).
- The melanin absorption curve is smoother. Melanin absorption is best at UV and blue wavelengths and gradually decreases as wavelength increases, still absorbing even infrared light. This is why melanin is so great at protecting our skin. Lasers that target melanin are used for hair, pigmented lesions, and tattoo removal. They operate in the red part of the visible spectrum where melanin still absorbs, but there is no competing absorption by hemoglobin. Examples are ruby 694 nm (*red*) and the more versatile alexandrite 755 nm (*red*), appropriate for a wider range of Fitzpatrick skin types.
- Water absorbs infrared light. Water absorption starts in the 800 to 900 nm range and increases as the wavelength increases, peaking at 2.94 μm which corresponds to the Er:YAG laser output.
- Lasers can also be used without targeting a specific chromophore, but simply for their general tissue ablative properties, such as the CO_2 or KTP lasers in a variety of otologic, larynx, or sinus surgery applications.

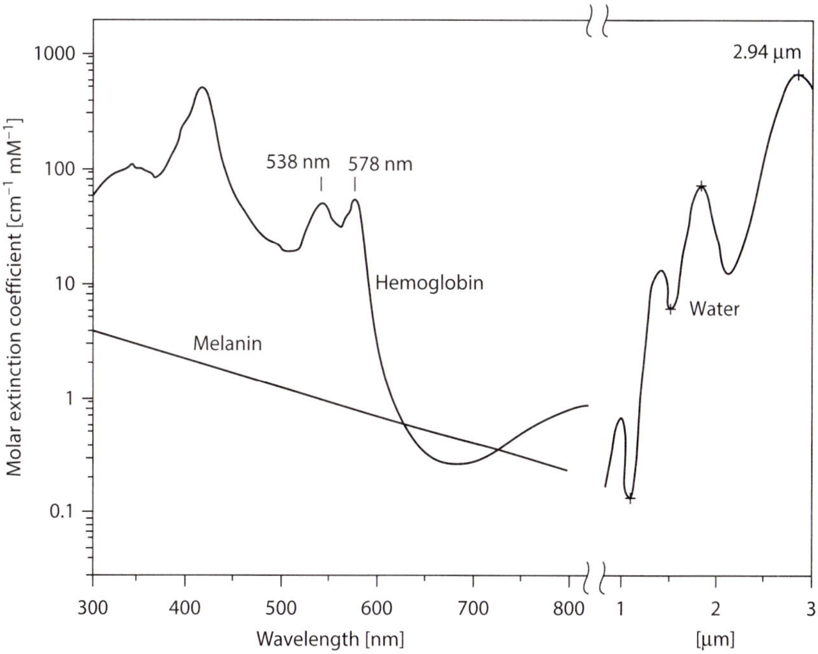

Figure 3-3 Absorption spectra of tissue chromophores. Lasers targeting vascular lesions exploit the two secondary absorption peaks of hemoglobin at 538 nm (*green*) and 578 nm (*yellow*). Lasers targeting melanin in pigmented lesions operate in the red visible light region (690-755 nm) where there is no competing absorption by hemoglobin. Lasers for facial rejuvenation target water which absorbs in the infrared region.

Commonly Used Medical Lasers

- *KTP (potassium titanyl phosphate, 532 nm—green)*: Absorbed well by hemoglobin. Used for pigmented dermal lesions and port-wine stains. Light can easily be delivered through a flexible fiberoptic bronchoscope for management of tracheobronchial lesions. KTP laser has been used in endoscopic sinus surgery and management of sinonasal polyps. Major advantage of the KTP laser in sinonasal surgery is excellent hemostasis.
- *Nd:YAG (neodymium yttrium aluminum garnet, 1.06 μm—near IR)*: Produces a layer of tissue coagulation and necrosis 4 mm deep, precise control is difficult. This laser allows good control of hemorrhage. It is used for palliation of obstructive esophageal and tracheobronchial lesions, photocoagulation of vascular lesions, and lymphatic malformations. Nd:YAG laser wavelength can be transmitted through optical fibers, allowing easy delivery via flexible endoscopes.
- *Er:YAG (erbium yttrium aluminum garnet, 2.94 μm—near IR)*: This laser wavelength is near the peak of water absorption, resulting in very shallow tissue penetration. It produces a clean incision with minimal thermal damage to adjacent tissue. Because of shallow penetration, hemostasis is difficult. Used for facial skin resurfacing and epidermal lesions, both benign and shallow premalignant (nonmelanoma) lesions.
- *CO_2 (10.6 μm—IR)*: This wavelength is invisible and needs a coaxial helium-neon (He-Ne) red laser as an aiming beam. CO_2 laser light is strongly absorbed by tissue with high water content. Tissue penetration is shallow. Precision and good hemostasis of small vessels are major advantages. This wavelength cannot be delivered via optical fiber;

however, specialized flexible waveguides (eg, OmniGuide, Lumenis) have been developed that allow delivery of this infrared wavelength directly to the tissues through a handpiece. The CO_2 laser is one of the most widely used lasers in otolaryngology with a wide range of applications in otology, laryngology, sinonasal surgery, and facial skin resurfacing.

- *Semiconductor (diode) lasers*: These lasers are available in multiple wavelengths. Advantage is their *portability*, lower cost, easy maintenance, and ability to include several wavelength options in one compact device. Laser properties, depth of tissue penetration, delivery methods, and applications are wavelength dependent. Semiconductor lasers have been used in a variety of otolaryngologic procedures including otology, laryngology, and facial cosmetic procedures.

Laser Skin Rejuvenation

- Lasers used for facial skin resurfacing operate in the infrared range (Er:YAG 2.94 μm, CO_2 10.6 μm), are well absorbed by water, and have shallow tissue penetration.
- Unlike dermabrasion, CO_2 laser allows precise control of depth of tissue penetration. CO_2 laser removes approximately 50 to 100 μm of surface tissue in one pass. CO_2 laser allows for "bloodless" skin resurfacing because small blood vessels in target skin are coagulated. Facial skin re-epithelializes within 2 weeks.
- Er:YAG mid-infrared laser is superbly absorbed by water, resulting in very shallow tissue penetration depth when used for skin resurfacing. Energy is absorbed in the epithelium; therefore, this laser is used for skin with mild to moderate signs of aging, predominantly contained within the epidermis. Er:YAG laser removes only about 25 to 30 μm of the skin surface. Some bleeding is encountered as the Er:YAG light is unable to coagulate the small vessels within the target skin. Skin re-epithelializes in 5 to 7 days.
- Nd:YAG laser can be designed to lase at 1.32 μm (eg, CoolTouch, Roseville, CA) and is used for nonablative skin rejuvenation. Water absorbs the 1.32 μm infrared light, but not very well. Enough heat is generated to produce a fibroblast reaction but skin is not ablated. Posttreatment pain is an issue. The wavelength range for nonablative skin rejuvenation lasers is approximately 1.30 to 1.45 μm, slightly too short to be well absorbed by water. Longer wavelengths would be much better absorbed by water, but would ablate the epidermis.
- *Perioperative considerations*: For herpes prophylaxis, valacyclovir 500 mg bid is started 24 hours before the procedure and continued until the tenth postoperative day. Some surgeons also use ciprofloxacin for *Pseudomonas* coverage. Lidocaine with epinephrine skin injections are used for analgesia before CO_2 laser skin resurfacing. Er:YAG laser is less painful and application of topical eutectic mixture of local anesthetics (EMLA) provides sufficient analgesia. After an ablative procedure, occlusive dressing or mupirocin 2% (Bactroban) is applied. After day 2, the postoperative care regimen involves washing the face with an antibacterial cleansing soap (Cetaphil), soaking the face in dilute acetic acid solution, and applying a Vaseline-based ointment until re-epithelialization occurs.
- *Complications of laser skin resurfacing*: Prolonged erythema, scarring, and hyperpigmentation may occur. Patients with Fitzpatrick skin types III or darker are at increased risk of pigmentary changes.
- *Contraindications to laser skin resurfacing*: Use of isotretinoin (Accutane) in the past 1 to 2 years as this could impair re-epithelialization, scleroderma, active acne, history of facial burns, or head and neck radiation therapy. Please refer to the "Facial Plastic Surgery" Chapter 55 for a discussion of additional facial rejuvenation techniques.

Laser Safety

- Most hospitals have a laser safety officer and a laser committee that develop guidelines for laser use, certify physicians in laser use, and ensure that safety protocols are implemented.
- Eye safety—Visible laser light is transmitted easily through the clear portions of the eye and can cause retinal burns. Infrared laser light is absorbed by water and can cause injury to the anterior chamber, that is, cornea and lens. The patient's eyes must be protected from laser light. Moist eye pads are acceptable. All operating room personnel must use wavelength-specific protective eyewear with sufficient optical density (OD). OD denotes how much light is attenuated by the lens at a given wavelength.
- Good suctioning is necessary to remove the laser plume.

Anesthesia and airway safety considerations

- Partial pressure of oxygen in the inhaled gas mixture is reduced to a minimum when lasing in the airway. Airway fires are possible with laser use in the upper aerodigestive tract.
- Wavelength-specific endotracheal tubes are available from various manufacturers. If these are not available, flexible metallic or insulated silicone endotracheal tubes should be used. PVC endotracheal tubes can ignite and cause an airway fire.
- Nitrous oxide should be avoided during laser surgery. The common inhalational agents such as enflurane, sevoflurane, and isoflurane are generally considered nonflammable.

Radiofrequency Surgery

Background and Physics

Radiofrequency (RF) energy is delivered to tissue where particles are ionized and a layer of plasma develops. The high-energy plasma particles are capable of causing bond dissociation in tissue at relatively low temperatures (40°C-100°C). This allows tissue removal, tissue shrinkage, or vessel coagulation without significant thermal damage.

Radiofrequency Ablation in Otolaryngology

- RF ablation has been used in otolaryngology for palliation of head and neck tumors, tonsillectomy, tongue base reduction in obstructive sleep apnea, turbinate reduction, palliation of microcystic lymphatic malformations, and others.
- RF ablation (Coblation) tonsillectomy (Smith & Nephew Inc, United Kingdom) was introduced in 2001 as an alternative technology for tonsillectomy. Multiple studies comparing Coblation tonsillectomy outcomes to other common techniques have found Coblation to be comparable, or possibly superior to electrocautery when considering postoperative pain and hemorrhage rates.[2]

Radiofrequency Ablation of the Tongue Base

- RF ablation of the tongue base is an established treatment for obstructive sleep apnea. An instrument is inserted into the tongue base near the foramen cecum and RF energy is delivered to the tissue. A controlled area of thermal damage is created which reduces the volume of bulky tongue base tissue as it heals.

- A 2008 meta-analysis found that radiofrequency surgery of the tongue base and soft palate in obstructive sleep apnea patients results in a 45% reduction in long-term (> 24 months) respiratory distress index (RDI).[3] Morbidity is low. Treatment can be repeated for additional benefit. Since OSA usually involves obstruction at multiple levels of the upper airway, RF tongue base ablation is usually combined with other OSA procedures. Please see elsewhere for more information on RF ablation of the tongue base.
- When operating on the tongue base, care should be taken to avoid injury to the neurovascular bundle which is located 2.7 cm deep and 1.6 cm lateral to the foramen cecum.[4]

References

1. Einstein A. *Zur Quantentheorie der Strahlung.* Physikalische Zeitschrift, Band 18, Seite 1917: 121-128.
2. Wilson YL, Merer DM, Moscatello AL. Comparison of three common tonsillectomy techniques: a prospective randomized, double-blinded clinical study. *Laryngoscope.* 2009;119(1):162-170.
3. Farrar J, Ryan J, Oliver E, Gillespie MB. Radiofrequency ablation for the treatment of obstructive sleep apnea: a meta-analysis. *Laryngoscope.* 2008;118(10):1878-1883.
4. Lauretano AM, Li KK, Caradonna DS, Khosta RK, Fried MP. Anatomic location of the tongue base neurovascular bundle. *Laryngoscope.* 1997;107(8):1057-1059.

Questions

1. Which of the following statements regarding laser physics and laser-tissue interaction is true?
   A. Visible spectrum lasers with longer wavelength have shallower tissue penetration.
   B. Tissue effect depends on *fluence*, which is the amount of energy deposited into tissue per unit area (J/cm²).
   C. When treating superficial pigmented skin lesions with a laser, the target chromophore is hemoglobin.
   D. CO_2 laser light (10.6 μm) is strongly absorbed by tissue with high-pigment (melanin) content.
   E. CO_2 laser light can be transmitted through an optical fiber, not through a waveguide.

2. Which of the following statements regarding laser and radiofrequency surgery is true?
   A. When radiofrequency energy is delivered to the tissues, a layer of plasma forms. These high-energy plasma particles are capable of dissociating molecular bonds at low temperatures (40°C-100°C).
   B. Postoperative pigmentary changes after laser skin resurfacing are more likely in patients with higher Fitzpatrick classes (III and above).
   C. Accidental eye exposure to the infrared CO_2 laser light (10.6 μm) can cause a corneal burn.
   D. The Nd:YAG laser (1.06 μm) produces a deep layer of tissue coagulation and necrosis. This makes it suitable for palliation of obstructive esophageal and tracheobronchial lesions, photocoagulation of bulky vascular lesions and lymphatic malformations.
   E. All of the above.

3. You are designing a new solid-state (diode) laser for treatment of superficial vascular lesions. Your target chromophore is hemoglobin. Please refer to Figure 3-3. Which of the following would be the best wavelength for this new laser?
   A. 595 nm
   B. 1.32 μm
   C. 755 nm
   D. 193 nm
   E. 10.6 μm

4. Which of the following lasers would be most appropriate for the treatment of superficial pigmented lesions, and why?
   A. CO_2, 10.6 μm, because it is absorbed by water and can be transmitted through a waveguide.
   B. Er:YAG, 2.94 μm, because it is highly absorbed by water and has very superficial tissue penetration.
   C. Alexandrite, 755 nm, because melanin absorbs light of this wavelength very well, and there is minimal competing absorption by hemoglobin at wavelengths longer than 600 nm.
   D. Pulsed dye (PDL), 595 nm, because this wavelength is near the peak absorption of hemoglobin.
   E. Holmium:YAG, 2.1 μm, because this near-infrared wavelength is absorbed by water, but can still be delivered via optical fiber.

5. During an operative procedure utilizing a laser, the following safety precautions should be implemented:
   A. All operating room personnel must wear wavelength-specific protective glasses, with adequate optical density.
   B. Patient's eyes must be protected with moist eye pads.
   C. When performing laser surgery in the aerodigestive tract, partial pressure of oxygen in the gas mixture should be reduced to a minimum, to decrease the likelihood of an airway fire.
   D. When performing laser surgery in the aerodigestive tract, it is preferable to use a wavelength-specific endotracheal tube or insulated silicone ET tube to reduce likelihood of an airway fire.
   E. All of the above.

Chapter 4
Anesthesia for Head and Neck Surgery

Overview

Optimal surgical outcomes result from a structured, multidisciplinary approach that begins before surgery and extends through recovery (often 30+ days). This process relies on:

- Proactive perioperative optimization of medical comorbidities.
- Standardized surgical and anesthetic protocols.

Achieving these goals requires collaboration among anesthesiologists, surgeons, internists, nurses, and other specialists. Anesthesiologists play a key role in:

- Coordinating perioperative care, particularly in head and neck surgery.
- Applying expertise in pharmacology, fluid management, airway control, and comorbidity optimization to support team-based decision-making.

Preoperative anxiety, especially about anesthesia, is common. To alleviate concerns, anesthesiologists should:

- Clearly explain the anesthetic process and procedural steps.
- Address patient and family questions to build trust and confidence.

Anesthetic agents are classified by primary effects:

- Hypnotics, amnestics, analgesics, and neuromuscular blocking agents (NMBAs).
- Many agents have overlapping properties and are used alone or in combination to optimize surgical conditions and patient safety.

Continuum of Depth of Sedation

The level of sedation is determined solely by the patient's response to stimuli, which varies and cannot always be predicted.

- It is not defined by a specific anesthetic agent, dosage, airway management technique, or device.
- Individual variability exists:

Table 4-1 Continuum of Depth of Sedation Assessment Guide Based on American Society of Anesthesiologists (ASA) Guidelines

	Minimal Sedation Anxiolysis	*Moderate Sedation/ Analgesia ("Conscious Sedation")*	*Deep Sedation/ Analgesia*	*General Anesthesia*
Responsiveness	Normal response to verbal stimulation	Purposeful response to verbal or tactile stimulation*	Purposeful response following repeated or painful stimulation*	Unarousable even with painful stimulus*
Airway	Unaffected	No intervention required	Intervention may be required	Intervention often required
Spontaneous Ventilation	Unaffected	Adequate	May be inadequate	Frequently inadequate
Cardiovascular function	Unaffected	Usually maintained	Usually maintained	May be impaired

*Reflex withdrawal from a painful stimulus is not considered a purposeful response.

  - Some patients may reach general anesthesia (GA) with minimal agents, for example, low-dose propofol and a nasal cannula, while others might remain minimally sedated despite an induction dose of propofol.
  - Sedation levels can also be combined with local anesthetics (LAs), nerve blocks, or nonsedating systemic analgesics to optimize surgical conditions and minimize risks.
- Monitored anesthesia care (MAC) is distinct from moderate sedation or specific pharmacologic protocols. It encompasses the anesthesiologist's expertise in assessing the patient, anticipating complications, and managing the transition to general anesthesia if necessary.
- It is imperative that anyone providing sedation is proficient in airway management and advanced life support skills and able to rescue patients whose level of sedation becomes deeper than initially intended, returning the patient to the level of sedation originally intended.

Airway Management

Among surgical specialties, otolaryngology uniquely entails sharing the airway with anesthesiology. Achieving a shared mental model before the day of surgery is therefore vital, encompassing the planned intubation technique, backup airway strategies, and any necessary airway devices. This collaborative approach ensures a well-coordinated, safe surgical plan that addresses potential challenges.

- *Pre-intubation:*
  - Fasting status: Preoperative fasting aims to minimize gastric contents and reduce the risk of regurgitation and pulmonary aspiration. Though rare in healthy patients, aspiration can lead to pneumonitis, pneumonia, and airway obstruction. According to ASA guidelines, otherwise healthy patients without significant comorbidities may consume clear liquids—including those containing simple or complex carbohydrates—until 2 hours before surgery. However, individuals taking medications that delay gastric emptying (eg, GLP-1 receptor agonists) should undergo a thorough

medication review and dosage adjustments preoperatively. Additional measures may include a gastric ultrasound to assess residual volume, rapid sequence induction (RSI) to reduce aspiration risk, or, in certain cases, case cancellation.
    - **Histamine-2 receptor antagonists**, ranitidine (Zantac) 150 mg PO or 50 mg IV and famotidine (Pepcid) 40 mg PO or 20 mg IV, can be administered as part of the premedication regimen. They are used to raise the pH of subsequently secreted gastric acid above the critical level of 2.5, thereby reducing the pulmonary sequelae should aspiration occur.
- *Intubation:* The otolaryngologist's nasal fiber optic examination provides extremely useful preoperative data to the anesthesiologist and provides excellent data for a discussion on the best approach to patients with anomalous airway anatomy. This discussion must be tempered with the acknowledgment that the original plan may fail and that multiple backup plans should also be put in motion. Including a surgical approach to the airway in the planning phase is essential. Airway tragedies have occurred with both an anesthesiologist and an otolaryngologist in attendance when they lacked communication and foresight. Additionally, all airway management equipment should be readily available; the use of a "difficult airway cart" and cognitive aid provides the most reliable solution.
- The use of nasal oxygenation, high-flow nasal oxygen, or nasal CPAP can provide a period of apneic oxygenation during prolonged airway manipulations. Additionally, high-flow nasal oxygenation, which delivers a degree of positive pressure, can provide suitable conditions for some short oral procedures.
- *Airway devices*: Often, otolaryngology procedures require specialized endotracheal tubes. These should be included in preoperative consultation with the anesthesiologist to ensure their availability and any changes in the anesthetic plan that they introduce. Neural integrity monitoring electromyogram tracheal (NIMS) tubes use is predicated on the lack of NMB at the time of monitoring. NIMS tubes do not preclude the use of NMB at other times during the procedure, but require a dynamic collaboration between the anesthesia and surgical teams.
- *Airway fires:* With the advent of electrocautery and lasers in surgery, the potential for airway fires has increased. The oxygen-enriched and/or nitrous oxide-enriched atmosphere created in the oropharynx will readily support combustion of flammable materials such as an endotracheal tube. The laser type and object material will determine how much time is necessary to ignite an object.
    - The lowest possible concentration of oxygen should be used (21%-40% FIO_2) that will maintain adequate patient oxygen saturation.
    - The placement of an endotracheal tube wrapped with reflective material to reduce the amount of energy absorbed is advantageous. Placement in the area surrounding the surgical field of saline-soaked pads and a methylene-blue-colored saline-filled cuff will also help dissipate excess heat energy.
    - Limiting the bursts to a short duration will help to reduce the risk of an airway fire.
    - Should an airway fire occur, fresh gas flow should be stopped, the endotracheal tube removed, any additional burning material extinguished, removed, and the patient reintubated immediately. A protocol should be devised and readily available to deal with such emergencies.
- *Extubation*: Over the recent years, there has been a substantial reduction in airway loss events during anesthetic induction. This has not occurred by chance but by active efforts on the part of the anesthesia community. Data collected for the fourth National Audit Project (NAP4) in the United Kingdom identified a surprising number of lost

airways after failed extubation. The cause they identified was the "failure to plan for failure." Therefore, the same planning and collaboration that now exists surrounding the induction phase of the anesthetic should also be applied to the emergence. Continuous end-tidal CO_2 monitoring should be available for all intubated patients outside of the perioperative setting and is now becoming routine monitoring for high-risk self-ventilating patients.

- *Airway security*: Any patient with a demonstrated or suspected difficult airway (can't intubate or can't ventilate) should be notified of their condition in writing. Importantly, their critical airway data should be transmitted to future providers to avoid unnecessary tragedies. The written notification that the patient receives is a first step in this process, but is best followed with a flag in the patient's record, written or electronic. The Medic Alert Foundation currently maintains an international difficult airway/intubation registry that has been endorsed by the Society for Airway Management. All providers can access this airway data log, and patients may opt into the bracelet identification system.
- Surgical patients who are extubated and transferred out of the postoperative care unit (PACU) are still at risk of losing their airway. Patients with acute airway events often present to the hospital, and patients with known difficult airways are often admitted by other services for treatment of other comorbid conditions. The existence of these classes of patients has engendered the establishment of difficult airway rescue teams (DART). These teams include anesthesiologists, otolaryngologists, nursing and technical staff. In institutions supporting these predetermined teams supplied with specifically designated equipment carts, many of these patients have been rescued in a timely manner.

Anesthetic Agents

Sedative Hypnotics and Amnestics

- Neurosynaptic function is reversibly inhibited by anesthetic agents, targeting membrane proteins, lipids, or the inhibitory neurotransmitter GABA.
- Multisynaptic pathways are often affected, with anesthetic agents potentially influencing multiple sites within the nervous system as well as various organ systems simultaneously.
- Sympathetic tone may be altered, leading to significant effects on autonomic regulation, particularly within the cardiovascular system leading to alterations in heart rate, blood pressure, and vascular tone, demonstrating the broad physiological impact of anesthetic agents.
- Each anesthetic drug has unique advantages and limitations, making no single agent ideal for all situations. Combining drugs such as benzodiazepines, opioids, propofol, ketamine, and etomidate allows for precise titration of the desired level of consciousness. These agents can also be paired with volatile anesthetic agents and gases, creating numerous combinations that can be customized based on patient comorbidities and surgical needs.
- Total intravenous anesthesia (TIVA) employs intravenous agents to both induce and maintain general anesthesia. This technique can be implemented manually, with the anesthesiologist determining bolus doses and infusion rates, or through a target-controlled infusion (TCI) pump, where a specific plasma or brain concentration is set and maintained. Mastery of TIVA requires a thorough understanding of pharmacokinetics, close monitoring of vital signs, and interpretation of processed electroencephalography to ensure optimal depth of anesthesia and patient safety

Table 4-2

	Class	Metabolism	*Pharmacokinetics/ Pharmacodynamics*	Dose	Advantages	Disadvantages	Considerations
Thiopental	Barbiturate (ultra-short acting)	• Hepatic metabolism, liver oxidation to active metabolite • Renally excreted	Half-life ($T_{1/2}$) 8 minutes	For induction: 3-5 mg/kg IV	• Acts in one arm-brain circulation time and lasts 5-15 minutes after bolus • Decrease ICP	• Accumulates with repeated administration • Cardiovascular and respiratory depression • Extravasation causes tissue necrosis	Not currently available in the United States.
Propofol	$GABA_A$ receptor agonist	• Hepatic metabolism • Renally excreted	Distribution half-life: 2-4 minutes Duration of action: 3-8 minutes	For induction: 1.5-2.0 mg/kg Procedural sedation: 0.5-1.0 mg/kg single bolus or 10-20 mg aliquots titrated	• Rapid onset • Rapid offset (short context-sensitive half time) • Anti-emetic • Safe in malignant hypothermia patients • Main agent for TIVA	• Causes vasodilation and negative inotropy • Apnea, airway obstruction, oxygen desaturation • Painful on injection	• White solution, oil-in-water emulsion made with soyabean oil and purified egg phosphatide, and lecithin. Safe for egg allergy patients. • *Food and Drug Administration* (FDA) black box warning, stating that "the agent should be administered only by those trained in the administration of general anesthesia and not involved in the procedure.

Etomidate	$GABA_A$ receptor agonist	Hepatic and plasma metabolism via hepatic/plasma esterase activity-renal excretion	• Short context-sensitive half-life • Terminal metabolic half-life 2-5 hours	Induction: 0.2-0.3 mg/kg	• Rapid onset due to high lipid solubility • Preserves ventilation drive, maintains cardiovascular stability, decreases intracranial pressure	Suppression of corticosteroid synthesis, leading to primary adrenal suppression	End-stage liver disease leads to increased volume of distribution and decreased clearance.
Ketamine	NMDA (*N*-Methyl-d-Aspartate) receptor antagonist)	• Hepatic metabolism, CYP450 • Diazepam inhibits CYP450, prolonging effects of ketamine • Renally excreted	Highly lipid soluble -elimination half-life 2 hours	Intravenous: 1-2 mg/kg Intramuscular: 5-10 mg/kg	• Causes dissociative anesthesia, patients are unresponsive to noxious stimuli but may appear awake • Pharyngeal and laryngeal reflexes intact • Maintain respiratory drive • Analgesic (opiate sparing postoperative analgesic or as an opiate sparing adjunct to general anesthesia) • Bronchodilation • properties	• Causes increased intracranial pressure (ICP), tachycardia dysphoric reaction • Alters EEG waves, important to note when utilizing TIVA	Recent data suggest that prolonged low-dose infusions (8-72 hours) are therapeutic in the treatment of depression and chronic pain syndromes.

(*Continued*)

Table 4-2 (*Continued*)

	Class	*Metabolism*	*Pharmacokinetics/ Pharmacodynamics*	*Dose*	*Advantages*	*Disadvantages*	*Considerations*
Dexmedetomidine	Selective alpha-2 adrenergic agonist	• Hepatic metabolism via *N*-glucoridation, *N*-methylation, and CYP2A • Mainly renally excreted, bile (4%)	• Can be given IV, IM, intra-nasal • Mean elimination half-life: 1.5-3 hours (IV) • IV infusions have linear concentration-dependent kinetics • Intranasal formulations have bioavailability of 65%, with great variability range: 35%-93%	• Used for premedication, procedural sedation, monitored anesthesia care, or off-label use as an adjunct to maintenance of general anesthesia	• Maintains ventilatory drive, useful during airway examinations or awake intubation • Useful as an adjunct during difficult extubation, particularly patients with agitation, delirium, or intoxication	• Minimal analgesic properties • Decreases HR, CO, circulating catecholamines in a dose-dependent manner • Requires a continuous infusion, taking time to take effect (10-minute loading dose 1 μg/kg/10 min, followed by continuous infusion (0.2-1 μg/kg/h) • Hypotension, bradycardia asystole if titrated too quickly	

Intravenous Anesthetics

Benzodiazepines provide amnesia, reduce anxiety, and increase the seizure threshold without undue respiratory or cardiovascular depression; however, anterograde amnesia can impede postoperative recovery. The three most commonly used benzodiazepines are diazepam (Valium), lorazepam (Ativan), and midazolam (Versed).

- **Midazolam**
  - Water soluble (reduces pain of injection associated with diazepam)
  - Approximately twice as potent as diazepam, with a more rapid peak onset (30-60 minutes)
  - Elimination half-time of 1 to 4 hours
  - Well-suited to shorter procedures where extubation is anticipated or for sedation during local anesthesia (1-2 mg IV in adults)
  - Produces a higher rate of postoperative delirium in the elderly and other at-risk populations (posttraumatic stress disorder patients)
- **Flumazenil (Romazicon)**
  - Benzodiazepine antagonist
  - The recommended dose is 0.2 mg IV over 15 seconds, which can be repeated every 60 seconds for four doses (1 mg total); more than 3 mg over 1 hour is advised.
  - Half-life ($t_{1/2}$) is 7 to 15 minutes, and a repeated dose may be required over an extended period when it is used to treat overdosing of long-acting benzodiazepines (lorazepam's $t_{1/2}$ is 9-16 hours).

Other Sedative Agents

- **Droperidol**
  - Butyrophenone.
  - In 2001, the FDA included a black box warning for droperidol, citing data of QT prolongation and torsade de pointes when given at higher doses of 2.5 to 7.5 mg. Subsequently, 0.625 to 1.25 mg of droperidol is occasionally used for its antiemetic properties.
  - Requires active ECG monitoring only.
  - Contraindicated in patients with prolonged QT intervals.
- **Haloperidol (Haldol)**
  - Butyrophenone
  - Long-acting antipsychotic medication that may be useful in treating acute delirium in the postoperative period.
  - Causes QT prolongation; routine use is not recommended.
- **Diphenhydramine (Benadryl)**
  - Antihistamine.
  - Sedative, anticholinergic, antiemetic properties.
  - Usual dose is 25 to 50 mg po, IM, or IV.
  - Blocks histamine release, used in conjunction with steroids and H_2 blockers as prophylaxis for potential allergic reactions.

Inhalation Agents

Inhalation agents, including volatile anesthetics and gases such as nitrous oxide, are administered via the lungs using a tracheal tube or supraglottic airway device.

- They reach the CNS by:
  - Diffusing across the alveolar-capillary membrane
  - Transport via blood after achieving a target alveolar concentration
- Factors affecting uptake and distribution:
  - Agent concentration
  - Minute ventilation

- Alveolar membrane diffusion capacity
- Blood-gas partition coefficient (solubility)
- Cardiac output and alveolar-arterial gradient
- Blood-brain partition coefficient

Potency (Minimal Alveolar Concentration)

- Minimal alveolar concentration (MAC) is the anesthetic concentration preventing movement in 50% of individuals during a surgical stimulus.
- Declines by ~6% per decade, with a 25% reduction for a 70 year old versus a 30 year old.
- MAC values are additive (eg, 0.5 MAC of two agents equals 1 MAC), allowing the combination of agents to balance efficacy and minimize side effects.

Table 4-3

Agent	*MAC*	*Blood-gas partition coefficient*	*Advantages*	*Disadvantages*	*Considerations*
Nitrous Oxide (N_2O)	104% (therefore, one MAC of N_2O cannot be delivered)	0.47	• Short-term adjunct to general anesthesia at 30% to 70% • Rapid onset and offset • Potentiation of volatile anesthetics via the second gas effect • Improved cardiac stability—Analgesia	• Associated with nausea and vomiting • Causes expansion of air-filled spaces (N_2O is 34 times more soluble than nitrogen, N_2O can double the volume of a compliant air-filled space in 10 minutes and triple it in 30 minutes • Potent greenhouse gas, 300 times global warming potential (GWP) of CO_2	• May cause a significant expansion of the closed middle ear space and potential disruption of a tympanic graft. Therefore, N_2O is not used during procedures involving air-filled closed spaces or when a patient is at risk of a pneumothorax. • Air-filled cuffs are also subject to this effect, and cuff pressure should be carefully monitored when nitrous oxide is in use.
Isoflurane (Halogenated methyl ethyl ether)	1.15%	1.4	• Quick onset and offset • Cheap • GWP similar to sevoflurane (510)	• Pungent ethereal odor • Rapid increases in isoflurane concentration lead to transient increases in HR, arterial BP, plasma levels of norepinephrine • Dilates coronary arteries	• Linked to a possible increase in postoperative cognitive dysfunction in the elderly and increased risk of neurodegeneration in pediatric patients. The FDA and the anesthetic community are actively investigating this.

(Continued)

Table 4-3 (*Continued*)

Agent	*MAC*	*Blood-gas partition coefficient*	*Advantages*	*Disadvantages*	*Considerations*
Sevoflurane (Fluorinated methyl isopropyl ether)	2.2%	0.74	• Nonpungent, ideal for inhalational inductions • Bronchodilator similar to isoflurane	• Mildly depresses myocardial contractility • Moderate environmental impact with GWP (130), shorter atmospheric lifespan than desflurane	
Desflurane (Fluorinated methyl ethyl ether)	6%	0.42	• Quick offset • Eliminated rapidly • Does not accumulate in adipose tissue	• Requires a heated vaporizer due to its lower partial pressure • Pungent odor, unsuitable for inhalation inductions • High GWP (2500), most harmful of the volatile agents with long atmospheric persistence	• Due to environmental concerns, many anesthesia departments are phasing out desflurane.

Neuromuscular Blocking Drugs

- Neuromuscular blocking drugs interrupt nerve impulse conduction at the neuromuscular junction allowing muscle relaxation, which is used to facilitate intubation of the trachea and to provide for optimum surgical working conditions.
- Classified as either depolarizing or nondepolarizing muscle relaxants:
  - Succinylcholine is the only clinically relevant available example of depolarizing muscle relaxants.
  - Vecuronium, atracurium, rocuronium, and cisatracurium are the most common nondepolarizing muscle relaxant examples.

Agent	*Onset (seconds)*	*Duration (minutes)*	*Metabolism*
Succinylcholine	30-60	5-10	Plasma cholinesterase
Rocuronium	60-90	45-70	Hepatic
Vecuronium	90-180	30-40	Hepatic
Atracurium	60-120	> 30	Spontaneous plasma degradation and plasma esterase
Cisatracurium	90-120	60-80	Spontaneous plasma degradation and plasma esterase

Monitoring of Neuromuscular Blockade

- Always confirm adequate anesthesia (using a spectral index [BIS] monitor, which is a form of processed electroencephalograph [EEG] monitoring) before administering additional neuromuscular blocking agents.
- Residual neuromuscular blockade remains a common problem postoperatively, carrying risks of hypoxia, airway obstruction, aspiration, and prolonged PACU stay.
- Quantitative neuromuscular monitoring (eg, acceleromyograpy or mechanomyography) is the gold standard for assessing blockade depth and preventing residual paralysis.
- Supramaximal electrical stimulation is delivered to a peripheral nerve, with the muscle response measured to gauge the degree of blockade (eg, measured by train-of-four [TOF], post-tetanic count [PTC]).
- Deep blockade of larynx and diaphragm requires complete (PTC = 0) or deep (PTC ≥1, TOF count = 0) neuromuscular block.

Traditional Reversal Agents

- Acetylcholinesterase inhibitors including neostigmine 40 to 75 μg/kg, edrophonium 1 mg/kg, and pyridostigmine 0.2 mg/kg facilitate impulse transmission at the neuromuscular junction by increasing acetylcholine.
- Anticholinergics (glycopyrrolate or atropine) should be coadministered to mitigate unwanted muscarinic side-effects (eg, bradycardia, secretions).
- TOF less than 0.4 or TOF greater than two twitch count required prior to administration of neostigmine to ensure effective reversal.
- Inadequate reversal or delayed dosing can lead to residual blockade, reinforcing the importance of ongoing monitoring.

Sugammadex (Bridion)

- Selective relaxant binding agent that encapsulates rocuronium or vecuronium molecules, rapidly reversing their effect.
- Allows optimal intubating conditions using rocuronium and easy reversal, avoiding the side effects of succinylcholine (eg, myalgias, hyperkalemia)
- If sugammadex is underdosed, not all rocuronium molecules are encapsulated, allowing unbound rocuronium to reenter the neuromuscular junction and cause residual paralysis.
- Redosing rocuronium after sugammadex administration can result in variable onset and offset of paralysis.
- Other considerations:
  - Excreted primarily unchanged in urine, so caution is advised in patients with renal impairment
  - May reduce oral contraceptive efficacy due to potential progesterone binding; advise supplemental contraception for 7 days postsurgery.
  - Currently, inadequate evidence is available to support use in pregnancy.

Analgesics

Analgesics are used synergistically with anesthetic agents to optimize surgical conditions and preemptively manage postoperative pain. Before initiating treatment, it is crucial to assess pain characteristics—acute or chronic—and determine its etiology. Assuming the cause of pain without proper evaluation risks misdiagnosis and patient harm. A thorough assessment, including patient consultation, ensures the selection of the most appropriate therapeutic approach.

Local Anesthesia

- **Local Anesthesia Overview**
  - Definition: Local anesthesia blocks sensation in a limited area without affecting consciousness.
  - Mechanism: LAs reduce sodium ion influx by binding to sodium channels, preventing nerve impulse propagation.
  - Classification: All clinically useful agents are either **aminoesters** or **aminoamides** and share key features: diffusibility, reversibility, water solubility, clinical stability, and minimal local tissue irritation.
- Aminoesters and Aminoamides
  - Basic structure: Consists of a tertiary amine, an intermediate bond (ester [R-COO-R] or amide [R-NHCO-R]), and an aromatic group.
  - Key properties influencing activity:
    1. Lipid solubility
       - Higher lipid solubility generally increases potency and duration.
    2. Degree of ionization
       - Governed by the Henderson–Hasselbalch equation; higher p*K*a = fewer nonionized (lipid-soluble) molecules at a given pH.
       - Infected (lower pH) tissues increase ionized drug fraction, reducing diffusion and anesthetic efficacy.
       - Alkalinization raises the nonionized fraction, enhancing membrane penetration.
       - Proximal nerve blocks in healthy tissue can bypass infections where pH is compromised.
    3. Protein binding
       - Greater protein binding correlates with longer-acting anesthetics.

Uptake, Metabolism, and Excretion

- Absorption
  - LAs typically diffuse from the injection site (eg, mucosa or subcutaneous tissue) into the bloodstream.
  - Rate of absorption depends on the drug's physicochemical and vasoactive properties, injection site, dosage, use of vasoconstrictors, nerve block factors, and patient pathology.
  - Rapid uptake can occur in specific areas—such as the larynx and trachea—resulting in blood levels close to intravenous administration.
- Metabolism
  - Amide LAs (eg, lidocaine) undergo liver metabolism starting with N-dealkylation.
  - Ester LAs (eg, procaine) are hydrolyzed by cholinesterases in the liver and plasma.
  - Both pathways rely on liver-produced enzymes, so liver dysfunction can reduce clearance.
- Excretion and toxicity
  - Renal excretion eliminates many catabolites of both ester and amide LAs.
  - Some metabolites retain parent drug activity and may contribute to toxicity if accumulation occurs.

Local Anesthetic Toxicity

- Causes: Rapid absorption, excessive dose, or inadvertent intravascular injection can quickly elevate blood levels.
- Symptoms:
  - CNS: Early excitatory signs (circumoral paresthesia, tinnitus, mental status changes), progressing to tonic-clonic seizures, and coma-producing respiratory depression and respiratory arrest.
  - Cardiovascular: Dose-related depression of contractility and vascular tone; high doses can cause profound cardiovascular collapse.
  - Management:
    - Initial seizure control with benzodiazepines such as diazepam or, less effectively midazolam, applying caution as they can exacerbate respiratory depression.
    - In the event of systemic toxicity, advanced cardiac life support (ACLS) should be initiated, following guidelines.
    - Lipid emulsion rescue: Begin with a 1.5 mL/kg bolus of 20% intralipid; repeat/infuse if needed (max 10 mL/kg over approx. 30 minutes). Please refer to http://www.lipidrescue.org/ for additional information.
- Epinephrine, additive to LA:
  - Prolongs block duration, reduces systemic absorption, and decreases bleeding
  - Concentrations: 1:100,000 (1 mg/100 mL) or 1:200,000 (1 mg/200 mL)
  - Adverse effects: Tachycardia, hypertension, and occasional hypertensive crisis (caution in patients taking monoamine oxidase inhibitors [MAOIs] or tricyclic antidepressants [TCAs]).
  - Toxicity: Nervousness, restlessness, sense of impending doom, potential arrhythmias, and seizures. These symptoms may progress to ventricular irritability and seizures.
- Allergic reactions:
  - Incidence: < 1% of all adverse reactions; often linked to preservatives (methylparaben, metabisulfite).
  - True allergy to LA is more common among ester derivatives.
  - Choosing the anesthetic technique for a patient with a history of LA allergy is not an infrequent clinical problem.
    - Management:
      - ◊ Clarify history: Distinguish toxic or vasovagal events from true allergy.
      - ◊ Some authorities have advocated provocative intradermal testing, but this should only be undertaken when prepared to treat anaphylaxis and can still be unreliable. Alternatively, some authors suggest using a preservative-free LA from the opposite class of the one suspected. If doubt still exists, one must consider alternative techniques, such as general anesthesia.
- Prilocaine and benzocaine can reduce hemoglobin to methemoglobin, which has a diminished ability to transport oxygen to the peripheral tissues.
  - A pulse oximeter cannot measure methemoglobin. If significant quantities of methemoglobin are present, the oxygen saturation will read 85% regardless of what the actual saturation is, and therefore may be grossly in error and unreliable.
  - Patients with glucose-6-phosphate deficiencies are more susceptible to methemoglobinemia.
  - The treatment of methemoglobinemia is intravenous administration of a 1% methylene blue solution to a total dose of 1 to 2 mg/kg.

Table 4-4

Aminoester	*Cocaine*	*Procaine Hydrochloride*	*Chloroprocaine*	*Benzocaine*
Class	Benzoic acid ester	Benzoic acid derivative, weak ester	Halogenated derivative of procaine, a weak ester	Ester of para-aminobenzoic acid similar to procaine.
Activity	Extremely potent as a topical anesthetic	Ineffective as topical	Ineffective as topical	Excellent topical anesthetic
Onset	5-10 minutes	2-5 minutes	2-5 minutes	5-10 minutes
Duration of action	30-60 minutes	30-90 minutes	30-60 minutes	30-60 minutes
Maximum dose	2-3 mg/kg	1000 mg	800 mg plain and 1000 mg with epinephrine	200 mg
Metabolism	Hydrolyzed by plasma cholinesterase	Rapidly hydrolyzed by plasma cholinesterase (may prolong succinylcholine effects)	Hydrolyzed more rapidly than procaine by plasma cholinesterase (may prolong succinylcholine effects)	Hydrolyzed by plasma cholinesterase
Uses	Topical application to mucosal surfaces (rarely used clinically)	Field and nerve blocks	Field, nerve blocks, and epidural	Topical airway anesthetic or as an ointment for wound dressings
Notable issues	• Cocaine is unique in producing vasoconstriction. • Blocks reuptake of norepinephrine and dobutamine at adrenergic nerve endings, causing tachycardia, hypertension, mydriasis, cortical stimulation, addiction, and sensitization of the myocardium to catecholamines. • Elective surgery in acutely intoxicated patients should be aborted. • It may precipitate hypertensive crisis by reducing catecholamine catabolism.	• Percent protein binding: 6%	• Low systemic toxicity	• Can cause methemoglobinemia. • Hurricaine solution contains 20% benzocaine in a flavored, water-soluble polyethylene glycol base. It provides rapid topical anesthesia to mucous membranes, but when used improperly toxicity is common and should be used with caution. Since 2006, the VA has banned its use. The FDA has stated that it should not be used in teething infants.

Table 4-5

Aminoamide	*Lidocaine*	*Mepivacaine*	*Prilocaine*	*Bupivacaine*	*Ropivacaine (single isomer of bupivacaine)*
Activity	Excellent topical anesthetic	Moderate to poor topical anesthetic	Excellent topical anesthetic	Poor topical anesthetic	Poor topical anesthetic
Onset	5-10 minutes	30 seconds-4 minutes	2-4 minutes	5-10 minutes	5-10 minutes
Duration of action	1-3 hours	1-4 hours (depending on location)	1-2 hours	3-10 hours	4-12 hours
Maximum dose	5 mg/kg plain and 7 mg/kg with epinephrine	6 mg/kg and in some texts 400 mg maximum adult dose	8 mg/kg but 600 mg maximum adult dose	2-3 mg/kg	1-3 mg/kg
Metabolism	Transformed by hepatic carboxylesterases and cytochrome P450 enzymes	Transformed by hepatic carboxylesterases and cytochrome P450 enzymes	Transformed by hepatic carboxylesterases and cytochrome P450 enzymes	Transformed by hepatic carboxylesterases and cytochrome P450 enzymes	Transformed by hepatic carboxylesterases and cytochrome P450 enzymes
Uses	Topical anesthesia for mucosal membranes. Also used for field blocks, nerve blocks, epidural, and spinal anesthesia.	Effective for infiltration and peripheral nerve blockade, producing a dense block. Commonly used for dental anesthesia.	Similar to lidocaine produces a dense block	Infiltration, peripheral nerve blockade, spinal, and epidural anesthesia. At lower concentrations, it produces a purely sensory block, and at higher concentrations it produces a sensory and motor block.	Infiltration, peripheral nerve blockade, and epidural anesthesia. Produces less motor blockade than bupivacaine.
Notable issues	• Percent protein binding: 64% • 0.5%-2% solutions used for injection into tissue	• Percent protein binding: 77% • 2% solution contains levonordefrin 1:20,000 (a sulfite), which can cause anaphylactic symptoms	• Percent protein binding: 55% • A known side effect of prilocaine is methemoglobinemia with dose equal to and greater than 600 mg.	• Percent protein binding: 95%	• Percent protein binding: 94%

(*Continued*)

Table 4-5 (*Continued*)

Aminoamide	*Lidocaine*	*Mepivacaine*	*Prilocaine*	*Bupivacaine*	*Ropivacaine (single isomer of bupivacaine)*
	• 4% can be used for trans-tracheal anesthesia, atomized or nebulized for airway anesthesia. IV lidocaine (1.5 mg/kg) can be given during intubation and extubation to blunt the response to tracheal stimulation. The practice of using lidocaine to suppress automaticity in ectopic myocardial foci has been supplanted by the use of amiodarone. • Class 1B antiarrhythmic agent, used for treating certain ventricular arrhythmias.		• EMLA cream, a mixture of lidocaine 2.5% and prilocaine 2.5% in an emulsion is effective in lessening the pain associated with venipuncture, catheter placement, and has been successfully employed in the harvesting of split-thickness skin grafts. Satisfactory anesthesia is achieved by placing the cream under an occlusive dressing at least 1 hour prior to the procedure and persists for 2 hours after removal. Weight-based dosing is extremely important as there have been many reports of toxicity in pediatric patients.	• Tightly bound to tissue and plasma protein and does not produce high blood levels when appropriately administered. However, toxic doses do not produce classic symptoms prior to cardiovascular collapse, so patients should be closely monitored during administration. Bupivacaine produces cardiac toxicity prior to CNS toxicity.	• Ropivacaine is tightly bound to tissue and plasma protein and does not produce high blood levels when appropriately administered. It is less cardiotoxic than bupivacaine at lower doses. Therefore, it is often used for continuous infusion catheters (1-4 days). Use with epinephrine has no advantages in block prolongation.

Local Anesthetic Agent

Aminoamide Agents

Liposomal formulation of bupivacaine (Exparel) acts as a depo and has a duration of up to 72 hours; therefore, unable to give additional LA during this time frame. This is an excellent agent for an opiate-sparing postoperative analgesia technique and also reduces the risk of postoperative nausea and vomiting. However, it is a poor choice for cases where postoperative nerve monitoring is required.

Opioids

The most commonly used perioperative opioids include fentanyl, morphine, and hydromorphone. Although they provide effective analgesia, sedation, and generally stable hemodynamics, they can cause CNS and respiratory depression, as well as nausea and vomiting. Elderly patients are especially prone to postoperative cognitive dysfunction. Opioids are often given during induction but are rarely used alone. Growing concern over relapse in patients on buprenorphine—particularly if it is tapered perioperatively—highlights the need for a coordinated plan among surgical, anesthesia, and addiction services. In light of the opioid epidemic, clinicians should limit opioid use and, wherever possible, adopt nonopioid pain management strategies.

Morphine

- Best titrated in incremental doses.
- Avoid use in patients with reactive airway disease because of its ability to cause histamine release along with increased central vagal tone.
- Common side effects include pruritus due to morphine-induced histamine release; this discomfort can sometimes surpass the patient's pain in severity.
- Active morphine metabolites (morphine-glucuronides) are excreted via the kidney and will accumulate in patients with renal failure. Therefore, doses subsequent to initial administration should be based solely on clinical need, not a dosing regimen.

Hydromorphone (Dilaudid)

- Five times more potent than morphine, therefore 0.2 mg of Dilaudid is as effective as 1 mg of morphine.
- Compared to morphine, hydromorphone causes less pruritus and nausea and vomiting. Therefore, it is an excellent drug of choice for patient-controlled analgesia (PCA) dosing.

Methadone

- Potent μ-receptor agonist, *N*-methyl-D-aspartate (NDMA) receptor antagonist, serotonin and norepinephrine reuptake inhibition.
- Rapid onset (6-8) minutes.
- Longest half-life (24-36 hours) of the clinically used opioids and is inversely associated with opioid tolerance (24 hours for opioid tolerant patient, 55 hours for opioid naïve patient). Incomplete cross-tolerance to other opioids makes the effect of a single dose of methadone highly unpredictable.
- Metabolized by hepatic P450 cytochrome enzyme, CYP2B6, CY3A4, patients with genetic polymorphisms of CYP4502B6 enzyme may experience variability in how they metabolize methadone.
- Potential attenuation of chronic postsurgical pain.
- Risk for patients with specific comorbidities including obstructive sleep apnea, liver or kidney dysfunction, and outpatient ambulatory surgical setting.
- Associated with numerous opioid-related adverse effects including postoperative nausea and vomiting, pruritus, ileus, sedation, and respiratory depression.

Codeine

- A methylated morphine.
- Hydrocodone is a codeine derivative.
- Usually given PO as a single agent or in combination with acetaminophen or ibuprofen, and are commonly prescribed for postoperative relief.
- When used as a combined medication, it is important to educate patients about avoiding toxic doses of acetaminophen or ibuprofen by escalating consumption of the combination tablet or adding additional NSAIDs.
- Metabolized by the CYP2D6 enzyme, significant genetic variability occurs in the number of this gene. Therefore, patients can vary from ultrafast metabolizers (1%-2% of patients) all the way to nonmetabolizers (5%-10% of patients) and will experience ultra-high active metabolite concentrations or no active metabolite, respectively. A patient history of their experience with this medication will often uncover this difference. Alternatively, a patient's first dose of this medication can be given in the recovery room and its effect assessed.

Fentanyl (Sublimaze), **sufentanil** (Sufenta), and **alfentanil** (Alfenta), the synthetic opioids, can be given as premedications, although in general they are given intravenously in small amounts at the induction of general anesthesia, titrated for conscious sedation or postoperative pain relief. All of these agents exhibit context-sensitive half-lives; therefore, the total dosing and time interval will determine their elimination time.

Remifentanil

- Ultra-short-acting selective micro-opioid receptor agonist.
- 15- to 30-fold more potent than alfentanil.
- Rapidly hydrolyzed by nonspecific plasma and tissue esterases, making onset and recovery rapid, with no cumulative effects, and its metabolism is unaffected by impaired renal clearance or hepatic function.
- Remifentanil infusion (0.1-0.5 μg/kg/min) is often used during TIVA to maintain the general anesthetic state, acting synergistically with propofol, reducing propofol requirement and providing a degree of akinesis.
- It does not provide any postoperative analgesia due to its rapid metabolism.

Pentazocine, butorphanol, and nalbuphine are combined agonist/antagonist drugs. They exhibit a ceiling effect with regard to analgesia and, therefore, may be less useful.

Naloxone

- Specific opioid antagonist.
- Provided in ampules of 0.4 mg/mL (400 μg/mL) but, unless an emergency situation exists, can be titrated in doses of 20- to 40-μg increments to achieve the desired level of arousal.
- Naloxone has been associated with flash pulmonary edema when administered rapidly in larger doses.

Meperidine (Demerol)

- Rarely used now to treat pain due to the risk of serotonin syndrome when combined with MAOIs, as well as other antidepressants, muscle relaxants, and benzodiazepines.
- Used at low doses (12.5-25 mg) in the treatment of postoperative shivering.

Ketamine (Please see section under IV anesthetics.)

Nonsteroidal Anti-inflammatory Drugs

Nonsteroidal anti-inflammatory drugs (NSAIDs) that can be administered either PO or IV are useful first-line agents, as per the WHO pain ladder. For postoperative pain control acetaminophen as a single agent or in combination with diclofenac is an excellent option that reduces patient opiate exposure risk.

Acetaminophen

- Dose: 650 mg PO or 1 g IV Q6h Maximal: 4 g/24 h
- Contraindications: Hepatic failure.
- Stable nondrinking cirrhotics have been shown to take this medication safely.

Ketorolac

- Dose: 30 mg IV Q8h Maximal: 60 mg/24 h
- Contraindications: Renal failure, reactive airway disease, active bleeding, or high risk for hematoma formation

Diclofenac

- Dose: 50 mg PO Q8h-Q12 or 75 mg Q12h
- Contraindications: Renal failure, reactive airway disease, active bleeding, or high risk for hematoma formation

Antisialogues

Table 4-6

Antimuscarinic agent	*Atropine sulfate*	*Scopolamine*	*Glycopyrrolate*
	Tertiary amine, therefore, easily crosses placenta and blood-brain barrier (BBB), acting centrally.	Tertiary amine, therefore easily crosses placenta and blood-brain barrier, acting centrally.	Quaternary amine, does not cross blood-brain barrier.
Dose	0.4-0.8 mg IM or IV	0.2-0.4 mg IM	0.2-0.4 mg IV
	Acts at peripheral muscarinic receptors to block the action of Ach, increasing heart rate and pupil size while reducing secretory gland activity, causing antisialagogue effect and anhydrosis	Similar to atropine, but has stronger antisialagogue and ocular activity. Crosses BBB more effectively than atropine to produce amnesia, drowsiness, fatigue, and non-REM sleep.	More potent and longer acting at peripheral muscarinic receptors than atropine.

Antiemesis

Nausea and vomiting are usually a protective physiological function against ingested toxins, but in the case of postoperative nausea and vomiting (PONV), it is deleterious. Occurring in about a third of untreated surgical patients, PONV may result in surgical wound dehiscence, delayed hospital stay, unanticipated hospital admissions, and increased aspiration rates.

Risk factors predicting the incidence of PONV include:

- Female sex
- History of PONV
- Type of procedure including otolaryngology procedures, particularly middle ear procedures
- Nonsmoker
- Age less than 40

A combination of these factors can produce a PONV risk reaching 75%. This process may be triggered directly via the medullary chemoreceptor trigger zone and indirectly through gastric enterochromaffin cells and the vestibular system, both of which are transmitted via efferent cranial nerves. These signals all culminate in activation of the vomiting center.

The most common cause of nausea in the PACU is PONV; however, other serious causes should always be part of the differential diagnosis, including gastric irritants or insufflation, hypoxia, hypotension, hypoglycemia, increased ICP, and myocardial infarction.

Pharmacologic therapies can target the multifactorial triggers of PONV, each reducing incidence by about 20% to 25%. However, meaningful risk reduction requires anticipatory planning rather than reactive rescue. A patient-specific, multimodal approach—minimizing emetogenic agents, suctioning blood, and using prophylactic strategies, reducing opioid use—offers optimal prevention.

Pharmacological Antiemetics

- Several classes of antiemetic agents antagonize the key neurotransmitter receptors involved in nausea and vomiting.
- Some agents act on multiple receptors but are typically classified by their primary mechanism of action.
- Five main receptor types mediate the vomiting reflex: M1 (muscarinic), D2 (dopamine), H1 (histamine), 5-HT3 (serotonin), and NK1 (neurokinin).

Table 4-7

Class	*Anticholinergic—M1 muscarinic receptor antagonist*	*Antihistamine*	*Dopamine receptor antagonists*	*Serotonin receptor antagonists*	*Neurokinin receptor antagonists*	*Glucocorticoids*	*Benzodiazepines*
Drug	Scopolamine	Diphenhydramine Promethazine	Phenothiazines—Prochlorperazine, chlorpromazine Butyrophenones—Droperidol Benzamides—Metoclopramide	Ondansetron, Palonosetron, Granisetron, Dolasetron	Aprepitant, Fosaprepitant, netupitant, Rolapitant		Dexamethasone
Use	Transdermal patch placed presurgery is usually well tolerated, providing 1 mg over 3 days.	Diphenhydramine (25-50 mg orally, 10-50 mg IV/IM), Promethazine (25 mg 12 hourly)	Promethazine (Phenergan) 25-50 mg and prochlorperazine (Compazine) 5-10 mg are commonly used as rescue antiemetics only. Droperidol used in low doses (0.625-1.25 mg) as a rescue antiemetic (QT prolongation incurred at higher doses and the FDA's black box warning of this effect).	Commonly used as prophylactic agent.	Particularly useful in prevention of delayed emesis.		

(*Continued*)

Table 4-7 (*Continued*)

Class	*Anticholinergic—M1 muscarinic receptor antagonist*	*Antihistamine*	*Dopamine receptor antagonists*	*Serotonin receptor antagonists*	*Neurokinin receptor antagonists*	*Glucocorticoids*	*Benzodiazepines*
Notes	Warn patients of side effects including dry mouth. Drowsiness, dry eyes, mydriasis, vision disturbance, photosensitivity, and dermatitis at site of application.	Sedation is a common side effect, can cause anticholinergic effects.	Phenothiazines antagonize D2 dopamine receptors, as well as M1 muscarinic and H1 histamine blocking effects. Main adverse effects of phenothiazines are extrapyramidal reactions including dystonia, tardive dyskinesia.	Can cause QT prolongation. Oral formulation comparable efficacy to intravenous.	Work best in conjunction with serotonin receptor antagonists and dexamethasone.		Dexamethasone has long been used during otolaryngological procedures to prevent PONV and airway edema. Caution required with risks of poor glucose control, possible deficiencies in wound healing as well as the other well-described side effects of steroidal therapy

Nonpharmacological Antiemetics

- Various methods have been suggested and studied, with acupuncture and acupressure holding the most promise.
- Isopropyl alcohol (eg, having the patient inhale alcohol from a skin preparation pack) may provide short-term effective treatment.

Postoperative Pain Management

A perioperative pain management plan should be tailored to each patient's unique factors, the anticipated or existing level of pain, and the planned procedure. While it is reasonable to develop a strategy based on these considerations, individual variability requires vigilant postoperative monitoring to ensure adequate analgesia and patient safety.

- Basic strategies for all patients should include acetaminophen, NSAIDS unless there are contraindications, and local or regional analgesia techniques when applicable.
- Opioids may be prescribed in oral or IV formulation on an as-needed basis postoperatively.
- Patient-controlled analgesia (PCA) has become a well-established method of delivering opiates to postoperative surgical patients. Hydromorphone has become the preferred agent as it produces less nausea and pruritus. PCA is generally well accepted by patients because it provides them with some degree of control over their situation and is adaptable to pediatric and geriatric patients.
- Ketamine or lidocaine infusions may be indicated for selected patients.
- Nonpharmacologic options include compression, elevation, acupuncture, and music. These are low-risk interventions that may offer some benefit. However, current evidence supporting their efficacy is limited, and further research is needed.

Fluid and Transfusion Management

- Growing body of evidence to recommend the use of cardiac output monitors in high-risk patients or those undergoing major surgery.
- Use of goal-directed fluid therapy using noninvasive and minimally invasive volume status monitors (eg, Delta CardioQ) has improved clinical outcomes in a large variety of cases, particularly during free-flap reconstruction surgeries.
- Careful preoperative optimization can help reduce the need for intraoperative blood transfusions and the use of vasopressors.

Other Considerations

- Preoperative limb marking helps prevent inadvertent IV placement in an extremity designated for flap harvest.
- Attention to positioning is also critical, especially when the anesthesia machine sits 180 degrees from the patient's head, resulting in the need for circuit extenders.
- Inadvertent intraoperative hypothermia (core temperature < 36°C) can increase perioperative blood loss, coagulopathy, and recovery time, as well as lead to postoperative shivering, delayed wound healing, and higher infection rates. Strategies for maintaining normothermia include keeping the ambient operating room temperature above

21°C, using forced-air warming devices (eg, Bair Hugger), and warming both IV fluids and irrigation solutions. However, caution is needed to avoid potential thermal injury from forced-air warmers.

Complications

This discussion of complications of general anesthesia is confined to those that are of relevance to otolaryngologists. However, one should not lose sight of the fact that anesthesia affects all organ systems, which may be a source of potential complications.

- Aspiration pneumonitis (Mendelson syndrome) may occur either during intubation or extubation of the trachea or with sedation and a loss of airway reflexes.
  - Gastric contents of greater than 200 mL with a pH less than 2.5 are associated with a high risk of aspiration syndrome.
  - Postaspiration respiratory tree lavage has not been demonstrated to reduce this syndrome. This syndrome is treated supportively and may require postoperative intubation, and can progress to acute respiratory distress syndrome.
  - Aspiration can also occur with a properly positioned, cuffed endotracheal tube.
  - Sodium citrate (Bicitra) 15 to 30 mL administered 30 minutes prior to induction of anesthesia is effective in raising the pH of gastric contents already present in the stomach and reducing the risk of aspiration pneumonitis.
- Many of the inhalation anesthetics are associated with sensitization of the myocardium to catecholamines. In the presence of excess endogenous or exogenous catecholamines, patients may develop cardiac arrhythmias (ventricular ectopy or fibrillation). It is therefore recommended that the dose of epinephrine administered not exceed 10 mL of a 1:100,000 solution (ie, 100 µg) in any 10-minute period when these anesthetics are in use.
- Malignant hyperthermia (MH) is a rare (incidence of 1:10,000-1:50,000 anesthetics) and potentially lethal entity.
  - Triggered by the potent inhalation agents and succinylcholine, and is associated with a genetic predisposition.
  - Once triggered, MH causes a massive increase in intracellular calcium and uncoupling of metabolic pathways, resulting in an extreme elevation of temperature, an increase in CO_2 production, metabolic acidosis, cardiac arrhythmias, and, if untreated, eventual cardiovascular collapse.
  - Dantrolene is the only directed therapeutic agent; it acts by blocking intracellular calcium release.
  - If a patient has a known history of MH or MH susceptibility, TIVA should be the anesthetic of choice, avoiding MH trigger agents on an anesthesia machine that has not had inhalational agents attached to it.

Block Techniques

- Specific nerve blocks or field blocks reduce patient's pain, thereby reducing the need for systemic analgesics and, in some cases, obviate the need for general anesthesia.
- These techniques improve patient safety and experience of the procedure.
- The majority of nerve blocks are currently preformed utilizing landmarks and increasingly under ultrasound guidance.

- Eliciting a paresthesia, once used as a technique to locate nerves, is to be avoided as this incurs a high risk of nerve injury.
- The specific goals of concomitant IV sedation must be kept clearly in mind when utilizing a block technique. Importantly, sedation should never substitute for an inadequate LA block.

Laryngoscopy, Tracheostomy

- The larynx and trachea receive their sensory nerve supply from the superior and inferior laryngeal nerves, which are branches of the vagus nerve.
- Anesthesia may be provided to the larynx by the topical application of local anesthesia (using a laryngeal syringe) to the mucous membrane of the pyriform fossa (deep into which runs the superior laryngeal nerve) and to the laryngeal surface of the epiglottis and the vocal folds (Figure 4-1).
- Local anesthesia of the larynx and trachea also may be accomplished by the percutaneous infiltration of local anesthetic solution around the superior laryngeal nerve and the transtracheal application of LA to the tracheal mucosa.
- For percutaneous infiltration, the superior laryngeal nerve is located as it pierces the thyrohyoid membrane (Figure 4-2).
- The transtracheal application of local anesthesia requires insertion of a 25-gauge needle through the cricothyroid membrane in the midline (Figure 4-3).

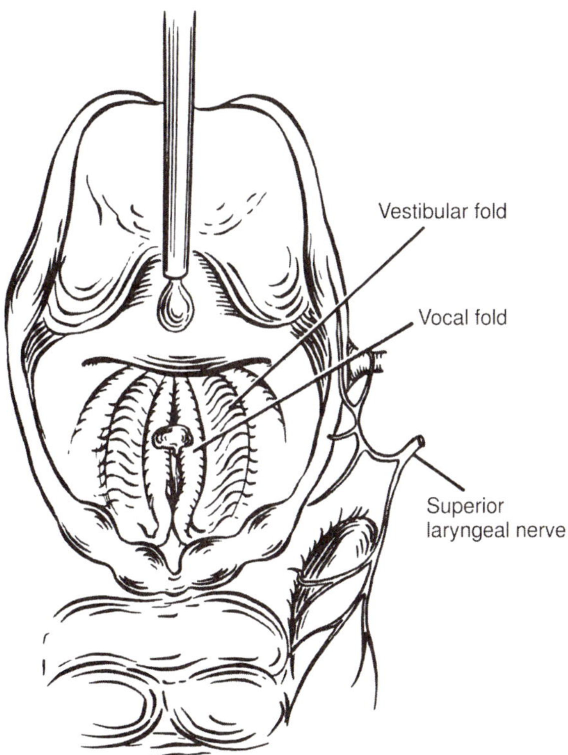

Figure 4-1 Topical anesthesia to the larynx.

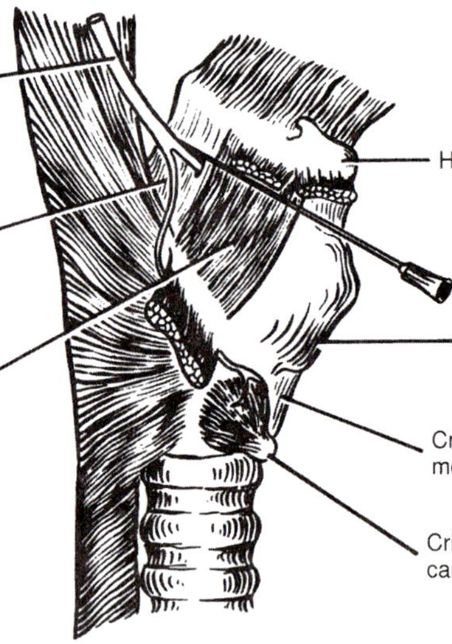

Figure 4-2 (1) Palpate the greater cornu of the hyoid bone. (2) Insert a 25-gauge needle approximately 1 cm caudal to this landmark. (3) The needle is inserted to a depth of approximately 1 cm until the firm consistency of the thyrohyoid membrane is identified. (4) Inject 3 mL of local anesthetic solution.

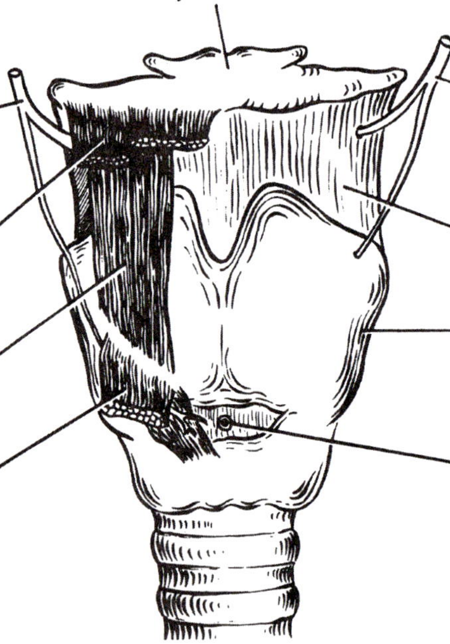

Figure 4-3 (1) Introduce the 25-gauge needle in the midline between the thyroid and cricoid cartilages. (2) Puncture the cricothyroid membrane. It is readily felt as a "pop." Free aspiration of air with the attached syringe verifies the intratracheal position of the needle tip. (3) Instill 4 mL of local anesthetic solution. In addition to anesthesia of the larynx and trachea (steps 1 and 2), the topical application of local anesthesia to the oropharynx is required for adequate visualization for laryngoscopy and tracheoscopy.

Reduction of Dislocated Temporomandibular Joint

In the common presentation of temporomandibular dislocation, the condyle rests on the anterior slope of the articular eminence (Figure 4-4). There is intense pain and severe spasm of the surrounding mandibular musculature. Reduction of this dislocation may frequently be accomplished by unilateral intracapsular injection of local anesthesia.

Reduction and Fixation of Mandibular Fracture

Complete anesthesia for reduction and fixation of a mandibular fracture requires adequate anesthesia of the maxillary and mandibular branches of the trigeminal nerve and superficial branches of the cervical plexus (Figure 4-5).

The mandibular branch of the trigeminal nerve is readily anesthetized near its exit from the skull through the foramen ovale (Figure 4-6). Anesthesia of the maxillary division of the trigeminal nerve may be accomplished in the pterygopalatine fossa near the foramen rotundum, where the nerve exits from the skull (Figure 4-7). The most frequent complication of

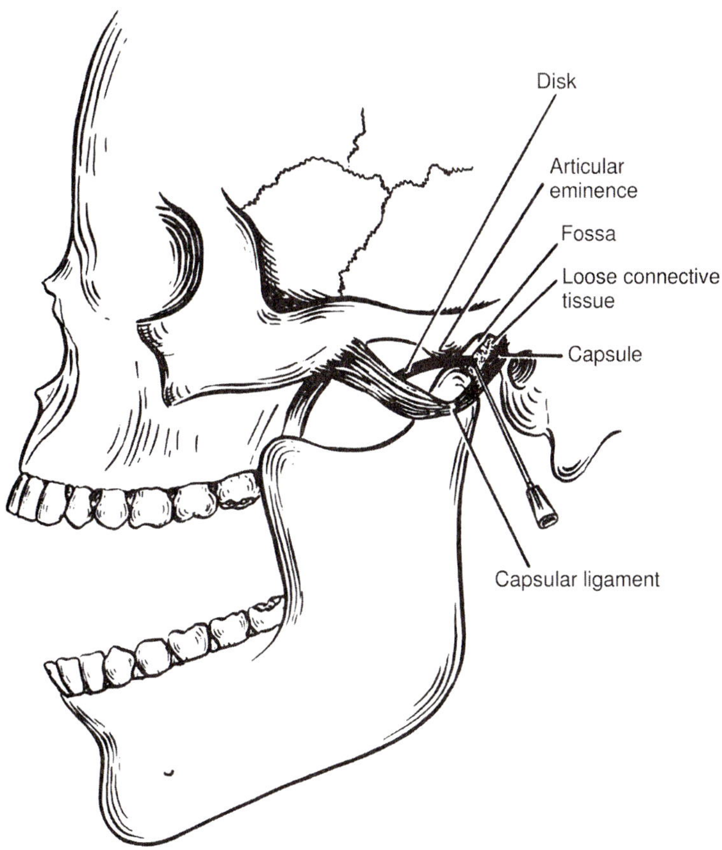

Figure 4-4 (1) With the head of the condyloid process locked anteriorly, the depression of the glenoid fossa is easily palpated. (2) The needle is inserted into the depression of the glenoid fossa and directed anteriorly toward the head of the condyloid process. (3) When the condyloid process is contracted, the needle is slightly withdrawn. (4) Instill 2 mL of local anesthetic solution into the capsule.

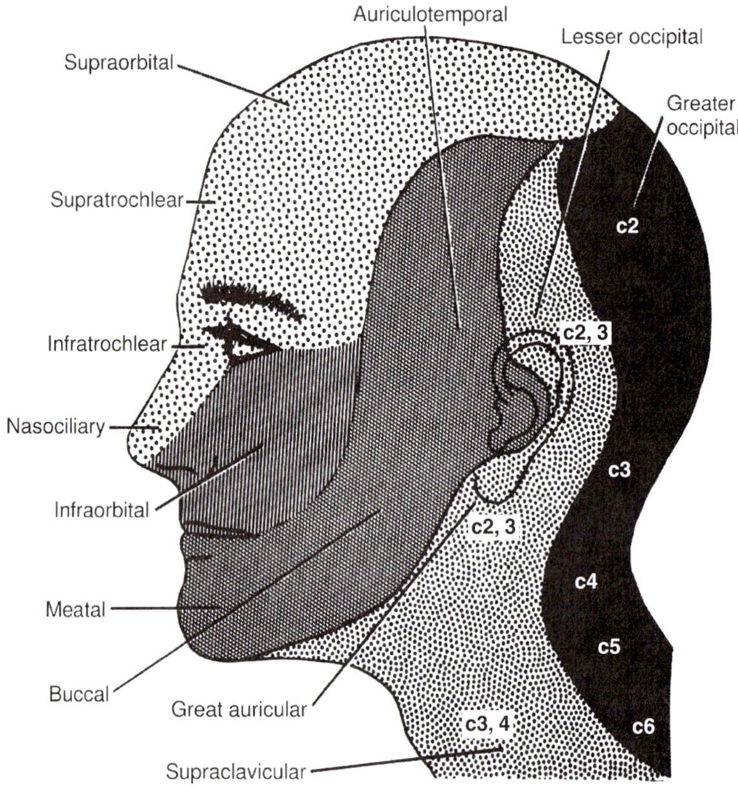

Figure 4-5 Cutaneous innervation of the head and neck.

mandibular and maxillary nerve block is hemorrhage into the cheek, which is usually managed conservatively. Subarachnoid injections and facial nerve blocks are two other rarely reported complications.

The superficial branches of the cervical plexus are easily blocked as they emerge along the posterior margin of the sternocleidomastoid muscle; infiltration is accomplished along the posterior margin of this muscle using 10 to 15 mL of anesthetic solution.

Otology

The sensory innervation of the external ear is illustrated in Figure 4-8. The middle ear receives its sensory innervation through the tympanic plexus (cranial nerves V3, IX, and X).

- V3—auriculotemporal nerve
- IX—Jacobson nerve
- X—auricular nerve

Myringotomy

For myringotomy, inject the cartilaginous and bony junction of the external auditory canal. Instead of introducing LA through the classic 12, 3, 6, and 9 o'clock infiltration, infiltrate at 12, 2, 4, 6, 8, and 10 o'clock. After the first injection, the subsequent injection sites are already

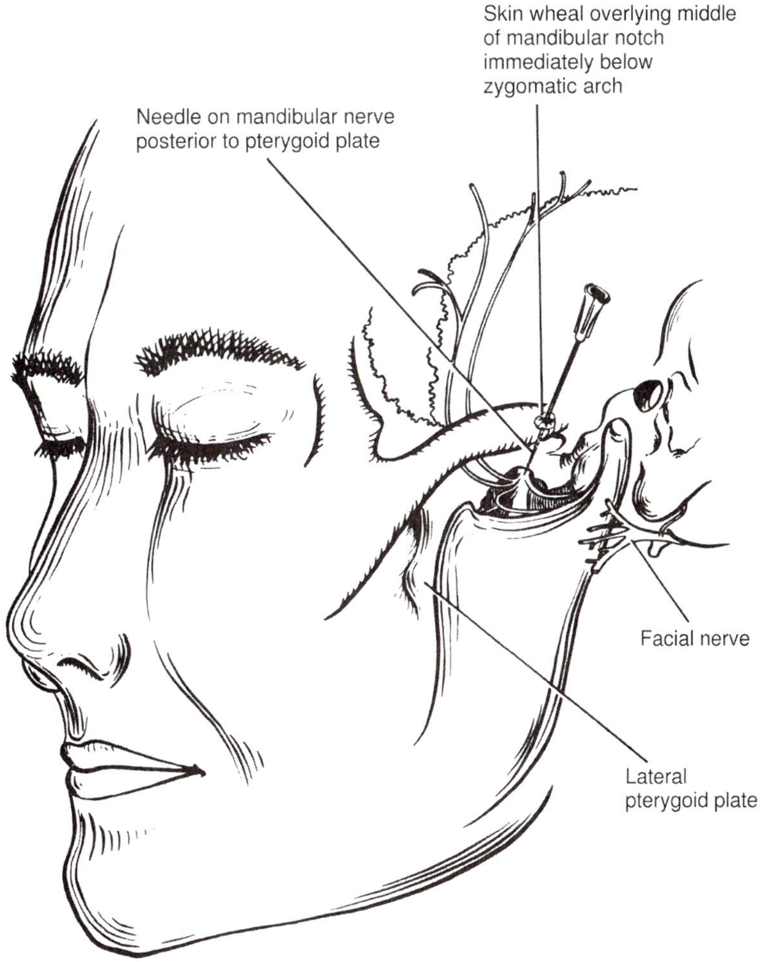

Figure 4-6 (1) A skin wheal is raised at the midpoint between the condyle and coronoid process of the mandible and just below the zygoma. (2) An 8-cm needle is introduced perpendicular to the skin until contact with the pterygoid plate occurs, usually at a depth of 4 cm. (3) The needle is withdrawn and then reinserted slightly posterior to a depth of approximately 6 cm. (4) When paresthesia in the mandibular division is elicited, the needle is fixed, and approximately 5 mL of anesthetic solution is administered.

anesthetized before the needle prick. For myringotomy alone, it is not necessary to infiltrate the skin of the bony canal wall, and no LA agent should infiltrate into the middle ear cavity. (See "Complications" later in text.)

Stapedectomy

In addition to the technique described for myringotomy, with stapedectomy, it is necessary to infiltrate the tympanomeatal flap. This technique ensures adequate anesthesia while providing vasoconstriction (1% lidocaine with epinephrine 1:100,000) for hemostasis.

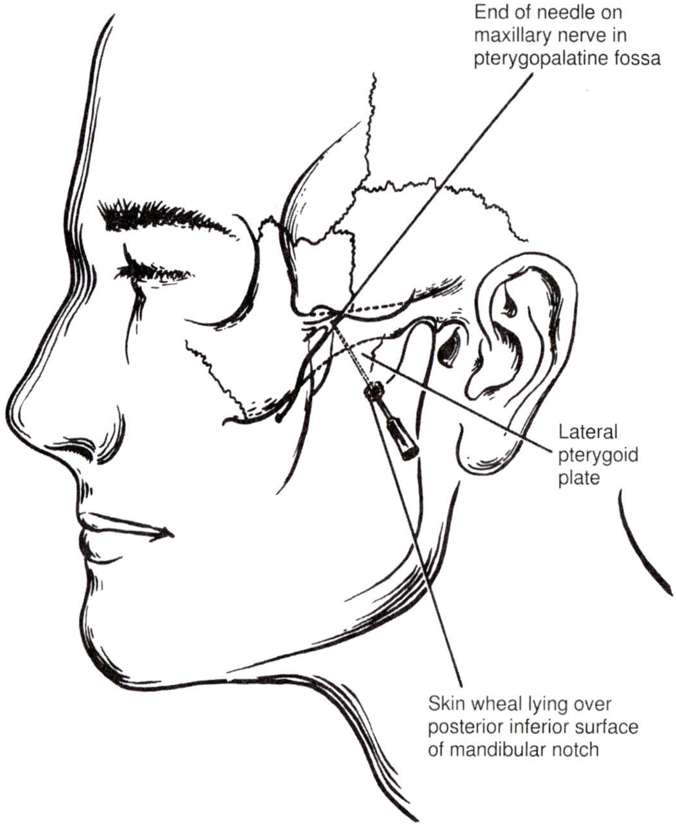

Figure 4-7 (1) A skin wheal is raised just over the posterior-inferior surface of the mandibular notch. (2) An 8-cm needle is inserted transversely and slightly anterior to a depth of 4-5 cm, where it comes into contact with the lateral pterygoid plate. (3) The needle is withdrawn slightly and directed in a more anterosuperior direction to pass anterior to the pterygoid plate into the pterygopalatine fossa. (4) The needle is advanced another 0.5-1.5 cm until paresthesia is elicited. A total of 5-10 mL of local anesthetic solution is deposited.

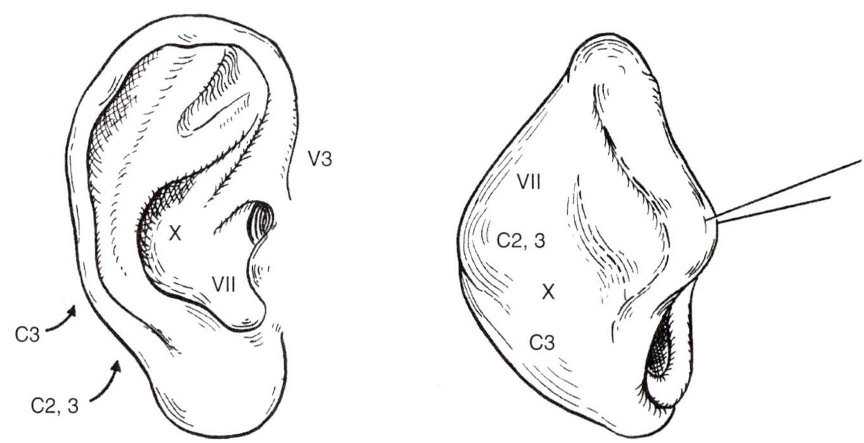

Figure 4-8 Sensory innervation of the external ear.

Complications

Two transient complications have been reported from LA infiltration for stapedectomy. These result from diffusion of the LA from the tympanomeatal flap to the middle ear cavity.

- Temporary facial nerve paralysis results from the LA coming into contact with the dehiscent facial nerve. Patience and reassurance for a few hours resolves the problem.
- Violent vertigo with nystagmus (similar to Ménière) can occur 45 minutes after infiltration. Provided no damage has been done to the vestibular labyrinth, this problem is secondary to the effect of lidocaine on the membranous labyrinth through the oval or round windows.

These complications are particularly distressing if they occur after an office myringotomy. Therefore, we recommend that there be no infiltration of LA into the skin of the bony canal wall. LA applied at the junction of the bony and cartilaginous canal is adequate and does not risk migrating into the middle ear cavity.

Tympanoplasty and Mastoidectomy (Canalplasty, Meatoplasty)

Tympanoplasty and mastoidectomy are usually performed under general anesthesia, although they may be done under local anesthesia. In addition to the stapedectomy infiltration, postauricular and conchal infiltration are necessary (see Figure 4-8) for sensory innervation. The skin of the anterior canal wall needs to be anesthetized if surgery is to include that anatomic site.

Nasal Surgery

Nasal Polypectomy Cocaine pledgets along the mucosal surfaces, as well as those in contact with the sphenopalatine ganglion, supply adequate anesthesia for polypectomy. Occasionally, it is necessary to supplement this anesthesia with infiltration, as for rhinoplasty.

Septoplasty and Rhinoplasty The sensory innervation of the septum and external nose is illustrated in Figures 4-9 to 4-13. In addition to local infiltration, as shown in Figure 4-13, cocaine pledgets along the mucosal surfaces and sphenopalatine ganglion are used for septoplasty and rhinoplasty. For the best hemostasis and anesthesia result, it is wise to wait at least 20 minutes before performing the surgery.

Sinus Surgery

Caldwell-Luc Operation To achieve good anesthesia for sinus surgery, one needs to block the infraorbital nerve, the sphenopalatine ganglion, and the posterior superior dental nerve. The posterior-superior dental nerve exists from the maxillary nerve adjacent to the sphenopalatine ganglion. To block the sphenopalatine ganglion and posterior-superior dental nerve, introduce local anesthesia through the greater palatine foramen via a curved needle.

Further topical anesthesia is with cocaine pledgets applied intranasally against the sphenopalatine ganglion. Local infiltration of the mucosa in the canine fossa supplies the hemostasis needed over the line of incision.

Ethmoid Sinuses The sensory innervation of the ethmoid sinuses is intertwined with that of the nose and septum. In addition, they are innervated by the anterior ethmoid nerve (branch of the nasociliary, V_1) and the posterior ethmoid nerve (branch of the infratrochlear, V_1).

Sphenoid Sinuses The sensory innervation of the sphenoid sinuses is from the pharyngeal branch of the maxillary nerve as well as the posterior ethmoid nerve.

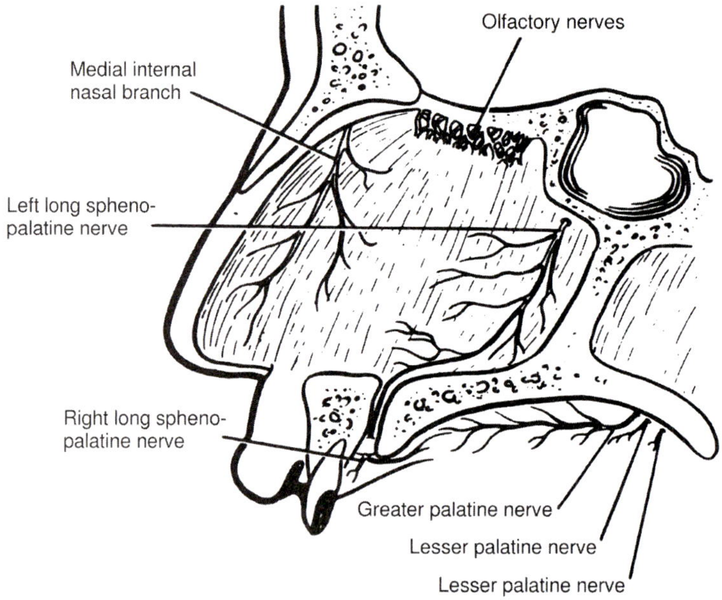

Figure 4-9 Sensory innervation of the internal nose.

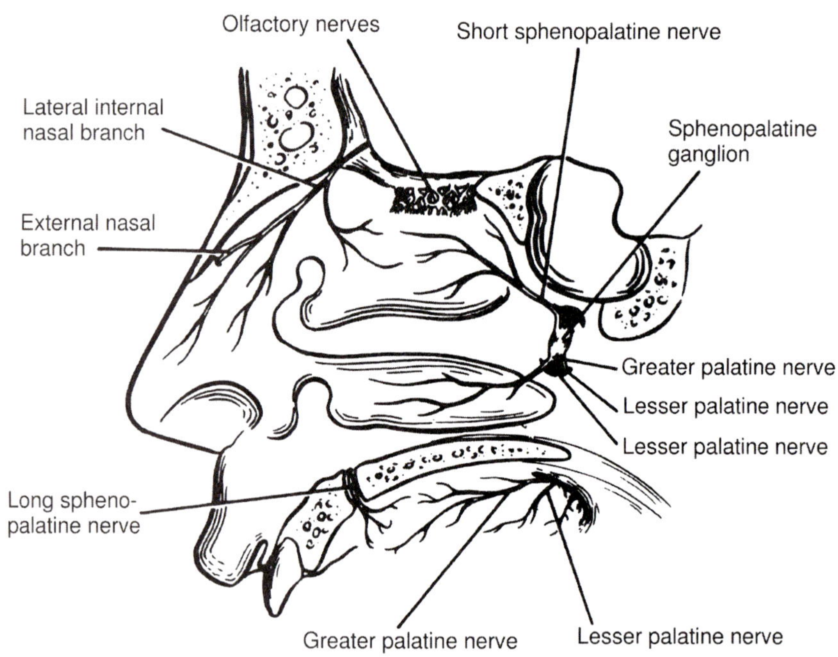

Figure 4-10 Sensory innervation of the nose.

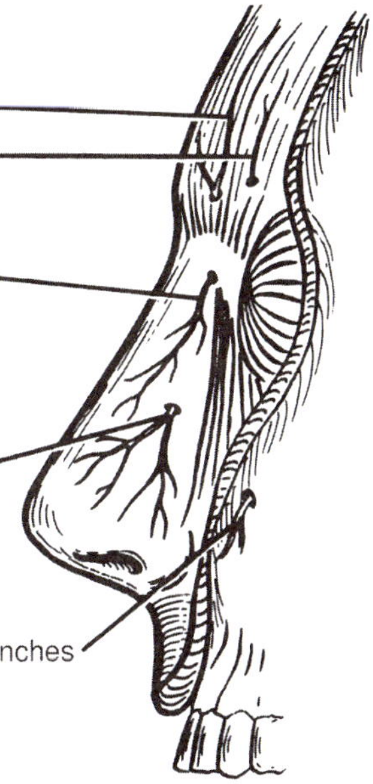

Figure 4-11 Sensory innervation of the nose.

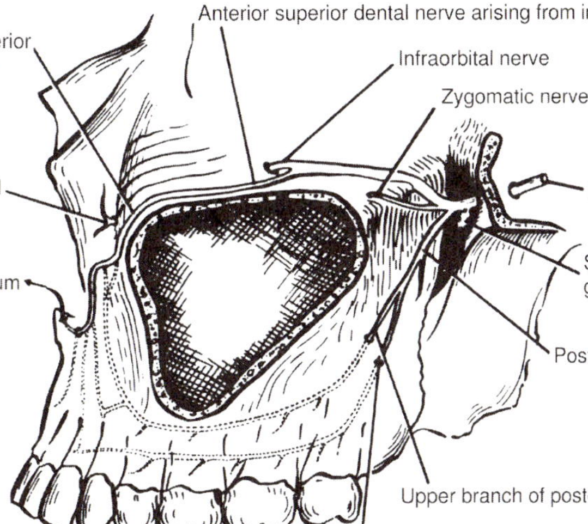

Figure 4-12 Sensory innervation of the nose.

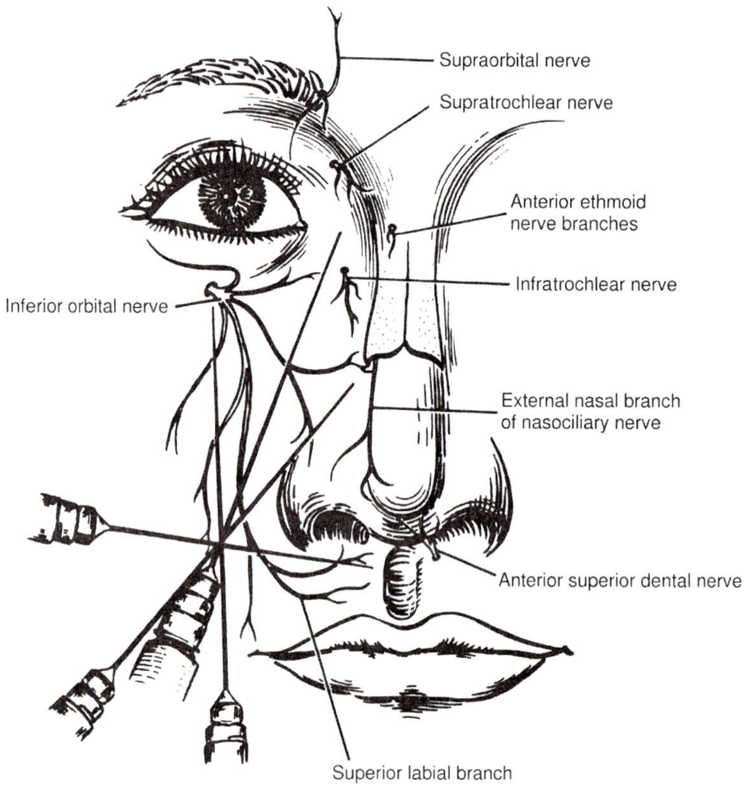

Figure 4-13 Infiltration for rhinoplasty.

Conclusion

Anesthesia for head and neck surgery can be among the most challenging and high-pressure experiences in the operating room. Although many of these procedures are considered "minor" based on anatomical involvement, the constant airway manipulation tests an anesthesiologist's ability to anticipate and mitigate serious complications. Because the airway is shared, close collaboration and clear communication between anesthesiologists and otolaryngologists are essential for ensuring patient safety and achieving optimal outcomes.

Bibliography

ASA perioperative surgical home. http://www.asahq.org/psh.

Barash PG, Cullen BF, Stoelting RK, Cahalan M, Stock MC, Ortega R. *Clinical Anesthesia*. 7th ed. Philadelphia, PA: Wolters Kluwer Health; 2013.

4th National Audit Project (NAP4): Major complications of airway management in the United Kingdom Report and Findings–March 2011.

MedicAlert Foundation difficult airway registry. http://www.medicalert.org/everybody/difficult-airwayintubation-registry.
Richard AJ, Stanley IS, Clifford AS, Brenda G. *Anesthesiologist's Manual of Surgical Procedures.* 4th ed. Philadelphia, PA: Wolters Kluwer Health/Lippincott Williams & Wilkins; 2009.

Questions

1. Which approach is **most** effective for reducing postoperative nausea and vomiting (PONV)?
   A. Rely solely on rescue antiemetics after symptoms begin.
   B. Provide a single agent if the patient reports minimal nausea.
   C. Employ a proactive, multimodal strategy including risk factor reduction and multiple antiemetics.
   D. Limit fluid intake to prevent nausea.

2. Which statement about neuromuscular blockade is most accurate?
   A. Rocuronium is contraindicated in malignant hyperthermia (MH)-susceptible patients.
   B. Deep neuromuscular blockade is mandatory for every head and neck surgical case.
   C. Neostigmine is ineffective for reversing nondepolarizing blockade.
   D. Sugammadex can rapidly reverse rocuronium, though it requires caution in patients with renal failure.

3. Which statement best describes the use of intravenous anesthetic agents in head and neck surgery?
   A. Total intravenous anesthesia (TIVA) with propofol and remifentanil is typically avoided due to hemodynamic instability.
   B. TIVA with propofol and remifentanil can provide stable hemodynamics and reduce PONV.
   C. Inhalational agents are always required for airway management in MH-susceptible patients.
   D. Ketamine is contraindicated in all head and neck procedures.

4. Which choice most accurately reflects the varying levels of sedation?
   A. Deep sedation maintains complete patient responsiveness and no risk to the airway.
   B. The sedation continuum ranges from minimal sedation through general anesthesia, each level requiring progressively more monitoring.
   C. Moderate sedation and general anesthesia are clinically indistinguishable.
   D. Minimal sedation involves loss of protective airway reflexes.

5. Regarding the use of local anesthetics (LAs), which statement is most accurate?
   A. LAs do not cross the blood-brain barrier.
   B. They rarely need vasoconstrictors to extend their duration of action.
   C. Amide LAs are metabolized by plasma cholinesterases.
   D. LA potency is mainly determined by lipid solubility.

Chapter 5
Surgical Hemostasis and Clotting Mechanisms

Introduction

The most important considerations for maintaining surgical hemostasis begin before the procedure starts. This chapter provides practical tools to approach patients before, during, and after the surgical procedure. Below is a summary explanation of normal hemostasis and its conceptualization into four basic components. Explanations are provided to illustrate the uses and limitations of the routine coagulation tests. Common coagulation disorders are briefly discussed. Perioperative management of anticoagulants, as well as the use of reversal agents, is discussed. Finally, we discuss topical and systemic hemostatic agents that may be used perioperatively and briefly discuss the impact of new biologic therapies on surgical hemostasis. The routine clinical application of these basic concepts of blood coagulation can enhance practice and benefit patients.

Basic Concepts of Hemostasis

Hemostasis is a term describing the complex processes that keep blood in its fluid state within the vasculature, yet allow it to clot to stop hemorrhage.

The Four Conceptual Components of Hemostasis

- The process of normal hemostasis can be divided conceptually into four basic components of the blood, listed as follows: (1) blood vessels (lined by endothelial cells), (2) platelets, (3) coagulation system, and (4) fibrinolytic system (Table 5-1).
- These components undergo a series of regulated events that lead to clot formation.

Primary Hemostasis

After endothelial injury in a blood vessel, four steps lead to the formation of a platelet plug.

1. Vasoconstriction
   - An injury to a blood vessel triggers vasoconstriction—the decrease in blood flow slows bleeding and promotes platelet adhesion.

Table 5-1 Four Conceptual Hemostasis Components

Component	*Composition/Reactions*
Blood vessel	Vessel wall; vasoconstriction extravascular proteins, eg, collagen and tissue factor
Platelet	Adhesion, release, aggregation
Coagulation system	All coagulation factors, vWF, and natural anticoagulant proteins, eg, protein C, AT3
Fibrinolytic system	Clot lysis, split products

AT3, antithrombin 3; vWF, von Willebrand factor.

2. Platelet adhesion
    - The initial contact interaction between platelets and *any nonplatelet surface* (the damaged vessel wall)
    - Mediated by a platelet surface glycoprotein receptor termed GPIb complex and the plasma protein, von Willebrand factor (vWF), which is expressed by damaged endothelial cells
3. Platelet activation/aggregation
    - A platelet membrane surface receptor, "the aggregation receptor," made up of two platelet surface proteins, GPIIb/GPIIIa, is expressed on activated platelets.
    - GPIIb/GPIIIa binds fibrinogen, which is expressed on other activated platelets expressing GPIIb/GPIIIa and form cross-links, leading to platelet aggregation.
4. Platelet release
    - Platelets are activated by the adhesion and release thromboxane A2, serotonin, and ADP, which activate other platelets and further slow blood flow.
    - The sequence vasoconstriction, platelet adhesion, platelet activation/aggregation, and release constitutes the process of primary hemostasis.
    - This process is independent of blood coagulation and occurs even in patients with hemophilia.

Primary hemostasis is insufficient to completely stop hemorrhage, which requires secondary hemostasis.

Secondary Hemostasis

- After primary hemostasis, a series of interdependent enzyme-mediated reactions initiates the formation of a stable fibrin clot, which replaces the unstable platelet plug.
- Secondary hemostasis involves both the intrinsic and extrinsic coagulation cascades.
- Tissue factor (TF) is released by the injured endothelium, which combines with activated factor FVII (FVIIa) to initiate the extrinsic clotting cascade.
- The exposed collagen and activated platelets (express HMK and PK) allow for the initiation of the intrinsic clotting cascade.
- Both pathways intersect at factor Xa and lead to the conversion of prothrombin (factor II) to thrombin (IIa) which then converts fibrinogen (I) to fibrin (Ia) to form a stable hemostatic clot.

- Next, as the blood vessel heals, proteins are released that activate plasmin (tissue plasminogen activator (tPA) or urokinase (uPA) to form plasminogen, which breaks down the stable clots and promotes further tissue healing, in a process called fibrinolysis.

Disorders of Hemostasis

Tables 5-2 through 5-5 list common and uncommon bleeding disorders by the conceptual component of hemostasis that is affected.

Blood Vessel Disorders

Can include disorders that cause fragility or alterations in the caliber of blood vessels, poor vascular repair pathways, vasculitis, and vascular malformations.

Primary Hemostasis Disorders

- Typical symptoms caused by disorders of primary hemostasis are mucosal bleeding (epistaxis, hematuria, bleeding gums) and petechiae.
- The most common inherited disorder of primary hemostasis is von Willebrand disease (deficient or dysfunctional vWF resulting in decreased ability to form a stable platelet plug), which is treated with desmopressin (DDAVP).

Secondary Hemostasis Disorders

- The most common symptoms caused by defects in secondary hemostasis are hematomas, hemarthrosis, and hemoperitoneum.
- The most common inherited disorder of secondary hemostasis is hemophilia A, an X-linked recessive disorder resulting in deficiency of factor VIII, treated with factor replacement.

Table 5-2 Common and Uncommon Blood Vessel Bleeding Disorders

Blood Vessel Bleeding Disorders	
Hereditary	Ehlers-Danlos syndrome
	Marfan Syndrome
	Cavernous Hemangioma (Kasabach-Merritt Syndrome)
	Osteogenesis imperfecta
	Hereditary hemorrhagic telangiectasia (Osler-Weber-Rendu)
	Ataxia telangiectasia
Acquired	Scurvy (Vitamin C deficiency)
	Amyloidosis
	IgA vasculitis (Henoch-Schönlein purpura)
	ANCA-associated vasculitis (GPA, EGPA)
	Kawasaki disease

Table 5-3 Common and Uncommon Platelet/Primary Hemostasis Disorders

Platelet Bleeding Disorders	
Hereditary	Bernard-Soulier syndrome Glanzmann thrombasthenia Storage pool disorders Chediak-Higashi Hermansky-Pudlak Wiskott-Aldrich syndrome Scott syndrome Gray platelet syndrome Platelet-type von Willebrand disease ADP receptor P2 defects Platelet thromboxane A2 (TXA2) receptor deficiency Platelet thromboxane synthase deficiency Platelet cyclo-oxygenase deficiency
Acquired	Essential thrombocythemia Polycythemia vera Myelodysplastic syndromes Pseudo-Bernard Soulier syndrome Type I Gaucher disease Acute megakaryoblastic leukemia Postcardiac bypass pump Thrombocytopenic thrombotic purpura (TTP) Idiopathic thrombocytopenic purpura

Table 5-4 Common and Uncommon Coagulation/Secondary Hemostasis Disorders

Coagulation Bleeding Disorders	
Hereditary	Hemophilia—FVIII, FIX, FXI All other clotting factor deficiencies von Willebrand disease Factor XIII deficiency Hypofibrinogenemia Dysfibrinogenemia
Acquired	Acquired specific factor inhibitors Acquired von Willebrand disease DIC Lupus anticoagulant, factor II deficiency Amyloidosis Acquired heparin-like anticoagulant

Table 5-5 Common and Uncommon Fibrinolytic Bleeding Disorders

Fibrinolytic Bleeding Disorders	
Hereditary	Deficiency of plasminogen activator inhibitor-1 Alpha-2 antiplasmin deficiency
Acquired	DIC Liver disease Postcardiac bypass pump

Disorders of Fibrinolysis

- When the process of fibrinolysis is unregulated, hyperfibrinolysis may occur which can cause bleeding.
- The most common form of hyperfibrinolysis is disseminated intravascular coagulation (see following discussion).

Disseminated Intravascular Coagulation

- Disseminated intravascular coagulation (DIC) is characterized by systemic intravascular activation of the coagulation cascade, consumption of coagulation factors, and widespread fibrin deposition, followed by deficient fibrinogen and platelets, excessive bleeding, and potential multiorgan failure.
- Most common underlying causes of DIC include:
  A. Sepsis
  B. Inflammation
  C. Trauma
  D. Cancer
  E. Obstetrical complications such as amniotic fluid embolism or placental abruption
- A diagnosis of DIC can be made by the clinical history, presentation, along with a combination of laboratory abnormalities including thrombocytopenia, prolonged prothrombin time (PT) and activated partial thromboplastin time (aPTT), elevated D-dimer (fibrin degradation product), and low levels of fibrinogen.
- Chronic low-grade DIC may be seen in patients with a history of malignancies.

Heparin-Induced Thrombocytopenia

- Heparin-induced thrombocytopenia (HIT) is a major complication that can occur with exposure to any form of heparin (rarer with LMWH).
- HIT is defined as a platelet drop of less than 150,000/μL or a 50% reduction from the baseline count, 5 to 14 days after the initial exposure to these drugs.
- Characterized by a precipitous drop in platelet counts and hypercoagulability, with approximately 50% of patients developing thromboembolic sequelae.
  - It may also be manifested as *delayed-onset HIT* occurring 9 to 30 days after the discontinuation of unfractionated heparin/low molecular weight heparin (UFH/LMWH) therapy.
- HIT is a highly prothrombotic state.
  - Most of the thromboses are venous in nature, but arterial thrombosis is seen as well.

- HIT is a clinical diagnosis supported by laboratory testing.
  - Identifying the typical platelet drop after exposure to UFH is crucial in the diagnosis of HIT.
  - Can be predicted using the "4T" score (thrombocytopenia, timing, thrombosis, other causes of thrombocytopenia not evident).
  - Clinical diagnosis may be challenging as other causes of thrombocytopenia including dilutional, drug-induced, postoperative bleeding, DIC, and sepsis need to be excluded and HIT may occur in conjunction with the other disorders.
- The incidence of HIT in patients exposed to UFH is 3% to 5% and it is up to 1% in patients exposed to LMWH with up to 600,000 cases and resulting in up to 90,000 deaths yearly.
  - More common in elderly patients and females.
  - Laboratory tests include functional activation assays and an antigen assay.
    A. The functional assays include heparin-induced platelet aggregation assay (HIPA) and serotonin release assay (SRA).
  - These are less sensitive and more specific.
    B. The Heparin-PF4 antibody assay is highly sensitive but less specific.
    C. Both types of assays should be performed if the diagnosis is in question.
  - Treatment of HIT includes prompt cessation of all heparin products.

Treatment of HIT

- Treatment should include immediate discontinuation of all forms of heparin and transition to other anticoagulants such as fondaparinux, argatroban, bivalirudin, or lepirudin.
  - These are direct thrombin inhibitors (DTI) that bind and inhibit free and clot-bound thrombin.
  - Any patients with HIT also on warfarin should discontinue warfarin immediately and be considered for reversal with Vitamin K as warfarin can worsen hypercoagulability by rapidly decreasing levels of protein C and protein S.
- LMWH is contraindicated in patients with HIT due to cross-reactivity to the antibodies.
- Post-HIT warfarin initiation must be postponed until the patient's platelet count has recovered to near-normal levels (< 150,000/μL).
- Warfarin should be started at a low dose (2.5-5 mg) overlapping with argatroban or lepirudin.
- Warfarin should be continued for 3 months if HIT is not associated with thrombosis.

Tests of Coagulation

Preoperative Screening

Preoperative clinical history and examination are the most important components of a preoperative evaluation of the patient's hemostatic ability.

History and Physical

- A careful bleeding history is a more reliable predictor of bleeding than coagulation laboratory tests.

A. Several retrospective reviews have repeatedly proven that routine coagulation screening tests do not predict bleeding risks in surgical patients, and specifically in patients undergoing tonsillectomy.
B. However, considerable variation occurs in the adequacy of a preoperative screening history and examination.

There are three simple questions to remember in taking a bleeding history.

1. "Have you ever had any surgery?"
   - Do not forget to ask about dental surgery.
   - When patients have undergone a prior surgery without bleeding problems, it serves as a "hemostatic stress test."
   - If the patient has had recent major surgery (within 1-2 years) without bleeding, and no active signs or symptoms of bleeding, one can feel confident that the chances of a hemostatic defect are exceedingly small.
2. "What do you take for pain?"
   - This is the simplest way to elicit information regarding the patient's use of nonsteroidal anti-inflammatory drugs (NSAIDs) and aspirin (ASA).
   - Additional over-the-counter drugs with possible hemorrhagic tendency are ginkgo biloba, garlic, ginseng, Cordyceps sinensis, flaxseed, echinacea, aloe vera, and hawthorn supplements.
3. "Is there a family history of bleeding or clotting?"
   - This question hopes to elicit a familial hemostatic defect that has not yet become clinically apparent, or may only emerge in the postoperative setting.

How to Use Screening Tests of Coagulation

- If coagulation tests are used, they should be performed in addition to a careful bleeding history.
- The following are the common screening tests of coagulation:
  A. Prothrombin time (PT), activated partial thromboplastin time (aPTT), and complete blood count (CBC and platelet count).
- The hemostasis components that coagulation tests measure are listed in Table 5-6.
- The PT and PTT coagulation tests are functional global assays.
- Global assays do not test for specific proteins or enzymes and are therefore insufficient measures to assess bleeding risk or assure hemostatic integrity.
  A. The bleeding time is insensitive to many hereditary disorders, such as von Willebrand disease.

Table 5-6 Testing the Four Hemostatic Components

Conceptual Hemostatic Component	*Coagulation Screening Tests*
Blood vessel	Bleeding time
Platelet	Bleeding time; CBC
Coagulation system	PT, aPTT, TT
Fibrinolytic system	Not measured

aPTT, activated partial thromboplastin time; CBC, complete blood count; PT, prothrombin time; TT, thrombin time.

B. The PT and aPTT are artificial reflections of normal hemostasis, often insensitive.
C. Some medications, like direct oral anticoagulants, do not consistently affect these screening tests.

When to Worry About Preoperative Coagulation Test Results

Approach to a Patient With Elevated aPTT or PT/INR

- Routine preoperative anesthesia evaluation or laboratory evaluation may reveal prolonged aPTT or PT or both.
- Elective surgeries should be postponed for further evaluation.
  A. Isolated prolongation of PT is usually seen in factor VII deficiency, due to vitamin K or liver disease.
  B. Prolongation of aPTT or both aPTT/PT reflects multiple factor deficiencies or if there is an acquired inhibitor.
  C. Extremely important to know whether the patient has a factor deficiency or an acquired inhibitor.
  D. This is accomplished by ordering *mixing study* laboratory test.
  E. If the mixing study corrects the PT or aPTT, it is suggestive of a factor deficiency.
  F. Mixing study will not be corrected if an inhibitor antibody is present.
  G. Diagnosis of some inhibitors may need incubation of the plasma mixture for several hours.
  H. Factor VIII and circulating lupus anticoagulants (LAs) are the most frequently encountered inhibitors.
- Acquired factor VIII inhibitor is dangerous and may cause large, rapidly expanding hematomas that may impinge on the trachea or on other vital structures resulting in death.
- LAs are antiphospholipid immunoglobulin G or M antibodies that prolong phospholipid-dependent coagulation in vitro and generally are not dangerous.
- LAs do not cause bleeding.
- LAs in some patients may cause thrombosis.
- These were first recognized in a patient with systemic lupus erythematosus, as such called lupus anticoagulant (LA), although it is more frequently encountered in patients without lupus.

Common Antiplatelet Agents and Anticoagulants in Surgical Patients

Understanding antiplatelet and anticoagulation medications in surgical patients is extremely important to prevent and treat postoperative complications, such as thromboembolism. This knowledge is also critical in patients undergoing surgery who are already on these medications but are undergoing a procedure with a high risk of bleeding. In general, each patient's situation should be considered when starting or stopping antiplatelet or anticoagulation medications. If a patient needs urgent surgery, it is recommended to involve other team members including prescribing physicians prior to discontinuing anticoagulant medications.

- Before a procedure, one should consider the risks of (1) bleeding and (2) thromboembolic events related to interruption of antithrombotic therapy.
- Although there are no official guidelines within otolaryngology defining high and low bleeding-risk procedures, several review articles have characterized common

Table 5-7 Otolaryngologic Procedure Bleeding Risks

High risk: • 30-d risk of major bleed >1.5% in nonanticoagulated patients • Risk of intracranial, intraocular, intrathoracic, or intraspinal bleeding	Thyroid/parathyroidectomy Laryngectomy Neck dissection Transoral surgery Tonsillectomy/adenoidectomy Free tissue transfer Nasal/sinus surgery Complex facial repair Tracheostomy Lateral skull base surgery PEG placement
Low to moderate risk: • 30-d risk of major bleed ≤1.5% in nonanticoagulated patients	Fine-needle aspiration Direct laryngoscopy (without biopsy) Esophagoscopy Vocal fold injection Tympanoplasty Excision of cutaneous basal and squamous cell carcinoma Dental procedures Lip laceration repair

Data adapted from American College of Chest Physicians Evidence Based Guidelines, International Society of Thrombosis and Hemostasis Guidance Statements, and Otolaryngology review articles.

otolaryngologic procedures to fit within the categories previously defined by the International Society on Thrombosis and Hemostasis and American College of Chest Physician Clinic Practice Guidelines which are defined in Table 5-7.

- A stratification of patient risk of thrombosis based on current guidelines is outlined in Table 5-8.
- Table 5-9 lists the current recommendations for perioperative management.

Antiplatelet Agents

- Antiplatelet drug therapy is widely prescribed and should be considered during preoperative evaluation for elective and emergent surgeries.
- *Antiplatelet agents*: aspirin, thienopyridines (ie, clopidogrel and ticagrelor).
- Acetylsalicylic acid (aspirin) (ASA) inhibits platelet aggregation and activation by irreversibly inhibiting cyclooxygenase (COX-1) which prevents thromboxane production.
  - At higher doses, ASA inhibits COX-1 and COX-2 which results in analgesia and an anti-inflammatory effect.
- Clopidogrel (Plavix) and prasugrel (Effient) inhibit platelet aggregation by irreversibly binding the P2Y12 receptor, inhibiting ADP activation of GPIIb/GPIIIa complex, whereas ticagrelor (Brilinta) reversibly inhibits this receptor.

Perioperative Management

- For patients with coronary stents requiring surgery, contact cardiologist and discuss the risks and benefits.
- The recommendations below reflect the most recently published guidelines regarding perioperative interruption of antiplatelet agents.

Table 5-8 Thrombotic Risks for Discontinuation of Antiplatelet Therapy

High Risk *>10% risk of ATE or VTE*	*Moderate Risk* *4%-10% risk of ATE or VTE*	*Low Risk* *<4% risk of ATE or VTE*
Atrial fibrillation with CHA_2DS_2VASc score ≥ 7	Atrial fibrillation with CHA_2DS_2VASc score of 5-6	Atrial fibrillation with CHA_2DS_2VASc score of 1-4 (and no previous stroke)
Atrial fibrillation associated with valvular heart disease, prosthetic valves, or rheumatic valvular heart disease	VTE within the past 3-12 months	Bileaflet aortic valve replacement without major risk factors for stroke
Recently (≤ 1 y) placed coronary stent	Recurrent VTE	Bioprosthetic valve
Recent (< 3 mo) stroke or TIA	Nonsevere thrombophilia (including heterozygous factor V Leiden mutation)	VTE > 12 mo prior
Recent (< 3 mo) VTE	Active cancer or recently treated cancer	
Acute coronary syndrome	Bileaflet aortic valve with stroke risk factors (ie, AFib, previous stroke/TIA, valve thrombosis, HTN, diabetes, CHF, or age ≥ 75 years)	
Nonstented percutaneous coronary intervention after myocardial infarction	Mechanical mitral valve without major stroke risk factors	
Antiphospholipid antibody, severe thrombophilia (including homozygous factor V Leiden, Protein C or S deficiency)		
Active cancer with high VTE risk (including myeloproliferative disorders)		

Afib, atrial fibrillation; ATE, arterial thromboembolism; CHA_2DS_2VASc, congestive heart failure, hypertension, age ≥ 75 years, diabetes mellitus, prior stroke or transient ischemic attack, vascular disease history, age ≥ 65 years, female sex; CHF, congestive heart disease; HTN, hypertension; TIA, transient ischemic attack; VTE, venous thromboembolism.

- ASA and clopidogrel should not be stopped for low-risk bleeding procedures.
  - Low-risk procedures include: endoscopy without biopsy, skin biopsy or other dermatologic procedures, ophthalmic procedures, and dental procedures
- For elective moderate- to high-bleeding risk procedures.
  - For patients on ASA and P2Y12 inhibitors with coronary stents placed within the past 3 months, it is recommended to continue both medications or to interrupt only one medication 7 to 10 days prior to surgery.
  - For patients on ASA and P2Y12 inhibitors with coronary stents placed between 3 and 12 months prior, it is recommended to hold the P2Y12 inhibitor but continue aspirin.
    - If ASA interruption is indicated due to high risk of bleeding, guidelines suggest it should be held for fewer than 7 days.
    - Clopidogrel can be stopped 5 days prior to elective noncardiac surgery.

Table 5-9 Antiplatelet and Anticoagulant Medications Perioperative and Reversal Information

	Mechanism of Action	*Half-Life*	*Recommended Time to Hold Preop*	*Resume Postop*	*Reversal Agent*
Antiplatelet Agents					
Acetylsalicylic acid/ Aspirin (ASA)	Irreversible COX-1 inhibitor	20 mins (effects last platelet lifespan of 7 days)	Do not hold	24 h	Platelet transfusion (4-5 Units) DDAVP TXA
Clopidogrel (Plavix)	Irreversible inhibition of P2Y12 receptor	6 h (effects last platelet lifespan of 7 days)	5 days	24 h	Platelet transfusion (10U q12 h × 48 h) DDAVP
Prasugrel (Effient)	Irreversible inhibition of P2Y12 receptor	7 hours (effects last platelet lifespan of 7 days)	7 days	24 h	Platelet transfusion (10U q12 h × 48 h) DDAVP
Ticagrelor (Brilinta)	Reversible inhibition of P2Y12 receptor	8 h	3-5 days	24 h	None
Unfractionated Heparin	Activation of antithrombin; inhibits factors IIa, IXa, Xa, XIa, and XIIa	1.5 h	IV: 4-6 h SQ: 8-12 h	24 h	Protamine Sulfate
Low Molecular Weight Heparin Enoxaparin (Lovenox)	Inactivation of factor Xa and thrombin via antithrombin activation	5-7 h	24 h	2-3 days	No FDA-approved agents Consider protamine sulfate (1 mg IV per 1 mg LMWH within past 8 h)
Fondaparinux (Arixtra)	Factor Xa inhibitor	17 h	36-48 h	6-24 h	No FDA-approved agents Consider Factor VIIa infusion for severe bleeding
Argatroban (Acova)	Direct thrombin inhibitor	50 mins	4 h	2-3 days	No FDA approved or recommended agents
Bivalirudin (Angiomax)	Direct thrombin inhibitor	25 mins	> 3 h	2-3 days	No FDA approved or recommended agents
Lepirudin (Refludan)	Direct thrombin inhibitor	1.5 h	10 h	2-3 days	No FDA approved or recommended agents

(*Continued*)

Table 5-9 Antiplatelet and Anticoagulant Medications Perioperative and Reversal Information (*Continued*)

	Mechanism of Action	*Half-Life*	*Recommended Time to Hold Preop*	*Resume Postop*	*Reversal Agent*
Direct Oral Anticoagulants					
Dabigatran (Pradaxa)	Direct thrombin inhibitor	12-14 h	48 h	2-3 days	Idaruizumab
Rivaroxaban (Xarelto)	Factor Xa inhibitor	9-11 h	48 h	2-3 days	Prothrombin complex concentrates Andexanet alfa
Apixaban (Eliquis)	Factor Xa inhibitor	9-11 h	48 h	2-3 days	Prothrombin complex concentrates Andexanet alfa
Edoxaban (Savaysa)	Factor Xa inhibitor	10-14 h	48 h	2-3 days	Prothrombin complex concentrates
Warfarin (Coumadin)	Vitamin K antagonist: inhibits factors II, VII, IX, X, and protein C, protein S	40 h	3-5 days if INR < 1.5	12-24 h	Vitamin K

h, hours; IV, intravenous; mins, minutes; SQ, subcutaneous; U, units.

- Ticagrelor can be stopped 3 to 5 days prior to elective noncardiac surgery.
- Prasugrel should be held 7 days prior to elective noncardiac surgery.
- It is recommended to restart antiplatelet medications within 24 hours postoperatively.

Reversal

- ASA reversal includes transfusion of 4 to 5 units of platelets and/or desmopressin (DDAVP) infusion (0.3 μg/kg).
- Recommended reversal for clopidogrel and prasugrel includes aggressive platelet transfusions (10 U q12 h × 48 h) and DDAVP infusion (0.3 μg/kg).
- Because ticagrelor reversibly binds to platelets, it cannot be reversed with platelet transfusion, as it remains active throughout the bloodstream and will bind to infused platelets.
- Historically, aminocaproic acid was administered for antiplatelet reversal, with potentially decreased hemorrhage-related mortality but also yielded increased risk of deep venous thrombosis (DVT).
- Emerging data suggest that tranexamic acid (TXA) may also be administered intravenously for reversal of antiplatelet agents.

Heparins

Standard or Unfractionated Heparin

- Heparin is a heterogeneous sugar molecule that leads to anticoagulation by binding to antithrombin (AT) which inactivates thrombin (factor IIa), thus inhibiting conversion of fibrinogen to a fibrin clot and inactivating factors IXa, Xa, XIa, and XIIa.

- Heparin is administered either intravenously (IV) or subcutaneously (SQ), with higher bioavailability with IV administration.
- Unfractionated heparin (UFH) also nonspecifically binds to various plasma proteins and platelets resulting in variability in anticoagulant response in different patients.
- The anticoagulant response to UFH is nonlinear—intensity and duration, rise disproportionately with increasing dose.
- Dosage of UFH varies based on the indication—treatment or prophylaxis.
  A. Treatment
    - Weight-based dosing of UFH is preferred over fixed dosing.
    - Dosing differs for acute coronary syndromes (ACS) and acute venous thromboembolism (VTE). ACS uses a low-intensity protocol while acute VTE uses a high-intensity protocol.
    - Hospitals often have pharmacy protocols for dosing and lab monitoring, which require a bolus dose followed by continuous infusion.
    - The initial bolus is an IV dose of 60 U/kg (not to exceed 5000 Units) followed by 12 to 15 U/kg continuous infusion for low-intensity or 18 U/kg continuous infusion for high-intensity regimens.
    - For ACS, an aPTT target therapeutic range is roughly 50 to 70 seconds, and for acute VTE target is 60 to 85 seconds.
    - Most hospitals have a measured UFH therapeutic range based on responsiveness of their aPTT reagent to a heparin concentration of 0.3 to 0.7 IU/mL (anti-Xa activity—see following discussion).

  B. Prophylaxis
    - Prophylaxis dose is generally administered SQ at a dose of 5000 units every 8 or 12 hours.
    - Prophylaxis dose is not monitored by aPTT, and should not prolong aPTT.

Perioperative Management

- It is recommended that IV heparin be held for 4 hours or more prior to procedures and resumed at least 24 hours after a procedure, although it may be held longer postoperatively if high risk of postoperative bleeding.
- Subcutaneous heparin can be held 8 to 12 hours prior to procedures.

Reversal

- Protamine sulfate binds to heparin to form a stable salt and neutralize UFH (https://www.ncbi.nlm.nih.gov/books/NBK547753/)
- 1 mg of protamine neutralizes approximately 100 units of UFH.
- An appropriate intravenous dosage should be calculated—based on the estimated heparin in the patient.
  - For example, a patient on 1000 U/h of UFH would require 10 mg of protamine.
- Administer intravenously over 1 to 3 minutes to avoid bradycardia and hypotension.
- The aPTT can be used to assess the effectiveness of protamine.
- The most common adverse effect of protamine is anaphylaxis, with reports from 0.06% to 10.6%, and patients should be monitored closely for developing symptoms.

Low Molecular Weight Heparin

- Low molecular weight heparins (LMWHs) are obtained by depolymerization of UFH yielding smaller fragments, making the extent of nonspecific binding to plasma proteins and platelets lower for LMWH than UFH.

- The ratio of anti-Xa/anti-IIa activity is more than 4 with LMWH and equal to 1 with UFH.
- Therefore, LMWH inhibits coagulation by activating AT, inactivating factor Xa and thrombin.

- The most commonly used LMWH in the United States is enoxaparin (Lovenox).
- Since LMWHs give reproducible anticoagulant effects, they have fixed dosing without monitoring in most patients.
- LMWHs do not prolong the aPTT.
- Anti-Xa assay *can be used* to monitor LMWH activity and is recommended:
  - In patients who weigh > 150 Kg
  - In patients with renal insufficiency
  - In patients who are pregnant
- The anti-Xa activity should be measured 4 hours after the subcutaneous administration with a therapeutic target of 0.6 to 1.0 IU/mL for enoxaparin.

Perioperative Management

- Guidelines recommend holding therapeutic LMWH for 24 hours prior to a procedure and giving only half the normal dose with the final administration prior to holding for all procedures.
- Resume 24 hours or more after a low bleeding-risk procedure, or 48 to 72 hours after a high bleeding-risk procedure.

Reversal

- Despite widespread use of LMWH, there are no FDA-approved reversal agents.
- The current American College of Chest Physician (ACCP) guidelines recommend using protamine for reversal of LMWH, although it only partially reverses the anti-Xa activity (~60%).
  - Dosing: 1 mg of protamine per 1 mg of LMWH in the past 8 hours.
  - After protamine is given, factor Xa levels should be checked every 3 hours if bleeding persists.

Other Parenteral Anticoagulants

Argatroban

- Synthetic direct thrombin inhibitor administered via continuous IV infusion that directly binds to the active site of thrombin and prevents it from breaking down fibrinogen
  - Dose-dependent effect
  - Half-life of 50 minutes
- Argatroban is metabolized in the liver and should be used with caution in mild hepatic insufficiency.
- Indicated for therapeutic anticoagulation in patients with renal dysfunction, on dialysis or extracorporeal membrane oxygenation (ECMO), and for patients in multisystem organ failure due to its strictly hepatic metabolism

Perioperative Management

- Discontinue 4 hours prior to surgery.
- Resume 2 to 3 days after surgery.

Reversal

- No approved or recommended reversal agent.

Bivalirudin

- Bivalirudin is a reversible direct thrombin inhibitor that is given via continuous IV infusion.
- With a short half-life (25 minutes), it is usually the preferred therapeutic anticoagulant in HIT in critically ill patients or those potentially needing surgery.
- Renally metabolized and should be avoided in patients with renal insufficiency.

Perioperative Management

- Discontinue 2 to 4 hours prior to surgery.
- Restart 2 to 3 days after the procedure.

Reversal

- There is no reversal agent for bivalirudin.

Fondaparinux

- Fondaparinux (Arixtra) is a synthetic selective inhibitor of factor Xa via activation of AT given subcutaneously that is an alternative to UFH and LMWH for VTE prophylaxis.
- It has an instant onset of action and only requires once-daily dosing, given its long half-life of 17 to 21 hours.
  - Dosing is typically 2.5 mg administered subcutaneously daily.
- It does not affect the aPTT, PT, or clotting time, and does not bind to thrombin.
- Drug levels can only be monitored by special anti-Xa assays
- Fondaparinux is recommended for VTE prophylaxis in cases of HIT.
  - Guidelines have also suggested benefits of using fondaparinux over heparins for VTE prophylaxis in patients with COVID-19, undergoing orthopedic procedures, obese patients, and in cancer patients undergoing surgery.

Perioperative Management

- Can be safely discontinued 48 hours prior to surgery.
- Should be resumed 12 to 24 hours postoperatively in low bleeding risk procedures, or 2 to 3 days in high-risk procedures.

Reversal

- There is no FDA-approved agent for the reversal of fondaparinux, but guidelines suggest administration of factor VIIa can be considered in cases of severe bleeding.

Lepirudin

- Irreversible direct thrombin inhibitor, synthetic form of hirudin, a natural anticoagulant produced by leeches.
- Can be administered IV or SQ.
- Half-life is approximately 1.5 hours.
- Lepirudin is renally metabolized and should be avoided in patients with renal insufficiency.
- Patients may develop anti-hirudin antibodies to this medication if administered for > 5 days.

Perioperative Management

- Discontinue 10 hours prior to surgery.
- Similar to other direct thrombin inhibitors, it may be restarted 2 to 3 days postoperatively.

Reversal

- There is no reversal agent for lepirudin.

Oral Anticoagulants

Direct Oral Anticoagulants

- Direct oral anticoagulants (DOACs) are non-vitamin K-dependent oral anticoagulants.
- DOAC is the term proposed by the International Society on Thrombosis and Hemostasis; it replaced novel anticoagulants (NOACS).
- There are currently several DOACs available for clinical use; the most common medications include: dabigatran (Pradaxa), rivaroxaban (Xarelto), apixaban (Eliquis), and edoxaban (Savaysa). Table 5-9 includes basic information about each.
- Dabigatran is a direct and competitive thrombin inhibitor, whereas the other three are factor Xa inhibitors (Citation: package inserts).
- The peak onset of action occurs 2 to 3 hours after dosing, and the half-life for these medications ranges from 9 to 14 hours in patients with normal kidney function.
- Their advantages are fixed dosing (except in patients with end-stage renal disease), and they do not require routine monitoring.
- Current FDA-approved indications for DOACs are nonvalvular atrial fibrillation, VTE prophylaxis after elective total knee arthroplasty (TKA) or total hip arthroplasty (THA), and treatment of VTE.
- Compared with warfarin, DOACs have minimal interactions with food and fewer interactions with other medications.
  - However, inhibitors of the protein CYP3A43, including antifungals (azoles), some antiepileptics, macrolide antibiotics, and some calcium channel blockers have interactions.
- They are contraindicated in pregnant and breastfeeding patients, and Warfarin remains the first-line in treatment of antiphospholipid syndrome, mechanical heart valves, and atrial fibrillation related to rheumatic heart disease.
- These medications are renally metabolized and may require dose adjustments in patients with kidney disease.

Perioperative Management

- In the preoperative setting for procedures with low to moderate bleeding risk, it is recommended to hold DOACs for 24 hours prior to surgery and resume the medication at least 24 hours after surgery.
- In procedures with high bleeding risk, DOACs are typically held for 48 hours prior to surgery (or up to 4 days preop in patients with kidney disease), and it is generally recommended that they are resumed 2 to 3 days after surgery.
- Given the rapid onset of action of these medications of 2 to 3 hours, it is important to weigh the ongoing risk of postoperative bleeding with the indications for anticoagulation, and this should involve conversations with the prescribing physicians.

Reversal

- One major concern when DOACs first emerged was the lack of direct reversal agents. More recently, several direct reversal agents have been developed and are FDA-approved or under review.

- The first-line and FDA-approved reversal agent for dabigatran is idaruizumab, a monoclonal antibody fragment that binds directly to dabigatran. Its onset of action is 10 to 30 minutes.
  - Idaruizumab is administered 5 g IV in 2 doses of 2.5 g given 15 minutes apart.
- Prothrombin complex concentrates (PCCs) (24 IU/kg) are recommended as first-line treatment of severe bleeding in patients using rivaroxaban, apixaban, and edoxaban.
- Andexanet alfa is a recombinant modified factor Xa molecule that binds to and sequesters factor Xa inhibitors. It is FDA-approved for the reversal of rivaroxaban and apixaban (factor Xa inhibitors) and is under FDA review as a reversal agent for the other oral factor Xa inhibitors.
  - Its onset of action is 2 to 5 minutes.

Warfarin

- The anticoagulant effect of warfarin results from the inhibition of the vitamin K-dependent clotting factors II, VII, IX, and X as well as protein C and protein S.
- The antithrombotic effect of warfarin to prevent clot expansion is not present until approximately the fifth day of therapy.
- This effect depends on the clearance of functional factor II (prothrombin), which has a half-life of approximately 50 hours in patients with normal hepatic function.
- The half-life of warfarin ranges from 20 to 60 hours with a mean of 40 hours.
- Do not use loading doses of warfarin (ie, 10 mg or more per day) as these are of limited value and may increase the patient's risk of bleeding.
- The anticoagulant effect of warfarin is measured by international normalized ratio (INR).
- In acute thrombosis (VTE/PE, etc.), a full 5-day overlap of warfarin with either UFH or LMWH is recommended until the target INR is achieved.

Perioperative Management

- In general, warfarin is held 3 to 5 days prior to surgery for most procedures when INR is lower than 1.5.
- Decisions to hold warfarin and bridging are dependent on the bleeding risk weighed against the risk of VTE (see following discussion).
- Typically, warfarin can be resumed within 12 to 24 hours postoperatively since it does not achieve anticoagulant effect for 24 to 72 hours after initiation and typically takes 4 to 6 days to achieve therapeutic doses.
  - Further discussion should be had in procedures with a high risk of postoperative bleeding.

Bridging

Assess the risk of thrombosis for holding warfarin.

- *Low risk:* Atrial fibrillation, PE/DVT over 3 months ago, cardiomyopathy, DVT prophylaxis, coronary artery disease, venous access device prophylaxis.
- *Intermediate risk:* Multiple low-risk factors, or less than 1 month on anticoagulation
- *High risk:* PE/DVT less than 3 months ago, transient ischemia/stroke of cardiac origin, mechanical heart valve hypercoagulable disorders, vascular access occlusion

  A. Low-risk patients
     - Atrial fibrillation, VTE/DVT over 3 months ago, cardiomyopathy, DVT prophylaxis, coronary artery disease, and venous access device prophylaxis.
     - No heparin bridging recommended.

B. Intermediate and high-risk patients
- *Intermediate risk:* Multiple low-risk factors, or less than 1 month on anticoagulation
- *High risk:* PE/DVT less than 3 months ago, transient ischemia/stroke of cardiac origin, mechanical heart valve hypercoagulable disorders, vascular access occlusion
- Bridging with LMWH or UFH is recommended.
  - If a patient is at high risk for clotting (eg, has a mechanical mitral valve) and requires a planned procedure, heparin can be used before and after the surgery until LMWH can be safely given.
  - Enoxaparin dosing for bridging is 1 mg/kg SQ bid or 1.5 mg/kg SQ qd.
- Day 5—Hold warfarin 5 days prior to surgery.
- Day 4—24 hours after stopping warfarin, start LMWH (or UFH) at full dose.
- Continue LMWH days 4 through 2.
- Day 1—24 hours before surgery—no LMWH.
- Day 0—Surgery.
- Postop Day 0—If no bleeding or low risk of bleeding, start warfarin (double the individual patient's normal dose).
- Postop Day 1—Start LMWH, continue warfarin at normal dose.
- Postop Day 2—Draw INR, continue LMWH, and warfarin until therapeutic INR × 2.

Reversal

- Supratherapeutic INR with warfarin therapy is extremely common in clinical practice.
- Although it can be rapidly reversed with administration of phylloquinone (vitamin K_1), management should be based on the level of the supratherapeutic INR if associated with bleeding.

No bleeding

- For elevation of INR up to 8, in a patient with no other bleeding risk factors:
  - Hold warfarin and follow INR closely until it decreases to less than 4.
- In patients with INR greater than 8 or with other risk factors for bleeding:
  - Hold warfarin and follow INR closely until it decreases to less than 4.
  - Orally administer Vitamin K at a dose of up to 2.5 mg.

Active Bleeding

- Warfarin should be stopped.
- 5 mg of Vitamin K can be given orally, intravenously, or subcutaneously.

Hemostatic Agents

A number of hemostatic agents have become widely used in the field of Otolaryngology. We briefly review each use below.

Aminocaproic Acid (Amicar)

- Epsilon aminocaproic acid (Amicar) competitively inhibits plasminogen, preventing fibrinolysis.
- FDA approved for treatment of hemorrhage caused by excessive fibrinolysis, including postcardiac surgery, management of hematologic disorders, and bleeding associated with placental abruption.

- Can be administered orally, IV, or topically.
- Adverse effects include risk of thrombosis and rhabdomyolysis.
- Within otolaryngology, it has shown potential to decrease blood loss and transfusion requirements in pediatric patients undergoing cranial vault surgery, and its use has been described in preventing postprocedural dental or oral bleeding in patients with bleeding disorders, and management of epistaxis in patients with hereditary hemorrhagic telangiectasia.
- Few studies have examined its use in post-tonsillectomy hemorrhage, with equivocal results.

Tranexamic Acid (TXA)

- Tranexamic Acid (TXA) inhibits plasminogen to stabilize preformed fibrin clots produced by secondary hemostasis and suppress fibrinolysis.
- It can be administered IV, orally, or topically and has a half-life of 2 hours.
  - It is excreted by the kidneys, and dosing adjustments are indicated in severe renal diseases.
- TXA has been shown to decrease mortality in cases of postpartum hemorrhage and traumatic brain injury and decrease the need for blood transfusions in trauma patients.
- Meta-analyses on this medication have risk of thrombosis, even in patients undergoing free-flap microvascular reconstruction.
- There is a theoretical increased risk of seizures with TXA; however, this adverse effect has not been established in multiple studies examining its safety.
- In otolaryngology, topical TXA has been shown to reduce oral bleeding after dental extractions, nebulized TXA can decrease blood transfusions in hemoptysis, and topical TXA-soaked nasal packing significantly improves time to hemostasis in epistaxis, even in patients with hereditary hemorrhagic telangiectasia (HHT).
  - A meta-analysis also demonstrates that both topical and systemic TXA reduce blood loss and field visualization in endoscopic sinus surgery. (PMID: 37259887)
  - Data are equivocal regarding the efficacy of TXA in post-tonsillectomy hemorrhage; however, it has a relatively low risk of adverse events and high potential benefits.

Commercially Available Topical Hemostatic Agents

Matrix Agents

Absorbable materials that create a physical framework and allow for adherence of platelets and coagulation factors to promote clot formation.

- Oxidized regenerated cellulose agents
  - Applied dry and used to pack an area for hemostasis
  - Used for control of capillary, venous, and small arterial hemorrhage by providing a matrix for platelet adhesion
  - Dissolves within 7 to 14 days
    - Surgicel (loosely knit fabric), Surgicel Nu-Knit (densely woven matrix that can be sutured in place), Surgicel Powder (assists with broad surface oozing), and Surgicel Fibrillar (resembles cotton wool and can be precisely placed)
  - Their absorption causes a low pH in surrounding tissues, potentially inhibiting thrombin and increasing infection risk.
- Gelatin matrix
  - Gelfoam, Surgifoam

  - Applied to bleeding surfaces to absorb a significant volume to concentrate coagulation factors
    - Swelling of matrix provides direct compression
  - Absorbed at 4 to 6 weeks

Biologic Agents

- Topical thrombin
  - Can be human, bovine, or recombinant form of thrombin reconstituted by mixing with normal saline and applied in liquid form via syringe.
  - Promotes platelet aggregation, converts fibrinogen to fibrin, and activates clotting factors.
    - Gelfoam Plus, Thrombin-JMI
  - Potential adverse effects include possible transmission of prion disease (human form), development of anti-thrombin antibodies (bovine form), or allergic reactions.
- Thrombin + gelatin matrix
  - Tamponade gelatin matrix swelling combined with hemostatic effects of thrombin which expands when applied to a bleeding surface.
  - Requires mixing of solutions prior to use; may be stored for 3 to 8 hours
  - Floseal (human thrombin + bovine gelatin), Surgiflo
  - Adverse effects: Anemia, prion/viral disease transmission, allergic reaction
  - Dissolves in 6 to 8 weeks
- Fibrin sealants
  - Tisseel, Evicel.
  - Frozen thrombin and fibrinogen solutions in separate chambers of a single outflow syringe, thawed in warm water bath prior to use and injected while mixed together.
  - Thrombin catalyzes formation of fibrin from fibrinogen and produces a stable clot.
    - Also contains additional agents that may help stabilize clot and inhibit fibrinolysis.
  - Used for diffuse venous oozing, may be applied to raw wound surfaces to create clot, and can be helpful to achieve hemostasis at vascular anastomoses.
  - Absorbed within 14 days; do not tend to cause immune or inflammatory responses.

Bone Wax

- Sterile combination of isopropyl palmitate, paraffin, and beeswax
- Can be directly applied to obstruct medullary vessels in bone
- Adverse effects: Associated with foreign body reaction and granuloma formation

Acknowledgement

We would like to thank Dr. John Godwin for his efforts on this chapter in prior editions.

Bibliography

1. Douketis JD, Spyropoulos AC, Murad MH, et al. Perioperative Management of Antithrombotic Therapy: An American College of Chest Physicians Clinical Practice Guideline. *Chest*. 2022;162(5):e207-243.
2. Douketis JD, Spyropoulos AC. Perioperative management of patients taking direct oral anticoagulants. *JAMA*. 2024;332(10):825-834.

3. Aldhaeefi M, Badreldin HA, Alsuwayyid F, et al. Practical guide for anticoagulant and antiplatelet reversal in clinical practice. *Pharmacy*. 2023;11(1):34.
4. Jamshaid W, Jamshaid M, Coulson C, Sharma N, Muzaffar J, Nieto H. A systematic review on the efficacy of tranexamic acid in head and neck surgery. *Clin Otolaryngol*. 2023;48(4):527-539.
5. Brown KGM, Solomon MJ. Topical haemostatic agents in surgery. *Br J Surg*. 2023;111(1):znad361.

Questions

1. Why is a bleeding history more likely to reveal a bleeding disorder than screening tests of coagulation?
   A. The PT/PTT tests do not measure fibrinolytic bleeding.
   B. The bleeding time often misses mild von Willebrand disease.
   C. Antiplatelet drugs such as Plavix may not affect the PT/PTT or bleeding time.
   D. A bleeding history is likely to uncover hemostatic stress such as dental extractions.
   E. All of the above.

2. Which of the following are true statements regarding the differences or similarities between standard UFH and LMWH?
   A. Both UFH and LMWH prolong the PTT.
   B. Only LMWH requires monitoring using the PTT or anti-Xa.
   C. Only LMWH requires dose adjustment in renal failure.
   D. A weight-based nomogram for UFH avoids the need for PTT monitoring.
   E. Only UFH is a polysaccharide with a specific binding site for AT-III.

3. Which of the following statements are true regarding typical HIT?
   A. The platelet drop in HIT is less than 100,000.
   B. The platelet drop in HIT is 50% or more from baseline.
   C. The drop in platelets is typically 24 hours after heparin exposure.
   D. The drop in platelets never occurs days after heparin is stopped.
   E. HIT is more common with the use of LMWH.

4. Which of the following statements are true regarding DIC?
   A. DIC is diagnosed by specific laboratory findings.
   B. DIC is only a clinical diagnosis.
   C. DIC can manifest clinically in overt and occult syndromes.
   D. DIC is always treated by heparin therapy to stop thrombosis.
   E. The D-dimer test is diagnostic of DIC.

5. A 35-year-old woman presents to the emergency room (ER) with a history of bruising easily over the past 1½ weeks. She also reports a large bruise over the right thigh associated with pain and difficulty walking, as well as a spontaneous bruise on her left forearm. She did not have a history of a fall or trauma prior to this. She did have an upper respiratory tract infection (URI) and was prescribed Augmentin 2 weeks prior. She denies bleeding from anywhere. She also denies history of excessive bleeding after a dental extraction or since childhood or menorrhagia. There is no family history of bleeding in her family. On laboratory evaluation her PT is 12.7, and aPTT is 58. CBC has a white blood cell (WBC)—6.7, Hgb—9.0,

platelet (PLT)—145. On physical examination, she has a large hematoma over her right thigh. Before surgical management of the hematoma, you would:

A. Call the laboratory to perform a bleeding time.

B. Obtain a 50:50 mixing study to evaluate the presence of factor deficiency or inhibitor.

C. Check for lupus anticoagulant.

D. Order a DIC panel.

Chapter 6
Related Neurology and Neurosurgery

Neurology

A. Headache syndromes
   i. Migraine
      a. aka trigeminovascular syndrome
      b. *Paroxysmal* headache (HA) associated with multiple signs and symptoms that can overlap with sinus symptoms
         1. Unilateral
         2. Throbbing pulsatile headache in the frontotemporal or orbital area
         3. Aura
            - Can arise before or during the HA
            - Usually visual but can be sensory or motor
         4. Pain builds over 1 to 2 hours and progresses posteriorly
         5. Headache lasts 4 to 72 hours
         6. Photophobia, phonophobia
         7. Nausea—80%, vomiting—50%, anorexia and food intolerance and light headedness
         8. Signs
            - Cranial/cervical tenderness
            - Horner syndrome
            - Conjunctival injection
            - Tachycardia or bradycardia
            - Hypertension or hypotension
            - Hemisensory changes or hemiparesis
            - Adie's-like pupil (light-near dissociation)
      c. Diagnosis
         1. Two of the following characteristics:
            - Unilateral location
            - Pulsating quality
            - Moderate to severe pain
            - Aggravated or caused by physical activity
         2. During the HA patient must have one of the following:
            - Nausea and/or vomiting
            - Photophobia and phonophobia

d. Imaging
   1. Diagnostic imaging is not necessary in patients with *stable* history of migraine headaches and a normal neurologic exam
e. Management recommendations
   1. CT is not recommended for headache evaluation when MRI is available, unless in an emergency situation
   2. Persistent over-the-counter (OTC) pain medication for the treatment of unrelenting headache is not advised as this symptom may indicate underlying brain pathology
   3. First-line treatment of migraine should not include opioid or butalbital-containing medications
   4. Lifestyle modifications
      - Avoidance of carrying heavy purses or bags over one shoulder
      - Avoidance of certain foods
      - Maintaining hydration status
      - Sleep hygiene
      - Limit stress
   5. Integrative medicine
      - Magnesium
      - Riboflavin
      - Coenzyme Q10
   6. Abortive medications
      - These medications aim to reverse or at least stop the progression of a headache.
      - Most effective when given within 15 minutes of symptom onset when the pain is mild.
      - Types
        (a) Triptans: selective serotonin receptor agonists
        (b) Ergot alkaloids: ergotamine, dihydroergotamine
        (c) Analgesics and nonsteroidal anti-inflammatory drugs (NSAIDs)
        (d) Combination medications
           - Acetaminophen, aspirin, and caffeine (ie, Excedrin)
           - Butalbital, aspirin, and caffeine (Fiorinal)
           - Isometheptene, dichloralphenazone, acetaminophen (Midrin, Duradrin, and others)
        (e) Antiemetics
   7. Prophylactic medications
      - Indication
        (a) More than two headaches per month
        (b) Duration of headache more than 24 hours
        (c) Significant disability for equal to or more than 3 days
        (d) Abortive therapy fails or is overused
        (e) Abortive medications used more than twice a week
      - Types
        (a) Antiepileptic drugs
        (b) Beta blockers
        (c) Tricyclic antidepressants
        (d) Ca^{2+} channel blockers
        (e) Botulinum toxin: up to nine treatment cycles for progressive improvement in symptoms

ii. Tension headache
   a. Most common type of recurring headache thought to be related to muscular factors and psychogenic forces (stressful event)
   b. Throbbing quality with onset more gradual than migraines; usually tension headaches are more constant and less severe
   c. Headaches can last up to 7 days
   d. Not associated with nausea or vomiting, photophobia and/or phonophobia
   e. Diagnostic criteria
      1. Two of the following must be present:
         - Tightening in frontal-occipital locations
           (a) Occipitonuchal
           (b) Bifrontal
         - Bilateral
         - Mild to moderate intensity
         - Not aggravated by physical activity
   f. Management
      1. Imaging is only required if headache pattern changes and is not a common primary headache disorder, such as migraine, cluster, or tension headache
   g. Treatment
      1. Massage, relaxation techniques
      2. Lifestyle modification: regular exercise, balanced meals, adequate sleep
      3. Trigger points injection/occipital nerve block
      4. NSAIDs
      5. Tricyclic antidepressants, muscle relaxers
iii. Cluster headache
   a. Group of headaches (known as histamine headaches) with multiple characteristics
      1. Severe unilateral pain that is orbital, supraorbital, or temporal.
      2. Each headache lasts 15 to 180 minutes and can occur 8 times a day or every other day.
      3. The HA may occur 1 to 8 times a day for as long as 4 months.
      4. HA are often nocturnal, during sleep or early morning hours.
      5. Associated with one or more of the following ipsilateral signs:
         - Conjunctival injection
         - Lacrimation
         - Nasal congestion
         - Rhinorrhea
         - Facial hydrosis
         - Miosis
         - Ptosis
      6. Two main forms of cluster headaches:
         - Episodic: at least 2 cluster headache phases that last 7 days to 1 year are separated by a cluster-free interval of 1 month or longer.
         - Chronic: cluster occurs more than once a year without remission or the cluster-free interval is less than 1 month.
   b. Management
      1. Pharmacologic approach
         - Abortive treatment
           (a) Oxygen
              - 8 L/min for 10 minutes or 100% by mask

(b) Triptans
- Stimulation of 5-HT1 (serotonin) receptors produce vasoconstrictive effect and may abort attack
- Intranasal administration effective

(c) Ergot alkaloids
- Stimulation of alpha receptors to cause vasoconstriction
- Most effective when given early in a cluster headache attack
- Intranasal administration is effective

- Preventive/prophylactic treatment
  (a) Calcium channel blockers
  - Verapamil considered most effective
  - Can be combined with ergotamine and lithium

  (b) Anticonvulsant
  - Topiramate and divalproex found to be most effective for prophylaxis.
  - Mechanism of action is unclear.

2. Surgical approach
   - Percutaneous radiofrequency ablation of the gasserian ganglion
     (a) 50% success rate
     (b) 20% have fair-to-good results
     (c) 30% failure rate
   - Gamma knife radiosurgery
     (a) Increased risk for disturbance in facial sensation
   - Occipital nerve block
     (a) Abortive procedure for cluster headache
   - Deep brain stimulation (DBS)
     (a) Electrodes placed in ipsilateral posterior inferior hypothalamus
     (b) Candidates for DBS are those patients who have chronic cluster headaches refractory to pharmacologic therapy
   - Stimulation of the pterygopalatine ganglion
     (a) Candidate for stimulation are select patients with chronic cluster headaches.

B. Facial Pain

i. Trigeminal neuralgia

a. Characteristics

1. Distinct, sudden, lancinating pain following the sensory distribution of the trigeminal nerve
2. Pain is most similar to an "electric shock" that worsens in less than 20 seconds and begins to fade to burning
   - Pain shoots from the corner of the mouth to the angle of the jaw in 60%.
   - Pain shoots from the upper lip or teeth to the eyebrow or area around the eye in 30%.
   - V1 involved in less than 5% of cases.
   - V2 and V3 distribution affected in 35% of patients.
3. Triggers: chewing, talking, smiling, drinking hot or cold fluids, touching, shaving, teeth cleaning, encountering cold air on the face
4. Common causes include vascular compression at the root entry zone or demyelination due to diseases like multiple sclerosis (MS)

b. Diagnosis
   1. No laboratory, radiographic or electrophysiologic studies are routinely needed for patients with characteristic history and normal neurologic exam.
   2. Criteria established by International Headache Society
      - Paroxysmal attacks of pain that last up to 2 minutes and involve a distribution of the trigeminal nerve (V1-V3).
      - Pain has at least one of the following characteristics: intense, sharp, superficial, or stabbing, or pain starts from specific trigger areas or by triggering factors.
      - Attacks are stereotyped in the individual patient.
      - No neurologic deficit based on clinical exam.
      - Pain is not attributed to another disorder.

c. Management
   1. Multiple treatment options
      - Pharmacologic therapy
        (a) 75% of patients have substantial relief and adequate control with medical therapy.
        (b) Carbamazepine best studied and only indicated drug by FDA.
           - Initial response to carbamazepine is diagnostic.
           - Side effects: ataxia (15%), dizziness (44%), drowsiness (32%), nausea (29%), vomiting (18%)
        (c) Lamotrigine and baclofen are second-line options; gabapentin has been shown to be effective, particularly with MS patients.
      - Percutaneous glycerol or thermal rhizotomy of the Gasserian ganglion
      - Balloon compression
      - Open cranial procedures (ie, microvascular decompression)
        (a) Most durable treatment
      - Radiation therapy (ie, gamma knife radiosurgery)

ii. Cranial neuropathy syndromes

a. Tolosa-Hunt syndrome
   1. Episodic unilateral orbital or retro-orbital pain with ophthalmoplegia
   2. Involvement of cranial nerves 3 to 6
   3. Thought to be due to a nonspecific granulomatous inflammation involving the posterior superior orbital fissure, orbital apex, and cavernous sinus
   4. Diagnosis of exclusion (MRI needed to rule out other pathologies)
   5. Symptoms last for an average of 8 weeks if untreated
   6. Treatment: steroids

b. Raeder syndrome
   1. First division of trigeminal nerve involved causing neuropathic pain or sensory loss; other divisions of trigeminal nerve can also be involved
   2. Sympathetic dysfunction also (miosis, ptosis) without anhidrosis
   3. Neuroimaging necessary to exclude other diagnoses
   4. Syndrome not specific to any underlying pathologic process

c. Gradenigo syndrome
   1. Apical petrositis: infection of petrous temporal bone
   2. Due to infection extending from middle ear and mastoid air cells into the pneumatized petrous apex via the perilabyrinthine air tract
   3. Involvement of Dorello canal and possibly the trigeminal nerve
   4. Abducens nerve palsy with possible orbital or retro-orbital pain

- d. Vernet syndrome
  1. Lesion (tumor, infection, fracture, thrombosis) of jugular foramen
  2. CN 9 to 11 effected: ipsilateral trapezius and sternocleidomastoid weakness, dysphonia, dysphagia, loss of taste over posterior one-third of tongue, depressed pharyngeal sensation
- e. Collet-Sicard syndrome
  1. Unilateral palsy of CN 9 to 12
  2. Lack of sympathetic dysfunction

iii. Stroke Syndromes

- a. **Rule of thumb:** acute neurologic deterioration with ipsilateral cranial nerve deficit(s) and contralateral sensory or motor dysfunction localizes the stroke to the brain stem (midbrain, pons, medulla)
- b. Dejerine-Roussy syndrome
  1. Stroke of the thalamus involving the (PCA)
  2. Contralateral sensory loss, contralateral dysesthesia (thalamic pain), ballistic or choreoathetoid movements, transient hemiparesis
- c. Weber syndrome
  1. Stroke of the caudal midbrain involving the posterior cerebral artery (PCA)
  2. Ipsilateral gaze weakness (oculomotor nerve palsy), contralateral weakness
- d. Benedikt syndrome
  1. Stroke of the tegmentum (midbrain floor) involving the posterior cerebral artery (PCA)
  2. Oculomotor nerve palsy, contralateral hemichorea, hemiathetosis (red nucleus damage)
- e. Raymond syndrome
  1. Stroke of the pons involving the paramedian branches of the basilar artery
  2. Ipsilateral lateral gaze weakness, contralateral weakness
- f. Foville syndrome
  1. Stroke of inferior medial pons involving the basilar artery
  2. Contralateral hemiparesis, ipsilateral facial palsy (CN7), lateral gaze palsy (CN6), reduced touch and position sense (medial lemniscus)
- g. Millard Gubler syndrome
  1. Stroke of the basis pontis (caudal pons) involving the basilar artery
  2. Contralateral weakness, ipsilateral lateral gaze weakness, and ipsilateral facial weakness
- h. Palatopharyngeal paralysis of Avellis
  1. Stroke of cephalad portion of nucleus ambiguous
  2. Paralysis of the palatal, pharyngeal muscles with sparing of laryngeal muscles
  3. Somatotopic organization of motor nucleus places laryngeal muscles caudal
- i. Dejerine anterior bulbar syndrome
  1. Stroke of paramedian medulla involving the basilar artery
  2. Sudden onset of reduced touch and position sense (dorsal column/medial lemniscus) of the contralateral side of body with contralateral hemiplegia, preservation of pain and temperature, with ipsilateral tongue weakness (CN12) and upbeat nystagmus, without facial droop
- j. Wallenberg syndrome
  1. Stroke of lateral medulla involving the vertebral artery
  2. Ipsilateral loss of facial sensation, ataxia, nystagmus/vertigo/nausea (vestibular nucleus involvement), dysphagia (nucleus ambiguous), Horner syndrome, contralateral hemisensory loss (spinothalamic tract)

iv. Seizure disorders
  a. Infantile spasms (West syndrome)
    1. Sudden flexor or extensor spasms of head, trunk, or limbs
    2. Associated with tuberous sclerosis (neurocutaneous syndrome)
    3. On EEG, see hypsarrhythmia
  b. Juvenile myoclonic epilepsy
    1. Myoclonic jerks that arise usually in the morning
    2. Patients have normal intelligence
    3. On EEG, see 4-6 Hertz (Hz) spike waves and polyspike discharges
  c. Benign focal epilepsy of childhood
    1. Generalized seizures at night, focal seizures during the day
    2. On EEG, see di- or triphasic sharp waves
  d. Petit Mal
    1. Frequent, blank staring spells
    2. On EEG see generalized, symmetric 3-Hz spike-wave discharge
  e. Gelastic seizures
    1. Involuntary laughter with alternating crying or sobbing spells; with precocious puberty when associated with hypothalamic hamartoma
    2. 25% associated with hypothalamic hamartoma
    3. 21% of patients with hypothalamic hamartoma have gelastic seizures
    4. hypothalamic hamartoma associated with other midline deformities (ie, callosal agenesis)
  f. Temporal lobe seizures
    1. Most common in adults
    2. Involves mesial temporal structures
    3. Associated with **auras** (hallucinations, sensory illusions, viscerosensory symptoms such as sensation over the abdomen or chest wall) and **automatisms** (stereotyped repetitive movement of the mouth, tongue, lips or jaw → lip smacking)
    4. Anterior temporal lobe resection is 80% effective
    5. On EEG, see focal temporal slowing or epileptiform sharp waves or spikes in the anterior temporal lobe region

v. Inflammatory disorders of the nervous system
  a. Multiple sclerosis
    1. Acquired relapsing demyelinating disease that is disseminated throughout the central nervous system in time and space
    2. Female predilection with peak presentation at 35 years of age
    3. Optic neuritis or trigeminal neuralgia are common symptoms
    4. Multiple patterns of presentation
      - Relapsing-remitting: most common; occasional symptoms that resolve on their own
      - Secondary progressive: begin as relapsing-remitting but then become progressively worse
      - Primary progressive: symptoms do not relapse and become progressive
      - Progressive with relapses: symptoms that resolve but when they return are worse than the prior symptom
      - Benign multiple sclerosis: patient with symptoms but remain functionally active for over 15 years

5. Radiographic signs
   - Dawson fingers: hyperintense lesions seen on MRI FLAIR sequence that are perpendicular to the ventricles
   - Open ring sing: enhancement is often incomplete on contrasted MRI studies
   - Lesions are often hyperintense on T2 MRI
6. Laboratory evaluation
   - IgG and albumin values from the serum and CSF should be measured to obtain the IgG index (a value greater than 0.7 is elevated)
   - Oligoclonal bands are often seen in CSF

b. Amyotrophic lateral sclerosis
   1. Disease of the upper and lower motor neurons
   2. Signs of anterior horn cell disease without sensory neuropathy
   3. Associated with Parkinson-like dementia complex
   4. Most patients die within 5 years of symptom onset

c. Progressive multifocal leukencephalopathy
   1. Due to activation of JC virus (papovavirus) in immunocompromised patients
   2. Reactivated virus attacks oligodendrocytes of subcortical white matter
   3. Usually affects the parietal-occipital lobes
   4. Seen in 4% of AIDS patients and patients with leukemia and lymphoma
   5. MRI findings: hyperintense on T2 and FLAIR sequences, nonenhancing
   6. Diagnosis confirmed by PCR analysis of JC virus RNA in CSF

d. Neuroborreliosis
   1. Neurologic symptoms that arise after tick bite from *borrelia burgdorferi*
   2. Most common symptom is painful sensory radiculitis
   3. Other symptoms: Bell palsy, limb paresis, oculomotor weakness, arthralgias, cardiomyopathy
   4. Treatment: penicillin or ceftriaxone

e. Meningitis
   1. Bacterial meningitis
      - Most common in the winter months
      - Glucose decreased, protein elevated, CSF leukocytosis, and elevated opening pressure
   2. Tuberculous meningitis
      - Secondary to infection elsewhere, usually lungs
      - Mortality rate higher than in bacterial meningitis
      - Early treatment prevents poor outcome
      - Involve skull base (basal meningitis)
      - Treatment: isoniazid, rifampin, pyrazinamide, ethambutol
        (a) Treatment given for 18 to 24 months
        (b) INH depletes B6, therefore its use mandates replacement
      - CSF profile: slight increase in ICP, pleocytosis with lymphocytic predominance, increased protein, decreased glucose.
      - CSF glucose should be normally 60% of serum glucose, usually 45 mg/dL or greater.
   3. Viral meningitis/encephalitis
      - CSF profile: lymphocytic pleocytosis, mild elevation in protein, normal glucose.
      - Peaks in the summer and fall seasons.
      - RNA viruses: enteroviruses, arboviruses, rhabdoviruses, arenaviruses.

- DNA viruses: HSV-1, HSV-2, VZV, CMV, HHV-6.
- Enteroviruses are the most common cause of viral meningitis.

vi. Gertsmann syndrome
  a. Syndrome due to lesion of dominant parietal lobe (inferior parietal lobule)
  b. Acalculia, agraphia without alexia, right and left confusion, finger agnosia (inability to distinguish fingers of the hand)
  c. Anosognosia (unawareness of the contralateral side of the body) involves the nondominant parietal lobe

vii. Central pontine myelinolysis
  a. Due to aggressive correction of chronic hyponatremia
  b. Symptoms: seizures, dysarthria, pseudobulbar palsy, dysphagia, hyperreflexia, quadriplegia, coma
    1. Can also occur without symptoms
  c. Diagnosis: confirm with MRI; CSF studies can show elevated myelin basic protein
  d. To avoid this condition, correct sodium by 12 mmol/L in 24 hours

viii. Vitamin deficiency
  a. Thiamine (B_1) deficiency
    1. Wernicke encephalopathy
      - Ophthalmoplegia, nystagmus, anisocoria, gait ataxia, confusion, coma, death
    2. Korsakoff psychosis
      - Confabulation, psychosis, amnesia
      - Mammillary bodies affected
    3. With treatment symptoms of Wernicke's involving the eyes improve; confusion improves to a varying degree; Korsakoff amnesia is left in about 80% of patients
  b. B_{12} deficiency
    1. Subacute combined degeneration of the spinal cord
      - Degeneration of posterior and lateral columns of the spinal cord
      - Decreased pressure, vibration, and touch sense
      - Weakness of the extremities, especially legs
      - Ataxia

ix. Neurodegenerative diseases
  a. Huntington disease
    1. Trinucleotide repeat (CAG) localized on chromosome 4.
    2. Autosomal dominant disease with complete penetrance.
    3. More common in males with symptoms beginning at age 35 to 40.
    4. Abnormal gene products cause damage to inhibitory pathway between motor cortex and subcortical structures causing hyperkinesia and choreoathetosis.
    5. Disease progresses to death within 20 years of symptom onset.
  b. Friedreich ataxia
    1. Trinucleotide repeat (GAA) located on chromosome 9.
    2. Frataxin gene not expressed in this disease; frataxin is an iron storage protein that is not expressed.
    3. Symptoms related to degeneration of spinal cord tracts, medulla, and deep nuclei → ataxia, dysarthria, areflexia.
    4. Symptoms begin between 10 and 15 years and disorder is deadly by middle age (40-50).

c. Alzheimer disease
   1. A type of dementia associated with language dysfunction, intellectual loss, and memory loss.
   2. Can be a rare cause of new-onset auditory hallucinations.
   3. Diagnosis based on history, physical exam, and brain imaging to exclude reversible causes of dementia.
   4. Several genes associated with AD → the E4 allele of the apolipoprotein E (chromosome 19) is associated with 25% to 40% of all cases.
   5. Degeneration of the nucleus basalis of Meynert causes decreased cholinergic input to frontal cortex.
   6. Treatment: Tacrine (central-acting acetylcholinesterase inhibitor) and donepezil (reversible acetylcholinesterase inhibitor) may slow cognitive decline.

x. Brain stem auditory evoked response (BAER)
   a. Can be measured from several important components of the auditory pathway
   b. Seven peaks in BAER
      1. Wave 1: auditory nerve
      2. Wave 2: cochlear nucleus
      3. Wave 3: superior olive
      4. Wave 4: lateral lemniscus
      5. Wave 5: inferior colliculus
      6. Wave 6: medial geniculate body
      7. Wave 7: auditory radiations/cortex
   c. BAER shows prolonged latency with structural lesion of the brain stem or auditory nerve.
   d. BAER is abnormal in 90% of patients with acoustic schwannoma and usually consists of delayed conduction from the auditory nerve to the caudal pons (wave 1-wave 3)
   e. BAER is abnormal in 33% of MS patients and usually involves increased latency between wave 3 and wave 5

Neurosurgery

A. Subarachnoid hemorrhage (SAH)
   i. Patients present with acute onset, "thunder clap" headache.
   ii. Most devastating complication related to vasospasm and delayed cerebral ischemia.
      a. "Triple H" therapy used to treat vasospasm: hypertension, hypervolemia, hemodilution; risks of treatment associated with hyponatremia, pulmonary edema, cerebral edema, and myocardial infarction.
      b. Balloon angioplasty and spasmolysis with verapamil via an endovascular route are also treatments for vasospasm.
   iii. Hunt & Hess grade is a prognostic scale based on presentation
      a. Grade 1: asymptomatic or mild headache with slight nuchal rigidity; 11% mortality
      b. Grade 2: moderate to severe headache with nuchal rigidity with no neurologic deficit other than cranial nerve palsy; 26% mortality
      c. Grade 3: drowsiness, confusion, mild focal deficit; 37% mortality
      d. Grade 4: stupor, moderate to severe hemiparesis; 71% mortality
      e. Grade 5: deep coma, decerebrate rigidity, moribund appearance; 100% mortality

iv. Modified Fisher scale is a radiographic score that predicts risk for vasospasm.
  a. Grade 0: no SAH or IVH
  b. Grade 1: focal or diffuse thin (< 1 mm) SAH, no IVH; positive predictive value (PPV) of 10%
  c. Grade 2: focal or diffuse thin (< 1 mm) SAH with IVH; PPV of 20%
  d. Grade 3: focal or diffuse thick (> 1 mm) SAH, no IVH; PPV of 30%
  e. Grade 4: focal or diffuse think (> 1 mm) SAH, with IVH; PPV of 40%

B. Carotid-Cavernous Fistula
  i. These fistulas are divided into traumatic or spontaneous.
  ii. Both traumatic and spontaneous fistulas present with retro-orbital pain, chemosis, pulsatile proptosis, ocular or cranial bruit, decreased visual acuity, diplopia, and rarely epistaxis and SAH.
  iii. Symptoms depend on the direction of venous flow and volume of blood flow through the fistula.
  iv. Four types of fistula
    a. Type A: direct, high-flow shunt between the internal carotid artery (ICA) and CS
    b. Type B: low-flow shunt between dural branches of intracavernous ICA and CS
    c. Type C: low-flow shunt; supply from the meningeal branches of external carotid artery (ECA) and CS
    d. Type D: low-flow shunt between the dural branches of the ICA and ECA with the CS
  v. Treatment
    a. Half of all low-flow fistulas spontaneously resolve.
    b. Mainstay of treatment is transarterial balloon occlusion for Type A fistulas.
    c. Transvenous balloon occlusion via the inferior petrosal sinus for Type B-D fistulas.

C. Dural arteriovenous fistulas
  i. Arteriovenous shunts involving dural vessels that usually arise because of thrombosis of a dural venous sinus (transverse sinus most common).
  ii. Presentation: includes pulsatile tinnitus, exophthalmos (due to increased drainage into venous system; ie, venous hypertension), visual symptoms, papilledema, hydrocephalus, and intracranial hemorrhage.
  iii. The presence of retrograde cortical venous drainage indicates the potential for intracranial hemorrhage and mandates URGENT TREATMENT because of the higher bleeding risk.
  iv. Hemorrhage in the setting of a DAVF has a high morbidity with about a 30% mortality.
  v. Borden Classification
    a. Venous drainage directly into dural venous sinus or meningeal vein; 2% have aggressive behavior (hemorrhage or neurologic deficit)
    b. Venous drainage directly into dural venous sinus or meningeal vein with venous reflux to normal subarachnoid veins; 39% have aggressive behavior
    c. Venous drainage directly into subarachnoid veins; 79% with aggressive behavior

D. Arteriovenous malformation (AVM)
  i. Lack intervening capillary network
  ii. Composed of feeding arteries, a nidus (shunting arterioles and interconnected venous loops), draining veins

iii. Increased flow through feeding arteries can cause the formation of aneurysms in the nidus
iv. Majority of AVMs are solitary (98%), 2% are multiple and can be associated with Osler-Weber-Rendu syndrome or Mason-Wyburn syndrome
v. Spetzler-Martin AVM grading system
   a. Composite score to assess surgical risk of resection, maximum score of 5 points associated with the highest morbidity
   b. Size of nidus
      1. < 3 cm = 1 point
      2. 3 to 6 cm = 2 points
      3. > 6 cm = 3 points
   c. Eloquence of surrounding brain
      1. Noneloquent = 0
         - Frontal lobe, nondominant temporal lobe, cerebellar hemispheres
      2. Eloquent = 1
         - Sensorimotor cortex, language cortex, visual cortex, internal capsule, thalamus, hypothalamus, brain stem, cerebellar nuclei, regions adjacent to these structures
   d. Venous draining
      1. Superficial = 0
      2. Deep = 1
vi. Treatment includes embolization, microsurgical resection, or radiosurgery.

E. Head trauma
   i. Herniation syndromes related to Monro-Kellie doctrine, which states that the cranial vault holds a constant volume that is the sum of brain parenchyma, CSF, and blood.
   ii. An increase in the volume of any one of these components will increase intracranial pressure (ICP).
   iii. Herniation syndromes
      a. Uncal herniation
         1. Herniation of the uncus through the tentorial incisura
         2. Pupil dilation with down and out appearance of the globe due to compression of the oculomotor nerve (CN3)
         3. Kernohan notch: mass effect on the contralateral cerebral peduncle causing ipsilateral hemiparesis; a "false-localizing" sign
      b. Central herniation
         1. Diencephalon and parts of the temporal lobes are squashed inferiorly under the tentorium cerebelli.
         2. Branches of the basilar artery can stretch and cause fatal bleeding if they rupture (Duret hemorrhage)
      c. Cingulate (subfalcine) herniation
         1. The medial frontal lobe is pushed under the falx cerebri.
         2. Pressure can be placed on the anterior cerebral arteries.
      d. Transcalvarial/external herniation
         1. Herniating brain contents outside the confines of the calvarium
         2. Usually due to skull fracture or as a therapeutic surgical procedure for raised ICP (craniectomy)
      e. Upward cerebellar herniation
         1. Increased pressure in the posterior fossa can push the cerebellum rostrally.

f. Tonsillar/downward cerebellar herniation
   1. Movement of the cerebellar tonsils through the foramen magnum.
   2. Coning of the tonsils can cause compression of the lower brain stem and upper spinal cord leading to respiratory and cardiac dysfunction.
   3. Fatal.

g. Medical treatment for elevations in ICP
   1. Raising the head of bed, reducing jugular venous pressure, hypertonic saline, mannitol, acute hyperventilation, chemically induced coma
   2. Mannitol and hyperventilation should be used with caution due to the risk of aggravating ischemia
      - Mannitol can deplete intravascular volume and hyperventilation can cause vasoconstriction.
      - Hypertonic saline (3%) can be used as a resuscitative fluid that can also reduce ICP acutely.
      - Nevertheless, once primary survey is complete, mannitol and hyperventilation are recommended to acutely reduce elevations in ICP, which may last up to 6 hours.
      - Other risks of mannitol: opens blood-brain barrier and can worsen vasogenic edema; can cause nonketotic hyperosmolar state with high associated mortality; overuse can cause hypertension and increased CBF if autoregulation is defective; high doses can cause acute renal failure (especially when there is sepsis or if serum osm > 320, underlying kidney disease, co-use of nephrotoxic drug)

iv. Dissection or thrombosis of vertebral artery

a. Injury due to transverse foramen fracture or blunt injury to the vessel.

b. Dissection or thrombosis can lead to infarction of the posterior fossa contents.

c. An occluded vessel has the potential for recanalization and subsequent distal embolization.
   1. The precise incidence of recanalization is unknown, but many favor sacrificing the involved artery via an endovascular approach if there is enough collateral circulation.

d. Other options include observation and beginning antiplatelet therapy.

e. Patient with dissection or pseudoaneurysm formation of the vertebral arteries or extracranial carotid arteries may pose a difficult treatment dilemma because optimal treatment has not been defined.
   1. Many authors agree to start heparin drip for 1 to 2 weeks, followed by bridge to warfarin for additional 4 to 12 weeks.
      - Most injuries heal within 6 weeks.

f. For patients with high hemorrhage risk, aspirin and/or plavix can be used as an alternative to anticoagulation because it is thought that there could be less risk for bleeding, although further studies need to clarify this point.

g. New stenting techniques with flow diversion technology can also be considered; stent placement would mandate the use of antiplatelet therapy as well.

F. Trigeminal neuralgia

i. Electric, shock-like pain that typically radiates in a V2 and/or V3 distribution; rarely have pain in a V1 distribution.

ii. Primary treatment includes carbamazepine and/or oxcarbazepine.

iii. Other treatments include peripheral alcohol injection, glycerol rhizolysis, radiofrequency thermocoagulation, and microvascular decompression.

iv. Typically, the superior cerebellar artery compresses the trigeminal nerve at the root entry zone.
v. Decompression of the nerve using telfa pledgets can cure this disease.
vi. MVD is not an appropriate treatment for MS patients.

G. Craniovertebral junction abnormalities
i. Chiari 1 malformation associated with tonsillar herniation 6 mm below the foramen magnum and crowding of the foramen magnum causing obstruction of cerebrospinal fluid flow into the cervical cistern
ii. Occipitocervical instability seen in Down syndrome (trisomy 21) and Klippel-Feil syndrome (complex genetic syndrome causing faulty segmentation with subsequent autofusion of the segments of the vertebral column; commonly affects the cervical spine)
iii. Platybasia is the abnormal flattening of the clivus with an associated skull base angle of over 143 degrees.
iv. Basilar invagination is the rostral migration of the odontoid process through the foramen magnum; associated with platybasia.
v. Rheumatoid arthritis (RA) associated with a number of abnormalities: patients are at risk for developing atlanto-occipital instability/atlantoaxial instability (AAI), superior migration of the odontoid process/cranial settling, and subaxial subluxation (SAS); any form of long-term instability can be associated with the formation of a reactive pannus that can compress the spinal cord.
vi. These conditions can cause myelopathy, obstructive hydrocephalus, and cranial neuropathies; therefore, decompression and stabilization are the mainstay of treatment.
   a. For irreducible lesions (nothing gained by cervical traction) → decompression at the site of encroachment (ventral or posterior) as well as stabilization are often required.
   b. For reducible lesions, immobilization alone with posterior spinal or craniospinal fusion without decompression is the mainstay of treatment.
vii. Late neurologic deterioration in patients with RA or Chiari is concerning for syrinx formation, but this is very rare.

H. Idiopathic intracranial hypertension (pseudotumor)
i. Papilledema and symptomatic elevation of ICP > 20 cm of H_2O without any imaging evidence of intracranial disease (other than sinus thrombosis)
   a. Some authorities disagree regarding the ICP threshold for diagnosis
   b. Most devastating complication: blindness from optic atrophy
   c. Young women of childbearing age who are obese are most commonly affected
   d. Work up: MRI brain with and without contrast and magnetic resonance venography (MRV); lumbar puncture (LP) with opening pressure > 25 cm of H_2O; ophthalmologic evaluation for visual fields, visual acuity, and papilledema.
   e. Risk of blindness not necessarily correlated with duration of symptoms, headache, papilledema, visual acuity
   f. Treatment: if medical therapy fails (weight loss, acetazolamide, furosemide) should pursue optic nerve sheath fenestration and/or CSF shunt

I. Spontaneous intracranial hypotension
i. Usually occurs from leakage of CSF outside the cranial cavity.
ii. Headaches resemble post-spinal tap headaches and are positional; caffeine and hydration can help treat these postural headaches.
iii. Diagnosis can be made with lumbar tap: dry tap or very low opening pressure.

iv. CSF profile does show elevated protein and pleocytosis.
v. B2 transferrin can also be sent to confirm if any collected fluid from the nares is suspicious for CSF.
vi. MR cisternography can localize the leak but standard MRI protocols are usually sufficient to localize the skull base defect.
vii. Contrasted MRI of the brain reveals dural enhancement over cerebral and cerebellar convexities, tentorium, and falx; this finding is reversible with the resolution of symptoms.
viii. Surgical closure of the fistula is needed for those patients with persistent CSF rhinorrhea or otorrhea.
   a. Clinical suspicion for pseudotumor cerebri should be high for patients presenting with spontaneous CSF leak.

J. Craniopharyngioma
   i. World Health Organization (WHO) Grade 1 tumor that can be found anywhere between the infundibulum and the pituitary gland
   ii. Arises from Rathke cleft
   iii. Bimodal distribution with peaks during childhood from age 10 to 14 and again during middle age
      a. Children most often present with adamantinomatous subtype, and adults usually present with papillary subtype
   iv. Imaging
      a. MRI findings reveal a sellar mass usually associated with suprasellar extension, contrast enhancement, calcification, T1 hyperintensity with tumors containing more protein, blood, or cholesterol (adamantinomatous subtype).
   v. If papillary, the tumor will be isointense to T1.
   vi. After surgery most will have predictable endocrine deficiency; these findings are most often seen in children.
      a. Most serious is obesity which develops in about 50% of patients.
         1. Patients are unable to control their appetite secondary to damage to hypothalamic satiety center
      b. 50% of patients will require GH replacement.
      c. Diabetes insipidus (DI) occurs in 90% of patients and is usually permanent.
      d. 90% of patients will require hydrocortisone and thyroid replacement therapy after surgery.

K. Pituitary adenoma
   i. Benign WHO Grade 1 tumors that can be functional or nonfunctional.
   ii. Microadenomas are less than 10 mm, and macroadenomas are greater than 10 mm in size.
   iii. 65% are functional and 35% are nonsecretory
      a. Prolactin secreting: 48%
      b. Growth hormone secreting: 10%
      c. ACTH secreting: 6%
      d. TSH secreting: 1%
   iv. Prolactinomas should most often be initially treated with bromocriptine or cabergoline, while patients with other functional adenomas should be offered surgery as their initial treatment strategy.
   v. Nonfunctional pituitary adenomas can be associated with endocrinopathies.
      a. Elevated prolactin can be due to stalk effect which occurs due to the tonic inhibition of dopamine (inhibits prolactin secretion).

b. Prolactin levels are usually less than 200 ng/mL in setting of stalk effect.
c. Secondary hypothyroidism can also occur due to the presence of the pituitary adenoma and its mass effect on the adenohypophysis.

vi. Unless symptomatic, benign nonfunctional tumors can be managed with serial imaging surveillance.

vii. Pituitary apoplexy
a. Hemorrhage of the pituitary gland and adenoma due to venous infarction.
b. Patients usually present with symptoms of subarachnoid hemorrhage, panhypopituitarism, as well as cranial neuropathies and visual changes because of mass effect on the neural elements of the cavernous sinus as well as the optic apparatus.

viii. Imaging
a. The morphology of adenomas is best appreciated on sagittal and coronal reconstruction views of axial MRIs.
b. Microadenomas
1. Adenomas are hypointense areas within the more hyperintense normal pituitary on T1-weighted images.
2. Normal gland enhances, which accentuates the hypointense signal of the tumor
c. Macroadenomas
1. Isointense to slightly hypointense on T1-weighted images
2. Hyperintense on T2-weighted images
3. Blood within the pituitary usually has a high signal on T1-weighted images

ix. Tumors that cause neurologic decline and nonprolactinomas should be treated with surgical excision; the authors endorse endoscopic-assisted transsphenoidal surgery as the modality of choice for their resection.
a. Postoperatively patients should be closely monitored every 6 hours for diabetes insipidus (urine specific gravity < 1.003; rising serum sodium > 145; and normal postoperative pituitary function.

L. Meningioma

i. Dural-based extra-axial tumors that are predominantly WHO Grade 1 and comprise up to 34.7% of all primary brain tumors.
a. Grade 2 and grade 3 tumors are less common and make up 7% and 2.4% of all meningiomas, respectively.

ii. Can be found in multiple locations in the skull base: olfactory groove, planum sphenoidale, tuberculum sellae, sphenoid wing, cavernous sinus, tentorial, diaphragma sellae, petroclival, foramen magnum, etc.

iii. Presentation usually related to the location of the meningioma.

iv. Imaging
a. Usually isointense on T1 and hyperintense on T2 MRI Homogeneous contrast enhancement
b. Dural tail: reactive process in the dura adjacent to a meningioma that causes contrast enhancement
c. CSF cleft sign: represents the tumor-brain interface between extra-axial lesions and parenchyma; usually hyperintense rim on T2
d. Mother-in-law sign: due to the highly vascular nature of meningiomas, angiography can show the stasis of contrast within the tumor during the venous phase.
e. Hyperostosis of surrounding bone

v. These tumors can encase critical neurovascular structures and cause compression of these elements.
vi. Decompression is critical → surgical management is the mainstay of treatment.
vii. Simpson grading: meningioma recurrence rate is dependent on extent of resection.
   a. Grade I
      1. Complete removal including resection of underlying bone and associated dura
      2. 9% symptomatic recurrence at 10 years
   b. Grade II
      1. Complete removal and coagulation of dural attachment
      2. 19% symptomatic recurrence at 10 years
   c. Grade III
      1. Complete removal without resection or coagulation of dura
      2. 29% symptomatic recurrence at 10 years
   d. Grade IV
      1. Subtotal resection
      2. 44% symptomatic recurrence at 10 years
   e. Grade V
      1. Decompression with or without biopsy
      2. 100% symptomatic recurrence at 10 years (small sample in original paper)
viii. The authors reserve radiation therapy for patients who have a tissue diagnosis and decompression of the cranial nerves has been achieved.

Bibliography

1. Lal D, Rounds A, Dodick DW. Comprehensive management of patients presenting to the otolaryngologist for Sinus pressure, pain, or headache. *Laryngoscope*. 2014.
2. Maarbjerg S, Gozalov A, Olesen J, Bendtsen L. Trigeminal neuralgia - a prospective systematic study of clinical characteristics in 158 patients. *Headache*. 2014.
3. van Gijn J, Kerr RS, Rinkel GJ. Subarachnoid haemorrhage. *Lancet*. 2007;369(9558):306-318.
4. Russin J, Cohen-Gadol AA. Editorial: What did we learn from the ARUBA trial? *Neurosurg Focus*. 2014;37(3):E9.
5. Brain Trauma Foundation, American Association of Neurological Surgeons, Congress of Neurological Surgeons, et al. Guidelines for the management of severe traumatic brain injury. XV. Steroids. *J Neurotrauma*. 2007;24 Suppl 1:S91-95.

Questions

1. A 35-year-old woman presents with the primary complaint of "sinus pain." She states that she has had severe pain around her eye that is associated with tearing, nasal congestion, and rhinorrhea; all of her symptoms are on the right side. Upon further questioning, she reveals that she has had these symptoms throughout most of her adult life and says that these symptoms are quite persistent for 2 to 3 weeks and then relapse; she is symptom-free for 1 to 2 months before the symptoms return. She believes most of her symptoms occur with changes in the weather and she does not complain of associated nausea, vomiting, or photophobia. What is her diagnosis?

A. Migraine headache
B. Chronic sinusitis
C. Allergic rhinitis
D. Cluster headache
E. Tension headache

2. A 45-year-old man presents to your clinic with left eye pain. On examination, he has no extraocular movement from his left eye. Other than a frozen eye and a slightly dilated pupil that does not normally constrict to light, he has a normal neurologic exam. An MRI shows abnormal enhancement of the anterior cavernous sinus, superior orbital fissure, and orbital apex without signs of mass effect or of a dural tail extending posteriorly or laterally. What is the diagnosis?
A. Raeder syndrome
B. Tolosa-Hunt syndrome
C. Gradenigo syndrome
D. Vernet syndrome

3. A 55-year-old man presents to clinic with a 1-year history of facial pain. He states that he has sharp, lancinating pain radiating down his mandible that is exacerbated by shaving, brushing his teeth, and by cool air touching his face. You correctly diagnose him with trigeminal neuralgia. What is the first-line treatment for trigeminal neuralgia?
A. Microvascular decompression
B. Thermal rhizotomy
C. Lamotrigine
D. Carbamazepine

4. A 29-year-old man presents with a history of a seizure disorder. He states that his seizures are associated with lip-smacking and odd sensations over his chest wall that lead to unconsciousness and generalized tonic-clonic activity. What is the seizure disorder that affects this patient?
A. Gelastic seizures
B. West syndrome
C. Temporal lobe seizures
D. Petit-mal seizures

5. A 65-year-old woman presents with headache, personality changes, anosmia, central scotoma of the right eye, optic nerve atrophy of the right eye, and left eye papilledema. She is diagnosed with Foster-Kennedy syndrome, and an MRI of her brain is ordered which reveals a large mass of the anterior cranial fossa most consistent with an olfactory groove meningioma. She undergoes an endoscopic, endonasal approach for the resection of the mass which involves coagulation of the ethmoidal arteries, removal of the crista galli and cribiform plate of the ethmoid bone, resection of the involved dura underlying the meningioma, and extirpation of the mass. What is the Simpson grade for the degree of resection of the meningioma?
A. Grade 1
B. Grade 2
C. Grade 3
D. Grade 4
E. Grade 5

Chapter 7
The Chest for ENT

A simple overview of lung function is the intention of this chapter. It is meant to outline basic aspects of respiratory physiology and function, but as with any organ system, it is but the tip of the iceberg.

Definitions

Lung volumes can be divided into primary volumes and capacities.

A. Primary volumes
   i. *Tidal volume (TV)*: Volume of gas that is either inspired or expired per respiratory cycle
   ii. *Residual volume*: Amount of gas that remains in the lungs at the end of a maximal expiratory effort
B. Capacities
   i. *Total lung capacity*: Amount of gas contained in the lung at the end of a maximal inspiratory effort
   ii. *Vital capacity*: Maximum volume of gas exhaled when a patient makes a forceful exhalation after inspiring to the total lung capacity
   iii. *Functional residual capacity*: Volume of gas that remains in the lung at the end of quiet exhalation

Dynamic lung volumes are as follows:

A. *Forced expiratory volume in 1 second (FEV_1)*: Volume of gas exhaled from the lung after initiation of a forceful exhalation following a maximal inspiration
B. *Forced expiratory volume in 1 second/forced vital capacity (FEV_1/FVC) ratio*: Ratio of the volume of gas exhaled from the lungs during the first second after forceful exhalation divided by the total volume of gas exhaled after forceful exhalation

Basic Tests of Pulmonary Function

Lung Volumes and Capacities

Figure 7-1 is an excellent way to understand the various lung volumes and capacities.

There are three points of reference: (1) total lung capacity which is at the point of maximal inspiratory effort; (2) the total volume at maximal voluntary expiration, or residual volume; and (3) the volume at the end of passive expiration, or functional residual capacity.

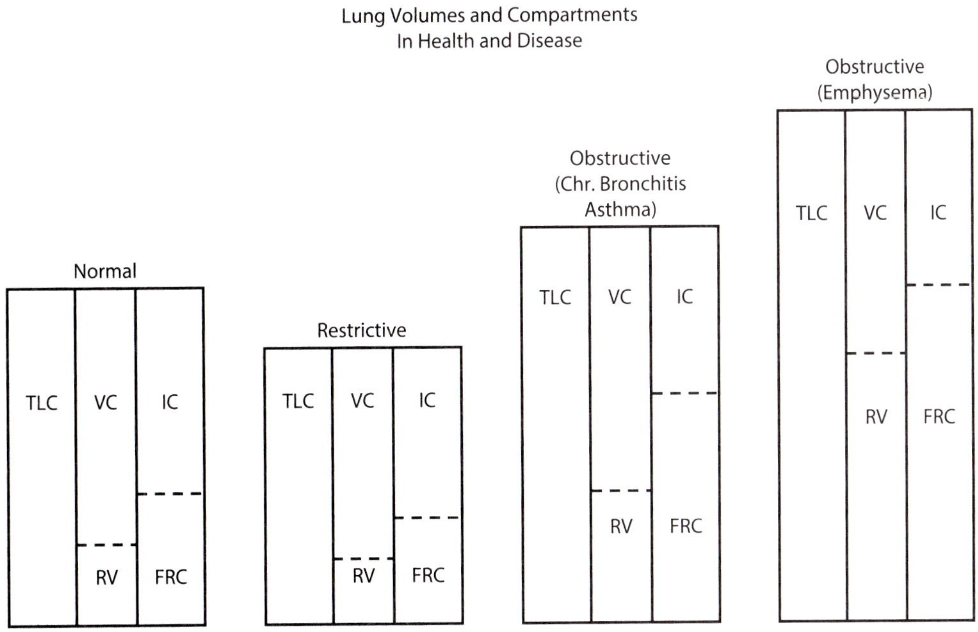

Figure 7-1 Lung compartments in normal health and in restrictive and obstructive diseases. Total lung capacity and residual volumes are generally the largest in emphysema.

This appears to be best reinforced and understood if one performs the maneuvers that are involved in achieving the volumes and capacities.

The lung volumes should be viewed in the context of two opposing forces that are seeking to expand or retract the lung.

Spirometry

The spirometer has a nitrogen or helium analyzer and allows the physician to obtain data concerning lung volumes, capacities, and dynamic lung volumes. It can help determine whether a patient has normal or abnormal lung function. The spirometer enables the physician to assess the abnormalities of function and place the individual into one of two major pulmonary disease categories: chronic airflow limitation (diseases such as asthma, chronic bronchitis, and pulmonary emphysema) or restrictive lung disease (diseases such as pulmonary fibrosis).

Flow Volume Loops

The maximal expiratory flow volume curve has been widely used by pulmonary laboratories for the past several years. In a spirometer tracing, volume is plotted against time (FEV_1 is the volume of gas exhaled during the first second after exhalation from a maximal inspiration). If the volume-time relation is normal, the flow rate is presumed to be normal; flow is never actually measured. In the flow volume loop, however, instantaneous flow is measured by means of a pneumotachograph, and flow is plotted against lung volume. Conditions that produce airflow limitation cause a reduction in measured flow rates throughout the patient's FVC maneuver.

Figure 7-2 illustrates a normal flow volume loop and a flow volume loop from a patient with chronic airflow limitation (such as chronic obstructive pulmonary disease [COPD]). Note that

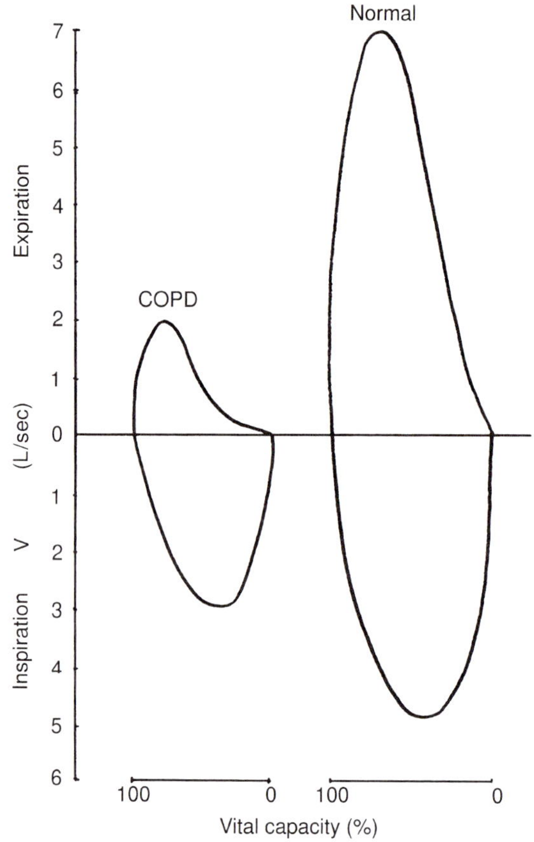

Figure 7-2 Flow volume loop. Note the reduction in flow.

the shape of the curve is concave in the normal patient but convex in the patient with limited flow. Note also that the flow volume loop characterizes the relations between flow and volume during the inspiratory portion of the respiratory cycle. The uses of this portion of the curve are discussed in a subsequent section of this chapter.

As with patients whose spirometry tracings indicate airflow limitation, bronchodilator medication is administered to patients with abnormal flow volume loops compatible with airflow limitation. Patients with reversible disease demonstrate a 15% to 20% improvement in the flow volume loop after bronchodilator administration. Patients with restrictive lung diseases have abnormal flow volume loops, but because they do not have an abnormality of the airways, their FEV_1/FVC ratio is usually normal. The slope of the expiratory loop in these patients is normal, in keeping with their normal airways.

Additional Uses of the Flow Volume Curve As noted, the flow volume curve can be used to evaluate inspiration as well as exhalation. This feature enables the pulmonary physiologist to evaluate the upper airway and assess the presence or absence of upper airway obstruction; this can also be a useful test for an otolaryngologist.

With inspiration, pleural pressure becomes more negative than the intraluminal pressure in the intrathoracic airways. Consequently, on inspiration, the caliber of the airways located within the chest increases. In the extrathoracic airways, such as the trachea, however, inspiration leads to a reduction in the intraluminal pressure, making atmospheric pressure greater than the pressure within the tracheal lumen. As a result, during inspiration, the caliber of the tracheal lumen tends to diminish because atmospheric pressure exceeds intratracheal pressure.

In patients with variable extrathoracic (upper airway) obstruction, the obstruction tends to narrow the tracheal lumen. On inspiration, this narrowing becomes more pronounced by the effect of inspiration, which also causes a reduction in the size of the tracheal lumen. Hence, on inspiration, patients with variably obstructing lesions of the upper airway show a reduction in inspiratory flow, so that the inspiratory curve often appears flattened. On exhalation, intratracheal pressure becomes greater than atmospheric pressure, which causes the tracheal lumen to expand. This expansion tends to negate the effect of a variably obstructing tracheal lesion, and the expiratory portion of the flow volume curve appears normal even if there is a variably obstructing lesion present. Thus, in a patient with a variably obstructing lesion of the upper airway, the inspiratory curve is flattened, whereas the expiratory curve appears normal. Figure 7-3 illustrates the curve produced by variably obstructing extrathoracic (upper airway) lesions.

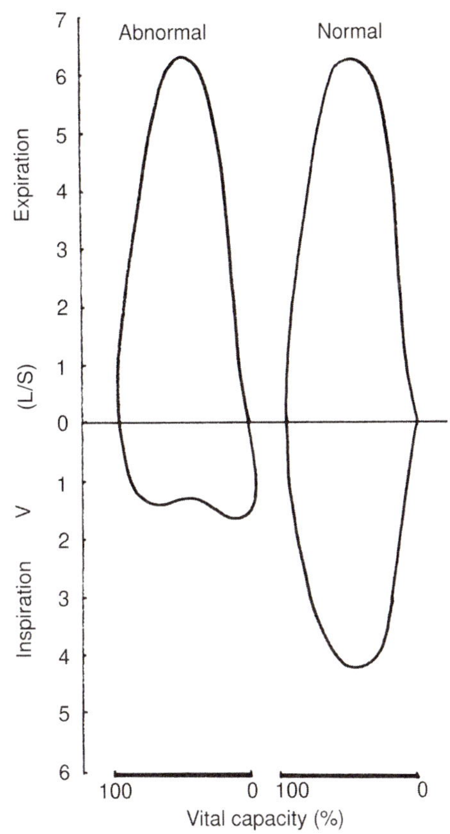

Figure 7-3 Extrathoracic obstruction.

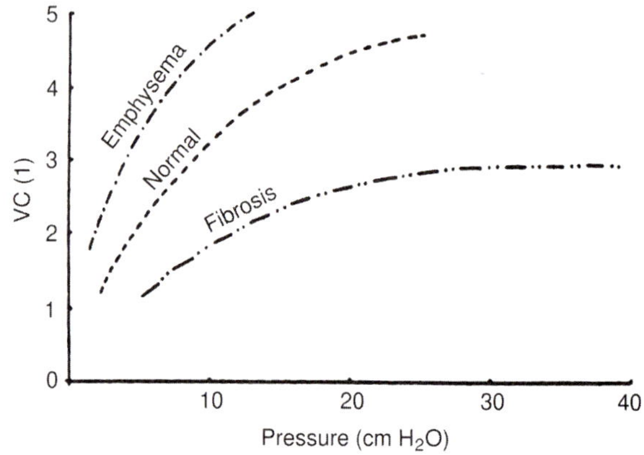

Figure 7-4 Compliance curve: pressure-volume relation.

Lung Compliance

Compliance is a measure of the distensibility, or elasticity, of the lung parenchyma. Elasticity refers to the ability of a structure to resist deformation. A rubber band is often referred to as an "elastic band"; it is an elastic structure, not because it can be stretched but because it reverts to its original length when released. Hence, elasticity is the property whereby the original shape is preserved.

Distensibility, on the other hand, is the ease with which shape can be altered. An elastic structure is not distensible, whereas a distensible structure does not possess elastic qualities. In the lung, distensibility refers to the ease with which changes in distending pressure change lung volume. A lung in which small distending pressures produce large changes in volume is a highly distensible (or highly compliant) lung. A lung in which high distending pressures are required to produce even small changes in lung volume is poorly distensible and poorly compliant. It is also a highly elastic (or "stiff") lung. Clinical examples are (1) the emphysematous lung, which is highly distensible, highly compliant, and poorly elastic secondary to the destruction of the elastic structures of the lung, and (2) the fibrotic lung, which is poorly compliant, poorly distensible, and very elastic or stiff owing to the increased deposition of collagen. Figure 7-4 illustrates compliance curves in patients with normal, highly compliant (emphysematous), or "stiff" (fibrotic) lungs.

Diffusing Capacity

The diffusing capacity refers to the quantity of a specific gas that diffuses across the alveolar-capillary membrane per unit of time. The diffusing capacity is often used to assess the size of the pulmonary capillary blood volume. In most pulmonary function laboratories, carbon monoxide is used to measure the diffusing capacity. This gas avidly binds to hemoglobin. In clinical practice, the diffusing capacity is thought to represent the volume of capillary blood into which carbon monoxide can dissolve. Diseases such as emphysema, which are characterized by a reduction in capillary blood volume, are associated with a low diffusing capacity.

Six-Minute Walk A simple test that measures a patient's exercise capacity and essentially measures the distance walked in 6 minutes. The more elaborate test is a cardiopulmonary stress test, which measures exhaled gases and oxygen consumption. It should be noted that there is a good correlation between the 6-minute test and the cardiopulmonary stress test, and in patients with COPD it correlates better than the conventionally measured FEV_1. It again emphasizes the need to incorporate the muscle pump or bellows into our understanding of the respiratory system.

Immune Function The appreciation of the lungs as an integral part of our immune mechanisms has been recognized since the late 18th century, but suffice it to say, we have made some progress in the understanding. The alveolar macrophage is the effector cell in controlling response to pathogens, but given the ongoing exposure of the alveolar membrane to these triggers, the mechanism of control of the response to triggers is equally important.

Drug-induced pulmonary toxicity is an area that may offer an insight into mechanisms that balance the processing of stimuli and mediate the response which could be as damaging.

Cough/Sinusitis and Asthma Sinonasal disease and asthma commonly serve as a cause of a cough that persists for many weeks. Vocal cord dysfunction may also lead to chronic cough.

Postulates about the association of sinusitis and asthma include the following:

A. Bacterial seeding
B. Enhanced β-blockade
C. Nasobronchial reflex
D. Eosinophil activation
E. Simple nasal obstruction

If one works through the algorithm of cough management and difficult-to-treat asthma, it is easy to appreciate the interactions between asthma, sinonasal disease, and gastroesophageal reflux disease. The three disease states and the use of angiotensin-converting enzyme inhibitors will be the causative etiology of a cough that persists for greater than 8 weeks in the setting of a normal chest X-ray. For a third of the time, more than one etiology will be responsible.

Work of Breathing The test used to assess a patient's ability to be weaned from mechanical ventilation can be used to help assess work of breathing. When a patient has been on ventilator support, the assessment for potential exhaustibility is assessed with a spontaneous breathing trial.

If the patient has a "rapid shallow breathing index" (RSBI) of less than 105 over a 30-minute period, he or she has an 85% chance of successful extubation. The *RSBI* is the frequency of breathing divided by the tidal volume measured in liters. The tachypnea as an indication of failure appears to be intuitive, but the reason for the tachypnea is not. The tachypnea is related to the assessment of the load per breath as a ratio of the maximal sustainable load, and the respiratory center adopts rapid shallow breathing as a protective mode to prevent respiratory muscle fatigue.

A real-life analogy would be to think of a distance runner who works his pace up to a point and then reduces it to "cruising," at which there is tolerance of respiratory effort that will not cause immediate fatigue. This phenomenon is a contributing factor to what is referred to as a second wind.

This becomes a clinical issue in the elderly patient with common comorbidities of pulmonary disease, cardiac disease, and obesity, where there is commonly an attendant component of deconditioning. This reduces the denominator, that is, the maximum workload, and hence increases dyspnea.

Blood Gases

Alveolar ventilation refers to the volume of gas in each breath that participates in gas exchange multiplied by the respiratory rate. Alveolar ventilation determines the level of arterial carbon dioxide; in the clinical setting, the adequacy of alveolar ventilation is assessed by measuring the arterial partial pressure of carbon dioxide (P_{CO_2}).

In clinical practice, the most common causes of hypoxemia are simple hypoventilation and ventilation-perfusion inequality. Other causes of hypoxemia include anatomic shunts and abnormalities of diffusion, but these problems are rarely found in clinical hypoxemia.

The otolaryngologist is often confronted with a patient whose blood gas measurements reveal hypoxemia, and it is important that the attending physician be able to distinguish patients who have intrinsic pulmonary disease from those with simple hypoventilation (such as may be produced by anesthetic administration) and normal lungs. One useful technique for evaluating the presence or absence of intrinsic lung disease is the determination of the alveolar-arterial (A-a) gradient. A simple way to calculate the A-a gradient is to assume that the alveolar oxygen tension is 148-arterial $Pco_2 \times 1.2$. If the alveolar oxygen tension is calculated and the arterial Po_2 measured, the A-a gradient can be estimated. If there is less than a 20 mm Hg gradient between alveolar and arterial oxygen tensions, it is likely that the lungs are normal and that alveolar hypoventilation is the sole abnormality producing the hypoxemia. Patients with normal lungs who have primary alveolar hypoventilation exhibit normal oxygen tensions when the cause of the alveolar hypoventilation is removed. A patient with a sedative overdose has normal oxygenation when the effects of the sedative on respiratory drive wear off.

Diseases that produce widened A-a gradients produce hypoxemia that cannot be corrected by simply increasing the level of alveolar ventilation. As stated, the most common cause of hypoxemia in these patients is maldistribution of alveolar ventilation and pulmonary blood flow. Diseases such as asthma, bronchitis, and emphysema impair ventilation because of abnormal airway flow. The reduction in flow produces abnormal ventilation-blood flow relations, which create the observed hypoxemia.

The rationale for the treatment of hypoxemia produced by ventilation-perfusion abnormalities is illustrated in Figure 7-5. If alveolus 1 has a reduction in ventilation due to airway narrowing, the alveolar oxygen tension in alveolus 1 decreases. The saturation of red blood cells (RBCs) in blood vessel I supplying alveolus 1 also decreases. Alveolus 2, which receives normal ventilation, has a normal alveolar oxygen tension. RBCs in the blood vessel II supplying alveolus 2 are normally saturated. Blood vessel III, which receives blood from vessels I and II, thus holds partially and fully saturated RBCs, so that the saturation of RBCs in III is

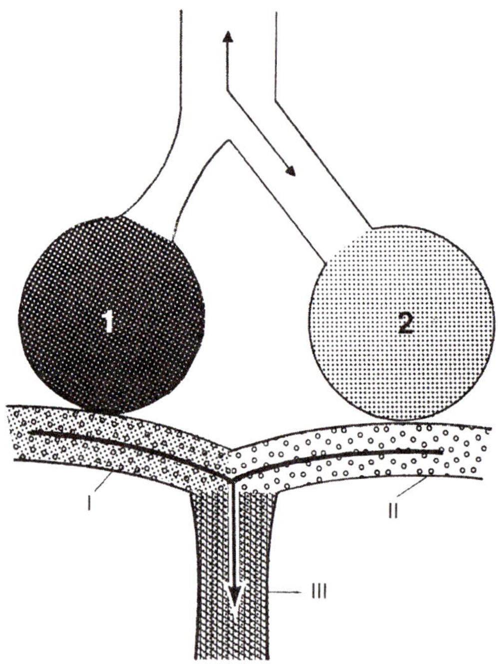

Figure 7-5 Ventilation perfusion mismatch. 1, 2, alveoli; I, II, III, blood vessels.

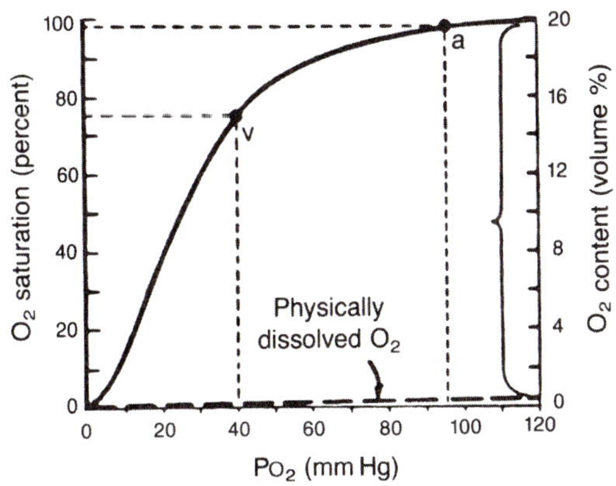

Figure 7-6 Oxyhemoglobin dissociation curve. O_2 saturation is given by the vertical axis on the left and O_2 content by the vertical axis on the right. Note the S shape of the curve and the location of the arterial point on the flat part of the dissociation curve and the venous point on the steep portion of the curve. The hemoglobin content of this blood is 15 g/dL, and the amount of O_2 carried in physical solution is much less than that bound to hemoglobin, as indicated by the bracket on the O_2 content axis.

reduced. Ventilation-perfusion abnormalities cannot be corrected by simple hyperventilation because hyperventilation does not increase the alveolar oxygen tension in alveolus 1 enough to increase the saturation of RBCs in vessel I. Hyperventilation may slightly increase the alveolar oxygen tension in alveolus 2, but the RBCs in blood vessel II are already fully saturated, and, therefore, the increase in alveolar oxygen tension cannot improve the saturation in the blood vessels supplying the alveolus. Thus, vessel III, supplied by vessels I and II, remains with less than optimal RBC saturation. On the other hand, if the inspired oxygen tension delivered to the patient is increased, the alveolar oxygen tension in alveolus 1 can be improved and the saturation of RBCs will increase. Samples of blood from vessel III will show an increase in saturation as well.

As shown in Figure 7-6, the shape of the oxyhemoglobin dissociation curve is such that small increments in oxygen tension may be associated with significant improvement in oxygen saturation if the increments occur on the steep slope of the dissociation curve. A higher inspired oxygen tension creates a situation in which the alveolar oxygen tension in alveolus 1 rises, thus raising the RBC saturation in vessel I. As already noted, RBCs in vessel II are fully saturated, but now vessel III has improved RBC saturation in RBCs emanating from vessel I, plus normally saturated blood from vessel II. It is evident that if the inspired oxygen tension delivered to the patient is increased, the alveolar oxygen tension in alveolus 1 can be improved and the saturation of RBCs will increase. Samples of blood drawn from vessel III will demonstrate an increase in saturation as well.

It is for these reasons that diseases characterized by ventilation-perfusion mismatching show improvement in hypoxemia when treated with higher inspired oxygen tensions. However, if there is a true anatomic shunt present in alveolus 1, so that blood vessel I does not come into contact with the alveolus, raising the inspired oxygen tension will have no effect on the hypoxemia because the RBC saturation in vessel I cannot be increased. True anatomic shunts do not respond to increases in inspired oxygen tension.

Pulmonary Volumes and Capacities

A. *TV*: Depth of breathing, volume of gas inspired or expired during each normal respiratory cycle, 0.5 L (average).
B. *Inspired reserve volume (IRV)*: Maximum that can be inspired from end-inspiratory position, 3.3 L (average).

C. *Expired reserve volume (ERV)*: Maximum volume that can be expired from end-respiratory level, 0.7 to 1.0 L (average).
D. *Reserved value (RV)*: Volume left in lungs after maximum expiration, 1.1 L (average).
E. *FEV_1*: Should be 80% or more of the predicted value from a normative chart.
F. *FVC*: Should be 80% or more of the predicted value from a normative chart. The FEV_1/FVC ratio should be more than 0.75 for younger patients and 0.70 for older individuals.
G. *Total lung capacity (6 L for men, 4.2 L for women)*: IRV + TV + ERV + RV (total volume contained in the lungs after maximum inspiration).
H. *Vital capacity (4.8 L for men, 3.1 L for women)*: IRV + TV + ERV (maximum volume that can be expelled from the lungs for effort following maximum inspiration).
I. *Functional residual capacity (2.2 L for men, 1.8 L for women)*: RV + ERV (volume in the lungs at resting expiratory level).
J. *Physiologic dead space (dead space of upper airway bypassed by tracheotomy, 70-100 mL)*: Anatomic dead space + the volume of gas that ventilates the alveoli that have no capillary blood flow + the volume of gas that ventilates the alveoli in excess of that required to arteriolize the capillary blood.

Mean Normal Blood Gas and Acid-Base Values

	Arterial blood	*Mixed venous blood*
pH	7.40	7.37
Pco_2	41 mm Hg	46.5 mm Hg
Po_2	95 mm Hg	40 mm Hg
O_2 saturation	97.1%	75.0%
HCO_3	4.0 mEq/L	25.0 mEq/L

Miscellaneous Information

A. Silo-filler disease (bronchiolitis obliterans) is a pathologic entity consisting of a collection of exudate in the bronchioles, obliterating the lumen. This complication often follows inhalation of nitrogen dioxide, exposure to open bottles of nitric acid, and exposure to silos. The diagnosis is based on a history of exposure, dyspnea, cough, and X-ray findings similar to those of miliary tuberculosis. Treatment is symptomatic. Prognosis is poor; most patients eventually succumb to this disease.
B. Bronchogenic cysts are congenital, arise from the bronchi, and are lined with epithelial cells. Furthermore, their walls may contain glands, smooth muscles, and cartilage. In the absence of infection, they may remain asymptomatic; otherwise, they give a productive cough, hemoptysis, and fever. The recommended treatment is surgical excision.
C. Blebs or bullae are air-containing structures resembling cysts, but their walls are not epithelium lined.
D. Anthracosilicosis is also called coal miner's pneumoconiosis.
E. Berylliosis is characterized by an infiltration of the lungs by beryllium. It is often found in workers at fluorescent lamp factories.
F. Bagassosis is characterized by an infiltration of the lungs by sugarcane fibers.

G. Byssinosis is characterized by an infiltration of the lungs by cotton dust.
H. Adenocarcinoma of the bronchus is the leading primary pulmonary carcinoma in women, and bronchogenic (squamous cell) carcinoma is most common in men.
I. Pancoast syndrome (superior sulcus tumor) is caused by any process of the apex of the lung that can invade the pleural layers and infiltrate between the lower cords of the brachial plexus, and may involve the cervical sympathetic nerve chain, phrenic, and recurrent laryngeal nerves. It is usually secondary to a benign or malignant tumor; however, a large inflammatory process may cause this syndrome as well. The symptoms are as follows:
   i. Pain in shoulder and arm, particularly in the axilla and inner arm
   ii. Intrinsic hand muscle atrophy
   iii. Horner syndrome (enophthalmos, ptosis of the upper lid, constriction of the pupil with narrowing of the palpebral fissure, and decreased sweating homolaterally)
J. Congenital agenesis of the lung has been classified by Schneider as follows:
   i. *Class I*: Total agenesis.
   ii. *Class II*: Only the trachea is present.
   iii. *Class III*: Trachea and bronchi are present without any pulmonary tissue.
K. Apnea after tracheotomy is due to carbon dioxide narcosis causing the medulla to be depressed. Prior to the tracheotomy, the patient was breathing secondary to the lack of oxygen. After the tracheotomy, this oxygen drive is removed, and hence the patient remains apneic. Treatment is to ventilate the patient until the excess carbon dioxide level is reduced. Mediastinal emphysema and pneumothorax are the most common complications of tracheotomy.
L. Hypoxemia is defined as less than 75% oxygen saturation or less than 40 mm Hg Po_2. A methemoglobin level of more than 5 mg/dL produces cyanosis.
M. Bronchogenic cyst is a defect at the fourth week of gestation. It constitutes less than 5% of all mediastinal cysts and tumors.
N. The bronchial tree ring is cartilaginous until it reaches 1 mm in diameter. These small bronchioles without cartilaginous rings are held patent by the elastic property of the lung. The bronchial tree is lined by pseudostratified columnar ciliated epithelium as well as nonciliated cuboidal epithelium.
O. The adult trachea measures 10 to 12 cm and has 16 to 20 rings. The diameter is approximately 20 mm × 15 mm.
P. The larynx descends on inspiration and ascends on expiration. It also ascends in the process of swallowing and in the production of a high-pitched note.
Q. The esophageal lumen widens on inspiration.
R. The total lung surface measures 70 m^2. The lung contains 300 million alveoli. It secretes 200 mL of fluid per day.
S. During inspiration, the nose constitutes 79% of the total respiratory resistance, the larynx, 6%, and the bronchial tree, 15%. During expiration, the nose constitutes 75% of the resistance; the larynx, 3%, and the bronchial tree, 23%.
T. Tracheopathia osteoplastica is a rare disease characterized by growths of cartilage and bone within the walls of the trachea and bronchi that produce sessile plaques that project into the lumen. There is no specific treatment other than supportive. It is of unknown etiology. The serum calcium is normal, and there are no other calcium deposits.
U. Calcification found in a pulmonary nodule implies that it is a benign nodule.
V. Middle lobe syndrome may be present.
W. The right upper lobe and its bronchus is the lobe that is most susceptible to congenital anomaly.

X. Cystic fibrosis (mucoviscidosis) is familial and may be autosomal recessive. The patient presents with multiple polyps, pulmonary infiltration with abscesses, and rectal prolapse. The pancreas is afflicted with a fibrocystic process and produces no enzymes. Trypsin is lacking in the gastric secretion. Ten to fifteen percent of the patients pass trypsin in the stool. There is general malabsorption of liposoluble vitamins. Treatment consists of a high-protein, low-fat diet with water-soluble vitamins and pancreatic extracts. Many patients die of pulmonary abscesses.

Y. A person ventilated with pure oxygen for 7 minutes is cleared of 90% of the nitrogen and can withstand 5 to 8 minutes without further oxygenation.

Mediastinum

A. Suprasternal fossa has these characteristics:
   i. It is the region in which the sternocleidomastoid muscles converge toward their sternal attachments. Bound inferiorly by the suprasternal notch, they have no superior boundary.
   ii. The deep cervical fascia splits into an anterior and a posterior portion. These portions are attached to the anterior and posterior margins of the manubrium, respectively.
   iii. The space between these fascial layers is the small suprasternal space containing (1) anterior jugular veins and (2) fatty connective tissues.
   iv. Behind this space lies the pretracheal fascia.
   v. Laterally on each side are the medial borders of the sternohyoid and sternothyroid muscles.

B. In the adult the innominate artery crosses in front of the trachea, behind the upper half of the manubrium. In the child it crosses over the level of the superior border of the sternum.

C. The trachea enters the mediastinum on the right side.

D. The trachea bifurcates at T4-T5 or about 6 cm from the suprasternal notch. As a person approaches 65 years of age or more, it is possible that the trachea bifurcates at T6.

E. To the left of the trachea are the aorta, left recurrent laryngeal nerve, and left subclavian artery. To the right of the trachea are the superior vena cava, azygos vein, right vagus, and right lung pleura.

F. The innominate and left carotid arteries lie anterior to the trachea near their origin. As they ascend, the innominate artery lies to the right of the trachea.

G. The pulmonary artery passes anterior to the bronchi and assumes a position superior to the bronchi at the hilus, with the exception that the right upper lobe bronchus is superior to the right pulmonary artery.

H. The left main bronchus crosses in front of the esophagus. It presses on the esophagus and together with the aorta forms the bronchoaortic constriction. The first part of the aorta is to the left of the esophagus. As it descends, it assumes a left posterolateral position to the esophagus.

I. The course of the esophagus is as shown in Figure 7-7. The esophagus has four constricting points:
   i. Cricopharyngeus muscle.
   ii. Aorta crossing.
   iii. Left main stem bronchus crossing.
   iv. Diaphragm ($a < b = c < d$). At the level of c the esophagus passes from the superior mediastinum to the posterior mediastinum.

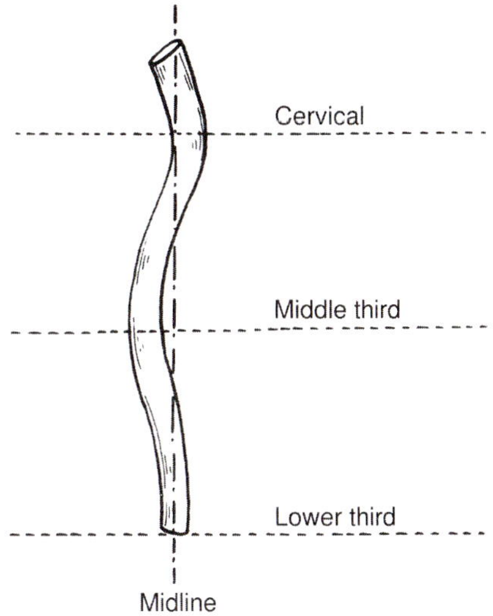

Figure 7-7 Course of the esophagus.

J. The following structures are found within the concavity of the aorta:
   i. Left main stem bronchus
   ii. Left recurrent laryngeal nerve
   iii. Tracheobronchial nodes
   iv. Superficial part of the cardiac plexus
K. The right main stem bronchus is wider, shorter, and follows a more vertical course than the left one.
L. The interior thyroid vein is immediately in front of the trachea in its infraisthmic portion.
M. Ten percent of the population has a thyroidea ima artery. It arises from either the innominate artery or the aorta and passes upward along the anterior aspect of the trachea.

Course of the Vagus

Left Side

A. It passes inferiorly between the left subclavian and the left carotid.
B. It follows the subclavian to its origin.
C. It passes to the left of the arch of the aorta.
D. It gives off the recurrent laryngeal nerve, which passes superiorly along the left border of the tracheoesophageal groove (between the esophagus and trachea).
E. The main vagus continues to descend behind the left main stem bronchus.

Right Side

A. It descends anterior to the subclavian where it gives off the recurrent laryngeal nerve that loops around the subclavian artery and ascends posteromedial to the right common carotid artery to reach the tracheoesophageal groove (between the esophagus and the trachea).

B. The main trunk descends posteriorly along the right side of the trachea, between the trachea and right pleura.
C. It descends posterior to the right bronchus.

Fascia of the Mediastinum

The space between the various mediastinal organs is occupied by loose areolar tissues. The fascial layers of the mediastinum are a direct continuation of the cervical fascia. A portion of the cervical fascia, the perivisceral fascia, encloses the larynx, pharynx, trachea, esophagus, thyroid, thymus, and carotid sheath contents. This space enclosed by this perivisceral fascia extends to the bifurcation of the trachea. Anteriorly it is bound by the pretracheal fascia. The pretracheal fascia is an important landmark in mediastinoscopy in that dissection should be done only beneath this layer.

Boundaries of the Mediastinum

See Figure 7-8.

A. *Lateral*: Parietal pleura
B. *Anterior*: Sternum
C. *Posterior*: Vertebrae
D. *Inferior*: Diaphragm
E. *Superior*: Superior aperture of the thorax

Superior Mediastinum The boundaries are as follows:

A. *Superior*: Superior aperture of the throat
B. *Anterior*: Manubrium with sternothyroid and sternohyoid muscles
C. *Posterior*: Upper thoracic vertebrae
D. *Inferior*: Manubrium to fourth vertebra

Structures of the superior mediastinum are the thymus, innominate veins, aorta, vagus, recurrent laryngeal nerve, phrenic nerve, azygos vein, esophagus, and thoracic duct.

Anterior Mediastinum It lies between the body of the sternum and the pericardium and contains the following:

A. Loose areolar tissues
B. Lymphatics

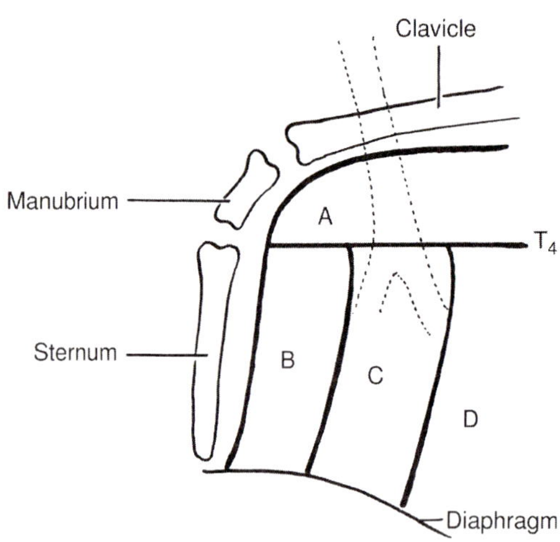

Figure 7-8 Various chambers of the mediastinum. A. superior mediastinum; B. anterior mediastinum; C. middle mediastinum; D. posterior mediastinum.

C. Lymph nodes
D. Thymus gland

Middle Mediastinum It contains the heart, ascending aorta, superior vena cava, azygos vein, bifurcation of the main bronchus, pulmonary artery trunk, right and left pulmonary veins, phrenic nerves, and the tracheobronchial lymph nodes.

Posterior Mediastinum Anteriorly lie the bifurcation of the trachea, the pulmonary vein, the pericardium, and the posterior part of the upper surface of the diaphragm. Posteriorly lies the vertebral column from T4 to T12. Laterally lies the mediastinal pleura.

The posterior mediastinum contains the thoracic aorta, azygos vein, hemizygous vein, cranial nerve X, splanchnic nerve, esophagus, thoracic duct, posterior mediastinal lymph nodes, and the intercostal arteries.

Lymph Nodes of the Thorax

See Figure 7-9.

A. Parietal nodes are inconsequential clinically. They are grouped into intercostal, sternal, and phrenic nodes.

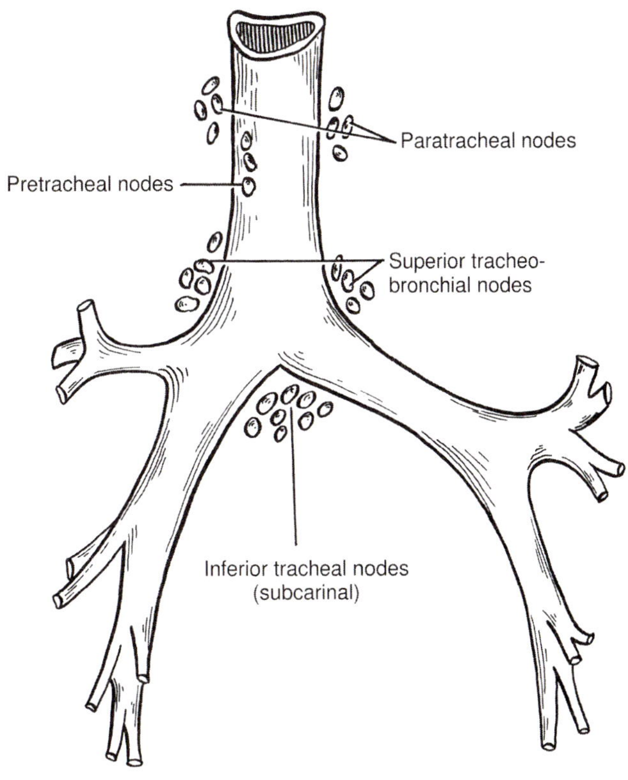

Figure 7-9 Thoracic lymph nodes.

B. Visceral nodes are of greater clinical importance. They are grouped as follows:
   i. Peritracheobronchial
      a. Paratracheal
      b. Pretracheal
      c. Superior tracheobronchial
      d. Inferior tracheobronchial
   ii. Bronchopulmonary (hilar nodes)
   iii. Anterior mediastinal or prevascular
   iv. Pulmonary
   v. Posterior mediastinal

Lymphatic Drainage of the Lung

Right Side

A. *Superior area (anteromedial area of the right upper lobe)*: Right paratracheal nodes
B. *Middle area (posterolateral area of right upper lobe, right middle lobe, and superior right lower lobe)*: Right paratracheal nodes and inferior tracheobronchial nodes
C. *Inferior area (lower half of right lower lobe)*: Inferior tracheobronchial nodes and posterior mediastinal nodes

Left Side

A. *Superior area (upper left upper lobe)*: Left paratracheal, anterior mediastinal, and sub-aortic nodes
B. *Middle area (lower left upper lobe and upper left lower lobe)*: Left paratracheal, inferior tracheobronchial, and anterior mediastinal nodes
C. *Inferior area (inferior part of the left lower lobe)*: Inferior tracheobronchial nodes. (Inferior tracheobronchial nodes drain into the right paratracheal nodes.)
   i. *Right upper lung*: Right neck
   ii. *Right lower lung*: Right neck
   iii. *Left lower lung*: Right neck
   iv. *Left upper lung*: Left neck
   v. *Lingular lobe*: Both sides of the neck

Purposes of Mediastinoscopy

Barium swallow and tracheogram are usually obtained before mediastinoscopy if indicated.

A. Histologic diagnosis
B. To determine which nodes are involved
C. To make the diagnosis of sarcoidosis

Mediastinal Tumors

One-third of all mediastinal tumors are malignant. Among the malignant ones, lymphoma is most commonly encountered.

A. *Superior mediastinum*: Thyroid, neurinoma, thymoma, parathyroid
B. *Anterior mediastinum*: Dermoid, teratoma, thyroid, thymoma
C. *Low anterior mediastinum*: Pericardial cyst

D. *Middle mediastinum*: Pericardial cyst, bronchial cyst, lymphoma, carcinoma
E. *Posterior mediastinum*: Neurinoma, enterogenous cyst

Superior Vena Cava Syndrome

A. *Etiology*: Malignant metastasis, mediastinal tumors, mediastinal fibrosis, vena cava thrombosis
B. *Signs and symptoms*: Edema and cyanosis of the face, neck, and upper extremities; venous hypertension with dilated veins; normal venous pressure of the lower extremities; visible venous circulation of the anterior chest wall

Endoscopy

Size of Tracheotomy Tubes and Bronchoscopes

Age	*Tracheotomy tubes*	*Bronchoscope (mm)*
Premature	No. 000 × 26 mm to No. 00 × 33 mm	3
6 months	No. 0 × 33 mm to No. 0 × 40 mm	3.5
18 months	No. 1 × 46 mm	4
5 years	No. 2 × 50 mm	5
10 years	No. 3 × 50 mm to No. 4 × 68 mm	6
Adult		7

Esophagoscopy

A. Size of the esophagoscope
B. *Child*: 5 mm × 35 mm or 6 mm × 35 mm.
C. *Adult*: 9 mm × 50 mm.
D. Average distance from incisor teeth to other areas during esophagoscopy (Figure 7-10).
E. *Left lung*: Lobes and segments.
  i. Upper division of upper lobe
    a. Apical posterior
    b. Anterior
  ii. Lower division of upper lobe
    a. Superior
    b. Inferior
  iii. Lower lobe
    a. Superior
    b. Anteromedial basal
    c. Lateral basal
    d. Posterior basal
F. *Right lung*: Lobes and segments
  i. Upper lobe
    a. Apical
    b. Posterior
    c. Anterior

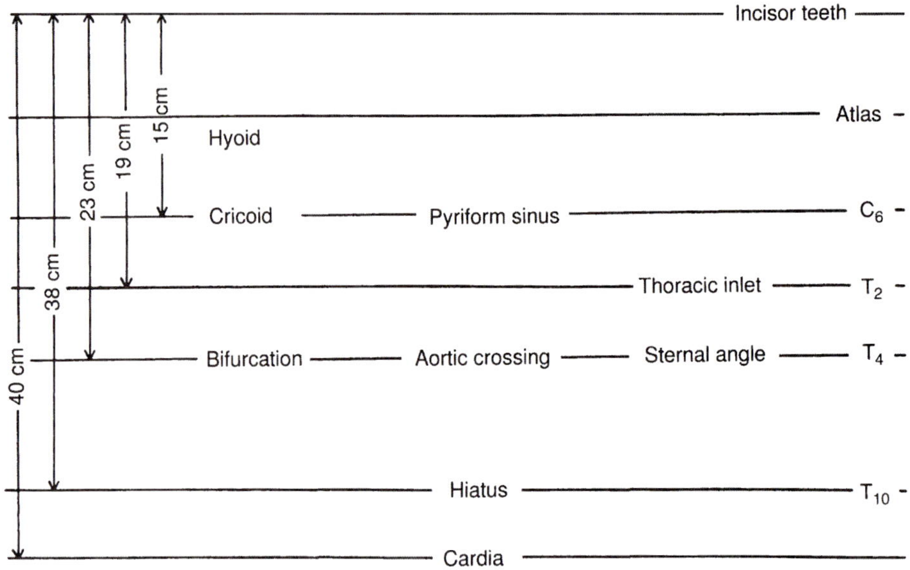

Figure 7-10 Relative landmarks for esophagoscopy.

- ii. Middle lobe
    - a. Lateral
    - b. Medial
- iii. Lower lobe
    - a. Superior
    - b. Medial basal
    - c. Anterior basal
    - d. Lateral basal
    - e. Posterior basal

G. Relative contraindications for esophagoscopy
- i. Aneurysm of the aorta
- ii. Spinal deformities, osteophytes
- iii. Esophageal burns and steroid treatment

H. Relative contraindications for bronchography
- i. Acute infection
- ii. Acute asthmatic attacks
- iii. Acute cardiac failure

I. Causes of hemoptysis (in order of decreasing frequency):
- i. Bronchiectasis
- ii. Adenoma
- iii. Tracheobronchitis
- iv. Tuberculosis
- v. Mitral stenosis
    - a. Foreign bodies
        1. *Right upper lobe bronchus*: Most common site
        2. *Left upper lobe bronchus*: Second most common site
        3. *Trachea*: Least likely site

4. *Cervical esophagus*: Most common site for esophageal foreign bodies
5. *Most common foreign bodies in children*: Peanuts, safety pins, coins
6. *Most common foreign bodies in adults*: Meat and bone

Vascular Anomalies

See Chapter 45. The normal great vessels are shown in Figure 7-11.

A. *Double aortic arch*: This anomaly is a true vascular ring. It is due to the persistence of the right fourth branchial arch vessel. The symptoms include stridor, intermittent dysphagia, and aspiration pneumonitis. The right posterior arch is usually the larger of the two arches.

B. *Right aortic arch with ligamentum arteriosus*: It is due to the persistence of the right fourth branchial arch vessel becoming the aorta instead of the left fourth arch vessel. This vessel crosses the trachea, causing an anterior compression.

C. *Anomalous right subclavian artery*: It is due to the right subclavian artery arising from the dorsal aorta, causing posterior compression of the esophagus. There is no constriction over the trachea.

D. *Anomalous innominate and/or left common carotid*: The innominate arises too far left from the aorta. It crosses the trachea anteriorly, causing anterior compression. The left common carotid arises from the aorta on the right or from the innominate artery. It also causes anterior compression of the trachea. In a variant of this anomaly, the innominate and the right common carotid arise from the same trunk, and when they divide, they encircle the trachea and esophagus, causing airway obstruction as well as dysphagia.

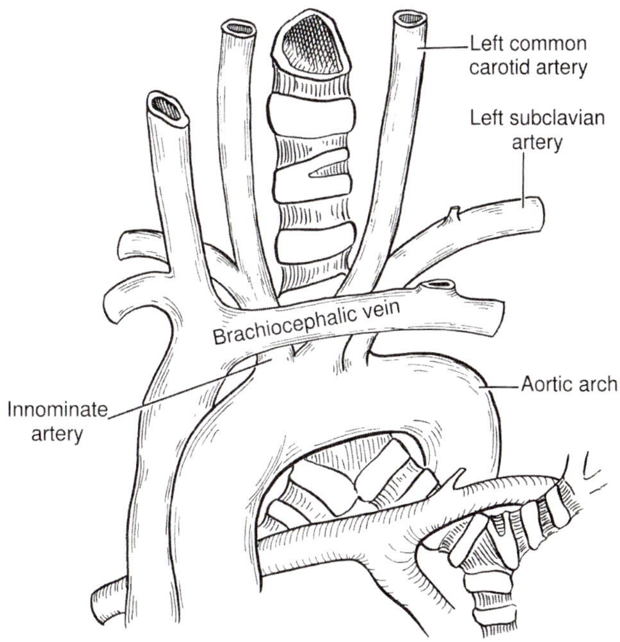

Figure 7-11 Normal great vessels.

E. Patent ductus arteriosus.
F. Coarctation of the aorta.
G. *Enlarged heart*: An enlarged heart, especially with mitral insufficiency, can compress the left bronchus.
H. *Dysphagia lusoria*: This term is used to include dysphagia caused by any aberrant great vessel. The common cause is an abnormal subclavian artery arising from the descending aorta.
I. *Anomalous innominate arteries*: They have been estimated to be the most common vascular anomaly. They cause anterior compression of the trachea. During bronchoscopy, if the pulsation is obliterated with the bronchoscope, the radial pulse on the right arm and the temporal pulse are reduced. In the case of a subclavian anomaly, the bronchoscope compressing the abnormal subclavian produces a decrease in the radial pulse, although the temporal pulse remains normal. A bronchoscope compressing a double aortic arch pulsation produces no pulse changes in either the radial or the temporal pulse.

Diseases Producing Limitation of Airflow

Pulmonary diseases that produce a reduction in the flow of air through airways more than 2 mm in diameter produce spirometric evidence for this limited airflow. Airflow limitation is reflected on the spirometer tracings as a reduction in FVC and FEV_1. In addition, the FEV_1/FVC ratio falls below the predicted normal value. Functional residual capacity is elevated, as is the RV. In more advanced cases, the total lung capacity is also increased.

An abnormal spirogram does not indicate the cause of disease, as asthma, chronic bronchitis, and emphysema all show evidence of airflow limitation. When a spirometric tracing reveals evidence of airflow limitation, the patient is normally given a bronchodilator (eg, metaproterenol) and the test is repeated.

Patients with reversible airflow limitation, such as asthma, most often demonstrate 15% to 20% improvement in dynamic lung volumes following administration of a bronchodilator. These patients are described as exhibiting "reversible airflow limitation."

Patients whose pre- and postbronchodilator tracings do not vary may have chronic bronchitis or emphysema, or may be in the throes of an asthmatic attack that is so severe that the response to the bronchodilator is muted. It is, therefore, not possible to eliminate asthma as a diagnostic possibility if the postbronchodilator study does not show reversibility.

Because the incidence of postoperative pulmonary complications increases with the severity of airflow limitation, it is important to perform spirometry on all patients who, based on history and physical findings, are likely to have pulmonary diseases characterized by obstruction of flow. If the spirogram is abnormal and indicative of obstruction, a bronchodilator should be given. If reversibility is demonstrated, the patient is given a bronchodilator prior to surgery to maximize his or her lung function preoperatively and reduce the incidence of postoperative complications.

Restrictive Lung Disease

The spirometric abnormality produced by patients with restrictive lung disease differs significantly from the curves produced by patients with chronic airflow limitation. Patients with restrictive lung disease exhibit a reduction in their total lung capacity. Diseases that produce restriction include diseases in which a functioning lung is replaced by granulomas or fibrosis (eg, sarcoid or interstitial fibrosis), diseases that lead to restricted expansion of the lungs as seen in primary neurologic disorders (amyotrophic lateral sclerosis) or primary muscle disorders (muscular dystrophy), diseases in which there is a reduction in the amount of functioning lung (pneumonectomy), and diseases in which there is a reduction in lung expansion (scoliosis and fibrothorax).

The spirometric tracing of a patient with restrictive lung disease demonstrates a reduction in FVC and FEV_1, but the FEV_1/FVC ratio is preserved. Whereas with chronic airflow limitation the values for functional residual capacity, RV, and total lung capacity are elevated, in restrictive lung diseases these values are reduced.

Patients with restrictive lung diseases do not demonstrate improvement after the administration of bronchodilators, as the defect in restrictive lung diseases does not lie in the airways per se.

Bibliography

Bates D. *Respiratory Function in Disease.* 3rd ed. Philadelphia, PA: W.B. Saunders; 1989.

Bickerman HA. Lung volumes, capacities, and thoracic volumes. In: Chusid EL, ed. *The Selective and Comprehensive Testing of Adult Pulmonary Function.* United Kingdom, UK: Futura Publishing Company; 1983:5.

Bone RC, Dantzker DR, George RB, et al. *Pulmonary and Critical Care Medicine.* Vol 1 and 2. St. Louis, MO: Mosby Year Book; 1993.

Cherniack N. *Chronic Obstructive Pulmonary Disease.* Philadelphia, PA: W.B. Saunders; 1991.

Comroe JH Jr. *Physiology of Respiration.* 2nd ed. Chicago, IL: Mosby Year Book; 1974.

Questions

1. Spirometric evidence of obstructive airways disease is based on
   A. Reduced FEV_1
   B. Reduced FEV_1/FEV ratio
   C. Both

2. Increased work of breathing could be due to
   A. Decreased pulmonary function
   B. Airway obstruction
   C. Decreased muscle function
   D. All of the above

3. A 6-minute walk distance is a good indicator of cardiopulmonary performance.
   A. True
   B. False

4. Amiodarone lung toxicity may provide a good model for understanding the immune function of the lung.
   A. True
   B. False

5. Flow volume loops can help distinguish between intra- and extrathoracic sites of airway obstruction.
   A. True
   B. False

Chapter 8
Related Ophthalmology for ENT

Orbit

A. The orbit forms a quadrilateral pyramid: roof, floor, medial wall, and lateral wall.
   i. *Roof*: Orbital process of the frontal bone, lesser wing of the sphenoid
   ii. *Floor*: Orbital plate of maxilla, orbital surface of zygoma, orbital process of the palatine bone
   iii. *Medial wall*: Frontal process of maxilla, lacrimal bone, sphenoid bone, lamina papyracea of the ethmoid bone
   iv. *Lateral wall*: Lesser and greater wings of the sphenoid, zygoma
B. The trochlea, a pulley through which runs the tendon of the superior oblique muscle, is located between the roof and the medial wall.
   i. The trochlea is the only cartilage in the orbit.
   ii. A displaced trochlea causes diplopia on downward gaze.
   iii. *Trochleitis* is the inflammation of the trochlea or the paratracheal region.
      - It causes pain and tenderness locally without extraocular movement deficit.
      - It is diagnosed with CT scan.
      - Treatments include oral NSAIDs, if nonresponding, oral or local steroid injection.
C. The anterior and posterior ethmoid foramina are situated at the junction between the frontal and ethmoid bones, on the frontal side of the suture line.
D. The inferior orbital fissure is in the floor of the orbit.
   i. It is bound by the greater wing of the sphenoid, orbital surface of the maxilla, and orbital process of the palatine bone.
   ii. It transmits the two branches of the CN V2 (infraorbital nerve and the zygomatic nerve), fine branches from the sphenopalatine ganglion to the lacrimal gland, infraorbital artery and vein, and ophthalmic vein branch.
E. The superior orbital fissure lies between the roof and the lateral wall of the nose. It is a gap between the lesser and the greater wings of the sphenoid bone.
   i. It transmits cranial nerves (CNs) III, IV, V1, VI, the superior orbital vein, ophthalmic vein, orbital branch of the middle meningeal artery, and recurrent branch of the lacrimal artery.
   ii. Compression of the structures in the superior orbital fissure by a bony fragment or mass causes *superior orbital fissure syndrome*, which presents with ophthalmoplegia, ptosis, fixed and dilated pupil without vision loss.

F. The optic canal runs from the middle cranial fossa into the apex of the orbit. It is formed by a curvilinear portion of the lesser wing of the sphenoid bone.
   i. The optic nerve and ophthalmic artery course through the optic canal.
   ii. *Orbital apex syndrome* is typically caused by a compressive lesion near the orbital apex.
      - complete ophthalmoplegia
      - Ptosis
      - fixed and dilated pupil
      - visual function impairment
      - ipsilateral upper face hypesthesia from CN II, III, IV, V1, and VI involvement.

G. The cavernous sinus is NOT a part of the orbit, nevertheless it is considered a crucial ophthalmic structure.
   i. It extends from the superior orbital fissure and is bordered by the sphenoid bone and temporal bone.
   ii. CN III, IV, V1, and V2 travel through the two dural layers of the lateral wall.
   iii. CN VI lies free in the cavernous sinus.
   iv. Sympathetic fibers travel along the internal carotid artery into the cavernous sinus, where they join CN V1 to enter the orbit.
   v. The superior and inferior ophthalmic veins drain into the cavernous sinus.
   vi. *Tolosa-Hunt syndrome* is an idiopathic inflammation of the cavernous sinus.
      - episodic orbital pain associated with one or more of CN III, IV or VI palsy.
      - nonspecific evidence of inflammation in the cavernous sinus on imaging.
      - The diagnosis is clinical.
      - responds to systemic steroids but may run a relapsing-remitting course.
   vii. *Carotid-cavernous fistula* (C-C fistula) can occur after head or facial trauma.
      - pulsatile exophthalmos
      - dilated and tortuous "cork-screw" conjunctival vessels
      - and periorbital bruit by auscultation are pathognomonic features
      - CTA, MRA, or color Doppler can assist in the diagnosis of the fistula, but cerebral angiography remains the gold standard
      - Some low risk C-C fistulas may close spontaneously and can be monitored closely.
      - Endovascular approaches have replaced open surgery to become the primary surgical treatment. Options include detachable balloon occlusion, coil or material embolization, covered stent graft placement and parental artery occlusion.
   viii. *Cavernous sinus thrombosis* is a life-threatening condition most often following central facial infections (such as abscess, cellulitis, sinusitis, pharyngitis, tonsillitis, otitis media, mastoiditis, dental infections), and is therefore septic.
      - Other causes are surgeries, trauma, or hypercoagulable states.
      - The ocular findings are found in almost all cases.
      - Periorbital edema, chemosis, ptosis, proptosis, pain with eye movement.
      - Partial or complete ophthalmoplegia can occur rapidly.
      - Nonreactive pupil and diminished facial sensation can also occur.
      - Immediate treatment with antimicrobial and antithrombotic agents is indicated.

Lids

A. The upper lid contains the following:
   i. Orbicularis oculi—innervated by CN VII
   ii. Levator palpebrae superioris—innervated by CN III
   iii. Müller muscle—innervated by sympathetic fibers

iv. Tarsal plate—made of thick connective tissue, houses the meibomian glands
v. Meibomian glands—open at the lid margins, produce meibum into the tear film.
- Hordeolum (or a stye) is an acutely inflamed meibomian gland.
- In chronic stage, the rubbery nodule on the lid is called a chalazion.

vi. Sweat glands—produce sweat on the skin
vii. Exocrine glands of Krause and Wolfring—produce aqueous tears on the conjunctiva

B. The lower lid contains the following:
i. Orbicularis oculi
ii. Lower lid retractors
iii. Tarsal plate
iv. Sweat glands
v. Meibomian glands
vi. Exocrine glands of Krause and Wolfring

C. Lateral palpebral ligament is also called lateral canthal tendon.
i. Unites the lateral ends of the tarsal plates.
ii. Fixes onto the orbital surface of the zygomatic bone.
iii. A displaced lateral canthal tendon may give rise to an inferiorly displaced canthus or slight ptosis.

D. The medial tarsal ends divide into superficial/anterior and deep/posterior heads.
i. The superficial heads unite and form the medial canthal tendon, which anchors the eyelids medially.
ii. If the medial canthal tendon loses its support, a rounding of the medial aspect of the eyelid leads to *pseudohypertelorism.*
iii. The deep heads form the muscular diaphragm over the lacrimal fossa, envelope the puncti, and swing back to attach to the posterior lacrimal crest, establishing the "lacrimal pump" mechanism.
iv. Disruption of this muscle attachment may result in epiphora.

E. The septum orbitale/orbital septum is the orbital periosteum extending into the lid to attach to the tarsal plates.
i. It separates the eyelid from the orbital contents.
ii. It keeps the orbital fat from entering the lid, which contains no subcutaneous fat.
iii. The superior orbital septum attaches to the levator apparatus with subsequent attachment to the tarsal plate.
iv. The inferior septum attaches directly to the tarsal plate.
v. Medially, the septum is fused with the palpebral ligament leading toward the posterior lacrimal crest.

F. The suspensory ligament of Lockwood
i. A continuous band of fibrous tissue slung beneath the eyeball from side to side.
ii. Its ends blend with the cheek ligaments and with the medial and lateral horns of the aponeurosis of the levator palpebrae superioris.

G. The lower lid retractors are the capsulopalpebral heads of the inferior rectus/inferior oblique complex.
i. Cause a slight retraction of the lower lid with forced openings.
ii. Fibers can be separately supplied by the sympathetic nerves and CN III.

H. Control of the eyelids
i. The upper lid is opened by levator palpebrae superior (CN III) and Müller muscle (sympathetic fibers).
ii. The lids are closed by the orbicularis oculi (CN VII).

iii. The ophthalmic division of CN V is responsible for the sensory innervation to the upper lid (V1 branch) and the lower lid (V1 and V2).
iv. *Entropion*: Turning in of the lid margin, most commonly from the lower lid retractor weakness and obicularis oculi override.
v. *Ectropion*: Turning out of the lid margin, commonly from tissue laxity from aging.
vi. *Horner syndrome*: Impaired sympathetic input, most commonly from injury of the superior cervical sympathetic trunk, giving rise to ipsilateral ptosis, miosis (anisocoria greater in the dark), and anhidrosis with apparent enophthalmos. The ptosis is caused by weakness or paralysis of Müller muscle, which can account for up to 2 mm of upper lid retraction.
vii. *Ptosis* often results from levator palpebrae dehiscence, CN III palsy secondary to diabetic microvascular disease and posterior communicating artery aneurysm, and myasthenia gravis. The underlying cause should be carefully identified to decrease morbidity and mortality.
viii. *Lagophthalmos* is the inability to close the eyelids completely. The causes include:
- Traumatic loss of lid tissue
- Cicatricial changes of lid skin secondary to thermal burn, chemical burn, and connective tissue disease
- Facial nerve palsy such as in unsafe chronic suppurative otitis media (CSOM), Bell palsy, skull base tumors and/or surgeries, parotid tumor and surgeries, and trauma
- Treatments are frequent lubrication (up to hourly) with preservative-free artificial tears is necessary to prevent cornea damage from prolonged exposure; taping the eyelids closed at night is preferred if possible; surgical treatments include tarsorrhaphy and lid weight.

Extraocular Muscles

A. The six extraocular muscles and their functions are as follows:
i. Lateral rectus (LR), to adduct
ii. Medial rectus (MR), to abduct
iii. Superior rectus (SR), to elevate (and intort)
iv. Inferior rectus (IR), to depress (and extort)
v. Superior oblique (SO), to intort (depress and abduct)
vi. Inferior oblique (IO), to extort (elevate and adduct)

B. There are six cardinal directions of gaze, in which the yoke (coupled) muscles work concertedly to maintain the same gaze in both eyes. In each of these gaze directions, one of the six extra muscles on each eyeball is positioned in the most advantageous orientation, therefore, becomes the main muscle in action. Of note, it is different from the primary function of each muscle (see A). In this scenario, assume both eyes are already in the designated gaze position and certain muscles are in a more advantageous position for action than others.
i. To the right, right LR and left MR
ii. To the left, right MR and left LR
iii. Up and to the right, right SR and left IO
iv. Down and to the right, right IR and left SO
v. Up and to the left, right IO and left SR
vi. Down and to the left, right SO and left IR

C. Innovation of the extraocular muscles
   i. The LR—CN VI
   ii. SO—CN IV
   iii. All the rest—CN III
D. *Extrocular muscle entrapment* in an inferior orbital fracture
   i. IR is the most commonly trapped muscle.
   ii. IO is the second most likely trapped muscle.
   iii. Symptoms: Diplopia and pain when looking up, nausea, bradycardia.
   iv. More likely in younger patients with nondisplaced fracture of the orbital floor, as opposed to an elderly patient with a large blowout fracture.
   v. Clinical diagnosis: To differentiate paralysis of the elevators from trapping of the IR or IO, the "forced duction test" is performed under local or general anesthesia. If the globe moves freely (compared to the unaffected opposite globe), there is no entrapment.
   vi. The entrapment itself may or may not be visible on imaging.
E. *Diplopia*
   i. The evaluation of diplopia is difficult and requires a detailed ophthalmologic examination (sensory motor test).
   ii. Monocular diplopia results from pathology in one eye such as cataract or refractive error.
   iii. Binocular diplopia results from misalignment of the two eyes in one or more gaze directions.
   iv. Binocular diplopia has a muscular or neurologic etiology.
   v. To diagnose true binocular diplopia, cover either eye; the diplopia resolves.
   vi. One or both eyes can be affected to cause binocular diplopia, such as in unilateral versus bilateral CN VI palsy. Cover uncover test of each eye should be performed.
   vii. Sometimes more than one extraocular muscle is involved, such as in CN III palsy, MR, IR, SR, and IO are all paralyzed.
   viii. Injury to the trochlea can occur during frontal sinus floor trephine or external ethmoidectomy, causing SO dysfunction and subsequent oblique diplopia.

Lacrimal System

A. The lacrimal gland (a serous gland predominantly) is in a fossa within the zygomatic process of the frontal bone.
   i. Lacrimal gland secretes tears through 17 to 20 openings.
   ii. Although the gland is developed at birth, secretion of tears does not take place until 2 weeks after birth.
   iii. The tear film comprises aqueous (lacrimal gland), mucous (goblet cells on the conjunctiva), and oil (meibomian glands on the lid margins).
B. The lacrimal sac (for tear drainage) lies in a fossa bound by the lacrimal bone, the frontal process of the maxilla, and the nasal process of the frontal bone.
   i. The lacrimal sac is about 12 mm long.
   ii. It collects drainage from the common canaliculus.
   iii. Superior and inferior canaliculi join to form the common canaliculus.
   iv. Each canaliculus has a vertical portion (~2 mm) and a horizontal portion (~8 mm).
   v. A punctum is the opening of the superior or inferior canaliculus at the lid margin.

C. The nasolacrimal duct drains the lacrimal sac and empties into the anterior portion of the inferior meatus. It is about 17 mm long.
   i. *Nasolacrimal duct obstruction* is a common cause of tearing.
   ii. The most common site of congenital obstruction is a stricture of the valve of Hasner, of the nasolacrimal duct, at the inferior meatus.
   iii. Acquired obstruction occurs primarily in the upper collecting system.
      - infection (dacryocystitis)—often with the formation of dacryoliths
      - trauma
      - retained foreign body (punctal plugs)
      - idiopathic, commonly seen in postmenopausal women.

D. Laceration of one or both canaliculi requires insertion of a silicone tube, which is looped between the inferior and superior puncti in the medial corner of the eye, brought through the nasolacrimal duct, and tied together within the nasal cavity. The laceration can be sutured over the tube, which is left in place for 6 weeks to 3 months.

The Globe

A. The cornea is a transparent, strong, and compact multilayered tissue in the center of the ocular surface.
   i. It consists of five basic layers: the epithelium, Bowman layer, stroma, Descemet membrane, and the endothelium.
   ii. A healthy normal cornea is avascular.
   iii. The density of the nerve fiber endings is 20 to 600 times higher than anywhere else, which explains the unusually high sensitivity.
   iv. The combined refractive power of the cornea and the tear film is about twice as much as that of the natural lens. Laser refractive surgery alters the refractive power by reshaping the cornea stroma with laser.
   v. Any cornea pathology, including dry eyes, can affect vision significantly.
   vi. *Herpes simplex* virus (HSV), typically HSV-1, can be a latent viral infection in CN V with a high recurrence rate.
      - It most frequently presents as *cold sore.*
      - It can cause severe ocular damage including *cornea scarring, neovascularization, uveitis, iris atrophy, glaucoma, and retinal necrosis.*
      - HSV ocular infection typically presents as a vesicular rash of the lids, conjunctival injection with severe pain.
      - Cornea dendrites are diagnostic.
      - The treatment of choice is oral acyclovir.
   vii. *Herpes Zoster* virus (VZV) can cause severe ocular damage like HSV.
      - The presentation typically includes vesicular rash in CN V1 distribution, conjunctival injection and pain.
      - The treatment of choice is oral valacyclovir.
      - Topical antiviral eyedrops are second-line treatment for resistant or high-risk HSV and VZV cases.
   viii. A corneal ulcer can be infectious or noninfectious.
      - Infectious corneal ulcer can be caused by bacteria, virus, fungus, and protozoa.
      - Sterile cornea ulcer can be neurotrophic or immune mediated.
      - Sometimes cornea transplant is necessary if perforation occurs.

B. The conjunctiva is a thin and vascular epithelial membrane that covers the anterior sclera and the inner surface of the eyelids.
   i. It houses many secretive glands as previously described in the eyelid section.
   ii. It is a very sensitive indicator of the inflammatory status of the eye due to the rich vasculature.
   iii. The limbal stem cells repopulate the cornea epithelium and serve as the barrier between the clear and avascular cornea epithelium and the opaque, highly vascular conjunctival epithelium.
   iv. In various *limbal stem cell deficiency* (LSCD) conditions, the border of the conjunctival epithelium and corneal epithelium is violated.
      - Pterygium—a triangular-shaped overgrowth of the conjunctiva onto the cornea as a result of UV exposure.
      - Chemical burn
      - Steven-Johnson syndrome
      - Ocular cicatricial pemphigoid—diagnosed by antibasement membrane antibody
      - Ocular graft versus host disease (oGVHD)—one of organ manifestation of GVHD
      - Contact lens overwear
      - Chronic ocular allergy
      - Trauma, including iatrogenic from previous ocular surgery
      - Previous ocular infectious diseases
      - Persistent corneal epithelial defects, scarring, inflammation, corneal melt, and corneal graft rejection can all result from LSCD, which can lead to chronic pain and vision loss.
      - The best treatment is an autologous limbal stem cell transplant with healthy limbal stem cells from either eye of the same patient. Allogeneic limbal stem cell transplantation (from cadaver or live donor) and cultured oral mucosa stem cells are possible for bilateral LSCD, with a lower success rate.
   v. *Viral conjunctivitis* is a very common ocular infection. Any common virus that causes upper respiratory infection can cause viral conjunctivitis.
      - It is most likely cause of conjunctivitis in the adult population.
      - The symptoms include red, irritated eye(s) with copious, viscous, watery discharge.
      - It often spreads from one eye to the other and runs a self-limited course.
      - Contrary to the common belief, treatment is usually not necessary.
      - The only exception is *endemic keratoconjunctivis* (EKC), which is caused by a group of adenoviruses, can cause cornea infiltrates and conjunctival symblepharon, and permanent damage to vision. Urgent ophthalmologic care is warranted in such a condition.
      - Bacterial conjunctivitis is relatively uncommon in immunocompetent adult population.

C. The sclera is composed of dense connective tissue for structural support.
   i. All extraocular muscles insert into the sclera.
   ii. The inflammation of the sclera can range from mild painless episcleritis to painful and blinding necrotizing scleritis.
   iii. Scleritis has strong associations with autoimmune disease, and the treatment often requires systemic treatments including NSAIDs, corticosteroids, and immunomodulatory agents.

D. The uvea is the continuous middle layer of the eye with a very rich blood supply. It is divided anatomically into the iris, the ciliary body, and the choroid.
   i. The iris is the only visible part of the uvea. It controls the amount of light entering the eye by changing the size of the pupil.
      - The circular sphincter pupillae muscle constricts the pupil following the parasympathetic input by way of CN III (see *diabetic CN III palsy*).
      - The radial dilator pupillae muscle widens the pupil following the sympathetic input by way of CN V1 (see *Horner syndrome*).
   ii. The most important function of the ciliary body is to produce the aqueous humor.
      - It drains anteriorly through the trabecular meshwork located at the iris roots.
      - The dysregulation of the aqueous humor production and drainage can lead to abnormal intraocular pressure, which is found in most types of *glaucoma*.
      - Ciliary body also controls accommodation, which is the ability to increase the refractive power of the eye to focus on near objects by changing the shape and position of the lens.
      - The ability to accommodate typically starts to decrease after age 40 and diminishes by age 60, which is called *presbyopia*. The mechanism of loss of accommodation is not fully understood.
      - In addition to the traditional bifocal or progressive glasses, multifocal contact lenses and multifocal intraocular lenses (implanted during a cataract surgery) have added to the mainstream options for presbyopia treatment.
      - Presbyopic laser refractive surgery and adjustable intraocular lens are under active research and clinical trials.
   iii. The choroid is the most vascular-rich structure in the eye.
      - It lies between the sclera and the entire retina.
      - It is responsible for oxygen supply and supports the metabolism of the outer layer of the retina.
      - The most common location for *ocular metastasis* is the choroid, from the most common primary malignancies, breast and lung cancers.
   iv. The inflammation of any part of the uvea is called *uveitis*, which is seen in a very wide variety of ocular and systemic inflammatory conditions.
      - *Anterior uveitis*—iris
      - *Intermediate uveitis*—the ciliary body, the anterior vitreous, and the peripheral retina
      - *Posterior uveitis*—the choroid and the posterior retina
      - *Panuveitis* involves all parts of the uvea.
      - *Retinal vasculitis* has a strong association with and is therefore often considered an integral part of uveitis.
      - *Uveitis* can result from trauma, infection (viral, bacterial, and parasitic), local or systemic inflammation (sympathetic ophthalmia, sarcoidosis, multiple sclerosis, Behcet disease, and all collagen vascular diseases).
      - There is a significant portion of uveitis considered idiopathic when all diagnostic tests appear negative.

E. The natural crystalline lens is a transparent biconvex structure that is enclosed in the lens capsule.
   i. From the outer layer in, the lens is divided into the cortex, the epinucleus, and the nucleus structurally.
   ii. The lens is suspended in position by fibrous strings called zonules of Zinn that originated from the ciliary body.

iii. The lens is nourished completely by the aqueous humor, as the fetal blood vessels to the lens completely regress before birth in normal development.
iv. The lens continuously grows in diameter and depth throughout life.
v. The major function of the lens is refractive.
vi. *Cataract* refers to the opacification of the lens which interferes with vision.
vii. Cataract formation is accelerated by normal aging, UV exposure, radiation, steroid use, trauma, infection, diabetes, and a number of congenital diseases.
viii. The only effective treatment of cataract is surgical removal with intraocular lens implantation.

F. The vitreous is a clear, viscous matrix occupying the posterior segment made of water, hyaluronic acid, and collagen fibers.
i. The vitreous occupies 80% of the globe volume.
ii. The vitreous is tightly attached to the vitreous base (at the most peripheral part of the retina), the retinal vessels, the optic nerve head, and the macula.
iii. With age, the vitreous shrinks and more liquified pockets form within.
iv. *Posterior vitreous detachment* refers to the separation of the vitreous from the retina, which can generate "floaters" or "spider web" in vision as a very common complaint. Occasionally, the separation traction can cause retina tears, which increases the risk of *retinal detachment.*

G. The retina is a neurosensory tissue that converts light into an electric signal.
i. There are two types of photoreceptors in humans, the rods and the cones.
ii. Different cones can selectively sense the red, green, and blue light, therefore responsible for color vision.
iii. The rods are responsible for night vision and peripheral vision.
iv. The central retina bordered by the superior and inferior temporal arcade vessels is called the macula.
v. The central 1.5 mm of the macula is the fovea, where only cones exist. The high density of cones in the fovea allows better visual acuity.
vi. Common retina pathologies that can be vision threatening:
- *Age-related macular degeneration*
- *Diabetic retinopathy*
- *Epiretinal membrane*
- *Macular hole*
- *Retinal detachment*

vii. *Usher syndrome* is one of the rare hereditary conditions.
- Characterized by neurosensory hearing loss and gradual vision loss from retinitis pigmentosa.
- Many gene mutations have been identified in Usher syndrome, most of which cause the loss of hair cells in the inner ear and the loss of rods and cones in the retina.
- The most common mutations found are MYO7A and CDH23 for Usher syndrome type I; USH2A for type II and CLRN1 for type III.

H. The optic nerve contains about 1 million axons of the retina ganglion cells, which transmit the visual signals to the brain.
i. The optic disc is the only visible portion of the optic nerve by direct observation.
ii. *Optic disc edema* is an important indicator of elevated intracranial pressure.
iii. *Optic neuritis* can be the presenting sign of multiple sclerosis.
iv. Various space-occupying lesions in the orbit or brain can cause compressive optic neuropathy.

v. Glaucoma is the most common optic neuropathy.
  - It affects 60 million people around the world.
  - It is the second leading cause of blindness after cataract.
  - The most common form of glaucoma is primary open-angle glaucoma (POAG) in the United States.
  - In POAG, the mechanism of elevated intraocular pressure has not been elucidated.
  - Treatment options include topical eyedrops, laser trabeculoplasty, and various surgical procedures, all of which aim at lowering the intraocular pressure.

Exophthalmos and Proptosis

A. Causes of exophthalmos and orbital proptosis include the following:
  i. Orbital tumor
    - Most common: *cavernous hemangioma, hemangiopericytoma, lymphoproliferative lesions, lacrimal gland tumor (adenoid cyst carcinoma and pleomorphic adenoma); optic nerve glioma, optic nerve sheath meningioma; schwannoma, neurofibroma, and melanoma.*
    - The diagnosis of a solid tumor is usually made with orbital imaging with CT or MRI. Open biopsy may require using a medial or lateral orbitotomy approach.
    - Vascular tumors may be better diagnosed on angiography. Aspiration or needle biopsy sometimes helps confirm the diagnosis.
    - Surgical approach is indicated for the risk of impending blindness, while radiation therapy may be indicated to retard the growth of the tumor.
    - Metastatic: Breast, prostate, melanoma, and lung cancer (in the order of frequency). A complete physical examination is indicated to diagnose the primary tumor. Orbital exenteration is usually not performed in favor of chemotherapy and radiation therapy.
  ii. *Orbital pseudotumor*, also called *idiopathic orbital inflammation.*
    - It can lead to proptosis, ocular motility limitation, and periorbital pain.
    - The diagnosis is based on careful history and imaging studies with CT or MRI.
    - Typically responsive to high-dose steroids, which is sometimes also used as a diagnostic tool.
    - New treatment of immunosuppressive or immunomodulating agents is promising.
  iii. *Orbital cellulitis/abscess*
    - Can sometimes cause proptosis without ophthalmoplegia.
    - When globe movement is reduced, presence of an orbital abscess must be suspected, and a CT or MRI scan obtained.
    - Most cellulitic conditions of the orbit originate from paranasal sinus disease, with surgical drainage via an anterior orbitotomy required.
    - Fungal orbital infection is a surgical emergency, such as mucormycosis and aspergillosis. Fungal infections can progress rapidly in immunocompromised individuals.
    - Infection of the lid anterior to the orbital septum generally remains localized to the lid (preseptal cellulitis); however, if posterior to the septum, it is by definition an orbital infection.

iv. Paranasal sinus mass
- Tumors of the paranasal sinuses may encroach upon the orbit—adenocarcinoma or squamous cell carcinoma.
- En bloc resection of the sinus tumor with orbital exenteration is usually indicated.
- Polypoid disease of the sinuses and frontal sinus osteoma may push into the orbit, causing proptosis.

v. *Granulomatosis with polyangiitis* (renamed from Wegener granulomatosis)
- A multisystem autoimmune disorder.
- It can be fatal if not treated promptly.
- Characterized by the classic triad of *necrotizing granulomatous vasculitis of the respiratory tract*, most characteristically the paranasal sinuses, *focal segmental glomerulonephritis,* and *necrotizing vasculitis of small vessels.*
- Ocular manifestations are seen in half of the patients, which include direct orbital extension from the paranasal sinuses, retro-orbital inflammation, dacryocystitis, scleritis, and peripheral ulcerative keratitis. Uveitis, retinitis, retinal vasculitis, and ischemic optic neuropathy can also occur.
- The diagnosis is established by clinical and laboratory findings. c-ANCA is often positive, and its quantity also correlates with the disease activity.
- Sometimes a tissue biopsy is necessary to establish the diagnosis.
- The treatment consists of corticosteroids and immunomodulating agents.

vi. Carotid-cavernous fistula is described previously.

vii. See following section for thyroid-associated orbitopathy.

Graves' Orbitopathy

A. Pathophysiology: *Graves' orbitopathy* (GO) is also known as thyroid-associated orbitopathy or thyroid eye disease.
   i. It is a chronic autoimmune disorder that also affects the skin, extraocular muscles, and the orbital fat via shared autoantigens.
   ii. Thyroid-stimulating hormone receptor (TSHR) is the primary autoantigen.
   iii. The level of thyroid-stimulating immunoglobulin (TSI), which activates the TSHR, is correlated with the activity of both thyroid disease and orbitopathy.
   iv. Orbital fibroblasts seem to be the major player in the development of orbitopathy. They generate more adipose tissue and increase the extraocular muscle volume by overproduction of collagen and extracellular matrix.
   v. Imaging studies with CT or MRI demonstrate a significant increase in volume of the extraocular muscles and/or orbital fat.
   vi. Although the majority of patients with GO also have *hyperthyroidism,* 5% to 10% of them are euthyroid and 10% have *hypothyroidism.*

B. Clinical presentation: An individual case of GO is best described by both activity (the inflammation status) and severity to guide management.
   i. GO typically consists of two clinic phases: the active inflammatory phase (lasting 1.5 to 3 years) and the cicatrizing recovery phase.
   ii. The common indications of inflammation activity include, but are not limited to, conjunctival injection and chemosis, lid redness and edema, and retrobulbar pain at rest with gaze.
   iii. The immunosuppressive therapy is only effective in the active phase.

iv. Surgical treatment is usually not recommended in the active phase.
v. The severity refers to the level of functional impairment resulting from GO.
vi. The most common signs of GO are proptosis (globe decompresses itself through the anterior orbit) and upper eyelid retraction with upper scleral show (from levator and/or Müller muscle inflammation or fibrosis).
vii. Ocular symptoms range from mild to severe, including foreign-body sensation; severe burning, pain, blurry vision, exposure keratopathy or even corneal ulcer from prolonged corneal exposure; various degrees of *strabismus;* and possible severe loss of vision from *compressive optic neuropathy*.
viii. The historic NO SPEC grading system by Werner only measures the severity of GO without consideration of the activity phase; therefore, it is no longer used.
ix. The two new systems, VISA (vision, inflammation, strabismus, and appearance) (more popular in North America) and EUGOGO (European Group of Graves' Orbitopathy) (more popular in Europe), are very detailed and more accurate for clinic grading.

C. Management of GO should be coordinated by a team consisting of the endocrinologist, ophthalmologist, and otolaryngologist.
i. Mild to moderate GO only requires supportive measures such as lubrication.
ii. During the active phase of severe GO, medical management is preferred. IV steroids, targeted immunotherapy to IL-6, and insulin-like growth factor receptor have all been shown to be effective.
iii. It is very important to be diligent with ocular surface protection during severe or actively progressing GO, as certain ocular surface damage can be irreversible.
iv. Of note, although rigorous management aiming to achieve euthyroid status should be carried out in all GO patients with thyroid dysfunction, more and more evidence shows that the course of GO is likely to be independent of medical or surgical antithyroid treatment.
v. Smoking and radioactive iodine have been shown to worsen GO.
vi. Methimazole, propylthiouracil, and thyroidectomy seem to be neutral to the progression of GO.
vii. During the cicatrizing phase, when the inflammation is less active, certain surgical interventions are indicated for severe GO (see section E).

D. The ocular damage from GO in each of the following categories can range from mild to severe.
i. Conjunctival injection (redness) due to exposure, desiccation, and inflammation. Conjunctival chemosis secondary to venous stasis.
ii. Corneal exposure and desiccation due to failure to close the lids over the cornea, leading to pain, redness, blurry vision, and corneal ulcer.
iii. Fixation of the extraocular muscles, causing strabismus, then ophthalmoplegia. The earliest limitation noted is typically in upward gaze.
iv. Compressive optic neuropathy leading to vision decrease, color vision loss, afferent pupillary defect, and even blindness.

E. The surgical treatments are usually implemented in the inactive phase as the structural changes are stabilized then.
i. The sequence is: Orbital decompression to reduce proptosis, strabismus surgery to improve diplopia, and lid surgeries to lessen lagophthalmos and cornea exposure. All the above procedures are also done to address disfigurement.
ii. Different orbital decompression surgeries usually involve various techniques including 1-wall, 2-wall, and 3-wall approach combined with orbital fat removal.

Currently, the treatment of choice is the endoscopic decompression of the medial orbit via an ethmoidectomy with removal of the lamina papyracea and a partial resection of the floor of the orbit.

iii. Strabismus surgeries are done for vision rehabilitation. Even if perfect binocular alignment is not achieved, the reduced degree of the misalignment of the two eyes could still allow prism correction (misalignment correction that is ground in glasses) that is otherwise impossible without surgery.

iv. Lid surgeries are done to reduce the upper and/or lower lid retraction, improve lagophthalmos, and minimize cornea exposure.

v. Sometimes blepharoplasty is performed on either or both lids to complete the functional and cosmetic rehabilitation.

Questions

1. The roof of the orbit consists of the orbital process of the frontal bone and the lesser wing of the sphenoid.
   A. True
   B. False

2. Lagophthalmos almost never results from parotid tumor excision.
   A. True
   B. False

3. Orbital decompression surgery should be performed during the active inflammatory phase of Graves' orbitopathy.
   A. True
   B. False

4. Bacterial conjunctivitis is much less common than viral conjunctivitis in healthy adults.
   A. True
   B. False

5. The acquired nasolacrimal duct obstruction commonly occurs at the level of the valve of Hasner.
   A. True
   B. False

Chapter 9
Fluids/Electrolytes/Nutrition

Malnutrition is a dietary deficiency that results from various environmental and medical conditions, such as mental health problems, social problems, GI disorders, and alcoholism, among others. This is defined as weight loss greater than 5% to 10% of ideal body weight, with preferential loss of adipose tissue over muscle. The resting energy expenditure is reduced. Improved caloric intake of nutritious food or nutritional supplements will often reverse malnutrition and starvation. Malnutrition can occur in specific scenarios; however, cachexia is a pathology commonly observed in patients with head and neck cancer. Cachexia is a multifactorial metabolic syndrome characterized by systemic sarcopenia, with or without loss of fat mass that accompanies a chronic disease (usually malignant), whereas malnutrition is a lack of adequate nourishment. While all cachectic patients suffer from malnutrition, cachexia is not always present in malnourished patients. Loss of adipose tissue in cachexia is a result of increased lipolysis by tumor or host products. Sarcopenia is mainly due to diminished synthesis of muscle protein and increased degradation of proteins; these amino acids are shunted into acute-phase response proteins in the liver resulting in liver hypertrophy.

At presentation, up to 50% of patients with head and neck cancer are already malnourished and it can be as high as 80% during radiotherapy or concurrent chemoradiation.[1]

- Associated with disease-mediated metabolic disorders, inflammatory responses (IL-1α, IL-1β, IL-6, and TNF), and insulin resistance.[2]
- Patients may experience either early satiety or food aversion.
- Other physical factors contributing to cachexia are as follows:
  - Mechanical obstruction
  - Dysphagia or odynophagia
  - Nausea or gastrointestinal disturbance

Cachexia is diagnosed as weight loss of more than 5% over the past 6 months or a BMI of less than 20 kg/m^2. Although no single marker can comprehensively measure the nutritional status, some have used albumin, prealbumin, and transferrin to assess nutritional status.

The importance of diagnosing and treating both malnutrition and cancer cachexia is evident in the increased perioperative morbidity when untreated. Poor wound healing, increased rates of sepsis, and increased rates of wound infections are seen with malnutrition. Increased complications from surgery, radiation, and chemotherapy are seen in patients with cancer cachexia. There is mounting evidence that cancer cachexia profoundly affects cardiac structure and function, causing significant impairment in patients who previously had no history of cardiac dysfunction. The implications of this for patients who undergo major surgical ablation may be profound, especially in the perioperative period. During therapy, weight loss is an independent poor prognostic sign. Morbidly obese patients can still be profoundly malnourished and weight loss during treatment is not necessarily healthy for them. This form of sarcopenic obesity may be difficult to diagnose and treat. Nutritional assessment and counseling by a certified nutritionist is a critical part of the evaluation of patients with head and neck cancer. Additionally, early intervention by a speech pathologist is important to determine if oral nutrition will be sufficient, or if alternative means will be necessary.

Patient Evaluation

History

- Document weight loss in the past 3 to 6 months
  (a) Intentional
  (b) Unintentional—Consider cancer cachexia
- Alcohol abuse
- Dysphagia or odynophagia
- Document anorexia

Physical Examination

- Loss of muscle mass, especially Type II fast twitch muscles such as biceps or quadriceps
- Temporal muscle fat pad loss, orbital fat loss
- Evidence of vitamin deficiencies such as dry scaling skin, cheilosis, or stomatitis

Anthropometric

- Body mass index (BMI) = weight (kg)/height (cm) × 100.
- Midarm circumference can be used to estimate skeletal muscle mass.

Laboratory Measures

- Albumin
  - 21-day half-life.
  - Levels less than 3.0 g/dL are associated with perioperative morbidity.
  - Low in malnutrition, infection, burns, fluid overload, hepatic failure, cancer, nephrotic syndrome.
- Transferrin (200-360 mg/dL)
  - 7-day half-life
  - Levels less than 150 mg/dL indicate malnutrition.
  - More accurately reflects short-term changes in protein nutritional status.
  - It may be calculated from the total iron-binding capacity (TIBC). Transferrin = (0.68 × TIBC) + 21.
  - Affected by iron status.
- Prealbumin (16-40 mg/dL)
  - 2 to 3 day half-life.
  - Can be used to assess nutritional status and the need for supplementation.
  - Low in malnutrition, infection, liver failure; increased in renal failure.
- C-reactive protein (CRP)
  - Elevated CRP helps determine if above proteins are reduced because of inflammatory process versus inadequate substrate.

  - More than 10 suggests physiological stress.
  - May affect the reliability of albumin and prealbumin as nutrition status surrogates.
- Anemia is associated with cancer cachexia.
- Serum glucose levels may help detect insulin resistance, seen in patients with cancer cachexia.
- A total lymphocyte count (TLC) of less than 1700/μL is a gross measurement of impaired humoral immunity and is associated with a fivefold increase in the risk of wound infection.
- The prognostic nutritional index (PNI) is predictive of complications and morbidity.

$$PNI = 158 - 16.6 \text{ (albumin)} - 0.78 \text{ (triceps skinfold)} - 0.20 \text{ (transferrin)} - 0.58 \text{ (delayed hypersensitivity)}$$

Risk:

Low = < 40
Moderate = 40–49
High = > 50

In general, physical examination is a better tool for diagnosing malnutrition; however, overall assessment must be synthesized between physical findings and serum markers. Subjective global assessment tools are fairly simple, inexpensive questionnaires that combine data from weight and dietary histories with physical examination observations to subjectively classify patients as well-nourished, moderately malnourished, or severely malnourished.

Summary

Unintentional weight loss may be due to a paraneoplastic syndrome, cancer cachexia. Anemia, hypoglycemia, and elevated CRP are hallmarks of this wasting syndrome. It is not treatable with nutritional supplementation alone, although this is an integral part of the therapy. There are no FDA-approved remedies for cancer cachexia, but current management strategies include corticosteroids and megesterol acetate (Megace). Future strategies may include nutraceuticals, omega-3 fatty acids in nutritional supplements, and targeted treatments using Ghrelin analogs. Preliminary data suggest that nonsteroidal anti-inflammatory drugs may be useful in dampening the inflammatory response associated with this condition. A nutritional consult is a critical part of evaluating patients. If patients are malnourished, nutritional supplements should be considered part of the treatment plan.

Refeeding Syndrome

Patients who have had negligible nutrient intake for 5 days may be at risk for refeeding syndrome, which occurs within 4 to 7 days of starting to refeed. Profound electrolyte imbalances may occur, especially hypophosphatemia, which may be accompanied by cardiac arrhythmias (most common cause of death), coma, confusion, and convulsions. During fasting, the main sources of energy are ketone bodies derived from fatty acids and amino acids. When the patient undergoes refeeding, augmented insulin secretion results in increased glycogen, fat, and protein synthesis that diminishes already dangerously low phosphate, potassium, and magnesium serum levels.

Glucose and thiamine levels often drop. The shifting of electrolytes and fluid balance increases cardiac workload. Increased oxygen consumption and inadequate oxygen delivery strain the respiratory system. These patients merit close monitoring. Replenishing vital electrolytes (potassium, phosphate, and magnesium) in a controlled setting is essential.

Nutritional Requirements

For the malnourished patient, the physician must determine the nutrient and caloric requirements needed.

- The average adult needs 30 to 35 kcal/kg/d.
- To avoid protein-calorie malnutrition, provide 6.25 g of protein per 125 to 150 kcal.
- Nitrogen balance should be assessed through serial laboratory and body weight assessments.

Nutritional Delivery Techniques

Enteral Feedings

Oral nutrition is preferred when possible, but many head and neck disorders, particularly head and neck cancer and its surgical or nonsurgical treatment, may preclude adequate nutrition due to dysphagia, aspiration, and discomfort. The use of feeding tubes often helps bypass areas of severe mucositis in patients undergoing radiation or chemoradiation therapy, and may be used postoperatively after major head and neck surgery if oral feeding is not advisable due to acute dysphagia or reconstructive concerns.

Routes of enteral feeding:

- Nasogastric (NG) tube
  - Advantage: easiest to place
  - Disadvantages: nasal and pharyngeal discomfort, esophageal reflux, risk of alar necrosis
- Gastrostomy (G) tube (usually percutaneous endoscopic gastrostomy, PEG)
  - Advantages: well-tolerated, relative ease of placement
  - Disadvantage: surgical procedure required, possibility of infection or intra-abdominal complication
- Jejunostomy (J) tube
  - Advantage: reduces gastroesophageal reflux and vomiting (important if complex reconstruction is present)
  - Disadvantages: do not allow for bolus feeding, same as other disadvantages of the G tube

Gastrostomy tube insertion reduces the use of swallowing musculature, resulting in poorer swallowing outcomes in patients with G tubes compared to nasogastric tubes.[3] Prophylactic enteral nutrition must be analyzed independently per patient, taking into consideration tumor site and stage, the patient's socio-economic status, and psychological characteristics. There is no consensus about whether prophylactic tube placement is appropriate, although this is commonly done in patients with more than 10% weight loss, severe pretreatment dehydration, aspiration, and dysphagia, and in patients who will be receiving intense multimodality treatment to the upper aerodigestive tract (eg, concurrent chemoradiation). Prophylactic G tube placement should be considered prior to initiation of radiation and chemoradiation, as interruption of treatment due to dehydration or malnourishment may lead to compromise in survival. Patients with feeding tubes have lower mean weight loss when compared to patients without feeding tubes.[4] Although both NG and G tubes have specific advantages and disadvantages, both are effective in maintaining nutritional status. Nevertheless, when possible, oral feeds should be preserved in properly selected patients to decrease the chances of late dysphagia, as patients who become dependent on enteral feeding during radiation are more likely to remain completely or partially dependent in the long term.

Parenteral Nutrition

This route of nutritional delivery provides for rapid nutritional replacement without being dependent on a functioning alimentary tract. Peripheral parenteral nutrition (PPN) is administered via a peripheral IV and is not adequate for complete nutritional supplementation. It is often given as a supplement consisting of 5% to 10% dextrose, 3.5% amino acids, and lipids to provide 1000 to 2000 cc/d.

Total parenteral nutrition (TPN) must be given via a dedicated central venous catheter. The indications are as follows:

- Nonfunctioning gastrointestinal (GI) tract
- Severe protein malnutrition with loss of normal GI function
- High-flow chyle leak after neck dissection with failure to respond to conservative measures (surgical intervention, dietary modification, octreotide, etc.)

TPN and PPN allow for rapid replacement of nutritional deficits (1-2 weeks) and do not depend on the GI tract function. The role of TPN and PPN is limited in patients with head and neck disorders due to the ability to supplement patients via enteral feeding.

Fluid, Electrolytes, and Acid-Base Balance

The "one size fits all" fluid therapy is often chosen for reasons of convenience. A prevailing practice has been to administer hypotonic maintenance intravenous fluids in both children and adults.[5] This has been associated with a high incidence of hospital-acquired hyponatremia, fluid overload, organ damage (lungs, brain, and kidneys), hyperchloremic metabolic acidosis (excess chloride administration), coagulation abnormalities, increased need for transfusion with blood products, and increased fatalities with certain solutions. Acutely ill patients may have hemodynamic (volume depletion) and nonhemodynamic stimuli (nausea, vomiting, hypoxemia, hypercapnia, cancer, cachexia) associated with an excess of vasopressin. Water excretion decreases with increased levels of plasma vasopressin, whereas solute excretion remains relatively constant; this way, fluid overload may aggravate hyponatremia.

Choosing the appropriate volume and composition of intravenous fluids requires great care. IV fluids can be classified according to the concentration of sodium plus potassium in the fluid, as being either isotonic (approximately equal to the plasma sodium concentration) or hypotonic (less than the plasma sodium concentration). The dextrose content of intravenous fluids does not affect the tonicity, since the dextrose is rapidly metabolized when it enters the bloodstream and should not produce hyperglycemia. The inappropriate use of intravenous (IV) fluids ranges from inadequate resuscitation, resulting in tissue hypoperfusion, to excessive fluid infusion leading to tissue edema and severe electrolyte derangement.

The average 70-kg male is composed of 60% (42 L) water. Of this 42 L, approximately two-thirds (28 L) is intracellular and one-third (14 L) is extracellular. The extracellular compartment can be further divided into the interstitial fluid (10 L) and the plasma (4 L). Various electrolytes are distributed among the different fluid compartments of the body (Table 9-1). No single rate of administration or composition of maintenance intravenous fluids is appropriate in all circumstances. Thus, intravenous fluids may be viewed as medications that must be analyzed individually and require careful dose adjustment that is specific to the disease state of each patient. The default maintenance solution for adults is 5% dextrose in a solution of 0.9% saline administered at a rate of 100 to 120 mL per hour. If the patient is stable, the goal is to promote a negative balance (Tables 9-2 and 9-3).

Table 9-1 Body Fluid Electrolyte Composition

Substance	*Extracellular fluid (mEq/L)*	*Intracellular fluid (mEq/L)*
Sodium	140	10
Potassium	4	150
Magnesium	1.7	40
Chloride	105	10
Bicarbonate	28	10
Phosphate/sulfate	3.5	150
Protein anions	15	40

Fluid Disturbances

- Overhydration (volume excess)
  (a) Polyuria
  (b) Urine Na greater than 30 mEq/L
  (c) Pulmonary edema
  (d) Distended neck veins
  (e) Ascites
  (f) Peripheral edema
  (g) Systolic hypertension
  (h) Elevated wedge pressure
- Dehydration (volume depletion)
  (a) Oliguria
  (b) Urine Na less than 10 mEq/L
  (c) Hypotension
  (d) Poor skin turgor
  (e) Sunken eyeballs
  (f) Thirst
  (g) Tachycardia
  (h) Hemoconcentration
  (i) Low wedge pressure

Table 9-2 Fluid Exchange

Routes		*Average daily volume (mL)*
Water Gains:	Oral fluids	800-1500
	Solid foods	500-700
	Water oxidation	250
Water Loss:	Urine output	800-1500
	Intestinal	250
	Insensible	500-700

Table 9-3 Fluid Requirements

Adults:		35 cc/kg/24 h
Children:	First 10 kg:	100 cc/kg/24 h or 4 cc/kg/h
	Second 10 kg:	50 cc/kg/24 h or 2 cc/kg/h
	Second > 20 kg:	25 cc/kg/24 h or 1 cc/kg/h
Fever		500 cc/24 h/C above 38.3°C (101°F)

Sodium

- Normal serum Na levels: 135 to 145 mEq/L
- Normal intake Na 1 mEq/kg/24 h
- **Hypernatremia (Na >150 mEq/L)**
  - Symptoms: Neurological abnormalities, such as confusion, disorientation, or seizures. The worst manifestation is a coma.
  - Etiology:
    - **Elevated serum sodium always implies a free water deficit**
    - *Lost free water*: Diabetes insipidus (either central or nephrogenic), insensible losses (endotracheal intubation, sweating, burns), diarrhea, vomiting, osmotic
    - Both central and nephrogenic DI give the following results:
      - ◊ **Low urine osmolality**
      - ◊ **Low urine sodium**
      - ◊ **Increased urine volume**
    - *Solute loading*: tube feeding, brainstem injury, inappropriate IV, Cushing syndrome.
  - Therapy: Depends on the fluid status, but the basic principle is to treat the underlying disorder and slowly rehydrate with hypotonic fluid, dextrose 5% in water (D5W), or oral water.
    - Rapid rehydration can lead to cerebral edema or congestive heart failure (CHF).
    - Do not correct at a rate of more than 12 mEq/L/day.
- **Hyponatremia (Na <130 mEq/L)**
  - Symptoms: Confusion, disorientation, seizures, or coma. There will be neither edema nor signs of dehydration. Hyponatremic encephalopathy develops in less than 48 hrs.
    - First step in the management of hyponatremia is to **assess volume status** to determine the cause and, therefore, the treatment.
    - Hypervolemic, hypovolemic, or euvolemic hyponatremia.
  - Etiology: Hypervolemic: CHF, nephrotic syndrome, cirrhosis; hypovolemic: iatrogenic (diuretics), water intoxication, GI loss (diarrhea), skin loss (burns). Euvolemic: syndrome of inappropriate antidiuretic hormone (SIADH), hypothyroidism, myxedema, sepsis, hyperglycemic osmotic effect (correct 2 mEq for every 100 mg of excess glucose to give a serum sodium that correctly reflects the sodium/fluid status).
  - Therapy: Depends on the fluid status of the patient. If hypervolemic (CHF, renal failure), then restrict fluid and use diuretics.
    - If hypovolemic, then rehydrate with normal saline.
    - If patient symptomatic, infuse hypertonic saline for rapid initial correction of 2mEq/L/h for 2 to 3 hours.
    - Do not correct serum sodium more than 10 to 12 mEq/L in the first 24 hours or more than 18 mEq/L in the first 48 hours.

- Check sodium frequently.
- In SIADH (as from malignancy), use demeclocycline as it blocks the effect of ADH at the kidney.

Potassium

- Normal serum K^+ levels: 3.5 to 5.0 mEq/L
- Normal intake
  (a) *Adults*: 40 to 60 mEq/24 h
  (b) *Children*: 2 mEq/kg/24 h
- **Hyperkalemia ($K^+ > 5.5$)**
  - Symptoms: Generally not associated with seizures or neurological symptoms, hyperkalemia can lead to **cardiac arrhythmia.**
    - First peaked T-waves, then loss of P waves, and then widened QRS complex resulting in arrhythmia and asystole.
    - Weakness, loss of deep tendon reflexes, confusion, and irritability.
  - Etiology: Increased potassium release from tissues, such as in rhabdomyolysis or hemolysis. Renal failure, metabolic acidosis, prolonged immobility, seizures, and Type IV renal tubular acidosis. Increased dietary potassium can only cause hyperkalemia if it is associated with renal insufficiency.
  - Therapy: If there are EKG changes or there is severe hyperkalemia (> 6.5), prompt intervention is warranted.
    - First administer calcium gluconate intravenously to stabilize the heart.
    - Follow with IV insulin and glucose (D50).
    - $NaHCO_3$: shifts potassium into cells and alkalinizes the urine.
    - Kayexalate (oral): takes 2 to 24 hours to take effect.
    - Loop diuretic.
    - Consider dialysis in severe cases.
- **Hypokalemia ($K^+ < 3.0$ mEq/L)**
  - Symptoms: anorexia, nausea, vomiting, ileus, muscular weakness, ECG changes ("u" waves, ST depression, prolonged QT, premature ventricular contractions, AV block, and cardiac arrest)
  - Etiology: decreased intake, GI loss, especially NG suction, vomiting, diarrhea, laxative abuse, diuretics, and steroid therapy
  - Therapy: Replete maximum rate of 40 mEq/h (monitoring)
    - Peripheral 20 mEq in 50 to 100 cc D_5W
    - Central 20 to 40 mEq in 50 to 100 cc D_5W

Remember serum pH will affect serum K^+ (acidosis will produce an increase in serum K^+, while alkalosis produces a decrease).

Calcium

- Normal serum Ca^{2+} levels: 8.5 to 10.6 mg/dL
- Normal intake
  (a) 1 to 3 g/24 h.
  (b) Total body stores 1 to 2 g.
  (c) Serum Ca^{2+} is 45% bound to albumin, 40% ionized, and 15% in organic ions.
  (d) Serum total Ca^{2+} decreases with decreasing serum protein; however, ionized Ca^{2+} remains constant.

- **Hypocalcemia (Ca^{2+} < 8 mg/dL)**
  - Symptoms: usually symptomatic below 7.5 mg/dL, numbness, tingling, headaches, cramps, Chvostek sign (facial nerve irritability), Trousseau sign (carpopedal spasm), arrhythmia, prolonged QT on EKG.
  - Etiology: hypoparathyroidism (iatrogenic most common), hypoalbuminemia, hypomagnesemia, vitamin D deficiency, pancreatitis, renal failure, malabsorption, pseudohypoparathyroidism.
  - Therapy: emergent Ca gluconate or chloride 1 g (10 cc of 10% solution = 1 ampule) intravenous pyelogram (IVP) over 10 to 15 minutes with cardiac monitor.
    - Remember to check Mg.
    - Chronic hypocalcemia replaces with Os-cal 1.5 to 3.0 g/d with vitamin D (calcitriol 0.25-2.0 μg/d); start 0.25 μg/d then may increase by 0.25 μg/d q2-4 weeks as needed.
    - Transient hypocalcemia (7-8) after thyroid surgery may not require treatment (Rx).
    - New rapid parathyroid hormone (PTH) assays may guide surgeons post-thyroidectomy with immediate post-thyroid PTH greater than 10 to 12 pg/mL at a very low risk of post-thyroidectomy hypocalcemia.
    - Correct hypoalbuminemia; when serum albumin is below 4.0 g/dL, for every 1 mg/dL decrease in albumin, increase the calcium level by 0.8 mg/dL.
- **Hypercalcemia (Ca^{2+} > 10.6)**
  - Symptoms: Mild elevations (< 11.5) often asymptomatic and may require no Rx. Kidney stones, osteoporosis/osteomalacia/fractures, GI disturbance (constipation and abdominal pain), and confusion.
  - Etiology: The most common by far is primary hyperparathyroidism; other causes are ectopic PTH production (malignancy), bony metastases, milk-alkali syndrome, vitamin D toxicity, granulomatous disease (sarcoid, TB), Paget disease, thiazides, parathyroid malignancy.
  - Therapy
    - Greater than 14: emergency level.
    - Hydration (normal saline 1-2 L q2h).
    - Diuretics, Furosemide: Only after hydration has been given.
    - Calcitonin: If hydration and furosemide do not control the calcium.
    - Biphosphonate (pamidronate), potent but slow (more than a week to take effect).
    - Steroids for granulomatous disease.
    - Treat the underlying disorder.

Magnesium

- Normal serum Mg levels: 1.6 to 2.5 mg/dL
- Normal intake 20 mEq/d
- **Hypomagnesemia Mg^{2+} less than 1.5 mg/dL**
  - Symptoms: It presents with hypocalcemia and cardiac arrhythmia; there is also muscle weakness and myoclonus.
  - Etiology: loop diuretics, alcohol withdrawal, parathyroidectomy, burns, decreased intake (ethyl alcohol [EtOH] abuse, TPN, malnutrition), and decreased GI absorption.
  - Therapy urgent, 1 to 2 g $MgSO_4$ (8-16 mEq) over 15 to 30 minutes, then 1 g IM q 4 to 6 h or Mg oxide (Uro-Mag) 2 tabs bid.
  - Important to correct low Mg if the patient is hypocalcemic.

- **Hypermagnesemia Mg^{2+} greater than 3 mg/dL**
  - Symptoms: muscular weakness and loss of deep tendon reflexes. Hypertension, nausea, vomiting, lethargy, weakness, ECG changes (aortic valve [AV] block, prolonged QT).
  - Etiology: It is rare to have hypermagnesemia without renal insufficiency. Overuse of magnesium-containing laxatives.
  - Therapy: Saline to promote diuresis. Urgent Ca gluconate 20 cc 10% solution IVP, eliminate exogenous sources, dialysis.

Acid-Base Disorders

The acid-base system is designed to maintain the pH at a level of 7.4 for optimal cellular function. A number of mechanisms including the respiratory system, renal system, extracellular buffers (primarily HCO_3^-), and intracellular buffers (proteins, phosphates, and hemoglobin) exist to control the pH within this narrow range (Table 9-4).

Excess hydrogen ion (acid) is eliminated by the lungs based on the reaction:

$$H^+ + HCO_3 = H_2CO_3 = CO_2 + H_2O$$

Most of the excess hydrogen is eliminated by this route, with a relatively small amount (~70 mEq) eliminated by the renal system. Both the pulmonary and renal systems make adjustments to compensate for the alterations in the acid-base balance (Table 9-4). There are four general categories of acid-base disorders: respiratory acidosis and alkalosis, and metabolic acidosis and alkalosis.

Respiratory Acidosis

Primary respiratory acidosis is characterized by an increase in the partial pressure of arterial CO_2 (Pco_2) secondary to disorders that limit pulmonary function. This is most commonly seen in diseases that limit the body's ability to eliminate CO_2 such as chronic obstructive pulmonary disease, impairment of central respiration (head injuries or drugs), or chest wall trauma that prevents adequate ventilation. The diagnosis is confirmed by an arterial blood gas that demonstrates a low pH and an elevated Pco_2. The lowered pH reflects the body's attempt to compensate for the rising Pco_2 as depicted in the above-mentioned formula. In chronic situations, the renal system may contribute to the compensation by retaining HCO_3^-. Treatment is centered on addressing the chronic hypoventilation and may include steroids, antibiotics, inhalers, reversal of respiratory suppression, and consideration of intubation/mechanical ventilation.

Table 9-4 Acid-Base Disturbances

Disturbance	*pH*	*H^+*	*Compensation*	*Examples*
Metabolic acidosis	Decrease	Increase	$Paco_2$ decreases by 1.3 mm Hg for each mEq/L decrease in HCO_3	Lactic acidosis, ketoacidosis
Metabolic alkalosis	Increase	Decrease	$Paco_2$ increases by 5-7 mm Hg for each mEq/L increase in HCO_3	Vomiting, NG tube suction, Cushing syndrome
Respiratory acidosis	Decrease	Increase	HCO_3 increases by 1 mEq/L for each 10 mm Hg increase in $Paco_2$	Hypoventilation, CNS lesion
Respiratory alkalosis	Increase	Decrease	HCO_3 decreases by 2 mEq/L for each 10 mm Hg decrease in $Paco_2$	Hyperventilation, fever/sepsis, hypoxemia

Respiratory Alkalosis

Primary respiratory alkalosis is characterized by hyperventilation that leads to a reduction in Pco_2. The two primary etiologies are direct stimulation of the central respiratory centers (aspirin, CNS tumors/trauma/cerebral vascular accident [CVA]) or indirect stimulation through hypoxia. It may also be seen in psychogenic hyperventilation, sepsis, errors in mechanical ventilation, and fevers. The diagnosis is confirmed by an arterial blood gas that demonstrates an elevated pH (> 7.45) with a low Pco_2 (< 35). Treatment is directed to the correction of the underlying disorder.

Metabolic Acidosis

Metabolic acidosis results from a variety of disorders that result in an excess acid load, decreased acid secretion, or excess bicarbonate loss. It is characterized by a low arterial pH (< 7.36) and a low HCO_3 (< 22). The reduction in arterial pH leads to a compensatory hyperventilation that decreases the Pco_2 and minimizes the change in arterial pH. Important in distinguishing among the many causes of a metabolic acidosis is the anion gap. The anion gap allows the clinician to classify the causes of metabolic acidosis into a high anion gap versus a normal anion gap (Table 9-5). The anion gap is calculated by subtracting the sum of the chloride and the bicarbonate from the sodium concentration. The usual value is 10 mEq/L.

Diagnosis is confirmed by an arterial blood gas that reflects a low pH and a lowering of the HCO_3^-. The anion gap should be calculated to help guide the determination of an etiology. Treatment is directed toward the underlying disorder. In many cases of mild metabolic acidosis (pH > 7.25), no treatment is necessary. The use of bicarbonate to treat metabolic acidosis is controversial, and in some patients with lactic acidosis and ketoacidosis, it may cause more harm than benefit. In selected situations (pH < 7.20, HCO_3^- < 10 mEq/L), some clinicians would use bicarbonate while addressing the underlying cause of the acidosis.

Metabolic Alkalosis

A metabolic alkalosis is caused by a primary elevation in plasma HCO_3^- above 27 mEq/L leading to an increased pH greater than 7.44. The increased pH stimulates a decrease in pulmonary ventilation. The drop in ventilation leads to an increase in the Pco_2, thereby attempting to minimize the alterations in the blood pH. The underlying causes of metabolic alkalosis are due to a loss of acid or excess alkali intake. Table 9-6 lists the most common causes of metabolic alkalosis. By far the most common cause is related to the loss of acids (HCl). In general, there is no classic clinical picture of metabolic alkalosis. Most commonly, the laboratory values will indicate an elevated serum bicarbonate (> 30 mEq/L). An arterial blood gas will then need to be obtained to assess

Table 9-5 Etiology of Metabolic Acidosis

- Normal anion gap
- Excess acid intake (HCl, NH_4Cl)
- Bicarbonate loss
  (a) GI tract (diarrhea, fistulas, NG tube)
  (b) Proximal renal tubular acidosis
  (c) Distal renal tubular acidosis
- Increased anion gap
- Ketoacidosis (diabetes mellitus, alcohol)
- Lactic acidosis
- Poisons (aspirin, ethylene glycol)
- Renal failure

Table 9-6 Etiology of Metabolic Alkalosis

• Acid loss (generally HCl)
• GI (vomiting, NG tube)
• Increased urine acidification
(a) Diuretics
(b) Aldosterone excess
(c) Bartter syndrome
• Excess alkali
(a) Alkali abuse
(b) Overtreatment of metabolic acidosis (ie, HCO_3^-)
• Severe potassium depletion

the acid-base status and rule out a metabolic alkalosis or the elevated bicarbonate may reflect a true respiratory acidosis with the elevated bicarbonate representing a compensatory response.

Once the metabolic workup confirms an elevated HCO_3^- with an alkalotic pH, the next step is to assess the patient's volume status. Most commonly, GI losses (vomiting, NG tube) will account for the metabolic alkalosis, and treatment can be focused on restoring an adequate volume, chloride, and potassium intake which will allow the body to self-correct the acid-base equilibrium. Obviously, the underlying disorder must be addressed while at the same time providing the necessary fluids and electrolytes that allow the renal system to excrete the excess bicarbonate. The amount of fluid and electrolytes will be guided by the patient's clinical response, but often several liters of normal saline and several hundred milliequivalents of potassium will be needed over several days.

References

1. Langius JAE, Doornaert P, Spreeuwenberg MD, Langendijk JA, Leemans CR, van Bokhorst-de van der Schueren MAE. Radiotherapy on the neck nodes predicts severe weight loss in patients with early stage laryngeal cancer. *Radiother Oncol J Eur Soc Ther Radiol Oncol*. 2010;97(1):80-85.
2. Tuca A, Jimenez-Fonseca P, Gascón P. Clinical evaluation and optimal management of cancer cachexia. *Crit Rev Oncol Hematol*. 2013;88(3):625-636.
3. Paleri V, Roe JWG, Strojan P, et al. Strategies to reduce long-term postchemoradiation dysphagia in patients with head and neck cancer: an evidence-based review. *Head Neck*. 2014;36(3):431-443.
4. Mekhail TM, Adelstein DJ, Rybicki LA, Larto MA, Saxton JP, Lavertu P. Enteral nutrition during the treatment of head and neck carcinoma: is a percutaneous endoscopic gastrostomy tube preferable to a nasogastric tube? *Cancer*. 2001;91(9):1785-1790.
5. Padhi S, Bullock I, Li L, Stroud M, National Institute for Health and Care Excellence (NICE) Guideline Development Group. Intravenous fluid therapy for adults in hospital: summary of NICE guidance. *BMJ*. 2013;347:f7073.

Questions

1. Disadvantages of TPN include all of the following, except
   A. Difficulty attaining nutritional requirements because of fluid overload
   B. Major infection or sepsis
   C. Central venous access if required
   D. Small bowel obstruction or paralytic ileus

2. What is the recommended daily energy intake and protein intake for HNSCC patients undergoing surgery or chemoradiation therapy?
   A. 30 kcal/kg/day and 1.0 g protein/kg/day
   B. 1.2 kcal/kg/day and 30 g protein/kg/day
   C. 10 kcal/kg/day and 1.2 g protein/kg/day
   D. 30 kcal/kg/day and 1.2 g protein/kg/day

3. How does cancer cachexia differ from starvation?
   A. There is decreased protein breakdown.
   B. Refeeding by any means replenishes some body mass and increases survival outcomes.
   C. There is approximately equal loss of muscle and fat.
   D. Metabolism is characterized by a slow catabolic mode to minimize energy expenditure.

4. Which of the following is the most important test to review when addressing hyperkalemia greater than 6.5 mEq?
   A. Myoglobin
   B. CPK
   C. EKG
   D. Creatinine

5. What are the indications for TPN?
   A. Nonfunctioning of GI tract
   B. Severe protein malnutrition with loss of normal gastrointestinal (GI) function
   C. Chyle leak after neck dissection
   D. All of the above

Chapter 10
Pharmacology and Therapeutics

Chemotherapy

- The reader is directed to Chapter 46—Chemotherapy and Immunotherapy for Head and Neck Cancer for review of chemotherapeutic drugs and their applications and indications.

Perioperative Drugs

- The reader is directed to Chapter 4—Anesthesia for Head and Neck Surgery for review of local anesthetics, narcotics, sedatives, and the various other perioperative drugs.

Allergy Medications

- The reader is directed to Chapter 58—Immunology and Allergy for review of antihistamines, decongestants, corticosteroids, mast cell stabilizers, leukotriene antagonists, and the treatment of anaphylactic conditions.

Antimicrobials

- The following tables summarize the main antimicrobials encountered in otolaryngology.

ANTIBACTERIALS

DNA

Classification	*Name*	*Spectrum*	*Mechanism of Action*	*Side Effects*
Fluoroquinolones (bactericidal)			Inhibit DNA gyrase and bacterial topoisomerase, promoting DNA strand breaks	Stevens-Johnson syndrome (SJS), QTc prolongation, arthropathy, tendonitis, tendon rupture
	Ciprofloxacin	GN bacilli, *Pseudomonas*, atypicals No anaerobic or GP coverage		
	Levofloxacin	*Pseudomonas*, MSSA, *Streptococcus sp.*, GN bacilli, atypicals		
	Moxifloxacin	MSSA, *Streptococcus sp.*, anaerobes, atypicals		
Nitrofuran	Nitrofurantoin (bacteriostatic, can be bactericidal at high concentrations)	Broad spectrum—GP and GN: *E. coli* and *S. saprophyticus*	Damages bacterial DNA	Pulmonary fibrosis, hemolytic anemia, neuropathies
Nitroimidazole (bactericidal)	Metronidazole	Anaerobes, GN: *B. fragilis*, *C. difficile*, protozoa Penetrates blood-brain barrier	Binds to cellular proteins and DNA	Headache, nausea, vaginitis, metallic taste, disulfiram-like reaction with alcohol, peripheral neuropathy
Folic Acid Inhibitors (bactericidal)	Trimethoprim	Broad spectrum—GP and GN: MSSA, CA-MRSA	Inhibits reduction of dihydrofolic acid to tetrahydrofolic acid	SJS/TEN, urolithiasis, cytopenia, hepatitis, hyperkalemia, increases warfarin levels
Sulfonamides (bacteriostatic)	Sulfamethoxazole	Broad spectrum—GP and GN: MRSA	Inhibits enzymatic conversion of pteridine and *p*-aminobenzoic acid (PABA) to dihydropteroic acid	Nausea, vomiting, diarrhea, hypersensitivity, hematologic effects (anemia, agranulocytosis, thrombocytopenia)

RNA

Classification	*Drug*	*Spectrum*	*Mechanism of Action*	*Side Effects*
Pseudomonic acid	Mupirocin (bacteriostatic; bactericidal at high concentrations)	Mostly GP	Inhibits RNA and protein synthesis	Contact dermatitis
Antimycobacterial (bactericidal)	Rifampin	Broad spectrum—GP + GN: *Pseudomonas*, *M. tuberculosis*	Blocks RNA transcription	Liver enzymes, rash, discoloration of teeth, urine, saliva, sweat, tears

Ribosome - 50S

Classification	*Drug*	*Spectrum*	*Mechanism of Action*	*Side Effects*
Macrolides (bacteriostatic)		Broad spectrum: *Streptococcus* sp., *Corynebacterium*, *Chlamydia* sp., *Legionella*, *Moraxella*, *H. pylori*	Irreversible binding to 50S ribosome to inhibit protein synthesis	QTc prolongation, reduced birth control effectiveness, drug-drug interactions
	Erythromycin			Avoid in liver disease, increases GI motility
	Clarithromycin	*H. influenza*		Adjust for CKD
	Azithromycin	*Mycoplasma*, *M. avium* complex, *H. influenza*		Avoid in hepatic disease
Lincosamide	Clindamycin (bacteriostatic; bactericidal at high concentrations against staphylococci, streptococci, anaerobes such as *B. fragilis*)	*Streptococcus* sp., MSSA, CA-MRSA, anaerobes	Irreversible binding to 50S ribosomal subunit	*C. difficile* infections, adjust with liver dysfunction
Oxazolidinone (bactericidal)	Linezolid	Resistant GP organisms	Binds to 50S ribosomal subunit	Cytopenia, serotonin syndrome, altered taste, tongue discoloration, optic neuritis
Phenicol (bacteriostatic)	Chloramphenicol	Broad spectrum GP + GN: *S. pneumoniae*, *N. meningitides*, *H. influenza*, *E. faecium*	Binds 50S subunit	Irreversible aplastic anemia, myelosuppression, neuritis, glossitis, gray baby syndrome

Ribosome - 30S

Classification	*Drug*	*Spectrum*	*Mechanism of Action*	*Side Effects*
Aminoglycosides (bactericidal)	(listed from most to least vestibulotoxic)	Aerobic GN bacilli: *Pseudomonas, Klebsiella, Serratia, Proteus, Acinetobacter, Enterobacter*	Binds to 30S ribosomal subunit	Vestibulocochlear toxicity, reversible nephrotoxicity
	Streptomycin			
	Gentamicin	Synergy with β-lactam to treat *Enterococcus* sp.; not as effective against *Pseudomonas*		
	Tobramycin	More active against *Pseudomonas*		
	Amikacin	Reserve for resistant *Pseudomonas* and *Acinetobacter* infections		Most cochleotoxic
Tetracyclines (bacteriostatic)		Broad: GP (MSSA, MRSA), GN, protozoa, spirochetes, mycobacteria, and atypical species	Binds reversibly to 30S ribosomal subunit	Hepatotoxicity, photosensitivity, tinnitus, pseudotumor cerebri, teeth discoloration Avoid in children, pregnancy Expired medication can cause Fanconi syndrome
	Doxycycline			
	Tetracycline			Adjust for CKD
	Minocycline			
	Demeclocycline			
Glycylcycline	Tigecycline (derivative of minocycline)	Very broad spectrum—reserve for ID or MDR organisms	Binds reversibly to 30S ribosomal subunit to inhibit protein synthesis	Nausea, vomiting, diarrhea, photosensitivity, teeth discoloration, fetal damage

Cell Wall Synthesis

Classification	*Drug*	*Spectrum*	*Mechanism of Action*	*Side Effects*
Penicillin* (bactericidal)			Binds PBPs inhibiting cell-wall synthesis	Interstitial nephritis, cytopenia Adjust for CKD
	PCN G, PCN V	GP cocci and rods, GN cocci, most anaerobes; NOT GN bacilli		
Anti-staphylococcal	Nafcillin, oxacillin, dicloxacillin	MSSA		Nafcillin and oxacillin metabolized by liver
Broad-spectrum, second generation	Ampicillin, amoxicillin	Above plus GN bacilli: *E. coli*, *P. mirabilis*, *Salmonella*, *Shigella*, *H. influenza*		30% incidence of rash in those with infectious mononucleosis (EBV)
Anti-pseudomonal, third generation	Carbenicillin, ticarcillin	GN organisms, indole-positive *Proteus*, *Enterobacter*, *Pseudomonas*		
Fourth generation	Piperacillin	Same as above plus *Klebsiella*, enterococci, *B. fragilis*, *Pseudomonas*		
PCN w/β-lactamase inhibitor	Amoxicillin/clavulanate Ticarcillin/clavulanate	Oxacillin-sensitive *S. aureus*, *H. influenza*, β-lactamase producing Enterobacteriaceae		β-lactamase inhibitors cause increased diarrhea
	Ampicillin/sulbactam	Same plus anaerobes (*B. fragilis*), *A. baumannii*		
	Piperacillin/tazobactam	As above		
Cephalosporins (bactericidal)			Binds PBPs inhibiting cell-wall synthesis	Cytopenia, anaphylaxis, pseudomembranous colitis Adjust for CKD
First generation	Cefazolin, cephalexin, cefadroxil	Most GP cocci, *E. coli*, *P. mirabilis*, *K. pneumoniae*		
Second generation	Cefaclor, cefuroxime, cefprozil	Less active against staphylococci; greater activity against GN bacilli: *H. influenza*, *M. catarrhalis*		

Cephamycin subgroup	Cefotetan, cefoxitin	*E. coli, P. mirabilis, Klebsiella, Bacteroides*		
Third generation	Cefdinir, cefixime, cefotaxime, cefpodoxime, ceftazidime, ceftriaxone, cefditoren	Therapy of choice for GN meningitis, less active against most GP; *E. coli, P. mirabilis, Proteus, Klebsiella, Enterobacter, Serratia, Citrobacter, Neisseria, H. influenza*		
	Cefotaxime, ceftriaxone	Usually active against pneumococci with intermediate susceptibility to PCN; Lyme disease, meningitis due to *H. influenzae*		
	Ceftazidime	Above plus *P. aeruginosa*; poor GP coverage		
Fourth generation	Cefepime	Pneumococci, MSSA, *Neisseria, H. influenza, Enterobacter*, indole-positive *Proteus, Citrobacter, Serratia, P. aeruginosa*		
Fifth generation	Ceftaroline	Like ceftriaxone with improved GP activity: MRSA, VISA		
β-lactamase inhibitor combination, new-generation	Ceftolozane/tazobactam	Broad spectrum against GN bacilli: *P. aeruginosa*, most ESBL; limited GP		
	Ceftazidime/avibactam	Broad spectrum: most Enterobacteriaceae, *P. aeruginosa, Acinetobacter*		
Carbapenems (bactericidal)		Broad spectrum: GN, anaerobes (*B. fragilis*), *P. aeruginosa*, GP (including MRSA)	Binds PBPs inhibiting cell-wall synthesis	*C. difficile*, seizures in high doses Adjust for CKD
	Imipenem/cilastatin, meropenem, doripenem			
	Ertapenem	Narrower spectrum: no *Pseudomonas, Acinetobacter* coverage; MRSA		

(*Continued*)

Cell Wall Synthesis (Cont.)

Classification	*Drug*	*Spectrum*	*Mechanism of Action*	*Side Effects*
Monobactam (bactericidal)	Aztreonam	GN: *Pseudomonas, Enterobacter*; no anaerobe or GP coverage	Inhibits mucopeptide synthesis of cell wall	Rare: TEN, eosinophilia Adjust for CKD
Glycopeptides (bactericidal)	Vancomycin	MSSA, MRSA, MRSE, *Streptococcus* sp., *Corynebacterium*, *E. faecalis* and *faecium*; oral: *C. difficile*	Inhibits late-stage cell wall synthesis	Vancomycin-induced renal failure, red man syndrome Adjust for CKD
Lipoglycoprotein (bactericidal)	Telavancin (derivative of vancomycin)	Useful in vancomycin-intermediate resistant bacteria	Inhibits late-stage cell wall synthesis and causes cell membrane depolarization	
Cyclic peptides	Bacitracin (bacteriostatic, - bactericidal depending on organism/ concentration)	GP	Inhibits peptidoglycan transport	Contact dermatitis

Cell Membrane Destabilizer

Classification	*Drug*	*Spectrum*	*Mechanism of Action*	*Side Effects*
Lipopeptide (bactericidal)	Daptomycin	GP: MSSA, MRSA; may have activity against VISA, VRSA	Depolarization of cell membrane	Constipation, nausea, headache, edema, myopathy, peripheral neuropathy
Polymyxin (bactericidal)	Polymyxin B, Polymyxin E	GN, MDR GN	Destabilizes membrane	Contact dermatitis, possible nephrotoxicity/ neurotoxicity Adjust for CKD

CA, community-acquired; CKD, chronic kidney disease; EBV, Epstein-Barr virus; ESBL, extended-spectrum beta-lactamase; GN, gram negative; GP, gram positive; ID, infectious disease; MDR, multiple drug resistant; MRSA, methicillin-resistant *S. aureus;* MRSE, methicillin-resistant *S. epidermidis;* MSSA, methicillin-sensitive *S. aureus*; PBP, penicillin-binding proteins; PCN, penicillin; SJS, Stevens-Johnson syndrome; TEN, toxic epidermal necrolysis; VISA, vancomycin-intermediate *S. aureus*; VRSA, vancomycin-resistant *S. aureus.*

*10% of the general population claims PCN allergy; 5%-10% of patients who report a PCN allergy are skin test-positive and only one-third of those will have a positive oral challenge; incidence of anaphylaxis from PCN is < 0.015%; cross-reactivity with first-generation cephalosporins is 1%-5%.

Antifungals

Classification	*Drug*	*Spectrum*	*Mechanism of Action*	*Side Effects*
Azoles			Disrupts ergosterol synthesis	GI, hepatotoxicity, P450 inhibitors
	Ketoconazole	Skin infections		
	Clotrimazole	Broad-spectrum, *Candida*		
	Fluconazole	*Candida, C. neoformans, B. dermatitidis, C. immitis, H. capsulatum*		CSF penetration Adjust for CKD
	Itraconazole	Same as above, plus *Aspergillus, Fusarium* sp., *Scedosporium* sp.		
	Voriconazole	Same as above		Care with slow metabolizers
	Posaconazole	Same as above plus *Mucorales*		
Polyene	Amphotericin B (fungistatic vs -cidal)	Same as above	Binds to ergosterol, disrupts fungal membrane	Infusion reactions, nephrotoxicity, hepatotoxic, cytopenia, neurotoxic, cardiotoxic
	Nystatin (fungistatic and -bactericidal)	*Candida, Trichophyton*		Contact dermatitis
Echinocandins	Caspofungin	*Aspergilla, Candida*	Inhibits cell wall synthesis	Hepatotoxic, cytopenia
Griseofulvin	Griseofulvin	*Trichophyton* sp., *Microsporum* sp.	Inhibits mitosis and microtubules	Leukopenia, jaundice, elevated liver function tests, photosensitivity, SJS/TEN
Allylamine	Terbinafine	*Trichophyton* sp., *Microsporum* sp., yeasts	Inhibits ergosterol synthesis	Headache, mood changes, neutropenia, taste disturbance, hepatic failure, SJS/TEN, ocular effects, smell disturbance, thrombotic microangiopathy

CKD, chronic kidney disease; CSF, cerebrospinal fluid; SJS, Stevens-Johnson syndrome; TEN, toxic epidermal necrolysis.

Antivirals

Classification	*Drug*	*Spectrum*	*Mechanism of Action*	*Side Effects*
Ciclovirs		HSV-1, HSV-2, CMV, varicella zoster	Blocks viral DNA synthesis	Cytopenia, SJS, CNS effects Adjust for CKD
	Acyclovir			
	Valacyclovir (prodrug of acyclovir)			
	Famciclovir (prodrug of acyclovir)			
	Ganciclovir and Valganciclovir	Congenital CMV		
Antimetabolite	Cidofovir	CMV retinitis, recurrent respiratory papillomatosis (off-label), resistant HSV	Blocks viral DNA synthesis	Possible carcinogen, alopecia, nephrotoxicity, cytopenia Adjust for CKD
Neuraminidase inhibitors		Influenza A and B	Inhibits virus neuraminidase enzyme, preventing release of viral particle	
	Oseltamivir			Headache, nausea, vomiting, rare neuropsychiatric issues
	Peramivir (IV)			Diarrhea, rash neuropsychiatric issues
	Zanamivir (inhaled)			Oropharyngeal edema/rash (allergy), bronchospasm, rash neuropsychiatric issues

CNS, central nervous system; CKD, chronic kidney disease; CMV, cytomegalovirus; HSV: herpes simplex virus; SJS, Stevens-Johnson syndrome.

Vaccines*

Target	*Type*		*Indications*	*Contraindications*
Streptococcus pneumoniae	Conjugate	PCV 15, 20, 21	4-dose series at 2, 4, 6, and 12–15 months (PCV 15 or 20), "catch up" dosing before PPSV 23 (PCV 15), unvaccinated adults 50 years or older (PCV 15, 20, or 21)	Allergic reaction to diphtheria vaccine
	Polysaccharide	PPSV 23	1 dose (at least 8 weeks after any prior PCV15 dose), adults 50 years or older	
Haemophilus influenza type B	Conjugate		≥ 6 weeks of age; 3-4 doses	
HPV	Protein subunit/conjugate	Bivalent (16,18) - Cervarix (not available in USA)		Latex allergy
		9-valent (6,11,16,18,31,33,45,52,58)-Gardasil-9	≥ 9 years of age; 2-3 doses over 6 months	Yeast hypersensitivity
MMR with/without Varicella	Live, attenuated		≥ 1 year of age; 2 doses (at least 1 month apart)	Severe immunodeficiency
Varicella-Zoster	Live	Var	2 doses (first dose 12-15 months, second dose 4-6 years)	Severe immunodeficiency
	Recombinant	Shingrix	2 doses ≥50 years of age	
Influenza	Nasal spray: live, attenuated; injection: subunit/conjugate	FluMist quadrivalent; trivalent or quadrivalent injection	≥ 6 months of age	Guillain-Barré syndrome
Pertussis	Subunit/conjugate	DTaP, Tdap	DTaP 5 doses 2 months-6 years; Tdap booster every 10 years and during each pregnancy	

DTap, diphtheria, tetanus, and acellular pertussis; HPV, human papillomavirus; MMR, measles, mumps, rubella; PCV, pneumococcal conjugate vaccine; PPSV, pneumococcal polysaccharide vaccine; Tdap, tetanus, diphtheria, acellular pertussis.

*Previous allergic reaction to previous vaccine administration or to a component of the vaccine is a contraindication to future doses of that vaccine; influenza and pertussis vaccinations are recommended during pregnancy, while other vaccines are not recommended.

Tetanus Vaccination History	*Clean, Minor Wounds*		*All Other Wounds*	
	DTap, Tdap, or Td	*TIG*	*DTap, Tdap, or Td*	*TIG*
Unknown or < 3 doses	Yes	No	Yes	Yes
> 3 doses	No (unless last dose >10 years ago)	No	No (unless >5 years since last dose)	No (unless severe immunodeficiencies including HIV)

DTap, diphtheria, tetanus, and acellular pertussis; HIV, human immunodeficiency virus; Tdap, tetanus, diphtheria, acellular pertussis; Td, tetanus and diphtheria.

Biologic Agents

- Medicinal agents originating from biologic source used to prevent and treat cancers or autoimmune diseases, which includes the use of antibodies, interleukins, and vaccines

Cetuximab

- Recombinant humanized monoclonal antibody approved for squamous cell carcinoma (SCC) of the head and neck.
- Mechanism includes selective binding of epidermal growth factor (EGF) receptor to competitively inhibit EGF resulting in cell growth inhibition, cellular apoptosis, and reduction of vascular endothelial growth factor (VEGF) production.
- Indicated in the initial treatment of locally or regionally advanced SCC and recurrent or metastatic SCC.
- May be used as monotherapy after platinum-based therapy for metastatic disease or in combination with platinum-based therapy or with radiation therapy.
- Most common side effects include rash, fatigue, and hypomagnesemia.

Pembrolizumab

- Monoclonal antibody that binds to programmed cell death protein 1 (PD-1).
- Interaction of PD-1 with its ligands (PD-L1 and PD-L2) serves as an immune checkpoint, preventing T cell-mediated immune response against the body's normal cells.
- Blocking this interaction, therefore, activates the immune system to attack cancer cells that express PD-L1.
- FDA indications include advanced head and neck SCC, melanoma, Merkel cell carcinoma, lung cancer, and lymphoma.
- Side effects include diarrhea, arthralgia, dermatitis, and hypothyroidism.

Rituximab

- Humanized monoclonal antibody used for the treatment of granulomatosis with polyangiitis (GPA; Wegener granulomatosis) and non-Hodgkin lymphoma.
- Mechanism of action involves binding of CD20 surface protein on B-cells, which allows natural killer cell-mediated destruction of B-cells through antibody-dependent cellular cytotoxicity and complement-dependent cytotoxicity.
- It also promotes CD20+ cell apoptosis.
- Indicated in the treatment of moderate to severe forms of GPA and has generally replaced the use of methotrexate and cyclophosphamide as the secondary treatment of this disease.
- Side effects include leukopenia, thrombocytopenia, and neutropenia with increased infection rates.

Infliximab

- Recombinant human-mouse IgG monoclonal antibody used to treat relapsing polychondritis.
- Mechanism through the neutralization of TNF-α, thereby reducing proinflammatory cytokine production, reduction of endothelial permeability, and reducing adhesion molecule release.
- Up to 50% of patients may have formation of antinuclear antibodies with use.

Tocilizumab

- Recombinant humanized monoclonal antibody targeting the interleukin-6-receptor, which inhibits transduction of inflammatory mediators that summon T and B cells.
- Initiated with glucocorticoid therapy as the glucocorticoid is tapered until tocilizumab is used as long-term monotherapy.
- Used to treat inflammatory autoimmune diseases such as giant cell arteritis (temporal arteritis), a large-vessel vasculitis that can also affect medium and small arteries.

Teprotumumab

- Monoclonal antibody that binds to the insulin-like growth factor-1 receptor (IGF-1R).
- Results in decreased fibroblast proliferation and decreased proptosis.
- FDA approved for thyroid eye disease.
- Adverse effects include muscle cramps, alopecia, hyperglycemia, and hearing loss.

Bevacizumab

- Monoclonal antibody that binds VEGF, preventing new blood vessel growth.
- FDA approved for renal carcinoma, glioblastoma, and lung cancer.
- Off-label use for recurrent respiratory papillomatosis and hereditary hemorrhagic telangiectasia.
- Adverse effects include gastrointestinal perforation, hemorrhage, renal injury, venous thromboembolism, and hypertension.

Dupilumab

- Monoclonal antibody that binds the alpha subunit of the IL-4 receptor, blocking the signaling of IL-4 and IL-13.
- FDA approved for CRS with nasal polyposis (CRSwNP), atopic dermatitis, asthma, and eosinophilic esophagitis.
- Clinical trials show a significant reduction in nasal polyp and nasal congestion scores compared to placebo (LIBERTY NP SINUS-24 and 52).
- Adverse effects are rare but include injection site reactions, dermatitis, psoriasis, eosinophilia, insomnia, toothache, gastritis, arthralgia, and conjunctivitis.

Omalizumab

- Monoclonal antibody that exclusively binds free IgE, resulting in immunoglobulin depletion and decreased expression of the high-affinity IgE receptor FcεRI on mast cells and basophils.
- FDA approved for CRSwNP, asthma, IgE-mediated food allergy, and chronic spontaneous urticaria.
- Clinical trials show a significant reduction in nasal polyp, nasal congestion, and SNOT-22 scores compared to placebo (POLYP 1 and 2).
- Adverse effects are rare but include possible anaphylaxis, local site reaction, and arteriothrombotic effects.

Mepolizumab

- Monoclonal antibody that binds IL-5 and blocks it from interacting with its receptor on eosinophils.
- The result is impaired eosinophil differentiation, maturation, migration, and survival.

- FDA approved for CRSwNP, asthma, eosinophilic granulomatosis with polyangiitis (Churg-Strauss Syndrome), and hypereosinophilic syndrome.
- Clinical trials show a significant reduction in nasal polyp and nasal congestion visual analog scores compared to placebo (SYNAPSE).
- Adverse effects include anaphylaxis, angioedema, injection site reaction, and arthralgia.

Corticosteroids

- Utilized in the treatment of a variety of inflammatory and immune-mediated disorders (eg, sarcoidosis), which can be administered topically or systemically.
- Common systemic corticosteroids include prednisone and dexamethasone.
- Unless systemic use is less than 5 days, a taper is typically required to prevent adrenal insufficiency from hypothalamic-pituitary-adrenal (HPA) axis suppression.
- Fluticasone and mometasone are commonly used topical corticosteroids, which do not require tapering despite prolonged use because there is little impact on the HPA axis.
- Available corticosteroids have differing potencies with the equi-efficacious doses listed below:

Hydrocortisone	1
Prednisone	4
Prednisolone	4
Methylprednisolone	5
Triamcinolone	5
Dexamethasone	25

- Prolonged systemic corticosteroid use can lead to hypertension, Cushing syndrome, blood sugar dyscrasias, mental status changes (anxiety, insomnia), glaucoma, cataract (posterior subcapsular) formation, decreased bone mineral density, avascular necrosis (AVN) most commonly of the femoral head, and peptic ulcer formation
  - AVN is the most litigated corticosteroid complication and is associated with prednisone doses in excess of 290 mg.
- Topically administered corticosteroids typically have few or no systemic adverse effects due to lack of systemic absorption.
- Intranasal corticosteroids (INCS):
  - Local adverse effects include epistaxis and, rarely, nasal septum perforation with intranasal administration.
  - Research has shown no significant effect on cataract formation or intraocular pressure.

INCS are indicated for the treatment of inflammatory conditions of the nose and paranasal sinuses including allergic and nonallergic rhinitis, vasomotor rhinitis, and chronic rhinosinusitis (CRS).

- Otologic topical steroids:
  - Several antibiotic and corticosteroid otic drops formulations are available.
  - Indicated in the treatment of infectious otitis externa or as a single modality therapy for eczematous otitis externa.
- The table below lists and compares several commonly employed topical nasal corticosteroids:

Drug	*Youngest Approved Age (yr)*	*Possible Growth Suppression in Children*	*Nasal Polyposis Indication*	*Pregnancy Approved*	*Scent*
Beclomethasone propionate	4	Yes	No	No	Yes
Budesonide	6	N/A	Yes	Yes	No
Ciclesonide	12	N/A	No	No	No
Flunisolide	6	N/A	No	No	Yes
Fluticasone propionate	4	No	Yes	No	Yes
Fluticasone furoate	2	No	No	No	No
Mometasone	2	No	Yes	No	No

- Preoperative systemic steroid use has been shown to decrease intraoperative bleeding, improve surgical field visualization, and decrease operative time (prednisone 30 mg PO daily for 5 days before surgery)

Anticholinergics

- Muscarinic acetylcholine receptor antagonists are commonly employed in head and neck conditions.
- Available in both topical and systemic formulations.

Nasal Preparations

- **Ipratropium bromide**
  - Available in 0.03% and 0.06% preparations
  - Decreases parasympathetic mediated nasal secretions
  - Rapid onset and low systemic absorption
  - Indications include virally mediated rhinitis, allergic and nonallergic rhinitis, and especially vasomotor rhinitis

Systemic Preparations

- Utilized for motion sickness, systemic secretion reduction, treatment of vagal reactions, and as part of advanced cardiac support during code events

- **Scopolamine**
  - Commonly employed in the treatment of motion sickness by blocking vestibular input to the central vestibular system which is responsible for the vegetative symptoms.
  - Both systemic and transdermal formulations have demonstrated efficacy with prophylaxis; neither has literature support for active symptom management and may impair central nervous system recovery from vestibular dysfunction.
- **Glycopyrrolate**
  - Quaternary amine (does not cross the blood-brain barrier) commonly used to reduce oral, pharyngeal, and respiratory secretions prior to endoscopy.
- **Atropine**
  - Typically used in the treatment of bradycardia or cardiac arrest events.
  - Adverse effects are mediated by the blockage of normal parasympathetic activity resulting in tachycardia, flushing, blurred vision, urinary retention, decreased gastrointestinal motility, constipation, mental status changes, and xerostomia.
  - "Blind as a bat, mad as a hatter, hot as a hare, dry as a bone."

Vasoconstrictors

- Decrease the size of mucous membranes and/or decrease bleeding via arteriolar vasoconstriction
- **Epinephrine (adrenaline)**
  - Potent agonist of α1, α2, β1, and β2 receptors; normal synthesis occurs in the adrenal medulla.
  - Vasoconstriction is mediated by α1 receptors.
  - β1 receptor agonism results in positive effects on cardiac inotropy, chronotropy, and dromotropy, while β2 agonism induces smooth muscle relaxation (coronary vasodilation and bronchodilation).
  - Can be administered topically (intranasal and aerosolized).
  - Topical use on the nasal mucosa produces pallor and shrinkage due to vasoconstriction (1:1000 or 1:2000 dilutions).
  - Onset is within 5 minutes, and the duration of action is less than 1 hour.
  - Commonly used with local anesthetics to increase the duration of activity by preventing interstitial drug washout and to decrease bleeding.
- **Ephedrine**
  - Induces the release of preformed stores of norepinephrine.
  - Longer action duration and less potent than epinephrine.
  - Can be administered topically or systemically.
- **Pseudoephedrine**
  - Commonly used analog employed as a systemic decongestant.
  - Regulations exist on over-the-counter (OTC) availability due to its use in methamphetamine synthesis.
- **Phenylephrine**
  - α1 agonist, sympathomimetic.
  - Commonly employed as a topical nasal decongestant.
  - Can be used as a vasopressor in critical care situations.

- **Cocaine**
  - Local anesthetic with vasoconstrictive properties.
  - Works by blocking the reuptake of catecholamines at synapses.
  - Topical use in the nose provides both anesthesia and vasoconstriction.
  - Both serum (3 hours) and urinary (6 hours) levels can be detected after topical use.
  - Maximum dose is about 2 to 3mg/kg; most prevalent preparation is a 4% solution.
- **Oxymetazoline**
  - A common α1 agonist used topically for nasal decongestion and epistaxis.
- Both phenylephrine and oxymetazoline used for longer than 3 to 5 days can result in tachyphylaxis (blunted response to the same dose of drug) and rebound nasal congestion (rhinitis medicamentosa) with cessation of use.

Treatment of Gastric Acidity

- Laryngopharyngeal reflux and gastroesophageal reflux disease are common problems evaluated by an otolaryngologist.
- Symptoms include hoarseness, dry cough, globus sensation, and throat clearing.
- Gastric acid can have significant deleterious effects on airway inflammation and healing after airway surgery.
- Treatment typically starts with lifestyle modifications and moves to medicinal therapy for recalcitrant disease.
- The goals of pharmacotherapy are to reduce gastric acid production (antihistamines and proton pump inhibitors), neutralize gastric acid (antacids), or clear gastric contents distally (promotility agents).

Antihistamines

- The H_2 histamine receptor promotes acid production from gastric parietal cells.
- Famotidine, nizatidine, and cimetidine are OTC H_2-receptor-specific antihistamines available for acid suppressive therapy.
- Ranitidine was recently withdrawn from the market due to contamination with the carcinogen NDMA.
- Cimetidine is a cytochrome P450 inhibitor; drug interactions should be investigated prior to the recommendation of this drug.

Proton Pump Inhibitors (PPI)

- PPIs block the production of gastric acid by inhibiting the production of hydrogen ions by the H^+/K^+ ATPase enzyme on the luminal surface of parietal cells.
- Available drugs include omeprazole, pantoprazole, lansoprazole, rabeprazole, and their enantiomers (esomeprazole, dexlansoprazole).
- These medications should be taken 1 hour before a meal to maximize effect.
- Long-term use can lead to several adverse effects including negative Ca^{2+} homeostasis (possible risk of fractures) and B_{12} deficiency (megaloblastic anemia).
- Other conditions that are at increased risk include *Clostridium difficile*-associated diarrhea and dementia development.
- Supplemental calcium intake is a reasonable recommendation if long-term treatment is to be considered.

Acid Neutralization

- Antacids neutralize gastric acid by providing hydroxide ions or congregate bases to bind with hydrogen ions.
  - Examples include aluminum hydroxide, magnesium hydroxide, sodium bicarbonate, and calcium carbonate.
  - Typically taken at or shortly after a meal once acid production has commenced.
  - Generally safe if taken in moderation, though caution should be exercised in patients with sodium sensitivity (eg, congestive heart failure).

Protective Barriers

- **Alginic acid**
  - A polysaccharide derived from brown algae that forms a viscous gum in the stomach and neutralizes postprandial acid (eg, Gaviscon).

Promotility Agents

- **Metoclopramide**
  - Dopaminergic antagonist that increases the tone of the lower esophageal sphincter, decreases the tone of the pyloric sphincter, and increases gastric antrum motility.
  - Side effects include possible extrapyramidal symptoms (dystonias) and cumulative effect with other dopamine antagonists (typical and atypical antipsychotics).

Hemostatic Agents

- **Desmopressin acetate** (ddAVP/arginine vasopressin)
  - Selective vasopressin V2 receptor agonist.
  - Results in secretion of von Willebrand factor and factor VIII.
  - Useful in patients with Hemophilia A (factor VIII deficiency), type I von Willebrand disease, or prolonged bleeding times (platelet dysfunction) from conditions such as renal insufficiency.
  - ddAVP can also stimulate the release of tissue-type plasminogen activator (fibrinolysis).
- **Aminocaproic acid**
  - Lysine analog that acts as a competitive binder to plasminogen
  - Can be given to counter fibrinolysis
- **Fibrin sealants**
  - Bovine and human thrombin combined with fibrin (eg, Tisseel, Hemaseel, Crosseal)
- **Gelatin hemostatic agents**
  - Purified gelatin (eg, Gelfoam)
- **Combination products**
  - Gelatin matrix combined with thrombin (eg, Floseal)
- **Oxidized regenerated cellulose**
  - Serves as a matrix for clot formation (eg, Surgicel and Surgicel Fibrillar)
- **Microfibrillar collagen**
  - Causes platelet aggregation and activation of clotting factors (eg, Avitene)
- **Cyanoacrylate**
  - Polymerizes when it contacts water-containing tissues (eg, Dermabond)

Ototoxicity

- Ototoxicity encompasses both cochlear and vestibular effects.
- The following table summarizes the main ototoxic medication classes.

Drug Class	*Duration*	*Primary Target*	*Site of Damage*
Aminoglycosides	Permanent	Drug specific	1. Inner row of outer hair cells (OHC) at the cochlear basal turn 2. Stria Vascularis
Platinum-based chemotherapeutics	Permanent	Cochlea	1. Inner row of OHCs at the cochlear basal turn 2. Stria Vascularis
Loop diuretics	Transient	Cochlea	Stria Vascularis
Quinine	Transient	Cochlea	1. Stria Vascularis 2. Organ of Corti
Salicylates	Transient	Cochlea	OHCs

Aminoglycosides (AGs)

- Results in bilateral, permanent high-frequency sensorineural hearing loss (SNHL).
- Toxicity is associated with serum levels above therapeutic target levels.
- Renal clearance makes renal dosing and kidney function monitoring essential.
- AGs chelate iron, causing free radical formation and subsequent cell damage starting with the inner row of OHCs.
- Proceeds in a basal to apical direction explaining the high-frequency SNHL seen early.
- Histopathologic findings include intermittent OHC loss and stria vascularis damage.
- A1555G mutation in the mitochondrial 12S ribosomal RNA imparts exquisite AG sensitivity, which is more common in certain Chinese populations.
- While all AGs damage both the cochlear and vestibular hair cells, many affect one or the other primarily.
- In order of vestibulotoxic to cochleotoxic AG severity:
  - Streptomycin, gentamycin, tobramycin, kanamycin, amikacin, neomycin (SGT KAN)
- Otic preparations of AGs carry a *significant* risk of inner ear toxicity if the tympanic membrane is *not* intact (must be able to visualize the entire TM prior to administration).
  - Middle ear AG administration is used in medical vestibular ablation for vestibular hyperfunction (eg, gentamycin injection for Meniere disease).

Platinum-based Chemotherapeutics

- Cisplatin and carboplatin are commonly used in the treatment of upper aerodigestive SCC.
- Dose-dependent ototoxicity, typically high-frequency SNHL between 4kHz and 8kHz.
- Histopathology is similar to AG damage.
- SNHL is seen in more than 50% of patients, and tinnitus is seen in 7%; few progress to have speech understanding deficits.
- Audiological recommendations include regular pre- and post-treatment audiograms to surveil for potential hearing loss.

Quinine and Chloroquine

- Quine and chloroquine are antimalarial treatments.
- Primarily cochleotoxic due to reversible vasculitis and ischemia of the inner ear with degenerative changes being found in the organ of Corti and stria vascularis.
- Neonates born to mothers taking these medications can exhibit bilateral SNHL even if the mother's hearing is normal.

Loop Diuretics

- Main examples are ethacrynic acid (1% of usage) and furosemide (~6% of usage), which work to block the action of the Na^+-K^+-$2Cl^-$ symporter in the ascending loop of Henle.
- Ototoxic effects from loop diuretics are typically transient.
- Mechanism is through electrolyte imbalances in the endolymph by blocking the H^+/K^+ ATPase enzyme.
- Toxicities can be minimized if parenteral administration is given over time versus a bolus.

Salicylates

- Aspirin (acetylsalicylic acid/ASA) and other salicylates produce reversible hearing loss and tinnitus.
- Occurs with doses greater than 2.7 g of ASA.
- Renally cleared; once systemically cleared, cochlear effects subside.

Dermatologic Agents

Minoxidil

- Direct vasodilator when given systemically.
- Topical preparation is FDA-approved to treat male pattern baldness.
- Mechanism of action is speculated to be through increased blood flow, oxygen, and nutrients to hair follicles.
- Adverse effects include local pruritus, irritation, and hypertrichosis.
- Available in 2% and 5% OTC preparations with the 5% formulation being more efficacious.

Finasteride

- Finasteride is an orally available 5α-reductase inhibitor (testosterone to dihydrotestosterone conversion) used in the treatment of androgenic alopecia.
- Hair regrowth is seen in 90% of patients.
- Few short-term adverse effects are known; long-term effects are unknown.

Vitamin A Analogs

- Tretinoin is a form of vitamin A used to improve the appearance of aging skin, particularly photoaged skin.
- Improves collagen synthesis in the papillary dermis, which can improve the appearance of rhytids.
- Used to help prepare skin prior to chemical peels (chemexfoliation).
- Potent teratogen: Strong counseling to avoid in pregnancy is warranted.
- Consider pharmacologic contraceptives if prolonged use in females of childbearing age is being planned.

Sunscreens

- Ultraviolet (UV) radiation skin exposure is associated with photoaging and skin cancer.
- UV radiation is separated into UVA (320-400 nm) and UVB (290-320 nm).
- UVB directly damages cells, while UVA causes indirect damage by the creation of reactive oxygen species.
- Broad-spectrum sunscreens block both UVA and UVB radiation.
- Sunscreen use has been shown to decrease the risk of skin photodamage, actinic keratosis, and SCC.
  - Data regarding basal cell carcinoma and melanoma are less clear
- Sunscreen should be applied 30 minutes before sun exposure and every 2 hours during UV exposure.
- The effectiveness of sunscreen can be estimated by the sun protection factor (SPF):
  - It takes 30 times longer for skin to burn with SPF 30 than without sunscreen.
- Active ingredients are either radiopaque inorganic compounds (zinc and titanium oxides) that block UV radiation or organic compounds (para-aminobenzoic acid) that absorb the UV radiation.
- Organic compounds tend to become less effective as UV exposure increases.
- Inorganic compounds have typically been available as thick pastes with a white appearance, but new formulations with nanoparticles are available with fewer cosmetic concerns.
- Inorganic compounds provide superior protection in general; although, consistent use of any sunscreen is superior to intermittent or inadequate use.

Botulinum Toxin

- Extremely potent neurotoxin produced by the bacterium *Clostridium botulinum.*
- Secreted exotoxin composed of one heavy and one light chain.
- The light chain selectively cleaves presynaptic SNARE proteins, preventing acetylcholine-containing vesicles from fusing with the nerve terminal membrane.
- Results in flaccid paralysis of affected neuromuscular junctions.
- Reinnervation occurs through the growth of collaterals within 3 months.
- Clinical indications include effacement of rhytids, treatment of facial dystonias, spasmodic dysphonia, bruxism, strabismus, achalasia, hyperhidrosis, and sialorrhea.
- Seven different serotypes exist (A-G), each targeting unique locations in vesicular and target SNARE proteins.
- Serotypes A (BOTOX) and B (MYOBLOC) are commercially available.

Antiemetics

- Most agents target receptors in the chemoreceptor trigger zone (CTZ) found in the floor of the ventricle or the emetic center in the lateral reticular formation in the medulla.
- Histamine and acetylcholine receptors are found in the lateral reticular formation, and dopamine receptors in the CTZ.
- Antihistamines include scopolamine and promethazine, which can be taken systemically or transdermally.

- Anticholinergics include diphenhydramine.
- Dopamine antagonists include prochlorperazine and metoclopramide.
  - Care must be taken in patients taking anti-dopaminergic agents (ie, typical or atypical antipsychotics) to prevent extrapyramidal symptoms.
- Selective serotonin agonists for the 5-HT_3 receptors are commonly used due to their very favorable side effect profile.
  - Ondansetron is the most common.
  - May prolong the QTc interval, leading to Torsades de Pointes.
  - Correct any significant electrolyte abnormalities prior to use systemically.

Mucolytics and Expectorants

- Mucolytic agents work by depolymerizing mucopolysaccharides and increasing their solubility.
- *N*-Acetylcysteine is an example; uses include thinning of secretions in asthma, paracetamol (acetaminophen) overdose, and renal protectant with the use of IV radiocontrast.
- Guaifenesin is an expectorant; its mechanism of action is poorly understood.
- Other agents include ammonium and iodide salts.

Selected Therapeutic Regimens

Bell Palsy

- Treatment: Systemic steroids should be administered within 72 hours of symptom onset (with option of additional antiviral therapy).
- Antiviral therapy alone is not recommended.

Cochlear Implant

- Age <5: Same pneumococcal vaccines as similarly aged children.
- Age 6-18: At least one previous dose of PCV15 or PCV20 and one dose of PPSV23 if PCV15 is used.
- Adults: At least one previous dose of PCV15, 20, or 21 and one dose of PPSV23 if PCV15 is used.

Deep Neck Infections

- Bacteriology: mixed, often with both aerobic (*Streptococcus, Staphylococcus*) and anaerobic bacteria (foul smelling, poorly detected in culture)
- Treatment: broad-spectrum IV antibiotics with blood and/or abscess culture with directed antibiotics

Necrotizing Fasciitis

- Type 1: polymicrobial including ≥ 1 anaerobic bacteria; typically, *Streptococcus* > *Staphylococcus* > *Enterococcus* >*Lactobacillus* > *Corynebacterium* and *E. Coli*, *Klebsiella* and *Bacteroides* for anaerobic
- Type 2: monomicrobial, typically Group A *Streptococcus* (30% incidence of toxic shock syndrome)

- Type 3: *Vibrio* species from sea life injuries (bite, sting, etc.)
- Treatment
  - Surgical debridement
  - Empiric antibiotic regimen: a carbapenem or piperacillin-tazobactam **plus** vancomycin or daptomycin **plus** clindamycin

Acute Otitis Externa (AOE)

- Bacteriology: *P. aeruginosa*, *S. aureus*; (less than 2% of AOE are fungal, viral, or eczema)
  - Treatment: antiseptic topicals (acetic acid/alcohol), topical antimicrobials (fluoroquinolones), aural toilet, and/or wick placement if canal is obstructed.
  - Nonototoxic if tympanic membrane integrity is in question.
  - Patients should be reassessed within 48 to 72 hours.

Acute Otitis Media (AOM)

- Bacteriology: *S. pneumoniae* (~50%, resistance varies), nontypeable *H. influenzae* (~45%, 33%-50% produce β-lactamase), *M. catarrhalis* (~10% of cases, >90% produce β-lactamase)
- Treatment
  - Observation for 48 hours offered for children 6 to 23 months with nonsevere unilateral AOM and for children 2 years or older with nonsevere unilateral or bilateral AOM.
  - Amoxicillin is first line.
  - PCN-allergic patients: Cefdinir, cefuroxime, cefpodoxime, or ceftriaxone are recommended.

Chronic Suppurative Otitis Media

- Bacteriology: mixed and includes *S. aureus*, *P. aeruginosa*, anaerobic bacteria, plus those commonly found in AOM
- Treatment: antimicrobial/antiseptic topical therapy (acetic acid/alcohol, fluoroquinolones) plus aural toilet

Acute Bacterial Rhinosinusitis

- Bacteriology: *H. influenzae*, *S. pneumoniae*, *M. catarrhalis*; rarely *S. pyogenes*, *S. aureus*, *P. aeruginosa* (often in cystic fibrosis), anaerobic (odontogenic sinusitis)
- Treatment (pediatrics)
  - Observation for 72 hours is an option for nonsevere symptoms.
  - Antibiotics and/or treatment escalation indicated for children with severe onset or worsening symptoms, or failure to improve within 72 hours.
  - First-line regimen: amoxicillin with or without clavulanate for a minimum of 10 days.
  - Nonsevere history of penicillin allergy: Cefdinir, cefuroxime, or cefpodoxime (third-generation cephalosporins) are recommended.
- Treatment (adults)
  - Watchful waiting or amoxicillin with or without clavulanate as first-line for 5 to 10 days
  - Penicillin-allergic: doxycycline, levofloxacin, or moxifloxacin

Acute viral rhinosinusitis

- Treatment: analgesics, nasal saline, topical intranasal corticosteroids

Chronic Rhinosinusitis

- Bacteriology: mixed, including *S. aureus, P. aeruginosa*, a large mix of aerobic and anaerobic bacteria
- Treatment: longer-duration antibiotics (at least 3 weeks)
  - Polymicrobial biofilms lead to resistance, may make treatment difficult with oral antibiotics alone; can add topical/systemic steroids, antibiotic irrigations, and surgery.

Acute Bacterial Tonsillitis/Pharyngitis

- Bacteriology: *S. pneumoniae*, group A β -hemolytic *Streptococcus* (*S. pyogenes*), *H. influenza*
- Treatment: penicillin

Tympanostomy Tube Otorrhea

- Treatment: topical antibiotic ear drops (fluoroquinolones) only without oral antibiotics

Xerostomia

- Seen commonly in patients with autoimmune salivary gland conditions (Sjögren syndrome) or postradiation sequelae.
- Conservative treatments include drinking small, frequent sips of water, use of sugar-free sialagogues, and use of cellulose-based salivary substitutes.
- Cholinergic agonists (parasympathomimetic) stimulate the saliva production when functioning parenchyma is present (eg, pilocarpine and cevimeline).
- Due to cholinergic systemic effects (diarrhea, hyperhidrosis, increased airway secretions), use is typically limited.

Aphthous Stomatitis

- Recurrent aphthous ulcers (ie, canker sores) are common, affecting between 20% and 50% of the population; however, etiology is unclear, and no definitive treatments exist.
- Topical corticosteroids: 0.05% clobetasol and 0.05% fluocinonide are more potent and effective than triamcinolone.
- Antimicrobial: Tetracycline antibiotic solutions reduce ulcer size, duration, and pain.
- Anti-inflammatory: Amlexanox paste 5% facilitates healing but does not reduce the frequency of outbreaks.
- Anesthetic: Viscous lidocaine at various concentrations can be used to help control pain.

Smoking Cessation

- Multiple medications are FDA approved as part of a comprehensive approach to tobacco cessation.
- Nicotine replacement therapies include transdermal patches and gums.
- Bupropion and varenicline are medicinal options that reduce nicotine craving and withdrawal symptoms.
- Bupropion inhibits dopamine and norepinephrine reuptake and blocks nicotinic acetylcholine receptors.
- Varenicline is a partial agonist at central nicotinic acetylcholine receptors.

Tinnitus

- No medicinal treatments have demonstrated long-term benefit in symptom reduction.
- Antidepressants, anticonvulsants, anxiolytics, and intratympanic medications have failed to demonstrate benefit in randomized controlled trials.

Chronic Cough

- No strong medication options for the persistent chronic cough exist.
- Opiates are the mainstay of the refractory, chronic cough; extended-release morphine demonstrates the highest efficacy (5 mg dose).
- Other centrally acting medications include amitriptyline, paroxetine, gabapentin, and carbamazepine and locally acting agents such as benzonatate; none have demonstrated effectiveness in clinical trials.

Cystic Fibrosis (CF)

- Autosomal recessive genetic disorder characterized by derangement of the CF transmembrane conductance regulator (CFTR) causing restricted chloride efflux and mucociliary dysfunction.
- More than 1000 mutations have been identified with the ΔF508 mutation accounting for nearly 70% of all cases.
- The G551D mutation accounts for 5% of cases and is related to reduced CFTR protein channel opening or opening probability.
- Historically, most treatments are designed as noncurative, symptomatic control of disease, but newer medications targeting specific mutations and heart-lung transplants have improved long-term survivability and quality of life.
- **Ivacaftor**
    - CFTR potentiator approved for CF patients over 4 months of age with the G551D mutation, thereby potentiating chloride channel opening and improving chloride transport across the channel pore.
    - Outcome studies have shown improved lung function and quality of life measures with a reduction in the number and severity of pulmonary exacerbations.
    - Common adverse reactions include oropharyngeal pain, headaches, upper respiratory tract infections, and cough.
- **Trikafta** (elexacaftor/tezacaftor/ivacaftor)
    - Approved for CF patients over 2 years of age with at least one ΔF508 mutation.
    - Triple therapy with the addition of elexacaftor and tezacaftor to ivacaftor, which increases the amount of CFTR protein that reaches the cell surface.

Bibliography

American Academy of Otolaryngology – Head and Neck Surgery. http://www.entnet.org/. Accessed January 2025.

Bachert C, Zhang N, Cavaliere C, Weiping W, Gevaert E, Krysko O. Biologics for chronic rhinosinusitis with nasal polyps. *J Allergy Clin Immunol.* 2020;145:725-739.

Center for Disease Control and Prevention, CDC.gov.

Flerlage J, Engorn B. *The Harriet Lane Handbook: A Manual for Pediatric House Officers.* Philadelphia, PA: Saunder. Elsevier; 2015.

Lee KJ. *Essential Otolaryngology: Head & Neck Surgery.* 12th ed. New York, NY: McGraw Hill, Medical Publishing Division; 2019.

Questions

1. Of the drugs listed, which is the least likely to cause sensorineural hearing loss?
   A. Tobramycin
   B. Amikacin
   C. Neomycin
   D. Streptomycin

2. Which biologic agent targets the alpha subunit of the IL-4 receptor, blocking the signaling of IL-4 and IL-13?
   A. Cetuximab
   B. Rituximab
   C. Dupilumab
   D. Mepolizumab

3. Which best describes botulinum toxin?
   A. The target of the drug is the enzymatic cleavage of SNARE proteins along the postsynaptic membrane.
   B. There are few clinical indications.
   C. Reinnervation occurs through collateral growth.
   D. Serotype B is the only serotype indicated for cosmetic use.

4. Which antibiotic can produce a rash in patients with Epstein-Barr virus mononucleosis?
   A. Cefdinir
   B. Amoxicillin
   C. Doxycycline
   D. Azithromycin

5. Which fluoroquinolone does not cover *Pseudomonas*?
   A. Ciprofloxacin
   B. Levofloxacin
   C. Moxifloxacin
   D. None of the above

Chapter 11
Head & Neck Manifestations of HIV and Granulomatous Diseases

Head and Neck Manifestations of HIV

Overview

- Human immunodeficiency virus (HIV) is a blood-borne and sexually transmitted infection that leads to acquired immunodeficiency syndrome (AIDS).
- An enveloped, single-stranded RNA virus that primarily infects CD4+ T lymphocytes (though it can infect other cells that express CD4, such as macrophages).

Clinical Presentation

- HIV can spread via blood, semen, vaginal fluid, or breast milk.
- Primary HIV infection can be asymptomatic or present as a viral prodrome occurring 2 to 4 weeks after exposure.
- Symptoms include fever, reactive cervical lymphadenopathy, pharyngitis, maculopapular rash, orogenital ulcers, and meningoencephalitis.
- Leukopenia and decreased CD4 count can also occur with associated opportunistic infections.

Diagnosis

- HIV is diagnosed via anti-HIV antibodies detected in serum. These are persistently present for 3 months following exposure.

Table 11-1 2014 CDC HIV Age-Specific Infection Stage

	Age on date of CD4 T-lymphocyte test					
	< 1 year		*1-5 years*		*6 years or greater*	
Stage	*Cells/μL*	*%*	*Cells/μL*	*%*	*Cells/μL*	*%*
1	≥ 1500	≥ 34	≥ 1000	≥ 30	≥ 500	≥ 26
2	750-1499	26-33	500-999	22-29	200-499	14-25
3	< 750	< 26	< 500	< 22	< 200	< 14

The stage is primarily based on CD4 count, and the percentage is considered only if the count is missing.

Center for Disease Control (CDC) Staging System

- Incorporates both clinical manifestations and CD4 count. It was initially designed for surveillance purposes, though it provides an adequate overview of a patient's clinical picture (Table 11-1)
- Classified into one of five stages (0, 1, 2, 3, unknown):
  Stage 0—HIV+ patient, with a previous negative HIV test within 6 months of seroconversion. These patients remain Stage 0 until 6 months after diagnosis.
  Stage 1—*Acute HIV infection*. Occurs within 2 to 4 weeks after HIV infection. Symptoms may include flu-like illness.
  Stage 2—*Clinical latency* (HIV inactivity or dormancy). Asymptomatic or chronic HIV infection.
  Stage 3—*Acquired immunodeficiency syndrome* (AIDS). Presence of AIDS-defining condition = Stage 3.
  Stage unknown—No information available on CD4 count and no information available on AIDS-defining conditions.

Management

- Consists primarily of medications that target specific viral enzymes and comprises a treatment regimen known as antiretroviral therapy (ART)
- Pre-exposure prophylaxis (PrEP)
  - For high-risk individuals, it reduces the risk of transmission of HIV via sexual activity by 90% and via intravenous drug use by 70%
- Post-exposure prophylaxis (PEP)
  - Reduces the risk of seroconversion after potential exposure to HIV
  - Must be initiated within 72 hours after potential exposure, and ideally within one hour of exposure

Epidemiology

- Approximately 39.9 million individuals living with HIV worldwide, in 2023.
- Up to 50% of immunosuppressed patients present with head and neck complaints.

Infectious/Inflammatory Conditions Associated With HIV

Salivary Gland

- HIV may affect any of the salivary glands, but the parotid gland is the most common due to the presence of intraparotid lymph nodes.
- Salivary gland lesions are particularly prevalent in the pediatric population.
- Parotid lesions are generally infectious, inflammatory, or neoplastic in nature.
- Diagnosis can be confirmed via fine-needle aspiration in the majority of cases.
- Diagnostic imaging with ultrasound, computed tomography (CT), or magnetic resonance imaging (MRI) is useful when clinically indicated.
- Approximately 75% of parotid lesions are benign lymphoepithelial cysts. About 6% represent neoplasms, and the remainder consists of infectious/inflammatory processes.

Benign Lymphoepithelial Cyst

- The most common parotid gland lesions seen in HIV-positive patients.
- Etiology is related to viral inflammation.
- May present as unilateral lesions, but imaging often reveals subclinical disease bilaterally. Benign lymphoepithelial cysts (BLECs) are bilateral in up to 80% of cases.
- Typically present asymptomatically, though compression of the parotid ducts can cause pain and sialadenitis.
- Cervical lymphadenopathy is present in up to 90% of cases.
- BLEC may be confused with papillary cystadenoma lymphomatosum (Warthin tumor)–both are cystic and bilateral.

Management

- No definitive surgical excision is required for BLEC.
- Treatment goals consist of decreasing the viral load with the use of ART, which causes regression of the cysts.
- Options include ART, serial aspiration for cosmesis, sclerotherapy, radiotherapy, and parotidectomy.

Diffuse Infiltrative Lymphocytosis Syndrome

- Clinically similar to Sjogren syndrome seen in HIV-positive patients.
- *Clinical presentation*: Diffuse parotid enlargement and sicca symptoms (ie, xerostomia and xerophthalmia).

Management

- Primarily symptom control with salivary substitutes and sialagogues.
- Dental caries are a potential complication, and referral to dentistry is warranted.

Oral Cavity

- The immunodeficiency caused by HIV results in opportunistic infections and inflammatory conditions.
- Due to the increased risk of malignancy in these patients, the index of suspicion must remain high, and nonresolving or suspicious lesions should be biopsied.

Oral Candidiasis

- Oral candidiasis is the most common oral cavity lesion seen in HIV/AIDS, though incidence has decreased since the introduction of ART.
- The most common causative organism is *Candida albicans.*
- There are four types of oral candida: pseudomembranous, atrophic, angular cheilitis, and hyperplastic.
- The diagnosis is confirmed by potassium hydroxide preparation or by periodic acid-Schiff stain.

Management

- CD4 count more than 200 cells/mm^3, topical antifungals such as nystatin mouthwash can be used.
- CD4 count less than 200 cells/mm^3, systemic antifungals such as fluconazole are recommended.
- HIV patients are at risk of developing fluconazole-resistant candidiasis following repeated courses of treatment.

Oral Hairy Leukoplakia

- As the name suggests, oral hairy leukoplakia (OHL) is a white, corrugated, hyperkeratotic lesion, which most commonly affects the lateral tongue.
- The lesions are asymptomatic.
- Epstein-Barr virus (EBV) is the causative agent, and the presence of EBV in the biopsy sample confirms the diagnosis.
- OHL has a strong association with HIV infection, and its presence in a previously healthy individual should warrant workup for HIV.

Management

- OHL does not require any specific management, as it does not harbor malignant transformation potential.
- However, one must be mindful that the differential diagnosis for OHL includes lichen planus, idiopathic leukoplakia, and carcinoma in situ, and thus observation is required for evolution.

Gingival and Periodontal Disease

- Gingival disease, especially when necrotizing or ulcerative, is highly suggestive of HIV infection.
- Presentation in a previously healthy patient should warrant serologic testing, imaging, and dentistry referral.
- When the degree of bony destruction is out of proportion with the amount of mucosal injury, malignant neoplasms and bacillary angiomatosis must be considered. Biopsy should be taken.

Management

- Initial management consists of topical therapy to cover bacterial and fungal etiologies, such as chlorhexidine and nystatin mouthwash.
- Frank necrotic tissue requires debridement.

Complicated Infections as a Result of HIV

- Like immunocompetent individuals, patients with HIV also have a high incidence of sinonasal and otologic infections.

- The microbiology of these infections is similar to that of immunocompetent patients, with the most common organisms represented by *Streptococcus pneumoniae, Haemophilus influenzae, and Moraxella catarrhalis.*
- For patients with relatively normal CD4 counts (> 200 cells/mm^3), the management of these infections is no different from that of an immunocompetent patient.
- AIDS patients are at risk of developing complicated infections of the middle ear, temporal bone, and paranasal sinuses from opportunistic organisms.
- Must maintain a high clinical suspicion for severe head and neck infections such as malignant otitis externa and invasive fungal sinusitis.
- Chronic otitis media, tympanic membrane perforations, conductive and sensorineural hearing loss have been reported to be more prevalent in HIV-positive children in Sub-Saharan Africa.

HIV-Associated Malignancies

- HIV-associated malignancies are categorized into AIDS-defining and non-AIDS defining.
- In the era of ART, the incidence of AIDS-defining malignancies has been declining. However, several other malignancies, including cancers of the lung, liver, kidney, anus, and head and neck have been on the rise.

Kaposi Sarcoma

- Kaposi sarcoma (KS) is an angioproliferative tumor caused by human herpes virus 8, commonly associated with HIV infection.
- The incidence of KS in HIV patients is approximately 5%.

Clinical Presentation

- AIDS-associated KS frequently presents in the head and neck in as many as 70% of cases.
- KS in AIDS patients commonly presents in the oral cavity, with the most frequent subsites consisting of the hard palate, gingiva, and tongue. These mucosal lesions may be associated with pain, ulceration, bleeding, and loose teeth.
- Cutaneous KS presents as a maculopapular violaceous lesion that does not blanche.

Workup

- Biopsy demonstrates slit-like vascular channels, extravasated erythrocytes, and spindle cell proliferation.
- Initial evaluation should aim to identify other mucosal, cutaneous, or visceral lesions.
- Immune status and CD4 count should be investigated.

Management

- The primary management goal in KS is to successfully treat the underlying cause. This can cause regression of the lesions. The role of surgery in KS is palliative.
- Other options for controlling lesions include external beam radiation, cryotherapy, laser excision, intralesional chemotherapy, and systemic chemotherapy.

Lymphoma

- Both non-Hodgkin lymphoma (NHL) and Hodgkin lymphoma (HL) occur at an increased frequency in HIV patients.
- Lymphomas are the second most common malignancy seen in HIV patients, with an incidence of up to 19%. The most common type is diffuse large B-cell lymphoma, followed by Burkitt lymphoma.
- Lymphoma in immunocompromised patients is commonly associated with Epstein-Barr Virus (EBV, also known as human herpes virus 5), and the same is true of HIV-associated lymphomas.
- EBV is detected in up to 50% of HIV-associated lymphoma cases.

Clinical Presentation

- Symptoms are consistent with lymphoma of other etiologies and include B symptoms (fever, night sweats, unexplained weight loss of greater than 10% body mass) as well as enlarging lymph nodes. Depending on the location of the mass, compressive symptoms may also be a presenting complaint.
- HIV-associated lymphoma tends to present at a later stage, with worse performance status, more frequent B symptoms, and higher Ann Arbor stage compared to HIV-negative patients.

Workup

- Fine-needle aspiration biopsy may be used, but open biopsy is preferable, as it is typically required to confirm the specific type of lymphoma.
- Cross-sectional imaging of the body is required for staging. PET is also used for staging.

Management

- The standard treatment consists primarily of chemotherapy with concurrent ART.
- Two chemotherapy regimens are used in diffuse large B-cell lymphoma:
    - R-CHOP—rituximab, cyclophosphamide, doxorubicin, vincristine, prednisone
- R-EPOCH—rituximab, etoposide, prednisone, vincristine, doxorubicin
- External beam radiotherapy is also used for locoregional control and palliation.

Primary Central Nervous System Lymphoma

- Primary central nervous system lymphoma (PCNSL) is commonly associated with HIV infection and/or immunodeficiency state.
- Presenting symptoms result from nerve compression or raised intracranial pressure.

Management

- Traditional chemotherapies for B-cell lymphomas (ie, R-CHOP) are not effective due to poor penetration through the blood-brain barrier.
- Methotrexate-based regimens have been the most successful to-date.

Burkitt Lymphoma

- Burkitt lymphoma is a type of B-cell lymphoma and is the fastest-growing tumor in humans, with a doubling time of 24 to 48 hours.
- HIV comprises the majority of immunodeficiency-related Burkitt lymphoma.
- The incidence of Burkitt lymphoma in HIV does not appear to correlate with low CD4 counts.

- The clinical presentation differs from that of the endemic form. It rarely presents as a jaw lesion and more commonly presents as a mass elsewhere in the head and neck or in the abdomen.

Management

- HIV-associated Burkitt lymphoma is treated with a combination of high-dose chemotherapy and ART.
- The prognosis is dependent on age. A series of adult HIV patients treated in this manner achieved a remission rate of 70% and a 2-year overall survival of 47%.

Hodgkin Lymphoma

- Hodgkin lymphoma is the most common non-AIDS-defining malignancy and presents distinctively in comparison to immunocompetent/HIV-negative individuals.
- Diagnosis is confirmed histopathologically by the presence of Reed-Sternberg cells.
- Tends to present at a more advanced stage and with a less favorable histopathologic type, specifically mixed cellularity and lymphocyte-depleted types. (In contrast, the nodular sclerosing type is the most common in HIV-negative patients).
- The 5-year overall survival is 41%, which is considerably worse than HL seen in HIV-negative patients.

Management

- Combination chemoradiotherapy
- ABVD (Adriamycin, bleomycin, vinblastine, dacarbazine)

Nonmelanotic Skin Cancer

- Nonmelanotic cutaneous malignancies are more common in immunosuppressed patients, and this is true of HIV patients as well.
- Additional risk factors for nonmelanotic skin cancer (NMSC) are the same as in immunocompetent individuals.

Management

- The management of NMSC in HIV-positive patients is consistent with standard management for these malignancies

Granulomatous Diseases of the Head and Neck

- What is a granuloma?
  a. A granuloma is created by a chronic immunologic process resulting clinically in localized nodular inflammation.
- What is the differential diagnosis of a granuloma in the head and neck?
  a. There is a significant range of symptoms caused by granulomatous diseases, not limited to the head and neck. A full history and physical examination should be performed for all patients with a granulomatous biopsy. Refer to Table 11-2.

Differential Diagnosis

See Table 11-2.

Table 11-2 Differential Diagnosis: Granulomatous Diseases of the Head and Neck

Autoimmune	*Unknown origin*	*Neoplastic*	*Infectious*	*Fungal/parasitic*	*Congenital*
Granulomatosis with polyangiitis	Sarcoidosis	Langerhans cell histiocytosis	Cat scratch disease	Histoplasmosis	Chediak-Higashi syndrome
Churg-Strauss (eosinophilic granulomatosis with polyangiitis)		Eosinophilic granulomatosis	Rhinoscleroma	Blastomycosis	Job syndrome
Relapsing polychondritis		Hand-Schuller-Christian disease	Leprosy	Rhinosporidiosis	
Systemic lupus erythematous		Letterer-Siwe disease	Nontuberculous mycobacteria	Coccidiomycosis	
Behcet disease		Fibrous histiocytoma	Tuberculosis	Aspergillus/Mucor	
		Lobular capillary hemangioma	Actinomycosis	Candidiasis	
			Syphilis	Leishmaniasis	

Autoimmune

Granulomatosis With Polyangiitis (GPA, Renamed From Wegener Granulomatosis)

- Small and medium-vessel vasculitis.
- Belongs to a larger group of necrotizing vasculopathy syndromes, all of which involve an autoimmune attack by abnormal circulating ANCA antibodies (anti-neutrophil cytoplasmic antibodies).
- Thought to be a T-cell-mediated hypersensitivity reaction.

Presentation

- Extremely variable.
- *Classic triad*: Airway necrotizing granulomas, systemic vasculitis, and focal glomerulonephritis.
- Most common presenting symptom is rhinitis.
- *Renal*: Rapidly progressive glomerulonephritis (75%).
- *Sinonasal*: Nasal congestion, crusting, rhinitis, epistaxis, septal perforation, and possible saddle nose deformity.
- *Otologic*: Conductive hearing loss from Eustachian tube dysfunction, middle ear effusion, and possible sensorineural hearing loss.
- *Oral cavity*: Gingival hypertrophy, gingivitis, tooth decay, nonspecific ulcerations
- *Ocular*: Pseudotumors, conjunctivitis, scleritis, episcleritis, uveitis, nasolacrimal obstruction.
- *Larynx:* Subglottic stenosis.
- *Pulmonary*: Cavitary lesions, nodules, infiltrates, pulmonary hemorrhage.

Histology

- Characteristic patchy necrosis surrounded by giant cells, causing necrotizing granulomas.
- Macrophages, inflammatory cells, and giant cells.
- True vasculitis, demonstrating granulomatous inflammation of vessel walls.

Workup/Diagnosis

- cANCA (cytoplasmic antineutrophil cytoplasmic antibodies) that react with proteinase (PR3) are associated with GPA but are not definitely sensitive or specific.
- Elevated ESR and CRP.
- Anemia, urine sediment (RBC casts or > 5 RBCs/HPF).
- Imaging—CXR, consider CT sinus as clinically indicated.
- Must have tissue biopsy demonstrating necrotizing granulomatous inflammation.

Treatment

- Induce remission with cyclophosphamide or rituximab in addition to high-dose corticosteroids.
- Maintenance with less toxic immunosuppressant therapy, such as methotrexate, azathioprine, leflunomide, or mycophenolate mofetil.
- Role of trimethoprim/sulfamethoxazole: (a) may help prevent relapse, especially in disease limited to the upper airway, (b) *Pneumocystis jiroveci* pneumonia (PJP) prophylaxis.

Churg-Strauss Syndrome (Eosinophilic Granulomatosis With Polyangiitis [EGPA])

- Allergic, granulomatous, small and medium-vessel vasculitis
- Necrotizing vasculopathy syndrome, in the same group as GPA

Presentation

- Extremely variable
- *Classic triad*: Asthma, systemic vasculitis, eosinophilia
- Occurs in patients with a history of airway allergic hypersensitivity
- Usually manifests in three stages:
  a. *Allergic stage*: Prodromal, allergic rhinitis and asthma, polyps, and nasal obstruction
  b. *Eosinophilic stage (aka Loeffler syndrome)*: Hypereosinophilia causes damage to respiratory and GI tracts, may experience weight loss, night sweats, asthma, cough, abdominal pain, and GI bleeding
  c. *Vasculitic stage*: Inflammation of vessels causes decreased perfusion of tissues and organs, may be severe and life-threatening. May develop thrombi, peritonitis, or perforation, or heart disease

Histology

- Fibrinoid, epithelioid, and eosinophilic extravascular granulomas with necrosis

Workup/Diagnosis

- Associated with pANCA (perinuclear antineutrophil cytoplasmic antibodies) that bind myeloperoxidase (MPO), positive in 50%
- Elevated eosinophils and granulomas in affected tissues
- American College of Rheumatology Criteria (1990); require 4/6
  a. Asthma
  b. Eosinophils more than 10% of the complete blood count with differential
  c. Mononeuritis multiplex or polyneuropathy
  d. Nonfixed pulmonary infiltrates
  e. Paranasal sinus abnormalities (rhinitis, sinusitis, polyps)
  f. Histological evidence of extravascular eosinophils

Treatment

- High-dose corticosteroids and immunosuppressive agents such as azathioprine or cyclophosphamide are the mainstays of treatment.

Lupus

- Caused by deposition of antibodies and immune complexes, Type 3 hypersensitivity reaction

Incidence/Epidemiology

- Typically occurs in young, female patients; more common in ethnic and minority groups, blacks, Hispanics, and Asians
- Associated with human leukocyte antigen (HLA) DR2 and DR3

Presentation

- Three subtypes.
- *Discoid lupus erythematosus (DLE)*: Least aggressive type, only affecting superficial tissues. Oral or cutaneous erythematous plaque lesions, alopecia. May develop scarring.
- *Subacute cutaneous lupus (SCL)*: Papulosquamous lesions that do not scar; mild systemic involvement.
- *Systemic lupus erythematosus (SLE)*: The most severe form of lupus. Typically present with malar butterfly rash. Hoarseness and pain may result from laryngotracheal perichondritis and true vocal fold thickening. May have nasal crusting, dryness, or septal perforation.

Workup/Diagnosis

- *DLE*: Clinical diagnosis alone (serology negative).
- *SCL*: Clinical diagnosis, inconsistent results from antinuclear antibodies (ANA), SS-A, and SS-B.
- *SLE*: Nonspecific tests are typically positive and used to establish initial diagnosis (ANA, SS-A, SS-B). Specific markers include anti-double-stranded DNA (ds-DNA) and Sm antigen (SmAg).
  a. ACR diagnostic criteria require 4/11 for SLE (acronym is "SOAP BRAIN MD"); **S**erositis, **O**ral ulcers, **A**rthritis, **P**ulmonary fibrosis, **B**lood dyscrasias, **R**aynaud/renal, **A**NA, **I**mmunologic (anti-Sm or anti-dsDNA), **N**europsychiatric, **M**alar rash, **D**iscoid rash

Treatment

- Typically consists of NSAIDs and corticosteroids.
- Other options include azathioprine, cyclophosphamide, and antimalarial agents such as hydroxychloroquine.

Behcet Disease

Presentation

- Recurrent aphthous ulcers on the oral mucosa and genitalia.
- Uveitis and ocular inflammation also present.
- May experience neurologic disease, brain stem or spinal cord involvement.
- Progressive sensorineural hearing loss.
- Vasculitis; affects vessels of all sizes, even as large as pulmonary artery.
- Venous thromboembolic events, arthritis, and renal and cardiac involvement are all possible.

Workup/Diagnosis

- Recurrent oral ulcers (three or more episodes per year) and two of genital ulcers, uveitis, skin lesions (erythema nodosum), or positive pathergy test (pustular response to skin trauma)

Treatment

- Interferon α-2a is effective in long-term treatment of severe uveitis.
- Steroid cream for topical treatment.
- Colchicine or Dapsone.
- Eye drops.

Idiopathic

Sarcoidosis

- Idiopathic, systemic noncaseating granulomatous disease of unknown origin; commonly affects lungs, hilar lymph nodes, and upper respiratory tract
- Most cases clear without treatment

Incidence/Epidemiology

- Predominates in females, third to fifth decades.
- 10 to 20 times more common in black patients in North America.

Presentation

- Often presents with hilar adenopathy on chest radiography or cervical adenopathy.
- 90% of patients have pulmonary involvement (hilar adenopathy, cough, dyspnea).
- *Laryngeal sarcoid*: Presents as supraglottic submucosal mass, usually in epiglottis, and possible vocal cord paralysis.
- *Sinonasal sarcoid*: May present with crusting, "cobblestone" mucosa, epistaxis, synechiae, stenosis, or cartilage destruction.
- *Salivary gland involvement*: Can range from asymptomatic parotid mass to **"Heerfordt syndrome"** or uveoparotid fever, an extrapulmonary manifestation of sarcoid consisting of uveitis, parotitis, fever, facial palsy, and sensorineural hearing loss.
- Cutaneous findings include erythema nodosum, Darier-Roussy (subcutaneous) nodules, and "lupus pernio."
- *Lupus pernio*: Chronic, red or purple indurated cutaneous plaques on nose, cheeks, ears, and hands that are pathognomonic for sarcoidosis.
- *Lofgren syndrome*: Acute form of sarcoidosis characterized by polyarthralgias, erythema nodosum, bilateral hilar Lymphadenopathy.
- Cardiac arrhythmia, neuropathy, sensorineural hearing loss, renal and hepatic involvement may also be present.

Histology

- Discrete noncaseating, epithelioid granulomas

Workup/Diagnosis

- *Lab*: Elevated angiotensin-converting enzyme (ACE) and urine/serum calcium levels are associated with sarcoidosis
- Serum protein electrophoresis (SPEP) may show polyclonal gammopathy
- Biopsy: Noncaseating granulomas with Langerhans cells

Treatment

- Most cases clear without medical treatment but may progress to long-term or even life-threatening disease.
- Average mortality rate is 5% in untreated cases.
- Usually treated with NSAIDs.
- Corticosteroids can be used for exacerbations of pulmonary and sinonasal disease.

- Severe disease may be treated with azathioprine, methotrexate, or leflunomide.
- Sinonasal surgery may improve symptoms but recurrence likely.
- Supraglottic lesions monitored conservatively; surgery reserved for obstructive lesions.

Neoplastic

Langerhans Cell Histiocytosis

- Classification for this group of disease is not well established; previously referred to as "Histiocytosis X."
- Rare disorders involve clonal proliferation of Langerhans cells, which are epidermal macrophages or dendritic cells.

Incidence/Epidemiology

- Poor prognosis if presenting in young patients

Subtypes

- Eosinophilic Granuloma
- Hand-Schuller-Christian disease
- Letterer-Siwe disease

Presentation

- Most commonly present as otitis media.
- Finding on nasal examination can include a mass, septal perforation, or epistaxis.

Histology

- Sheets of polygonal histiocytes.
- Variable number of eosinophils, plasma cells, and lymphocytes.
- Langerhans cell nucleus is pale and deeply grooved, and cytoplasm may demonstrate Birbeck granules on electron microscopy (tennis racket-shaped organelles with the nuclear cytoplasm).

Workup/Diagnosis

- Histological diagnosis by tissue biopsy
- Immunohistochemistry–CD1 positive, S100 positive

Treatment

- *Solitary lesion*: May be excised or treated with limited radiotherapy.
- *Multiple lesions*: Chemotherapy often employed, agents include alkylating compounds, antimetabolites, or vinca alkaloids. Can be combined with steroids.

Infectious

Cat Scratch Disease

Incidence/Epidemiology

- Caused by *Bartonella henselae*—an intercellular, pleomorphic, gram-negative bacteria
- Often seen in children

Presentation

- Patients have a history of cat exposure (scratch or bite).
- Tender adenopathy occurring within 3 to 14 days in the region of exposure (axillary, cervical, or submandibular).

- May or may not present with a vesicle or pustule at site of scratch within a week.
- *Bacillary angiomatosis*: May occur in patients with HIV. It is caused by *B. henselae* or *B. quintana*. Patients present with cutaneous papules and subcutaneous nodules or on mucous membranes. Other organs such as the spleen, bone, and liver may be affected.

Histology

- Necrotizing granulomatous lymphadenitis with stellate microabscesses seen on biopsy.

Workup/Diagnosis

- (1) History of cat exposure with (2) presence of inoculation site and (3) lymphadenopathy; (4) Excisional biopsy showing suppurative and granulomatous lymphadenitis.
- Polymerase chain reaction (PCR) may confirm the presence of bacteria.
- Enzyme-linked immunosorbent assay (ELISA) can be used for detecting early antibodies to the bacteria.

Treatment

- Usually self-limited, supportive treatment.
- Azithromycin, rifampin, or trimethoprim-sulfamethoxazole may be used in immunocompromised patients.
- Bacillary angiomatosis should be treated as this disease is progressive and fatal.

Leprosy

Incidence/Epidemiology

- Caused by *Mycobacterium leprae*: Obligate intracellular parasitic, acid-fast bacillus

Presentation

- Slow evolution of bacterial infection.
- Bacteria are thermolabile and grow optimally at 27°C to 33°C.
- Common areas of infection include cold peripheral tissues including fingers, nose, testicles, feet, and earlobes.
- Patients present with loss of peripheral sensation.
- Skin lesions can be hypopigmented or erythematous macules; eyebrow and eyelash loss can also occur.
- Early symptoms may include nasal and paranasal sinus involvement including saddle nose deformity, epistaxis, and nasal congestion.
- Late symptoms may include CNS (nerve paralysis), eye (pain, photophobia, glaucoma, blindness), laryngeal (stridor, hoarseness, ulceration) involvement.

Workup/Diagnosis

- Biopsy is required for diagnosis.
- PCR may be performed on nasal smears, skin biopsy, and blood specimens.

Treatment

- Long-term dapsone alone or in combination with clofazimine and rifampin

Nontuberculous Mycobacteria

Incidence/Epidemiology

- Caused by *Mycobacterium avium-intracellulare* complex, *M. scrofulaceum, M. kansasii, M. fortuitum,* and *M. bohemicum*

Presentation

- Patients present with corneal ulceration, cervical lymphadenopathy, and possibly mastoiditis.

- Adenitis is slow growing in the submandibular or periauricular region without systemic signs of infection.
- This mass is often nontender and does not respond to antibiotics.
- It may cause overlying skin changes or spontaneous fistulization.

Workup/Diagnosis

- Stains for acid-fast are only positive in 20% to 50% of patients.
- Diagnosis is typically suggested by clinical course and physical findings.

Treatment

- Excision of lymph node
- Recurrence may occur with incision and drainage alone

Tuberculosis

Incidence/Epidemiology

- Caused by *Mycobacterium tuberculosis*: acid-fast positive bacillus
- Inhaled into lungs and rarely affected the head and neck
- Common in areas where AIDS is prevalent

Presentation

- Most common head and neck presentation is cervical lymphadenopathy.
- Nodes are firm, matted, bilateral, and nontender.
- Nodes are most commonly found in the posterior triangle and supraclavicular area.
- Can also present in the larynx, typically in the posterior glottis as granulation and ulceration cause hoarseness, odynophagia, dysphagia, and stridor.
- Laryngeal involvement can present with edema, hyperemia, nodularity, ulcerations, and obliteration of anatomic landmarks.
- Epiglottis can become characteristically turban shaped.
- Otologic manifestation includes painless, odorless, watery to thick, cheesy otorrhea with multiple, small tympanic membrane perforations.
- Ossicular chain may or may not be eroded by granulation tissue.
- Other manifestations include septal perforation, involved salivary gland, and tonsillar tissue.

Workup/Diagnosis

- Purified protein derivative test (positive if 15 mm or larger induration).
- Chest X-ray or chest CT.
- PCR of sputum or cultures or biopsy can also be diagnostic.
- Consider excisional biopsy if other tests are negative.

Treatment

- Respiratory isolation should be started.
- Consider contacting the local public health department.
- Isoniazid, rifampin, pyrazinamide, and ethambutol for 2 months, followed by repeat smear and culture to determine the remainder of treatment course which can last for up to 9 months.
- *En bloc* lymph node excision may be needed for chronically draining nodes.

Actinomycosis

Incidence/Epidemiology

- Caused by *Actinomyces* species, most commonly *Actinomyces israelii* in humans—branching, filamentous anaerobic rods

Presentation
- Chronic granulomatous and suppurative disease.
- Most commonly occurs following dental manipulation, trauma, or infection.
- 50% have head and neck or cervicofacial manifestation is consistent with a mass.
- May also present in the thorax, abdomen, or pelvis.
- In the head and neck, it can present as a mass in the sinuses, mastoid, major salivary glands, and thyroid.
- Mass often has purple discoloration to overlying skin and may spontaneously fistulize.
- Mass is slow growing or may present rapidly as a suppurative infection and abscess formation.

Histology
- Multifilamented, anaerobic.
- Sulfur granules can be present and represent neutrophils and organisms.

Treatment
- Surgical debridement.
- IV penicillin G for 2 to 6 weeks followed by 6 to 12 months of oral penicillin.
- Tetracycline, doxycycline, or clindamycin is used in penicillin-allergic patients.

Syphilis

Incidence/Epidemiology
- Caused by *Treponema pallidum*—spirochete bacterium
    a. *Primary stage:* Presents with a painless chancre at inoculation site approximately 3 weeks after exposure.
    b. *Second stage*: Contagious stage, approximately 4 to 10 weeks after primary lesion. General malaise, fever, arthralgias, and skin and mucosal lesions.
    One-third remain latent, one-third go into remission, and one-third progress to tertiary syphilis. The latent phase may last up to 30 years.
    c. *Tertiary stage*: May occur years after infection, may involve CNS (neurosyphilis), major vessels (aortitis), or produce gumma in various places including the temporal bone.
- Spreads via sexual transmission

Presentation
- Gumma are inflammatory granulomas with an intervening zone of epithelioid and multinucleated cells and a peripheral zone with fibroblasts and capillaries.
- Gumma develops in bone, skin, and the liver.
- Head and neck symptoms include generalized lymphadenopathy, laryngitis, vocal fold paralysis, dysphasia, and oral ulcers.
- Granulomas may also be found in the oral cavity and nasal cavity.
- Septal perforation can be found in the bony septum.
- May cause fluctuating high-frequency sensorineural hearing loss, tinnitus, and vertigo (otosyphilis). Hearing loss may progress to profound levels. Patients may present with a positive Hennebert sign and may exhibit Tulio phenomenon.

Histology
- Dense chronic inflammation with many plasma cells

Workup/Diagnosis
- Serologic tests such as rapid plasma reagin (RPR) on serum or Venereal Disease Research Laboratory (VDRL) on cerebrospinal fluid (CSF) can be sensitive for screening patients. Seroreactivity can correlate with disease progression.
- Specific fluorescent treponemal antibody absorption (FTA-ABS) testing.
- Direct visualization of spirochetes through dark-field examination.

Treatment

- IM Benzathine penicillin, one dose is used for early syphilis; three weekly injections are used to treat late latent stage syphilis; 10 to 14 days of IV penicillin is recommended for treatment of tertiary syphilis.
- Steroids if otologic symptoms are present.
- Cases should be reported to the public health department.

Fungal

Histoplasmosis

Incidence/Epidemiology

- Caused by *Histoplasma capsulatum,* a dimorphic fungus found in the Ohio and Mississippi River Valleys.
- Airborne transmission of avian or bat droppings.
- Presence of oral histoplasmosis in a previously healthy individual should prompt HIV testing, as it is an AIDS-defining illness.

Presentation

- Can range from asymptomatic to severe infection.
- Can affect immunocompetent and immunocompromised patients.
- Immunosuppression is a strong risk factor for disseminated disease.
- Otolaryngologic presentations include painful ulceration of the lips, gingiva, tongue, pharynx, and larynx.
- Sore throat, painful mastication, hoarseness, gingival irritation, and weight loss.
- The disease may progress to involve the heart and CNS.

Workup/Diagnosis

- Cultures are performed on Sabouraud medium. Blood culture should be obtained in all cases.
- Skin testing—rarely useful diagnostically as positive test does not predict active disease.
- Antibody tests—complement fixation, latex agglutination.
- Polymerase chain reaction.
- Antigen testing—urine and serum antigen detection via complement fixation.

Treatment

- Itraconazole is used for the treatment of mild disease.
- Amphotericin B is used for severe disease including CNS involvement.

Blastomycosis

Incidence/Epidemiology

- Caused by *Blastomyces dermatitidis* endemic to central United States and southern parts of the Canadian Prairie provinces.
- This organism is inhaled in soil dust or in old homes.

Presentation

- Patients may be asymptomatic.
- Lung is the most common site of infection, presenting with acute or chronic pneumonia.
- Skin lesions are the second most common presentation after lung, found on the face and limbs and are initially verrucous with scarring.
- Triad of symptoms includes cutaneous disease, pulmonary involvement, and constitutional symptoms in immunocompromised patients.
- Genitourinary symptoms may also be present: prostatitis, epididymo-orchitis.
- Rarely can blastomycosis present in the larynx, parotid, and paranasal sinuses.

Histology
- Pseudocpitheliomatous hyperplasia
- Single birefringent, broad-based bud

Workup/Diagnosis
- Sputum culture on Sabouraud medium
- Antigen testing—serum and urine antigen detection
- Serologic testing—enzymatic and antigen-mediated radioimmunoassay

Treatment
- Itraconazole is the general treatment option.
- Amphotericin B is used if immunocompromised or CNS involvement.

Congenital

Chronic Granulomatous Disease (CGD)

Incidence/Epidemiology
- Due to hereditary defects in the immune system. These typically involve neutrophils and monocytes (phagocytes). This condition is characterized by recurrent bacterial and fungal infections and granuloma formation.
- 66% are X linked, 33% are autosomal recessive.
- Chediak-Higashi syndrome and Job syndrome are included within this spectrum of disorders.
- Chediak-Higashi syndrome is an autosomal recessive disorder presenting with neuropathy, neutropenia, oculocutaneous albinism, and malignancy.
- Job syndrome is characterized by increased levels of IgE and eosinophilia. Patients usually present with multiple *Staphylococcus* abscesses.

Presentation
- Multiple, chronic infections by catalase-positive organisms, gram-negative bacteria and fungi.
- Patients present with eczema, osteomyelitis, abscesses, and granulomas.
- Can affect single- or multiple-organ systems. The lung is the most common site of involvement; however, lymphatic, hepatic, skeletal, gastrointestinal, and genitourinary systems can also be affected.

Diagnosis
- Patients suspected of having CGD should undergo neutrophil function testing.
- Genetic testing for known gene mutations.

Treatment
- Antimicrobial prophylaxis: most commonly trimethoprim-sulfamethoxazole for antibacterial, itraconazole for antifungal.
- Vaccination with BCG is contraindicated in CGD. Live vaccines should be avoided.
- Other treatments include interferon gamma, granulocyte colony-stimulating factor (G-CSF), and granulocyte-macrophage colony-stimulating factor to stimulate neutrophils.
- Hematopoietic cell transplantation is the only established curative therapy for CGD, although gene therapy trials are currently underway.

Appendix A The World Health Organization Clinical Staging System for HIV, 2007

Adults and adolescents	Children
Clinical Stage 1 (Asymptomatic)	
Asymptomatic Persistent generalized lymphadenopathy	Asymptomatic Persistent generalized lymphadenopathy
Clinical Stage 2 (Mild Symptoms)	
Moderate unexplained weight loss (< 10% of presumed or measured body weight) Recurrent respiratory tract infections, sinusitis, tonsillitis, otitis media, and pharyngitis) Herpes zoster Angular cheilitis Recurrent oral ulceration Papular pruritic eruptions Seborrhoeic dermatitis Fungal nail infections	Unexplained persistent hepatosplenomegaly Recurrent or chronic upper respiratory tract infections (otitis media, otorrhoea, sinusitis, tonsillitis) Herpes zoster Linear gingival erythema Recurrent oral ulceration Papular pruritic eruption Fungal nail infections Extensive wart virus infection Extensive molluscum contagiosum Unexplained persistent parotid enlargement
Clinical Stage 3 (Advanced Symptoms)	
Unexplained severe weight loss (> 10% of presumed or measured body weight) Unexplained chronic diarrhea for longer than 1 mo Unexplained persistent fever (above 37.6°C intermittent or constant, for longer than 1 mo) Persistent oral candidiasis Oral hairy leukoplakia Pulmonary tuberculosis (current) Severe bacterial infections (such as pneumonia, empyema, pyomyositis, bone or joint infection, meningitis, or bacteremia) Acute necrotizing ulcerative stomatitis, gingivitis, or periodontitis Unexplained anemia (< 8 g/dL), neutropenia (< 0.5×10^9/L), or chronic thrombocytopenia (< 50×10^9/L)	Unexplained moderate malnutrition not adequately responding to standard therapy Unexplained persistent diarrhea (> 14 days) Unexplained persistent fever (> 37.5°C) Persistent oral candidiasis (after first 6 weeks of life) Oral hairy leukoplakia Lymph node tuberculosis Pulmonary tuberculosis Severe recurrent bacterial pneumonia Acute necrotizing ulcerative gingivitis or periodontitis Unexplained anemia (< 8 g/dL), neutropenia (< 0.5×10^9/L) or chronic thrombocytopenia (<50 × 109/l) Symptomatic lymphoid interstitial pneumonitis Chronic HIV-associated lung disease, including bronchiectasis

(*Continued*)

Clinical Stage 4 (Severe Symptoms)	
HIV wasting syndrome	Unexplained severe wasting, stunting, or severe malnutrition not responding to standard therapy
Pneumocystis pneumonia	Pneumocystis (jirovecii) pneumonia
Recurrent severe bacterial pneumonia	Recurrent severe bacterial infections (such as empyema, pyomyositis, bone or joint infection, meningitis, but excluding pneumonia)
Chronic herpes simplex infection (orolabial, genital, or anorectal of > 1-mo duration or visceral at any site)	Chronic herpes simplex infection (orolabial or cutaneous of more than 1 month's duration or visceral at any site)
Esophageal candidiasis (or candidiasis of trachea, bronchi, or lungs)	Esophageal candidiasis (or candidiasis of trachea, bronchi, or lungs)
Extrapulmonary tuberculosis	Extrapulmonary tuberculosis
Kaposi sarcoma	Kaposi sarcoma
Cytomegalovirus infection (retinitis or infection of other organs)	Cytomegalovirus infection (retinitis or infection of other organs with onset at age more than 1 mo)
Central nervous system toxoplasmosis	Central nervous system toxoplasmosis (after the neonatal period)
HIV encephalopathy	HIV encephalopathy
Extrapulmonary cryptococcosis including meningitis	Extrapulmonary cryptococcosis, including meningitis
Disseminated nontuberculous mycobacterial infection	Disseminated nontuberculous mycobacterial infection
Progressive multifocal leukoencephalopathy	Progressive multifocal leukoencephalopathy
Chronic cryptosporidiosis (with diarrhea)	Chronic cryptosporidiosis (with diarrhoea)
Chronic isosporiasis	Chronic isosporiasis
Disseminated mycosis (coccidiomycosis or histoplasmosis)	Disseminated endemic mycosis (extrapulmonary histoplasmosis, coccidioidomycosis, penicilliosis)
Recurrent nontyphoidal Salmonella bacteremia	Cerebral or B-cell non-Hodgkin lymphoma
Lymphoma (cerebral or B-cell non-Hodgkin) or other solid HIV-associated tumors	HIV-associated nephropathy or cardiomyopathy
Symptomatic HIV-associated nephropathy or symptomatic HIV-associated cardiomyopathy	
Invasive cervical carcinoma	
Atypical disseminated leishmaniasis	

Bibliography

Gulati S, Krossnes B, Olofsson J, Danielsen A. Sinonasal involvement in sarcoidosis: a report of seven cases and review of literature. *Eur Arch Otorhinolaryngol.* 2012;269(3):891-896.

Lynch JP 3rd, Hoffman GS. Wegener's granulomatosis: controversies and current concepts. *Compr Ther.* 1998;24(9):421-440.

Marsot-Dupuch K, Quillard J, Meyohas MC. Head and neck lesions in the immunocompromised host. *Eur Radiol.* 2004;14:E155-E167.
Montone KT. Infectious diseases of the head and neck. *Am J Clin Pathol.* 2007;128:35-67.
World Health Organization. *WHO Case Definitions of HIV for Surveillance and Revised Clinical Staging and Immunological Classification of HIV-Related Diseases in Adults and Children.* Switzerland: World Health Organization; 2007.

Questions

1. Which malignancy is associated with HIV infection and/or immunocompromised state?
   A. Kaposi sarcoma
   B. Primary CNS lymphoma
   C. Plasmablastic lymphoma
   D. All of the above

2. Which diagnosis does not require subsequent investigation into HIV status?
   A. Oral histoplasmosis
   B. Oral hairy leukoplakia
   C. Necrotizing gingivostomatitis
   D. Oral candidiasis

3. Which disease is often associated with a bony septal perforation?
   A. Tuberculosis
   B. Leprosy
   C. Syphilis
   D. Blastomycosis
   E. Langerhans histiocytosis

4. An 8-year-old patient presents with a history of several weeks of a violaceous, submandibular mass showing sulfur granules on fine-needle aspiration. What is your definitive management?
   A. PO antibiotics only
   B. IV antibiotics only
   C. Surgical curettage only
   D. Surgical curettage and IV, then PO antibiotics
   E. Conservative management

5. Which of the following is not one of the five diagnostic criteria for cat scratch disease?
   A. History of exposure to a cat
   B. Inoculation site
   C. Fever
   D. Adenopathy
   E. Biopsy showing necrotic granuloma
   F. Warthin-Starry-Sky stain showing intracellular pleomorphic gram-negative bacillus

Part 2
Otology/Neurotology/Audiology

Chapter 12
Anatomy of the Ear

A. The temporal bone forms part of the side and base of the skull. It constitutes two-thirds of the floor of the middle cranial fossa and one-third of the floor of the posterior fossa. There are four parts to the temporal bone:
   i. Squamosa
   ii. Mastoid
   iii. Petrous
   iv. Tympanic
B. The following muscles are attached to the mastoid process:
   i. Sternocleidomastoid
   ii. Splenius capitis
   iii. Longissimus capitis
   iv. Digastric
   v. Anterior, superior, posterior, auricular (The temporalis muscle attaches to the squamosa portion of the temporal bone and not to the mastoid process.)
C. The auricle (Figure 12-1) is made of elastic cartilage, the cartilaginous canal of fibro-cartilage. The cartilaginous canal constitutes one-third of the external auditory canal (whereas the eustachian tube is two-thirds cartilaginous), and the remaining two-thirds is osseous. Innervation of the auricle is outlined in Figure 12-2.
D. The skin over the cartilaginous canal has sebaceous glands, ceruminous glands, and hair follicles. The skin over the bony canal is tight and has no subcutaneous tissue except periosteum.

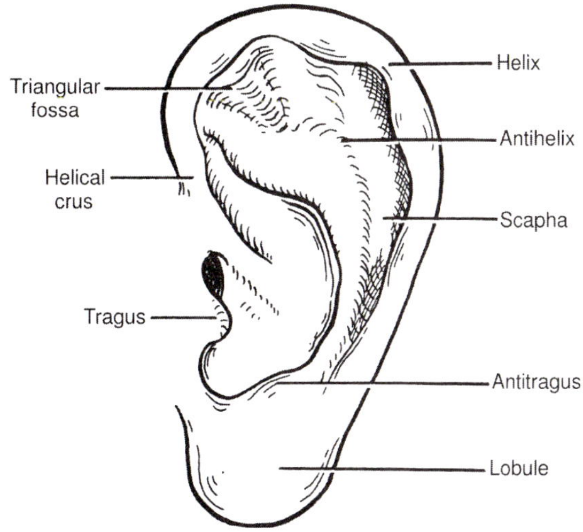

Figure 12-1 Auricle.

E. Boundaries of the *external auditory canal* are:

Anterior	Mandibular fossa
	Parotid
Posterior	Mastoid
Superior	Epitympanic recess (medially)
	Cranial cavity (laterally)
Inferior	Parotid

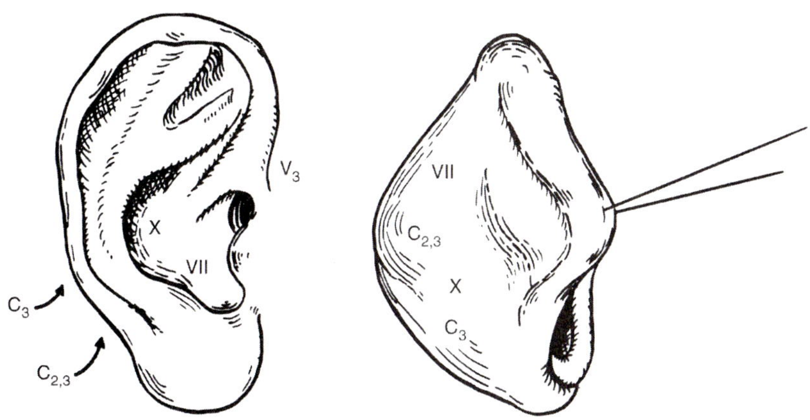

Figure 12-2 Sensory innervation of the auricle. C_3, via greater auricular nerve; $C_{2,3,}$ via lesser occipital nerve; X, auricular branch; V_3, auriculotemporal nerve; VII, sensory twigs.

The anterior portion, floor, and part of the posterior portion of the bony canal are formed by the tympanic part of the temporal bone. The rest of the posterior canal and the roof are formed by the squamosa.

F. Boundaries of the *epitympanum* are:

Medial	Lateral semicircular canal and VII nerve
Superior	Tegmen
Anterior	Zygomatic arch
Lateral	Squamosa (scutum)
Inferior	Fossa incudis
Posterior	Aditus

G. Boundaries of the *tympanic cavity* are:

Roof	Tegmen
Floor	Jugular wall and styloid prominence
Posterior	Mastoid, stapedius, pyramidal prominence
Anterior	Carotid wall, eustachian tube, tensor tympani
Medial	Labyrinthine wall
Lateral	Tympanic membrane, scutum (laterosuperior)

H. The *auricle* is attached to the head by
   i. Skin
   ii. An extension of cartilage to the external auditory canal cartilage
   iii. Ligaments
      a. Anterior ligament (zygoma to helix and tragus)
      b. Superior ligament (external auditory canal to the spine of the helix)
      c. Posterior ligament (mastoid to concha)
   iv. Muscles
      a. Anterior auricular muscle
      b. Superior auricular muscle
      c. Posterior auricular muscle

I. Notch of Rivinus is the notch on the squamosa, medial to which lies the Shrapnell membrane. The tympanic ring is not a complete ring, with a dehiscence superiorly.

J. *Meckel cave* is the concavity on the superior portion of the temporal bone in which the gasserian ganglion (V) is located.

K. *Dorello canal* is between the petrous tip and the sphenoid bone. It is the groove for the VI nerve. *Gradenigo syndrome,* which is secondary to petrositis with involvement of the VI nerve, is characterized by:
   i. Pain behind the eye
   ii. Diplopia
   iii. Aural discharge
L. The suprameatal triangle of *Macewen triangle* is posterior and superior to the external auditory canal. It is bound at the meatus by the spine of Henle, otherwise called the *suprameatal spine.* This triangle approximates the position of the antrum medially. *Tegmen mastoideum* is the thin plate over the antrum.
M. *Trautmann triangle* is demarcated by the bony labyrinth, the sigmoid sinus, and the superior petrosal sinus or dura.
   Citelli angle is the *sinodural* angle. It is located between the sigmoid sinus and the middle fossa dura plate. Others consider the superior side of Trautmann triangle to be Citelli angle.
   Solid angle is the angle formed by the three semicircular canals.
   Scutum is the thin plate of bone that constitutes the lateral wall of the epitympanum. It is part of the squamosa.
   Mandibular fossa is bound by the zygomatic, squamosa, and tympanic bones.
   Huguier canal transmits the chorda tympani out of the temporal bone anteriorly. It is situated lateral to the roof of the protympanum.
   Huschke foramen is located on the anterior tympanic plate along a nonossified portion of the plate. It is near the fissures of Santorini.
   Porus acusticus is the "mouth" of the internal auditory canal. The canal is divided horizontally by the *crista falciformis.*
N. There are three parts to the inner ear (Figure 12-3).
   i. *Pars superior*: Vestibular labyrinth (utricle and semicircular canals)
   ii. *Pars inferior*: Cochlea and saccule
   iii. Endolymphatic sac and duct
O. There are four small outpocketings from the perilymph space:
   i. Along the endolymphatic duct
   ii. Fissula ante fenestram
   iii. Fossula post fenestram
   iv. Periotic duct
P. There are four openings into the temporal bone:
   i. Internal auditory canal
   ii. Vestibular aqueduct
   iii. Cochlear aqueduct
   iv. Subarcuate fossa
Q. The *ponticulum* is the ridge of bone between the oval window niche and the sinus tympani.
R. The *subiculum* is a ridge of bone between the round window niche and the sinus tympani.
S. *Körner septum* separates the squamosa from the petrous air cells.
T. Only one-third of the population has a pneumatized petrous portion of the temporal bone.

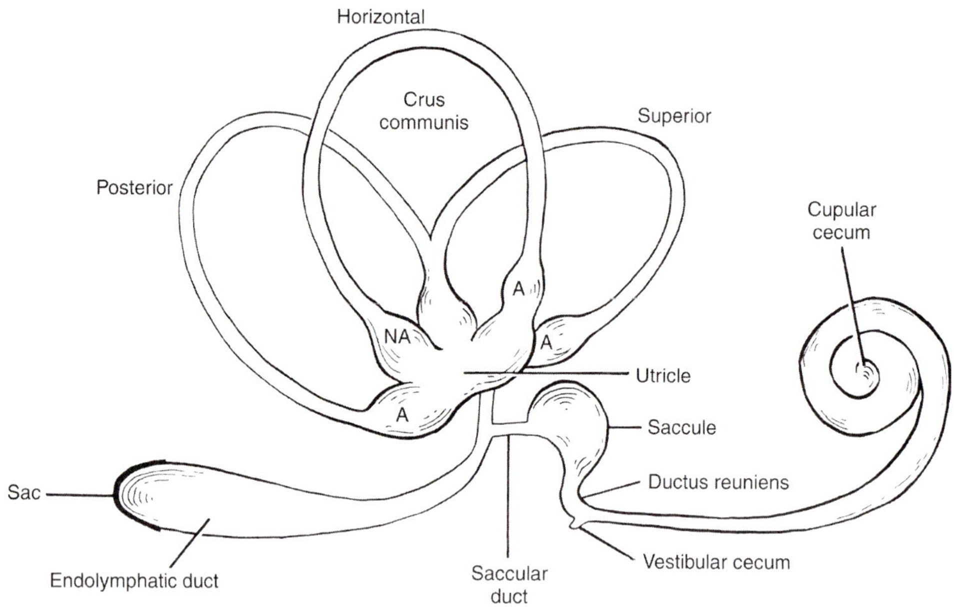

Figure 12-3 Membranous labyrinth. A, ampulated end; NA, nonampulated end.

U. *Scala communis* is where the scala tympani joins the scala vestibuli. The helicotrema is at the apex of the cochlea where the two join (Figure 12-4).
V. The *petrous pyramid* is the strongest bone in the body.
W. The upper limit of the internal auditory canal diameter is 8 mm.
X. The *cochlear aqueduct* is a bony channel connecting the scala tympani of the basal turn with the subarachnoid space of the posterior cranial cavity. The average adult cochlear aqueduct is 6.2-mm long.

Inner Ear

See Figure 12-4.

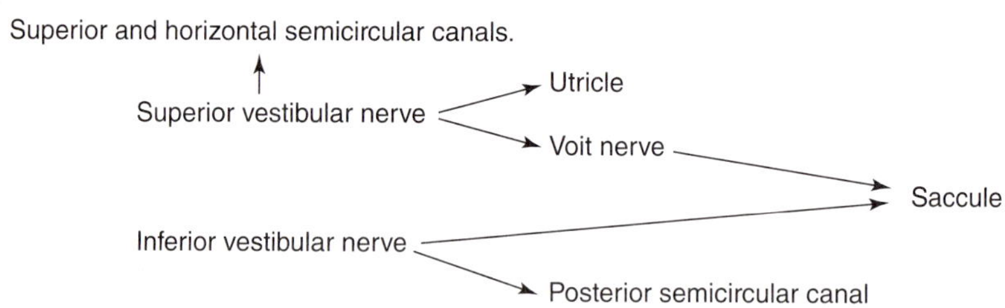

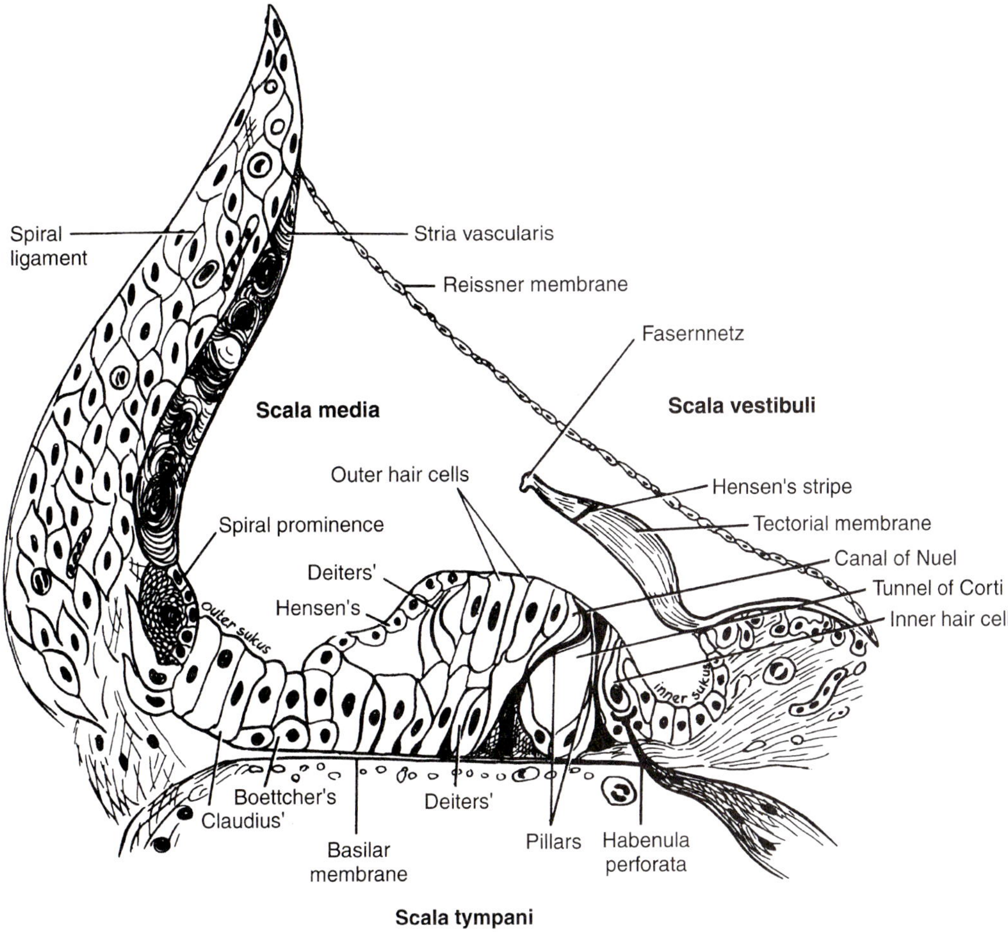

Figure 12-4 Organ of Corti.

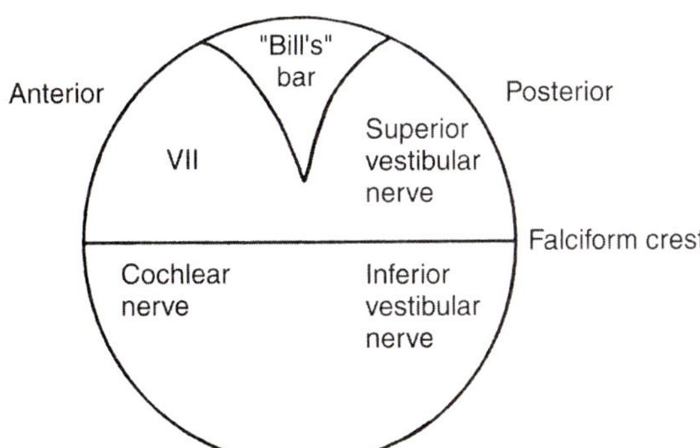

Figure 12-5 Cross-section of internal auditory canal.

Blood Supply

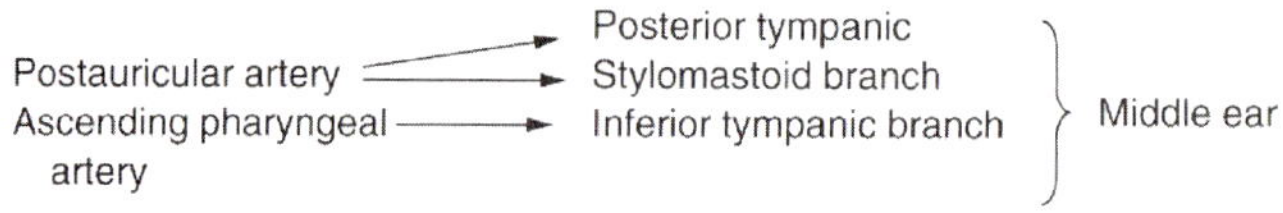

The long process of the incus receives the least blood supply and hence is the most frequently necrosed.

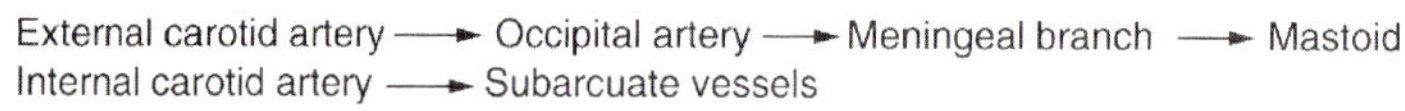

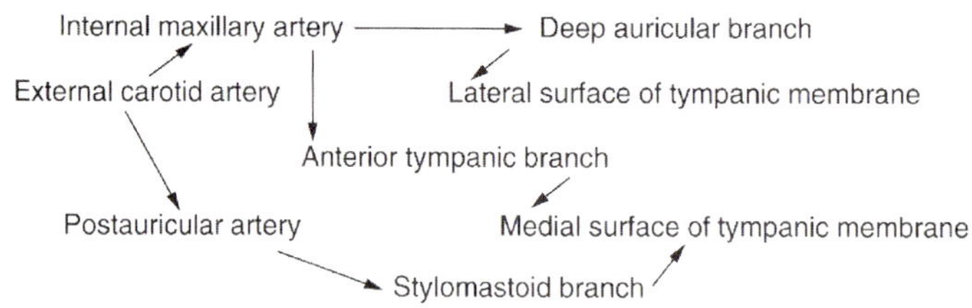

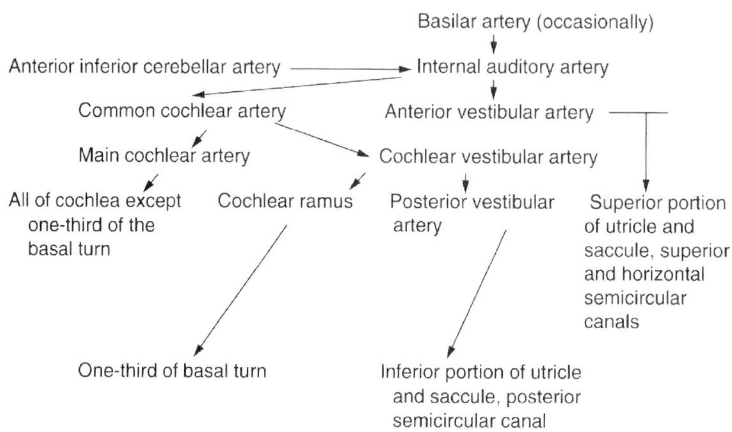

Middle Ear

Tympanic plexus = V_3, IX, and X
V_3 → Auriculotemporal nerve
IX → Jacobson nerve
X → Auricular nerve

Tympanic Membrane

See Figure 12-6.
The tympanic membrane has four layers:

A. Squamous epithelium
B. Radiating fibrous layer

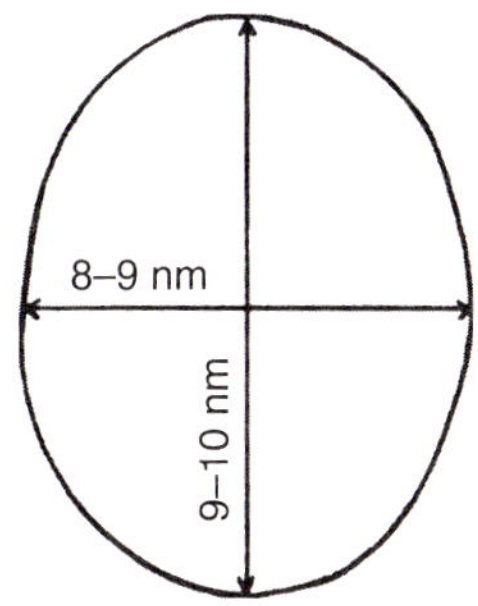

Figure 12-6 Measurements of tympanic membrane.

C. Circular fibrous layer
D. Mucosal layer

Average total area of tympanic membrane: 70 to 80 mm^2
Average vibrating surface of tympanic membrane: 55 mm^2

Venous Drainage

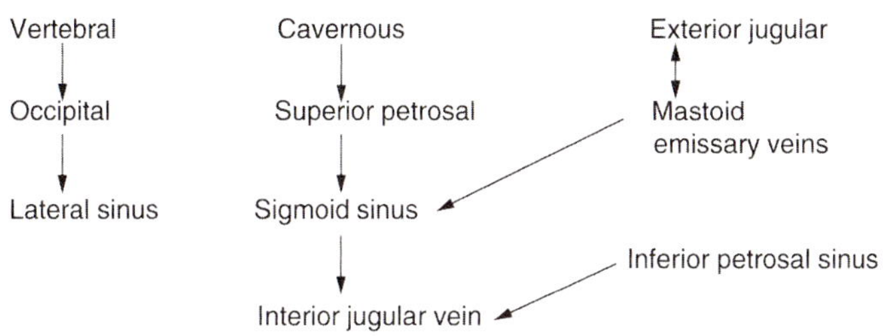

Ossicles

Malleus

A. Head
B. Neck
C. Manubrium
D. Anterior process
E. Lateral or short process

Incus

A. Body
B. Short process
C. Long process (lenticular process)

Stapes

A. Posterior crus
B. Anterior crus
C. Footplate (average 1.41 mm × 2.99 mm)

Ligaments

Malleus

A. Superior malleal ligament (head to roof of epitympanum)
B. Anterior malleal ligament (neck near anterior process to sphenoid bone through the petrotympanic fissure)
C. Tensor tympani (medial surface of upper end of manubrium to cochleariform process)
D. Lateral malleal ligament (neck to tympanic notch)

Incus

A. Superior incudal ligament (body to tegmen)
B. Posterior incudal ligament (short process to floor of incudal fossa)

Stapes

A. Stapedial tendon (apex of the pyramidal process to the posterior surface of the neck of the stapes)
B. Annular ligament (footplate to margin of vestibular fenestram)
   i. *Malleal*: Incudal joint is a diarthrodial joint.
   ii. *Incudo*: Stapedial joint is a diarthrodial joint.
   iii. *Stapedial*: Labyrinthine joint is a syndesmotic joint.

Middle Ear Folds of Significance

There are five malleal folds and four incudal folds:

A. *Anterior malleal fold*: Neck of the malleus to anterosuperior margin of the tympanic sulcus
B. *Posterior malleal fold*: Neck to posterosuperior margin of the tympanic sulcus
C. *Lateral malleal fold*: Neck to neck in an arch form and to the Shrapnell membrane
D. *Anterior pouch of von Troeltsch*: Lies between the anterior malleal fold and the portion of the tympanic membrane anterior to the handle of the malleus
E. *Posterior pouch of von Troeltsch*: Lies between the posterior malleal fold and the portion of the tympanic membrane posterior to the handle of the malleus

Prussak space (Figure 12-7) has the following boundaries:

A. *Anterior*: Lateral malleal fold
B. *Posterior*: Lateral malleal fold
C. *Superior*: Lateral malleal fold
D. *Inferior*: Lateral process of the malleus
E. *Medial*: Neck of the malleus
F. *Lateral*: Shrapnell membrane

The *oval window* sits in the sagittal plane.

The *round window* sits in the transverse plane and is protected by an anterior lip from the promontory. It faces posteroinferiorly as well as laterally.

The tensor tympani inserts from the cochleariform process onto the medial surface of the upper end of the manubrium. It supposedly pulls the tympanic membrane medially, thereby

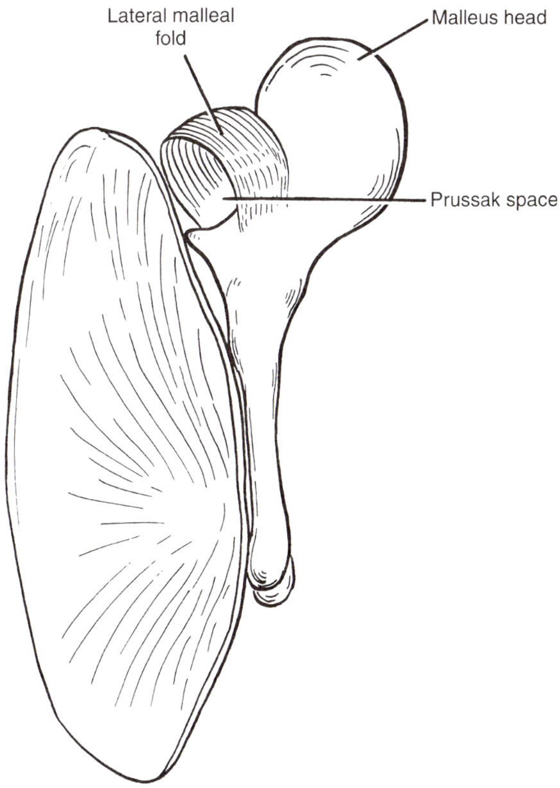

Figure 12-7 Prussak space.

tensing it. It also draws the malleus medially and forward. It raises the resonance frequency and attenuates low frequencies.

The stapedius muscle most frequently attaches to the posterior neck of the stapes. Occasionally, it is attached to the posterior crus or head and rarely to the lenticular process. It is attached posteriorly at the pyramidal process. It pulls the stapes posteriorly, supposedly increases the resonant frequency of the ossicular chain, and attenuates sound.

Eustachian Tube

A. It is 17 to 18 mm at birth and grows to about 35 mm in adulthood.
B. At birth, the tube is horizontal and grows to be at an incline of 45 degrees in adulthood. Thus, the pharyngeal orifice is about 15 mm lower than the tympanic orifice.
C. It can be divided into an anteromedial cartilaginous portion (24 mm) and a posterolateral bony (11 mm) portion. The narrowest part of the tube is at the junction of the bony and the cartilaginous portions. (Reminder: The external auditory canal is one-third cartilaginous and two-thirds bony.)
D. The cartilaginous part of the tube is lined by pseudostratified columnar-ciliated epithelium, but toward the tympanic orifice, it is lined by ciliated cuboidal epithelium.

E. It opens by the action of the tensor palati (innervated by the third division of the V nerve) acting synergistically with the levator veli palatini (innervated by the vagus). In children, the only muscle that works is the tensor palati because the levator palati is separated from the eustachian tube cartilage by a considerable distance. Therefore, a cleft palate child with poor tensor palati function is expected to have eustachian tube problems until the levator veli palatini starts to function.
F. In a normal individual, a pressure difference of 200 to 300 mm H_2O is needed to produce airflow.
G. It is easier to expel air from the middle ear than to get it into the middle ear (reason for more tubal problems when descending in an airplane).
H. A pressure of −30 mm Hg or lower for 15 minutes can produce a transudate in the middle ear. A pressure differential of 90 mm Hg or greater may "lock" the eustachian tube, preventing opening of the tube by the tensor palati muscle. It is called the critical pressure difference.
I. If the pressure differential exceeds 100 mm Hg, the tympanic membrane may rupture.
J. A Valsalva maneuver generates about 20 to 40 mm Hg of pressure.
K. The lymphoid tissues within the tube have been referred to as the tonsil of Gerlach.
L. The tympanic ostium of the tube is at the anterior wall of the tympanic cavity about 4 mm above the most inferior part of the floor of the cavity. The diameter of the ostium is 3 to 5 mm. The size of the pharyngeal ostium varies from 3 to 10 mm in its vertical diameter and 2 to 5 mm in its horizontal diameter.

Figures 12-8 to 12-22 are temporal bone horizontal sections from HF Schuknecht's Research Laboratory at the Massachusetts Eye and Ear Infirmary.

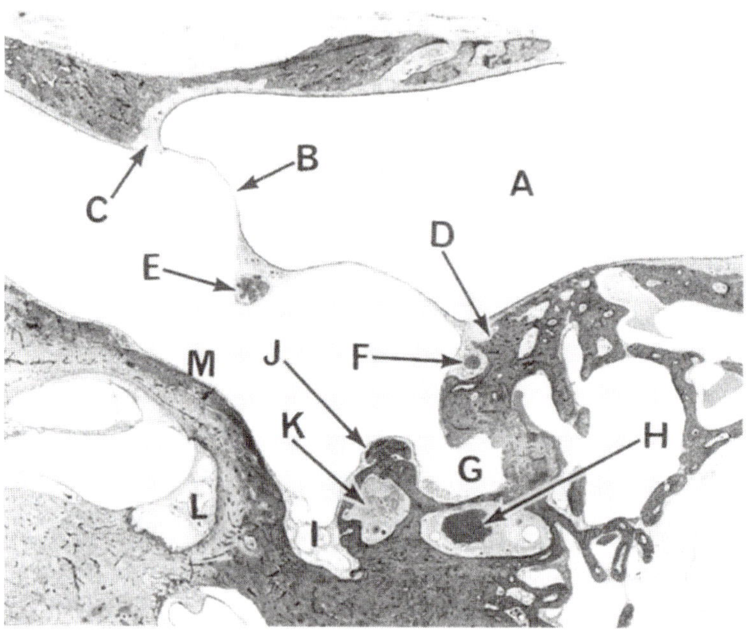

Figure 12-8 A, external auditory canal; B, tympanic membrane; C, fibrous annulus; D, tympanic sulcus; E, malleus handle; F, chorda tympani; G, facial recess; H, facial nerve; I, sinus tympani; J, pyramidal process; K, stapedius muscle; L, round window; M, promontory.

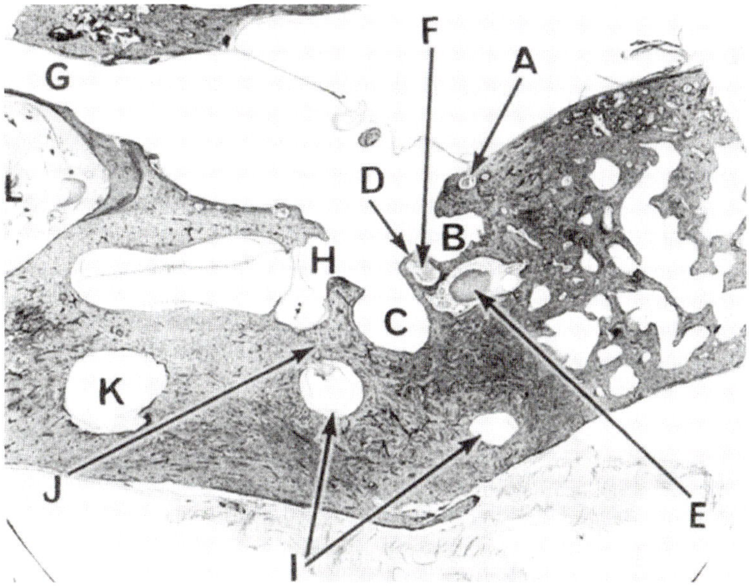

Figure 12-9 A, chorda tympani; B, facial recess; C, sinus tympani; D, pyramidal process; E, facial nerve; F, stapedius muscle; G, eustachian tube; H, round window niche; I, posterior semicircular canal; J, microfissure with no known significance; K, internal auditory meatus; L, carotid canal.

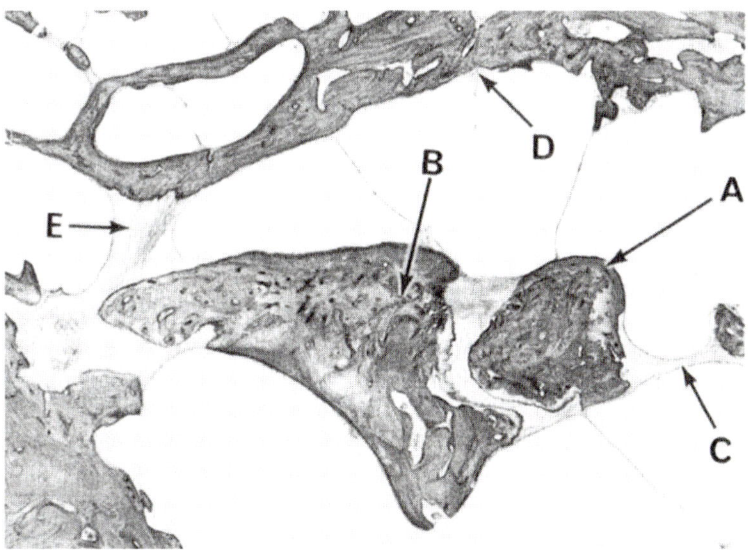

Figure 12-10 A, malleus head; B, incus body; C, anterior malleal ligament; D, lateral wall of the attic; E, posterior incudal ligament.

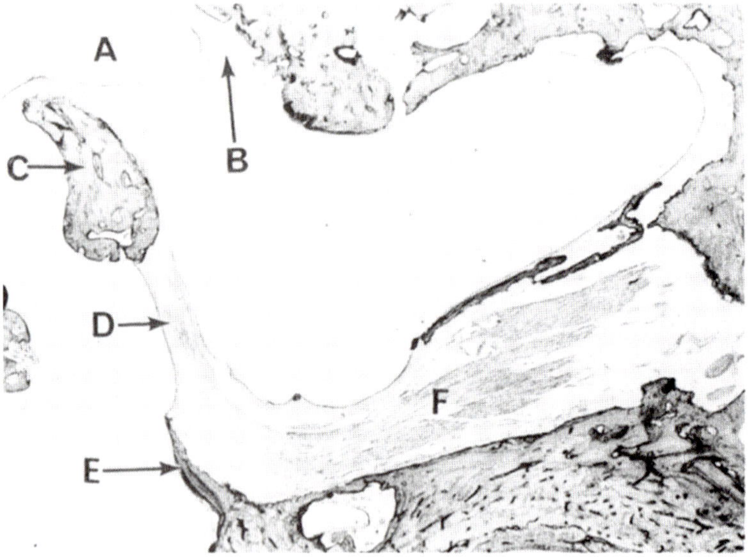

Figure 12-11 A, external auditory canal; B, fibrous annulus; C, malleus; D, tendon of tensor tympani; E, cochleariform process; F, tensor tympani muscle.

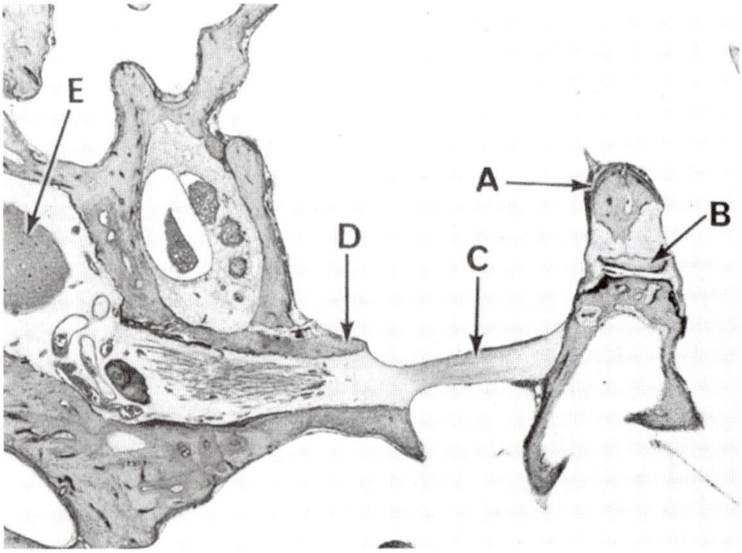

Figure 12-12 A, incus; B, lenticular process; C, stapedius tendon; D, pyramidal process; E, facial nerve.

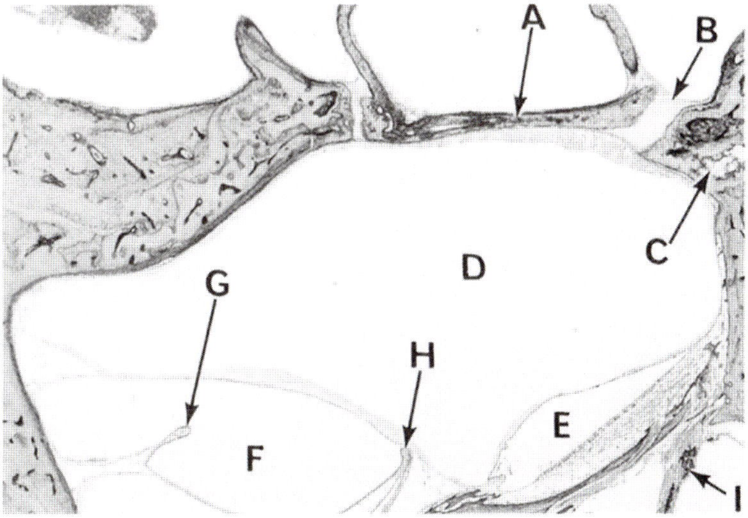

Figure 12-13 A, stapes footplate; B, annular ligament; C, fissula ante fenestram; D, vestibule; E, saccule; F, utricule; G, inferior utricular crest; H, utriculoendolymphatic valve; I, saccular nerve.

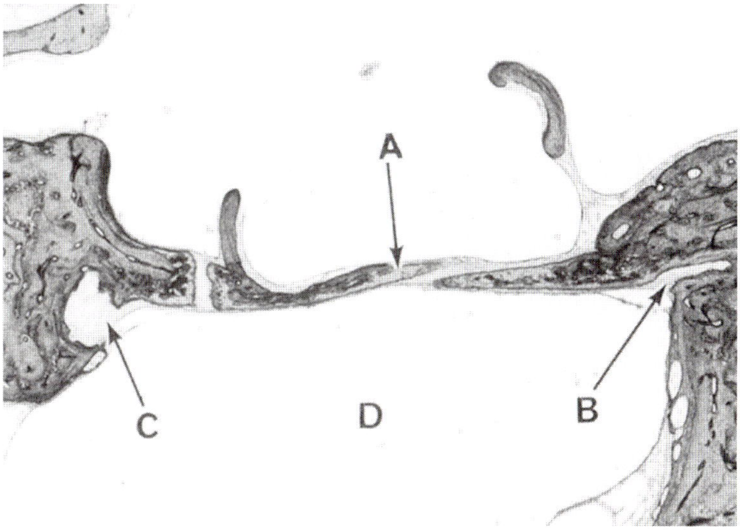

Figure 12-14 A, stapes footplate; B, fissula ante fenestram; C, fossula post fenestram; D, vestibule.

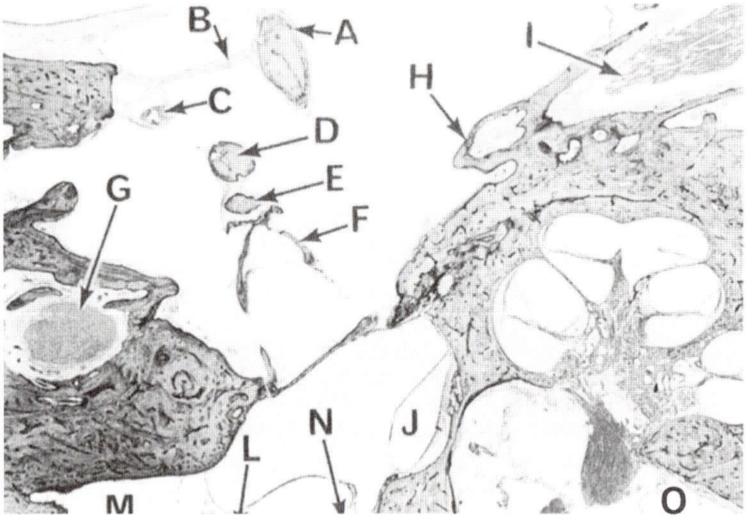

Figure 12-15 A, malleus; B, tympanic membrane; C, chorda tympani; D, incus; E, lenticular process; F, stapes; G, facial nerve; H, cochleariform process; I, tensor tympani; J, saccule; L, inferior utricular crest; M, lateral semicircular canal; N, sinus of endolymphatic duct; O, internal auditory canal.

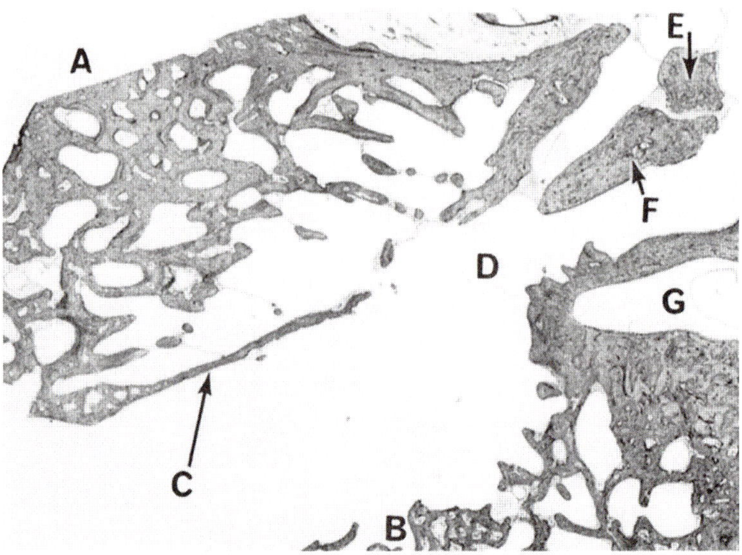

Figure 12-16 A, squamosa part of the temporal bone; B, petrous part of the temporal bone; C, Körner septum; D, aditus; E, malleus; F, incus; G, lateral semicircular canal.

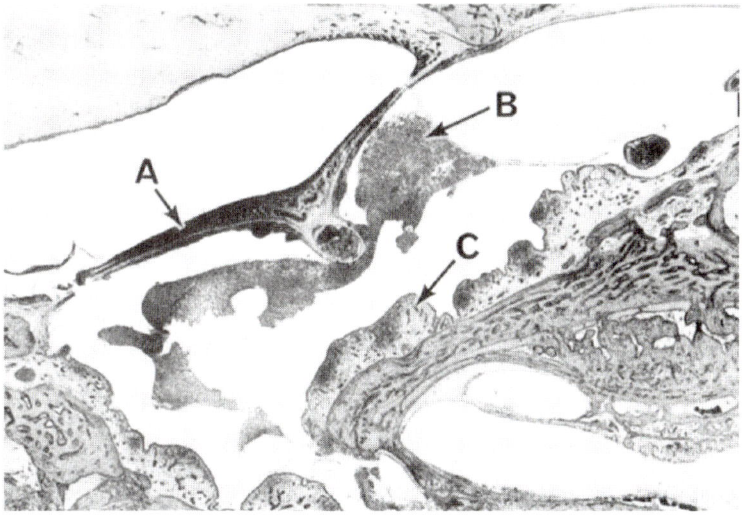

Figure 12-17 Acute otitis media. A, tympanic membrane; B, purulent material; C, thickened middle ear mucosa.

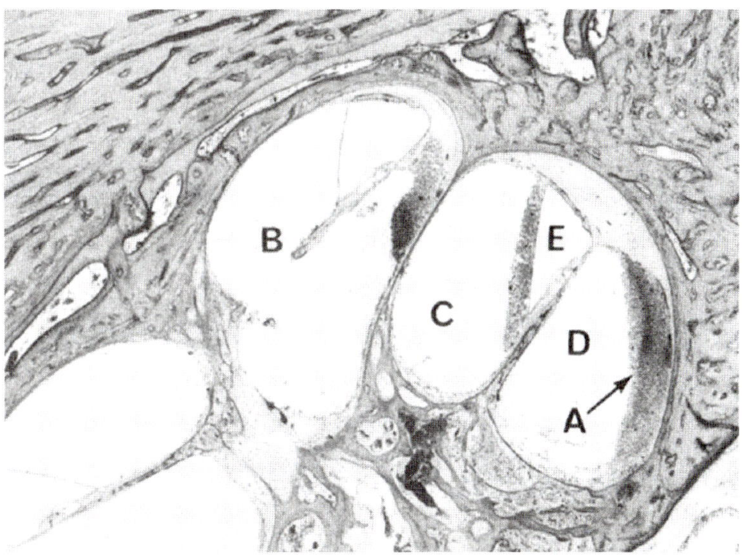

Figure 12-18 Acute labyrinthitis. A, leukocytes; B, helicotrema; C, scala vestibuli; D, scala tympani; E, scala media.

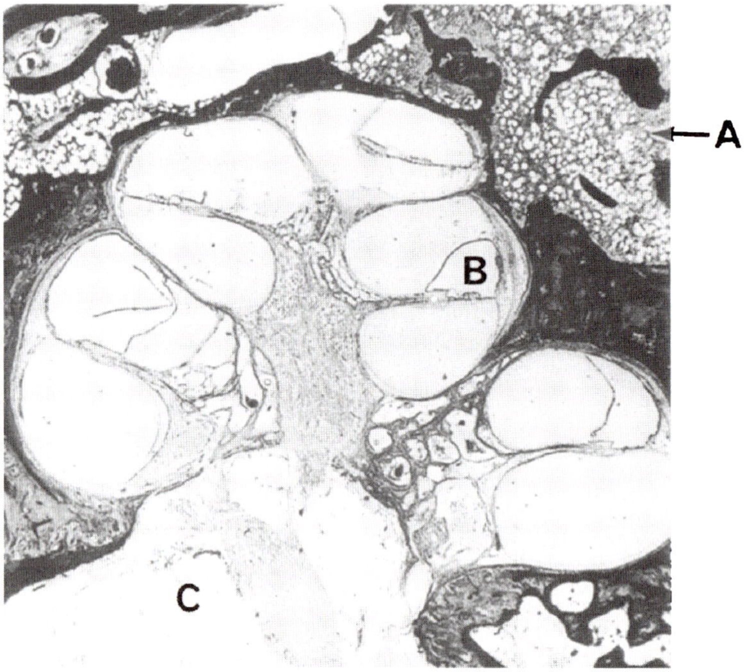

Figure 12-19 Congenital syphilis. A, leutic changes in the otic capsule; B, endolymphatic hydrops; C, internal auditory canal.

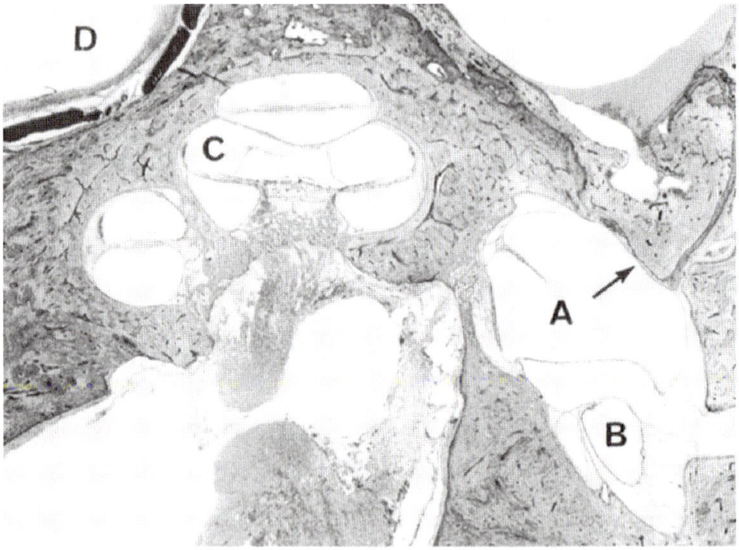

Figure 12-20 Ménière disease. A, enlarged saccule against footplate; B, utricule; C, "distended" cochlear duct; D, carotid artery.

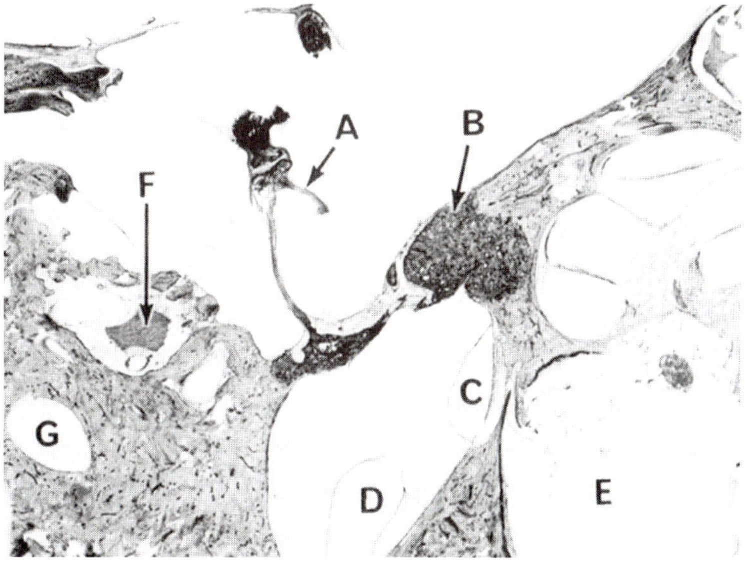

Figure 12-21 Otosclerosis. A, stapes; B, otosclerotic bone; C, saccule; D, utricle; E, internal auditory canal; F, facial nerve; G, lateral semicircular canal.

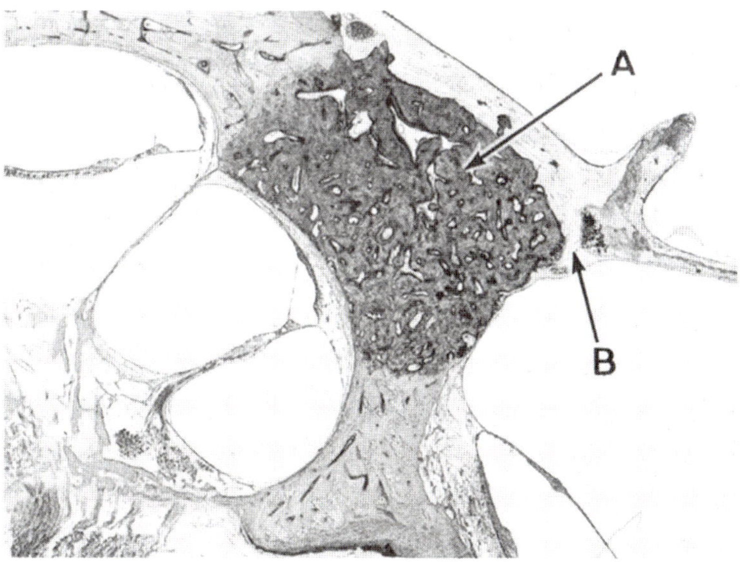

Figure 12-22 Otosclerosis. A, histologic otosclerosis without involving the footplate; B, annular ligament.

Embryology of the Ear

Auricle

During the sixth week of gestation, condensation of the mesoderm of the first and second arches occurs, giving rise to six hillocks (hillocks of His). The first three hillocks are derived from the first arch, and the second arch contributes to the last three (Figure 12-23).

First arch:	First hillock → Tragus (1) Second hillock → Helical crus (2) Third hillock → Helix (3)
Second arch:	Fourth hillock → Antihelix (4) Fifth hillock → Antitragus (5) Sixth hillock → Lobule and lower helix (6)

Seventh week: Formation of cartilage is in progress.
Twelfth week: The auricle is formed by fusion of the hillocks.
Twentieth week: It has reached adult shape, although it does not reach adult size until age 9.

The concha is formed by three separate areas from the first groove (ectoderm) (see Figure 12-23).

A. *Middle part of the first groove*: Concha cavum
B. *Upper part of the first groove*: Concha cymba
C. *Lowest part of the first groove*: Intertragus incisor

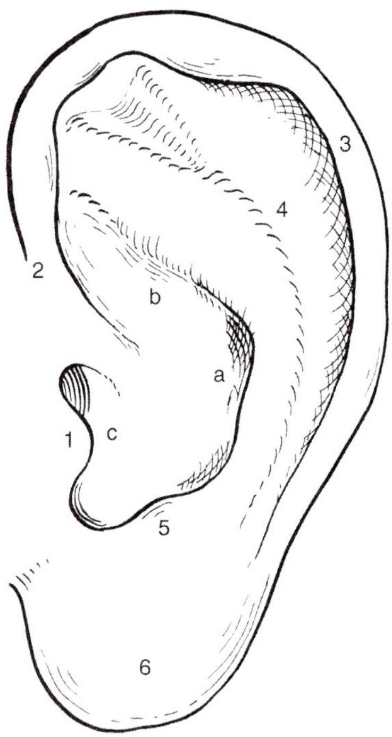

Figure 12-23 Embryology of the auricle.

External Auditory Canal

During the eighth week of gestation, the surface ectoderm in the region of the upper end of the first pharyngeal groove (dorsal) thickens. This solid core of epithelium continues to grow toward the middle ear. Simultaneously, the concha cavum deepens to form the outer one-third of the external auditory canal. By the 21st week, this core begins to resorb and "hollow out" to form a channel. The innermost layer of ectoderm remains to become the superficial layer of the tympanic membrane. Formation of the channel is completed by the 28th week. At birth, the external auditory canal is neither ossified nor of adult size. Completion of ossification occurs around age 3, and adult size is reached at age 9.

Eustachian Tube and Middle Ear

During the third week of gestation, the first and second pharyngeal pouches lie laterally on either side of what is to become the oral and pharyngeal tongue. As the third arch enlarges, the space between the second arch and the pharynx (first pouch) is compressed and becomes the eustachian tube. The "outpocketing" at the lateral end becomes the middle ear space. Because of the proximity to the first, second, and third arches, the V, VII, and IX nerves are found in the middle ear. By the 10th week, pneumatization begins. The antrum appears in the 23rd week. It is of interest that the middle ear is filled with mucoid connective tissue until the time of birth. The 28th week marks the appearance of the tympanic membrane, which is derived from all three tissues.

Ectoderm → Squamous layer
Mesoderm → Fibrous layer
Entoderm → Mucosal layer

Between the 12th and the 28th weeks, four primary mucosal sacs emerge, each becoming a specific anatomic region of the middle ear.

Saccus anticus → Anterior pouch of von Troltsch
Saccus medius → Epitympanum and petrous area
Saccus superior → Posterior pouch of von Troltsch, part of the mastoid, inferior incudal space
Saccus posterior → Round window and oval window niches, sinus tympani

At birth, the embryonic subepithelium is resorbed, and pneumatization continues in the middle ear, antrum, and mastoid. Pneumatization of the petrous portion of the temporal bone, being the last to arise, continues until puberty.

The middle ear is well formed at birth and enlarges only slightly postnatally. At age 1, the mastoid process appears. At age 3, the tympanic ring and osseous canal are calcified.

The eustachian tube measures approximately 17 mm at birth and grows to 35 mm in adulthood.

Malleus and Incus During the sixth week of embryonic development, the malleus and incus appear as a single mass. By the eighth week, they are separated, and the malleoincudal joint is formed. The head and neck of the malleus are derived from Meckel cartilage (first arch mesoderm), the anterior process from the process of Folius (mesenchyme bone), and the manubrium from Reichert cartilage (second arch mesoderm). The body and short process of the incus originate from Meckel cartilage (first arch mesoderm) and the long process from

Reichert cartilage (second arch mesoderm). By the 16th week, the ossicles reach adult size. On the 16th week, ossification begins and appears first at the long process of the incus. During the 17th week, the ossification center becomes visible on the medial surface of the neck of the malleus and spreads to the manubrium and the head. At birth, the malleus and incus are of adult size and shape. The ossification of the malleus is never complete, so that part of the manubrium remains cartilaginous. (The lenticular process is also known as "sylvian apophysis" or "os orbiculare.")

Stapes

At 4.5 weeks, the mesenchymal cells of the second arch condense to form the blastema. The VII nerve divides the blastema into stapes, interhyale, and laterohyale. During the seventh week, the stapes ring emerges around the stapedial artery. The lamina stapedialis which is of the otic mesenchyme appears to become the footplate and annular ligament. At 8.5 weeks, the incudostapedial joint develops. The interhyale becomes the stapedial muscle and tendon; the laterohyale becomes the posterior wall of the middle ear. Together with the otic capsule, the laterohyale also becomes the pyramidal process and facial canal. The lower part of the facial canal is said to be derived from Reichert cartilage.

During the 10th week, the stapes changes its ring shape to the "stirrup" shape. During the 19th week, ossification begins, starting at the obturator surface of the stapedial base. The ossification is completed by the 28th week except for the vestibular surface of the footplate, which remains cartilaginous throughout life. At birth, the stapes is of adult size and form.

Inner Ear

During the third week, neuroectoderm and ectoderm lateral to the first branchial groove condense to form the otic placode. The latter invaginates until it is completely submerged and surrounded by mesoderm, becoming the otocyst or otic vesicle by the fourth week. The fifth week marks the appearance of a wide dorsal and a slender ventral part of the otic vesicle. Between these two parts, the endolymphatic duct and sac develop. During the sixth week, the semicircular canals take shape, and by the eighth week, together with the utricle, they are fully formed. Formation of the basal turn of the cochlea takes place during the seventh week, and by the 12th week, the complete 2.5 turns are developed. Development of the saccule follows that of the utricle. Evidently, the pars superior (semicircular canals and utricle) is developed before the pars inferior (sacculus and cochlea). Formation of the membranous labyrinth without the end organ is said to be complete by the 15th week of gestation.

Concurrent with formation of the membranous labyrinth, the precursor of the otic capsule emerges during the eighth week as a condensation of mesenchyme precartilage. The 14 centers of ossification can be identified by the 15th week, and ossification is completed during the 23rd week of gestation. The last area to ossify is the fissula ante fenestram, which may remain cartilaginous throughout life. Other than the endolymphatic sac which continues to grow until adulthood the membranous and bony labyrinths are of adult size at the 23rd week of embryonic development. The endolymphatic sac is the first to appear and the last to stop growing.

At the third week, the common macula first appears. Its upper part differentiates into the utricular macula and the cristae of the superior and lateral semicircular canals, whereas its lower part becomes the macula of the saccule and the crista of the posterior semicircular canal. During the eighth week, two ridges of cells as well as the stria vascularis are identifiable. During the 11th week, the vestibular end organs, complete with sensory and supporting cells, are formed.

During the 20th week, development of the stria vascularis and the tectorial membrane is complete. During the 23rd week, the two ridges of cells divide into inner ridge cells and outer ridge cells. The inner ridge cells become the spiral limbus; the outer ones become the hair cells, pillar cells, Hensen cells, and Deiters cells. During the 26th week, the tunnel of Corti and canal of Nuel are formed.

The neural crest cells lateral to the rhombencephalon condense to form the acoustic-facial ganglion, which differentiates into the facial geniculate ganglion, superior vestibular ganglion (utricle, superior, and horizontal semicircular canals), and inferior ganglion (saccule, posterior semicircular canal, and cochlea).

At birth, four elements of the temporal bone are distinguishable: petrous bone, squamous bone, tympanic ring, and styloid process. The mastoid antrum is present, but the mastoid process is not formed until the end of the second year of life; pneumatization of the mastoid soon follows. The tympanic ring extends laterally after birth, forming the osseous canal.

Clinical Information

A. Congenital microtia occurs in about 1:20,000 births.
B. The auricle is formed early. Therefore, malformation of the auricle implies a malformation of the middle ear, mastoid, and VII nerve. On the other hand, a normal auricle with canal atresia indicates abnormal development during the 28th week, by which time the ossicles and the middle ear are already formed.
C. Improper fusion of the first and second branchial arches results in a preauricular sinus tract (epithelium lined).
D. Malformation of first branchial arch and groove results in:
   i. Auricle abnormality (first and second arches)
   ii. Bony meatus atresia (first groove)
   iii. Abnormal incus and malleus (first and second arches)
   iv. Abnormal mandible (first arch)
E. When the maxilla is also malformed, this constellation of findings is called Treacher Collins syndrome (mandibular facial dysostosis).
   i. Outward–downward slanted eyes (antimongoloid)
   ii. Notched lower lid
   iii. Short mandible
   iv. Bony meatal atresia
   v. Malformed incus and malleus
   vi. Fishmouth
F. Abnormalities of the otic capsule and labyrinth are rare because they are phylogenetically ancient.
G. An incidence of 20% to 30% dehiscent tympanic portion of the VII nerve has been reported.
H. The incidence of absent stapedius tendon, muscle, and pyramidal eminence is estimated at 1%.
I. Twenty percent of preauricular cysts are bilateral.
J. In very young infants, Hyrtl fissure affords a route of direct extension of infection from the middle ear to the subarachnoid spaces. The fissure closes as the infant grows. Hyrtl fissure extends from the subarachnoid space near the glossopharyngeal ganglion to the hypotympanum just inferior and anterior to the round window.

Bibliography

Anson B, Donaldson JA. *Surgical Anatomy of the Temporal Bone.* 3rd ed. Philadelphia, PA: WB Saunders; 1980.

Eggston AA, Wolff D. *Histopathology of the Ear, Nose and Throat.* Baltimore, MD: Williams & Wilkins; 1947.

May M. Anatomy of the facial nerve (spacial orientation of fibres in the temporal bone). *Laryngoscope.* 1973;83:1311.

Questions

1. Development of the membranous portion of the inner ear is complete by which embryologic time frame?
   A. Week 8
   B. Week 15
   C. Week 28
   D. Week 34

2. Which of the following nerves does not innervate the middle ear?
   A. V_3
   B. IX
   C. X
   D. VII

3. Which structure may be responsible for the spread of infection from the middle ear to the subarachnoid space in infants?
   A. Huguier canal
   B. Petrotympanic fissure
   C. Hyrtl fissure
   D. Foramen of Huschke

4. Normal development of the auricle with external canal atresia suggests a developmental abnormality during which embryologic time frame?
   A. Week 8
   B. Week 28
   C. Week 14
   D. Week 34

5. Which of the following attaches to the mastoid process?
   A. Sternocleidomastoid
   B. Splenius capitis
   C. Longissimus capitis
   D. Digastric
   E. All of the above

Chapter 13
Audiology and Electrical Response Audiometry

Acoustics

- *Sound*: energy waves of particle displacement, both *compression* (more dense) and *rarefaction* (less dense) within an elastic medium; triggers sensation of hearing by vibrating the tympanic membrane.
- *Amplitude of sound*: extent of vibratory movement from rest to the farthest point from rest in compression and rarefaction phases of energy waves
  - Sounds with higher amplitudes are perceived as louder than sounds with lower amplitude.
- *Intensity of sound*: amount of sound energy through an area per time; refers to sound strength or magnitude.
- *Sound pressure*: sound force (related to acceleration) over a surface per unit time.
- *Decibel (dB)*: unit to express intensity of sound; logarithm of the ratio of two sound intensities.
- *Frequency*: number of cycles (complete oscillations) of a vibrating medium per unit of time; psychoacoustic correlate is pitch.

$$\text{Period} = \text{Time for completion of one cycle}$$

- *Hertz (Hz)*: in acoustics, unit to express frequency (formerly cycles per second or cps).
  - Human ear is capable of hearing from approximately 20 to 20,000 Hz.
- *Pure tone*: single-frequency sound; rarely occurs in nature.
- *Complex sound*: sound comprising more than one frequency.
- *Noise*: aperiodic complex sound; can also mean any unwanted sound

Examples:

- White noise (containing all frequencies in the audible spectrum at average equal amplitudes)
- Narrow band noise (white noise with frequencies above and below a center frequency filtered out or reduced)
- Speech noise (white noise with frequencies > 3000 and < 300 Hz reduced by a filter).

- *Resonant frequency*: frequency at which a mass vibrates with the least amount of external force.
  - Determined by elasticity, mass, and frictional characteristics of the medium.
  - Natural resonance of external auditory canal is approximately 3000 Hz; of middle ear, 800 to 5000 Hz, mostly 1000 to 2000 Hz; of tympanic membrane, 800 to 1600 Hz; of ossicular chain, 500 to 2000 Hz.

The Decibel Scale

- A logarithmic expression of the ratio of two intensities.
  - Nonlinear
    - Energy increase from 5 to 7 dB is far greater than the increase from 1 to 3 dB
  - A relative measure
    - 0 dB does not indicate the absence of sound.
- Can be expressed with different reference levels: sound pressure level (SPL), hearing level (HL), and sensation level.

Sound Pressure Level (SPL)

- Most common measure of sound strength, usually referenced to micropascals (can also be referenced to dynes per centimeter squared or microbars).
- Sound pressure is related to sound intensity.
- The formula for determining the number of decibels is

$$\text{dB Intensity} = 10 \log I_o/I_r$$

where

I_o = intensity of output sound being measured
I_r = intensity of reference

However, intensity is proportional to pressure squared, as

$$I \propto p^2$$
$$\therefore \text{dB SPL} = 10 \log (p_o^2/p_r^2)$$

or

$$\begin{aligned}\text{dB SPL} &= 10 \log (p_o/p_r)^2 \\ &= 10 \times 2 \log (p_o/p_r) \\ &= 20 \log (p_o/p_r)\end{aligned}$$

where

p_o = pressure of the output of sound being measured
p_r = pressure of the reference, usually 20 μPa

Hearing Level (HL)

- HL is used as the reference on clinical audiometers.
- 0 dB HL at any frequency = average lowest intensity perceived by normal hearing listeners 50% of the time.
- HL referent is to ears with normal hearing sensitivity (Table 13-1), was developed because the ear is not equally sensitive to all frequencies.

Table 13-1 Number of dB SPL Needed to Equal 0 dB HL at Different Frequencies for TDH-49 and TDH-50 Earphones

Frequency (Hz)	*dB SPL*
125	47.5
250	26.5
500	13.5
1000	7.5
1500	7.5
2000	11.0
3000	9.5
4000	10.5
6000	13.5
8000	13.0

Adapted by Dr. Shoup (13th edition) with permission from American National Standard Specifications for Audiometers. ANSI S3.6–1996. New York, NY: American National Standards Institute, Inc.; 1996.

Sensation Level (SL)

- The SL referent is to a specific individual's threshold.
- dB SL refers to the number of decibels above the threshold for that same stimulus.
- Example:
  - Person's threshold = 20 dB HL at 1000 Hz
  - Sensation level of toneburst presentation = 50 dB HL
  - Resulting presentation level of toneburst = 70 dB HL

The Auditory System

Outer Ear

- Comprised of three major parts: the pinna, the external auditory canal or ear canal, and the tympanic membrane or eardrum.
- Pinna: the visible part of the ear that collects sound waves and directs them into the ear canal.
- External auditory canal: an inch-long resonance chamber that ends at the tympanic membrane or eardrum.
- Tympanic membrane: a thin membrane separating the outer ear from the middle ear, vibrates when sound waves reach it.

Middle Ear

- Air-filled space between the eardrum and oval window of the cochlea that houses the ossicular chain.
  - Ossicular chain comprised of three small bones: the malleus, incus, and stapes (smallest bone in the body).

- Middle ear dimensions (average adult): approximately 5/8 inch high (15 mm), 1/8 to 3/16 inch wide (2-4 mm), 1/4 inch deep, and 1 to 2 cm^3 in volume.
- Primary function: transform acoustic energy from the medium of air to the medium of liquid by means of sound waves traveling from the tympanic membrane along the ossicular chain to the oval window.
  (a) *The area effect of the tympanic membrane*: ratio of the vibrating portion of the tympanic membrane to that of the stapes footplate results in a 17:1 increase in sound energy by concentrating it into a smaller area.
  (b) *Lever action of the ossicular chain*: As the eardrum vibrates, the ossicular chain is set into motion about an axis of rotation from the anterior process of the malleus through the short process of the incus. Because the handle of the malleus is approximately 1.3 times longer than the incus long process, the force (pressure) received at the stapes footplate, through the use of leverage, is greater than that at the malleus by about 1.3:1. Thus, the transformer ratio of the middle ear is approximately 22:1 (the combination of the area effect of the tympanic membrane and the lever action of the ossicles: $17 \times 1.3 = 22$) which translates to approximately 25 dB.
  (c) *The natural resonance and efficiency of the outer and middle ears:* Enhances sound transmission for 500 to 3000 Hz.
  (d) *The phase difference between the oval window and the round window*: When sound energy impinges on the oval window, a traveling wave is created within the cochlea progressing from the oval window, along the scala vestibuli and the scala tympani, to the round window. The phase difference between the two windows results in a small change (~4 dB) in the normal ear.

Inner Ear

- Cochlea: primary hearing function of the inner ear; transforms the signal from mechanical energy into hydraulic energy and then ultimately, at the hair cells, into bioelectric energy. As the footplate of the stapes moves in and out of the oval window, a traveling wave is created (Bekesy's traveling wave theory) and moves the basilar and tectorial membranes. Because these two membranes have different hinge points, this movement results in a "shearing" motion that bends the hair cell stereocilia. This bending depolarizes the hair cells, which, in turn, activate afferent electrical nerve impulses.
- Basilar membrane: varies in stiffness and mass; energy wave travels from base to apex until it reaches a maximum point of displacement.
- Outer hair cells (OHCs): motile, react mechanically to the incoming signal by shortening and lengthening according to their characteristic (best) frequency. Under strong efferent influence, the OHCs are part of an active feedback mechanism, adjusting the basilar membrane's physical properties so that a given frequency maximally stimulates a specific narrow group of inner hair cells (IHCs). This effect is the "cochlear amplifier."
- IHCs: trigger most of afferent nerve responses; 95% of all afferent fibers innervate the IHCs.
- Cochlear organization: nonlinear tonotopic arrangement (basal end for high frequencies, apical end for low frequencies) that acts as a compression circuit by reducing a large range of acoustic inputs into a much smaller range, allowing the auditory system to process a wide range of intensities represented by the nonlinear, logarithmic decibel scale.

Central Pathway

- Mnemonic for the simplified sequence of these auditory structures is ECOLI: *E*ighth nerve, *C*ochlear nucleus, *O*livary complex, *L*ateral lemniscus, and *I*nferior colliculus.

- Eighth nerve: Once nerve impulses are initiated, signals continue along the auditory pathway from the cochlear spiral ganglion cells to the modiolus, where the fibers form the cochlear branch of the eighth nerve.
- Cochlear nucleus: The fibers pass to the cochlear nucleus at the pontomedullary junction of the brain stem, the first truly central connection. All fibers synapse at the ipsilateral cochlear nucleus.
- Olivary complex: The majority of fibers cross through the acoustic stria and trapezoid body to the contralateral superior olivary complex in the lower pons of the brain stem. This crossing is the first point of decussation where signals from both ears interact to allow binaural function.
- Lateral lemniscus: Fibers ascend to the nuclei of the lateral lemniscus in the pons.
- Inferior colliculus: Fibers ascend from lateral lemniscus to the inferior colliculus in the midbrain.
- The medial geniculate body in the thalamus is the last auditory nucleus before the cortex. From there, the nerve fibers radiate to the auditory cortex.

Tuning Fork Tests

- Standard part of the otologic examination.
- Can provide useful screening and confirmatory information.
- Should NOT replace audiometric test results.
- Most useful: 512 Hz fork (can also use 1024 Hz and 2048 Hz).
- Least useful: frequencies below 512 Hz due to resulting somatosensory stimulation that may confuse the patient and compromise findings.
- Essential to strike the fork gently to avoid creating overtones.
- See Table 13-2 for a summary of these tests and interpretation of results.

Weber Test

- Purpose: test of lateralization.
- Procedure:
  - Strike tuning fork and place stem on patient's midline of the skull.
  - Ask patient where the tone is louder: in the left ear, in the right ear, or at midline.

Rinne Test

- Purpose: Determine whether a major conductive component, or air-bone gap, is present.
- Procedure:
  - Strike tuning fork and place stem on patient's mastoid, then 2 inches (5 cm) lateral to the external ear canal opening.
  - Ask patient if tone sounds louder with the fork on the mastoid or just outside the ear canal.

Bing Test

- Purpose: Uses presence or absence of the occlusion effect to screen for possible conductive pathology.
- Procedure:

Table 13-2 Summary of Tuning Fork Tests

Test	*Purpose*	*Fork Placement*	*Normal Hearing*	*Conductive Loss*	*Sensorineural Loss*
Weber	To determine conductive versus sensorineural loss in unilateral loss	Midline	Midline sensation; tone heard equally in both ears	Tone louder in poorer ear	Tone louder in better ear
Rinne	To compare patient's air and bone conduction hearing	Alternately between patient's mastoid and entrance to ear canal	Positive Rinne: tone louder at ear	Negative Rinne: tone louder on mastoid	Positive Rinne: tone louder by ear
Bing	To determine if the occlusion effect is present	Mastoid	Positive Bing: tone is louder with ear canal occluded	Negative Bing: tone is not louder with ear canal occluded	Positive Bing: tone is louder with ear canal occluded
Schwabach	To compare patient's bone conduction to that of a person with normal hearing	Mastoid	Normal Schwabach: patient hears tone for about as long as the tester	Prolonged Schwabach: patient hears tone for longer time than the tester	Diminished Schwabach: patient stops hearing the tone before the tester

  - Strike tuning fork and place stem on patient's mastoid while opening and closing patient's ear canal with a finger.
  - Ask patient if tone sounds louder with the ear canal open or closed.

Schwabach Test

- Purpose: compares the patient's bone conduction hearing to that of a normal listener (usually the examiner). This test is not commonly conducted and requires that the hearing of the examiner/normal listener be confirmed as normal.
- Procedure:
  - Strike tuning fork and place stem alternately on patient's mastoid and examiner's mastoid.
  - When the patient no longer hears the sound, the examiner listens to the fork to see whether the tone is still audible.

Standard Audiometric Evaluation

Test Battery Approach

- Case history.
- Otoscopy: Visually assess pinna and ear canal.
- Pure tone audiometry: Assess frequency-specific hearing sensitivity (air conduction, and, if needed, bone conduction).
- Speech audiometry: Assess speech reception threshold and word recognition score.
- Immittance/impedance measures: Assess function of the tympanic membrane and muscle reflexes (tympanometry and acoustic reflexes).
- Otoacoustic emissions (OAE): Assess cochlear function.

Purpose of Evaluation

- Characterize hearing sensitivity:
  - Degree of hearing loss
  - Configuration of hearing responses
  - Type of hearing loss: conductive, sensorineural, mixed, or neural/auditory dyssynchrony
- Recommend management/treatment options:
  - Need for medical or surgical intervention, including implantable devices
  - Nonsurgical intervention, such as hearing aids, assistive devices, aural (re)habilitation, communication strategies
- Determine need for further testing

Pure Tone Audiometry

Air Conduction

- Air conduction results: degree of hearing loss due to disruption of sound transmission at any level of the auditory system resulting in a conductive, sensorineural, or mixed disorder.
- Determines pure tone thresholds with insert phone, headphone, or soundfield transducer by finding the lowest intensity at which the patient responds at least 50% of the time.
- 250 to 8000 Hz frequencies are typically assessed; inter-octave frequencies (eg, 1500 Hz) if 20 dB or more difference between octave frequency thresholds.
- 125 Hz is measured when low-frequency hearing exists.
- 3000 and 6000 Hz are typically included to provide a more complete profile of the hearing status.
- Extended high frequencies between 9000 and 20,000 Hz may be included for:
  - Assessment of early detection of hearing loss at high frequencies for specific concerns such as excessive noise exposure
  - Ototoxic monitoring
  - Tinnitus in presence of normal hearing

Bone Conduction

- Bone conduction results: degree of hearing loss due to inner ear, nerve or central damage
- Determines pure tone thresholds with bone oscillator by finding the lowest intensity at which patient responds at least 50% of time
- 250, 500, 1000, 2000, 3000, and 4000 Hz frequencies are typically assessed
  - Lower frequencies may elicit vibrotactile responses at louder levels

Air–Bone Gap

- Difference between air and bone conduction thresholds, reflects the contribution of reduced transmission or conduction of sound through outer and/or middle ears to decreased hearing sensitivity.

Masking

- Necessary when signal to test ear is strong enough to stimulate the non-test ear by sending vibrations through the skull: *crossover*.
  - Crossover in air conduction with supra-aural earphones occurs as low as 40 dB HL.
  - Crossover in air conduction and bone conduction occurs as low as 0 dB HL.
- Noise introduced into non-test ear to prevent that ear from detecting signals intended for test ear.

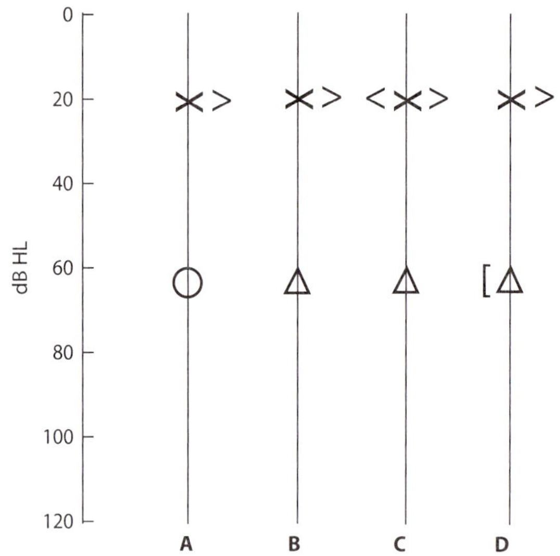

Figure 13-1 Examples of applying the rules that determine the need for masking and the results after having masked. A. Right air conduction threshold, unmasked, is 45 dB poorer than left bone conduction threshold and must be verified by masking. B. Right air conduction threshold masked (no change with masking). C. Right bone conduction threshold, unmasked, shows an air–bone gap greater than 10 dB. D. Right bone conduction threshold, masked (shifted with masking).

- Reduction in sound energy as it travels from one side of the skull to other is *interaural attenuation (IAA), varies* by individual due to characteristics of the skull.
  - IAA air conduction:
    - Supra-aural headphones = 40 to 65 dB depending on frequency and patient characteristics
    - Insert earphones = 50 to 70 dB depending on frequency and patient characteristics
  - IAA bone conduction = 0 to 10 dB depending on frequency and patient characteristics
- Preferred masker used for pure tones is narrow-band noise; preferred masker for speech is speech-spectrum noise.

Two rules of when to mask (see examples in Figure 13-1):

A. *Air conduction*: If air conduction threshold of test ear exceeds bone conduction threshold of the non-test ear by 40 dB or more for supra-aural earphones and 55 dB or more for insert earphones.

B. *Bone conduction*: If an air–bone gap greater than 10 dB exists between unmasked bone conduction threshold and air conduction threshold in either ear.

To better determine the integrity of the auditory system, pure tone results should be interpreted in conjunction with speech audiometry, tympanometry, and acoustic reflex test results.

Speech Audiometry

- Ideally presented using recorded material; can be presented with monitored live voice (MLV) in special situations, however MLV results are not as repeatable and the stimuli are not as well controlled as for recorded speech.

Speech Awareness/Detection Threshold (SAT/SDT):

(a) The lowest level in dB HL at which an individual detects/responds to the presence of speech.

(b) Sometimes appropriate when assessing small children, persons with physical or mental disabilities, those with a language barrier, or any time a speech recognition threshold (SRT) cannot be obtained.

(c) SAT/SDT results should be within 10 dB of a pure tone threshold anywhere across the conventional audiogram (250-8000 Hz), and will typically be obtained at a slightly lower threshold than the pure tones since speech is a complex stimulus.

Speech recognition threshold (SRT):

(a) Lowest level in dB HL at which a patient can repeat spondaic words (spondees) in 50% of presentations.
(b) Spondee: two-syllable compound word that is pronounced with equal stress on both syllables (eg, railroad, sidewalk, and eardrum).
(c) SRT measured primarily to confirm/cross-check pure tone thresholds and should be within 10 dB of the pure tone average (PTA, the average of air conduction thresholds at 500, 1000, and 2000 Hz). In a falling or rising audiometric pattern, a best two-frequency PTA may better corroborate the SRT.

Word (speech) recognition score (WRS):

(a) Expressed as a percentage of correct words.
(b) Typically, a phonetically balanced word list is presented at a suprathreshold level to assess a patient's ability to understand speech.
(c) Presentation level may vary depending on audiogram results and patient-reported symptoms. A common practice is to present the words at 30 to 40 dB HL above the patient's SRT. However, if a person has reduced loudness tolerance, the maximum score is sometimes obtained at a lower SL. Conversely, in sloping or falling configurations, a higher SL may yield one's maximum score.
(d) Interpretation is as follows:

90%-100% correct	Normal
76%-88% correct	Good/Slight difficulty
60%-74% correct	Fair/Moderate difficulty
40%-58% correct	Poor
≤40% correct	Very poor

- Interpretation regarding communication difficulty must take into account not only the score but also the absolute presentation level of the stimuli. The level of average conversational speech is 50 to 60 dB HL. In a 25-dB hearing loss, a presentation level of 30-dB SL means that the test words are presented at 55 dB HL, a level we are likely to encounter in normal conversational speech. In a 45-dB loss, 30-dB SL means a presentation level of 75-dB HL, a higher level than we normally encounter. Therefore, two individuals with different degrees of hearing loss may have the same score but have marked differences in how well they understand daily conversation.

Immittance Measures

Tympanometry

- An objective test that measures the mobility (compliance) of the middle ear at the tympanic membrane as a function of applied air pressure in the external ear canal.
  - Compliance: expressed as acoustic admittance in millimho (mMho) or as the admittance of an equivalent volume of air in cm^3 or mL, and pressure is expressed in dekapascals (daPa)
  - Peak: point of maximum compliance of the middle ear as the pressure changes
  - Maximum compliance: pressure at which the eardrum is most mobile, occurs when the pressure in the external ear canal equals the pressure in the middle ear

Table 13-3 Normative Values of Static Acoustic Admittance, TW, and Equivalent Ear Canal Volume for Children and Adults

Age (year)	*Admittance (mL)*	*TW (daPa)*	*EC Vol (mL)*
3-10	0.25-1.05	80-160	0.3-0.9
Adults (>18)	0.3-1.7	50-114	0.9-2.0

Data from Margolis RH, Hunter LI. Acoustic immittance measurements. In: Roeser RJ, Valente M, Hosford-Dunn H, eds. *Audiology Diagnosis*. New York, NY: Thieme; 2000.

- Normative data:
  - Due to maturational changes in the ear canal, tympanic membrane, and middle ear system, normative data are age specific.
    - Results can be quantified through normative values shown in Table 13-3 Static acoustic admittance: metric of middle ear mobility.
    - Tympanometric width (TW): gradient or steepness of the tympanogram; the poorer the compliance, the broader the TW.
    - Equivalent ear canal volume: estimate of the volume of space between the probe tip and the tympanic membrane; will include the size of the middle ear cavity in cases of tympanic membrane perforation or patent PE tube.
- Interpretation of results: Five types of tympanograms, illustrated in Figure 13-2C.
  - *Type A*: normal middle ear pressure and mobility, with a clearly defined peak of maximum compliance. Peak is in a normal range of compliance with pressure between −100 to +100 daPa in adults (see Figure 13-2A).

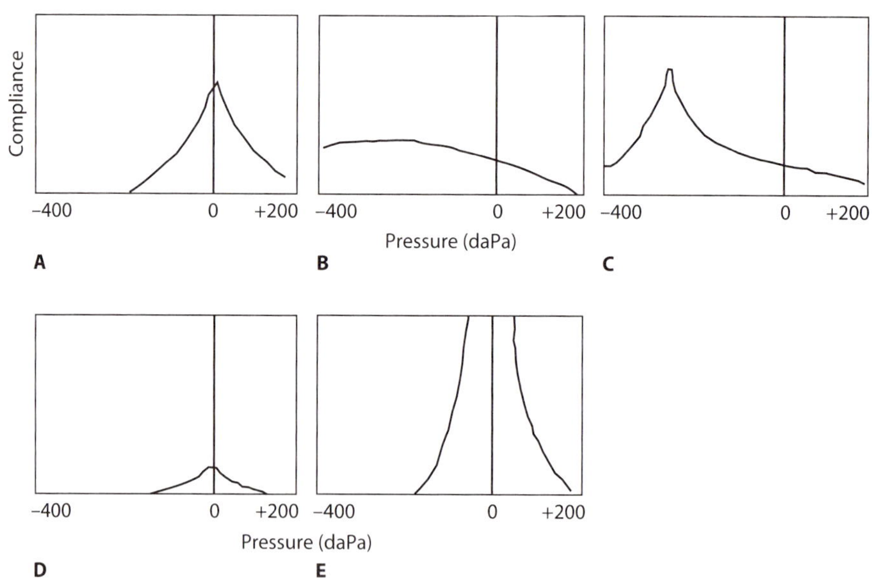

Figure 13-2 **A.** Type A, normal range of compliance and pressure, normal middle ear function. **B.** Type B, poor middle ear compliance across pressures. **C.** Type C, abnormal negative middle ear pressure. **D.** Type A_s, abnormally low compliance. **E.** Type A_d, abnormally high compliance.

- *Type A_s*: type A with abnormally shallow or low peak; restricted mobility. This type may be seen in otosclerosis, scarred tympanic membrane, or fixation of the malleus (see Figure 13-2D).
- *Type A_d*: type A with abnormally deep or high peak; "loose" or hypercompliant middle ear system.
  - Seen in flaccid tympanic membrane or in disarticulation, even partial, of the ossicular chain (see Figure 13-2E).
  - Flaccid eardrum: little or no hearing loss
  - Disarticulation: substantial conductive hearing loss, worse at the high frequencies
- *Type B*: flat or very low, rounded peak.
  - Normal ear canal volume: suggests little or no mobility and is consistent with fluid in the middle ear.
  - Large ear canal volume: suggests patent pressure equalizing (PE) tube or a perforation in the tympanic membrane (see Figure 13-2B).
  - Small ear canal volume: suggests obstruction such as cerumen or foreign object in ear canal or the probe may be plugged or against the ear canal wall.
- *Type C*: compliance peak in region of negative middle ear
- Consistent with a retracted tympanic membrane and a malfunctioning eustachian tube or simply a child sniffling (see Figure 13-2C).

Acoustic reflex threshold testing

- An objective measure of the lowest stimulus level that elicits the stapedial reflex.
- With the pressure set to hold the tympanic membrane at its maximum compliance, pure tone stimuli are presented; whether the signals go to one ear or to both, the stapedial reflex occurs bilaterally in response to loud sounds.
- Testing is performed with either ipsilateral or contralateral recording, or both.
  - Pathway is determined by the stimulation-recording arrangement.
    - A. Ipsilateral recording (stimulus and recording in the same ear)
      - i. Acoustic nerve
      - ii. Ipsilateral ventral cochlear nucleus
      - iii. Trapezoid body
      - iv. Ipsilateral facial motor nucleus *or* ipsilateral medial superior olive
      - v. Ipsilateral facial nerve
      - vi. Ipsilateral stapedius muscle
    - B. Contralateral recording (stimulus in opposite ear from the recording)
      - i. Acoustic nerve
      - ii. Ipsilateral ventral cochlear nucleus
      - iii. Contralateral medial superior olive
      - iv. Contralateral facial motor nucleus
      - v. Contralateral facial nerve
      - vi. Contralateral stapedius muscle
- Acoustic reflexes typically occur around 70 dB SL.
  - Normal acoustic reflex thresholds range from 70- to 100-dB HL for pure tones.
  - In the presence of any significant conductive pathology or hearing loss in the recording ear, the reflex will likely be absent.
  - If there is a hearing loss, whether conductive or sensorineural, in the stimulated ear greater than 65-dB HL, the reflex will likely be absent (Figure 13-3).

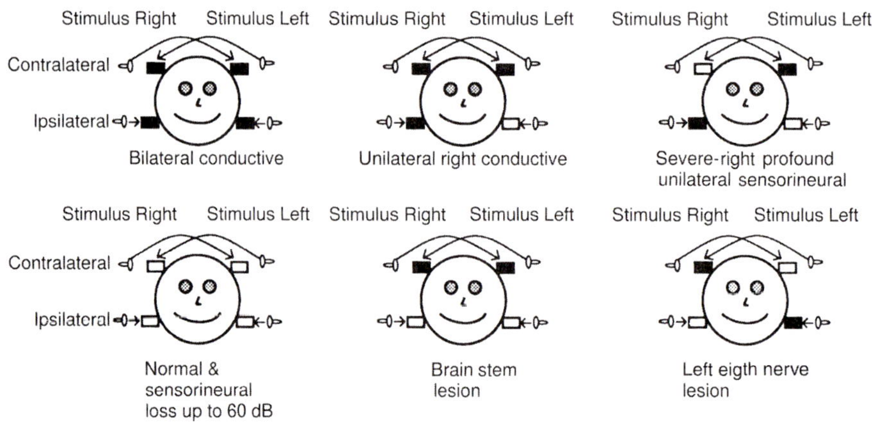

Figure 13-3 Acoustic reflex patterns. A. Reflex present at normal level. B. Reflex absent/elevated.

Otoacoustic Emissions

- Acoustic signals generated by the cochlear OHCs and transmitted out through the middle ear to the ear canal where they can be recorded by a sensitive microphone in a quiet environment.
- Otoacoustic emissions (OAEs) are an epiphenomenon, that is, not a process of hearing but a byproduct of it.
  - Efficient, objective, noninvasive "window" into cochlear function.
- Can be used to screen hearing, estimate cochlear (outer hair cell) response by frequency, and differentiate between sensory and neural hearing losses.
- Do not require behavioral responses; however, requires patient to be relatively still and quiet throughout testing.
- May be contraindicated in cases of middle ear dysfunction and/or significant debris in the ear canal due to the degradation of signal transmission to the cochlea and from the cochlea. Present OAEs indicate intact OHC function, but absent OAEs do not necessarily indicate OHC malfunction, unless normal middle ear status is confirmed.
- Clinical application of OAEs:
  - To distinguish between cochlear versus extracochlear pathologies
  - To help identify inorganic hearing loss
  - To screen for hearing loss
  - To monitor for changes in hearing in cases of ototoxicity and high noise exposure
  - To cross-check behavioral audiometry and estimated thresholds obtained via ABR or ASSR

Types of OAEs

A. Evoked OAEs (EOAEs): Generated in response to an acoustic stimulus
   i. Transient evoked OAEs (*TEOAEs):*
      a. Occur in response to transient, low-level (below 30 dB) signals such as clicks or very brief tonebursts. The normal TEOAE response has the same frequency components of the stimulus.

b. TEOAEs can be analyzed by octave band for presence or absence of cochlear response across the frequency range, but only provide a present or absent response for whether cochlear hearing is better or worse than the 30 to 40 dB range at each octave band, generally up through 4000 Hz.
c. Present TEOAEs: Cochlea has either normal function through the OHCs or has no more than approximately a 30-40-dB HL sensorineural hearing impairment.
   ◊ Present TEOAEs in the presence of confirmed sensorineural hearing loss (SNHL) may indicate a purely extracochlear pathology.
d. Absent TEOAEs: indicate a SNHL greater than 30 to 40 dB HL

ii. Distortion product OAEs (*DPOAE)s:*
a. Occur in response to two simultaneous brief pure tones of different frequencies (F_1 and F_2). In response to F_1 and F_2 stimuli, the healthy cochlea then produces several distortion products at frequencies different from the stimuli. The most prominent distortion product is usually at the frequency $2F_2$-F_1.
b. A DPOAE is a single tone evoked by two simultaneously presented pure tones.
c. Stimulus levels typically 55 to 65-dB SPL but intensity functions may be tested by varying the input intensities.
d. Usually easiest to obtain a distortion product (DP) from the human cochlea when the stimulus (or primary) frequencies, F1 and F2, are separated by ratio of 1:1.2, for example, 2000 and 2400 Hz.
e. By using different combinations of primary tones, different distortion-product frequencies can be generated, thereby allowing objective assessment of a large portion of the basilar membrane.
f. Of the several interactions of the stimulus tones, the interaction 2F1-F2 (or the cubic difference tone), usually produces the most detectable distortion product whose frequency is lower than either of the two stimulus frequencies.
g. Reflects cochlear status nearer F2 as opposed to F1 or the DP.
h. DPOAEs can be obtained in persons with more OHC loss and in response to higher frequency stimuli than can TEOAEs.
i. Help estimate presence of hearing loss by frequency, but not precise thresholds; absent DPOAEs with normal middle ear function generally indicate at least a 40-dB cochlear hearing loss depending on stimulus intensity.

B. Spontaneous OAEs (*SOAEs*): Approximately 35% to 60% of normally hearing individuals have spontaneous otoacoustic emissions, that is, generated with no external stimulus. SOAEs are rarely used clinically due to low specificity in identifying cochlear dysfunction.
C. Stimulus-frequency OAEs (SFOAEs): occur in response to ongoing stimuli; have no current clinical applications.

Hearing Loss

Characterized by degree, type, and audiometric configuration.

The Audiogram

- A graphic representation of a person's sensitivity to pure tones as a function of frequency.
- Frequency: Indicated by numbers across the top of the audiogram.

Table 13-4 Commonly Used Audiogram Symbols

Left Ear	*Interpretation*	*Right Ear*
X	Unmasked air conduction	O
□	Masked air conduction	Δ
>	Unmasked bone conduction	<
]	Masked bone conduction	[
↘	No response (NR)	↙
S	Sound field	S

Data from Guidelines for audiometric symbols. Committee on Audiologic Evaluation. American Speech-Language-Hearing Association, *ASHA Suppl.* 1990 Apr;(2):25-3.

- Intensity in decibels HL (dB HL): Indicated by numbers along the side of the audiogram.
- The most commonly used audiogram symbols are shown in Table 13-4.

Degree of Hearing Loss

- Scales of hearing ability based on pure tone thresholds: See Table 13-5.
- Different scales are used for children, who are still developing speech and language, and adults who have already acquired speech and language.

Table 13-5 Scales of Hearing Impairment and Impact on Communication

Degree of Hearing Loss	
A common classification system for use with children	
0-15 dB HL	Within normal limits
15-25 dB HL	Slight
25-30 dB HL	Mild
30-50 dB HL	Moderate
50-70 dB HL	Severe
70+	Profound
Data from Northern JL, Downs MP. *Hearing in Children*. 5th ed. Hagerstown, MD: Lippincott-Raven; 2002.	
A common classification system for use with adults	
0-25 dB HL	Within normal limits
26-40 dB HL	Mild
41-55 dB HL	Moderate
56-70 dB HL	Moderate to severe (or moderately severe)
71-90 dB HL	Severe
91+	Profound

Data from Roeser R, Buckley KA, Stickney GS. Pure tone tests. In: Roeser RJ, Valente M, Hosford-Dunn H, eds. *Audiology Diagnosis*. New York, NY: Thieme; 2000.

- Percentage of hearing loss:
  - rarely used clinically
  - can be used for medico-legal purposes
  - often based on an individual's thresholds at the speech frequencies of 500, 1000, 2000, and 3000 Hz
  - Should not be confused with word recognition score
- Descriptive terminology is more commonly utilized in most other situations (eg, "mild to severe"), such as understanding the impact of hearing loss on communication (see Table 13-5).
- "Hearing impaired": Hearing impaired refers to anyone with a hearing loss.
- "deaf": applies only to those with profound, SNHL (usually > 90-dB HL and for whom hearing is nonusable even with a hearing aid).
- "Hard-of-hearing": refers to the wide range of hearing loss between normal and deaf.

Hearing Loss Configuration

- Important information for determining possible etiology and functional impact on speech perception and aural performance.
- Possible configurations:
  - Flat (see Figure 13-4)
  - Rising (see Figure 13-5)
  - Sloping (see Figure 13-6)
  - Falling (Figure 13-7)
  - Notched (Figure 13-8)
  - Saucer-shaped (Figure 13-9)

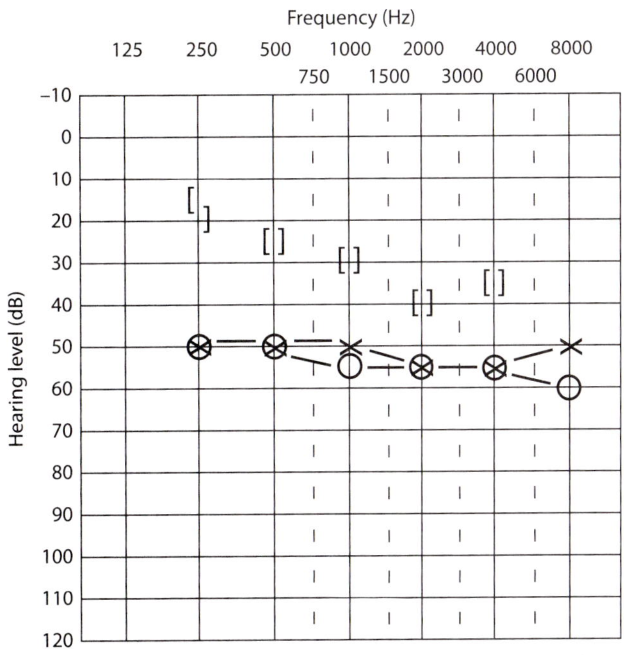

Figure 13-4 Bilateral mixed hearing loss in flat configuration.

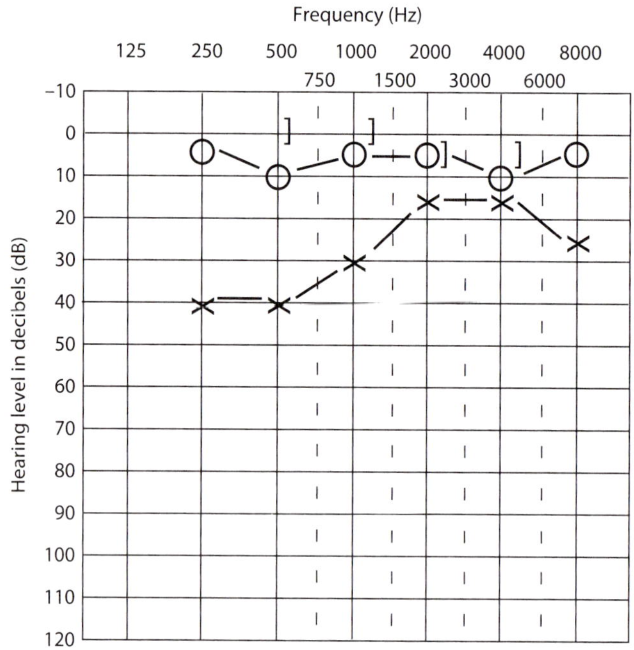

Figure 13-5 Conductive loss in the left ear in rising configuration.

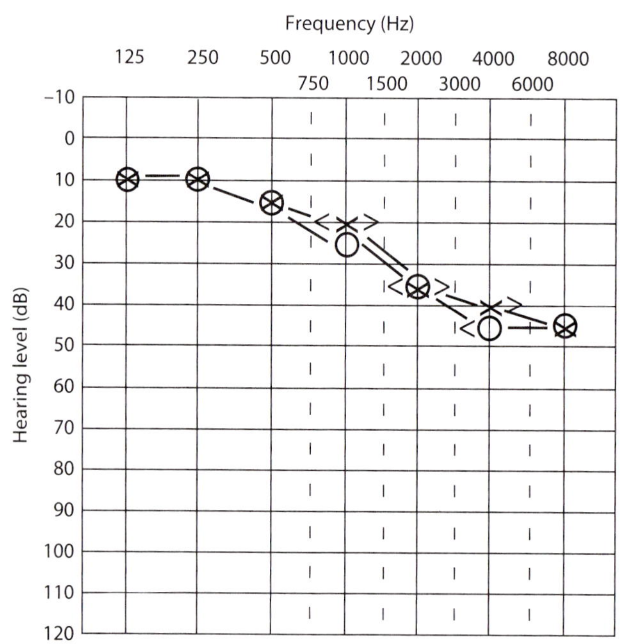

Figure 13-6 Sensorineural hearing loss in sloping configuration.

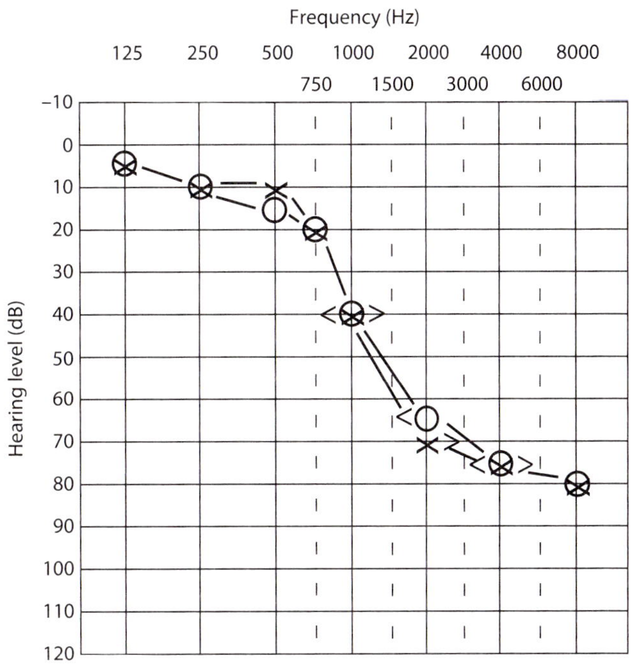

Figure 13-7 Sensorineural hearing loss in falling configuration.

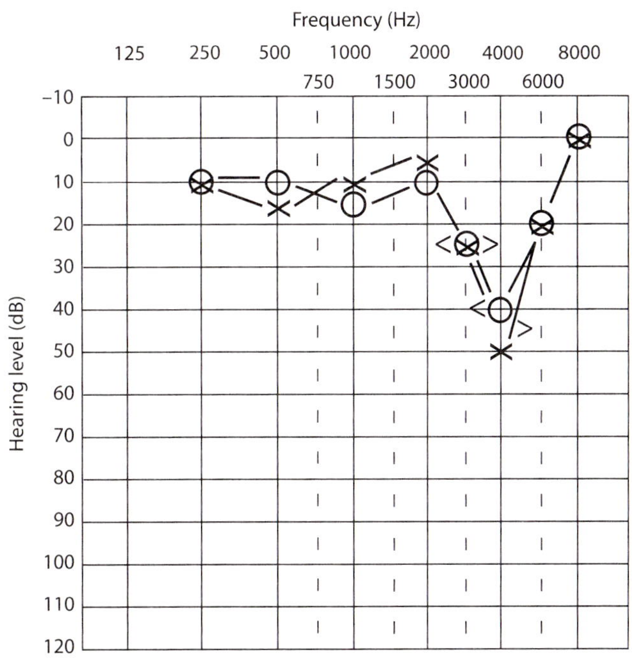

Figure 13-8 Sensorineural hearing loss in notched configuration.

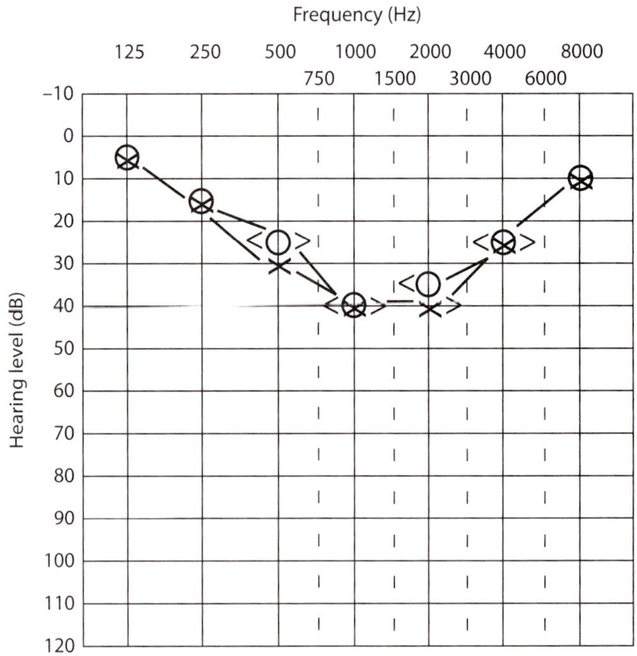

Figure 13-9 Sensorineural hearing loss in saucer-shaped configuration.

Types of Hearing Loss

Sample audiograms of the types of hearing loss—conductive, sensorineural and mixed—can be found in Figures 13-4 to 13-10.

Normal Hearing

- All air conduction thresholds in both ears are within normal limits (≤ 25-dB HL for adults and ≤ 15 dB HL for children; Figure 13-10).

Conductive Hearing Loss

- Hearing loss only by air conduction, with normal bone conduction thresholds, indicating outer or middle ear pathology impairing sound transmission to the inner ear (Figure 13-5).
- Often abnormal tympanometry results (Type B, Type As, Type Ad), but can also have normal tympanometry results.
- Caused by a disorder of external and/or middle ear.
- Generally does not exceed 60 dB HL.
- Pathologies that increase middle ear stiffness primarily affect low frequencies (eg, effusion).
- Pathologies that decrease middle ear stiffness produce a flat loss (eg, ossicular chain interruption; exception: partial ossicular discontinuity can produce a predominantly high frequency loss).
- Pathologies that only alter mass are infrequent and primarily affect high frequencies.
- Sufficient effusion combines stiffness and mass, producing a loss in both low and high frequencies, often with a characteristic peak at 2000 Hz.

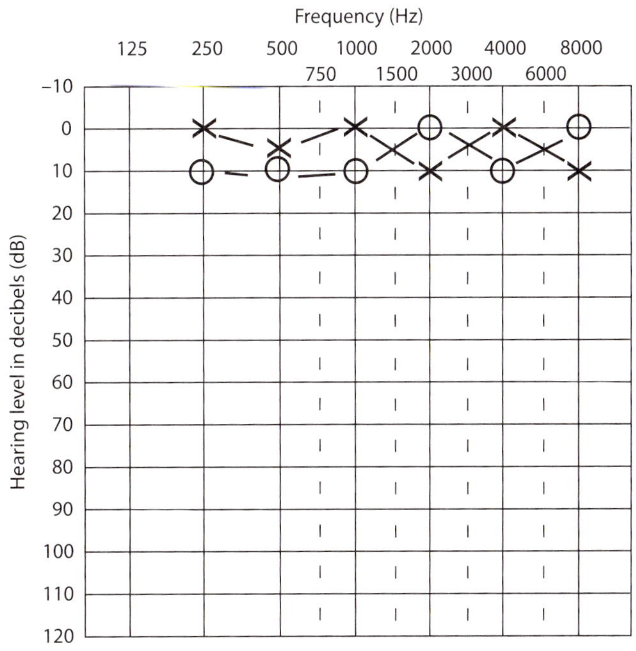

Figure 13-10 Normal hearing.

Sensorineural Hearing Loss

- Hearing loss by air and by bone conduction of similar degree, indicating pathology of the cochlea (sensory), nerve (neural), and/or auditory central nervous system (neural) (Figure 13-6).
- Caused by a disorder of the cochlea and/or eighth nerve.
- Can range from mild to profound.

Mixed Hearing Loss

- Combination of conductive and sensorineural hearing losses.
- Hearing loss by both air and bone conduction, but air conduction hearing is worse than bone conduction, indicating a conductive pathology overlaid on sensorineural pathology.

Central Hearing Loss

- Caused by a disorder of the auditory system in brain stem or higher
- May or may not appear as hearing loss on pure tone audiogram or yield abnormal results on conventional speech audiometric tests
- May cause patients to report disproportionate difficulty in understanding or processing speech relative to the audiogram

Auditory Neuropathy Spectrum Disorder

- Characterized by present outer hair cell responses as reflected by OAEs or the cochlear microphonic, and absent or characteristically abnormal brain stem responses as reflected in the acoustic reflexes or auditory brain stem response.
- May or may not appear as hearing loss on pure tone audiogram or yield abnormal results on conventional speech audiometric tests.

- Patients may present with disproportionate difficulty in understanding or processing speech in quiet and/or in noise relative to the audiogram.
- May be due to selective loss of inner hair cells, derangement of communication at the synapse between the hair cell and VIII CN, or dyssynchronous neural firing in the auditory pathways.

Site-of-Lesion Testing

- Tests that can help identify whether the site of the lesion is cochlear or retrocochlear for cases of SNHL.
- Can include both objective and behavioral measures.

Behavioral Tests

- Performance intensity function:
  - Assesses degradation in word recognition when presented at high-intensity levels and creates a performance intensity function (PI-PB).
  - Normal hearing or conductive hearing loss: PI-PB will rise to a high score and remain high with increases in intensity.
  - Sensorineural hearing loss: word recognition and PI-PB may peak and then decrease at higher levels).
    - Decrement in word recognition is not considered clinically significant unless positive for "rollover."
  - The rollover ratio = (PB max − PB min [beyond peak score])/PB max.
    - Positive "rollover": ratio of 0.30 or greater, indicative of an eighth nerve lesion and possible retrocochlear pathology.
- Sensitivity of this test is noted to be poor and should be supported with other objective testing and imaging

Physiologic Tests

- Acoustic reflex decay:
  - Measures whether stapedius muscle contraction is maintained during a continuous signal 10 dB above acoustic reflex threshold for 10 seconds. Contralateral stimulation is typically used.
  - "Positive" result indicative of retrocochlear involvement: Inability to maintain the contraction (loss of half of the amplitude of the reflex in 5 seconds, typically at 1000.

Electrical Response Audiometry

- ERA and auditory evoked potentials (AEP) are used interchangeably.
- Recorded while being evoked by a sound stimulus.
- "Objective" evaluation because the subject is not required to actively participate in the assessment.
- Short-latency automatic components are favored for threshold estimation
- Long-latency components are generally used to surmise the cognitive processing capacity of the brain and are often called event-related potentials (ERPs).

Auditory Evoked Potentials

- Electrical response from the nerve fibers in the auditory pathway to an auditory stimulus.
- Summation of electrical activity produced by thousands of nerve fibers within the auditory pathway and can be recorded through superficial electrodes.

- Components of each response:
  - Corresponds to the electrical activity of a specific neural generator site within the auditory pathway.
  - Primarily categorized by latency, the time after a stimulus onset that a response appears.
    - The longer the latency, the farther along the pathway the neural generator lies.
  - Characterized by amplitude.
    - Responses with more peripheral generator sites have smaller amplitudes than those from the cortex.
  - May be further classified as exogenous or endogenous responses.
    - Exogenous responses: influenced by external factors such as the evoking stimulus (ie, stimulus intensity), are not influenced by patient attention or processing of the stimulus.
    - Endogenous responses: influenced by internal cognitive processes rather than stimuli's acoustic variables, responses are altered by patient attention, expectancy, identification of significance, decision-making, and processing of the stimulus.
- Transient potential versus steady-state potential
  - Transient potentials: elicited by a rapidly changing stimulus such as a rapid on/off. The final measure of which is a summation of the multiple discrete responses elicited with each change in stimuli.
    - All early AEPs are transient responses.
  - Steady-state potentials: elicited by an ongoing stimulus with periodic variations in stimuli, responses follow the time course of the modulation.
- Numerous auditory evoked potentials have been identified; however, only a few are used routinely in clinical settings. Other AEPs are used primarily in research settings.

List of available AEP tests (not all are widely used clinically):

- Electrocochleography (ECoG or ECochG)
- Auditory brain stem response (ABR)
- Auditory steady-state response (ASSR), auditory steady-state evoked potential (ASSEP)
- Cortical electric response audiometry (CER or CERA), N1-P2 response
- Middle-latency response (MLR)
- Auditory-late response (ALR)
- P300
- Electroneurography (ENoG)
- Somatosensory evoked potential (SSEP)
- Electromyography (EMG)
- Cervical vestibular evoked myogenic potentials (cVEMP)—see Vestibular chapter
- Ocular vestibular evoked myogenic potentials (oVEMP)—see Vestibular chapter
- NRT—see Cochlear Implant chapter

Electrocochleography

- Generated response from the cochlea and the proximal portion of CN VIII.
- Three main components:
  1. Cochlear microphonic
     a. The first component to be identified; however, it is not used diagnostically in ECOG.
     b. Alternating stimuli is typically used to eliminate the cochlear microphonic (CM) in this response so that the SP can be more easily identified.

2. Summating potential
   a. Occurs immediately after the CM and persists for the duration of the stimuli.
   b. The summating potential (SP) is believed to be the product of outer hair cells and the non-linear element of cochlear transduction.
   c. Can be diminished in cases of SNHL due to outer hair cell damage.
   d. A large SP can indicate endolymphatic hydrops, or Meniere disease.
3. Action potential (AP)/compound action potential (CAP)
   a. The AP in ECOG is equivalent to the Wave I of the ABR.
   b. The AP reflects the synchronous activity of the nerve fibers at the basal end of the cochlea.

- The SP/AP wave complex reflects cochlear mechanics, particularly the movement of the basilar membrane and Reisser's membrane. Normal movement of these membranes is dependent on maintenance of a normal pressure gradient between the endolymph and the perilymph.
- ECOG measurements can be recorded using a special electrode placed on or near the tympanic membrane (TM). There are three main electrode types that could be used.
  - **Tiptrode:** Consists of a foam insert earphone covered in gold foil placed in the ear canal, similar to typical inserts used in behavioral audiometry.
  - **TMtrode:** Consists of a silver wire encased in a silastic tube with a soft gel tip. This is placed directly on the TM or the floor of the ear canal, as close to the TM as possible. Placement of this electrode type will greatly impact the amplitude of the response. Because it is placed closer to the generator site, the TMtrode produced a large amplitude response compared to the Tiptrode.
  - **Needle electrode:** The needle electrode is inserted through the tympanic membrane (or via surgical opening) onto the cochlear promontory, near the round window niche. This electrode type produces the highest response amplitudes due to proximity to the generator site; however, due to the invasiveness of the procedure, use of the needle electrode is limited to intraoperative applications.
- Testing is completed using an alternating click stimulus to obtain two to three repeatable waveforms for each ear. These waveforms are then averaged together to get one summated waveform that is labeled by the SP (the leading shoulder of the peak) and the AP (the main peak). A baseline at the start of the AP must also be identified to determine the amplitude of the response.
- Clinically useful in the differential diagnosis of Meniere disease, perilymphatic fistula, and third window disorders such as superior semicircular canal dehiscence (SSCD). It can also be useful in intraoperative monitoring of cochlear and auditory nerve status.
- Clinical indications for ordering EGOG testing: symptoms of episodic dizziness or vertigo, fluctuating hearing loss, aural fullness, and tinnitus.
- The primary diagnostic measure of ECOG is the SP/AP amplitude ratio (significance varies based on the electrode used).
  - Tiptrode: > 0.5 (50%) = abnormal
  - TMtrode: > 0.4 (40%) = abnormal
  - Needle electrode: > 0.3 (30%) = abnormal
- An abnormal SP/AP ratio suggests cochlear function on the date of testing, specifically indicating an imbalance of the endolymph/perilymph ratio within the cochlea.
  - Meniere disease: An overproduction and/or under-reabsorption of endolymph resulting in a higher pressure of endolymph relative to perilymph. The sensitivity of ECOG to Meniere disease is estimated to be 55% to 65%. Sensitivity increases if patient is symptomatic on the day of testing, particularly with hearing loss and aural fullness.

  - Perilymphatic fistula: Perilymph leaks from the cochlea (often at the round window), resulting in a higher pressure of endolymph relative to perilymph.
  - Superior canal dehiscence: The third window reduces the pressure in the scala vestibuli and scala tympani as pressure equalizes around the helicotrema. This reduces the perilymphatic pressure, shifting the pressure gradient such that endolymph is "greater" than perilymph.
- Contraindications for ECOG include abnormal middle ear status and SNHL that exceeds 50 to 60 dB HL, as amplitude of the response may be reduced, and could potentially result in false positive findings.

Auditory Brain Stem Response (ABR)

- Response is a product of the synchronous discharge of signals from the peripheral and central neurons of the auditory pathway.
- Not a test of hearing sensitivity, rather a measure of auditory system function from the outer ear through the lower brain stem.
- Consists of five primary positive peaks that occur at predictable time intervals from 1.4 to 6 ms after stimulus onset.
- Each of the five waveforms is thought to have distinct neural generator sites:
  - Wave I: Distal portion of CN VIII
  - Wave II: Proximal portion of CN VIII
  - Wave III: Caudal (lower) brain stem near trapezoid body and superior olivary complex
  - Wave IV: Superior olivary complex/lateral lemniscus, with likely contributions from the cochlear nucleus and lateral lemniscus
  - Wave V: Lateral lemniscus as it enters the inferior colliculus
- Depending on the application, the components of the ABR that are analyzed as diagnostic indicators include:
  - Morphology of the waveform presence/absence of waves
    - Normal ABR recordings at high intensities should contain well-defined peaks and the presence of at least waves I, III, and V for each ear.
    - In adults:
      - ◊ Wave I is larger than Wave II.
      - ◊ Wave I and III are usually about the same size, but III may be larger.
      - ◊ Wave V will typically be the largest.
    - In Infants:
      - ◊ Waves I and III may be larger in amplitude than wave V.
      - ◊ Wave I can reach adult latencies at 3 to 4 months. Wave II and V continue to mature and don't reach normal measures until about 18 months of age.
    - The following are variations of normal morphology:
      - ◊ Waves IV and V may be combined into a single peak, known as a IV/V complex.
      - ◊ Wave V may be on the descending slope of a high-amplitude wave IV.
      - ◊ Wave II and IV may be absent or small in amplitude.
  - Absolute wave latency
    - Absolute latency is the measure of the occurrence of peak relative to the onset of the stimulus.
    - Absolute latency measures of the click ABR waveform are the primary basis for ABR interpretation because they are reliable and robust.
    - Expected latency of wave components in response to high intensity stimuli are as follows:
      - ◊ Wave I = 1.5 ms
      - ◊ Wave II = 2.5 ms

        - ◊ Wave III = 3.5 ms
        - ◊ Wave IV = 4.5 ms
        - ◊ Wave V = 5.5 ms
    - Interwave latency
        - Interwave (interpeak) latency is a measure of the time between peaks.
        - I-III interwave latency should be about 2.0 ms.
        - III-V interwave latency should be about 2.0 ms.
        - I-V interwave latency should be about 4.0 ms.
    - Lowest stimulus level at which a response is present.
- ABR stimulus
    - Stimulus type, frequency, intensity, polarity, and rate can influence the ABR response.
    - Click stimulus:
        - Broadband stimulus with fast onset/offset and brief duration, which is important to generate a synchronous response.
        - Does not generate frequency-specific responses in threshold ABR.
        - Represents the high frequency region of 2000 to 4000 Hz only due to earlier activation of the basal portion of the cochlea, and temporal delays resulting in amplitude reduction and phase cancellation at the apical end of the cochlea.
        - Produces a predictable ABR waveform in normal individuals, and it has been used to generate the majority of the ABR normative data that is used clinically.
    - Toneburst stimulus
        - Frequency-specific stimulus that can be used to estimate hearing levels.
        - Balances the rapid onset required for neural synchrony while maintaining the spectral content of the signal. This is important because to maintain frequency specificity, a longer signal duration is needed; however, if the signal duration is too long, neural synchrony needed to elicit a response is lost.
        - Most commonly used air conduction toneburst stimuli: 500 Hz, 1000 Hz, 2000 Hz, and 4000 Hz.
        - Response is not as robust at click stimulus because the onset is not as sharp.
        - Waveforms show increased variability in morphology and prolonged latencies relative to the click ABR waveform.
        - Latencies may be longer due to stimulating a more apical region of the cochlea.
        - Early waveforms may be harder to identify; however, this is usually not an issue, as the primary diagnostic value when using toneburst stimuli is the presence or absence of wave V.
    - Chirp stimulus
        - An upward sweeping stimulus, where low-frequency components of the stimulus are presented first followed by high frequencies.
        - Developed in attempt to capture both high- and low-frequency components of the response.
        - Wave V is generated at approximately the same time for each frequency range, creating a "summed" response that reflects activity from the entire cochlea.
        - Both broadband and toneburst chirp stimuli—called chirp octave bands—have been developed.
        - The peak-equivalent SPL for chirp stimuli is about the same as the click, and for toneburst stimuli, thus threshold measures obtained with a chirp stimulus are the same as with a traditional toneburst/click stimulus.
        - Larger amplitude is noted compared to the click and toneburst stimulus response due to more widespread activity in the cochlea.

- Stimulus polarity
  - Indicates the direction of the initial displacement of the transduced diaphragm upon stimulus presentation—inward or outward.
  - The inward/outward movement of the traduced diaphragm directs the physiologic response of the cochlea in specific ways, evident in the cochlear microphonic response.
  - Types of stimulus polarity: rarefaction, condensation, and alternating.
    - ◊ Rarefaction stimulus: generated slightly shorter latency and higher amplitude for early ABR wave components relative to condensation stimulus.
    - ◊ Alternating stimulus polarity eliminates any components of the response that are being generated by cochlear mechanics, such as the CM, rather than a neural response.
  - Polarity-related effects of waveform can identify presence or absence of auditory neuropathy spectrum disorder (ANSD) or other auditory desynchrony disorders.

- Predictable change in waveform characteristics, in addition to patient history provides diagnostically significant information about the type of hearing loss.
  - ABR characteristics of conductive hearing loss
    - Prolonged absolute latencies of all waves, with normal interwave latencies
    - Present wave V, within normal limits in response to bone conduction stimuli
  - ABR characteristics of sensory (cochlear) hearing loss
    - As a result of cochlear recruitment, wave V will still fall into normal range, or close to it, at high intensity levels.
    - As intensity of stimulus is reduced, wave V amplitude is prolonged.
    - Depending on severity of the hearing loss, wave I may be absent or present with prolonged latency.
    - Wave I-V interwave latency could be slightly shorter than normal because of prolonged wave I latency.
    - Absent wave V, or only present at elevated presentation levels in response to bone conduction stimuli.

Clinical Application of ABR

- Neurodiagnostic ABRs:
  - Evaluates the integrity of the auditory neural pathways as a diagnostic tool used primarily to indicate auditory nerve and brain stem lesions.
  - Used to identify pathologies affecting cranial nerve VIII and/or other locations along the auditory pathway through the lower brain stem and contribute to the differential diagnosis in cases of retrocochlear lesions and neurological conditions such as multiple sclerosis.
  - Clinical indications for neurodiagnostic ABR include:
    - Asymmetric SNHL
    - Abnormal/absent acoustic reflexes
    - Abnormally poor word recognition
    - Known neurological conditions/disease
    - Unilateral tinnitus/aural fullness
    - Sudden SNHL
    - Dizziness/vertigo
    - Neurofibromatosis type II
  - The stimulus used for a neurodiagnostic ABR is typically a high-intensity Click stimulus.
  - The presence of high-frequency SNHL will affect the ABR waveform, and hearing thresholds should be considered in ABR interpretation. If hearing loss at 4000 Hz

exceeds 70 dB HL, there is a greater likelihood that you will not be able to obtain clear and replicable ABR waveforms.
- ABR interpretation is based on
  1. Absolute latencies of wave I, III, and V
  2. Interpeak latencies of waves I-III, waves III-V, and waves I-V
  3. Interaural wave V latency differences
     - If hearing loss is present, a correction formula, to subtract 0.1 ms from the measured wave V absolute latency for each 10 dB HL of hearing loss above 50 dB HL at 4000 Hz.
     - A significant interaural wave V latency difference is greater than 0.4 ms OR greater than 0.3 ms if applying hearing loss correction formula.
- In general, retrocochlear lesions could result in:
  - Prolongation of absolute wave latencies
  - Prolongation of interwave latency intervals
  - Degradation of waveform morphology, and/or absence of waves, particularly the later waves
- Lesion size and location will affect the degree to which the waveform is altered.
- The most sensitive index for tumor identification was a combination of abnormal wave V interaural latency differences and abnormally prolonged wave I-V interwave interval.
- In cases of demyelinating conditions such as multiple sclerosis, prolonged wave III-V and reduced wave V amplitude may be seen.
- Severe brain stem involvement, such as with stroke, trauma, or congenital defect, can result in the absence of later waves with intact wave I.
- Limitations of neurodiagnostic ABR:
  - The ABR is most sensitive to tumors greater than or equal to 2 cm. Depending on the size and location of a tumor, it is possible to have a normal ABR response.
  - In cases of sensorineural hearing loss, it may not be possible to determine if abnormal waveform morphology is due to a true extracochlear pathology or cochlear hearing loss.

• Threshold ABRs:
  - Used to infer auditory sensitivity in individuals when behavioral testing cannot be reliably performed.
    - That is, infants, difficult-to-test children, patients with developmental disabilities, and cases of inorganic hearing loss
  - Auditory thresholds can be estimated from the lowest intensity level where wave V is present and replicable.
  - Waveform latency information from air conduction ABR and results from bone-conduction ABR can provide insight into the nature of the hearing loss.
  - To obtain an accurate, clear, and repeatable result free of artifact, the patient must be in a natural sleep state or under sedation.
  - Click threshold
    - Click stimuli are generally used during threshold ABR procedures to assess overall integrity of the auditory system, as it is not frequency specific.
    - Finding a click threshold is sometimes completed to satisfy newborn hearing screening requirements. This can be manually completed by an audiologist, or an automated version of the click ABR can be completed by a newborn hearing screening technician. It is important to note an automated ABR (AABR) simply gives a pass/fail result and does not truly find threshold of the response. Further diagnostic testing is indicated when a failed response is noted.

    - A rarefaction click stimuli and condensation click stimuli should both be completed at higher intensities to distinguish between **cochlear microphonic (CM)** and true neural response.
        - ◊ CM is not a neural response; it is an immediate response generated from the cochlear outer hair cells.
        - ◊ CM latency is roughly 0.2 to 0.4 ms.
        - ◊ CM waveform response mimics the duration and waveform characteristics of the stimulus.
    - Inversion of the ABR waveform in response to a change in stimulus polarity indicates that the generator site is cochlear rather than neural. The presence of a CM with no neural-based waveform components is consistent with ANSD and/or CN VIII deficiencies.
    - It is important to distinguish between stimulus artifact and noise versus a cochlear microphonic when an inversion is noted. To do this, a recording is completed with a "pinched tube" to eliminate or drastically reduce the sound reaching the cochlea, without eliminating any potential artifact from the stimulus. A "pinched tube" waveform should be essentially flat, suggesting the previous response is truly the CM.
    - If waveform inversion is observed, the degree of hearing loss, if any, cannot be determined with an ABR regardless of what stimuli are used.
- ○ Air conduction toneburst
    - Frequency-specific threshold estimation of air conduction thresholds can be obtained using toneburst stimuli presented through insert earphones.
    - The primary waveform component identified is wave V.
    - Wave V latency should increase and amplitude should decrease as intensity is decreased.
    - Wave V latency is increased for lower frequency stimulus.
- ○ Bone conduction thresholds
    - Similar to pure-tone testing, type of hearing loss can be determined with ABR through the use of bone conduction stimuli.
    - Bone conduction results, however, are slightly different from air conduction results, both with click and toneburst stimuli.
    - Due to the limitations of the bone oscillator, the frequency range of a bone conduction click stimulus is thought to be in the range of 1000 to 2000 Hz which is lower compared to air conduction click stimuli.
    - Wave V latency in bone conduction responses may be slightly prolonged compared to air conduction Click due to the frequency range and stimulation of more apical region of the cochlea.
    - Bone conduction response will be less synchronous and therefore result in overall poorer waveform morphology.
    - To better reduce artifacts, alternating stimulus polarity should be used in bone conduction ABRs.
- ○ Once a threshold is determined, obtained value must be converted into the estimated hearing level (eHL).
    - Correction factors used to determine eHL vary from each clinic and for each evoked potential system.
- ○ Patient factors can influence the ABR response.
    - Age
        - ◊ Wave morphology and latencies are different in infants compared to older children and adults.

- ◊ ABR response typically matures by 18 months of age; however, corrected age should be considered in infants with history of prematurity.
- Gender
  - ◊ Females have slightly shorter latencies and larger amplitudes than males.
  - ◊ Females may also have slightly shorter interwave latencies.
- Body temperature
  - ◊ Both low temperature and high temperature can impact wave latencies and should be considered in the interpretation of wave I-V interpeak latencies for very ill patients.
- Muscle artifact
  - ◊ Excessive muscle movement can introduce artifact into the ABR waveform and obscure the morphology.
  - ◊ This is why patients must be in a natural sleep or sedated state for best results; however, if patients are able to lay still and relaxed for the duration of the testing, a full sleep state is not required.
- Medications
  - ◊ ABR is not generally affected by sedatives, muscle relaxants, or anesthetics.
  - ◊ Acute alcohol ingestion and prolonged alcohol abuse can increase wave latencies. Alcohol withdrawal may also increase wave amplitude.

Auditory Steady State Response (ASSR)

- Response uses a continuous (steady-state) frequency-specific, pure tone stimulus that activates the cochlea and CNS.
- It is generated by a mixture of amplitude modulation and rapid modulation of carrier frequencies (CF) of 500, 1000, 2000, and 4000 Hz.
- An automated algorithm specific to the AEP system being utilized is used to analyze the response.
- ASSR is used clinically to estimate frequency-specific hearing levels.
- Similar to ABR testing, ASSR requires patient to be in a natural sleep or sedated state.
- Advantages of ASSR
  - ASSR can estimate severe to profound hearing loss levels that cannot be obtained with ABR.
  - ASSR is an automated analysis, reducing the potential for clinician-related error.
  - ASSR is generally faster than ABR as multiple responses can be obtained simultaneously.
- Disadvantages of ASSR
  - Not as reliable as ABR, as ASSR may produce an artifactual response.
  - Limited information on anatomical site of lesion is provided with ASSR.
  - Difficult to obtain bone conduction responses with ASSR.
  - ASSR is unable to distinguish between cochlear hearing loss and ANSD.

Middle latency response (MLR)

- An early cortical potential generated from the thalamus, primary auditory cortex.
- MLR response has a 10 to 50 ms latency.
- MLR requires less neural synchrony compared to the ABR.
- Components of the MLR waveform include:
  - Na = the first large negative deflection (troth) following wave V of the ABR response
  - Pa = the first positive deflection (peak) following the wave V of the ABR
  - Nb = the second negative deflection (troth)
  - Pb = the second positive deflection (peak)

- Clinical Applications:
  - Evaluation of the auditory pathway above the brain stem.
  - Assess degree of dyssynchrony in auditory neuropathy.
  - Evaluate for nonorganic hearing loss.
  - Identify central auditory processing disorders (CAPDs).
  - Localize lesions at the thalamocortical and primary auditory cortex.
  - Approximate frequency-specific auditory sensitivity up to the cortical level.
  - Evaluate effectiveness of electrical stimulation for cochlear implants.
- Affected by age, sedation, and alertness of patient.
- In cases of CAPD, a prolonged Na latency and a smaller Na-Pa amplitude may be noticed.

P300

- A cortical processing potential generated from primary auditory and association cortex.
- Uses an oddball paradigm, meaning one stimulus is continually presented frequently while a second, distinct stimulus is presented infrequently.
- Response is influenced by patient attention and arousal state.
- Used to assess central processing disorders and cognitive status.
- Not commonly used in a clinical setting.

Auditory Late Response (ALR)

- A cortical potential generated from primary auditory and association cortex.
- The latency of this response is 80 to 300 ms.

Mismatch negativity

- A cortical processing potential believed to be generated from the primary auditory cortex
- Uses oddball paradigm to elicit a response

Electroneuronography (ENOG)

- A noninvasive, objective measure of facial nerve function.
- In this test, the brachial motor component of the facial nerve is electronically stimulated causing the nerve to respond farther along the pathway.
- ENOG provides information about the nerve integrity and the extent of damage that has occurred in instances of injury or infection affecting the facial nerve.
- ENOG could be affected by the process of Wallerian degeneration and, therefore, should not be scheduled within 72 hours of injury occurrence. If completed too soon, results may yield false-negative findings.
- Interpretation of the ENOG is based on a comparison of the affected side versus the unaffected side.
- The primary wave components are the N1, P1, and N2.
  - P1 typically occurs between 5 and 8 ms after stimulation.
- The main diagnostic measure of the ENOG response is the P1-N2 interpeak amplitude.
- Using the P1-N2 interpeak amplitude, a percent denervation is calculated, which indicates the percentage of neural fibers on the impaired side that are not responding. This measure can be used to predict patient recovery and to direct medical intervention.
- $\%\ \text{denervation} = 100 - |\text{amplitude}_{\text{impaired}}/\text{amplitude}_{\text{normal}}| \times 100$

- General prognostic guidelines are as follows:
  - 50% to 70% denervation = very good
  - 71% to 90% denervation = good
  - 91% to 98% denervation = less than satisfactory
  - > 98% denervation = poor
- Serial testing every 3 to 5 days for 21 days should be completed to assess for nerve regeneration over time.

Table 13-6 Classification of Auditory Evoked Potentials Auditory Electrophysiology: A Clinical Guide by Atcherson & Stoody

Common Name	*Latency Range (msec)*	*Analysis Method*	*Physiologic Description*	*Anatomical Generator*	*Stimulus Response*	*Exogenous or Endogenous*
ECochG	0-2	Time	Neurogenic	Hair cells, auditory nerve	Steady state, transient	Exogenous
ABR	1-10	Time	Neurogenic	Auditory nerve, brainstem	Transient	Exogenous
FFR	N/A	Time, frequency	Neurogenic	Brainstem	Steady state	Exogenous
MLR	15-35	Time	Neurogenic	Cortical	Transient	Exogenous
LAEP (LLR)	50-250	Time	Neurogenic	Cortical	Transient	Primarily exogenous
MMN	150-300	Time	Neurogenic	Cortical	Transient	Primarily exogenous
P300	250-400	Time	Neurogenic	Cortical	Transient	Primarily exogenous
N400	350-500	Time	Neurogenic	Cortical	Steady state	Exogenous
ASSR	10-30	Frequency, phase	Neurogenic	Brainstem, subcortical, cortical	Steady State	Primarily exogenous
VEMP	12-27	Time	Myogenic	Vestibulocolic reflex	Transient	Exogenous

Evaluation of Difficult-to-Test and Pediatric Patients

Behavioral Testing

- Generally preferable to physiologic procedures alone because behavioral approaches test hearing

Physiologic Measures

- Testing some aspect of auditory function.
- Necessary when behavioral testing cannot be completed or when patient age does not allow for behavioral testing.
- Behavioral and physiologic testing in combination follows the cross-check principle (objective and subjective information).

Behavioral Techniques Recommended method depends on the neurodevelopmental age of the patient.

Behavioral Observation Audiometry

- Reliance on *behavioral observation audiometry* (BOA) should be minimal because the response obtained typically is suprathreshold.
  - Intra- and intersubject variability is high and reliability is poor.
- Not the gold standard for obtaining information about hearing sensitivity.
- Cessation of sucking (pacifier, breastfeeding, bottle feeding) has been shown to be more reliable than other behaviors in terms of a "response."
- Should be utilized as a last resort when other methods are not appropriate and not used in isolation to determine hearing sensitivity.
- Attempted on patients who are unable to be operantly conditioned to provide reliable responses to sound.
- Utilized for patients who are neurodevelopmentally 6 months of age or younger.

Test Set-up/Conditions

- Patient in center of sound booth.
- Do not provide visual or somatosensory cues as sound is being presented.
- **Stimulus:** Speech, warbled tones, or pediatric noise are presented into the sound field through loudspeakers or through earphones.
- **Responses**: Eye widening, pause in activity, and/or (subtle) head turn toward the side of the sound.
- Intensity of the signals is varied until search of response to the lowest level stimuli is obtained.
- Typically, the minimal response level (MRL) to sounds obtained with BOA is higher than true auditory threshold.

Visual Reinforcement Audiometry (VRA):

- Utilized for patients who are neurodevelopmentally 6 to 30 months of age and have adequate physical strength and control of head movement.

Test Set-up/Conditions

- Patient in center of sound booth
- Do not provide visual or somatosensory cues as sound is being presented
- **Stimulus:** Speech, warbled tones, or pediatric noise are presented into the sound field through loudspeakers or through earphones
  - Ultimately, tonal frequencies (warbled tones or pediatric noise) are preferable to broadband signals (speech or narrowband noise) because a broadband signal could miss a loss in part of the frequency range
- **Transducers:** Insert earphones, supra-aural headphones, speakers
  - *Insert earphones* are preferred.
  - *Supra-aural headphones* can cause collapsing ear canals and restrict head turns, but can be used if inserts are not tolerated.
  - *Speakers* may be used if the infant or child will not tolerate earphones but will not yield ear-specific information.
    - 1 or 2 speaker set up can be utilized; 2 speaker set up is preferred.

Procedure

- Patient is operantly conditioned to turn his/her head to look at a toy/video when a sound is presented.
  - Clinician initially trains the patient by pairing sounds with reinforcers until sound alone elicits patient response.

  - When the child turns his/her head in response to a sound, the toy will become animated, or a video clip will play to reinforce the response.
  - After a few trials, reinforcement converts the reflexive action into a conditioned response.
- Intensity of the signals is varied until lowest consistent conditioned response level is obtained. Normative data are given in Table 13-7.

Conditioned Play Audiometry (CPA):

- Utilized for patients who are neurodevelopmentally 30 months of age or older
  - At this age, most children can be conditioned to make a voluntary response through a game.
- **Transducers:** Insert earphones, supra-aural headphones, bone oscillator, speakers (in rare circumstances)
  - At this age, most children will have tolerance for ear-specific transducers.
  - On the occasion that the child has the appropriate developmental capacity for CPA but does not tolerate ear-specific transducers, this test could be completed in the sound field with speakers (non-ear specific).

PROCEDURE

- Listening game where each time a tone is presented, the child responds by playing the game, for example, dropping blocks in a bucket.
  - Second tester or assistant can be used to assist in the game.
  - Child must be conditioned at suprathreshold levels prior to testing to ensure they can reliably complete the task.

Table 13-7 Normative Data and Expected Response Levels for Infants[a]

Age	*Noisemakers (~SPL)*	*Warbled Pure Tones (dB HL)*	*Speech (dB HL)*	*Expected Response*	*Startle to Speech (dB HL)*
0-6 wk	50-70	75	40-60	Eye widening, eye blink, stirring or arousal from sleep, startle	65
6 wk-4 mo	50-60	70	45	Eye widening, eye shift, eye blinking, quieting; beginning rudimentary head turn by 4 mo	65
4-7 mo	40-50	50	20	Head turn on lateral plane toward sound; listening attitude	65
7-9 mo	30-40	45	15	Direct localization of sounds to side, indirectly below ear level	65
9-13 mo	25-35	38	10	Direct localization of sounds to side, directly below ear level, indirectly above ear level	65
13-16 mo	30-25	30	5	Direct localization of sound on side, above and below	65
16-21 mo	25	25	5	Direct localization of sound on side, above, and below	65
21-24 mo	25	25	5	Direct localization of sound on side, above, and below	65

[a]Testing done in a sound room.
Data from Northern J, Downs M. *Hearing in Children*. 5th ed. Hagerstown, MD: Lippincott-Raven; 2002.

- The game activity itself is the reinforcer.
- Intensity of the various signals is varied until lowest repeatable response level is obtained.

Speech Audiometry

- For prelingual infants/children, a SAT or SDT may be obtained to speech stimuli.
- SRT may be obtained by using spondee picture cards or objects (eg, an airplane or toothbrush) for responses (pointing) or by conventional methods (verbal repetition).
- Word recognition may be tested using a standardized picture-pointing task until the child is old enough to repeat words clearly.

Physiologic Techniques

Immittance Measures (Tympanometry/Acoustic Reflexes) Child must be somewhat compliant as these measures are impacted by vocalizations/physical movements making results uninterpretable.

- Generally completed with a 226 Hz probe tone.
- 1000 Hz probe tone is recommended for 6 months of age and younger as it is more sensitive to middle ear changes and produces more valid results.
- **Gross Impressions Based on Immittance Measures:**
    - **Note:** Gross impressions of hearing can be made, but NOT diagnosis of hearing loss in isolation.
    - **Tympanograms:** Flat tympanograms can suggest slight to moderate conductive hearing loss but provides no information on sensorineural status.
    - **Acoustic reflexes:** Can be present at elevated levels with conductive hearing loss, but absent reflexes can be suggestive of severe to profound hearing loss or a central pathology
        - Caveats: Auditory neuropathy spectrum disorder (ANSD)/retro-cochlear pathologies

Auditory Brain Stem Response (ABR) or Auditory Steady State Response (ASSR)

- Electrophysiologic assessment tools like ABR or ASSR help estimate hearing sensitivity.
    - Typically, in the range of 500 to 4000 Hz, when frequency-specific stimuli (tone-bursts) are utilized.
    - Click stimuli are not frequency specific but sometimes utilized as a rough estimate of threshold in the 2000 to 4000 Hz frequency range.
    - ABR can be performed by bone conduction, if air conduction results are abnormal to determine presence of conductive hearing loss.
- Complicated by need for sedation/anesthesia in older infants and toddlers, or any patient who cannot remain still and quiet during testing

Otoacoustic Emissions (OAEs)

- Presence of TEOAEs ensures that cochlear hearing could not be worse than a mild hearing loss.
- DPOAEs can sometimes be recorded/have measurable amplitudes in the presence of even moderate to severe hearing loss depending on stimulus levels.
    - However, note that a present amplitude alone is not sufficient for assuming a present/acceptable response.
        - Responses must meet amplitude and signal-to-noise ratio criteria.
- Requires substantially less time than ABR/ASSR.
- OAE testing requires that the patient be relatively still and quiet for a short duration.

- A common limitation in children is presence of a middle-ear disorder, which usually precludes recording any type of OAE.
  - OAEs can be present in cases of negative middle ear pressure but are most often absent in the presence of middle ear fluid/flat tympanograms.
- In rare cases, persons may have hearing loss on behavioral testing, normal middle ear function, abnormal ABR, but normal OAEs; these findings may indicate auditory neuropathy/dyssynchrony.

History Interview The following should be addressed for children/infants:

- Detailed birth history
  - Gestational age, NICU stay (ie, mechanical ventilation, IV antibiotics, jaundice)
- Medical history
  - Related medical conditions (ie, cytomegalovirus [CMV]), history of recurrent OME, diagnosed neurodevelopmental disorders
- Speech and language development
  - Is the child meeting auditory, expressive language, receptive language, and motor milestones?
- Does the child respond similarly to age-matched peers?
  - Is communication development like their age-matched peers?
- Family history of pediatric hearing loss
  - Genetic-linked hearing loss (congenital versus progressive onset)

Identification of Infant Hearing Impairment

- Early hearing loss detection and intervention (EHDI) in infants is crucial.
  - Children with late-identified hearing loss show deficits in the following areas:
    - Communicative, cognitive, and socio-emotional developmental
    - Lower educational and occupational levels later in life
- An EHDI program includes universal neonatal hearing screening (UNHS), particularly valuable because nearly 50% of congenital hearing losses have no associated risk indicator (many presumably recessive traits) (Table 13-7).
- EHDI programs target congenital permanent hearing loss in one or both ears.
  - Some monitor infants at risk for late-onset hearing loss, as recommended by the Joint Committee on Infant Hearing (JCIH).
- In 2007 (upheld in 2019 update), the JCIH endorsed these principles for an EHDI program:
- All neonates have hearing screening via a physiologic measure (ABR and/or OAE) during their birth admission, and if not possible, then before 1 month of age.
  - Either technology is acceptable for well babies.
  - Only ABR should be used in screening of infants in the NICU.
- For those who do not pass the birth admission screen or subsequent rescreenings (either before discharge or as outpatients), appropriate audiologic and medical evaluations to confirm the presence of hearing loss should be in progress before 3 months of age.
- Infants with confirmed permanent hearing impairment must receive intervention services before 6 months of age.
- All infants who pass newborn screening but who have a risk indicator (see Table 13-8) for hearing loss, or communicative delays should have ongoing audiologic and medical surveillance and monitoring.
  - Including indicators associated with late-onset, progressive, or fluctuating hearing loss or auditory neural dysfunctions.
- These items make up the 1-month (screening)-3 (diagnosis)-6 (intervention) guideline.
  - 2019 position statement called for a potential shift to a 1-2-3 guideline to promote even earlier intervention for this population.

Table 13-8 Risk Indicators Associated With Permanent Congenital, Delayed-Onset, or Progressive Hearing Loss in Childhood

1. §Caregiver concern regarding hearing, speech, language, or developmental delay.
2. §Family history of permanent childhood hearing loss.
3. Neonatal intensive care of > 5 d or any of the following regardless of length of stay: ECMO, §assisted ventilation, exposure to ototoxic medications (gentamycin and tobramycin) or loop diuretics (furosemide/Lasix), and hyperbilirubinemia that requires exchange transfusion.
4. §In utero infections, such as CMV, herpes, rubella, syphilis, and toxoplasmosis.
5. Craniofacial anomalies, including those that involve the pinna, ear canal, ear tags, ear pits, and temporal bone anomalies.
6. Physical findings, such as white forelock, that are associated with a syndrome known to include a sensorineural or permanent conductive hearing loss.
7. §Syndromes associated with hearing loss or progressive or late-onset hearing loss, such as neurofibromatosis, osteopetrosis, and Usher syndrome; other frequently identified syndromes include Waardenburg, Alport, Pendred, and Jervell and Lange-Nielson syndromes.
8. §Neurodegenerative disorders, such as Hunter syndrome, or sensory motor neuropathies, such as Friedreich ataxia and Charcot-Marie-Tooth syndrome.
9. Culture-positive postnatal infections associated with sensorineural hearing loss, §including confirmed bacterial and viral (especially herpes viruses and varicella) meningitis.
10. Head trauma, especially basal skull/temporal bone fracture§ that requires hospitalization.
11. §Chemotherapy.

Risk indicators marked with a "§" are of greater concern for delayed-onset hearing loss.
Data from Joint Committee on Infant Hearing, 2007.

Pseudohypacusis

- Pseudohypacusis = false or exaggerated hearing loss (FEHL)
  - Hearing behaviors discrepant with audiologic test results, inconsistent/invalid test results, or an alleged loss of hearing sensitivity in the absence of organic pathology
- "Functional" and "nonorganic" hearing loss are not synonymous with pseudohypacusis.
  - When these terms are applied to hearing, they mean that there is no problem with the hearing system or that the deficit is not as great as presented.
- As with other diagnostic questions, a battery approach is advisable.
- Pseudohypacusis can be deliberate, unintentional, or a mix of both; the difference is difficult to know because those are states of mind.
  - Psychological labels, such as malingering/conversion disorder, as well as a judgmental posture, should be avoided.
- FEHL is twice as common in children as in adults, and, among children, twice as prevalent in females as in males.
  - The typical age in children is 11 years.
- A FEHL should not be dismissed lightly, particularly in children, because it is often associated with a psychosocial disorder and may require prompt intervention.
- Signs of possible pseudohypacusis are as follows:
  - *Pretest interview*: Patient seems to have no difficulty understanding but presents a moderate, bilateral hearing loss during testing.

- *Referral source*: A compensation case; eligibility determination for goods or services.
- *Patient history*: Patient can name a specific incident that caused the hearing loss and stands to gain in some way as a result, for example, money, avoidance of some burdensome duty or task, or excuse for poor performance.

- Performance on routine tests:
  - Characteristic behaviors
    - Leaning or cocking the head to the side of the signal
    - Straining, looking confused or wondering, especially upon signal presentation
    - Half-word responses during the SRT ("ear" for "eardrum")
    - Responding during speech audiometry with a questioning intonation as if uncertain
  - Test–retest reliability worse than 5 dB:
    - Inattentiveness on the part of the patient must first be ruled out, and reinstruction and retesting may be necessary.
    - Factors affecting attention can be pain, mental confusion, advanced age, or other substantial psychomotor limitations.
  - Disparity between the PTA and the SRT greater than 10 dB is one of the most common inconsistencies.
    - Agreement of the two measures should be within 10 dB.
    - However, SRT–PTA disagreement due to audiogram configuration must be ruled out.
      - ◊ With rising or sloping patterns, the two-frequency average (the average of the two best/lowest thresholds of 500, 1000, and 2000 Hz) may better agree with the SRT.
    - An invalidly elevated SRT may be detected by obtaining a word recognition score at or near the voluntary SRT (eg, SRT + 10 dB).
      - ◊ If a good word recognition score is obtained at threshold, the SRT was invalid.
    - Presence of acoustic reflexes with audiometric air–bone gaps.
  - In unilateral or asymmetrical hearing losses:
    - A difference greater than 65 dB between test ear and nontest ear unmasked results or absence of response (unmasked) in the poorer ear.
    - In air conduction testing, cross-hearing (crossover) should occur at no more than about 65 dB (may be 75 dB for insert earphones) above opposite-ear bone conduction thresholds.
    - Bone conduction testing
      - ◊ No air–bone gap in the worse ear even without masking the better ear, because cross-hearing should occur at no worse than 10 dB above opposite-ear bone conduction thresholds.

Physiologic Tests for Pseudohypacusis

Acoustic Reflex Testing The presence of the acoustic reflex at 5 dB or less above voluntary auditory thresholds strongly suggests some degree of pseudohypacusis (see Immittance Measures under Evaluation of Difficult-to-Test and Pediatric Patients).

Otoacoustic Emissions OAEs can be very helpful by providing objective information about cochlear function

- The presence of TEOAEs indicates that cochlear hearing could not be worse than approximately 30- to 40-dB HL for each octave band response present.
- DPOAEs can help determine probable audiometric configuration including higher-frequency information.

Auditory Brain Stem or Auditory Steady State Response

- Objective and can estimate hearing sensitivity
- Time-consuming and not always as readily available as other tests

Counseling

- Gentle approach is advisable such as "These tests suggest that maybe I didn't make it clear to you that you had to respond even if you barely heard the sound rather than when it was easy to hear. Let's try that test again."

Behavioral Tests for Pseudohypacusis

Stenger Test

- Excellent test for unilateral or asymmetrical hearing losses in which the difference between ears is at least 30 dB.
- When two tones of the same frequency are presented simultaneously to both ears, the patient will perceive the tone only in the ear in which the tone is louder.
- Performing the Pure Tone Stenger test:
    - Simultaneously present a tone 5 dB above threshold to the good ear and an identical tone 5 dB below the voluntary threshold to the poor ear.
    - If the patient responds, the test is negative because the patient heard the tone in the good ear. If the patient does not respond, the test is positive (for nonorganic hearing loss).
- Speech Stenger may be performed in the same manner using spondee (SRT) words in place of pure tones

Ototoxicity Monitoring

- For patients receiving ototoxic medications (eg, cisplatin, long-term aminoglycosides):
    - High-frequency audiometry, generally for stimuli 10,000 to 20,000 Hz is performed along with pure-tone audiometry in the conventional frequency range.
- Detecting threshold changes in the high-frequency threshold range provides the physician the opportunity to change the medication protocol.
    - If protocol cannot be changed, the audiologist can work with the patient on communication strategies/fit amplification as the hearing loss progresses.
- Significant ototoxic change is either:
    (1) a threshold shift of 20 dB or greater at any one test frequency
    (2) threshold shifts of 10 dB or greater at any two adjacent frequencies, or
    (3) loss of response at any three consecutive frequencies where thresholds were previously obtained.
- Utilize immittance measures (tympanometry) to rule out changes in middle ear status and their effect on hearing sensitivity.
- OAEs may also help detect early ototoxic changes, but no standardized significant change criteria have been established.
    - Reduction in OAE amplitudes can sometimes be seen before threshold shifts are seen with standard.
- Ototoxicity monitoring may include a variety of considerations:
    - Patient age, baseline hearing status, general health status, specific drug and dosing employed, concomitant medications, treatment schedule, and kidney and liver function.

Central Auditory Processing/Auditory Processing Disorders

- Auditory processing is the active, complex set of operations performed by the auditory nervous system on auditory inputs.
  - Auditory processing is not only central; auditory signals are acted upon throughout the auditory system.
    - Including the peripheral portion from the outer ear through the cochlea and eighth nerve
  - **Peripheral hearing loss must be ruled out before evaluating for CAPD/APD**
- Central auditory processing disorder (CAPD)/auditory processing disorder (APD) is suspected when:
  - Individual has greater difficulty understanding speech in quiet or noise than would be expected from hearing sensitivity.
  - Individual has difficulty processing auditory signals that cannot be explained by peripheral hearing results.
- Some behaviors typical of persons, especially children, who have CAPD/APD:
  - Frequently misunderstanding or misinterpreting what is said
  - Attention deficiency
  - Difficulty discriminating among speech sounds leading to reading, spelling, and other academic problems
  - Unusual difficulty in background noise
  - Reduced auditory memory
  - Reduced receptive and expressive language skills
  - General difficulty learning through the *auditory* channel
- Additional procedures
  - Ipsilateral and contralateral acoustic reflexes and ABR, which help to assess the integrity of the brain stem
  - CAP/APD test battery:
    - Tests administered depend on a test's efficacy for the patient's symptomatology and age.
    - CAP tests are presented monotonically (stimulation of one ear at a time) or dichotically (stimulation of both ears by different stimuli).
    - Tests are designed to make demands on the auditory system:
      - ◊ Understanding degraded speech (filtered; time-altered; competing speech or noise presented ipsilaterally, contralaterally, or binaurally; part of the signal to one ear and another to the opposite ear)
- If a CAP disorder is found, management should be based on the pattern of results from the test battery, and may include:
  - Optimizing the auditory experience
    - Increasing signal-to-noise ratio (signal well above noise)
    - Good acoustic environment (low noise and reverberation)
    - Enhanced speech input (strong, clear, and somewhat slowed)
  - Treatment
    - Assistive listening devices (FM, infrared), which provide good signal versus noise characteristics (see "Assistive Devices")
    - Auditory therapy
    - Low-gain traditional amplification

Noise-Induced Hearing Loss (NIHL) and Industrial Audiology

- Exposure to excessively strong sounds may destroy auditory cells, resulting in hearing loss.
  - Described as "noise-induced," but any sound—noise, speech, music—of sufficient intensity can damage hearing.
- Hazardous noise exposure can be occupational and/or recreational.
- Typically, hearing loss begins in a notch pattern in the 3000- to 6000-Hz region.
  - With repeated exposure broadens to the other frequency regions giving a shallower notch
- A sign of early damage in hunters/shooters is an asymmetrical 4000-Hz notch loss.
  - Often worse in the ear opposite the shoulder from which the gun is fired.
- Classification of NIHL
  - Temporary threshold shift (TTS)
  - Permanent threshold shift (PTS)
  - Acoustic trauma resulting from one or relatively few exposures to a very high sound level, such as an explosion
- Four factors contribute to the effects of noise:
  - Sound level (in dB SPL)
  - Spectral composition
  - Time distribution of the exposure during a working day
  - Cumulative noise exposure over days, weeks, or years
- Occupational noise exposure
  - The United States Occupational Safety and Health Administration (OSHA) has established guidelines for permissible noise exposure levels for a working day, assuming constant, steady-state noise and a 20-year work life (Table 13-9).
  - Since occupational noise is not always constant, a time-weighted average takes into account both level and duration, and that average is a level that, if constant for an 8-hour day, would have the same effect as the measured dose.
  - Hearing conservation program has four main components:
    - Assess the level and cumulative dose of noise exposure in a given setting using a sound level meter and dosimeter.
    - Control the amount of overexposure in a given setting by reducing the amount of noise created by the source, reducing the amount of noise reaching an individual's ears by constructing barriers, or by changing job procedures or schedule.

Table 13-9 OSHA Permissible Noise Exposures

Duration (h/d)	*SPL (on dBA scale, slow response)*
8	90
6	92
4	95
2	100
1	105
0.5	110
≤ 0.25	115

Reproduced with permission from United States Department of Labor, Occupational Safety and Health Administration. 29 CFR. Part 1910.95. Occupational noise exposure, 1981.

- If sound cannot be brought within safe levels, provide ear protection devices and information to motivate their proper use.
- *Monitor hearing*: pre-employment testing with periodic follow-up tests, usually annually.

- Ear protection devices
  - Recommended for both occupational and recreational use
  - Earmuffs, custom-fitted earplugs, or disposable earplugs provide 20 to 40 dB of sound attenuation
  - Effectiveness increases with proper fit
  - Passive (nonelectric): Some passive devices, such as valves, are amplitude sensitive to allow relatively normal hearing
    - They pass moderate sound levels but reduce high sound levels, although not always to a safe level.
    - Typically, does not distort speech, but not 100% effective.
    - Active (electric): Typically limit output to 85-dB SPL
  - To offset the blockage effect of the ear protectors, some units include slight amplification to hear usual conversation and environmental sounds.
  - Can distort speech.
  - Can be effective for specific circumstances where speech understanding is not needed.
- By informing, counseling, and motivating persons to protect their hearing, audiologists and otolaryngologists can make an enormous impact on preventing hearing impairment.

Management of Permanent Hearing Loss

Ways to assist persons with permanent hearing loss:

- Providing high-quality and appropriately fit amplification
- Maximizing auditory skills
- Enhancing use of visual cues
- Counseling on realistic expectations and appropriate education
- The goal is to have the individual function to the best of their abilities and be a full, productive, independent, well-adjusted member of society

Hearing Aids

- ***Function:*** Hearing aids amplify sound to make speech more audible to enable an individual to communicate more effectively.
- Basic terms of hearing aid function:
  - *Frequency response range*: The range of useful amplification across frequency
  - *Gain:* Amplification or the acoustic energy added to input sound (the difference between the input and output)
  - *Maximum power output*: The highest sound level a hearing instrument can produce
- ***Components:*** All hearing instruments have a microphone (typically multiple), an amplifier, and an output receiver powered by a battery.
- ***Styles:*** Behind-the-ear (BTE), receiver-in-the-canal (RIC), in-the-ear (ITE), in the canal (ITC), and completely in canal (CIC) aids.
  - The larger the instrument, the greater the array of circuit capabilities that can be incorporated

- ***General output limiting strategies***
  - *Peak clipping*: constant gain until the hearing aid's maximum power output is reached, above which the amplitude peaks are "clipped off."
    - Results in distortion
    - Not utilized in modern-day technology
  - *Compression limiting*: Automatic gain reduction (compression) at a preset level; whether input or output compression, the purpose is to limit the output with less distortion.
  - *Wide dynamic range compression*: gain decreases as input increases over a relatively wide range of sound input
    - Purpose is to compensate for the loss of cochlear OHCs
    - Utilized in all modern-day technology
- ***Digital signal processing***
  - Advantage of digital circuitry is the array of features and capabilities that can be incorporated in a small housing.
    - Gain, frequency response, and MPO, as well as other features, can be programmed according to the individual's audiometric data and preferences.
    - Multiband compression (different gain and output for separate frequency bands) can be used because hearing loss often differs across frequencies.
  - Additional advantages of digital processing include:
    - Great flexibility in setting all parameters, especially helpful for unusual audiometric configurations
    - Robust feedback reduction
    - *Multimemory*: different sets of performance saved in the hearing aid from which the wearer can select for different listening situations
    - *Datalogging*: accumulating information, such as average time per day of usage and percentage of time spent in different acoustic environments

Additional Fitting Considerations

"Open fit" Hearing Aids

- Behind the ear component sits over the pinna, and a thin wire delivers the sound into the ear canal, leaving the canal open.
  - Excellent for high-frequency hearing loss because open fittings amplify just the high frequencies while allowing other sounds to pass into the canal normally without amplification.
  - High risk of feedback (whistling) if the hearing loss is not appropriate for this type of fit.
- Directional microphones to improve signal-to-noise ratio
  - Standard for modern-day technology
  - Requires multiple microphones
- A "telecoil" for telephone listening without feedback whistle
- Direct Bluetooth connectivity
  - Wireless streaming
  - Native apps for patient-led adjustments to sound quality
  - Some have location services for "find my device" features

Bone Conduction Devices

- Used in cases of: unilateral or bilateral atresia, chronic purulent drainage, otitis externa, SSD
- Nonsurgical:
  - Can be worn on the head with a soft band to hold the bone oscillator in place

- Surgical:
  - Output is connected to a metal post-surgically embedded through skin into the skull or attaches to a magnet surgically implanted in the skull.
  - BAHS typically have slightly higher gain than conventional bone conduction hearing aids because of closer mechanical coupling.

Single-sided Deafness/Asymmetric Hearing Loss

- Cochlear implants approved for SSD in 2019 (see Cochlear implant chapter 18).
- Bone Conduction Device (see above)
- CROS (contralateral routing of signal) is for unaidable hearing loss in one ear and good hearing in the other ear
  - Sound on the poor side is picked by a microphone and routed to the good ear.
- BiCROS (bilateral CROS) is for bilateral hearing loss, but one ear is unaidable.
  - CROS system on the unaidable side
  - Conventional aid is on the better side

Tinnitus Masker

- A tinnitus masker has a noise generator in a hearing aid case to drown out the tinnitus.
  - For persons with tinnitus and hearing loss, a hearing aid itself may help mask the tinnitus.

Verification and Validation of Hearing Aid Fitting

Electroacoustic analysis Performance of a hearing aid should be verified in a hearing aid test box to ensure it is functioning correctly.

Real-Ear Measurements and Prescriptive Fitting

- This is the gold standard for hearing aid fittings.
- Ear canal sizes vary, and thus the performance of a hearing aid in an analyzer chamber (coupler) differs from that in an individual's ear canal.
  - When devices are verified in a test box, real ear coupler difference (RECD) can be utilized to account for the difference between the coupler and the actual ear canal size.
- A probe tube microphone measures sound very close to the tympanic membrane
  - This accounts for the (real ear) effects of the outer ear and canal and the loss of the natural gain produced by the ear canal resonance near 2700 Hz.
- Real-ear instruments include fitting formulas or "prescriptions" of gain and output for achieving maximum audibility of speech without being uncomfortable.
  - The instruments display a formula's target of optimum gain and frequency response for a particular patient's hearing loss.
    - Devices are adjusted to meet formula targets.
  - There are multiple formulas that have minor differences, and no one formula is best for all patients
- Validated questionnaires can also be used pre- and post-fitting to ensure the hearing aids are addressing patient needs.

Cochlear Implants

This topic is covered in Chapter 18.

Assistive Devices

- A hearing-impaired individual's lifestyle may be improved by a variety of assistive devices, whether or not hearing aids are used.
- Assistive listening devices:

  - Telephone amplifiers
  - FM or induction loop (telecoil) systems for large areas, such as classrooms, conference halls, and houses of worship
  - Remote microphones
  - Bluetooth TV connectors
- Visual or vibratory assistive devices:
  - Alarm clocks, smoke detectors, security systems, baby-cry detectors, and doorbells
  - Closed-caption television decoders (TV and recorded or DVD movies)
  - Text telephones (TT, also known as TTD and TTY); persons who cannot use a telephone can type and receive messages via telephone
  - Captioned telephones

Intervention, Training, and Education

- Pediatrics
  - When hearing loss is present before communication is established, early intervention is crucial to take advantage of the "sensitive" period of fastest communication growth from birth to age 3.
  - From 3 to 21 years of age, federal and state mandates require that children have a "free, appropriate education" in the "least restrictive environment."
    - Important to educate families to seek the appropriate accommodations in their educational environments
  - Communicative and educational options overlap and include auditory-oral, visual (sign and finger spelling), or a combination ("total communication").
  - Consider the family's communicative system and desires and presence of other limiting conditions.

- All age groups:
  - Auditory training: provided there is usable hearing, promotes listening skills, such as sound recognition and comprehension
    - Provided individually or in groups
    - Available in person or through online formats
  - Speech reading: integrating another person's lip movements, facial expressions, body gestures, situational cues, and linguistic factors
  - Counseling: give information (facts about communication, hearing loss, hearing aids, etc.) and also address psychosocial issues (acceptance of one's situation, parental guilt and anger, one's self-image, social adjustment, and so on)
  - Vocational guidance: States have agencies that can help with career choices and preparation.

Bibliography

Guidelines for audiometric symbols. Committee on Audiologic Evaluation. American Speech-Language-Hearing Association. *ASHA Suppl.* 1990 Apr;(2):25-23.

Joint Committee on Infant Hearing. Year 2019 Position Statement

Margolis RH, Hunter LI. Acoustic immittance measurements. In: Roeser RJ, Valente M, Hosford-Dunn H, eds. *Audiology Diagnosis*. New York, NY: Thieme; 2000.

Northern JL, Downs MP. *Hearing in Children*. 5th ed. Hagerstown, MD: Lippincott-Raven; 2002.

Roeser R, Buckley KA, Stickney GS. Pure tone tests. In: Roeser RJ, Valente M, Hosford-Dunn H, eds. *Audiology Diagnosis*. New York, NY: Thieme; 2000.

Questions

1. Which of the following is not an auditory evoked potential test?
   A. Auditory steady state response test
   B. Transient otoacoustic emission test
   C. Electrocochleography test
   D. Middle latency response

2. Tympanograms include all of the following *except*:
   A. Static acoustic immittance
   B. Equivalent ear canal volume
   C. Peak
   D. Cochlear microphonic

3. Speech audiometry is useful in which of the following situations?
   A. Cross-check of pure tone results
   B. Assess for retrocochlear pathology
   C. Assist with decision-making for treatment options (Hearing aids, Cochlear implants, etc.)
   D. Identify Pseudohypacusis
   E. All of the above

4. Which of these tests requires voluntary patient responses?
   A. Cortical response tests
   B. Conditioned play audiometry
   C. Auditory brain stem response
   D. Acoustic reflex test

5. All of these factors contribute to the effects of noise *except*:
   A. Cumulative hearing aid use over days, weeks, or years
   B. Sound level (in dB SPL)
   C. Spectral composition
   D. Time distribution of the exposure during a working day

Chapter 14
The Vestibular System and Balance Disorders

Anatomy and Physiology

A. The Osseous labyrinth is housed within the petrous temporal bone and comprises the vestibule, the cochlea, and the semicircular canals (SCCs). Cochlea and saccule constitute the pars anterior. The three SCCs and the utricle constitute pars posterior.
B. The vestibule sits in front of the posterior half of the fundus of the internal auditory canal (IAC).
   i. The ampullary end of the posterior SCC abuts the posterior wall and is the most inferior point in the vestibule.*
   ii. The oval window, the ampullary end of the lateral SCC, and the nonampullary end of the lateral SCC create three openings in the lateral wall.
   iii. Elliptical recess in the vestibule houses the utricle (horizontal orientation).
   iv. Spherical recess in the vestibule houses the saccule (vertical orientation).

**This is why posterior canal BPPV is the most frequently encountered type of BPPV. Check these links for animation videos of a posterior canalithiasis and right and left Epley maneuvers.*
Benign Paroxysmal Positional Vertigo (BPPV) https://www.youtube.com/watch?v=mXmlFPJyvZA BPPV Treatment - Right Epley Maneuver https://www.youtube.com/watch?v=hDP-ACWl7YI BPPV Treatment - Left Epley Maneuver https://www.youtube.com/watch?v=fDXf9M67RBE

A. The SCCs are located in the pars posterior of the labyrinth.
   i. The canals contain perilymph and the semicircular ducts.
   ii. The ampullated ends of the SCC house the sensory epithelium of the semicircular ducts or crista ampullaris.
B. The vestibular aqueduct originates in the vestibule and courses posteriorly toward the sigmoid sinus. It contains the endolymphatic duct and sac. The latter opens on the posterior fossa dura below Donaldson line.
   i. The endolymphatic duct is formed by union of the utricular and saccular ducts.
   ii. The utricular duct has a membranous fold in the medial wall of the utricle. It is called the valve of Bast and is implicated in Ménière's disease pathology according to some hypotheses (see pathogenesis).
C. The cochlear aqueduct originates in scala tympani close to the round window, and then courses posteriorly parallel to the inferior wall of the IAC.

D. Perilymph is postulated to derive from CSF. The electrolyte composition of perilymph is closer to CSF than endolymph.
E. Endolymph is high in potassium and low in sodium concentration.
F. Endolymph is produced at the level of the stria vascularis in the cochlea and can be derived from perilymph through Reissner membrane.
G. Vestibular dark cell, present in the ampullated ends of the semicircular ducts, the utricle, and the common crus maintain homeostasis of the endolymph by using the sodium/ATPase pump to pump potassium into the endolymphatic space. This creates a high positive endolymphatic potential. Several disease states including Ménière's disease can cause degeneration of the dark cells. Gentamicin is selectively toxic to the vestibular dark cells.
H. Endolymph has a radial flow through the cochlea and flows longitudinally into the endolymphatic sac in case of increased pressure. When it supersedes the storage capacity of the sac, hydrops may develop.
I. The endolymphatic sac is the only immunologically active organ of the inner ear. It contains high endothelial veins and fenestrated blood capillaries.
J. The membranous labyrinth contains endolymph and is comprised of the anterior labyrinth, or cochlear duct and ductus reuniens, and saccule and posterior labyrinth, or semicircular ducts and utricle.
K. The vestibular labyrinth consists of the semicircular ducts, the utricle, and the saccule.
L. The semicircular ducts lie eccentrically in the bony semicircular canal. *The membranous dilations called ampullae house the neurosensory epithelium (crista ampullaris).

*During ear surgery, an inadvertent opening of the SCC or a fistula from a cholesteatoma through SCC should be immediately recognized to avoid suctioning the perilymph and eccentric lying semicircular duct.

A. Crista ampullaris contains two types of cells:
   i. Type I broad shape, engulfed in multiple chalyx-like afferents. Their apex contain actin and actinomyosin.
   ii. Type II cylindrical shape with one simple afferent fiber at their base. Their apical pole contains stereocilia and a longer kinocilium.
      a. Cilia project into an amorphous membrane called the cupula.
      b. Movement of the endolymph initiated by movement of the head, causes the cilia to move.
         1. If they bend toward the kinocilium, the cell is depolarized/activated.
         2. If they bend away from it, they are inhibited/ hyperpolarized
         3. The orientation of the stereocilia relative to the kinocilium is different in the horizontal semicircular duct compared to the posterior and superior semicircular canal duct, which has implications for Ewald second and third laws of vestibular physiology (see below).

Ewald laws:

1. *Stimulation of the semicircular canal causes movement of the eyes in the plane of the stimulated canal: tonic movements (slow phase of nystagmus and segmental and axial tilts) are in the direction of the endolymph movement.*
2. *In the horizontal semicircular canals, an ampullopetal endolymph movement causes a greater stimulation than an ampullofugal one. Ampullopetal flow is utriculopetal.*
3. *In the vertical semicircular canals, the reverse is true. Ampullopetal flow is utriculofugal.*

iii. In the utricle and saccule, the neuroepithelium is contained within the macula and has the same two types of cells described above.
   a. The stercocilia project into the otolithic membrane which contains an amorphous layer. The otoliths lie atop the amorphous layer.
      1. A head tilt or an acceleration (in the horizontal plane for the utricle, in the vertical plane for the saccule) causes a sliding of the amorphous membrane and bending of the stereocilia bending them and causing them to depolarize or hyperpolarize depending on their orientation toward the kinocilium.
      2. Unlike in the semicircular ducts, in the utricle macula there are two populations of hair cells on either side of a line called striola with the kinocilium oriented toward that line. In the saccule, the kinocilium is away from the stereocilia

B. Innervation of the labyrinth
   i. The vestibular nerve is associated with the cochlear division centrally and forms with it the VIII cranial nerve.
   ii. Nerve fibers arise from the ganglion of Scarpa and are central to the cochlear nerve at the brainstem.
   iii. It organizes into a superior branch and inferior branch in the internal auditory meatus (IAC) as it is rotating and changing orientation into a posterior location within the IAC.
   iv. Superior branch innervated the utricular macula and the superior and horizontal crista ampullaris.
   v. Inferior branch innervates the saccular macula and the posterior crista ampullaris.
   vi. The posterior ampullary nerve is also called singular nerve. Singular nerve resection used to be a treatment for recalcitrant BPPV, but it was associated with significant adverse hearing outcomes.
   vii. Nerve of Oort or vestibulocochlear anastomosis is a variable communicating branch between the inferior vestibular nerve and the cochlear nerve.

- *The acousticofacial bundle (Fig 14-1) is constituted by the facial nerve, the cochlear, and vestibular nerves.*
- *Cochlear and vestibular nerves are indistinguishable at the level of the brain stem.*
- *Distinction between the two mostly happens at the porus: this is important to remember in retrosigmoid and retrolabyrinthine approaches.*
- *The acousticofacial bundle undergoes a rotation as it courses from the CPA to the porus: the facial nerve is initially anterior to the acoustic nerve but then distally becomes anterior superior with the cochlear nerve anterior inferior.*
- *Vestibular nerves (superior and inferior) are posterior within the IAC and are the nerves we see when we open the IAC via a translabyrinthine approach.*
- *Bill bar separates the facial nerve from the superior vestibular nerve at the level of the fundus.*
- *Crista falciformis separates the facial nerve from the cochlear nerve at the level of the fundus.*

A. Vascularization of the labyrinth
   i. Membranous labyrinth is supplied by the labyrinthine artery which is a branch of the basilar artery of the anterior inferior cerebellar artery and then enters the IAC and gives usually the following three branches.
      a. Vestibular or anterior vestibular artery branch: follows the same trajectory and irrigates the same structures as the superior vestibular nerve: utricle, superior, and horizontal SCC.*

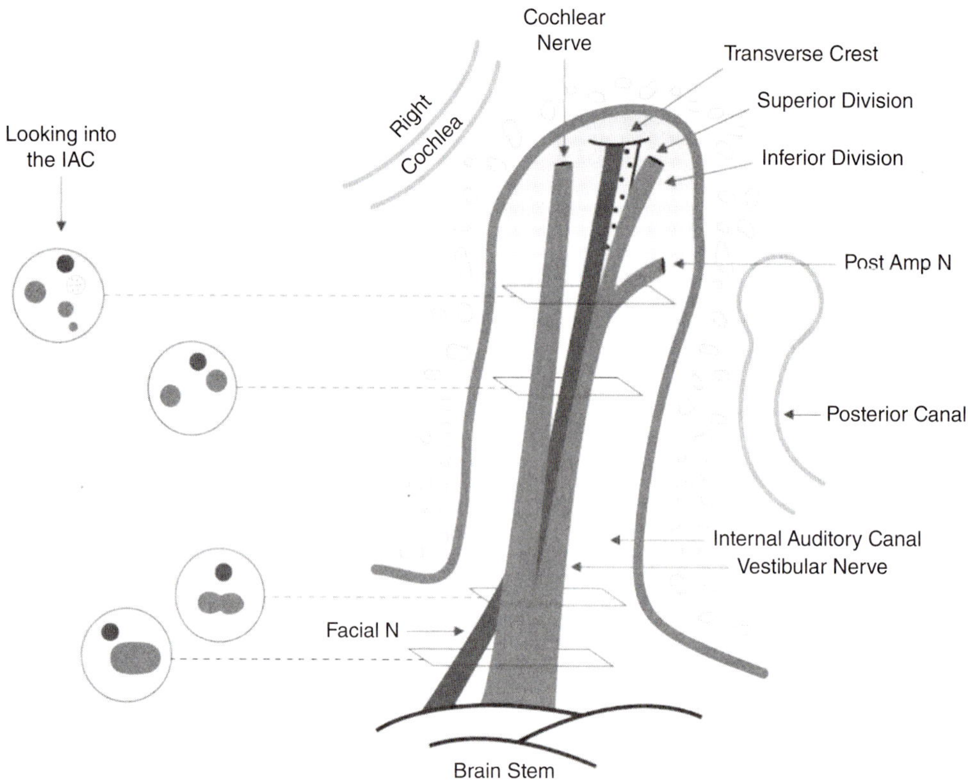

Figure 14-1 Disposition of the acousticofacial bundle (cochlear, vestibular, and facial nerves) from the brain stem to the fundus (posteroinferior view).

b. Posterior vestibular or vestibulocochlear artery: supplies most of the saccule and posterior SCC.
c. Cochlear artery proper.

> **Syndrome of Lindsay Heminway or occlusion of the anterior vestibular artery: symptoms similar to an acute vestibular neuronitis. The patient can also develop a posterior canal BPPV after a few weeks because the posterior ampulla is preserved. Rare because there rarely is an isolated stroke to this small artery.*

A. What does the vestibular system do?
   i. The vestibular system is responsible for balance and gaze stabilization.
   ii. The semicircular ducts sense rotational movement and otolith organs (utricle and saccule) detect linear movement but also acceleration.
   iii. Both components of the labyrinth work best when there is gravity. Microgravity environment/experiments gave us a lot of insight into the functioning of the vestibular system.

Table 14-1 Pairing of Semicircular Canals and Oculomotor Muscles

	Excitatory Pathway	*Inhibitory Pathway*
Superior SCC	• Bilateral superior recti • Contralateral inferior oblique	• Bilateral inferior recti • Contralateral superior oblique
Posterior SCC	• Ipsilateral superior oblique • Bilateral inferior recti	• Ipsilateral inferior oblique • Bilateral superior recti
Lateral SCC	• Contralateral lateral rectus • Ipsilateral medial rectus	• Contralateral medial rectus • Ipsilateral lateral rectus

iv. Semicircular ducts are functionally paired.
   a. Lateral ducts are paired.
   b. Posterior duct on one side is paired with the superior/anterior duct of the opposite side.
   c. We recognize three planes of rotational movement: lateral, right anterior left posterior (RALP), and left anterior right posterior (LARP).
   d. Head movement leads via inertia to a movement of the endolymph and a deflection of the cupula.
   e. Because of the pairing, the vestibular system acts in a push/pull mechanism, where stimulation of one side leads to inhibition of the other side
      1. Of note, at baseline, resting state and without any head movements, the hair cells within the semicircular ducts are firing. A movement of the head toward one side leads to a depolarization and increased firing rate of the hair cells on that side and an inhibition of the hair cells of the opposite side.
      2. While an inhibition of the firing rate can lead to zero, there is no upper limit to the amount of stimulation the excited side can produce from a firing rate standpoint. This means that a head movement occurring at a high velocity, the contralateral side cannot provide adequate information. This is the basis of the head impulse test which detects a corrective saccade whenever the head is thrusted toward the affected side.
   f. The semicircular ducts are also paired with oculomotor muscles (Table 14-1).

v. Ewald laws:
   a. First law: Stimulation of the semicircular canal causes movement of the eyes in the plane of the stimulated canal: tonic movements (slow phase of nystagmus and segmental and axial tilts) are in the direction of the endolymph movement.
   b. Second law In the *horizontal* semicircular canals, an *ampullopetal* endolymph movement causes a *greater stimulation* than an ampullofugal one. Ampullopetal flow is utriculopetal.
   c. Third law: In the *vertical* semicircular canals, the reverse is true. Ampullopetal flow is utriculofugal.

vi. The semicircular ducts play the greatest role in the vestibuloocular reflex. The otolith organs are more important in keeping upright posture and in detecting acceleration/movement, and affect the vestibulospinal reflex and modulate the tone of the truncal muscles. They are also responsible for detecting head and body tilt. Deficiencies in the otolithic pathways can lead to unusual symptoms such as head floating, dissociation.

vii. In a sudden vestibular deafferentation, there is a dramatic change in the firing rate of hair cells in the crista ampullaris of one membranous labyrinth. The contralateral healthy side is still firing at baseline, but the difference between the two sides is interpreted as a movement toward that side. This leads to an activation of the VOR with a slow-phase movement toward the affected ear and a corrective fast phase toward the healthy ear: the nystagmus beats away from the affected ear.

viii. Several compensation strategies occur acutely after an acute unilateral deafferentation:
   a. Alexander law: slow phase of the nystagmus is greatest when gaze is directed toward the healthy ear or another way to say it is the fast phase of the nystagmus is strongest when the gaze is directed toward the healthy ear, weakest when gaze is directed toward the affected ear.
   b. Cerebellar clamp mechanism a few days after the event: the cerebellar inhibits the received afferences from the healthy sides to reduce the difference between the two sides. Currently, patients start feeling improvement in the symptoms with reduction in the spinning. This is static compensation.
   c. Longer-term dynamic compensation takes time and includes significant changes that occur at the level of the vestibular nuclei in the pons. Bechterew phenomenon illustrates that compensation. A vestibular deafferentation on one side following a fully compensated contralateral lesion (labyrinthectomy, vestibular nerve section, etc.) will still lead to an observable typical nystagmus (fast-phase beating toward the contralateral side which is not healthy in this case).

ix. In episodic fluctuating disorders such as Ménière's disease, the nystagmus direction can change during an attack:
   a. At the onset of the attack, nystagmus beats toward the affected ear.
   b. As the attack progresses, the affected side becomes paretic (similar to a unilateral vestibular lesion/neuronitis), and nystagmus beats toward the normal ear.
   c. As the attack subsides, there is a recovery nystagmus beating toward the affected ear.

B. Central vestibular system and higher vestibular function
   i. The peripheral vestibular system detects and conveys information on velocity of head/body movement (crista ampullaris) and acceleration of head and body (maculae). The final position of the head and body is determined through the neural integrator within the reticular formation which projects into the vestibular nuclei and is responsible for determining the final position command for the conjugate eye movements.
   ii. Vestibular nuclei in the pons: receive cerebellar, reticular, cortical, cross-commissural, spinal proprioceptive and visual afferences
      a. Superior (Bechterew nucleus): relay for conjugate ocular reflexes mediated by the SCCs
      b. Lateral (Deiters nucleus): control of ipsilateral vestibulospinal reflexes
      c. Medial (Schwalbe nucleus): coordination of eye, head, and neck movements with connections to the medial longitudinal fasciculus
      d. Descending (spinal vestibular nucleus): integration of signals from the vestibular nuclei, the cerebellum, and reticular formation
   iii. The general pathway past the vestibular nuclei consists of: bilateral projection of vestibular nuclei to midbrain tegmentum, thalamus, and cortex in the parietoinsular vestibular area (PIVC) which is ill defined in humans.
   iv. Vestibulocerebellum: vermis, fastigial nucleus, and nodulus and flocculus modulate the pathway:

a. Coordinate movements of head and eyes
b. Motor learning, adaptation, and compensation

v. The vestibulothalamic and vestibulocortical pathways are responsible for the sensation and perception of head movements.
vi. The vestibulocular pathways are responsible for the control of the vestibular ocular reflex as well as for gaze stabilization, saccades, smooth pursuits, and optokinetic nystagmus.
vii. The vestibulospinal pathways are responsible for the motor commands to the muscles of the neck, upper torso, and lower limbs to maintain balance. These pathways are modulated by cortical and cerebellar efferents.
viii. Hippocampus and parahippocampus, where the vestibular function interacts with cognitive function and influences spatial memory, orientation, and navigation.

Classification of the Vestibular Symptoms and Disorders

A. When evaluating a patient for dizziness, it is important to identify whether this is a vestibular disorder first in opposition to a balance disorder, sensory ataxia, cerebellar ataxia, ocular condition, or hemodynamic problem.
B. The Barany Society published a standardized symptom classification document (Bisdorff et al, Classification of Vestibular symptoms: Towards an international classification of Vestibular disorders. *J Vest Res.* 2009;19:1-13) which gives more clarity to the symptoms we need to look for:
C. Internal vertigo where vertigo is an illusion of movement: spontaneous versus triggered, spinning versus nonspinning (rocking, swaying)
   i. Triggers are: positional, head motion, visual, sound, Valsalva maneuver, orthostatic or other
   ii. Dizziness defined as a sense of spatial disorientation: spontaneous versus triggered
   iii. Vestibulovisual symptoms
   iv. External vertigo
   v. Oscillopsia with or without head movement
   vi. Visual lag
   vii. Visual tilt
   viii. Movement-induced blur
D. Postural Instability
   i. Unsteadiness
   ii. Directional pulsion (drop attacks)
   iii. Balance associated near falls
   iv. Balance associated falls
E. Next, the clinician needs to determine whether the problem is peripheral or central and what pathophysiology is implicated (timing, acute versus chronic, continuous versus paroxysmal versus fluctuating) and whether this is a problem related to the semicircular canal pathways or the otolithic pathways.
F. Rocking sensation is rarely coming from the inner ear and usually orients toward central problems.
G. Head-floating sensation is typically related to disruption of otolithic pathways and can be seen in vestibular migraine.

H. The TiTrate approach described in Newman-Toker DE, Edlow JA. TiTrATE: A novel, evidence-based approach to diagnosing acute dizziness and vertigo. *Neurol Clin.* 2015 Aug;33(3):577-99, viii. doi: 10.1016/j.ncl.2015.04.011. PMID: 26231273; PMCID: PMC4522574. differentiates:
   i. New episodic disorders that can be triggered such as BPPV or spontaneous such as a cardiac arrhythmia.
   ii. New continuous disorders such as post-gentamicin vestibular deafferentation versus spontaneous such as a posterior fossa stroke.
   iii. Chronic persistent such as an uncompensated vestibular hypofunction with symptoms triggered by head movement versus chronic cerebellar ataxia.

I. Associated otologic or neurologic symptoms are important to elicit as well as family history of similar symptoms or known vestibular pathology. Head trauma, medications, previous otologic, or neurosurgical procedures as well as a history of chemotherapy and radiation can be pertinent.

J. A history of childhood motion sickness in a subject presenting with episodic vestibular symptoms increases the odds of a vestibular migraine diagnosis by 100-fold.

K. A targeted examination is very important. Table 14-2 shows differentiating characteristics of peripheral spontaneous nystagmus versus those of central origin.

L. Additional elements on the physical exam to look for include:
   i. Head impulse test (HIT): a positive HIT with corrective saccades in one or both directions suggests a vestibular hypofunction on that side
   ii. After head shake nystagmus: not always localizing but can indicate a lesion opposite to the direction of the nystagmus
   iii. Presence of skew deviation: raises concern for a medullary infarct

M. Vestibular testing can be used to complement the evaluation but is rarely necessary to establish a diagnosis. Uses of vestibular testing include:
   i. Confirm diagnosis
   ii. Map extent of lesion: one, two semicircular canals; is there utricular or saccular involvement?
   iii. Degree of compensation seen on video head impulse testing or rotary chair findings

Table 14-2

Peripheral Lesion (labyrinth and VIII Nerve)	*Central Lesion (Brain stem, Cerebellum, Cerebrum)*
Intense	Less intense
Diminishes with visual fixation	Can diminish with or without fixation, can increase in intensity with visual fixation
Direction fixed	Direction changing or gaze evoked
Horizontal rotary	Purely vertical or torsional or pendular
Follows Alexander law: more intense when gaze is in the direction of fast gaze	Does not follow Alexander law

iv. Determine characteristics of positional nystagmus when it is subtle, or associated with multiple canal involvement with BPPV or detection of central positional nystagmus
v. Determine candidacy to vestibular rehabilitation
vi. Evaluate vestibular function in case a destructive procedure is contemplated or following a destructive procedure (such as intratympanic gentamicin)

Laboratory Vestibular Testing

Electronystagmography/Videonystagmography (ENG/VNG)

A. Records the eye movement directly with infrared video cameras and but also with electrodes to measure the corneoretinal potential related to conjugate eye movements. The potential is traced as an upward or a downward deflection with various slope which depicts a slow movement and a fast movement of the eye. By convention, an upward deflection on the horizontal channel depicts a movement of the eyes toward the right and a downward deflection as a movement to the left.
B. Components of the ENG/VNG include:
  i. Looking for spontaneous nystagmus and gaze-evoked nystagmus.
  ii. Looking at positional nystagmus with the Dix-Hallpike positions or with the supine roll test.
  iii. Fistula testing as indicated by the clinic.
  iv. Bithermal or monothermal caloric testing or ice caloric in case of absent responses with the initial testing. It is preferred to use water in the caloric testing because it is more sensitive than air.
    a. Evaluates the function of the lateral semicircular canal.
    b. It is a test of low frequency of the vestibular system.
    c. The water or air is used at a cold and warm temperature (relative to body temperature) for 30 seconds with water and up to 60 seconds for air.
    d. When no responses are recorded, an ice caloric is indicated to look for any evidence of residual function.
    e. The caloric response relies on gravity and convection current with minimal direct thermal effect.
      1. Cold caloric (water/air) causes a downward movement of the endolymph which leads to ampullofugal flow in the lateral SCC. This leads to a deflection of hair cells away from kinocilium and hypoperpolarization of those cells. The end result is a slow phase toward the involved side with a compensatory fast saccade away from the irrigated ear.
      2. Warm caloric (water/air) causes an upward movement of the endolymph leading to ampullopetal flow in the lateral SCC, a depolarization of the hair cells and slow phase eye movement toward the contralateral ear with a fast compensatory phase toward the irrigated ear.
      3. COWS: Cold Opposite Warm Same.
    f. Jongkees formula
      1. Relative vestibular reduction equals the absolute difference in response provoked by bithermal stimulation on each side divided by the total response on all four experiments.
      2. $RVR = (RC + RW - LC - LW)/TR$, where RVR is relative vestibular reduction, TR total response, RC right cold caloric response, RW right ward caloric response, LC left cold caloric response, and LW left warm caloric response.

3. RVR of more than 25% is generally considered a weakness in the caloric response.
4. An absolute response on each side of less than 12 degrees per second is also considered a hypofunction.
5. Barany criteria for bilateral vestibular hypofunction are even more strict and require a total response on each side for both caloric experiments to be below 6 degrees per second.

g. Directional preponderance
   1. Looks at relative difference between all right-beating nystagmus and all left-beating nystagmus divided by the total response.
   2. (RW + LC) – (LW + RC) divided by total response.
   3. Unclear clinical utility of directional preponderance. In some studies, it may be stronger preponderance in case of a central lesion and lower preponderance in case of a peripheral lesion with the threshold generally considered to be 30%.

h. Pitfalls:
   1. EAC pathology
   2. TM pathology
   3. TM perforation
   4. Otologic surgery on one side with mastoidectomy may change the dissipation of temperature and affect the symmetric response in the absence of vestibular hypofunction.

C. Interpretation
   i. Peripheral findings
      a. Direction fixed spontaneous nystagmus
      b. Unilateral caloric weakness with more than 25% asymmetry
      c. Bilateral caloric weakness with a history in favor of a labyrinthine pathology
      d. Positional nystagmus with latency and short duration and fatigable
      e. Spontaneous nystagmus suppressible with visual fixation
   ii. Central findings
      a. Gaze evoked nystagmus/abnormal fixation suppression
      b. Isolated bilateral caloric weakness
      c. Abnormal oculomotor testing
      d. Hyperactive caloric response
      e. Pervasive caloric response or inverted caloric response: left beating nystagmus with left warm stimulation for example

Rotational Chair Testing

A. Tests the vestibular system at multiple frequencies higher than the caloric testing.
B. Evaluates the VOR response and both labyrinths simultaneously; it can be difficult to use to localize lesion.
C. Off-vertical axis rotation (OVAR) used to assess otolithic organs.
D. Multiple protocols include:
   i. Sinusoidal harmonic acceleration where gain and phase and asymmetry are measured
      a. Gain refers to the speed of slow-phase eye velocity compared to the velocity of the chair. Low gain can be a sign of bilateral vestibular loss.
      b. Phase measures the lead or the lag of maximum chair velocity compared to the maximum slow-phase eye movement velocity.

1. Phase lead is typically seen in uncompensated peripheral vestibular hypofunction but also if the vestibular nuclei are selectively damaged.
2. Phase lag is usually seen in cerebellar disorders.

ii. Symmetry
  a. Compares left and right peak slow-phase velocity
  b. Shows weakness on affected side in acute setting; improves with compensation
  c. Cannot be used in isolation to localize insult

E. Step velocity test where gain and time decay is measured.
  i. Gain as stated above.
  ii. Time decay is the amount of time it takes for the postrotary nystagmus to reach a velocity that is 67% of the peak velocity.
    a. Fast time decay usually indicates a peripheral uncompensated vestibular hypofunction.
    b. Slow decay is usually seen in conditions associated with motion sensitivity including vestibular migraine

Video Head Impulse Test (vHIT)

A. Lightweight goggles with built-in high-speed camera (> 250 Hz) for capturing eye movements; gyroscope measures head rotation.
B. New format without goggles not widely available yet but consists of a remote camera that would capture the head rotation and saccadic eye movements: interesting for children or patients with anatomical problems that would affect the wearing of the goggles.
C. Measures high-frequency VOR function when performing Halmagyi (head thrust) maneuver.
D. The test measures gains in each of three-dimensional HIT (lateral, RALP, LARP) with a gain below 0.75 (0.8 in some centers) considered weak.
E. The test also detects the presence of refixation saccades. They are overt (visible to the naked eye) in the acute phase of a peripheral vestibular deafferentation.
F. As compensation progresses, the gain starts normalizing and the saccades become synchronous and more covert.
G. Maximum head impulse velocity ~150 to 200 degree/s. Beyond that, the results are unreliable due to goggle slippage.

Vestibular-Evoked Myogenic Potentials (VEMPs)

A. This test is designed to measure function of the utricle and the saccule. It can be done using two kinds of stimulus.
  i. Air conduction (AC): Brief (0.1 ms), loud (SPL > 90 dB) 500 Hz tone burst presented in ear to evoke short latency myogenic potentials for evaluating otolith function (utricle and saccule)
  ii. Bone conduction (BC) using a mastoid oscillator (B81 better than B71) or a minishaker when there is middle ear pathology to circumvent the air conduction
    a. BC testing is less sensitive than AC for third-window pathology
    b. Absent oVEMPs responses on BC are not always indicative of utricular dysfunction because this response is very small to start with

B. Cervical VEMP (cVEMP)
  i. Is a test of saccular function and inferior vestibular nerve
  ii. We are looking at the Ipsilateral inhibitory response from tonically contracted sternocleidomastoid (SCM) muscle
  iii. Tracing: positive (inhibitory) peak ~13 ms followed by negative trough ~23 ms

        iv. Pathway: saccule → inferior vestibular nerve → vestibular nuclei → medial vestibulospinal tract (ipsilateral) → spinal accessory nuclei (CN XI) → sternocleidomastoid muscle
    C. Ocular VEMP (oVEMP)
        i. Contralateral response from inferior oblique/rectus muscles during upward gaze
        ii. Tracing: negative (excitatory) peak ~10 ms, positive peak ~16 ms
        iii. Evaluates utricle (sensitive to horizontal accelerations) and the superior branch of the vestibular nerve
        iv. Pathway: utricle → superior vestibular nerve → vestibular nuclei → medial longitudinal fasciculus → oculomotor nuclei (iii) → inferior oblique muscle
    D. VEMPs metrics used to evaluate function include
        i. Peak to peak amplitude asymmetry: EMG rectification of muscle contraction is important for this metric to be reliable
        ii. Thresholds
        iii. Latency
        iv. Frequency tuning shift: check cVEMP response at 1000 kHz and oVEMPs response at 4000 kHz
            a. Larger cVEMP response at 1000 kHz has been described in hydrops/Ménière's disease.
            b. Present oVEMP response at 4000 kHz has been described as a soft marker of superior semicircular canal dehiscence. It has also been reported in the setting of headaches.
    E. Absent responses may be due to middle ear pathology but they have also been described with age without it being a marker of pathology.
    F. cVEMP and oVEMP are used as electrophysiologic marker of a third window/superior semicircular canal dehiscence syndrome: decreased threshold response in cVEMP and augmentation of oVEMP amplitude response (> 17 μV)
    G. Absent response can be seen in vestibular migraine and Ménière's disease.

Subjective Visual Vertical (SVV)

    A. Tests perception of verticality without external reference points
        i. More than 2 to 3 degrees error is pathologic and in line with an asymmetric vestibular function
        ii. Sensitive for utricular dysfunction and central otolithic pathway up to the level of the brain stem in the acute stage
    B. Equipment can be expensive. DIY version exists: the bucket test

Computerized Dynamic Posturography (CDP)

    A. Cannot identify the source of the problem
    B. Complementary to rest of the testing
    C. Gives information regarding functional impairment
    D. Centre of pressure (COP) data on a force plate are used to evaluate performance
    E. Comprised of three tests
        i. Sensory organization test (SOT): Assesses the subject's ability to use visual, vestibular, and proprioceptive cues to maintain balance in various conditions:
            a. Condition 1: eyes open, fixed surface, and fixed visual surround
            b. Condition 2: eyes closed and fixed surface
            c. Condition 3: eyes open with fixed surface and sway-referenced visual surround
            d. Condition 4: eyes open on sway-referenced support surface

e. Condition 5: eyes closed on sway-referenced support surface
f. Condition 6: eyes open on sway-referenced support surface and visual surround

ii. Motor control test (MCT):
a. Evaluates automatic motor reflex responses to a sudden, unexpected forward or backward translation of the support surface.
b. It provides a lot of information regarding nonvestibular causes of imbalance.

iii. Adaptation test (ADT):
a. Assesses the ability to use motor strategies to "adapt" to unexpected perturbations of the support surface (toes up and toes down rotation of the platform).
b. Amplitude of sway is measured after each surface rotation. (Table 14-3-14-6)

Table 14-3 Clinical Classification of Vestibular Disorders

	Clinical Classification	
	Acute Peripheral Deafferentation	*Acute Central Deafferentation*
Symptoms	Severe external vertigo, ataxia, imbalance, nausea, and vomiting	Severe external or internal vertigo or dizziness or ataxia, imbalance, nausea, and vomiting
	Positive head impulse test	Negative head impulse test
	Direction fixed spontaneous nystagmus	Gaze-evoked nystagmus refixation on cover/uncover test
	No skew deviation	
Clinical Exam findings	After head shake nystagmus beating to the opposite side of the expected lesion (depending on HIT)	After head shake nystagmus can be present and nonlocalizing. Can also be vertical or rotary in central lesions (cross coupling)
	Skull-base vibration induced nystagmus in line with the after head shake Abnormal visual vestibulo-ocular reflex (VVOR) and VOR suppression: in favor of a lesion of the vestibulocerebellum	
Vestibular laboratory findings	Abnormal caloric testing on videonystagmography (VNG): more than 25% asymmetry	Caloric testing normal or showing hyperactive response
	Low gain and phase lead on rotary chair (sinusoidal harmonic acceleration protocol)	Normal or high gain. Normal phase or phase lag
	Low gain and fast time decay on step velocity protocol	Normal or high gain. Normal time decay or slow decay
	Low gain < 0.75 and overt saccades on videoHead impulse testing (vHIT)	Normal or high gain on vHIT. Absence of saccades
	Unilateral absent response on vestibular evoked myogenic potential (VEMPs)	Variable pattern on cervical and ocular VEMPs
	Abnormal subjective visual vertical	Other VNG findings including gaze-evoked nystagmus, vertical nystagmus, abnormal oculomotor testing, abnormal VVOR and VOR suppression tests

Table 14-4 Classification According to Type of Presentation

	Type of Presentation		
	Bilateral Vestibular Loss	*Paroxysmal stimulation of the vestibular system*	*Acute/Subacute unilateral failure of the vestibular function*
Symptoms	Oscillopsia with head motion, postural instability in low-vision environment and on uneven ground, deficits in spatial memory	Spontaneous attacks of vertigo and postural imbalance	External vertigo, movement-induced blur, visual lag, postural instability, oscillopsia, especially with head movement
Clinical exam findings	Positive head impulse test bilaterally	Spontaneous nystagmus of variable duration: vestibular paroxysmia, Meniere disease, vestibular migraine)	Spontaneous nystagmus direction fixed, follows Alexander law
	Positive Romberg and modified Romberg Loss of dynamic visual acuity (drop of more than 2 lines on Snellen Chart during head shaking)	Tuning fork exam may elicit a hearing loss in affected side in case of Meniere disease: Weber test would lateralize to the opposite ear, and air conduction is greater than bone conduction in affected ear	Positive HIT
	Loss of dynamic visual acuity (drop of more than 2 lines on Snellen Chart during head shaking)		After head shake nystagmus beating toward the unaffected side
			Skull-base vibration induced nystagmus beating toward the unaffected side
Vestibular laboratory findings	Caloric testing shows low responses of less than 6 degree/second on bithermal conditions on each side	Generally normal VNG when examined in the interictal state	See peripheral versus central
	Low gain below 0.6 on lateral videoHIT bilaterally with overt saccades	Discrepancy between caloric responses showing a hypofunction and normal vHIT has been described in Meniere disease	See peripheral versus central
	Abnormal computerized dynamic visual acuity	Absent oVEMP or cVEMPs have been described in Meniere disease and vestibular migraine	See peripheral versus central
	Rotary chair shows low gain below 0.1 on sinusoidal harmonic acceleration protocol and phase lead above 68 degrees	Positional nystagmus (horizontal, low amplitude, sometimes direction changing with supine roll position) has been described in vestibular migraine	
		Always test the hearing with an audiogram and look for low-frequency sensorineural hearing loss suggestive of Meniere disease	

Table 14-5 Classification According to Affected Pathway

	Localization Classification	
	Semicircular Canal Pathway	*Otolith Pathway*
Symptoms	Spinning external or internal vertigo, deviation of perceived straight ahead, postural imbalance, visual lag, movement induced blur, oscillopsia	Falls, drop attacks, directional pulsion, sensation of linear motion or head tilt, head floating, dizziness, dissociation
Clinical exam findings	Positive head impulse test	Head-heave test for utricular function
	Positive Romberg	
	Loss of dynamic visual acuity with head shaking in bilateral involvement	
	Positive after head shake nystagmus or skull-base vibration-induced nystagmus	
Vestibular laboratory findings	Caloric response asymmetry of more than 25% if lateral SCC affected	Abnormal ocular VEMPs (utricle)
	Abnormal VOR function tests including rotary chair depending on acuity of the lesion	Abnormal cervical VEMPs (saccule)

Table 14-6 Differential Diagnosis Adapted From the Vestibular Disorders Association Triage Protocol

			Timing and Triggers		
Timing	*Seconds*	*Seconds to Hours*	*Minutes to Hours*	*Minutes to Days*	*Hours to Constant*
Triggers	Rolling over in bed, getting in and out of bed, bending over, looking upward	Head movement, busy, dark environment, soft or uneven surfaces, history of acute event at onset	Spontaneous/episodic; may increase with head movement	Spontaneous/episodic. Possibly increase with head movement	May have association with head and visual movement
Symptoms	Brief external vertigo. No auditory symptoms, no other neurologic symptoms. Nausea and vomiting	Unsteadiness, oscillopsia, variable hearing loss, and tinnitus	External vertigo, hearing disturbance, ear fullness, tinnitus, progressive fluctuating hearing loss, nausea and vomiting	Possible visual aura, photophobia, phonophobia headaches, environmental triggers	Vague sensation of dizziness, internal or external vertigo
Possible diagnosis	BPPV	Vestibular hypofunction/neuronitis/labyrinthitis	Meniere disease	Vestibular migraine	Many possibilities including central and multifactorial, PPPD

Benign Paroxysmal Positional Vertigo

A. Recurrent episodes of *positional* vertigo
B. Short-lived vertigo lasting less than a minute generally and induced by a specific head position (not just head motion)
C. No interictal symptoms
D. Posterior semicircular canal most frequently involved
E. Pathophysiology:
    i. Canalithiasis: utricular otoliths degenerate and fall into the endolymph within the posterior semicircular canal ampullary region. Head movement leads to movement of the endolymph and contained debris which deflects the cupula
    ii. Cupulolithiasis: a less frequent occurrence is when the otliths get stuck against the cupula.
F. According to Ewald laws, in the setting of posterior canal BPPV, we will observe:
    i. Upbeat torsional geotropic nystagmus that is elicited in the Dix-Hallpike supine position to the affected side. There is a variable latency before onset of symptoms and nystagmus. The nystagmus typically lasts less than a minute.
    ii. Reversal of the nystagmus into downbeat and torsional nystagmus away from the affected ear when patient is seated: this nystagmus is generally less intense.
    iii. In cupulolithiasis cases, the onset of the symptoms and nystagmus is immediate and the duration is longer and the symptoms are generally more severe.
G. Risk factors: idiopathic, posttraumatic, postvestibular neuronitis.
H. Migraine headaches and low vitamin D levels seem to be associated with higher prevalence of BPPV.
I. Patients with vestibular migraine and Ménière's disease tend to have more frequent occurrence of BPPV.
J. Atypical forms of BPPV:
    i. Horizontal canal BPPV: diagnosed with the supine roll test
        a. Canalithiasis: geotropic horizontal direction-changing nystagmus with more intense nystagmus on the side of the BPPV
        b. Cupulolithiasis (heavy cupula): apogeotropic horizontal nystagmus, direction changing with less intense nystagmus on side of the BPPV
    ii. Superior canal BPPV very rare. A true superior canal BPPV would cause a downbeat apogeoptropic nystagmus with torsion away from the ear being tested with reversal of nystagmus upon sitting up.
        a. Low threshold to obtain imaging since downbeat nystagmus can be seen in Chiari malformation, cerebellar disease
        b. Positional downbeat nystagmus has been reported in superior semicircular canal dehiscence
K. Differential diagnosis of horizontal canalithiasis BPPV is light cupula. Other than otolith falling from the tectorial membrane into the semicircular ducts endolymphatic space, other pathologies can lead to a "light cupula scenario": alcohol or bleeding or inflammation changing the density of endolymph, debris from metabolism of orolith leading to light debris that make cupula float, macular dysfunction, density mismatch between endolymph and perilymph leading to deformation of the duct. Vestibular migraine has been implicated in light cupula presentation by stimulating the trigeminovascular pathway of the inner ear and leading to inflammation within the endolymph.

L. Treatment of BPPV according to the most recent AAOHNS Clinical Practice Guideline (2017)
   i. Canalith repositioning maneuver: Epley for posterior canalithiasis, Semont for posterior canal cupulolithiasis, logroll or Gufoni maneuver for horizontal canalithiasis and cupulolithiasis, forced head hanging maneuver or reverse Epley for superior canal BPPV
   ii. Observation is also something to consider if patient is difficult to treat with PT
   iii. Referral to vestibular rehabilitation
   iv. Habituation exercises such as Brandt-Daroff exercises
   v. Surgical treatment including posterior canal occlusion, singular neurectomy, vestibular neurectomy, or labyrinthectomy are extremely rarely needed
   vi. In cases of recalcitrant or frequently recurrent BPPV, consider central causes, screen for migraine or migraine variants, and consider migraine preventive treatment

Vestibular Neuronitis: Acute Presentation and Compensation Process

A. Frequent cause of peripheral vestibulopathy
B. If there is an associated hearing loss, we can use the term labyrinthitis
C. Sudden onset of external vertigo with neurovegetative symptoms
D. Superior vestibular nerve is most frequently affected
E. Pathophysiology: reactivation of the herpes simplex or the herpes zoster viruses within the ganglion of Scarpa. As seen above, an occlusion of the anterior vestibular artery can cause similar symptoms as well
F. Initial acute vertigo symptoms last a few days until the cerebellar clamp mechanism occurs
G. Clinical exam shows typical direction fixed nystagmus beating away from the affected ear
H. Dynamic compensation may take several weeks or months during which symptoms or postural instability of VOR deficiency (visual lag, movement-induced blur) may prevail
I. Causes of delay of compensation or decompensation of previously compensated hypofunction
   i. Cervical pain
   ii. Headaches
   iii. Central comorbidities
   iv. Sedatives and vestibular sedatives medications such as meclizine or benzodiazepines
J. Typical findings on vestibular testing include
   i. Calorics show hypofunction with more than 25% asymmetry on affected side
   ii. VideoHIT shows low gains and overt saccades. See Figure 14-2.
   iii. Rotary chair shows acutely low gain and phase lead on sinusoidal harmonic acceleration protocol, and low gains and fast time decay of step velocity protocols. See Figure 14-3.
K. Treatment:
   i. Acute: treat the vertigo and the neurovegetative symptoms with antihistamines, vestibular sedatives, antinausea medication
      a. No clear evidence for antivirals
      b. Steroid in the acute setting is optional. Some studies suggest it reduces the long-term level of caloric hypofunction
   ii. Chronic: vestibular rehabilitation

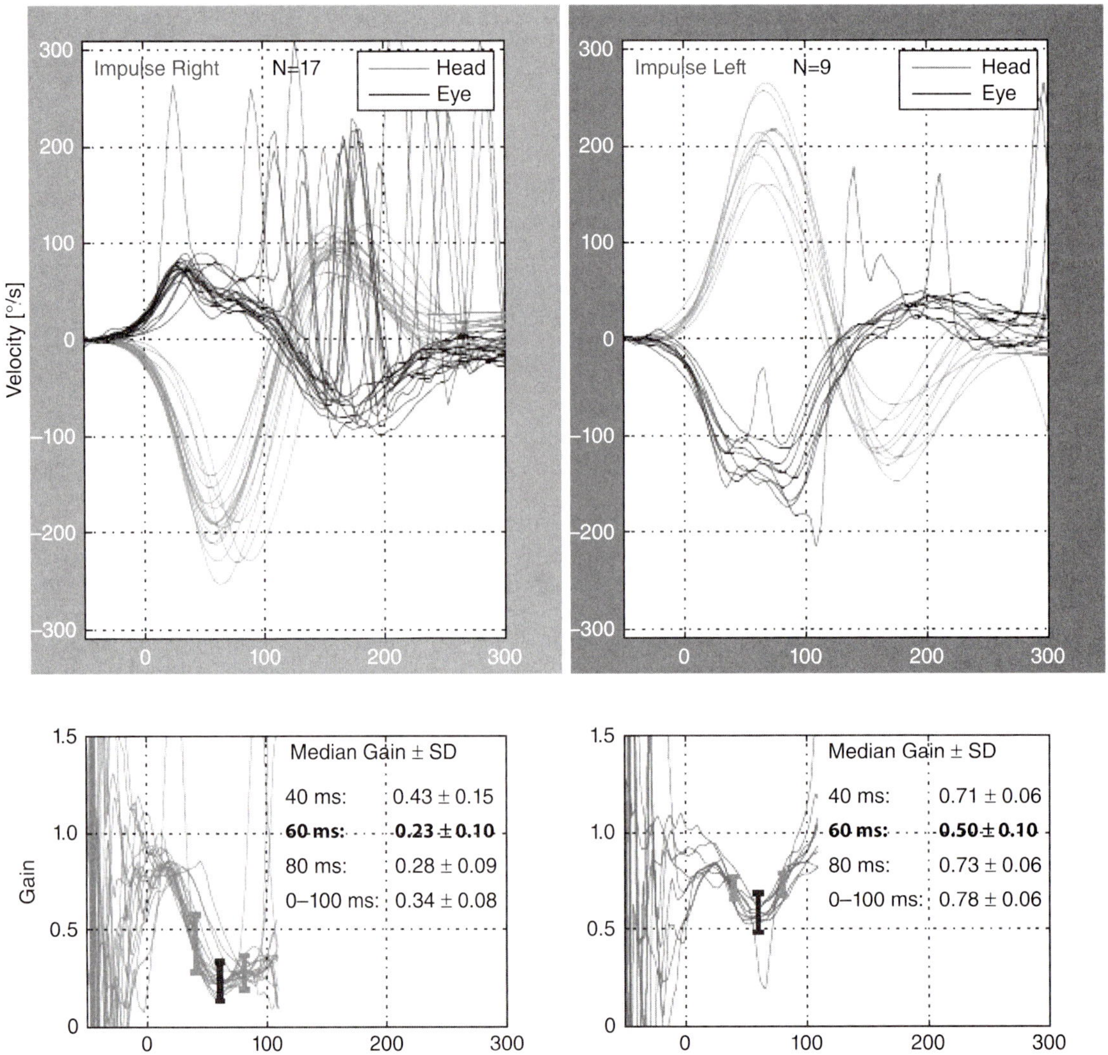

Figure 14-2 VideoHead Impulse testing in right vestibular neuronitis.

L. Differential diagnosis:
   i. First episode of recurrent vestibulopathy
   ii. Consider retrocochlear pathology including intravestibular/intralabyrinthine schwannoma
   iii. In the acute setting, a unilateral hearing loss can be a red flag for a pseudovestibular neuronitis related to a stroke in the caudal cerebellum, insular cortex or lesions in the pons or along the root entry zone of the acoustic nerve. Other red flags include:
      a. Severe headaches
      b. Severe postural imbalance
      c. Lack of improvement within 48 hours

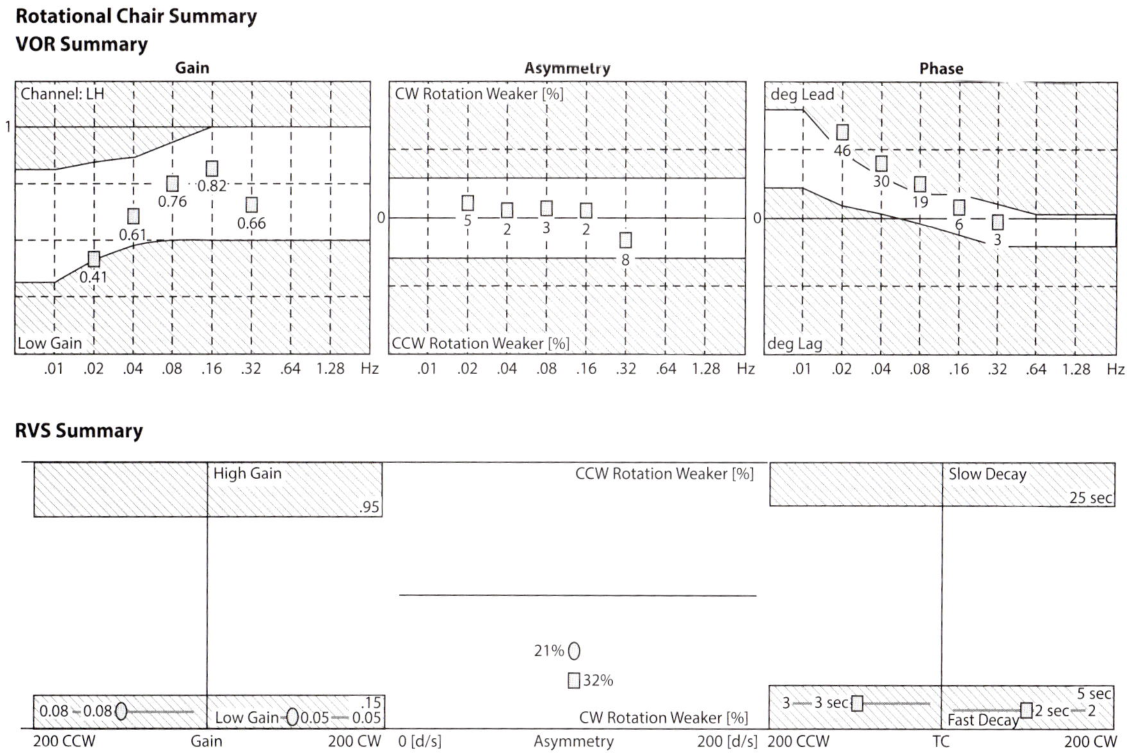

Figure 14-3 Rotary chair testing showing an uncompensated vestibular hypofunction. Top panel showing results of sinusoidal harmonic acceleration with low gain and phase lead. Bottom panel shows low gain and fast time decay.

d. Normal head impulse testing
e. Nonlocalizing after head shake nystagmus or cross coupling of after head shake nystagmus or other exam findings not in line with a clear-cut peripheral deafferentation

Bilateral Vestibular Hypofunction

A. Very disabling
B. Oscillopsia with head movement and postural instability in the dark or on uneven surfaces are hallmark symptoms
C. Causes:
   i. Idiopathic: isolated without hearing loss and with normal imaging
   ii. Toxic: aminoglycosides, platins
   iii. Infectious: meningitis
   iv. CANVAS: neurodegenerative disorder including cerebellar atrophy, bilateral vestibular areflexia, and neuropathy
   v. Genetic: Usher syndrome (type 1 mostly) associated with retinitis pigmentosa and congenital hearing loss

The Barany society recently defined diagnostic criteria for definite and probable bilateral vestibular hypofunction.

Definite Bilateral Vestibular Hypofunction

A. Chronic vestibular syndrome with the following symptoms:
   i. Unsteadiness when walking or standing plus at least of 2 or 3
   ii. Movement-induced blurred vision or oscillopsia during walking or quick head/body movements and/or
   iii. Worsening of unsteadiness in darkness and/or on uneven ground
B. No symptoms while sitting or lying down under static conditions
C. Bilaterally reduced or absent angular VOR function documented by
   i. Bilaterally pathological horizontal angular VOR gain less than 0.6, measured by the video-HIT or scleral-coil technique and/or
   ii. Reduced caloric response (sum of bithermal max peak SPV on each side less than 6 degree/s and/or
   iii. Reduced horizontal angular VOR gain less than 0.1 upon sinusoidal stimulation on a rotatory chair (0.1 Hz, V_{max} = 50 degree/s) and a phase lead greater than 68 degrees (time constant < 5 s) (Figures 14-4, 14-5, 14-6)
D. Not better accounted for by another diagnosis

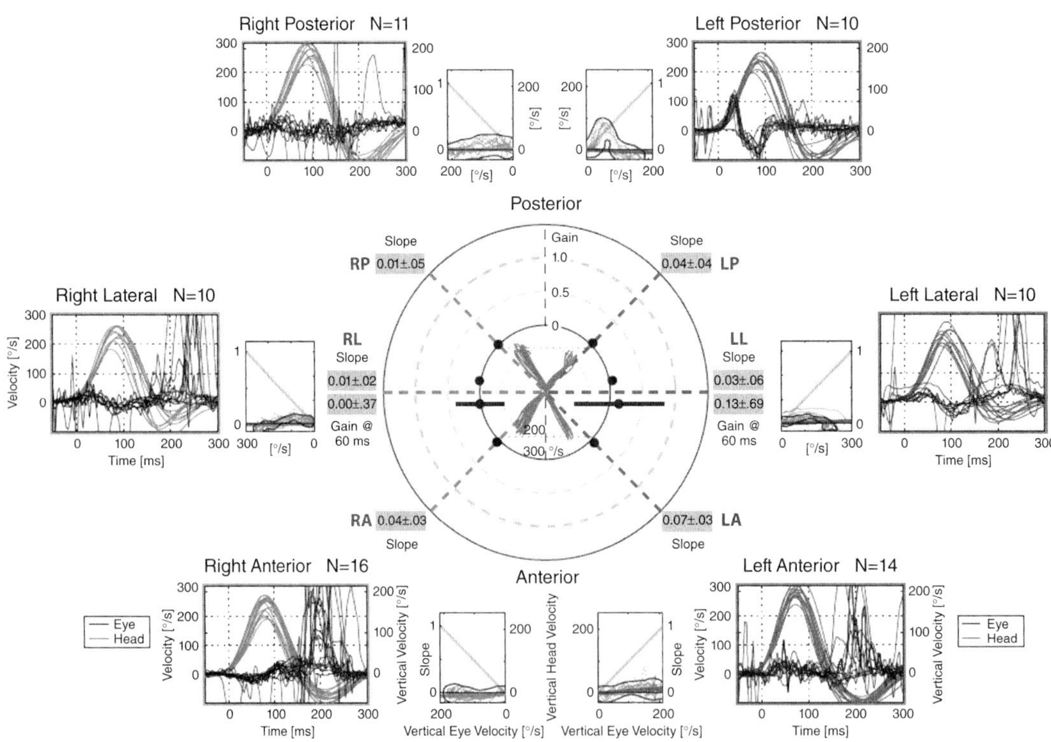

Figure 14-4 (vHIT) showing all six HIT gains below 0.6 bilaterally along with bilateral saccades.

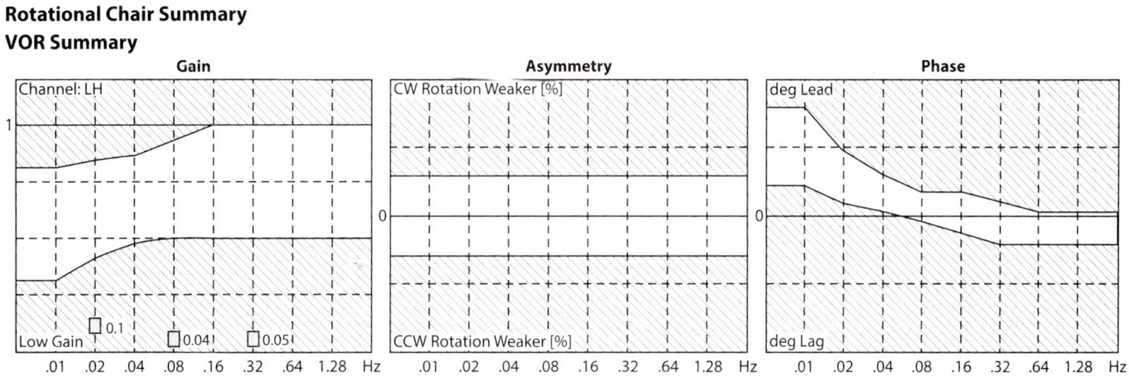

Figure 14-5 Rotary chair Sinusoidal harmonic acceleration showing very low gains below 0.1 and incalculable phase lead.

Diagnostic criteria of probable BVH are similar to above, except that criterion C is bilateral pathological horizontal bedside head impulse tests.

For better understanding of symptom characterization in the setting of BVH, please read the following article published in NEJM.

Bilateral Vestibular Hypofunction Recovery: Living without a balance mechanism NEJM (https://www.nejm.org/doi/full/10.1056/NEJM195203202461207)

A. Treatment
   i. Rehabilitation protocols focusing on substitution strategies.
   ii. Vestibular implants are not clinically available for routine clinical care of those patients. Various trials in the United States and Europe show modest results.

Presbyvestibulopathy

A. Individual variability in age-related degeneration of the vestibular organs
B. Barany Society criteria for presbyvestibulopathy

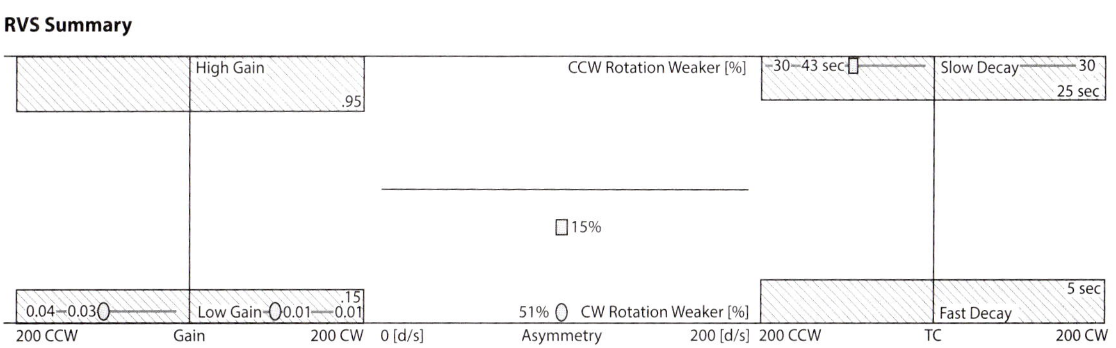

Figure 14-6 showing reduced time decay below five seconds bilaterally on step velocity rotary chair testing.

i. Chronic vestibular syndrome of at least 3 months duration with at least two of the following symptoms:
   a. Postural imbalance or unsteadiness
   b. Gait disturbance
   c. Chronic dizziness
   d. Recurrent Falls

ii. Mild bilateral peripheral vestibular hypofunction documented by at least one of the following:
   a. VOR gain measured by videoHIT between 0.6 and 0.8 bilaterally.
   b. VOR gain between 0.1 and 0.3 upon sinusoidal stimulation on a rotary chair (0.1 Hz, V_{max} = 50-60 degree/sec)
   c. Reduced caloric response (sum of bothermal maximum peak SPV on each side between 6 and 25 deg/sec)

iii. Age greater than or equal to 60

iv. Not better accounted for by another diagnosis

C. It may be associated with other causes of dizziness such as BPPV, and other causes of age-related imbalance such as neuropathy or arthritis.

Ménière's disease

A. Ménière's disease criteria have changed a bit since the initial 1995 AAOHNS criteria.

See Table 14-7.

A. Pathophysiology of Ménière's disease:

i. Endolymphatic hydrops (ELS) is correlated with Ménière's disease but no evidence to support it as a primary cause. It can be correlated to ictal symptoms with hydrops causing rupture of Reissner membrane and mixing of endolymph and perilymph with depolarization of hair cells and vertigo and hearing loss

ii. Postulated mechanisms of ELS development
   a. Structural obstruction of the endolymphatic duct with reduced absorption of endolymph
      1. anatomic variation of vestibular aqueduct
      2. Anteromedially displaced lateral sinuses
      3. Obstruction of ductus reuniens
      4. Dysfunction of utricularendolymphatic valve of Bast
   a. Disruption of posterior cerebral circulation with ischemia of stria vascularis
   b. Fluid homeostasis disorder related to disruption of water and sodium homeostasis including aquaporin receptor dysfunction
   c. Allergy which affects the endolymphatic sac, the sole immunologically active structure of inner ear
   d. Immune dysregulation:
      1. Autoimmune inner ear disease, Cogan syndrome have similar presentations as bilateral Ménière's disease at times
      2. Autoinflammatory mechanisms: specific proinflammatory cytokine profiles have been identified
   e. Genetic: familial type of Ménière's disease with cross-linkage studies showing multiple loci associated with immune regulation and inflammation as well as vasopressin/aquaporin receptors and sodium channels

Table 14-7 Various Criteria for Ménière's Disease

1995 AAO-HNS Criteria *(Otolaryngol H Neck Surg. 1995;113:181-185)*	***2015 ICVD Criteria*** *(J Ves Res. 2015;25:1-7)*	***2020 AAO-HNS Criteria*** *(Otolaryngol H Neck Surg. 2020; 162:415-434)*
Definite Ménière's Disease		
2 spontaneous vertigo attacks lasting more than 20 minutes	> 2 spontaneous vertigo attacks lasting more than 20 minutes and less than 12 hours	Two or more spontaneous vertigo episodes lasting between 20 minutes and 24 hours
Audiometrically documented hearing loss on at least one occasion	Audiometrically documented hearing loss in the low to mid frequencies. Thresholds must be at least 30 dB worse in the affected ear at two contiguous frequencies below 2000 Hz when compared to contralateral ear	Audiogram with low to midfrequency hearing loss on at least one occasion before, during or after one of the episodes of vertigo
Tinnitus or aural fullness in the affected ear	Fluctuating otologic symptoms (hearing loss, or tinnitus or aural fullness) within 24 hours of the vertigo episode	Fluctuating otologic symptoms: hearing loss, tinnitus, aural fullness
Other causes excluded	Not better accounted for by another vestibular disorder	Other causes excluded by other tests
Probable Ménière's Disease		
One spontaneous episode of vertigo lasting more than 20 minutes	> 2 spontaneous vertigo attacks lasting more than 20 minutes and less than 24 hours	2 spontaneous vertigo attacks lasting more than 20 minutes and less than 24 hours
Tinnitus or aural fullness in the affected ear	Fluctuating aural symptoms	Fluctuating aural symptoms
Audiometrically documented hearing loss on at least one occasion		
Other causes excluded	Other causes excluded	Other causes excluded

f. Migraine as a cause of Ménière's disease through activation of trigeminovascular pathway which can lead to inflammation within the labyrinth

g. Metabolic and infectious causes

B. Endophenotypes of Ménière's disease
   i. Type 1 idiopathic
   ii. Type 2 delayed post-trauma or surgery
   iii. Type 3 familial
   iv. Type 4 associated with autoimmune disorders
   v. Type 5 associated with migraine pathology

A. Audiological staging of Ménière's disease
   i. Stage I 4 TONE PTA (0.5, 1, 2 and 3 kHz) less than 26 dB
   ii. Stage II PTA between 26 and 40 dB
   iii. Stage III PTA between 41 and 70 dB
   iv. Stage IV PTA more than 70 dB

B. Patterns of presentation of Ménière's disease:
   i. Rarely bilateral at onset. Fifteen percent may develop bilateral disease over the course of the disorder
   ii. Hearing loss first (even decades prior) followed by classic attacks: delayed hydrops presentation
   iii. Monosymptomatic vertigo attacks followed by classic presentation
   iv. Simultaneous audiovestibular presentation at onset
   v. Atypical forms
      a. Lermoyez disease: vertigo onset is characterized by recovery of hearing and resolution of otologic symptoms that preceded the vertigo
      b. Tumarkin crisis: sudden loss of vestibulospinal reflex with loss of tone of the truncal extensor muscles leading to a sudden fall/drop attack. More frequently related to a sudden change of pressure along the utricular macula and less frequently along the saccular macula. The latter results in a lateropulsion type of drop attack

C. Treatment
   i. Conservative
      a. Vestibular suppressants for acute vertigo attacks: including antihistamines, benzodiazepine, and oral steroids
      b. Low salt diet: no specific target. Aim below 2 g/day and educate regarding importance of avoiding fluctuating levels of intake
      c. Diuretics:
         1. Triamterene/Hydrochlorothiazide 37.5 mg/25 mg QD
         2. Spironolactone and acetazolamide have been described
      d. Betahistine: 16 mg tid but can be increased to much higher doses as tolerated. (non-FDA approved.)
   ii. Surgical and procedural therapies
      a. If medical strategies fail, rule out other conditions including migraine variant before moving to aggressive measures, and after ruling out vestibular migraine and treating any associated migraine pathology, consideration for more aggressive approaches.
      b. In-office procedures include
         1. Nonablative intratympanic steroid injections
         2. Ablative intratympanic gentamicin injections.
      c. If hearing is preserved and functional, an endolymphatic sac decompression/shunt procedure can be offered (shunt with or without silastic, decompression, ligation). The new AAOHNS 2020 guideline does not offer any recommendation for or against this procedure citing lack of enough supporting evidence either way.
      d. In patients with significant hearing loss and no response to conservative measures, intratympanic gentamicin is typically the next step.
      e. Vestibular neurectomy has been used in refractory vertigo with serviceable hearing. The 2020 guidelines do not address it.
      f. In patients with refractory vertigo and nonserviceable hearing, a labyrinthectomy can be discussed.

D. Rehabilitation of auditory and vestibular function
   i. Traditional hearing aids can help in early stages of hearing loss.
   ii. If there is unilateral significant hearing loss, a CROS or BiCROS hearing aid can be used.

   iii. Cochlear implantation for unilateral or bilateral severe to profound sensorineural hearing loss can be considered.
   iv. Vestibular rehabilitation is recommended in case of chronic imbalance related to the actual disorder or the treatment of it by gentamicin or labyrinthectomy.
   v. Avoid vestibular rehabilitation in acute settings because it may aggravate symptoms.

Vestibular Migraine

A. Accounts for almost 20% of diagnoses of new dizziness complaints in a neurotology clinic.
B. The prevalence of VM in adults in the United States is estimated to be around 2.7%.
   i. Estimated prevalence of BPPV is 1.6% and that of Ménière's disease is 0.2% to 0.5%.
C. In 2012, the Barany Society defined diagnostic criteria for vestibular migraine and probable vestibular migraine (Table 14-8).
D. Endophenotypes of vestibular migraine
   i. Long duration of attacks
   ii. Absence of migraine headaches and cochlear symptoms during the attacks
   iii. Presence of cochlear symptoms (ear fullness, hearing loss, tinnitus) during the vestibular episodes
   iv. Presence of cochlear symptoms and migraine headaches during the episodes
   v. Presence of migraine headaches but no cochlear symptoms during the episodes
E. Migraine with brain stem aura (formerly called vertebrobasilar migraine) is slightly different from vestibular migraine. The criteria determined by the International Classification of Headache Disorders, third edition are followed.
   i. Episodes of migraine fulfilling the ICHD-3 criteria for migraine with aura and criterion B below

Table 14-8 Vestibular Migraine Diagnostic Criteria

Vestibular Migraine	*Probable Vestibular Migraine*
A. At least five episodes with vestibular symptoms of moderate or severe intensity, lasting 5 minutes to 72 hours	A. At least five episodes with vestibular symptoms of moderate or severe intensity, lasting 5 minutes to 72 hours
B. Current or previous history of migraine with or without aura according to the International Classification of Headache Disorders (ICHD)	B. Only one of the criteria B and C for vestibular migraine is fulfilled (migraine history or migraine features during the episode)
C. One or more migraine features with at least 50% of the vestibular episodes: 1. headache with at least two of the following characteristics: one-sided location, pulsating quality, moderate or severe pain intensity, aggravation by routine physical activity 2. photophobia and phonophobia 3. visual aura	C. Not better accounted for by another vestibular or ICHD diagnosis
D. Not better accounted for by another vestibular or ICHD diagnosis	

- ii. Auras with both of the following:
  - a. At least two of the following fully reversible brainstem symptoms
    1. Dysarthria
    2. Vertigo
    3. Tinnitus
    4. Hypoacusis
    5. Diplopia
    6. Ataxia not attributable to sensory deficit
    7. Decreased level of consciousness (Glasgow Coma scale ≤ 13)
  - b. No motor or retinal symptoms

F. Migraine with aura ICHD-3 criteria consist of the following:
- i. A. At least two attacks fulfilling criteria B and C
- ii. B. One or more of the following fully reversible aural symptoms: visual, sensory, speech and/or language, motor, brain stem, retinal
- iii. At least three of the following six characteristics
  - a. At least one aural symptom spreads gradually over more than 5 minutes
  - b. Two or more aura symptoms occur in succession
  - c. Each individual aura symptom lasts 5 to 60 minutes
  - d. At least one aura symptom is unilateral
  - e. At least one aura symptom is positive
  - f. The aura is accompanied or followed within 60 minutes by headache
- iv. Not better accounted for by another ICHD-3 diagnosis

G. Associated vestibular comorbidities and atypical presentation
- i. BPPV: Be careful regarding light cupula and positional nystagmus seen in migraine that is not true BPPV.
- ii. Ménière's disease: There is a subset of patients who fulfill both criteria for vestibular migraine and for Ménière's disease.
- iii. Visual vertigo and rocking dizziness are symptoms that have been associated with migraine. See below for motion-modulated oscillatory vertigo and persistent postural perceptual dizziness.
- iv. Nonotologic drop attacks.
- v. Vestibular syncope.

H. Pathophysiology: still uncertain with evidence pointing toward a mixed central and peripheral vestibulopathy picture. Postulated mechanisms:
- i. Activation and sensitization of the nociceptive brain stem centers cause the headaches.
- ii. Dizziness and spatial disorientation from hyperactivity within the thalamocortical network.
- iii. VOR dysfunction or vestibular hypersensitivity with migraine features may result from the altered activity of the vestibular system.
- iv. Neuroinflammation in the labyrinth due to alteration to the trigeminovascular system.

I. Treatment
- i. Lifestyle modification including dietary changes, identifying triggers
- ii. Blue light blockers which help with subjects who are very photosensitive or whose symptoms can be triggered by visual stimulation
- iii. Optimize sleep and screen for sleep disorders including sleep apnea
- iv. Stress management as needed
- v. Abortive treatment during episodes:
  - a. Consider triptans or the newer gepants for headaches
  - b. Consider promethazine, antihistamines, benzodiazepines for the vertigo symptoms

Table 14-9 General Guidelines Regarding First-Line Treatment for Vestibular Migraine

Medication	*Target Population for First Line*
Beta-blocker	Young male patient *Caution with asthma and diabetes*
Topiramate	Young female patient *Caution with kidney stones*
Tricyclic	Older patients paradoxically *Caution with dementia/BPH*
SNRI (venlafaxine)	Any age *Caution with blood thinners and hypertension* *Can cause insomnia (5%)*
Calcium channel blockers	Good as a second line except for familial hemiplegic migraine

vi. Preventive treatment: typically initiated when patients are having more than episode a week. See Tables 14-9 and 14-10:
   a. Nutraceuticals: magnesium, riboflavin, coenzyme Q10
   b. Tricyclic antidepressants
   c. Selective serotonin reuptake inhibitors and serotonin and norepinephrine reuptake inhibitors

Table 14-10 Pharmacologic Treatment of VM (Medication, Dose, and Side Effects)

Medication	*Dose*	*Side Effects*	*Rationale*
Nortriptyline	20-50 mg qhs	Dry mouth, constipation, grogginess, weight gain	Use if sleep disorder and if significant motion sensitivity due to anticholinergic effect
Propranolol	120-240 mg/day	Fatigue, mood change, decreased libido	Avoid in asthma. Consider in patients with anxiety, essential tremor but also hypertension
Topiramate	25-200 mg/day	Fatigue, cognitive dysfunction (newer formulations have fewer side effects), closed-angle glaucoma (rare), decreased appetite	Consider in overweight patients or if there is a suspicion of increased intracranial hypertension
Venlafaxine	37.5-75 mg qd	Fatigue, nausea, insomnia, weight gain, hypertension, GI issues (rare serotonin syndrome)	Consider if significant anxiety
Riboflavin	400 mg/day	-	
Magnesium oxide or other equivalent supplements	400-800 mg/day	GI issues	
Feverfew	50-300 mg q12h	-	
Coenzyme Q10	100 mg per day		

d. Antiseizure medications
e. Beta-blockers
f. Calcium channel blockers
g. Monoclonal antibodies anti-CGRP (approved for migraine headaches at this time)
    1. One randomized clinical trial showed some benefit for monthly galcanezumab injections in controlling symptoms of vestibular migraine
h. Botox according to the PREEMPT protocol for the headaches if patient fulfills criteria of chronic migraine

vii. Avoid vestibular rehabilitation in uncontrolled vestibular migraine patients, especially VOR rehab. Can consider motion desensitization protocols including grounding strategies and sensory retraining protocols. Vestibular rehabilitation will also help treat comorbidities such as BPPV.

Recurrent Vestibulopathy Not Otherwise Specified

A. Long thought to be a transitional state toward Ménière's disease or vestibular migraine.
B. Majority of patients have good clinical course with infrequent attacks and limited disability.
C. Long-term follow-up in rare cohorts does not show clear-cut progression toward Ménière's disease or vestibular migraine in the vast majority of subjects.
D. Symptomatic treatment and continued close observation are recommended.

Persistent Postural Perceptual Dizziness

A. Cause of chronic dizziness that is due to maladaptation following a vestibular or non-vestibular illness or psychological distress
B. Can coexist with other vestibular conditions with 25% of patients fulfilling criteria for vestibular migraine
C. Barany Society criteria are listed below:
    i. One or more symptoms of dizziness, unsteadiness, or nonspinning vertigo are present on most days for 3 months or more. Symptoms may wax and wane and do not need to be continuous.
    ii. Persistent symptoms occur without specific provocation but are exacerbated by three factors:
        a. Upright posture
        b. Active or passive motion without regard to direction or position, and,
        c. Exposure to moving visual stimuli or complex visual patterns
    iii. The disorder is precipitated by conditions that cause vertigo, unsteadiness, dizziness, or problems with balance including acute, episodic, or chronic vestibular syndromes, other neurologic or medical illnesses, or psychological distress.
        a. When the precipitant is an acute or episodic condition, symptoms settle into the pattern of criterion A as the precipitant resolves, but they may occur intermittently at first, and then consolidate into a persistent course.
        b. When the precipitant is a chronic syndrome, symptoms may develop slowly at first and worsen gradually.

   iv. Symptoms cause significant distress or functional impairment.
   v. Not better accounted for by another diagnosis.

D. www.neurosymptoms.org contains helpful publicly available information regarding PPPD.
E. PPPD patients describe symptoms of dissociation such as head floating and brain fog.
F. They may develop cervical stiffness and pain and headaches secondary to reduction of their head movement.
G. They can develop fatigue and deconditioning.
H. They can develop anxiety.
I. Treatment includes:
   i. SSRI/SNRI to reduce the brain hypersensitivity that is responsible for most symptoms.
   ii. Physical therapy to work on reconditioning and grounding, and sensory retraining but also on neck stiffness.
   iii. Cognitive behavioral therapy is used in cases where there is significant anxiety.

Mal de Debarquement

A. Chronic rocking dizziness that happens following passive motion exposure: typically internal oscillatory symptoms and rarely external.
B. Central maladaptive dysregulation of the VOR.
C. Functional MRI findings suggest long-range cortical, insular, limbic, and cerebellar connectivity changes.
D. It is a type of motion-modulated oscillatory vertigo (MMOV).
E. PPPD is also a type of MMOV.
F. Nonmotion triggered (NmMMOV) that occurs spontaneously without exposure to passive motion has a strong association with migraine.
G. Clinical exam is normal.
H. Vestibular function testing is either normal or noncontributory.
I. Treatment:
   i. Physical therapy to desensitize to readapt the VOR.
   ii. Psychotropic medications including SNRI/SSRI, benzodiazepines have been used with no great evidence for either.
J. Barany Society criteria for diagnosis of MDDS
   i. Nonspinning vertigo characterized by an oscillatory perception ("rocking," "bobbing," or "swaying") present continuously or for most of the day.
   ii. Onset occurs within 48 hours after the end of exposure to passive motion.
   iii. Symptoms temporarily reduce with exposure to passive motion.
   iv. Symptoms continue for greater than 48 hours.
      a. MDDS in evolution: symptoms are ongoing but the observation period has been less than 1 month.
      b. Transient MDDS: symptoms resolve at or before 1 month and the observation period extends at least to the resolution point.
      c. Persistent MDDS: symptoms last for more than 1 month.
   v. Symptoms not better accounted for by another disease or disorder.
K. The two other entities that have similar features to MDDS include PPPD and Mmmov.
   i. Hypersensitivity to complex visual motion stimuli may occur in NmMMOV and MDDS but is a defining feature in PPPD.
   ii. Motion exposure is not a precipitant in NmMMOV and PPPD.

iii. Passive motion improves symptoms in MDDS and NmMMOV but worsens symptoms in PPPD.
iv. Upright posture aggravates symptoms in all three entities.
v. Physical therapy has a less predictable response in NmMMOV and MDDS.

Superior Semicircular Canal Dehiscence Syndrome

A. Superior semicircular canal dehiscence syndrome was described by Minor in 1998.
B. Communication between the middle fossa dura and the superior aspect of the superior SCC.
   i. Thinner bone covering the lateral skull base including over the superior SCC.
   ii. Second hit is typically accepted as inciting event: increased pressure, trauma, labor.
C. Symptoms:
   i. Tullio phenomenon: sound-induced vertigo and oscillopsia
   ii. Valsalva-induced vertigo and oscillopsia
   iii. Hyperacusis
   iv. Autophony
   v. Pulsatile tinnitus
   vi. Sensitivity to internal body noises. Some patients also have a low-frequency conductive hearing loss. In that case, acoustic reflexes are usually preserved in contrast with otosclerosis where stapedial reflexes are absent.
D. Physical exam:
   i. Normal otoscopy.
   ii. Hennebert sign: ipsilateral torsional downbeat nystagmus.
   iii. Nasal Valsalva ("blow air into the ears against pinched nostrils") ipsilateral torsional downbeat nystagmus.
   iv. Glottic Valsalva contralateral torsional downbeat nystagmus.
   v. Release of Glottic Valsalva: ipsilateral torsional downbeat nystagmus.
   vi. Presentation of pure tones from 125 to 4000 kHz via headphones: ipsilateral torsional downbeat nystagmus.
   vii. Positional downbeat nystagmus similar to a superior canal BPPV can be seen due to unplugging of the canal, without reversal of nystagmus upon sitting up.
   viii. Skull base vibration induced nystagmus at 100 Hz with horizontal nystagmus beating toward the affected ear. At 500 Hz mastoid vibration can cause an excitatory torsional vertigo nystagmus in the plane of the affected SSCD.
   ix. Weber lateralizes to the ipsilateral ear even when placed on the medial malleolus in some cases.
E. Audiometric and vestibular function tests
   i. Low-frequency conductive hearing loss with suprathreshold bone line
   ii. Normal stapedial reflexes and tympanograms
   iii. 500 Hz air-conducted stimulus cervical VEMPs show responses at lower thresholds of 65 dB
   iv. Increased amplitude of ipsilateral ocular VEMPs using 500 Hz air conduction stimuli or bone conduction vibration
   v. Electrocochleography shows increased SP/AP
F. Diagnosis of superior semicircular canal dehiscence syndrome requires:
   i. Third window symptoms
   ii. Electrophysiologic third window: VEMPs or ECochG

iii. High-resolution temporal bone CT scan in the parasagittal planes showing the dehiscence

G. Treatment
   i. Resurfacing
      a. Middle fossa
      b. Transmastoid
   ii. Plugging
      a. Middle fossa
      b. Transmastoid
   iii. Plugging typically has better outcomes and lower risk of recurrence than resurfacing regardless of the approach (transmastoid versus middle fossa). Plugging carries a slightly higher risk of hearing loss and postoperative reduction in vestibular function.
   iv. Round window plugging.

Other Third Window Syndromes

A. Posterior canal dehiscence: much rarer than SSCD
   i. Often asymptomatic
   ii. Can present with third window symptomatology
   iii. Can be associated with sudden hearing loss and delayed hydrops picture due to proximity of the vestibular aqueduct and the intracranial pressure on exposed membranous labyrinth

B. Horizontal canal dehiscence typically seen in the setting of cholesteatoma or is iatrogenic

C. Enlarged Vestibular aqueduct: associated with syndromic and nonsyndromic causes of congenital hearing loss.
   i. Vestibular symptoms are more subtle and typically start occurring in the second decade of life.
   ii. Always check thyroid levels to rule out Pendred syndrome.

D. Traumatic perilymphatic fistula:
   i. Mechanisms: barotrauma, penetrating trauma (qtip), surgical/iatrogenic trauma, physical exertion
   ii. Range of symptoms from episodic to continuous along with Tullio phenomenon and Valsalva-induced symptoms as well as variable fluctuating or significant hearing loss
   iii. Physical exam findings
      a. Positive Hennebert sign/positive fistula sign slow deviation of the eyes away from the stimulated ear with a few fast phase beats toward the ear

E. Audiometric assessment

F. Treatment
   i. Conservative with bed rest, head elevation, avoiding increasing intracranial pressure (laxatives, antitussives)
   ii. Surgical exploration and plugging of round window and oval window if symptoms persist or hearing worsens

G. Vestibular atelectasis
   i. Combination of third window (sound and pressure induced) vertigo or nystagmus and bilateral vestibulopathy.
   ii. Collapse of the membranous labyrinth is the cause: calorics can be absent or show weakness with preserved high-frequency function measured by videoHIT. There is no functional loss of hair cells but mechanical impediment of signal transduction.

iii. Third window symptoms are due to contact of collapsed membranous labyrinth with stapes footplate.
iv. Treatment:
a. Conservative
b. Physical therapy for the bilateral vestibular hypofunction
c. Intratympanic gentamicin in debilitating cases with significant vestibular hypofunction

H. Otosyphylis
i. Manifestation of congenital syphilis or tertiary syphilis.
ii. Has been reported in secondary syphilis.
iii. Hennebert sign was first described in otosyphylis with gummatous lesions of the membranous labyrinth creating synechia between the vestibule and the stapes footplate.
iv. High index of suspicion is necessary.
v. If patient tests positive, rule out other STDs including HIV.
vi. Treatment consists of symptomatic treatment as well as antimicrobial treatment.

Vestibular Paroxysmia

A. Short spontaneous episodes of vertigo lasting seconds and typically less than a minute, and may occur up to 100 times per day. Some episodes can be triggered by head movement.
B. Staccato-like tinnitus/typewriter tinnitus may be associated with it.
C. Thought to be due to a focal demyelination of the vestibular nerve at the level of the brain stem/root entry zone/cisternal portion.
D. Physical exam:
i. Unlikely to observe during clinic visit but typical finding is a horizontal rotatory irritative nystagmus toward the affected ear
ii. Hyperventilation for 3 minutes can trigger a similar nystagmus
iii. Variable findings on vestibular testing: hyperresponsive labyrinth as well as hypofunction
E. Imaging: presence of neurovascular conflict is very sensitive but is not a diagnostic criterion because a lot of patients with the neurovascular conflict on MRI are asymptomatic.
F. Treatment is part of the diagnostic algorithm and response to treatment by a sodium channel blocker is part of the Barany Society criteria.
i. Carbamazepine 200 to 800 mg po per day
ii. Oxcarbazepine 300 to 900 mg po per day
iii. Major side effects of the above include drowsiness and hyponatremia
iv. Lacosamide is a third option
v. Microvascular decompression: has fallen out of favor

Controversial Causes of Vertigo

A. Cervicogenic dizziness
i. No evidence of impairment of neck proprioception specifically associated with symptoms of vertigo or dizziness.
ii. Almost every vestibular condition can be associated with head motion sensitivity and increase in neck muscle tension.

iii. Vestibular migraine is by the far the most common cause of a combination of neck pain and vestibular symptoms.
iv. Theoretical prospects: cervical pain may elicit vasovagal and cardioinhibitory reflexes which can cause symptoms of spatial disorientation or imbalance.

B. Spontaneous perilymphatic fistula
i. Similar symptoms to traumatic perilymphatic fistula without inciting traumatic event.
ii. Ménière's disease patients can report short pressure or noise-induced vertigo sensations related to the hydrops of the membranous labyrinth (saccule) coming into contact with the stapes footplate.
iii. May be overdiagnosed.
iv. Surgical exploration has been advocated with plugging of the oval window and round window niches.

Central Vestibular Disorders

A. Anatomical topography of the lesion typically divides vestibular disorders into peripheral (labyrinthine and vestibular nerve disorder affecting first- and second-order neurons) and central (upstream from the vestibular nuclei).

B. Some central lesions can cause a pseudovestibular neuronitis picture such as a multiple sclerosis lesion in the pons within one of the vestibular nuclei, or a ponto-medullary infarction affecting the anterior inferior cerebellar artery (AICA). Other neurologic symptoms typically are a giveaway but the head impulse test can be positive suggesting a vestibular deafferentation.

C. The vestibular network gets integrated in the cognitive functions within the cortex and the hippocampal and limbic system.
i. Multisensory motion perception, attention, spatial memory and navigation are examples of higher vestibular function.

D. Higher vestibular dysfunction can be related to a cortical lesion or subcortical lesions in the vestibular pathways. Cognitive dysfunction related to a peripheral vestibular disorder is also a type of higher vestibular dysfunction.
i. Room tilt illusion: spinning vertigo followed by rapid or gradual return/uprighting. Seen in lower brain stem infarctions or in cases of vestibular epilepsy
ii. Bilateral vestibular hypofunction patients have oscillopsia, postural instability, and have deficits of spatial memory and navigation, and hippocampal atrophy. There are no deficits of nonspatial memory.

E. Other examples of central vestibular disorders
i. Disorders associated with cortical lesions
a. Cortical vertigo
b. Pusher syndrome
c. Room tilt illusion
d. Spatial hemineglect
e. Spatial memory deficits
f. Vestibular epilepsy

F. Disorders associated with thalamic lesion
a. Thalamic astasia
b. Pusher syndrome

G. Disorders associated with brainstem lesions

a. Lateropulsion
b. Ocular tilt reaction
c. Paroxysmal ataxia/dysarthria
d. Pseudoneuritis
e. Room tilt illusion
f. Skew-torsion
g. Vestibular migraine

H. Disorders associated with cerebellar lesions

a. Downbeat nystagmus
b. Episodic ataxia type 2
c. Ocular tilt reaction
d. Positional vertigo/Positional nystagmus
e. Pseudovestibular neuronitis
f. Upbeat nystagmus

Bibliography

Basura GJ, Adams ME, Monfared A, et al. Clinical Practice Guideline: Ménière's Disease. *Otolaryngol Head Neck Surg*. 2020;162(2_suppl):S1-S55.

Brandt T, Strupp M, Dieterich M. Towards a concept of disorders of "higher vestibular function". *Front Integr Neurosci*. 2014;8:47.

Dlugaiczyk J. Rare disorders of the vestibular labyrinth: of Zebras, Chameleons and Wolves in Sheep's Clothing. Seltene Erkrankungen des vestibulären Labyrinths: von Zebras, Chamäleons und Wölfen im Schafspelz. *Laryngorhinootologie*. 2021;100(S01):S1-S40.

Goebel JA, ed. *Practical Management of the Dizzy Patient*. 2nd ed. Philadelphia, PA: Lippincott; 2008:137-152.

ICVD Consensus Documents - The Barany Society. The Barany Society. https://www.thebaranysociety.org/icvd-consensus-documents/

Clinical Vignette

A 56-year-old female patient presents to your clinic 6 months after the onset of dizziness and disequilibrium. Eight months before the onset of these symptoms, she had a severe episode of vertigo lasting 3 to 4 days and she was off-balance for a few weeks following that. While her initial complaint improved, she developed another type of dizziness, where she would feel lightheaded as well as disoriented when she is moving or sitting upright. She does have discrete episodes of vertigo, rapid heartbeat, faintness, cold sweats with anxiety and wonders if she is having panic attacks. Her episodes are present most of the day and she notes that she is swimmy headed and has a brain fog most of the day as well. She does describe a history of migraines and has 2 to 3 migraine headaches a month. She also describes circumoral paresthesias and electric-like shock sensation in her scalp (allodynia) that happens sporadically. Furthermore, she feels that laying down improves most of her symptoms but any movement of herself or around her will trigger her symptoms again. She also avoids going over bridges or into crowded places because visually busy environments make her worse.

On physical exam, she has no localizing signs, and her vestibular exam is normal except for excessive sway on modified Romberg.

MRI comes back normal. Vestibular functional tests were not completed due to excessive discomfort.

The above vignette is a classic case of PPPD. While patient has migraines as well, there is no clear indication of vestibular migraine. The inciting event was most likely a neuronitis that caused a maladaptive strategy at the level of the CNS.

Questions

1. A 34-year-old female patient presents with a complaint of recurrent positional vertigo. Her current symptoms started a week ago and she has daily positional vertigo lasting 10 seconds every time she looks up or lies in bed. On physical exam, the Dix-Hallpike maneuver shows an upbeat torsional geotropic nystagmus on the left side with a latency of 2 seconds and duration of ten seconds. Which part of the inner ear is stimulated to explain the nystagmus and which structure in the ear is the origin of the stimulus?
   A. Posterior canal ampulla; otolith from the utricle
   B. Lateral canal ampulla; otolith from the saccule
   C. Posterior canal ampulla; otolith from the saccule
   D. Lateral canal ampulla; otolith from the utricle

2. What type of symptoms would not be caused by an otolith dysfunction?
   A. Sensation of falling
   B. Chronic rocking dizziness
   C. Oscillopsia
   D. Drop attack
   E. Imbalance

3. A 50-year-old female patient presents with a 2-day history of external vertigo that started two weeks after a upper respiratory tract infection (URI). She has had continued spinning sensation with nausea and vomiting, and has only started to feel somewhat better but is still very off-balance. On physical exam, she has a left beating nystagmus in all directions of gaze, stronger when her gaze is to the left. Which important vestibular physiologic law does this illustrate?
   A. Ewald first and third laws
   B. Ewald second law
   C. Alexander law
   D. Barany law
   E. Flourens law

4. A 40-year-old male patient with a 2-year history of dizziness and imbalance that is mostly triggered by noise and coughing and lifting heavy objects. It lasts only a few seconds. He also complains of right autophony for the past few months. Physical exam is totally normal except for an ankle Weber lateralizes to the right. His audiogram shows a low-frequency conductive hearing loss in the right ear. What is the next best diagnostic exam?
   A. CT scan temporal bone
   B. Ocular vestibular evoked myogenic potential
   C. MRI of the brain with posterior fossa exam
   D. Syphilis IgG
   E. Videohead impulse test

5. A 47-year-old male patient with episodes of vertigo lasting 30 minutes to 2 hours associated with right aural fullness and right tinnitus. He has fluctuating hearing loss in his right ear between the episodes. He does have a history of migraines. He denies current migraines. He denies photophobia, phonophobia with the episodes but does have frontal throbbing headaches with the episodes. His clinical exam is unremarkable. His audiogram shows a mild low-frequency hearing loss with a threshold of 30 dB on 250 Hz and 500 Hz but otherwise normal. His episodes occur 2 to 3 times a month. Which of the following is an appropriate treatment for this patient?
   A. Low salt diet
   B. Migraine diet
   C. Lifestyle modification and intratympanic steroid injections
   D. Endolymphatic sac decompression
   E. Propranolol 120 mg bid

Chapter 15
Congenital Hearing Loss

Introduction

a. Deafness is the most common sensory defect (1 in 1000-2000 births; there are roughly 4 million births in the United States per year).
b. Early identification allows appropriate intervention as soon as indicated.
c. Fifty percent of congenital hearing loss is due to nongenetic factors.
   i. Environmental (25% of all congenital hearing loss cases)
      1. Infections (TORCH)
      2. Ototoxicity
      3. Prematurity
      4. Extracorporeal membrane oxygenation (ECMO)
      5. Hypoxia
   ii. Idiopathic (25% of all congenital hearing loss cases)
d. Fifty percent of congenital hearing loss is due to genetic factors.
   i. Seventy percent of genetic cases are nonsyndromic.
      1. Seventy-five percent to 80% of nonsyndromic deafness is inherited through autosomal recessive (AR) patterns.
      2. Eighteen percent to 20% of nonsyndromic deafness is inherited through autosomal dominant (AD) patterns.
      3. One percent to 3% of nonsyndromic deafness is classified as X-linked, or chromosomal disorders.
   ii. Thirty percent of genetic cases are syndromic.
      1. The majority of these cases are passed on through AR or X-linked inheritance.

Environmental Factors

Infections

Toxoplasmosis

- Organism: Protozoan parasite *Toxoplasma gondii*
- Epidemiology: In United States, around 1/10,000 births
- Primary infection: Occurs through ingestion of oocytes and ova. Common sources include consuming undercooked meat or the handling of contaminated soil, water, and cat feces.
- Infant transmission: vertical transmission or primary infection in neonatal period.

- Symptoms: Asymptomatic in majority of patients. If symptomatic, triad includes (a) chorioretinitis, (b) hydrocephalus, and (c) intracranial calcifications.
- Diagnostics:
  - Serology: IgM and IgG antibody tests
  - CSF studies: microscopic visualization of parasite
  - Amniocentesis: PCR
- Cochlear histopathology: encysted organisms within the inner ear causing tissue necrosis and inflammatory changes.
- Treatment: Pyrimethamine and sulfadiazine; treatment is capable of preventing hearing loss.

Rubella

- Organism: Togavirus
- Epidemiology: In vaccine era, rubella incidence below 1 per 1,000,000 births. Congenital rubella syndrome (CRS) incidence below 1case per 5,000,000 births
- Primary infection: Aerosol
- Symptom (CRS): congenital cataract, cardiovascular anomalies, mental retardation, retinitis, SNHL
- Infant transmission: vertical transmission or primary infection in neonatal period
- Diagnostics: PCR identification of IgG and IgM
- Cochlear pathology: degeneration of the organ of Corti, adhesion between the organ of Corti and Reissner membrane, rolled-up tectorial membrane, cochlea–saccule degeneration
- Treatment: supportive care

Cytomegalovirus (CMV)

- Organism: β-herpesvirus
- Epidemiology: the most common viral cause of congenital sensorineural hearing loss (SNHL). Congenital CMV (cCMV) affects up to 3% of all newborns. Eighty-percent to 90% of infants with congenital cCMV are asymptomatic at birth. As many as 15% of these infants will develop late sequelae.
- Primary infection: direct contact with urine, blood, or bodily fluids.
- Infant transmission: vertical transmission or primary neonatal infection.
- Symptom: microcephaly, intrauterine growth restriction, hepatosplenomegaly, chorioretinitis, jaundice, petechiae, thrombocytopenia, hyperbilirubinemia, SNHL
- Prevention: CMV hyperimmunoglobulin in pregnant women with primary CMV
- Diagnostics:
  - Prenatal: Greater than 21 weeks of gestation and greater than 6 weeks after infection → Nucleic acid PCR
  - Neonate: Less than 3 weeks → PCR of saliva, urine, or both
- Cochlear pathology: atrophy of the stria vascularis
- Treatment:
  - Symptomatic: 6 months of valganciclovir and hearing screens every 6 months for 3 years, then annually for additional 2 to 3 years
  - Asymptomatic: no treatment; continued audiometric screening
  - Asymptomatic with mild SNHL: no treatment; continued audiometric screening

Herpes Simplex Virus (HSV)

- Organism: HSV-1 and HSV-2; Herpesviridae
- Epidemiology: 1/3200 births

- Primary infection: contact
- Symptom: skin, eye, and mucous membrane lesions, CNS disease (seizures, spasticity, blindness, learning disabilities), constitutional symptoms
- Infant transmission: 85% peripartum; 10% postnatal; 5% in-utero
- Diagnostics: Screening not recommended; if infection suspected, then direct viral culture from blood or lesion.
- Treatment:
  - Skin, eye, mucous membranes: intravenous acyclovir for 14 days
  - CNS or disseminated disease: intravenous acyclovir for 21 days

Syphilis

- Organism: *Treponema pallidum*, gram-negative spirochete
- Epidemiology:
  - Tamari and Itkin estimated that hearing loss occurred in
    - Seventeen percent of congenital syphilis
    - Twenty-five percent of late latent syphilis
    - Twenty-nine percent of asymptomatic patients with congenital syphilis
    - Thirty-nine percent of symptomatic neurosyphilis
  - Karmody and Schuknecht estimated hearing loss occurred in up to 38%
- Primary infection: contact
- Symptoms:
  - Early (infantile): Severe and bilateral SNHL. These children usually have multisystem involvement and hence a fatal outcome.
  - Late (Tarditive): Progressive SNHL of varying severity and time of onset. Hearing losses that have their onset during early childhood are usually bilateral, sudden, severe, and associated with vestibular symptoms. The symptom complex is similar to that of Méniére disease. The late-onset form (sometimes as late as the fifth decade of life) has mild hearing loss.
- Infant transmission: vertical
- Diagnostics: histologic exam of placenta for spirochetes; in high-risk clinical scenarios (a) long bone radiographic exam; (b) lumbar puncture for cell count, protein, and VDRL
- Cochlear histopathology: Osteitis with round cell infiltration is noticed. With tertiary syphilis, gummatous lesions may involve the auricle, mastoid, middle ear, and petrous pyramid.
- Treatment: Steroids and penicillin
- Other: Two clinic signs are associated with congenital syphilis that deserve special mention: Hennebert sign and Tulio phenomenon. Hennebert sign consists of a positive fistula test without clinical evidence of middle ear or mastoid disease or a fistula. It has been postulated that the vestibular stimulation is mediated by fibrous bands between the footplate and the vestibular membranous labyrinth. Hennebert sign may also be present in Méniére disease. Another explanation is that the vestibular response is due to an excessively mobile footplate. The nystagmus in Hennebert sign is usually more marked on application of a negative pressure.

Tullio phenomenon consists of vertigo and nystagmus on stimulation with high-intensity sound, such as the Bárány noise box. This phenomenon occurs not only in congenital syphilis but also in patients with a semicircular canal fistula or dehiscence and in postfenestration patients if the footplate is mobile and the fenestrum patent. It can also be demonstrated in chronic otitis media should the patient have an intact tympanic membrane, ossicular chain, and a fistula—a rare combination.

For Tullio phenomenon to take place, a fistula of the semicircular canal and intact sound transmission mechanism to the inner ear (ie, intact tympanic membrane, intact ossicular chain, and mobile footplate) must be present. The pathophysiology is that the high-intensity noise energy transmitted through the footplate finds the course of least resistance and displaces toward the fistula instead of the round window membrane.

Other Infectious Etiologies

- **Zika virus:** A flavivirus transmitted by mosquitoes. Associated with microcephaly and SNHL.
- **Human immunodeficiency virus (HIV):** Can present with either conductive hearing loss from otitis media or SNHL secondary to opportunistic infection.

Ototoxicity

- Medications: aminoglycosides, chemotherapeutics, loop diuretics
- Predisposing factors: prematurity, diabetes, genetics
  - Mitochondrial gene mutation predisposes patients to aminoglycoside ototoxicity. Mutation occurs on 12S ribosomal RNA; 1555A>G.

Hypothyroidism

- Cretinism consists of retarded growth, mental retardation, and mixed hearing loss
- Seen in conjunction with congenital deafness.

Kernicterus

- Twenty percent of kernicteric babies have severe deafness secondary to damage to the dorsal and ventral cochlear nuclei and the superior and inferior colliculi nuclei.
- High-frequency hearing loss occurs.
- Indication for exchange transfusion is usually a serum bilirubin greater than 20 mg/dL.

Genetic Factors

Note: The genetic nomenclature for inheritable hearing loss follows a standardized methodology. Specific gene loci implicated in the development of congenital hearing loss are labeled DFN—for "DeaFNess." The loci are subcategorized to reflect their inheritance pattern: DFNA signifies AD inheritance, while DFNB signifies an AR inheritance. The number behind this notation reflects the sequential order of discovery within each gene locus family. For instance, DFNA1 was the first DFNA locus discovered, DFNA2 the second, etc. It should be noted that the DFN nomenclature solely reflects the pattern of inheritance for that particular locus and does not indicate if the corresponding phenotype is syndromic or non-syndromic. Furthermore, unique gene variances allow individual genes to be inherited in either AD or recessive fashion. For this reason, certain genes will be given both DFNB and DFNA distinctions.

Nonsyndromic

- Seventy percent of genetic hearing loss.
- AR inheritance is the most common form (~80%).
  - Gene loci nomenclature: DFNB
  - At least 30 loci identified

- Notable loci
  - DFNB1
    - ◊ Chromosome 13q12
    - ◊ Protein: GJB2 (gap junction beta 2)/connexin 26 GJB6/connexin 30
    - ◊ Function: transmembrane protein subunit of intercellular gap junctions. Facilitates transfer of proteins, ions, and signaling molecules between adjoining cells
    - ◊ Other: most common AR inherited cause of genetic hearing loss. Accounts for almost 50% of patients with nonsyndromic deafness and as many as 40% of all hearing loss cases
  - DFNB2
    - ◊ Chromosome 11q13
    - ◊ Protein: MYO7A
    - ◊ Function: expressed only in the Organ of Corti. Bridges the stereocilia to the extracellular matrix

- AD next most common (~20%)
  - Gene loci nomenclature: DFNA
  - 40 loci identified
  - Examples
    - DFNA1
      - ◊ Chromosome: 5q31
      - ◊ Protein: DIAPH
      - ◊ Function: regulation of actin polymerization in hair cells of the inner ear

- X-linked next most common form (1-3%)
  - Gene loci nomenclature: DFNX
  - Seven loci identified

Syndromic

- 30% of genetic hearing loss

More Common Autosomal Dominant Syndromic Disorders

Branchio-Oto-Renal Syndrome

Branchio-oto-renal syndrome is estimated to occur in 2% of children with congenital hearing impairment. The syndrome involves branchial characteristics including ear pits and tags or cervical fistula, and renal involvement ranging from agenesis and renal failure to minor dysplasia. Seventy-five percent of patients with branchio-oto-renal syndrome have significant hearing loss. Of these, 30% are conductive, 20% are sensorineural, and 50% demonstrate mixed forms. Mutations in *EYA1,* a gene of 16 exons within a genomic interval of 156 kB, have been shown to cause the syndrome. The encoded protein is a transcriptional activator. The gene has been located on chromosome 8q.

Neurofibromatosis

Neurofibromatosis (NF) presents with café-au-lait spots and multiple fibromas. Cutaneous tumors are most common, but the central nervous system (CNS), peripheral nerves, and viscera can be involved. Mental retardation, blindness, and sensorineural hearing loss can result from CNS tumors.

Neurofibromatosis is classified as types 1 and 2. NF type 1 is more common with an incidence of about 1:3000 persons. Type 1 generally includes many café-au-lait spots, cutaneous neurofibromas, plexiform neuromas, pseudoarthrosis, Lisch nodules of the iris, and optic gliomas. Acoustic neuromas are usually unilateral and occur in only 5% of affected patients.

Hearing loss can also occur as a consequence of a neurofibroma encroaching on the middle or inner ear, but significant deafness is rare. The expressed phenotype may vary from a few café-au-lait spots to multiple disfiguring neurofibromas. Type 1 is caused by a disruption of the *NF1* gene (a nerve growth factor gene) localized to chromosome 17q11.2.

NF type 2, which is a genetically distinct disorder, is characterized by bilateral acoustic neuromas, café-au-lait spots, and subcapsular cataracts. Bilateral acoustic neuromas are present in 95% of affected patients and are usually asymptomatic until early adulthood. Deletions in the *NF2* gene (a tumor suppressor gene) on chromosome 22q12.2 cause the abnormalities associated with neurofibromatosis type 2. Both types of neurofibromatosis demonstrate AD inheritance with high penetrance but variable expressivity. High mutation rates are characteristic of both types of disorder.

Osteogenesis Imperfecta

Osteogenesis imperfecta is characterized by bone fragility, blue sclera, conductive, mixed, or sensorineural hearing loss, and hyperelasticity of joints and ligaments. This disorder is transmitted as AD disorder with variable expressivity and incomplete penetrance. Two genes for osteogenesis imperfecta have been identified, *COLIA1* on chromosome 17q and *COLIA2* on chromosome 7q. The age at which the more common tarda variety becomes clinically apparent is variable. van der Hoeve syndrome is a subtype in which progressive hearing loss begins in early childhood.

Otosclerosis

Otosclerosis is caused by proliferation of spongy-type tissue on the otic capsule, eventually leading to fixation of the ossicles and producing conductive hearing loss. Hearing loss may begin in childhood, but most often becomes evident in early adulthood and eventually may include a sensorineural component.

Otosclerosis appears to be transmitted in an AD pattern with decreased penetrance, so only 25% to 40% of gene carriers show the phenotype. The greater proportion of affected females points to a possible hormonal influence. Recent statistical studies suggest a role for the gene *COLIA1* in otosclerosis, and measles viral particles have been identified within otosclerotic foci, raising the possibility of an interaction with the viral genome.

Stickler Syndrome

Cleft palate, micrognathia, severe myopia, retinal detachments, cataracts, and marfanoid habitus characterize Stickler syndrome clinically. Significant sensorineural hearing loss or mixed hearing loss is present in about 15% of cases, whereas hearing loss of lesser severity may be present in up to 80% of cases. Ossicular abnormalities may also be present.

Most cases of Stickler syndrome can be attributed to mutations in the *COL2A1* gene found on chromosome 12 that cause premature termination signals for a type II collagen gene. Additionally, changes in the *COL 11A2* gene on chromosome 6 have been found to cause the syndrome.

Treacher Collins Syndrome

Treacher Collins syndrome consists of facial malformations such as malar hypoplasia, downward slanting palpebral fissures, coloboma of the lower eyelids (the upper eyelid is involved in Goldenhar syndrome), hypoplastic mandible, malformations of the external ear or the ear canal, dental malocclusion, and cleft palate. The facial features are bilateral and symmetrical in Treacher Collins syndrome.

Conductive hearing loss is present 30% of the time, but sensorineural hearing loss and vestibular dysfunction can also be present. Ossicular malformations are common in these patients. Inheritance is AD with high penetrance. However, a new mutation can be present in as many as 60% of cases of Treacher Collins syndrome.

The gene responsible for Treacher Collins syndrome is *TCOF1* which is located on chromosome 5q and produces a protein named treacle, which is operative in early craniofacial development. There is considerable variation in expression between and within families, suggesting other genes can modify the expression of the treacle protein.

Waardenburg Syndrome

Waardenburg syndrome (WS) accounts for 3% of childhood hearing impairment and is the most common form of AD congenital deafness. There is a significant amount of variability in expression in this syndrome. There may be unilateral or bilateral sensorineural hearing loss in patients, and the phenotypic expressions may include pigmentary anomalies and craniofacial features. The pigmentary anomalies include: white forelock (20%-30% of cases), heterochromia irides, premature graying, and vitiligo. Craniofacial features that are seen in Waardenburg syndrome include dystopia canthorum, broad nasal root, and synophrys. All of the above features are variable.

There are four different forms of Waardenburg syndrome, which can be distinguished clinically. Type 1 is characterized by congenital sensorineural hearing impairment, heterochromia irides, white forelock, patchy hypopigmentation, and dystopia canthorum. Type 2 is differentiated from type 1 by the absence of dystopia canthorum, whereas type 3 is characterized by microcephaly, skeletal abnormalities, and mental retardation, in addition to the features associated with type 1. The combination of recessively inherited WS type 2 characteristics with Hirschsprung disease has been called Waardenburg-Shah syndrome or WS type 4.

Sensorineural hearing loss is seen in 20% of patients with type 1 and in more than 50% of patients with type 2. Essentially, all cases of type 1 and type 3 are caused by a mutation of the *PAX3* gene on chromosome 2q37. This genetic mutation ultimately results in a defect in neural crest cell migration and development. About 20% of type 2 cases are caused by a mutation of the *MITF* gene (microphthalmia transcription factor) on chromosome 3p. Waardenburg syndrome has also been linked to other genes such as *EDN3*, *EDNRB*, and *SOX10*.

More Common Autosomal Recessive Syndromic Disorders

The most common pattern of transmission of hereditary hearing loss is AR, comprising 80% of cases of hereditary deafness. Half of these cases represent recognizable syndromes.

Jervell and Lange-Nielsen Syndrome Jervell and Lange-Nielsen syndrome is a rare syndrome consisting of profound sensorineural hearing loss and cardiac arrhythmias. The genetic defect is caused by a mutation affecting a potassium channel gene that leads to conduction abnormalities in the heart.

Electrocardiography reveals large T waves and prolongation of the QT interval, which may lead to syncopal episodes as early as the second or third year of life. The cardiac component of this disorder is treated with beta-adrenergic blockers such as propranolol. An electrocardiogram should be performed on all children with early-onset hearing loss of uncertain etiology.

Genetic studies attribute one form of Jervell and Lange-Nielsen syndrome to homozygosity for mutations affecting a potassium channel gene (*KVLQT 1*) on chromosome 11p15.5, which is thought to result in delayed myocellular repolarization in the heart. The gene *KCNE1* has also been shown to be responsible for the disorder.

Pendred Syndrome Pendred syndrome is believed to be the most common syndromic form of congenital deafness. It includes thyroid goiter and profound sensorineural hearing loss. Hearing loss may be progressive in about 10% to 15% of patients. The majority of patients present with bilateral moderate to severe high-frequency sensorineural hearing loss, with some residual hearing in the low frequencies.

The hearing loss is associated with abnormal iodine metabolism (defect in tyrosine iodination) resulting in a euthyroid goiter, which usually becomes clinically detectable at about 8 years of age. The perchlorate discharge test shows abnormal organification of nonorganic iodine in these patients and is needed for definitive diagnosis. Radiological studies reveal that most patients have Mondini aplasia or enlarged vestibular aqueduct.

Mutations in the *PDS* gene, on chromosome 7q31, have been shown to cause this disorder. The *PDS* gene codes for the pendrin protein, which is a sulfate transporter. Recessive inheritance is seen in many families, whereas others show a dominant pattern with variable expression. Treatment of the goiter is with exogenous thyroid hormone.

Usher Syndrome Usher syndrome has a prevalence of 3.5 per 100,000 people; it is the most common type of AR syndromic hearing loss. This syndrome affects about one-half of the 16,000 deaf and blind persons in the United States. It is characterized by sensorineural hearing loss and retinitis pigmentosa (RP). Genetic linkage analysis studies demonstrate three distinct subtypes, distinguishable based on severity or progression of the hearing loss and the extent of vestibular system involvement.

Usher type 1 describes congenital bilateral profound hearing loss and absent vestibular function; type 2 describes moderate hearing losses and normal vestibular function. Patients with type 3 demonstrate progressive hearing loss and variable vestibular dysfunction and are found primarily in the Norwegian population.

Ophthalmologic evaluation is an essential part of the diagnostic workup, and subnormal electroretinographic patterns have been observed in children as young as 2 to 3 years of age, before retinal changes are evident fundoscopically. Early diagnosis of Usher syndrome can have important rehabilitation and educational planning implications for an affected child. These patients may benefit from a cochlear implant.

Linkage analysis studies reveal at least five different genes for type 1 and at least two for type 2. Only type 3 appears to be due to just one gene.

Sex-Linked Disorders

X-linked disorders are rare, accounting for only 1% to 2% of cases of hereditary hearing impairment.

Alport Syndrome Alport syndrome affects the collagen of the basement membranes of the kidneys and the inner ear, resulting in renal failure and progressive sensorineural hearing loss. The renal disease may cause hematuria in infancy, but usually remains asymptomatic for several years before the onset of renal insufficiency. The hearing loss may not become clinically evident until the second decade of life. Dialysis and renal transplantation have proven important therapeutic advances in the treatment of these patients.

COL4A5, which codes for a certain form of type IV collagen, has been identified as the gene locus for this syndrome. Genetic mutation results in fragile type IV collagen in the inner ear and kidney resulting in progressive hearing impairment and kidney disease.

These collagens are found in the basilar membrane, parts of the spiral ligament, and stria vascularis. Although the mechanism of hearing loss is not known, in the glomerulus there is focal thinning and thickening with eventual basement membrane splitting. Assuming a similar process occurs in the ear, it has been suggested that mechanical energy transmission is likely affected by loss of integrity of the basilar and tectorial membranes.

Norrie Syndrome Classic features of Norrie syndrome include specific ocular symptoms (pseudotumor of the retina, retinal hyperplasia, hypoplasia and necrosis of the inner layer of the retina, cataracts, phthisis bulbi), progressive sensorineural hearing loss, and mental disturbance. One-third of the affected patients have onset of progressive sensorineural hearing loss beginning in the second or third decade.

A gene for Norrie syndrome has been localized to chromosome Xp11.4, where studies have revealed deletions involving contiguous genes. A number of families have shown variable deletions in this chromosomal region.

Otopalatodigital Syndrome Otopalatodigital syndrome includes hypertelorism, craniofacial deformity involving supraorbital area, flat midface, small nose, and cleft palate. Patients are short-statured with broad fingers and toes that vary in length, with an excessively wide space between the first and second toe. Conductive hearing loss is seen due to ossicular malformations. Affected males manifest the full spectrum of the disorder, and females may show mild involvement. The gene has been found to be located on chromosome Xq28.

Wildervanck Syndrome Wildervanck syndrome is comprised of the Klippel-Feil sign involving fused cervical vertebrae, sensorineural hearing or mixed hearing impairment, and cranial nerve VI paralysis causing retraction of the eye on lateral gaze. This syndrome is seen most commonly in females because of the high mortality associated with the X-linked dominant form in males. Isolated Klippel-Feil sequence includes hearing impairment in about one-third of cases. The hearing impairment is related to bony malformations of the inner ear.

Mohr-Tranebjaerg Syndrome (DFN-1) DFN-1 is an X-linked recessive syndromic hearing loss characterized by postlingual sensorineural deafness in childhood followed by progressive dystonia, spasticity, dysphagia, and optic atrophy. The syndrome is caused by a mutation thought to result in mitochondrial dysfunction.

It resembles a spinocerebellar degeneration called Friedreich ataxia, which also may exhibit sensorineural hearing loss, ataxia, and optic atrophy. The cardiomyopathy characteristic of Friedreich ataxia is not seen in Mohr-Tranebjaerg.

X-linked Charcot-Marie-Tooth (CMT) X-linked CMT is inherited in a dominant fashion and is caused by a mutation in the connexin 32 gene mapped to the Xq13 locus. Usual clinical signs consist of a peripheral neuropathy combined with foot problems and "champagne bottle" calves. Sensorineural deafness occurs in some.

Multifactorial Genetic Disorders

Some disorders appear to result from a combination of genetic factors interacting with environmental influences. Examples of this type of inheritance associated with hearing loss include clefting syndromes, involving conductive hearing loss, and the microtia/hemifacial microsomia/Goldenhar spectrum.

Goldenhar Syndrome or Oculoauriculovertebral Dysplasia Oculoauriculovertebral dysplasia (OAVD) has an incidence of 1 in 45,000. It includes features such as hemifacial micro, otomandibular dysostosis, epibulbar lipodermoids, coloboma of upper lid, and vertebral anomalies that stem from developmental vascular and genetic field aberrations. It has diverse etiologies and is not attributed to a single genetic locus.

Autosomal Chromosomal Syndromes

Trisomy 13 can have significant sensorineural hearing loss.

Turner syndrome, monosomic for all or part of one X chromosome, presents generally in females as gonadal dysgenesis, short stature, and often a webbed neck or shield chest. They will also have sensorineural, conductive, or mixed hearing loss, which can be progressive and may be the first evidence of the syndrome in prepubertal females.

Mitochondrial Disorders

Hearing loss can occur as an additional symptom in a range of mitochondrial syndromes. A mutation in the mitochondrial genome can affect energy production through adenosine triphosphate (ATP) synthesis and oxidative phosphorylation. Tissues that require high levels of energy are particularly affected. Typically, mitochondrial diseases involve progressive neuromuscular degeneration with ataxia, ophthalmoplegia, and progressive hearing loss.

Disorders such as Kearns-Sayre; mitochondrial encephalopathy, lactic acidosis, and stroke (MELAS); myoclonic epilepsy with ragged red fibers (MERRF); and Leber hereditary optic neuropathy are all mitochondrial disorders. All of these disorders have varying degrees of hearing loss.

Several other mitochondrial mutations have been found to produce enhanced sensitivity to the ototoxic effects of aminoglycosides. Screening for these mutations would be indicated in maternal relatives of persons showing hearing loss in response to normal therapeutic doses of aminoglycosides.

Inner Ear Structural Malformations

By week 9 of gestation, the cochlea reaches adult size (2¾ turns). Arrest in normal development or aberrant development of inner ear structures may result in hearing impairment. Depending on the timing and nature of the developmental insult, a range of inner ear anomalies can result. Computerized temporal bone imaging techniques reveal that about 20% of children with congenital sensorineural hearing loss have subtle or severe abnormalities of the inner ear. About 65% of such abnormalities are bilateral; 35% are unilateral. Based on temporal bone histopathologic studies, inner ear malformations have typically been classified into five different groups.

Michel Aplasia Complete agenesis of the petrous portion of the temporal bone occurs in Michel aplasia, although the external and middle ear may be unaffected. This malformation is thought to result from an insult prior to the end of the third gestational week. Normal inner structures are lacking, resulting in anacusis. Conventional amplification or cochlear implantation offers little assistance. Vibrotactile devices have proven beneficial in some patients. AD inheritance has been observed, but recessive inheritance is also likely.

Mondini Aplasia Mondini aplasia involves a developmentally deformed cochlea in which only the basal coil can be identified clearly. The upper coils assume a cloacal form and the interscalar septum is absent. The endolymphatic duct is also usually enlarged. It is postulated that the deformity results from developmental arrest at approximately the sixth week of gestation because of the underdeveloped vestibular labyrinth. This anomaly can be inherited in an AD fashion and may not be bilateral. It has been described in several other disorders including Pendred, Waardenburg, Treacher Collins, and Wildervanck syndromes. Association of Mondini aplasia with nongenetic etiologies, such as congenital cytomegalovirus (CMV) infection, has been reported. CMV infection may account for more than 40% of deafness of unknown etiology.

A related anomaly and more severe syndrome, the CHARGE association consists of coloboma, heart disease, choanal atresia, retarded development, genital hypoplasia, ear anomalies including hypoplasia of the external ear, and hearing loss. These individuals have a Mondini type deformity and absence of semicircular canals.

Often accompanying the Mondini dysplasia is abnormal communication between the endolymphatic and perilymphatic spaces of the inner ear and subarachnoid space. It is usually caused by a defect in the cribriform area of the lateral end of the internal auditory canal. Presumably because of this abnormal channel, perilymphatic fistulae are more common in this disorder.

The presence of neurosensory structures in most cases warrants an aggressive program of early rehabilitative intervention, including conventional amplification.

Scheibe Aplasia (Cochleosaccular dysplasia or Pars Inferior dysplasia) The bony labyrinth and the superior portion of the membranous labyrinth, including the utricle and semicircular canals, are normally differentiated in patients with Scheibe aplasia. The organ of Corti is generally poorly differentiated with a deformed tectorial membrane and collapsed Reissner membrane, which compromises the scala media. Scheibe aplasia is the most common form of inner ear aplasia and can be inherited as an AR nonsyndromic trait.

The deformity has been reported in temporal bones of patients with Jervell and Lange-Nielsen, Refsum, Usher, and Waardenburg syndromes as well as in congenital rubella infants.

Conventional amplification with rehabilitative intervention is beneficial in many of these children.

Alexander Aplasia In Alexander aplasia, cochlear duct differentiation at the level of the basal coil is limited with resultant effects on the organ of Corti and the ganglion cells. Audiometrically, these patients have a high-frequency hearing loss with adequate residual hearing in the low frequencies to warrant the use of amplification.

Enlarged Vestibular Aqueduct Syndrome An enlarged vestibular aqueduct has been associated with early-onset sensorineural hearing loss, which is usually bilateral and often progressive and may be accompanied by vertigo or incoordination. This abnormality may also accompany cochlear and semicircular canal deformities. The progressive hearing loss is apparently the result of hydrodynamic changes and possibly labyrinthine membrane disruption. Familial cases have been observed, suggesting AD inheritance, but recessive inheritance is also possible. The deformity has also been found in association with Pendred syndrome.

Enlarged vestibular aqueduct syndrome (EVAS) is defined as a vestibular aqueduct measuring 1.5 mm or greater as measured midway between the operculum and the common crus on CT scan. Coronal CT scan is the best view for evaluating it in children. Enlarged vestibular aqueducts can also be seen on high-resolution magnetic resonance imaging (MRI).

EVAS may present as fluctuating sensorineural hearing loss. Conservative management, including avoidance of head trauma and contact sports, has been the mainstay of treatment. Surgery to close the enlarged structure frequently results in significant hearing loss and is not indicated. Patients with EVAS who develop profound hearing loss are suitable cochlear implant candidates.

Semicircular Canal Malformations Formation of the semicircular canals begins in the sixth gestational week. The superior canal is formed first and the lateral canal is formed last. Isolated lateral canal defects are the most commonly identified inner ear malformations on temporal bone imaging studies. Superior semicircular canal deformities are always accompanied by lateral semicircular canal deformities, whereas lateral canal deformities often occur in isolation.

These types of abnormalities account for roughly 20% of congenital deafness. In general, these disorders can be associated with genetic disorders, but more often occur independently.

Hereditary Deafness

Hereditary deafness can also be classified as follows:

A. Hereditary (congenital) deafness without associated abnormalities (AD, AR, or sex linked)
B. Hereditary congenital deafness associated with integumentary system disease (AD, AR, or sex linked)
C. Hereditary congenital deafness associated with skeletal disease (AD, AR, or sex-linked)
D. Hereditary congenital deafness associated with other abnormalities (AD, AR, or sex linked)

Hereditary Deafness Without Associated Abnormalities

Stria Atrophy (Hereditary, Not Congenital)

A. Autosomal dominant.
B. The sensorineural hearing loss begins in middle age and is progressive.
C. Good discrimination is maintained.
D. Flat audiometric curve.
E. Positive short increment sensitivity index (SISI) test.
F. Bilaterally symmetrical hearing loss.
G. Patient never becomes profoundly deaf.

Otosclerosis (Hereditary, Not Congenital)

Described in Chapter 23.

Hereditary Congenital Deafness Associated With Integumentary System Disease

Albinism With Blue Irides

A. Autosomal dominant or recessive
B. Sensorineural hearing loss

Ectodermal Dysplasia (Hidrotic)

Note that anhidrotic ectodermal dysplasia is sex-linked recessive, with a mixed or conductive hearing loss.

A. Autosomal dominant
B. Small dystrophic nails
C. Coniform teeth
D. Elevated sweat electrolytes
E. Sensorineural hearing loss

Forney Syndrome

A. Autosomal dominant
B. Lentigines
C. Mitral insufficiency
D. Skeletal malformations
E. Conductive hearing loss

Lentigines

A. Autosomal dominant
B. Brown spots on the skin, beginning at age 2
C. Ocular hypertelorism

D. Pulmonary stenosis
E. Abnormalities of the genitalia
F. Retarded growth
G. Sensorineural hearing loss

Leopard Syndrome

A. Autosomal dominant with variable penetrance
B. Variable sensorineural hearing loss
C. Ocular hypertelorism
D. Pulmonary stenosis
E. Hypogonadism
F. Electrocardiographic (ECG) changes with widened QRS or bundle branch block
G. Retardation of growth
H. Normal vestibular apparatus
I. Lentigines
J. Skin changes progressively over the first and second decades

Piebaldness

A. Sex linked or autosomal recessive
B. Blue irides
C. Fine retinal pigmentation
D. Depigmentation of scalp, hair, and face
E. Areas of depigmentation on limbs and trunk
F. Sensorineural hearing loss

Tietze Syndrome

A. Autosomal dominant
B. Profound deafness
C. Albinism
D. Eyebrows absent
E. Blue irides
F. No photophobia or nystagmus

Waardenburg Disease (Also Described Earlier)

A. Autosomal dominant with variable penetrance
B. Contributes 1% to 7% of all hereditary deafness
C. Widely spaced medial canthi (present in all cases)
D. Flat nasal root in 75% of cases
E. Confluent eyebrow
F. Sensorineural hearing loss—unilateral or bilateral (present in 20% cases)
G. Colored irides
H. White forelock
I. Areas of depigmentation (10% of the patients)
J. Abnormal tyrosine metabolism
K. Diminished vestibular function (75% of the patients)
L. Cleft lip and palate (10% of the patients)

Hereditary Congenital Deafness Associated With Skeletal Disease

Achondroplasia

A. Autosomal dominant
B. Large head and short extremities
C. Dwarfism
D. Mixed hearing loss (fused ossicles)
E. Saddle nose, frontal and mandibular prominence

Apert Disease (Acrocephalosyndactyly)

A. Autosomal dominant
B. Syndactylia
C. Flat conductive hearing loss secondary to stapes fixation
D. Patent cochlear aqueduct histologically
E. Frontal prominence, exophthalmos
F. Craniofacial dysostosis, hypoplastic maxilla
G. Proptosis, saddle nose, high-arched palate, and occasionally spina bifida
H. Occurs in about 1:150,000 live births

Atresia Auris Congenital

A. Autosomal dominant
B. Unilateral or bilateral involvement
C. Middle ear abnormalities with seventh nerve anomaly
D. Internal hydrocephalus
E. Mental retardation
F. Epilepsy
G. Choanal atresia and cleft palate

Cleidocranial Dysostosis

A. Autosomal dominant
B. Absent or hypoplastic clavicle
C. Failure of fontanelles to close
D. Sensorineural hearing loss

Crouzon Disease (Craniofacial Dysostosis)

A. Autosomal dominant
B. Hearing loss in one-third of cases
C. Mixed hearing loss in some cases
D. Cranial synostosis
E. Exophthalmos and divergent squint
F. Parrot-beaked nose
G. Short upper lip
H. Mandibular prognathism and small maxilla
I. Hypertelorism
J. External auditory canal sometimes atretic

K. Congenital enlargement of the sphenoid bone
L. Premature closure of the cranial suture lines, sometimes leading to mental retardation

Engelmann Syndrome (Diaphyseal Dysplasia)

A. Autosomal dominant; possible recessive
B. Progressive mixed hearing loss
C. Progressive cortical thickening of diaphyseal regions of long bones and skull

Hand–Hearing Syndrome

A. Autosomal dominant
B. Congenital flexion contractures of fingers and toes
C. Sensorineural hearing loss

Klippel-Feil (Brevicollis, Wildervanck) Syndrome

A. Autosomal recessive or dominant
B. Incidence in female subjects greater than in male subjects
C. Sensorineural hearing loss along with middle ear anomalies
D. Short neck due to fused cervical vertebrae
E. Spina bifida
F. External auditory canal atresia

Madelung Deformity (Related to Dyschondrosteosis of Leri-Weill)

A. Autosomal dominant
B. Short stature
C. Ulna and elbow dislocation
D. Conductive hearing loss secondary to ossicular malformation with normal tympanic membrane and external auditory canal
E. Spina bifida occulta
F. Female to male ratio of 4:1

Marfan Syndrome (Arachnodactyly, Ectopia Lentis, Deafness)

A. Autosomal dominant
B. Thin, elongated individuals with long, spidery fingers
C. Pigeon breast
D. Scoliosis
E. Hammer toes
F. Mixed hearing loss

Mohr Syndrome (Oral-Facial-Digital Syndrome II)

A. Autosomal recessive
B. Conductive hearing loss
C. Cleft lip, high-arched palate
D. Lobulated nodular tongue
E. Broad nasal root, bifid tip of nose

F. Hypoplasia of the body of the mandible
G. Polydactyly and syndactyly

Osteopetrosis (Albers-Schonberg Disease, Marble Bone Disease)

A. Autosomal recessive (rare dominant transmission has been reported)
B. Conductive or mixed hearing loss
C. Fluctuating facial nerve paralysis
D. Sclerotic, brittle bone due to failure of resorption of calcified cartilage
E. Cranial nerves II, V, VII involved sometimes
F. Optic atrophy
G. Atresia of paranasal sinuses
H. Choanal atresia
I. Increased incidence of osteomyelitis
J. Widespread form: may lead to obliteration of the bone marrow, severe anemia, and rapid demise
K. Hepatosplenomegaly possible

Oto-Facial-Cervical Syndrome

A. Autosomal dominant
B. Depressed nasal root
C. Protruding narrow nose
D. Narrow elongated face
E. Flattened maxilla and zygoma
F. Prominent ears
G. Preauricular fistulas
H. Poorly developed neck muscles
I. Conductive hearing loss

Oto-Palatal-Digital Syndrome

A. Autosomal recessive
B. Conductive hearing loss
C. Mild dwarfism
D. Cleft palate
E. Mental retardation
F. Broad nasal root, hypertelorism
G. Frontal and occipital bossing
H. Small mandible
I. Stubby, clubbed digits
J. Low-set small ears
K. Winged scapulae
L. Malar flattening
M. Downward obliquity of eye
N. Downturned mouth

Paget Disease (Osteitis Deformans)

A. Autosomal dominant with variable penetrance
B. Mainly sensorineural hearing loss but mixed hearing loss as well

C. Occasional cranial nerve involvement
D. Onset usually at middle age, involving skull and long bones of the legs
E. Endochondral bone (somewhat resistant to this disease)

Pierre Robin Syndrome (Cleft Palate, Micrognathia, and Glossoptosis)

A. Autosomal dominant with variable penetrance (possibly not hereditary but due to intrauterine insult)
B. Occurs in 1:30,000 to 1:50,000 live births
C. Glossoptosis
D. Micrognathia
E. Cleft palate (in 50% of cases)
F. Mixed hearing loss
G. Malformed auricles
H. Mental retardation
I. Hypoplastic mandible
J. Möbius syndrome
K. Subglottic stenosis not uncommon
L. Aspiration a common cause of death

Pyle Disease (Craniometaphyseal Dysplasia)

A. Autosomal dominant (less often autosomal recessive).
B. Conductive hearing loss can begin at any age. It is progressive and secondary to fixation of the stapes or other ossicular abnormalities. Mixed hearing loss also possible.
C. Cranial nerve palsy secondary to narrowing of the foramen.
D. Splayed appearance of long bones.
E. Choanal atresia.
F. Prognathism.
G. Optic atrophy.
H. Obstruction of sinuses and nasolacrimal duct.

Roaf Syndrome

A. Not hereditary
B. Retinal detachment, cataracts, myopia, coxa vara, kyphoscoliosis, retardation
C. Progressive sensorineural hearing loss

Dominant Proximal Symphalangia and Hearing Loss

A. Autosomal dominant
B. Ankylosis of proximal interphalangeal joint
C. Conductive hearing loss early in life

Treacher Collins Syndrome (Mandibulofacial Dysostosis; Franceschetti-Zwahlen-Klein Syndrome)

A. Autosomal dominant or intrauterine abuse
B. Antimongoloid palpebral fissures with notched lower lids
C. Malformation of ossicles (stapes usually normal)
D. Auricular deformity, atresia of external auditory canal
E. Conductive hearing loss

F. Preauricular fistulas
G. Mandibular hypoplasia and malar hypoplasia
H. “Fishmouth”
I. Normal IQ
J. Usually bilateral involvement
K. May have cleft palate and cleft lip
L. Arrest in embryonic development at 6 to 8 weeks to give the above findings

van Buchem Syndrome (Hyperostosis Corticalis Generalisata)

A. Autosomal recessive
B. Generalized osteosclerotic overgrowth of skeleton, including skull, mandible, ribs, and long and short bones
C. Cranial nerve palsies due to obstruction of the foramina
D. Increased serum alkaline phosphatase
E. Progressive sensorineural hearing loss

van der Hoeve Syndrome (Osteogenesis Imperfecta)

A. Autosomal dominant with variable expressivity.
B. Fragile bones, loose ligaments.
C. Blue or clear sclera, triangular facies, dentinogenesis imperfecta.
D. Blue sclera and hearing loss are seen in 60% of cases and are most frequently noted after age 20. The hearing loss is conductive and is due to stapes fixation by otosclerosis. Hearing loss can also be due to ossicular fracture. (Some use the term van der Hoeve syndrome to describe osteogenesis imperfecta with otosclerosis. Others use the term interchangeably with osteogenesis imperfecta regardless of whether or not otosclerosis is present.)
E. The basic pathologic defect is “abnormal osteoblastic activity.”
F. When operating on such a patient, it is important to avoid fracture of the tympanic ring or the long process of the incus. It is also important to realize that the stapes footplate may be “floating.”
G. The sclera may have increased mucopolysaccharide content.
H. These patients have normal calcium, phosphorus, and alkaline phosphatase in the serum.
I. Occasionally, capillary fragility is noted.

Hereditary Congenital Deafness Associated With Other Abnormalities

Acoustic Neurinomas (Inherited)

A. Autosomal dominant
B. Progressive sensorineural hearing loss during the second or third decade of life
C. Ataxia, visual loss
D. No café au lait spots

Alport Syndrome (Also Described Earlier)

A. Autosomal dominant.
B. Progressive nephritis and sensorineural hearing loss.
C. Hematuria, proteinuria beginning the first or second decade of life.

D. Men with this disease usually die of uremia by age 30. Women are less severely affected.
E. Kidneys are affected by chronic glomerulonephritis with interstitial lymphocytic infiltrate and foam cells.
F. Progressive sensorineural hearing loss begins at age 10. Although it is not considered sex linked, hearing loss affects almost all male but not all female subjects. Histologically, degeneration of the organ of Corti and stria vascularis is observed.
G. Spherophalera cataract.
H. Hypofunction of the vestibular organ.
I. Contributes to 1% of hereditary deafness.

Alström Syndrome

A. Autosomal recessive
B. Retinal degeneration giving rise to visual loss
C. Diabetes, obesity
D. Progressive sensorineural hearing loss

Cockayne Syndrome

A. Autosomal recessive
B. Dwarfism
C. Mental retardation
D. Retinal atrophy
E. Motor disturbances
F. Progressive sensorineural hearing loss bilaterally

Congenital Cretinism (See Earlier)

Congenital cretinism must be distinguished from Pendred syndrome.

A. About 35% present with congenital hearing loss of the mixed type (irreversible).
B. Goiter (hypothyroid).
C. Mental and physical retardation.
D. Abnormal development of the petrous pyramid.
E. This disease is not inherited in a specific Mendelian manner. It is restricted to a certain geographic locale where a dietary deficiency exists.

Duane Syndrome

A. Autosomal dominant (some sex-linked recessive)
B. Inability to abduct eyes, retract globe
C. Narrowing of palpebral fissure
D. Torticollis
E. Cervical rib
F. Conductive hearing loss

Fanconi Anemia Syndrome

A. Autosomal recessive
B. Absent or deformed thumb

C. Other skeletal, heart, and kidney malformations
D. Increased skin pigmentation
E. Mental retardation
F. Pancytopenia
G. Conductive hearing loss

Fehr Corneal Dystrophy

A. Autosomal recessive
B. Progressive visual and sensorineural hearing loss

Flynn-Aird Syndrome

A. Autosomal dominant
B. Progressive myopia, cataracts, retinitis pigmentosa
C. Progressive sensorineural hearing loss
D. Ataxia
E. Shooting pains in the joints

Friedreich Ataxia

A. Autosomal recessive
B. Childhood onset of nystagmus, ataxia, optic atrophy, hyperreflexia, and sensorineural hearing loss

Goldenhar Syndrome (Also Described Earlier)

A. Autosomal recessive
B. Epibulbar dermoids
C. Preauricular appendages
D. Fusion or absence of cervical vertebrae
E. Colobomas of the eye
F. Conductive hearing loss

Hallgren Syndrome

A. Autosomal recessive
B. Retinitis pigmentosa
C. Progressive ataxia
D. Mental retardation in 25% of cases
E. Sensorineural hearing loss
F. Constitutes about 5% of hereditary deafness

Hermann Syndrome

A. Autosomal dominant
B. Onset of photomyoclonus and sensorineural hearing loss during late childhood or adolescence
C. Diabetes mellitus
D. Progressive dementia
E. Pyelonephritis and glomerulonephritis

Hurler Syndrome (Gargoylism)

A. Autosomal recessive
B. Abnormal mucopolysaccharides are deposited in tissues (when mucopolysaccharides are deposited in the neutrophils, they are called Adler bodies); middle ear mucosa with large foamy gargoyle cells staining PAS-positive
C. Chondroitin sulfate B and heparitin in urine
D. Forehead prominent with coarsening of the facial features and low-set ears
E. Mental retardation
F. Progressive corneal opacities
G. Hepatosplenomegaly
H. Mixed hearing loss
I. Dwarfism
J. Cerebral storage of three gangliosides: GM_3, GM_2, and GM_1
K. Beta-galactosides deficient

Hunter Syndrome

Signs are the same as for Hurler syndrome, except that they are sex linked.

Jervell and Lange-Nielsen Syndrome (Also Described Earlier)

A. Autosomal recessive
B. Profound bilateral sensorineural hearing loss (high frequencies more severely impaired)
C. Associated with heart disease (prolonged QT interval on ECG) and Stokes-Adams disease
D. Recurrent syncope
E. Usually terminates fatally with sudden death
F. Histopathologically, PAS-positive nodules in the cochlea

Laurence-Moon-Bardet-Biedl Syndrome

A. Autosomal recessive
B. Dwarfism
C. Obesity
D. Hypogonadism
E. Retinitis pigmentosa
F. Mental retardation
G. Sensorineural hearing loss

(Recessive) Malformed Low-Set Ears and Conductive Hearing Loss

A. Autosomal recessive
B. Mental retardation in 50% of cases

(Dominant) Mitral Insufficiency, Joint Fusion, and Hearing Loss

A. Autosomal dominant with variable penetrance
B. Conductive hearing loss, usually due to fixation of the stapes
C. Narrow external auditory canal
D. Fusion of the cervical vertebrae and the carpal and tarsal bones

Möbius Syndrome (Congenital Facial Diplegia)

A. Autosomal dominant, possible recessive
B. Facial diplegia
C. External ear deformities
D. Ophthalmoplegia
E. Hands or feet sometimes missing
F. Mental retardation
G. Paralysis of the tongue
H. Mixed hearing loss

(Dominant) Saddle Nose, Myopia, Cataract, and Hearing Loss

A. Autosomal dominant
B. Saddle nose
C. Severe myopia
D. Juvenile cataract
E. Sensorineural hearing loss that is progressive, moderately severe, and of early onset

Norrie Syndrome (Also Described Earlier)

A. Autosomal recessive
B. Congenital blindness
C. Progressive sensorineural hearing loss in 30% cases

Pendred Syndrome (Also Described Earlier)

A. Autosomal recessive.
B. Variable amount of bilateral hearing loss secondary to atrophy of the organ of Corti. A U-shaped audiogram is often seen.
C. Patients are euthyroid and develop diffuse goiter at the time of puberty. It is said that the metabolic defect is faulty iodination of tyrosine.
D. Positive perchlorate test.
E. The goiter is treated with exogenous hormone to suppress thyroid-stimulating hormone (TSH) secretion.
F. Normal IQ.
G. Unlike congenital cretinism, the bony petrous pyramid is well developed.
H. Constitutes 10% of hereditary deafness.

Refsum Disease (Heredopathia Atactica Polyneuritiformis)

A. Autosomal recessive
B. Retinitis pigmentosa
C. Polyneuropathy
D. Ataxia
E. Sensorineural hearing loss
F. Visual impairment usually beginning in the second decade
G. Ichthyosis often present
H. Elevated plasma phytanic acid levels
I. Etiology: neuronal lipid storage disease and hypertrophic polyneuropathy

(Recessive) Renal, Genital, and Middle Ear Anomalies

A. Autosomal recessive
B. Renal hypoplasia
C. Internal genital malformation
D. Middle ear malformation
E. Moderate to severe conductive hearing loss

Richards-Rundel Syndrome

A. Autosomal recessive
B. Mental deficiency
C. Hypogonadism (decreased urinary estrogen, pregnanediol, and total 17-ketosteroids)
D. Ataxia
E. Horizontal nystagmus to bilateral gazes
F. Sensorineural hearing loss beginning during infancy
G. Muscle wasting during early childhood and absence of deep tendon reflexes

Taylor Syndrome

A. Autosomal recessive
B. Unilateral microtia or anotia
C. Unilateral facial bone hypoplasia
D. Conductive hearing loss

Trisomy 13 to 15 (Group D); Patau Syndrome

A. Low-set pinnae
B. Atresia of external auditory canals
C. Cleft lip and cleft palate
D. Colobomas of the eyelids
E. Micrognathia
F. Tracheoesophageal fistula
G. Hemangiomas
H. Congenital heart disease
I. Mental retardation
J. Mixed hearing loss
K. Hypertelorism
L. Incidence is 0.45:1000 live births
M. Usually die early in childhood

Trisomy 16 to 18 (Group E)

A. Low-set pinnae
B. External canal atresia
C. Micrognathia, high-arched palate
D. Peculiar finger position
E. Prominent occiput
F. Cardiac anomalies
G. Hernias
H. Pigeon breast
I. Mixed hearing loss

J. Incidence is 0.25:1000 to 2:1000 live births
K. Ptosis
L. Usually die early in life

Trisomy 21 or 22 (Down Syndrome; G Trisomy)

A. Extra chromosome on no. 21 or no. 22
B. Mental retardation
C. Short stature
D. Brachycephaly
E. Flat occiput
F. Slanted eyes
G. Epicanthus
H. Strabismus, nystagmus
I. Seen in association with leukemia
J. Subglottic stenosis not uncommon
K. Decreased pneumatized or absent frontal and sphenoid sinuses
L. Incidence is 1:600 live births

Turner Syndrome

A. Not inherited; possibly due to intrauterine insult
B. Low hairline
C. Webbing of neck and digits
D. Widely spaced nipples
E. XO; 80% sex-chromatin negative
F. Gonadal aplasia
G. Incidence is 1:5000 live births (Klinefelter syndrome is XXY)
H. Ossicular deformities
I. Low-set ears
J. Mixed hearing loss
K. Large ear lobes
L. Short stature
M. Abnormalities in the heart and kidney
N. Some with hyposmia

(Dominant) Urticaria, Amyloidosis, Nephritis, and Hearing Loss

A. Autosomal dominant
B. Recurrent urticaria
C. Amyloidosis
D. Progressive sensorineural hearing loss due to degeneration of the organ of Corti, ossification of the basilar membrane, and cochlear nerve degeneration
E. Usually die of uremia

Usher Syndrome (Recessive Retinitis Pigmentosa With Congenital Severe Deafness) (Also Described Earlier)

A. Autosomal recessive.
B. Retinitis pigmentosa giving rise to progressive visual loss. The patient is usually completely blind by the second or third decade.

C. These patients are usually born deaf secondary to atrophy of the organ of Corti. Hearing for low frequencies is present in some patients.
D. Ataxia and vestibular dysfunction are common. Usher syndrome, among all congenital deafness syndromes, is most likely to include vestibular symptoms.
E. It constitutes 10% of hereditary deafness.
F. Usher syndrome is classified into four types:
   i. *Type I*: Profound congenital deafness with the onset of retinitis pigmentosa by age 10; has no vestibular response; constitutes 90% of all cases of Usher syndrome
   ii. *Type II*: Moderate to severe congenital deafness with the onset of retinitis pigmentosa in late teens or early twenties; normal or decreased vestibular response; constitutes 10% of all cases
   iii. *Type III*: Progressive hearing loss; retinitis pigmentosa begins at puberty; constitutes less than 1% of all cases (types I, II, and III are autosomal recessive)
   iv. *Type IV*: X-linked inheritance; phenotype similar to that of type II

Well Syndrome

A. Nephritis
B. Hearing loss
C. Autosomal dominant

External Ear Deformities

Middle and external congenital deformities have been classified, but this classification is less commonly used than that for inner ear development anomalies.

Class I

A. Normal auricle in shape and size
B. Well-pneumatized mastoid and middle ear
C. Ossicular abnormality
D. Most common type

Class II

A. Microtia
B. Atretic canal and abnormal ossicles
C. Normal aeration of mastoid and middle ear

Class III

A. Microtia
B. Atretic canal and abnormal ossicles
C. Middle ear and mastoid poorly aerated
   i. The external deformity does not necessarily correlate with middle ear abnormality.
   ii. Patients with a congenitally fixed footplate have the following characteristics that differentiate them from patients with otosclerosis:
      a. Onset during childhood
      b. Nonprogressive
      c. Negative family history

d. Flat 50 to 60 dB conductive hearing loss
e. Carhart notch not present
f. Schwartz sign not present

Neonatal Screening

Early hearing detection and intervention (EHDI) has been a growing initiative since it was first proposed as part of the congressional report in the 1960s. Over the next four decades continued policy advancements eventually culminated in adoption of universal newborn hearing screening (UNHS). In its current form, this is implemented through the EHDI 1-3-6 Benchmark plan. This plan identifies who to screen and when. According to the proposal:

- By 1 month: all infants should be screened. Rescreening may be performed no later than the time of discharge.
- By 3 months: all infants who do not pass the initial hearing screening should undergo medical and audiologic evaluation.
- By 6 months: all infants with confirmed permanent hearing loss should receive early intervention as soon as possible, but no later than 6 months.

There are exceptions to these recommendations, including:

- Infants readmitted in first month of life with conditions known to be risk factors for hearing loss should undergo rescreening prior to discharge.
- Infants should not be screened more than the recommended times, as the probability of obtaining an erroneous "pass" increases with each screen.
- Ongoing surveillance of development milestones at home in all patients.

There are two audiologic methods used for hearing screen: automated ABR (AABR) and transient evoked otoacoustic emissions (TEOAE). Furthermore, two screening protocols have been described for well-infants. The one-step protocol allows for either OAE or AABR screening to be performed. If the initial screening is failed, a repeat screening can be performed with the same technologic modality no later than the time of discharge. In the two-step protocol, OAE testing is performed as initial screen followed by ABR as rescreening. Screening protocols for NICU infants are slightly different, as the Joint Committee on Infant Hearing recommends only AABR to be used. Implementation of AABR, through either the one or two-step protocols, has been found to result in fewer false positives and lower referral rates. However, AABR is more costly and time-consuming than TOAE. Patients who fail initial screening should undergo confirmation of hearing loss through a thorough audiologic and otolaryngologic evaluation.

Evaluation of Failed Screening and Additional Workup

Confirmation of suspected congenital hearing loss starts with a thorough history and physical including a detailed family history. Clinicians are advised to look for hereditary traits that may be associated with syndromic hereditary hearing impairment, such as white forelock of hair, premature graying, different colored eyes, kidney abnormalities, night blindness, severe farsightedness, childhood cardiac arrhythmias, or a sibling with sudden cardiac death.

All infants of suspected hereditary hearing impairment should undergo supplemental audiologic testing. For infants and younger patients, electrophysiologic tests such as the sleep-deprived or sedated auditory brain stem response (ABR), automated steady state responses (ASSR), stapedial reflex, and otoacoustic emission (OAE) can be done. Age-appropriate audiometry can supplement these aforementioned tests depending on the age of the patient. An audiogram that is U-shaped or cookie bite should alert the clinician to hereditary hearing loss. Vestibular function tests can be helpful in the diagnosis of patients with Usher syndrome.

Depending on the history and physical findings, additional diagnostics, such as imaging or laboratory studies, may be indicated. All children diagnosed with hearing loss should have a urinalysis to assess for proteinuria and hematuria as well as serial ophthalmologic screenings. Other tests should be ordered as clinically indicated. These tests include thyroid function tests, electrocardiogram, electroretinograms, renal ultrasound, and perchlorate discharge test.

Radiographic studies should be ordered on a case-by-case basis. A CT scan can help to visualize cochlear abnormalities, internal auditory canal aberrations, and cochlear dysplasia. MRI with gadolinium enhancement is the study of choice in patients with a family history of NF type 2. These studies can be invaluable when planning surgical intervention, particularly when planning cochlear implantation. MR is also used when the hearing loss is progressive but the CT scan is normal. Risk of radiation from CT scanning needs to be taken into account as well. At completion of an intensive and sometimes expensive evaluation, the specific etiology of a hearing loss still may remain uncertain.

Referral to a genetic counselor can be made in select situations. Infants who have confirmed hearing loss with a suspected environmental (nongenetic) cause of hearing loss should forgo genetic evaluation in favor of laboratory or imaging workup. Such patients should undergo screening for TORCH infections or directed diagnostics that reflect the underlying clinical suspicion. In patients where no environmental cause is found, or none is suspected, the option of genetic counselling and genetic testing should be offered. If syndromic hearing loss is suspected, targeted gene testing can be performed. If nonsyndromic hearing loss is suspected, *GJB2* and *GJB6* or next-generation sequencing (NGS) can be offered. NGS is a new technology allowing for assessment of numerous genes within a single panel.

The range of recurrence risk for future offspring cited for a family with an only child, who has an unexplained hearing loss, is 10% to 16%. Each additional normal hearing child born to such a family would decrease the probability that the disorder has a genetic etiology and thus decrease the recurrence risk. Likewise, if another child is born to the same family and has a hearing impairment, then the recurrence risk increases because the possibility of a genetic component causing the hearing loss is increased.

Conclusion

Diagnosis, prognosis, and estimation of recurrence risk are components of a complete genetic evaluation of a child with suspected genetic hearing loss. Precise diagnosis with a diligent search for etiology should be undertaken. Review of clinical and laboratory data by a clinician skilled in pattern recognition can lead to identification of a syndrome or family pattern useful in predicting the likely clinical course of the disorder. An accurate diagnosis also enhances the accuracy of recurrence-risk estimates. Future studies of genetic basis of hearing loss may lead to treatment options, such as gene therapy, to provide auditory rehabilitation to these patients.

Bibliography

Karmody C, Schuknecht HF. Deafness in congenital deafness. *Arch Otolaryngol.* 1966;83:18.

Loundon N, Marlin S, Busquet D, et al. Usher syndrome and cochlear implantation. *Otol Neurotol.* 2003;24:216-221.

Merchant SN, McKenna MJ, Nadol JB Jr, et al. Temporal bone histopathologic and genetic studies in Mohr-Tranebjaerg syndrome (DFN-1). *Otol Neurotol.* 2001;22:506-511.
Morton NE. Genetic epidemiology of hearing impairment. *Ann NYAS.* 1991;630:16-31.
Tamari M, Itkin P. Penicillin and syphilis of the ear. *Eye Ear Nose Throat Mon.* 1951;30:252, 301, 358.

Questions

1. Match the following auditory tests with their appropriate patient age range.
   A. Visual reinforcement audiometry
   B. Conditioned play audiometry
   C. Behavioral observation audiometry
      I. 0 to 6 months
      II. 6 months to 2 years
      III. 2 to 5 years

2. A patient with congenital hearing loss and CT imaging revealing absence of the lateral semicircular canal is most likely to present with which other syndromic features?
   A. Coloboma, patent ductus arteriosus
   B. Blue sclera, fragile bones
   C. Progressive nephritis
   D. Prolonged QT intervals

3. A newborn presents with congenital hearing loss. What are the chances that it is due to Connexin 26 mutation?
   A. 70%
   B. 35%
   C. 15%
   D. 50%
   Answer B

4. Which of the following is FALSE with regard to embryologic development of the inner ear?
   A. In general, the earlier the arrest in development of the otic placed, the more severe the nature of the inner ear dysfunction.
   B. Michel aplasia refers to complete labyrinthine aplasia and is the most severe form of inner ear maldevelopment.
   C. Mondini dysplasia is the most common form of inner ear maldevelopment and is associated with syndromic presentations.
   D. Enlarged vestibular aqueduct (EVA) almost always results in maximal SNHL early in childhood.
   E. Conventional amplification is a reasonable option in some of the less severe variants of otic placode arrest, including Scheibe dysplasia.

5. Which antibiotic class presents with increased ototoxic effects due to inheritance of mitochondrial mutations?
   A. Macrolides
   B. Cephalosporins
   C. Tetracyclines
   D. Aminoglycosides

Chapter 16
Tinnitus

Objective

- Observer can hear the tinnitus, much less common than subjective
  - Vascular—typically corresponds to pulse (aka, pulse synchronous tinnitus); may be venous, arterial, or combination (arteriovenous) source or secondary to high output cardiac state, tumors, other; (pulse synchronous tinnitus may also be subjective)
    - Pathogenesis:
      - ◊ Venous sources
        - * Jugular bulb: High riding and large, turbulent flow, dehiscent jugular plate at the level of middle ear
        - * Sigmoid sinus: diverticulum, turbulent flow, dehiscent sigmoid plate
        - * Other venous structures: aberrant condylar vein, superior petrosal sinus, inferior petrosal sinus; aberrant vein contacting labyrinthine structures
      - ◊ Arterial sources
        - * Carotid artery: cervical carotid dissection, aneurysm, or stenosis; aberrant carotid artery; carotid body tumor; dehiscent carotid plate within the middle ear
        - * Persistent stapedial artery: derived from internal carotid artery, passes through obturator foramen of stapes superstructure
      - ◊ Arteriovenous (AV) malformations and dural AV fistulas
        - * May be associated with venous drainage leading to enlarged cortical veins (high rate of bleeding)
        - * Often associated with sigmoid/transverse sinus and prior craniotomy
      - ◊ Tumors
        - * Paraganglioma, middle ear adenoma, choristoma, facial nerve neuroma, hemangioma
        - * Any tumor (or encephalocele) contacting the ossicular chain or TM may lead to pulse synchronous tinnitus (subjective or objective)
        - * High cardiac output states: anemia, thyrotoxicosis, pregnancy, beriberi, etc.
    - Diagnosis: auscultation with stethoscope, Toynbee tube, palpation of periauricular tissue
      - ◊ CT angiography
      - ◊ MRA/MRV
      - ◊ Formal cerebral angiography (small risk of stroke)

    - Treatment: based on etiology and severity of symptoms
        - ◊ Selective embolization, surgical resection/clipping, and radiosurgery are options for dural AV fistulas and malformations.
        - ◊ Surgical excision or combination of surgery and radiosurgery may be used for tumors.
        - ◊ High output states should be medically corrected.
        - ◊ Anatomic vascular abnormalities may or may not be amenable to intervention.
- Nonvascular—typically presents as clicking sensation
    - Palatal myoclonus—rapid (50-200 beats per minute) irregular clicking caused by eustachian tube opening and closing from palatal musculature contraction.
        - ◊ Symptoms often worse during times of stress.
        - ◊ Diagnosed by prolonged tympanogram showing movement with palatal contraction; may visualize palate with nasopharyngoscope as well; Toynbee tube may be used to auscultate rhythmic sound.
        - ◊ Treated with muscle relaxants or Botox in refractory cases.
        - ◊ Often associated with central nervous system disease; MRI of posterior fossa should be performed to assess.
    - Stapedial or tensor tympani muscle spasm
        - ◊ Can be heard as clicking or crackling noise
        - ◊ Diagnosis similar to above, but without observed palatal muscle contractions
        - ◊ Treated with muscle relaxants or sectioning of tendons if refractory
    - Patulous eustachian tube—symptoms worsen with respiration and are often described as roaring sensation; autophony;
        - ◊ Can be diagnosed by TM movement with respiration, but not always visualized. Prolonged tympanometry may also be helpful.
        - ◊ Placement of head in dependent position for relief of symptoms.
    - May be associated with temporomandibular joint disorders, normal swallowing that leads to TM movement (latter may be heard as single click with Toynbee tube)

Subjective

- Incidence: 10% of population.
- Can arise due to numerous conditions, many of which are poorly understood.
- Most commonly occurs secondary to hearing loss.
    - Presbycusis, noise-induced hearing loss, acoustic neuroma, and Meniere disease are commonly associated problems.
- Most pharmacologic agents that induce tinnitus are reversible.
    - Partial list includes aspirin, aminoglycosides, loop diuretics, caffeine, and alcohol.
- Characteristics:
    - Buzzing, clicking, humming, chirping, or hissing type sounds are commonly described.
    - Roaring quality may be associated with Meniere disease.
    - Pulsatile or pulse-synchronous sounds may be described, despite not being audible to observer.
        - Encephalocele against ossicles may cause pulsatile tinnitus.
        - Idiopathic intracranial hypertension.
            - ◊ Common in obese, middle-aged females
            - ◊ Associated visual disturbances and headache

- Sounds may be intermittent or continuous.
  - SBUTT: Sudden, brief, unilateral, tapering tinnitus; common in normal individuals
- Pathogenesis:
  - Most likely occurs due to functional abnormalities of the auditory portion of the central nervous system (CNS)
  - Neural plasticity may cause reorganization in the auditory nuclei in response to a more peripheral event. This may then induce a hyperactive state, causing tinnitus. Possible peripheral events include:
    - ◊ Decreased or abnormal peripheral input (hair cell loss, etc.).
    - ◊ A pathological insult may lead to decreased or abnormal spontaneous time pattern firing of auditory nerve fiber.
      - * This may be the cause in cases of nerve compression in acoustic neuromas and vascular loops.
- Other CNS centers likely play a role in the perception of tinnitus.
  - Cranial nerve centers (trigeminal) influence the auditory system
  - Amygdala, the limbic system, and other centers dealing with emotion may play a role as well
  - May explain why some individuals with normal audiograms may develop tinnitus
- Diagnosis:
  - Complete history to evaluate for potential sources of trauma, ototoxicity, noise exposure, etc.
  - Otomicroscopy to evaluate the ear canal, tympanic membrane, and middle ear space.
    - ◊ Debris, wax, hair, foreign body, and other materials may cause tinnitus.
  - Standard audiometric testing should be done to evaluate hearing thresholds and word recognition scores.
  - Otoacoustic emission testing may be performed to document outer hair cell function.
  - Tinnitus matching may be performed in contralateral ear to characterize frequency and volume of tinnitus.
    - ◊ No correlation between tinnitus characteristics and patient aggravation level.
    - ◊ Approximately 50% of patients studied have tinnitus amplitude of 5 dB.
  - If vascular etiology is considered, work up as above.
- Treatment:
  - Avoidance of noise/medication/other source of potential injury
  - Counseling patients plays a major role in tinnitus treatment.
    - ◊ Patients should be screened for anxiety and depression as these often exacerbate tinnitus symptoms.
    - ◊ All medications should be reviewed.
    - ◊ Dietary triggers such as high salt diet, alcohol intake, and caffeine should be discussed.
  - Over time, approximately 25% of patients have near symptom resolution, 50% report significant improvement, and 25% remain stable.
  - Bedside masking (whether actual masking device versus fan or radio between stations) should be used in those bothered by bedtime symptoms.
  - Hearing aid—first line of treatment in patients with associated hearing loss.
    - ◊ Return of previously lost sounds may mask tinnitus.

    - ◊ If tinnitus is refractory, one can use masking device (or tinnitus instrument) in hearing aids.
      - * Creates sound stimulus in hopes of masking tinnitus
      - * Can also be used independently of hearing aids
    - ◊ Use of masking device in hearing aid increases likelihood of tinnitus control from 25% to 55%.
  - Tinnitus retraining therapy—combination of counseling and broadband sound exposure habituates patient to tinnitus
    - ◊ Patients are exposed to 16 hours of broadband noise per day.
    - ◊ Noise is initially presented low but slowly increases to a level where the tinnitus is just still audible to the patient.
    - ◊ Ideally over a year a patient will either no longer hear tinnitus or be undisturbed by it.
  - Biofeedback therapy—requires patient cooperation in undergoing therapy with psychologist (cognitive behavioral therapy)
    - ◊ Uses various triggers such as increased temperature or pulse for patient to recognize increased focus on tinnitus. Using these triggers, patients can learn to focus attention away from tinnitus.
    - ◊ Significant overlap with stress reduction.
  - Neuromodulators—special auditory devices that deliver a combination of tones, music, and other sounds, based on a patient's unique tinnitus characteristics, in an effort to effect change in auditory neural pathways
  - Transcranial magnetic stimulation—repetitive treatments, designed to alter perception of tinnitus; still investigational with little supportive data in terms of efficacy
  - Cochlear implant placement—unilateral placement is being offered in some centers for disabling tinnitus; in conjunction with single-sided deafness, may represent emerging treatment option; ~75% effective at substantially reducing tinnitus.
  - Medication
    - ◊ Treatment of underlying anxiety and depression can help patients contend with tinnitus.
    - ◊ Various supplements, such as melatonin, lipoflavanoids, niacin, among others, have been suggested for tinnitus treatment.
    - ◊ Psychotropic medications, including low-dose antidepressants, antianxiety medications, selective serotonin reuptake inhibitors (SSRIs), and benzodiazepines have also been used for tinnitus treatment.

Bibliography

1. Aage M. Tinnitus. In: Jackler R, Brackmann D, eds. *Neurotology*. 2nd ed. Philadelphia, PA: Elsevier Mosby; 2005:182-193.
2. Galazyuk AV, Wenstrup JJ, Hamid MA. Tinnitus and underlying brain mechanisms. *Curr Opin Otolaryngol Head Neck Surg*. 2012 Oct;20(5):409-415.
3. Sismanis A. Pulsatile tinnitus: contemporary assessment and management. *Curr Opin Otolaryngol Head Neck Surg*. 2011 Oct;19(5):348-357.
4. Snapp HA, Schubert MC. Habilitation of auditory and vestibular dysfunction. *Otolaryngol Clin North Am*. 2012 Apr;45(2):487-511.

Questions

1. Which of the following is true with regard to tinnitus matching?
   A. Tinnitus frequency is correlated with patients' aggravation with symptoms.
   B. Tinnitus intensity is correlated with patients' aggravation with symptoms.
   C. Tinnitus frequency is correlated with likelihood of resolution.
   D. Tinnitus intensity is correlated with likelihood of resolution.
   E. None of the above.

2. A 40-year-old man presents with 4-month history of bilateral tinnitus. He is curious about the prognosis. You tell him approximately ____ of patients will either have resolution or improvement in symptoms.
   A. 75%
   B. 50%
   C. 25%
   D. <1%

3. Which of the following best describes tinnitus retraining therapy?
   A. Continuous sound stimulus to eliminate perception of tinnitus
   B. Use of an amplification device to amplify previous hearing loss frequencies
   C. Broadband sound exposure for portions of the day to habituate patient to tinnitus
   D. Use of various physiological triggers to help focus attention away from tinnitus

4. Which of the following is NOT a potential cause of objective pulsatile tinnitus?
   A. Dural AV fistula
   B. Idiopathic intracranial hypertension
   C. Carotid dissection
   D. Persistent stapedial artery

5. A patient presents with persistent rapid clicking in the right ear. On exam, you also notice palatal spasm. The next appropriate action would be to
   A. Botox
   B. CT scan temporal bone with contrast
   C. MRI head with and without contrast
   D. Muscle relaxants
   E. Lyme disease titers

Chapter 17
Hearing Rehabilitation: Surgical and Nonsurgical

Part 1: Hearing Amplification

Hearing Aid Basics

Components of a Hearing Aid

- **Microphone** picks up sound and converts it into electrical signals.
- **Amplifier/signal processor** is the heart of a digital hearing aid. A variety of digital signal processing (DSP) techniques can be used to process sound, identify and selectively amplify speech, recognize and suppress ambient noise, etc.
- **Receiver** converts the processed electrical signals back to acoustic energy and delivers sound to the ear, acting as a loudspeaker.
- **Power source** is usually a zinc-air disposable battery, with some having a rechargeable nickel metal hydride or silver-zinc battery.

Hearing aid components are housed in a custom-made acrylic shell. Analog hearing aids converted sound waves into electrical signals, but are no longer available from major, reliable manufacturers. Current hearing aids are digital, which convert sound waves into numerical codes.

Electroacoustic Properties of Hearing Aids

- Hearing aids are characterized by three parameters: frequency response, gain, and output sound pressure level 90 (OSPL-90).
- Frequency response of a typical hearing aid extends up to 8 to 10 kHz; however, some hearing aids have an extended high-frequency response.
- Gain is the ratio of output power to input power. Gain depends on the input frequency and input intensity.
- OSPL-90, or saturated sound pressure level (SSPL-90). Describes how much sound energy is generated by the hearing aid when the input level is at 90 dB.
- Nonlinear processing (compression)—hearing aid amplifies softer sounds more and louder sounds less. This method allows for more comfortable listening in ears with sensorineural hearing loss with much *recruitment* (narrowed dynamic range).
- Directional microphones enhance the signal-to-noise ratio and allow better understanding of speech in noisy environments. Many hearing aids allow the user to switch between directional and omnidirectional microphones.
- Some digital hearing aids use DSP techniques to recognize different listening environments and optimize their performance in real time. These devices can suppress feedback and amplify speech selectively while suppressing ambient noise.

- Two major parameters predict patients' success with hearing aids. These are *word recognition scores* and *dynamic range*. Patients with word recognition scores of at least 50% and a wide dynamic range are usually successful hearing aid users.
- Dynamic range is the difference between the uncomfortable loudness level (UCL) and the speech reception threshold (SRT).
- Dynamic range = UCL − SRT.
- MCL (most comfortable level) approximately bisects the dynamic range.
- The narrower the dynamic range of an ear, the more difficult to fit a comfortable hearing aid.

Styles of Hearing Aids

The four basic styles of hearing aids are:

- **BTE** (behind the ear)
- **ITE** (in the ear)
- **ITC** (in the canal)
- **CIC** (completely in the canal)
- Several variations of these basic styles are offered by various manufacturers, such as mini-BTE, invisible in the canal (IIT), half-shell (HS) which is a smaller version of the ITE, and others.
- Each of these styles incorporates some degree of venting. Large venting makes a hearing aid more comfortable by eliminating the occlusion effect and enhancing hearing in noise. Occlusion effect results from reverberation of low frequencies in a closed ear canal. Large venting allows low frequencies to escape the ear canal. Large venting, unfortunately, is contraindicated in ears with significant low-frequency hearing loss.)
- Open-fit hearing aid is essentially a BTE-style aid with a modified earmold that is open, soft, not custom fitted, and eliminates the occlusion effect, making it a comfortable first choice for new hearing aid wearers. Because of the large venting, it is not suitable for patients with significant low-frequency hearing loss.
- RITE (receiver in the ear) is a BTE-style aid with the receiver (speaker) positioned through the acoustic tube into the ear canal. This design takes advantage of the general principle that sound is perceived as more natural if delivered closer to the tympanic membrane. This feature is common today and can be recognized by the narrow acoustic tube with a wire inside.
- Extended-wear hearing aids. These CIC-style hearing aids are placed in the ear canal by an audiologist and worn continuously for a few months. When the battery needs to be replaced, the device is removed and replaced by the audiologist.
- Other helpful hearing aid features may include built-in programmable tinnitus masking technology, Bluetooth connectivity to other electronic devices, and connectivity to FM systems in lecture halls and other public spaces.

Implantable Hearing Devices

- Implantable hearing systems have been used primarily for the rehabilitation of moderate to severe sensorineural hearing loss, but also for certain types of conductive and mixed hearing loss. These systems can be partially or fully implantable. Two technologies are currently available: electromagnetic and piezoelectric.
- In *electromagnetic* implantable hearing devices, a floating mass transducer is surgically attached to the ossicular chain, usually the incus. Examples are the partially implantable Vibrant Soundbridge (Med-El, GmbH, Austria), FDA approved in 2000,

and Maxum (Ototronix, St. Paul, MN), FDA approved in 2001. The fully implantable Carina (Cochlear Ltd, Australia) is not FDA approved.

- In **piezoelectric** implantable hearing devices, a driver is implanted to mechanically vibrate the ossicular chain. A piezoelectric crystal changes shape (bends) in response to a changing electric field. A driver containing a piezoelectric crystal can convert electrical signals into mechanical vibrations of the ossicular chain. One example is the fully implantable Esteem (Envoy Medical Corp, White Bear Lake, MN), which requires removal of the incus and was FDA approved in 2010.
- Most patients perceive a benefit in sound fidelity of implantable hearing devices over conventional hearing aids. Occlusion effect is eliminated, and feedback problems are significantly reduced. One clear advantage is the ability to hear while bathing, swimming, or sleeping.
- Disadvantages of implantable hearing systems are the complexity of the surgical procedure for device placement, high cost, lack of insurance coverage, need for surgical battery replacement, and limited magnetic resonance imaging (MRI) compatibility. Some systems require an iatrogenic ossicular discontinuity to reduce feedback problems.
- The *osseointegrated bone conduction hearing devices* are indicated for rehabilitation of mixed and conductive hearing loss. They can also be used for unilateral deafness which is discussed separately.
- The titanium implant/abutment complex is surgically placed in the bone behind the affected ear, above the temporal line, and is allowed to osseointegrate. One style, termed percutaneous (Ponto by Oticon Medical, Somerset, NJ, and Baha by Cochlear Ltd, Australia), has the abutment protruding through an opening in the skin. The processor is then attached to the abutment.
- Another style, termed transcutaneous (Bonebridge by MED-EL, Austria; Osia by Cochlear Ltd, Australia; and Sentio by Oticon Medical, Somerset, NJ), has the implant as well as the vibrating abutment, placed under the skin, with the sound processor placed externally, magnetically attracted to the implant.
- The system collects sound as a hearing aid, processes the sound electronically, and delivers it to the cochlea via **bone conduction** (Figure 17-1). The advantage of this system over conventional hearing aids is that any conductive hearing loss component is effectively bypassed while amplification is provided only for the sensorineural

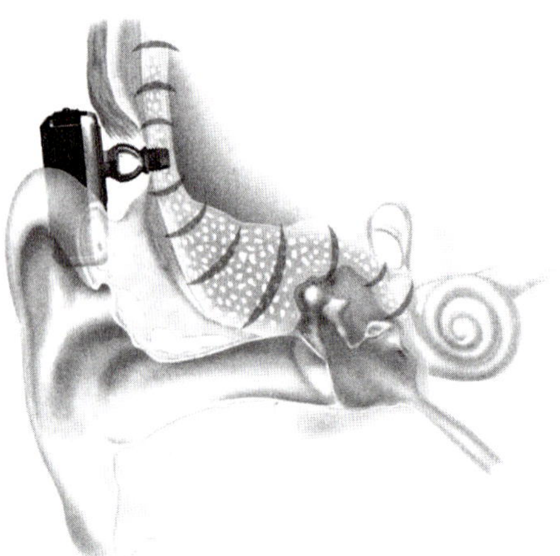

Figure 17-1 This osseointegrated system (Baha) delivers sound to the cochlea via the bone conduction mechanism. *(Picture provided courtesy of Cochlear™ Americas, © 2012 Cochlear Americas.)*

component. The greater the conductive component of hearing loss, the greater the advantage of this bone conduction system over conventional hearing aids.

- The bone conduction system is a good hearing rehabilitation method for mixed hearing losses with a significant conductive component, for ears with draining mastoid cavities, and for ears with conductive losses that are not amenable to surgical correction or standard amplification (ie, severe microtia and/or congenital atresia with severe ossicular malformations).
- *Cochlear implants* (Advanced Bionics, Valencia, CA; Cochlear Ltd, Australia; and MED-EL, Austria) are another implantable device, using electricity to stimulate the spiral ganglion cells of the auditory nerve. They are indicated for moderate to profound sensorineural hearing loss in adults, and severe to profound sensorineural hearing loss in children as young as nine months old, all in individuals with limited benefit from amplification.

Options for Single-Sided Deafness

- In patients with unilateral hearing loss that is not aidable by conventional hearing aids due to the severity of hearing loss and poor word recognition, several hearing rehabilitation options exist.
- *CROS (contralateral routing of signal) hearing aids*: The patient wears hearing aids in both ears. The hearing aid on the deaf ear collects sounds and transfers the sound information to the receiver worn on the contralateral better-hearing ear via radio waves. A system that delivers some additional amplification to the better-hearing ear is termed Bi-CROS.
- *Osseointegrated bone conduction hearing device* is an option for rehabilitation of single-sided deafness when the pure tone average in the better ear is 20 dB HL or better. The only-hearing ear should not have any significant hearing loss. Acoustic signals are collected from the deaf side, processed, and delivered via bone conduction to the contralateral healthy cochlea.
- *Cochlear implants* can also be used for the rehabilitation of single-sided deafness. Studies indicate good hearing performance in noise, no interference with the hearing ear, good sound localization, and relief of tinnitus in the deaf ear.[1,2]

Part 2: Ossiculoplasty

Mechanics of the Ossicular Chain

- The middle ear structures (tympanic membrane, ossicular chain, oval and round windows) collectively provide an **impedance matching** mechanism between the air-filled external environment and the fluid-filled labyrinth, ensuring that acoustic energy is not significantly attenuated as it enters the inner ear.
- The *ideal transformer model* predicts that the middle ear provides about 28 dB of gain, which offsets the losses due to impedance mismatch. This gain results from two lever mechanisms. First, the ratio of the size of the physiologically active portion of the tympanic membrane and oval window is about 20, resulting in a 26 dB gain. Second, the ratio of the length of the malleus and incus is 1.3, resulting in a modest 2 dB gain.
- Actual experimental measurements of middle ear pressure gains average only about 23 dB. Middle ear gain is frequency dependent and peaks around 1 kHz.
- Ideal middle ear prosthesis is lightweight, made of a biocompatible material, easy to trim, handle, and adjust, stable in the middle ear, and MRI compatible.
- Common ossicular prosthesis materials are: plastipore, hydroxyapatite, HAPEX (hydroxyapatite with polyethylene), and titanium.

Malleus-Incus Defect

- *Partial ossicular reconstruction prosthesis* (PORP) replaces part of the ossicular chain, such as the malleus-incus complex. This prosthesis spans the distance between the stapes suprastructure and the tympanic membrane, or between the stapes and undersurface of the malleus, if the manubrium is still intact.
- A thin layer of cartilage is often placed between the prosthesis head and the tympanic membrane to reduce the chance of prosthesis extrusion. The tragus is a common source of cartilage for ossicular reconstruction.
- Generally good hearing results are obtained with partial prostheses with most studies reporting at least two-thirds of patients reaching air–bone gaps of 20 dB or less.[3]

Total Ossicular Defect

- *Total ossicular reconstruction prosthesis* (TORP) replaces the entire ossicular chain and spans the middle ear cleft between the stapes footplate and the tympanic membrane (Figure 17-2).
- A thin layer of cartilage is often placed between the prosthesis head and the tympanic membrane to reduce the chance of prosthesis extrusion in ears with eustachian tube dysfunction.
- A *footplate shoe* can be used to stabilize the total prosthesis on the stapes footplate. The shoe can be built-in or placed concomitantly by the surgeon.
- Generally good hearing results are obtained with total ossicular prostheses, with most studies reporting at least half of patients reaching a postoperative air–bone gap of 20 dB or less.[3]

Incus Defect

- Incus defects can be reconstructed using native incus interposition or a synthetic prosthesis. A variety of prostheses are available to span the gap between the malleus and stapes (Figure 17-3). Small gaps in the IS joint can be bridged with calcium phosphate bone cement (Otomimix, Olympus Corp, Japan).

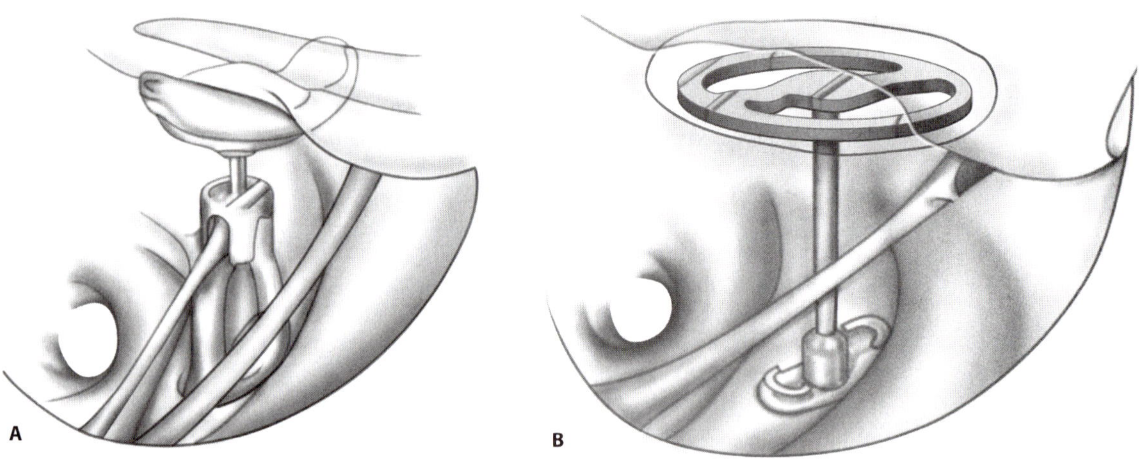

Figure 17-2. A. Partial prosthesis placed over the stapes capitulum; **B.** Total prosthesis placed on the footplate. *(Illustrations provided courtesy of Grace Medical, Inc.)*

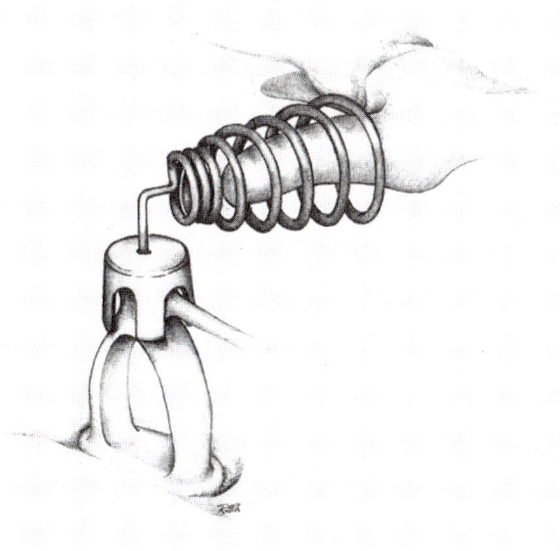

A

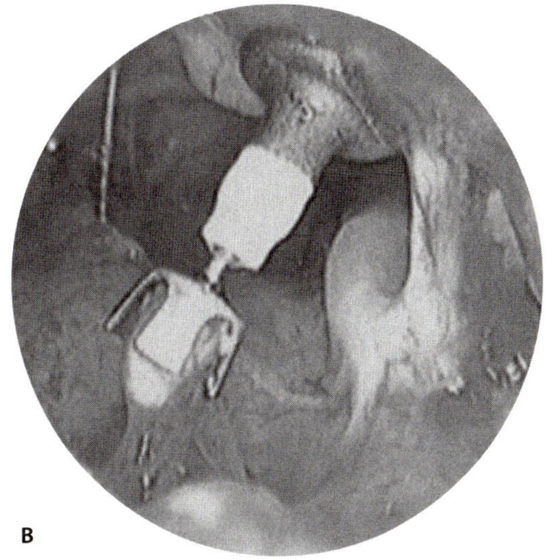

B

Figure 17-3 Examples of incus replacement prostheses: **A.** K-Helix reestablishes continuity between the eroded incus and healthy stapes; **B.** Wedge incus strut replaces the entire incus. *(Illustration and photo provided courtesy of Grace Medical, Inc.)*

- The most common native ossicle reconstruction technique is *incus interposition*, generally used in cases involving discontinuity at the incudostapedial joint (IJ) due to incus long process erosion. The native incus is removed, turned, and replaced to reestablish continuity between the malleus and stapes. Incus can be sculpted with a drill as desired before repositioning. Generally good hearing results are obtained in experienced hands, with 66% of ears brought to within 20 dB of the bone conduction line, with hearing results remaining stable over time.

Stapes Defect

- When the stapes becomes fixed due to otosclerosis, it can be replaced with a prosthesis to restore mobility to the ossicular chain.
- Stapedectomy—removal of stapes suprastructure and a portion or all of the stapes footplate.
- Stapedotomy—removal of stapes suprastructure and fenestration of the footplate to accommodate the prosthesis.
- *Indications for stapedectomy*: (a) conductive hearing loss with an air–bone gap of at least 25 to 30 dB, sufficient to produce a negative Rinne test with the 512-Hz tuning fork; (b) normal otoscopic examination; (c) acoustic reflex either biphasic or absent.
- Stapedectomy is performed on the worse-hearing ear in cases of bilateral otosclerosis. If hearing is similar in both ears, the patient is asked to identify which ear is better, and again, stapedectomy is performed on the worse-hearing ear as identified by the patient.

Special Situations

- Patients with osteogenesis imperfecta have brittle bones. While stapedectomy can improve hearing in these patients, care must be taken not to fracture the tympanic ring while curetting the scutum or fracture the incus while crimping the prosthesis. Should an incus fracture occur, the surgeon may need to place a malleo-vestibulo prosthesis instead, which spans the footplate to the manubrium.

- In rare patients with otosclerosis and Ménière disease, endolymphatic hydrops creates an increased risk that the saccule may be punctured as stapedectomy is performed, resulting in a degree of sensorineural hearing loss or a completely deaf ear. A hearing aid or osseo-integrated bone conduction system should be considered in place of surgery.[4]
- A blind patient may have more trouble compensating for minor vestibular deficits which can occur with stapedectomy.[4] Similarly, a patient with contralateral peripheral vestibulopathy may not tolerate even minor vestibular complications. A hearing aid should be considered. If peripheral vestibulopathy is suspected, caloric testing is indicated before considering stapedotomy.
- Patients with a mixed hearing loss should be counseled that hearing aids will likely be necessary even if the stapedectomy is successful in closing the air–bone gap to overcome the sensorineural component.
- **Stapedectomy surgical steps** generally include: elevation of the tympanomeatal flap, curetting the scutum for exposure of the footplate and facial nerve, separating the IS joint, testing mobility of the lateral chain and stapes separately, dividing the stapedius tendon, removing the stapes suprastructure, removing or fenestrating the footplate, placing an oval window covering if needed, placing and securing the prosthesis, testing prosthesis mobility, replacing the tympanic membrane to its normal anatomic position. The order of steps may vary among surgeons.

Stapedectomy Intraoperative Complications

- If a tympanic membrane perforation occurs, it is repaired with an underlay fascia graft.
- A markedly thickened footplate can complicate the procedure, but it can be drilled out and a prosthesis placed safely. A floating footplate can occur during efforts to remove it and can make the task nearly impossible. Options include fenestrating the floating footplate using a laser or aborting the procedure, allowing the footplate to refixate, then attempting the surgery at a later date.
- The tympanic segment of the facial nerve is examined before stapes surgery as it courses superior to the oval window. Mild dehiscence and overhang of the facial nerve can be managed by bending the prosthesis wire or drilling the inferior cochlear promontory. If severe facial nerve overhang is encountered, it is prudent to abort the procedure and recommend a hearing aid.[4]
- Rarely is a persistent stapedial artery seen coursing between the stapes crura, which is a contraindication for stapes surgery. The surgery should be aborted and the patient offered a hearing aid.

Stapedectomy Delayed Complications

- Persistent conductive hearing loss may be due to unrecognized lateral chain ankylosis in the epitympanum, incus subluxation, prosthesis that is too short, inadequately crimped prosthesis, or rarely superior canal dehiscence syndrome.
- Recurrent conductive hearing loss can occur due to necrosis and shortening of the long process of incus, displaced prosthesis, or reparative granuloma (1-2 weeks after surgery).
- Vertigo is sometimes seen for a few days after stapedectomy. This may be due to perilymph loss from suctioning.[4] If vertigo persists, the ear may be reexplored. A perilymph fistula or an excessively long prosthesis may be the cause.
- Sensorineural hearing loss can occur after stapedectomy. Historically, incidence is about 1% to 2% after primary stapedectomy and higher after revisions. Temporary threshold shifts can occur after stapes surgery as well.

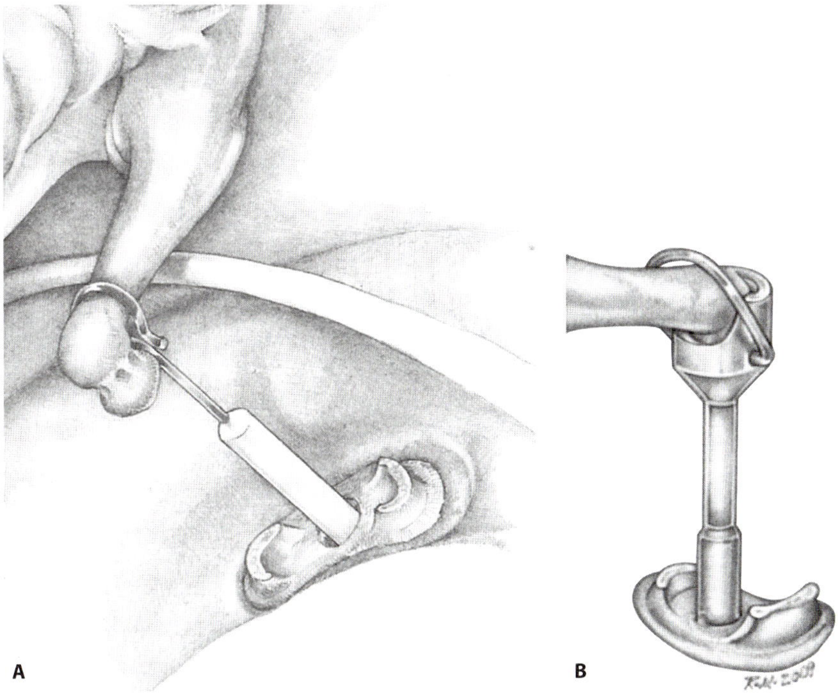

Figure 17-4 Designs of stapes prostheses: **A.** piston-style; **B.** bucket handle. *(Illustrations provided courtesy of Grace Medical, Inc.)*

- Serous labyrinthitis is thought to occur during the healing process after stapedectomy. Sensorineural hearing loss above 2 kHz and mild disequilibrium may occur. This type of postoperative labyrinthitis usually resolves within a few days without permanent sequelae.
- Stapes prosthesis designs are either *piston style* or *bucket handle* (Figure 17-4). The bucket handle is simply flipped over the distal incus for stability, and the piston prosthesis can be mechanically or laser/heat crimped to the incus if made of nitinol.
- Large series show comparable hearing results with stapedectomy and stapedotomy, with results stable over time. Air–bone gap closure within 10 dB is expected in the majority of primary stapedectomies, and closure within 20 dB in nearly all cases.[5]

Ossicular Chain Reconstruction in a Modified Mastoid Cavity

- Same principles are generally applied to ossicular reconstruction in a modified mastoid cavity.
- Middle ear volume in a mastoid cavity is smaller, and the middle ear cleft is shallower, making ossicular reconstruction more challenging.
- Ossicular chain reconstruction in a mastoid cavity can be done at the time of creation of the cavity or it can be staged, depending on the extent of mucosal disease and surgeon preference.
- There are a variety of shorter PORPs and TORPs available to span the distance between the stapes and tympanic membrane (ie, Goldenberg cap), or between the oval window footplate and the tympanic membrane.

References

1. Ghazal SD, Armine K, Margaret TD, Matthew LC. Cochlear implantation outcomes in adults with single-sided deafness: a systematic review and meta-analysis. *Otol Neurotol.* 2023 April;44(4): 297-309.
2. Dylan AL, Joshua AL, Shaun AN. et al. Cochlear implantation for treatment of tinnitus in single-sided deafness: a systematic review and meta-analysis. *Otol Neurotol.* 2020 Sep;41(8):e1004-e1012.
3. Slater PW, Rizer FM, Schuring AG, Lippy WH. Practical use of total and partial ossicular replacement prostheses in ossiculoplasty. *Laryngoscope.* 1997 Sep;107(9):1193-1198.
4. Lee KJ, Usawicz. Middle Ear Surgery. In: Lucente FE, ed. *Highlights of the Instructional Courses.* Mosby Year Book; 1994, Vol. 7, 315-318.
5. Kisilevsky VE, Dutt SN, Bailie NA, Halik JJ. Hearing results of 1145 stapedotomies evaluated with Amsterdam hearing evaluation plots. *J Laryngol Otol.* 2009 Jul;123(7):730-736.

Questions

1. Which of the following is not an indication for an osseointegrated bone conduction hearing device?
   A. Mixed hearing loss with a significant conductive component
   B. Conductive hearing loss with absent or either biphasic acoustic reflex, normal otoscopy, and an air-bone gap of 25 to 30 dB
   C. Ears with draining mastoid cavities
   D. Conductive hearing loss that is not amenable to surgical correction
   E. Unilateral profound sensorineural hearing loss

2. Which of the following has not been shown in patients with single-sided deafness and cochlear implantation?
   A. Good hearing performance in noise
   B. Relief of ipsilateral tinnitus
   C. Good sound localization
   D. Risk of contralateral sensorineural hearing loss as a result of cochlear implantation
   E. No interference with the hearing ear

3. Which of the following is a strict contraindication for stapedectomy or stapedotomy?
   A. Widely dehiscent facial nerve without overhang
   B. Severely thickened footplate
   C. Persistent stapedial artery
   D. Active serous effusion
   E. History of Meniere disease
   F. C and D
   G. D and E

4. Which of the following is true regarding venting in a hearing aid?
   A. Very few hearing aids incorporate venting.
   B. Large venting improves hearing in noise but is contraindicated in ears with significant high-frequency hearing loss.
   C. Large venting makes a hearing aid more comfortable by eliminating the occlusion effect.
   D. Occlusion effect results from the reverberation of high frequencies in an open ear.
   E. Open-fit hearing aids, with large venting, are suitable for patients with significant low-frequency hearing loss.

5. Which of the following is not a potential complication with stapes surgery?
   A. Tympanic membrane perforation, repaired with an underlay fascia graft.
   B. Sensorineural hearing loss occurs in 10% to 12% after primary stapedectomy and higher after revisions.
   C. A floating footplate can occur, which can be managed by fenestrating the floating footplate using a laser or aborting the procedure, allowing the footplate to refixate, then attempting the surgery at a later date.
   D. Temporary sensorineural hearing loss above 2 kHz with mild disequilibrium can occur, thought to be the result of serous labyrinthitis during the healing process after surgery.
   E. Recurrent conductive hearing loss can occur due to necrosis and shortening of the long process of incus, displaced prosthesis, or reparative granuloma (1-2 weeks after surgery).

Chapter 18
Cochlear Implants

Overview

- A cochlear implant (CI) is a surgically implanted device used for hearing rehabilitation of adults and children with advanced sensorineural hearing loss (SNHL) and/or poor speech discrimination who gain limited benefit from conventional hearing aids.
- At a fundamental level, a CI is a transducer that transforms acoustic energy into an electrical signal, which is used to stimulate surviving spiral ganglion cells of the auditory nerve.
- There are currently three FDA-approved CI manufacturers: Advanced Bionics Corporation (Valencia, CA, USA), Cochlear Corporation (Lane Cove, Australia), and Med-El GmbH (Innsbruck, Austria).
- Over the last three decades, advancements in surgical technique, electrode design, and improved speech processing strategies have led to increasingly better outcomes in CI recipients. As a result, FDA candidacy criteria have gradually expanded from initially only implanting postlingual deafened adults with profound bilateral SNHL to now implanting adults and children with greater degrees of residual hearing (Table 18-1). Furthermore, a growing proportion of patients are undergoing CI for off-label or nontraditional indications including single-sided deafness, retro-cochlear hearing loss, asymmetrical SNHL in adults and children with at least one ear that is better than the performance cut-off for age, and children less than 9 months of age.

Cochlear Implant Design

External Components

- Microphone—placed near the earhook and receives natural acoustic information and converts it to an analog electrical signal, which is sent to the behind-the-ear (BTE) or single unit off-the-ear sound processor.
- Sound processor—alters the signal through the processes of amplification, compression, and filtering. The analog signal is digitized via Fourier analysis, making it possible to convey timing, frequency, and intensity information in a way that is meaningful to the central nervous system.

Table 18-1

	Cochlear Implant Candidacy Guidelines			Cochlear Nucleus Hybrid System Candidacy Guidelines
	Adult	*Children (2-17 y)*	*Children (9-24 mo)*	*Adults Only (≥ 18 y)*
Hearing threshold	**Moderate to profound** SNHL in both ears (> 40 dB)	**Severe to profound** SNHL (> 70 dB)	**Profound** SNHL (> 90 dB)	Normal to moderate hearing loss (thresholds better than 60 dB HL) in the low frequencies (≤ 500 Hz) *and* severe to profound mid to high-frequency hearing loss, PTA (2,3,4 kHz) ≥ 75 dB HL in the ear to be implanted *and* moderately severe to profound mid to high-frequency hearing loss, PTA (2,3,4 kHz) ≥ 60 dB HL in the contralateral ear
Word Recognition	Limited benefit from binaural amplification defined by **≤ 50% sentence recognition in the ear to be implanted** (or ≤ **60%** by **CMS** criteria) and ≤ **60% in the contralateral ear** or binaurally.	Limited benefit from binaural amplification defined by **≤ 20%-30%** word recognition scores	Limited benefit from binaural amplification trial based on MAIS	Aided CNC word recognition score **between 10% and 60%** (inclusively) in the ear to be implanted. Contralateral ear equal to or better than that of the ear to be implanted but not more than 80% correct.

CMS, Centers for Medicare and Medicaid Services; MAIS, Meaningful Auditory Integration Scale; SNHL, sensorineural hearing loss.

- Radiofrequency (RF) transmitter antenna—sends the processed signal transcutaneously to the implanted receiver-stimulator.
- External magnet—aligns with the internal magnet to facilitate transcutaneous RF signal transmission.
- Battery.

Internal Components

- Internal magnet
- Internal RF Antenna
- Receiver/Stimulator—translates the electrical signal into rapid electrical impulses that are distributed to the individual wires within the electrode array
  - Continuous-Interleaved-Sampling (CIS) is the most common signal processing strategy used. The CIS strategy minimizes problems associated with channel interaction by presenting nonsimultaneous (or interleaved) brief, rapid impulses across the electrode array. As a result, the tonotopic organization of the cochlea is better represented.

- Electrode array—designed to be placed within the scala tympani. Contains individual wires that transmit data for each respective channel along the implanted multichannel electrode. The electrodes stimulate the spiral ganglion cells located in Rosenthal canal, which in turn propagate signal along the auditory nerve to the brain for further processing.
  - Standard electrode arrays contain 12 (MED-EL), 16 (Advanced Bionics), or 22 (Cochlear) electrode contacts, though some studies have found that the majority of users have less than 10 perceptually unique channels active at any one time.
  - Multiple electrode designs are available from each company to enhance the ability of the surgeon to preserve residual hearing and minimize insertion trauma. Electrodes have been made shorter, thinner, and more flexible. Surgeons can choose the electrode array best suited for the patient.

Candidacy Evaluation

Medical Assessment

- A thorough otologic medical history should attempt to determine the etiology of the hearing loss, though not always possible. Factors that may lead to cochlear ossification or scarring should be elicited, such as a history of meningitis, temporal bone fracture, otosclerosis, labyrinthitis, and prior vestibular schwannoma resection.
- Duration of deafness is valuable to understand as very long-standing severe or profound hearing loss may predict a poorer outcome.
- Patients with chronic otitis media may require staged surgery based on the experience of the surgeon, where infection, perforation, or cholesteatoma is initially treated and the implant is inserted during a staged second operation
- Recurrent acute otitis media (RAOM) should not be allowed to unduly delay implantation, particularly in children.
  - Cochlear implants can safely coexist with pressure equalizing (PE) tubes.
  - Children who are still susceptible to RAOM may keep PE tubes in place prior to undergoing surgery without placing the success of the CI or the patient at undue risk.
  - Replacement of PE tubes after CI is also acceptable for treatment of RAOM.
- Pertinent nonotological medical history that may result in poor wound healing include previous radiation to the area, immunodeficiency, poorly controlled diabetes mellitus, tobacco use, malnutrition, a prominent history of allergic hypersensitivity reactions, or widespread dermatological disease.
- Neurocognitive decline in the elderly (eg, dementia) or cognitive developmental delay in children and adults may reduce implant performance but are generally not considered contraindications.

Radiologic Assessment

- The goal of imaging is to ensure no contraindications to cochlear implantation exist and to facilitate safe surgical planning.
- **Magnetic resonance imaging (MRI)**
  - Superior modality for confirming the presence of the cochlear nerve since it allows direct visualization of the nerve. The cochlear nerve is best imaged on heavily T2-weighted MRI (eg, CISS, FIESTA) in the parasagittal plane.

- Gold standard for determining cochlear patency because it is able to distinguish between fluid versus cochlear fibrosis versus ossification.
- Useful in identifying retrocochlear pathology, such as vestibular schwannoma, that may interfere with signaling to the brain stem and auditory cortex.
- Spares the patient ionizing radiation but is more time-consuming and costly compared to CT.
- Provides the patient with their last opportunity to obtain high-quality brain imaging without artifact.

- **High-resolution computed tomography (HRCT)**
  - Useful in diagnosing bony cochlear malformations.
  - Useful in confirming presence of a cochlear nerve in cases of a narrow internal auditory canal (IAC) (< 3 mm) where MRI resolution is limited in its ability to adequately identify and separate nerves. In this setting, HRCT is used to evaluate the bony cochlear nerve canal (BCNC), whereby a closed BCNC supports the diagnosis of cochlear nerve deficiency/aplasia.
  - Provides details on the surgical anatomy, which may help execute safe surgery. Potential surgical obstacles include:
    - Poorly pneumatized mastoid and/or facial recess
    - Extremely anterior sigmoid sinus
    - High-riding jugular bulb
    - Aberrant facial nerve course, particularly either anterior or medial displacement of the proximal mastoid segment
    - Inner ear malformation with risk of CSF gusher (increased in the setting of a thin cribriform area between the modiolus [eg, IP3 deformity], a widened internal auditory canal, or enlarged vestibular aqueduct).

Audiometric Assessment

- In children, the method of candidacy testing is dependent upon age and level of cognitive development. In very young children, candidacy testing relies on otoacoustic emissions, auditory brainstem responses, behavioral testing, and parental questionnaires. In older children, behavioral audiometry and age-appropriate speech perception testing are performed. In most children, a minimum of a 3-month hearing aid trial should be completed before implantation. Evidence-based pediatric minimum speech test battery guidelines have been developed and published.
- In adults, candidacy evaluation should follow published adult minimum speech test battery guidelines that rely on speech perception testing using Arizona Biomedical Sentences (AzBio), Consonant-Nucleus-Consonant (CNC) monosyllabic words, and/or Bamford-Kowal-Bench Speech-in-Noise test (BKB-SIN).
- Sentence testing is performed in the unilateral and binaural best-aided condition with properly fitted hearing aids. Additional background noise is commonly used to better simulate real-world listening environment.

Psychological Assessment

- Performed for exclusionary reasons to identify subjects who have severe cognitive impairment, undetected psychosis, or unrealistic expectations.
- Valuable information related to the family dynamics and other factors in the patient's milieu that may affect implant acceptance and performance is assessed.
- Identification of mild dementia can help with planning and structuring an effective rehabilitation plan for after implantation. The relationship between cognition and hearing loss is complicated and not yet well understood.

Current Audiometric Selection Criteria

Adults

- FDA criteria exist for each device, but are not consistent across devices or companies. Insurance companies also have varied criteria, but are generally similar to FDA guidelines (Table 18-1).
- Audiometric testing protocols are not standardized (eg, some centers use AzBio in quiet and others test in noise), and thus patients may be considered a candidate in one center but not another. The goal of testing is to identify candidates who will benefit from implantation. FDA and insurance company guidelines are generally felt to be restrictive and understandably lag current practice and evidence. Most large centers in the United States find AzBio testing in noise and CNC word scores to be most helpful for counseling patients. In general, candidates have the following characteristics:
  - Bilateral moderate-to-profound SNHL
  - Aided sentence scores less than or equal to 50% in the ear to be implanted and less than or equal to 60% in the best-aided condition (usually binaural hearing aids).
  - Centers for Medicare and Medicaid Services (CMS) has stricter criteria: Bilateral moderate to profound sensorineural hearing loss and binaural aided sentences less than or equal to 60%.
  - Single-sided deafness, described as severe to profound (PTA of > 80 dB) with a CNC score of 5% or less in the ear to be implanted and normal or near normal in the contralateral ear (PTA of ≤ 30 dB).

Children

- Criteria for children are even less standardized than that for adults due to young age and evolving cognitive and language abilities.
- More than or equal to 9 months of age based on the FDA but earlier implantation has been demonstrated to be safe and may result in improved language outcomes.
- Little to no benefit from hearing aids over a 3 to 6 month trial period.
  - Trial period waived for children who had meningitis with radiographic evidence of ossification.
- Bilateral profound SNHL (for patients 12-24 months old); severe-to-profound SNHL (for patients > 24 months old).
- Aided open-set word recognition scores less than or equal to 30% in children capable of testing.
  - Multisyllabic lexical neighborhood test (MLNT) or lexical neighborhood test (LNT) are commonly used tests.

Special situations

- **Auditory neuropathy spectrum disorder (ANSD)**
  - Patients with ANSD have normal otoacoustic emissions but an absent auditory brain stem response. Pure tone thresholds range from normal to severe.
  - Reliable open-set speech recognition can be achieved with CI in ANSD.
- **Single-sided deafness (SSD)**
  - CI for SSD has been FDA approved for certain manufacturers, and an increasing number of commercial payors are covering this service.
  - CI for SSD has been shown to reduce or alleviate tinnitus, improve sound localization, and enhance quality of life in many patients.

- **Neurofibromatosis type II with bilateral vestibular schwannomas or sporadic vestibular schwannomas**
  - Historically, this patient population was not considered for cochlear implantation; however, more recent experience demonstrates that many CI recipients achieve open-set speech recognition. When an intact cochlear nerve exists, outcomes with a CI are generally superior to auditory brain stem implants (ABIs). If the CI does not work, an ABI is still an option.
- **Other retrocochlear or CNS disorders**
  - Patients with superficial siderosis, pachymeningitis, neurosarcoidosis, history of CNS radiation, brain stem lesions, or similar present as unique situations. The decision to proceed or not is difficult, particularly because the results are unpredictable. However, successful restoration of hearing is possible, thus making the attempt reasonable.

Contraindications

- Complete labyrinthine aplasia
- Complete cochlear ossification
- Cochlear Aplasia
- Absent cochlear nerve

Preoperative Considerations

Vaccinations for Prevention of Meningitis

- The Centers for Disease Control and Prevention (CDC) has specific recommendations for age-appropriate vaccination of adult and pediatric implant candidates and recipients.
  - https://www.cdc.gov/vaccines/vpd/mening/public/dis-cochlear-faq-gen.html
- **Prevnar 13 (PCV13)**—In children, must ensure the patient receives this as part of their routine childhood vaccination. If the vaccination was missed, the appropriate catch-up schedule should be used. PCV13 is given to children less than 2 years old. If a child with cochlear implants did not get the recommended doses when they were less than 2 years old, additional doses of PCV13 may be needed.
- **Pneumovax (PPSV23)**—Given to children when more than or equal to 2 years old (not effective prior) at least 8 weeks after they have completed the PCV13 series. Adults should receive one dose of PCV13 followed by one dose of PPSV23 if they have not previously received these vaccines.

Side Selection

- The selection of which ear to implant must be determined on an individual basis, and should take into account the amount of residual hearing, otologic history, duration of deafness, and any pertinent imaging or anatomical findings.
- In adults, the better-hearing ear generally does better with CI. However, if there is residual functional hearing in the better hearing ear, it may be advantageous to implant the worse hearing ear and continue to use a hearing aid in the better hearing ear. This is termed the "**bimodal condition**."
- In children born with bilateral deafness, early bilateral implantation ensures the "better ear" will always be implanted and all the potential advantages of binaural hearing obtained

- In prelingual patients with a long period of auditory deprivation (> 10 years), the better ear is often chosen because these patients generally have poor outcomes and have little useful residual hearing.
- In patients with cochlear malformations, the less dysplastic ear is often implanted first because it is generally safer, with fewer surgical risks, and better postoperative audiometric outcomes are seen (likely due to the probability of the cochlea having a more normal arrangement of stimulatable substrate).

Device and Electrode Selection

- Patients generally choose the device that best fits their needs after being counseled on all three FDA-approved devices.
  - Device performance and reliability is generally comparable between all three implant manufacturers, despite variations in component design and sound processing strategies.
  - Some devices have magnets more compatible to MRI scanning and may be preferred when periodic scans are anticipated.
- Electrode arrays are broadly characterized as having a perimodiolar (pre-curved) or straight (lateral wall) configuration.
- **Perimodiolar** electrode arrays are pre-curved which brings the electrodes closer to the modiolus. By minimizing the distance between the stimulating electrodes and the receiving neural cell groups, theoretical advantages of the perimodiolar configuration include lower energy requirements, reduction in channel interactions, and more discrete neural population stimulation. However, they are more difficult to insert, have a higher risk of tip fold over, and may have a higher incidence of intracochlear trauma.
- **Straight (lateral wall)** electrode arrays passively follow the outer cochlear wall and can be implanted more easily and less traumatically, providing a better opportunity to preserve residual low-frequency hearing. The surgeon can choose the depth of insertion during surgery, and there is a larger variety of manufactured electrode lengths from which to choose.

Bilateral Pediatric Cochlear Implantation

- For prelingual deafened children, there has been a trend toward early, bilateral cochlear implantation to permit optimal auditory development, language acquisition, and integration into society.
- The importance of early implantation is to capture the "window of opportunity" from birth to 2 years of age where there is high neural plasticity and peak language receptivity.
  - If this window is missed, **cross-modal plasticity** is observed whereby the brain reorganizes its resources by allocating the cortical areas originally designed for auditory purposes, for other modalities such as vision or somatosensation.
- Simultaneous versus sequential implantation
  - Simultaneous implantation results in better speech and language outcomes compared with sequential implantation with a long (> 12 months) interimplant delay.
  - Simultaneous implantation is less resource consuming for rehabilitation and spares the child a second anesthetic.
  - Logistical issues (hospital policy, insurance reimbursement, uncertain outcomes, parent reluctance) may affect the decision of whether to implant simultaneously or sequentially.
  - Results with sequential implantation with a short (< 12 months) interimplant delay are comparable with simultaneous implantation.

- Benefits of bilateral implantation
  - By implanting both ears, a greater number of spiral ganglion cell populations are being stimulated, thus guaranteeing that the better ear (eg, the one with greater neural survival) will be implanted. Additionally, one implant may compensate for contralateral frequency gaps resulting from asymmetric spiral ganglion cell population losses, and thus bilateral implantation could provide complementary cues and support better performance.
  - Bilateral implantation reduces the risk that a child will go "off air," resulting in auditory deprivation because having a second device allows patients greater latitude during times when the device malfunctions, batteries die, etc.
  - Bilateral implantation allows for enhanced **speech perception** (in quiet and noise) and **sound localization**, attributed to:
    - **Head shadow effect**: occurs when the head acts as an acoustic barrier, effectively shielding one ear from contralateral competing background noise. Patients with bilateral implants can preferentially utilize the ear with a more optimal signal-to-noise ratio to improve overall speech understanding in noisy environments.
    - **Binaural summation**: a result of central processing that occurs when the brain receives redundant information from each ear, allowing it to draw more meaningful acoustic information from those two sources than it could from a single ear's input.
    - **Squelch effect** (also known as the "cocktail party effect"): the ability to focus one's listening attention on a single talker among competing background noise due to central processing of interaural timing, level, and spectral differences.
    - **Improved sound localization**: The brain uses differences in interaural time and intensity to determine the direction from which a sound is coming.

Preserving Hearing During Cochlear Implantation

- In the past, patients were counseled that they would lose all residual hearing as a result of CI surgery. However, advances in CI technology (including thinner more flexible electrodes) and refinements to surgical technique (including atraumatic, "soft surgery" principles) have resulted in the ability to preserve residual low-frequency hearing in many patients undergoing CI surgery.
- Preserving low frequency (typically < 1 kHz) residual hearing allows for **electroacoustic stimulation (EAS),** which confers distinct advantages in speech perception in noise and music appreciation. Generally, hearing thresholds must be less than 80 dB HL to be considered functionally aidable.
  - Patients may wear a hearing aid to boost their low-frequency residual hearing in the same ear with the cochlear implant (termed the **"hybrid strategy"**).
- Principles of atraumatic "soft surgery" for hearing preservation cases:
  - Use of flexible electrodes, which require less insertion force, preserve residual hearing, and reduce intracochlear scarring.
  - Use of a round window insertion (versus cochleostomy) is preferred.
  - Electrode array is inserted very slowly.
  - Avoidance of suctioning perilymph.
  - Preserving the integrity of the ossicles and avoidance of overpacking around the implant.
  - Use of perioperative steroids.
- Mechanisms for acute mechanical inner ear injury during electrode insertion include:
  - Fracture of the osseous spiral lamina or spiral ligament.
  - Trauma to the lateral wall at the first basal turn of the cochlea.

    - Deflecting the tip of the array toward the basilar membrane resulting displacement of the basilar membrane or fracture of the interscalar partition with subsequent electrode excursion into the scala media or even the scala vestibuli.
    - Deep insertions, which result in trauma due to the narrower radius of turn and smaller scalar cross-sectional diameter.
- Potential benefits of minimizing electrode trauma during implantation
    - Preserving low-frequency residual hearing in patients allows for more natural hearing due to concurrent electroacoustic stimulation (EAS) strategies and greater music appreciation.
    - Less intracochlear fibrosis and ossification making revision surgery less problematic and may permit patient participation in future developments such as cellular regeneration.
    - Lower risk of device related otogenic meningitis.
    - Improved performance in the electric-only condition due to better neural preservation.
- Depth of insertion remains a controversial topic. The benefits of deep insertion include the ability to stimulate lower frequencies and a greater population of surviving nerve fibers or spiral ganglion cell populations, theoretically allowing for better frequency coverage. However, the intracochlear trauma sustained with deep insertions may offset certain advantages, and therefore using shorter electrodes may improve overall performance. Current focus is on individualizing electrode position through intraoperative testing, cochlear duct measurements and even live testing during surgery under local anesthesia.

Operative Technique

Surgical Steps

- Cochlear implantation is typically performed under general anesthesia without muscle relaxation to allow for facial nerve monitoring.
- *Incision*: A postauricular skin incision is designed to provide adequate exposure to the mastoid and place the receiver-stimulator device.
- *Mastoidectomy*:
    - A mastoidectomy with facial recess approach is performed in the vast majority of cases.
    - Careful thinning of the posterior EAC is important for exposure for working through the facial recess.
    - The posterior and inferior mastoid cavities are not saucerized because the bony overhangs are helpful in retaining the electrode array coiled within the mastoid.
    - Preservation of the incus buttress and care not to damage the incus is critical in patients with significant residual hearing.
- *Exposing round window*:
    - The round window niche is visualized through the facial recess.
    - Removal of bone around the round window niche will allow direct visualization of the round window membrane.
    - Occasionally, the round window niche is posteriorly positioned and is not well visualized through the facial recess or is obscured by ossification. In these situations, it is important not to be misdirected by hypotympanic air cells.
- *Securing the implant*: The receiver–stimulator can be secured in a shallow well created in the outer cortex of the skull. Alternatively, a tight subperiosteal pocket under the temporalis muscle may be created to secure the implant. A trough is usually drilled for the electrode.

- *Electrode insertion*: The electrode array is inserted into the scala tympani, either via the round window (most common) or through a cochleostomy positioned anteroinferior to the round window. It is inserted in a slow controlled motion, adhering to atraumatic "soft surgery" principles (see earlier discussion), which is especially important for hearing preservation.
- *Closure*: After insertion of the active electrode array, the cochlear opening is sealed with small pieces of fascia or muscle. The postauricular incision is closed in a layered fashion and a mastoid dressing is applied.

Special Surgical Situations

- **Cochlear malformations**
  - The majority of cochlear malformations can be implanted with the standard transmastoid-facial recess approach.
  - Alternative surgical approaches may be indicated depending on the malformation:
    - **Double posterior labyrinthotomy technique** is used for common cavity deformity.
    - **Suprameatal approach** is indicated in cases of an underdeveloped mastoid, narrow facial recess, anomalous facial nerve, or very anterior sigmoid sinus. In this approach, a tympanomeatal flap is elevated to visualize the round window.
    - **Subtotal petrosectomy** (canal wall down with EAC overclosure) is done for unfavorable anatomy prohibiting standard approach, uncontrollable CSF leak, or revision surgery for recurrent meningitis secondary to persistent CSF leak.
    - **Intentional scala vestibuli insertions** can be done for cochlear hypoplasia with absent round window or for cases of limited scala tympani ossification after meningitis or otosclerosis.
  - There is a higher incidence of an anomalous facial nerve course in patients with cochlear malformations.
    - Most common aberrant course observed is anteromedial displacement of the second genu and vertical segment into the region of the oval or round window.
  - Patients with inner ear malformations are at greater risk of both pre- and postimplantation meningitis.
- **Cochlear ossification**
  - Occurs in approximately one-half of patients deafened by neonatal meningitis.
  - Most cases of ossification are mild and only affect the first few millimeters of the basal turn. Management involves creation of a cochleostomy anterior to the round window with drilling of the new bone followed by conventional implantation.
  - For more advanced ossification, options include performing a partial electrode insertion, inserting into the scala vestibuli, or performing a more elaborate drill-out approach and using a split electrode.
  - Split electrodes (ie, two distinct electrodes) have been designed so that one electrode can be partially inserted in the drilled-out tunnel of the basal turn and the second electrode is inserted into a cochleostomy developed just anterior to the oval window.

Intraoperative Testing

- **Impedance Testing**
  - Assesses the electrode-tissue interface by measuring the resistance met across a closed circuit loop.
  - Can help confirm device integrity and potentially alert the surgeon to tip fold-over or extracochlear electrode placement.

- Can detect damage to an individual lead wire (eg, open circuit failure yielding high impedances) or a breach of insulation between two separate wires (eg, short circuit failure yielding low impedances).
- If greater than 3 or 5 individual electrode failures occur within an array, it may be a sign of impending device deterioration requiring future revision surgery.
- Transimpedance matrix measurements can detect electrode tip fold-over.

- **Neural response telemetry (NRT)** is a tool used to measure **electrically evoked compound action potential (ECAP).**
  - ECAP evaluates the patient's neural response to electrical stimulation following CI.
  - Determining ECAP thresholds may be helpful in children because they serve as a starting point for electrode stimulation levels for initial CI programming. In adults, behavioral level testing remains the preferred method of mapping.
- **Electrocochleography (ECoG)** records electrical potentials generated by the cochlea in response to acoustic stimulation.
  - May be used intraoperatively to assess for impending or active trauma for purpose of acoustic hearing preservation.
- **Plain film radiograph** (profile and modified Stenvers views)
  - Used to confirm correct intracochlear placement and ensure absence of buckling or tip fold-over
  - Can serve as a baseline should electrode migration be suspected later
- **Intraoperative fluoroscopy**
  - May be used when implanting complex cochlear anomalies to help determine the insertion angle, depth, and cochleostomy position.
  - Helpful in avoiding an intrameatal implantation, which is possible in common cavity, cochlear hypoplasia, and incomplete partition cochlear malformations.

Complications

Intraoperative Complications

- **Injury to tegmen ± dural tear**
  - Risk of CSF leak and meningitis
  - Repair with fascia underlay graft. Additionally, may add bone pate
  - May proceed with implantation
- **Violation of EAC**
  - Risk of electrode array extruding through the skin of the EAC and/or infection
  - A bony defect alone can be repaired with bone pate. If skin is violated, a cartilage or fascia graft should be used to reinforce the area.
- **Tympanic membrane tear**
  - Risk of infection.
  - Management involves cartilage or fascia tympanoplasty with concurrent implantation.
- **Facial nerve injury**
  - Rare (< 1%). Continuous facial nerve monitoring is commonly employed.
  - Injury may occur by direct transection or heat transfer from the drill.
  - Direct injury identified intraoperatively should be managed with nerve decompression and/or primary repair.
  - Postoperative facial paralysis should be observed in the recovery room followed by oral steroids if it does not resolve.

- **Malpositioned or damaged electrodes**
  - Kinking or electrode shorts may be identified on intraoperative imaging or electrophysiological testing, and requires the electrode to be removed and reinserted.
  - Surgical trauma may damage electrodes leading to device failure.

Early Complications

- **Taste disturbance (Dysgeusia)**
  - Usually temporary but may be permanent in 3% of cases.
  - The chorda tympani nerve can be preserved in almost all cases but may require dividing in rare cases where the round window niche cannot be well visualized.
- **Tinnitus**
  - Cochlear trauma from electrode insertion may cause new tinnitus or exacerbate existing tinnitus, although in most cases this is short lived. In fact, most studies show that cochlear implants may suppress tinnitus in a large percentage of cases.
- **Vestibular dysfunction**
  - Temporary vestibular symptoms are not uncommon after cochlear implantation, especially in the elderly. Vestibular rehabilitation is recommended.
  - Benign paroxysmal positional vertigo may occur and responds to standard treatment.

Late Complications

- **Wound infection or skin flap breakdown**
  - Historically, skin flap breakdown was the most common complication, but smaller devices and use of a more limited incision has decreased its incidence. Management initially includes antibiotics. Devices can sometimes be rescued but usually require removal and reimplantation after 3 to 6 months if unresponsive to medical treatment. Cochlear implants may become infected in a delayed fashion similar to other prosthetic implants such as hips and knees.
- **Device failure**
  - Occurs in ~4% of cases over lifetime of the device. Usually due to spontaneous electrical malfunction or trauma.
  - Explantation with reimplantation using a new electrode can be performed safely and without decrement to performance.
  - During surgery for cochlear reimplantation, the electrode is cut at the facial recess and initially left in place while the old device is removed and the new receiver/stimulator is placed. This is done to prevent premature collapse of the intracochlear tunnel created by the fibrous capsule that forms around the electrode after implantation, which would result in incomplete insertion. Once the new device is secured in place, the old electrode array is removed and the new one is immediately inserted through the same tract.
- **Cerebrospinal Fluid Leak**
  - Multiple potential causes for this rare complication:
    - Dura is exposed and violated during creation of the bony well or placement of tie-down sutures (if used).
    - Unsealed cochleostomy after electrode insertion.
    - **Oval or Round window fistula:** occurs in the setting of defective partitioning between the IAC fundus and cochlea which allows CSF to come into direct contact with the round and oval windows. Continuous CSF pressure erodes the stapes footplate or leaks around the electrode.
  - Management includes revision surgery to pack the leak. A lumbar drain or eustachian tube obliteration with ear canal overclosure may be useful adjunct measures to manage a leak.

- **Meningitis**
  - Incidence of bacterial meningitis in children with CIs is 30 times greater than the incidence in normal hearing children.
  - *Streptococcus pneumoniae* (62%) is the most common cause of meningitis. Other etiologies include *Hemophilus influenza, Staphylococcus, Group A Streptococcus, Pseudomonas,* and viral.
  - Risk factors for meningitis include use of an electrode positioner (*no longer used*), inner ear malformations, and CSF leak.
  - Retrograde bacterial spread via cochleostomy or oval window fistula may lead to recurrent meningitis.
  - Uncomplicated cases of acute otitis media should be promptly treated on an outpatient basis with oral antibiotics and close follow-up. Inpatient IV antibiotics may be considered in severe or persistent cases of acute infection.
- **Facial nerve stimulation**
  - Increased incidence in patients with cochlear otosclerosis, otic capsule fractures, cochlear anomalies, or in patients requiring high levels of stimulation due to long duration of auditory deprivation.
  - Management involves selective deactivation of individual electrodes.
  - In cases of intractable stimulation, revision surgery with explantation is indicated.
- **Device or electrode migration**
  - Receiver–stimulator migration may occur with head trauma or when not properly recessed in a bony well, or not snuggly fit into a tight subperiosteal pocket.
  - Electrode migration presents with fluctuating or inconsistent thresholds requiring frequent re-programming. More common in patients with cochlear malformations since the implant is not confined by the normal scalar anatomy.
  - Initial objection to implanting very young children were partially based on perceived potential for electrode migration or extrusion secondary to skull growth. However long-term studies have shown no migration of the electrode array over time, confirming the stability of the electrode despite concerns of the effects of skull growth.

Device Programming

- The initial stimulation is scheduled around 2 to 4 weeks after surgery though some centers have also begun offering early activation, often the next day or same week after surgery.
- Magnet strength for transmitter determined.
- Electrical threshold and comfort levels determined.
- Map created.
- Sound quality improves over the first 3 to 6 months after activation as the brain adapts to the new auditory signal.
- Most adults have 2 to 5 programming sessions in the first year, then annually or as needed. Increasingly this can be done remotely, allowing the patient to remain at home.
- Device programming in severely malformed cochleae, particularly common cavities, is challenging due to the unpredictable and scattered arrangement of the malformed neural elements along the outer wall of the cochlea which do not follow the normal tonotopic distribution.

Outcomes

Outcomes in Adults

- The cochlear implant can reliably restore excellent access to sound with thresholds as measured on an audiogram typically around 25 dB HL.
- Open-set sentence recognition scores in postlingual deafened adults commonly exceed 75% with current speech-processing strategies.
- Adult CI recipients report a restored capability to communicate on the telephone (attained by roughly 60%), the ability to converse without the necessity of lip-reading, improvement in tinnitus, and improvement in preimplantation depression.
- Prelingually deafened adults who communicate primarily with sign language may achieve sound awareness but rarely meaningful open-set word recognition. Preoperative explanation of goals and expectations is critical to a successful outcome in this population.
- Duration of deafness and preoperative speech perception scores can predict 80% of the variance in speech perception outcomes seen among CI recipients.
- Standard hearing test results fail to capture the true benefit of CI. To date there is limited disease-specific quality of life data, but more tools are being developed.

Outcomes in Children and Adolescents

- Adolescents with progressive SNHL who outgrow their hearing aid technology are excellent candidates and perform similar to adults with progressive loss.
- Prelingually deafened adolescents have a higher risk of becoming non-users of the device. Extensive preoperative discussions are needed to make a good decision and avoid this outcome.
- Postlingual deafened children have been shown to often achieve 90%+ word understanding after implantation.
- Prelingual deafened children (majority of pediatric deaf patients) make slower progress toward oral communication and with more variable outcomes.
  - Earlier implantation in children generally yields more favorable results, and many centers routinely implant children under 12 months of age.
- Children with bilateral cochlear implants do not perform worse on functional balance testing when compared with children with a unilateral implant.
- Pediatric CI is an extremely beneficial and cost-effective intervention. Many children implanted prior to age 3 (and an even higher percentage of children implanted prior to 18 months old) will eventually achieve age-appropriate speech recognition and production. Current expectations are for most children to transition into mainstream schooling in the early elementary years. Depending on the individual child they may need more or less support from deaf and hard of hearing services (eg, FM system, notetaker) to be successful. Not all children will be able to develop adequate oral language skills and will also need a manual language such as American Sign Language (ASL) to excel.

Outcomes in Hearing Preservation Surgery

- The rate of partial hearing preservation using conventional length electrode users ranges from 50% to 90%. It is important to understand how "hearing preservation" is defined when comparing studies.
- Short electrode arrays were designed to preserve low frequencies by not extending into and disturbing the apical cochlear neural elements where the low frequencies reside. These have been shown to preserve residual hearing in more than 90% of patients at the time of surgery. However, for an unknown reason, there is potential for delayed hearing loss,

typically in the first 3 to 6 months. Reimplantation with a standard array in these patients who lose their residual hearing will usually provide higher levels of speech recognition.

Outcomes in Cochlear Malformations

- The severity of inner ear dysplasia is thought to inversely correlate with speech perception performance.
- Patients with mild to moderate cochlear anomalies (eg, Mondini deformity) may potentially achieve same eventual audiometric outcome with CI as in children with radiographically normal ears, but it may take a longer period of time and more intensive habilitation with a speech-language pathologist.
- Patients with severe anomalies (common cavity, cochlear hypoplasia) typically have poor speech performance but the sound perception may still serve as a benefit.
- An intraoperative cerebrospinal fluid (CSF) gusher does not significantly impact speech perception outcome.

Outcomes in Single-Sided Deafness

- Tinnitus suppression is reported in 80% to 90% of patients.
- Significant improvements in speech perception, sound localization, and quality of life are consistently reported.
- Device wear time is associated with speech outcomes for adults with SSD. A minimum of 8 hours per day is recommended.
- A prolonged duration of single-sided deafness in postlingual adults does not appear to have the same deleterious effects on speech outcomes compared to in younger patients with bilateral deafness. Therefore a long duration of deafness in an adult with postlingual onset should not be precluded from considering cochlear implantation. In contrast, adults with congenital SSD onset should be counseled on guarded CI outcomes.

Outcomes in Patients with Vestibular Schwannoma

- Speech testing outcomes in patients with vestibular schwannoma are highly variable and depends on tumor size and management strategy.
- Most patients with observed or radiated vestibular schwannomas obtain open-set speech perception, whereas approximately 50% of patients who underwent microsurgical resection had this outcome.
- Cochlear ossification—that would prevent or complicate full electrode insertion—can occur within several months after microsurgery, with the translabyrinthine approach demonstrating the greatest risk followed by retrosigmoid approach and finally the middle fossa approach.
- Preservation of the cochlear nerve is required for successful cochlear implantation in patients undergoing microsurgery. Promontory stimulation testing can aid with determining the presence of a cochlear nerve in patients without measurable pure tone thresholds, though the usefulness of the test is controversial due to the presence of both false-negatives and false-positives.

Future Technology

- Fully implanted cochlear implants have been developed and are undergoing clinical trials. These show promise for eventually eliminating the need for an external sound processor and providing near-constant hearing in many environments.

- Drug eluting arrays to mitigate postimplant inflammation.
- Use of neurotrophic factors to prevent further neural degeneration and promote neural ingrowth providing improved electrode-to-neuron coupling.
- Electrocochleography (ECoG) provides real time electrical feedback during electrode placement to help the surgeon limit trauma and optimize depth of insertion.
- Robotic electrode insertion to minimize insertion variability and reduce intracochlear trauma.
- Use of pulsed optical stimulation to overcome issues with current spread seen with electrical stimulation and improve spatial selectivity of stimulation.

Bibliography

Carlson ML, Driscoll CL, Gifford RH, et al. Implications of minimizing trauma during conventional cochlear implantation. *Otol Neurotol.* 2011 Aug;32(6):962.

Carlson ML, Sladen DP, Haynes DS, et al. Evidence for the expansion of pediatric cochlear implant candidacy. *Otol Neurotol.* 2015 Jan 1;36(1):43-50.

Gifford RH, Dorman MF, Skarzynski H, et al. Cochlear implantation with hearing preservation yields significant benefit for speech recognition in complex listening environments. *Ear Hear.* 2013 Jul;34(4):413.

Houston DM, Miyamoto RT. Effects of early auditory experience on word learning and speech perception in deaf children with cochlear implants: implications for sensitive periods of language development. *Otol Neurotol.* 2010 Oct;31(8):1248.

Jiang ZY, Odiase E, Isaacson B, Roland PS, Kutz Jr JW. Utility of MRIs in adult cochlear implant evaluations. *Otol Neurotol.* 2014 Oct 1;35(9):1533-1535.

Questions

1. Low Pitches are detected in the
   A. Cochlear apex
   B. Reissner membrane
   C. Outer hair cells
   D. Cochlear base
   E. Supporting cells

2. Temporal coding (timing) of information is limited to frequencies
   A. Above 8000 HZ
   B. Below 500 HZ
   C. Beyond the range of audio ability
   D. Ultra-high frequencies
   E. At uncomfortable levels

3. Cochlear implants are not appropriate for
   A. Postlingual deafness
   B. Ossified cochleas
   C. Congenitally deformed cochleas
   D. Prelingual deafness
   E. Michel deformity

4. When low-frequency hearing is present, spectral information is best transmitted by
   A. Telephone
   B. Hearing aid
   C. Cochlear implant
   D. Tactile aid
   E. Middle ear implant

5. Essential components of a cochlear implant system are
   A. Microphone
   B. Processor
   C. Electrode array
   D. Transmission link
   E. All of the above

Chapter 19
Facial Nerve Paralysis

Anatomy and Physiology

The facial nerve is a mixed nerve containing:

1. Motor fibers from the motor nucleus within the pons to the posterior belly of the digastric muscle, stylohyoid muscle, stapedius muscle, and muscles of facial expression. Upper face receives bilateral central innervation; therefore, an upper motor neuron lesion will spare the upper face. A lower motor neuron lesion will involve the entire hemiface.
2. Parasympathetic fibers arising from the superior salivary nucleus within the pons. Preganglionic, parasympathetic afferent fibers form two nerves:
   a. *Greater superficial petrosal nerve.* Branches off the main trunk at the geniculate ganglion, synapses at the pterygopalatine ganglion, and provides input to lacrimal, nasal, and palatine glands.
   b. *Chorda tympani nerve.* Branches off the main trunk along the mastoid/vertical segment, joins the lingual nerve, synapses at the submandibular ganglion, and provides input to sublingual and submandibular glands.
3. Special sensory afferent fibers travel in the lingual nerve to the chorda tympani nerve and provide taste to the anterior two-thirds of the tongue, and travel to the nucleus solitarius.
4. Afferent fibers also provide sensation from the concha, external auditory canal, and earlobe.

The facial nerve is divided into six segments:

1. *Intracranial segment* (17-24 mm) from brain stem to internal auditory canal (IAC).
2. *Meatal segment* (8-10 mm) from the fundus of the IAC, running in the anterosuperior quadrant, to the meatal foramen.
3. *Labyrinthine segment* (4 mm) from the meatal foramen to the geniculate ganglion. The meatal foramen is the narrowest segment of the intratemporal bony channel, and the nerve is most susceptible to inflammation at this point.
4. *Tympanic segment* (11 mm) from the geniculate ganglion to the second genu.
5. *Mastoid/vertical segment* (13 mm) from the second genu to the stylomastoid foramen.
6. *Extratemporal segment* from the stylomastoid foramen, divides into the temporal, zygomatic, buccal, marginal mandibular, and cervical branches to innervate the muscles of facial expression.

Etiology of Facial Paralysis

There are hundreds of etiologies of facial paralysis with the most common causes being:

1. Viral reactivation
2. Lyme disease
3. Trauma
4. Postsurgical cases
5. Benign or malignant tumors

The most common causes of synchronous, bilateral facial paralysis are:

1. Lyme disease
2. Möbius syndrome
3. Neurofibromatosis type 2
4. Cavernous brain stem hemangioma and other brain stem pathologies
5. Bilateral temporal bone fractures
6. Guillain-Barré syndrome
7. HIV

Assessment of Facial Paralysis

Assessment of facial paralysis begins with a detailed history and physical exam. The physical exam includes a thorough head and neck exam with attention to otologic findings, cranial nerves, and palpation of the parotid gland and neck. In some cases, additional workup is required and may include laboratory testing, imaging, audiogram, and electrophysiologic testing.

Facial paralysis may be classified into flaccid facial paralysis (FFP), postparalysis facial palsy (PPFP), characterized by hypertonicity and synkinesis, and mixed facial paralysis (MFP) with elements of flaccidity and hypertonicity. Facial function is documented with the following:

1. Complete set of photographs, with eight standard expressions including patient at rest, brows elevated, gentle eye closure, tight eye closure, small smile, large smile, pucker, and saying "eeee" along with the basal view of nose.
2. Video clip of eight standard expressions and articulation of plosives.
3. Facial nerve examination of patient at rest and during movement with documentation of:
   a. *Static parameters*. Brow height, palpebral fissure width, oral commissure position, nasolabial fold depth.
   b. *Dynamic parameters*. Brow elevation, gentle and full eye closure, oral commissure excursion, nasolabial fold depth and orientation with smile, lower lip movement.
   c. *Synkinesis parameters*. Evaluate for ocular, midfacial, mentalis, and platysmal synkinesis.

Comprehensive intake and analysis of facial nerve patients may include:

1. Clinician-graded scales of facial function. There are numerous instruments available.
   a. House-Brackmann and Sunnybrook are most frequently employed.
   b. Automated assessments of facial function are emerging in the literature (eg, electronic facial paralysis assessment [eFACE]).

2. Patient-reported outcome measures.
   a. Quality of life assessment (eg, facial clinimetric evaluation [FaCE] instrument)
   b. Synkinesis assessment questionnaire (SAQ)
   c. Nasal obstruction and septoplasty effectiveness (NOSE) scale
3. Quantitative facial measurements.
   a. Facial assessment by computer evaluation (FACE-gram).
4. Layperson assessment.

Treatment of Acute Facial Paralysis

Viral-Associated Facial Paralysis

Viral-associated facial paralysis is the most common cause of facial paralysis. Facial paralysis involves all zones of the face (upper, middle, and lower), may be complete or incomplete, and should be fully evolved within 72 hours of onset. Bell palsy is thought to be caused by herpes simplex virus reactivation within the geniculate ganglion. The incidence of Bell palsy is 15 to 30 per 100,000 people. Ramsay Hunt syndrome or *herpes zoster oticus* is caused by varicella-zoster virus reactivation and is characterized by auricular vesicles, sensorineural hearing loss, and vestibular symptoms, in addition to facial paralysis. Workup for viral-associated facial paralysis is minimal. Routine imaging and labs are not indicated, aside from Lyme titer in Lyme-endemic areas. Treatment includes:

1. Oral steroids within 48 to 72 hours.
   a. 10-day course with at least 5 days at high dose, (eg, prednisone 60 mg for 5 days followed by a 5-day taper.)
2. Antivirals may provide a benefit when combined with oral steroids.
3. Meticulous eye care with drops, ointment, and nightly eye taping.
4. Consider electrodiagnostic testing in patients with acute facial paralysis within 12 days of onset.
   a. If electroneuronography (ENoG) is less than 10% compound action potentials and needle electromyography (EMG) demonstrates no voluntary motor units, patient may be a candidate for surgical facial nerve decompression, though this remains controversial.
5. May offer facial nerve physical therapy to patients at risk for prolonged recovery.

Lyme-Associated Facial Paralysis

Lyme-associated facial paralysis develops acutely, may be bilateral, and is often associated with severe headaches, fever, rash, arthralgias, and fatigue. Lyme testing should be performed on patients presenting with acute facial paralysis in Lyme-endemic areas. Treatment includes:

1. Antibiotics against *Borrelia burgdorferi*.
2. Meticulous eye care with drops, ointment, and nightly eye taping.
3. Combined treatment with steroids may lead to worse outcomes

Trauma and Temporal Bone Fractures

All patients require a formal trauma workup. It is important to determine whether temporal bone fracture is otic capsule sparing or otic capsule involving. Workup and treatment include:

1. Imaging with fine-cut temporal bone CT scan to determine if fracture involves the otic capsule and whether bony spicules are impinging on the facial nerve.
2. Obtain audiogram when possible.
3. Consider surgical exploration for immediate-onset facial paralysis.

4. Delayed-onset facial paralysis may be followed by serial ENoG, with consideration for facial nerve decompression if ENoG falls to less than 10% compound action potentials.
5. Meticulous eye care with drops, ointment, and nightly eye taping, with consideration for early placement of platinum eyelid weight.

Postsurgical Facial Paralysis

Postsurgical facial paralysis may occur expectedly after facial nerve sacrifice or unexpectedly after skull base, otologic, parotid, mandibular, or facial plastic surgery.

1. If the nerve was not visualized during surgery, and the status of continuity is not known:
   a. Obtain ENoG.
   b. Surgical exploration is recommended, unless ENoG establishes continuity of the nerve.
   c. If nerve is transected, repair with tension-free primary neurorrhaphy.
   d. If cable grafting is required, the following options are often utilized:
      1. *Great auricular nerve*. Avoid when concern for cervical metastasis.
      2. *Sural nerve*. May be harvested endoscopically and provides excellent length.
      3. *Medial antebrachial cutaneous nerve*. Branching pattern is advantageous for coaptation with multiple distal branches of facial nerve.

Acute Otitis Media and Facial Paralysis

Facial paralysis may occur in the setting of acute otitis media. Conservative treatment is recommended, and recovery of facial function is expected:

1. Broad-spectrum antibiotics.
2. Consider CT scan.
3. Perform myringotomy and obtain cultures. May consider placement of PE tube.
4. The use of steroids is controversial.

Treatment of Persistent Flaccid Facial Paralysis

Along with aesthetic and psychosocial consequences, FFP results in functional impairment, including lack of eye closure, ocular irritation, speech and articulation difficulty, and oral incompetence. When treating FFP, the face is divided into three zones, and each zone is considered separately when developing an individualized treatment plan.

1. *Upper face*. Forehead, brow, upper eyelid, lower eyelid
2. *Midface*. Nasal valve, nasolabial fold, oral commissure
3. *Lower face*. Lower lip, chin, neck

Upper Face

1. *Brow ptosis correction*. Correction of brow ptosis improves facial asymmetry, corrects visual field defects, and prevents ocular irritation from desquamation of skin cells onto cornea.
   a. May be performed in the office setting under local anesthesia.
   b. Direct brow lift removes an ellipse of skin above the brow and can predictably elevate the brow; however, the resulting scar may be noticeable.
   c. The "power brow" lift uses two or three monofilament sutures passed through the eyebrow and secured to a reconstruction plate at the level of the hairline.
   d. Ultratine (Endotine Inc., Coapt, Palo Alto, CA) brow lift uses biodegradable polymeric device to elevate the brow after subperiosteal dissection.

2. *Upper eyelid*. Treatment of paralytic lagophthalmos relieves ocular discomfort, prevents exposure keratitis, corneal abrasion, and loss of vision, and improves palpebral fissure width asymmetry. There are several options to treat the lagophthalmos:
   a. May be performed in the office setting under local anesthesia.
   b. Platinum weight is preferred over gold weight because of its thinner profile and decreased incidence of capsule formation. Eyelid weight is attached to the tarsal plate and centered between the mid-pupillary line and medial limbus.
   c. Platinum chain is designed to conform to contour of tarsal plate.
   d. Eyelid spring is designed to achieve a natural blink; however, there are high revision rates (approximately 100%).
   e. Tarsorrhaphy provides corneal protection; however may result in unfavorable aesthetic results and visual field defects. Tarsorrhaphy is an option when unable to achieve adequate closure with lid loading and/or lower eyelid repositioning techniques, or in patients with corneal anesthesia or corneal ulcer.
3. *Lower eyelid*. Treatment of lower eyelid relieves ocular discomfort and improves ectropion, retraction, and scleral show.
   a. Tarsal strip procedure/lower lid tightening creates a tarsal strip via lateral canthotomy with cantholysis. The tarsal strip is suspended to orbital periosteum to improve lower lid malposition.
   b. Fascia lata sling from nasal bone to superior orbital rim may be used in cases of severe lower lid malposition.

Midface

1. *Nose*. External nasal valve collapse and nasal obstruction may occur in flaccid facial paralysis.
   a. Fascia lata sling technique is used for nasal valve correction. A preauricular incision is extended to the temporal region, and a separate incision is created in the alar crease. Fascial lata strip is tunneled from ala and secured to temporalis fascia with permanent sutures.
2. *Nasolabial fold*. Effacement and malposition of the nasolabial fold creates facial asymmetry and contributes to external nasal valve collapse.
   a. Fascia lata technique for modification of nasolabial fold may be combined with nasal valve and oral commissure correction for three-ribbon static suspension of the flaccid face.
   b. Strip of fascial lata is attached to a dermal tab along the planned nasolabial fold and secured to temporalis fascia with permanent sutures.
   c. Minimal nasolabial incision technique is an option for younger patients to avoid the long, linear scar along the nasolabial fold.
3. *Static smile restoration*. Reserved for poor operative candidates or patients with poor prognosis.
   a. Fascia lata suspension of the oral commissure improves facial asymmetry, oral incompetence, and speech and articulation issues.
4. *Dynamic smile restoration*. One of the major goals of facial reanimation is to restore a dynamic smile. Options for dynamic smile restoration include:
   a. Regional muscle transfer (see Regional Muscle Transfer section below)
      1. Provides single-stage surgery with potential for immediate results.
      2. Considered second-line therapy due to insufficient smile excursion and associated facial contour deformities.
      3. Option for patients who desire dynamic reanimation but are not candidates for free muscle transfer.

b. Nerve transfer (see Nerve Transfer section below)
    1. Coaptation of the distal facial nerve to an alternative motor nerve.
    2. Performed when the proximal facial nerve is unavailable, but distal facial nerve branches and viable facial musculature are both present, prior to muscle and motor endplate atrophy.
    3. Patients with FFP and no signs of recovery after 6 months, even with an intact facial nerve, are candidates for nerve transfers.
    4. Ideally, the procedure is performed before 18 months after denervation, with better results seen after shorter time of denervation.

c. Free muscle transfer (see Free Muscle Transfer section below)
    1. Gold standard for dynamic smile reanimation in children and adults with muscle and motor endplate atrophy.
    2. Gracilis muscle is most frequently used due to the lack of donor site morbidity, consistent neurovascular pedicle anatomy, and ability for two-team approach during muscle harvest.

Regional Muscle Transfer

1. Temporalis transfer
    a. Involves rotating a strip of temporalis muscle over zygomatic arch and securing to the oral commissure.
    b. May cause temporal hollowing and/or increased midfacial bulk.
    c. Orthodromic temporalis transfer involves detaching the temporalis tendon and coronoid process and securing tendon to the oral commissure.
2. Masseter transfer
    a. Infrequently used secondary to horizontal vector pull and midfacial contour defect.

Nerve Transfer

1. Masseteric (V3)-to-facial nerve transfer
    a. Most widely employed nerve transfer.
    b. Provides a powerful source of axons, is in close proximity to distal facial nerve branches, and has low donor site morbidity.
    c. Does not provide spontaneous smile.
2. Hypoglossal (XII)-to-facial nerve transfer
    a. Use has decreased over the past decade in favor of alternative motor nerve sources with fewer complications.
    b. Associated with hemi-tongue atrophy, speech and swallowing difficulties, synkinesis/mass movement.
    c. Split hypoglossal transfer technique decreases tongue-related morbidity.
    d. May be combined with other facial reanimation procedures to provide facial tone.
3. Contralateral facial nerve (VII)-to-facial nerve transfer
    a. Sural nerve cable graft coapted to distal branches of unaffected facial nerve, tunneled under the upper lip, and coapted to distal branches of affected facial nerve.
    b. May be performed as one- or two-stage procedure.
    c. Potential for spontaneous smile.
    d. Fewer axons are available compared to other nerve transfers, and results are inconsistent.
4. Spinal accessory nerve (XI) and cervical rootlets
    a. Have been described but are less frequently employed.

Free Muscle Transfer

1. One-stage gracilis free muscle transfer
   a. Gracilis driven by ipsilateral masseteric branch of trigeminal nerve (V3).
   b. Indications: unavailable contralateral facial nerve, consider in patients greater than 40 years old, patient preference for single-stage surgery with faster results.
   c. Provides initial movement within 4 to 6 months, a reliably strong muscle contraction, and oral commissure excursion.
   d. Success rate of 92%.
   e. Lack of spontaneous smile
2. Two-stage gracilis free muscle transfer
   a. Gracilis driven by contralateral facial nerve.
   b. First stage involves endoscopic harvest of the sural nerve and cross-face nerve grafting.
   c. Tinel's sign, or tapping on the tip of the nerve graft to produce tingling in midface of unaffected side, is used to follow axon growth clinically.
   d. Second-stage muscle transfer 6 to 9 months later.
   e. Indications: younger patients, patients who desire a spontaneous smile.
   f. Provides initial movement within 6 to 9 months after muscle transfer. Oral commissure excursion is decreased compared to one-stage gracilis.
   g. Success rate 80%.
   h. Potential for spontaneous smile.
3. Dual innervation of gracilis free muscle transfer
   a. Gracilis driven by both contralateral facial nerve via cross-face nerve grafting and ipsilateral masseteric nerve.
   b. The goal is to provide the strength and reliability of a one-stage procedure with the spontaneity of a two-stage procedure.
   c. More data are needed to establish indications and long-term outcomes.

Lower Face

1. *Lower lip*. Paralysis of the depressor labii inferioris (DLI) causes lower lip asymmetry and may lead to speech and articulation difficulty and/or oral incompetence.
   a. Treat with contralateral lower lip weakening using botulinum toxin.
   b. Lip weakening may be made permanent by resection of DLI fibers.
   c. Digastric muscle transfer is described to re-establish mimetic movement on the paralyzed side, but is less commonly employed due to the ease of contralateral weakening techniques.

Physical Therapy

Patients with persistent FFP are offered facial nerve physical therapy before and after surgical interventions. Physical therapy involves:

1. Soft-tissue stretching and active assistive movement exercises to improve circulation.
2. Eyelid stretching techniques to break cross-covalent linkage of the levator palpebrae superioris and improve eye closure.
3. Emphasis on decreasing compensatory movement on contralateral side to improve overall symmetry.
4. Optimization of dynamic movement from regional muscle transfer, nerve transfer, or free muscle transfer.

Treatment of Post-Paralysis Facial Palsy

PPFP may lead to extreme discomfort and functional impairment from severe synkinesis and hypertonicity. The treatment of PPFP begins with physical therapy. Chemodenervation and other procedures are often added to the physical therapy regimen.

Physical Therapy

Essential to optimize outcomes in patients with PPFP. Physical therapy focuses on patient education, soft tissue massage, neuromuscular retraining (NMR), and biofeedback. Rehabilitation techniques for PPFP include:

1. *Facilitation.* For the treatment of PPFP without synkinesis. Involves soft-tissue stretching and NMR with biofeedback, emphasizing slow, controlled facial movements.
2. *Movement control.* For the treatment of PPFP with synkinesis. Involves aggressive soft-tissue stretching, NMR with biofeedback, and relaxation and meditation techniques.

Chemodenervation

Botulinum toxin is administered on affected side to prevent involuntary movement and/or on unaffected side to improve facial symmetry and function.

1. *Paralyzed brow.* Administration of botulinum toxin to contralateral forehead decreases contralateral brow elevation, improving dynamic facial symmetry.
2. *Ocular synkinesis.* Patients develop involuntary eye closure with other facial movements. This leads to visual field defects and may be particularly bothersome. Administration of botulinum toxin to affected orbicularis oculi improves static symmetry and dynamic function. Care is taken to avoid excessive weakening and associated lagophthalmos.
3. *Epiphora or Bogorad syndrome.* Administration of botulinum toxin to lacrimal gland decreases excessive tearing.
4. *Mentalis synkinesis.* Administration of botulinum toxin directly into mentalis dimpling smooths out the chin.
5. *Lower lip weakness.* Administration of botulinum toxin to contralateral DLI balances lower lip position (see treatment for Lower Lip in FFP).
6. *Platysmal synkinesis.* Platysma frequently receives inappropriate proportion of regenerating axons following facial nerve insult. Downward pull of hyperinnervated platysma muscle counteracts oral commissure excursion. Administration of botulinum toxin in multiple places along platysmal bands improves aesthetic and functional issues.

Myectomy

Myectomies remove a portion of hyperactive muscle to improve facial function.

1. *Depressor anguli oris (DAO) myectomy.* A portion of the DAO is resected via a transoral approach to help decrease downward pull on the oral commissure.
2. *Buccinator myectomy.* A portion of the buccinator is resected to decrease lateral pull on the oral commissure. This can be combined with DAO resection.
3. *Ocular myectomy.* The inferolateral portion of oculi muscle may be removed in patients with severe ocular synkinesis not controlled with Botulinum toxin.

Selective Neurectomy

Selective neurectomy, also called selective neurolysis, is a procedure to cut synkinetic nerves to improve midfacial tightness and oral commissure excursion.

Bibliography

Bhama PK, Hadlock TA. Contemporary facial reanimation. *Facial Plast Surg*. 2014;30:145-151.

Boahene K. Facial reanimation after acoustic neuroma resection: options and timing of intervention. *Facial Plast Surg*. 2015;31:103-109.

Gaudin RA, Jowett N, Banks CA, Knox CJ, Hadlock TA. Bilateral facial paralysis: a 13-year experience. *Plast Reconstr Surg*. 2016;138:879-887.

Robinson MR, Baiungo J, Hohman M, et al. Facial rehabilitation. *Operative Techniques in Otolaryngology*. 2012;23:288-296.

Questions

1. Which segment of the facial nerve is the narrowest and most susceptible to inflammation?
   A. Meatal segment
   B. Labyrinthine segment
   C. Tympanic segment
   D. Mastoid segment

2. Ramsay Hunt syndrome is characterized by the following EXCEPT
   A. Vesicles
   B. Vertigo
   C. Sensorineural hearing loss
   D. Third nerve palsy

3. Which is a common cause of synchronous, bilateral facial paralysis?
   A. Viral reactivation
   B. Cholesteatoma
   C. Mobius syndrome
   D. Geniculate ganglion hemangioma/vascular malformation

4. Treatment of facial paralysis in the setting of acute otitis media should initially include
   A. No systemic therapy
   B. Observation
   C. Myringotomy
   D. Middle fossa decompression

5. Which procedure has the potential to restore a spontaneous smile?
   A. Masseteric (V)- to-facial nerve transfer
   B. Split hypoglossal (XII)-to-facial nerve transfer
   C. Temporalis transfer
   D. Two-stage gracilis free muscle transfer

Chapter 20
Disorders of the Temporal Bone and Noninfectious Disorders of the Ear

External Ear

- Trauma
  - Lacerations: simple with or without involved cartilage; stellate from blunt trauma; partial or total avulsion
    - Treatment: deep cleaning, debridement, surgical repair; may require stage or flap reconstruction; systemic antibiotics. Consider bolster to prevent hematoma
    - Complications: perichondritis, cartilage necrosis
  - Hematoma—typically occurs from blunt trauma
    - Treatment: incision and drainage with through-and-through sutures and bolster dressing
      - ◊ Systemic antibiotics (consider fluoroquinolones)
    - Complications: cauliflower/wrestler's ear, perichondritis
  - Frostbite—exposure to subfreezing temperature and wind leading to disruption of endothelial layer with extravasation of erythrocytes, platelet aggregation, and sludging
    - Symptoms: pain, burning, discoloration; reduced pliability; loss of sensation
    - Treatment: slow warming; antibiotics; anticoagulants; debridement of necrotic tissue after demarcation. No pressure or pressure dressing to the ear.
  - Bites—lobe of ear is most common site
    - Treatment: meticulous cleaning; systemic antibiotics; surgical repair and/or debridement.
      - ◊ Human bites have greater propensity for infection.
  - Keloids and hypertrophic scars—increased rates in African American and Hispanic populations (up to 30%)
    - Treatment: steroid injection, surgical excision, pressure dressing, rarely radiation therapy
- Chondritis, perichondritis, and cellulitis—typically secondary to blunt or penetrating trauma; extension of infectious otitis externa
  - Superficial infections commonly *Staphylococcus spp;* perichondritis and chondritis commonly *Pseudomonas spp*
    - Rule out: relapsing perichondritis, cutaneous lymphoma, gouty tophus
    - Symptoms: pain, erythema, induration typical with chondritis and perichondritis; cartilage deformity ("cauliflower ear") seen in chronic or recurrent infections and advanced/untreated cases; fevers, chills, elevated white count in severe cases

- Treatment: mild—oral anti-staphylococcal and anti-streptococcal antibiotics
  - ◊ Severe infection/immunocompromised patient: IV therapy
  - ◊ Perichondritis/chondritis: oral fluoroquinolone if abscess not present; abscess—incision and drainage with oral fluoroquinolone for 2 to 4 weeks; bolster placement as needed

- Herpes zoster oticus (HZO)—most commonly in elderly and immunocompromised; reactivation of virus within ganglion nerve cells
  - Signs/symptoms: otalgia, vesicles in conchal bowl and/or external ear canal (EAC), tinnitus, vertigo, decreased lacrimation, sensorineural hearing loss (SNHL) with loss of stapedial reflex
  - HZO with facial paralysis—Ramsay Hunt Syndrome (RHS); 60% regain function after complete paralysis
  - Diagnosis: Tzank smear with multinucleated giant cells, viral titers
  - Treatment: valacyclovir 1000 mg Q8H for 7 days; oral prednisone (1 mg/kg/day) for facial nerve involvement or SNHL; surgical decompression of facial nerve not advocated in RHS
- Carcinoma of the external ear
  - 6% of skin cancers involve the ear.
  - Lymphatic drainage—anterior auricular nodes: lateral pinna and anterior canal wall; postauricular nodes: superior and upper posterior pinna, posterior canal wall; superficial and deep cervical nodes: lobule and floor of external ear canal.
  - Metastasis associated with depth of invasion.
  - Staging:
    - Skin and Pinna
      - ◊ TX—Primary tumor cannot be assessed.
      - ◊ T0—No evidence of primary tumor.
      - ◊ Tis—Carcinoma in situ.
      - ◊ T1—Tumor 2 cm or less.
      - ◊ T2—Tumor larger than 2 cm but smaller than 5 cm.
      - ◊ T3—Tumor larger than 5 cm.
      - ◊ T4—Tumor invades deep extradermal structures (bone, muscle, cartilage).
    - University of Pittsburgh staging system for SCC involving the temporal bone
      - ◊ T1—Tumor limited to external auditory canal without bone or soft tissue extension
      - ◊ T2—Tumor with limited external auditory canal bony erosion or less than 0.5 cm soft tissue involvement
      - ◊ T3—Tumor eroding full-thickness bony external auditory canal with less than 0.5 cm soft tissue involvement, or tumor involving the middle ear and/or mastoid
      - ◊ T4—Tumor eroding the medial wall of middle ear or beyond, or greater than 0.5 cm soft tissue involvement, or patient with facial nerve paresis or paralysis
    - Regional lymph nodes:
      - ◊ NX—Regional lymph nodes cannot be assessed.
      - ◊ N0—No regional lymph node metastasis.
      - ◊ N1—Regional lymph node metastasis.
  - Basal cell carcinoma—most common malignancy of the ear (45%)
    - Symptoms: erythematous lesion with raised margins; silvery scales common, occurs on the pinna and in the external canal
    - Treatment: biopsy, topical agents, wide local excision; may require cartilage excision, skin graft, or local flaps

- Squamous cell carcinoma
  - Symptoms: pain, bloody discharge, polyp with granular appearance, facial nerve paralysis, hearing loss
  - Treatment: biopsy, wide surgical excision, may require parotidectomy, sleeve resection of ear canal, or temporal bone resection; postoperative radiation for advanced cases
- Malignant melanoma—7% of head and neck sites involve the ear
- Other tumors of the ear: adenoid cystic carcinoma, adenocarcinoma, adenoma, pleomorphic adenoma

External Ear Canal

- Infectious diseases
  - Acute otitis externa (AOE) (swimmer's ear, tropical ear)—risk factors include immunosuppression, canal manipulation, narrow EAC, obstructive pathology (eg, exostoses), prior radiation
    - Etiology: swimming/water exposure, tropical/humid climates, canal trauma, chronic dermatologic conditions, occlusive devices (eg, hearing aids)
    - Most commonly bacterial—*Pseudomonas aeruginosa*
    - Signs/symptoms: pain ("tragal sign"), pruritus, otorrhea (often purulent), cellulitic changes, preauricular, or cervical lymphadenopathy
    - Treatment: frequent aural toilet, dry ear precautions, pain control; topical therapy with acidifying agent (acetic acid, diluted vinegar), moderate to severe disease treated with topical therapy (fluroquinolone +/− steroid, neomycin, tobramycin if TM intact); severe canal edema may require otowick and oral antibiotics
  - Fungal otitis externa (FOE)—similar to bacterial otitis externa, fungal elements visible on examination (eg, hyphae, fungal ball or "wet newspaper")
    - *Aspergillus* most common, *Candida* and *Penicillium* also seen
    - Treatment: acidifying agents (boric acid, gentian violet), dry ear precautions and frequent aural toilet, topical antifungal agents (eg, clotrimazole, CSF powder), systemic therapy for refractory disease
  - Chronic otitis externa (COE)—risk factors include chronic skin conditions, external beam radiation, allergen exposure
    - Signs/symptoms: pruritus, discomfort without otalgia, aural fullness, thickening of the skin with erythema, keratosis, cicatricial narrowing with canal obliteration in late state (medial canal fibrosis)
    - Rule out malignancy with biopsy as needed
    - Treatment: dry ear precautions, frequent debridement, topical lubrication (baby oil) or acidification (acetic acid), steroids for pruritis; canalplasty for stenosis/medial canal fibrosis
  - Malignant otitis externa (MOE)—primarily seen in immunocompromised hosts (uncontrolled diabetes, HIV, transplant, elderly)
    - Skull base osteomyelitis (SBO): MOE progressing to involve skull base and lower cranial nerves (CN VII most common); EAC infection spreads to stylomastoid and jugular foramina via fissures of Santorini and tympanomastoid suture line; high morbidity, mortality 5% to 20%

- Signs/symptoms: deep-seated otalgia often out of proportion to exam findings, otorrhea, EAC edema, granulation tissue at bony-cartilage suture (hallmark of disease), "picket fence" fevers due to septic thrombophlebitis of sigmoid sinus
- Imaging
  - ◊ Technetium (Tc-99) scintigraphy to confirm diagnosis
    - * Concentrates in areas of osteoblastic activity
    - * High sensitivity for bone infection
    - * Single photon emission computed tomography (SPECT) more sensitive than planar imaging
    - * Tc-99 remains in bone after infection resolves—not used to track disease
  - ◊ Gallium-67 or Indium-111 labeled leukocyte scan
    - * Shows areas of inflammatory cell activity
    - * Sensitivity increased with Tc-99 scan
    - * Used to follow treatment response
    - * Scan every 4 weeks during treatment
  - ◊ MRI with gadolinium
    - * Helpful in delineating soft tissue involvement
    - * Useful for identifying osteomyelitis along skull base
    - * Can also be used to follow after treatment
  - ◊ High resolution CT without contrast
    - * Bony erosion and soft tissue abnormalities; significant bone erosion required before abnormal
- Treatment: address underlying medical issues (e.g., aggressive glucose control), EAC debridement, and biopsy to rule out malignancy
  - ◊ Surgical intervention only for debridement of bony sequestrum
  - ◊ Hyperbaric oxygen therapy unproven
    - * Antibiotic therapy: oral fluoroquinolone first-line therapy
      - ▪ Parenteral antipseudomonal aminopenicillins if unable to take fluoroquinolones
      - ▪ Typical treatment duration of 6 weeks
      - ▪ Treatment continues until clinical exam is normal
      - ▪ Can use MRI and/or Gallium-67 scan to determine resolution

- Noninfectious diseases
  - ○ Seborrheic dermatitis, psoriasis
    - Psoriasis affects 2% to 5% of the population. In 18% with systemic psoriasis, ear is affected. Scalp and postauricular sulcus often affected.
    - Eczema—external otitis, the most common dermatologic condition of the external canal, may be associated with dandruff.
    - Symptoms: itching; weeping; dry, scaly, fissured skin; crusting and flaking; recurrent external otitis; canal stenosis
    - Treatment: frequent cleaning to prevent accumulation, 1% hydrocortisone solution or lotion, betamethasone for acute treatment
  - ○ Keratosis obturans
    - Primarily seen in adults (30-60 years)
    - Rapid accumulation of keratin debris; wax casts; plugged external auditory canal; painless erosion and expansion of external canal; may be associated with drainage, foul odor, and secondary external otitis

    - Can lead to conductive hearing loss secondary to mechanical obstruction and/or TM thickening
    - Pathology: chronic inflammation and poor epithelial migration
    - Treatment: frequent cleaning; topical 1% hydrocortisone; betamethasone for acute treatment
  - Cholesteatoma of the ear canal
    - Keratin accumulation in the external canal associated with osteitis and bone necrosis; usually occurs on the floor of the external canal; commonly associated with pain and keratin invasion of bone
    - Pathology: invasion of bone by epithelium and secondary necrosis versus focal bone injury with secondary invasion of epithelium
    - Treatment: frequent cleaning of the external auditory canal; topical steroids; may require surgical debridement of osteitic bone. May require canal wall down mastoidectomy if extensive bone erosion.
  - Osteoma
    - Pedunculated bone mass developing along tympanosquamous and tympanomastoid suture lines; occluding osteoma may require surgical removal.
  - Exostoses
    - Lamellar thickening of bone of external ear canal associated with cold air/water exposure, commonly involving the anterior and posterior canal walls. Exostoses may cause canal stenosis, cerumen impaction, retention of moisture and skin, and rarely hearing loss.
    - Treatment: canaloplasty and possible skin graft
  - Foreign bodies
    - Insects, nuts, beans, gum, putty, beads, toys, etc. Avoid irrigation—vegetable matter will expand; blind instrumentation may cause bleeding or swelling of the ear canal and may impale the foreign material through the eardrum.
    - Treatment: local anesthetic block, microscopic examination, and instrumentation for removal of foreign body; mineral oil or antibiotic solution may facilitate removal. Depending on status of canal after removal, topical antibiotic may be required.
- Myringitis
  - Acute bullous myringitis—inflammation of the lateral surface of the TM and medial EAC often secondary to upper respiratory infections, occurs with serous otitis media in 30% to 40%
    - Symptoms: severe otalgia, bullae on the TM, serosanguinous otorrhea with bullae rupture, conductive or mixed hearing loss
    - Pathology: *Streptococcus pneumoniae, Hemophilus influenza, Moraxella catarrhalis*; *Mycoplasma pneumoniae* was considered common in past but unproven
    - Treatment: analgesics, topical antibiotics with incision and drainage of bullae for pain relief as needed; treat AOM/SOM accordingly
  - Chronic (granular) myringitis—loss of normal epithelium with replacement by granulation tissue
    - Symptoms: painless, foul-smelling otorrhea; aural fullness; pruritus; conductive or mixed hearing loss; often asymptomatic; can progress to blunting of the TM or acquired stenosis of the EAC leading to medial canal fibrosis
    - Treatment: numerous topical agents used with variable success (antibiotics, desiccating agents, chemical cautery, acidification); surgical debridement with tympanoplasty/canalplasty in obliterative or refractory disease

Middle Ear and Mastoid

- Trauma
  - Temporal bone fractures, basilar skull fractures
    - Epidemiology: Most common cause is motor vehicle accidents, followed by assault.
      - ◊ 70% occur in second to fourth decades of life with a male/female ratio of 3:1
    - Classification: transverse, longitudinal, and mixed based on orientation of fracture line to petrous ridge axis
      - ◊ Modern classification is based on whether the fracture involves or spares the otic capsule.
        - Created due to poor correlation between temporal bone sequelae and traditional fracture classification. For example, transverse fractures originally thought to be associated with SNHL but modern data show longitudinal fractures are three times more likely to have associated SNHL.
        - Only 5.8% of temporal bone fractures involve the otic capsule.
    - Diagnosis:
      - ◊ Otoscopic evaluation often reveals hemotympanum, which is the most common cause of initial conductive hearing loss.
        - If present, audiometric evaluation should be repeated in 6 to 8 weeks to allow resolution.
      - ◊ Bedside tuning fork exam (dependent on level of patient consciousness).
      - ◊ High-resolution CT (HRCT) of the temporal bone to evaluate fracture location, ossicular integrity, and otic capsule involvement.
      - ◊ Audiometry is required for diagnosis.
        - Conductive hearing loss can occur from hemotympanum, TM perforation, and ossicular discontinuity. Incudostapedial joint subluxation, followed by incus dislocation and stapes crura fracture, are most common ossicular disruptions.
        - SNHL is most severe with otic capsule involvement. Nonotic capsule fractures involving SNHL have been suggested to occur from intralabyrinthine hemorrhage and membranous labyrinth injury.
        - Hearing loss pattern is often mixed.
  - Middle ear trauma
    - Foreign body can puncture TM resulting in a wide variety of injuries.
      - ◊ Simple TM perforation without ossicular injury leads to temporary CHL; these typically heal without surgical intervention.
      - ◊ Ossicular injury can occur from malleus handle fracture, incudostapedial joint subluxation, incus dislocation, and stapes subluxation.
        - Middle ear exploration is warranted after recovery from any vestibular insults (see below).
        - On pneumatic otoscopy, TM may be hypermobile.
      - ◊ Penetrating trauma can also enter the vestibule through the oval window.
        - When acute vestibular complaints occur with hearing loss need to consider perilymphatic fistula. This can also occur with stapes subluxation.
        - Treated with bedrest, minimization of straining (stool softeners), and anti-vertiginous agents. Surgery is avoided if possible during the healing phase.
    - Audiometric evaluation is required to determine type and severity of hearing loss.
    - HRCT temporal bones imaging modality of choice to determine the integrity of the ossicles and labyrinth.

- Infectious
  - Acute otitis media (AOM)
    - Risk factors: environmental (eg, day care, secondhand smoke), anatomic (eg, cleft palate, craniofacial anomalies), genetic syndromes (Trisomy 21), socioeconomic status, premature birth, adenoid hypertrophy, or functional obstruction of the Eustachian tube (ET)
    - ET shorter, more horizontal in children resulting in impaired clearance
    - Symptoms: otalgia, irritability, fever, ear tugging, poor sleep, otorrhea/otorrhagia in cases of suppurative OM (see following discussion)
    - Physical exam: bulging and erythematous TM, limited movement on pneumatic otoscopy, air-fluid level in middle ear (purulent)
    - Pathogens: *S. pneumoniae* most common, penicillin resistance increasing due to alterations of (penicillin) binding proteins in cell wall; *H. influenza* and *M. catarrhalis* are common
    - Treatment: pain control (narcotics rarely required), urgent myringotomy rarely necessary and requires sedation in young children but can be helpful in severe cases with unresolving otalgia, children less than 2 years can be observed without antibiotic therapy for 48 to 72 hours especially if mild symptoms and treated for failure to improve (80% of AOM improve within 72 hours without antibiotics)
      - ◊ Antibiotics
        - Amoxicillin 80 to 90 mg/kg/day divided BID
        - Length of treatment controversial (7-10 days typical; > 10 days no advantage in reducing failure rates or duration of middle ear effusion)
        - Amoxicillin should *NOT* be used in patients receiving amoxicillin in past 30 days or PCN allergic patients
        - Amoxicillin-clavulanic acid recommended for children receiving amoxicillin in past 30 days, concurrent purulent conjunctivitis, or history of recurrent AOM unresponsive to amoxicillin; 90 mg/kg/day of amoxicillin and 6.4 mg/kg/day clavulanate
        - PCN-allergic patients: clindamycin, trimethoprim-sulfamethoxazole
        - Ceftriaxone IM: patients unable to take oral medications or mild-delayed hypersensitivity to amoxicillin
  - Recurrent acute otitis media (RAOM)
    - Common in children less than 2 years, highest incidence 6 to 12 months
    - Similar risk factors as AOM (see earlier discussion)
    - Signs and symptoms: same as AOM; may have a sterile effusion between episodes without acute inflammation
    - Diagnosis: ≥ 3 episodes in 6 months or less than 4 episodes in 12 months; must be asymptomatic between episodes
    - Treatment: antibiotics as above for acute infections, prophylactic treatment not recommended; tympanostomy tubes (+ adenoidectomy for sleep disordered breathing, age > 4 years, or repeat tympanostomy tube placement)
  - Chronic suppurative otitis media (CSOM) +/− cholesteatoma
    - Epidemiology: Often in areas with limited health resources and low socioeconomic status; most common in children less than 2 years old; risk factors include RAOM, AOM in early childhood, chronic secretory OM
    - Risk factors: population predisposition (native Americans, Inuit, Native Australians and New Zealanders), nasopharyngeal reflux, chronic middle ear or TM dysfunction

- Etiology: biofilm formation allowing increased antibiotic resistance and frequently polymicrobial, ET dysfunction leading to TM retraction (tubotympanic vs atticoantral)
- Signs/symptoms: aural fullness and hearing loss (audiogram typically low-frequency CHL/MHL), chronic or recurrent malodorous otorrhea; exam shows TM perforation, inflammation and edema of middle ear mucosa with polypoid degeneration, granulation tissue/aural polyps in the pars flaccida associated with TM retraction and cholesteatoma; complicated CSOM can cause facial nerve paresis/paralysis, vertigo due to labyrinthine fistula, intracranial extension
- Diagnosis made on physical exam; HRCT temporal bones useful in surgical planning, complicated CSOM, cholesteatoma, revision surgeries; MRI with contrast in cases of suspected intracranial complications
- Biopsy granulation tissue unresponsive to topical therapy to rule out malignancy
- Treatment—primary goal is safe, dry ear
  - ◊ Topical therapy with fluroquinolone (*P. aeruginosa*) +/− steroid for severe inflammatory middle ear disease or granulation tissue
  - ◊ Oral antibiotics for complicated cases, severe canal involvement, or facial cellulitis
  - ◊ Surgery: goals of surgery included removal of cholesteatoma and granulation tissue, restore continuity between the middle ear cleft and mastoid cavity in cases of antral obstruction
    - ∗ Tympanoplasty: 80% to 90% success rate; success rates are not increased with concomitant mastoidectomy
  - ◊ Tympanomastoidectomy: cases with suspected or diagnosed cholesteatoma, otorrhea refractory to medical therapy
  - ◊ ET treatment: no modality has proven long-term efficacy; options include balloon tuboplasty, laser tuboplasty, stenting

○ Chronic otitis media with effusion (COM, COME)

- 90% of children have OME by age 4 with highest incidence in children 1 to 2 years old; also seen in adults
- Etiology: ET dysfunction reduces middle ear clearance of transudate from middle ear mucosa, glycoproteins increase fluid viscosity, can become superinfected (AOM, RAOM); increased risk in smokers, history of nasopharyngeal or head and neck radiation, adenoid hypertrophy
- At-risk populations: cleft palate, craniofacial syndromes, Trisomy 21, immunocompromised
- Signs/symptoms: aural fullness, hearing loss (CHL/MHL), mild otalgia but often asymptomatic; visible middle ear effusion (mucoid vs serous) or air-fluid level with intact TM and impaired mobility on pneumatic otoscopy
- Treatment:
  - ◊ Clinical practice guidelines—updated 2015
  - ◊ Watchful waiting appropriate in children without HL, speech delay, developmental delay, TM damage
  - ◊ No role for antibiotics, steroids, antihistamines, or decongestants
  - ◊ Re-evaluate every 3 months, if complications or hearing loss develop, tympanostomy tubes should be placed
  - ◊ Adenoidectomy—same as RAOM; Cochrane review demonstrated reduction in rate of COME; can be performed primarily in children with chronic adenoiditis, nasal obstruction, or sleep disordered breathing
  - ◊ Chronic ET dysfunction may lead to requirement for cartilage tympanoplasty with or without cartilage-embedded tube

- Tuberculous otitis media
  - Increasing incidence due to multidrug resistant strains, immunocompromised populations (HIV/AIDS, organ transplant), immigration from endemic regions
  - Etiology: hematogenous or lymphatic spread from primary pulmonary disease, direction of extension through ET; middle ear involvement without pulmonary disease rare
  - Signs/symptoms: multiple TM perforations, cloudy otorrhea, polypoid granulation tissue in the middle ear; COM unresponsive to medical therapy/failed middle ear/mastoid surgery; can be associated with nontender cervical adenopathy (scrofula)
  - Diagnosis: positive acid-fast bacilli stain, chest X-ray if positive, skin testing with PPD
  - Pathogen: *Mycobacterium tuberculosis*; atypical *mycobacterium* uncommon
  - Treatment: medical therapy with multidrug regimen (involvement of infectious disease specialists recommended); surgery uncommon in primary therapy but may be needed for tympanoplasty and/or ossiculoplasty following treatment

Complications of Otitis Media

- Extracranial (intratemporal) complications
  - Hearing loss
    - Conductive/mixed hearing loss
      - ◊ Acute and/or chronic OM due to fluid in the ME
      - ◊ Can also cause direct damage to the ossicular chain
      - ◊ Incudostapedial (IS) joint most commonly involved due to distal incus erosion (watershed zone)
    - Sensorineural hearing loss
      - ◊ Uncommon
      - ◊ Pathogenesis unknown but several theories exist— inflammatory substances that cross round window causing serous labyrinthitis; effusion impairs oxygen transport to inner ear; direct extension of bacteria into inner ear through oval and/or round window
  - Vestibular dysfunction—pathogenesis unknown but likely similar to SNHL
  - Tympanic membrane perforation—spontaneous rupture in approximately 5% of AOM; spontaneous resolution in 90% of cases
  - Acute coalescent mastoiditis
    - Local inflammation over mastoid process (pain, erythema, tenderness, fluctuance, auricular protrusion) due to purulent fluid in the mastoid air cell system
    - Often with symptoms of systemic toxicity (fever, lethargy, etc.); leukocytosis common on laboratory testing
    - Only 30% of cases of acute mastoiditis have a history of recurrent AOM
    - HRCT temporal bones demonstrates opacification of the middle ear and mastoid with bony erosion of the mastoid septae, can also demonstrate subperiosteal abscess
    - Pathogens: *S. pneumoniae* most common, others include *S. pyogenes, S. aureus, H. influenza*
    - Treatment: IV antibiotics first-line therapy +/– myringotomy
      - ◊ If myringotomy performed obtain culture for directed therapy
      - ◊ Empiric therapy with third-generation cephalosporin or antipseudomonal aminopenicillin

            ◊ If no improvement after 24 to 48 hours consider surgical intervention
                * Mastoidectomy and myringotomy with/without ventilation tube
                * Drain subperiosteal abscess if present
    - Facial nerve paralysis
        - Etiology: due to congenital dehiscence of fallopian canal or erosion of bone secondary to disease process
        - Usually involves tympanic segment (30% of the population has congenital dehiscence)
        - Imaging not required unless useful for surgical planning
        - Treatment
            ◊ AOM: antibiotic therapy (PO vs IV), myringotomy with or without ventilation tube; prednisone 1 mg/kg/day for 7 days
            ◊ COM: IV antibiotics with transition to PO following surgery and culture-directed therapy; tympanomastoidectomy with proximal and distal decompression of the fallopian canal for obvious neural sheath abnormalities; recovery to HB I-II/VI in 52% to 83%
    - Labyrinthine fistula—7% to 10% of cases, lateral semicircular canal most commonly affected
        - Etiology: similar to facial nerve paralysis
        - Signs/symptoms: vertigo or dizziness, and Tullio phenomenon and/or Hennebert sign, SNHL
        - HRCT temporal bones, only 60% of confirmed fistulas visible on preoperative imaging; definitive diagnosis at surgery
        - Management remains controversial—canal wall down with exteriorization of disease versus canal wall up with complete removal and repair of fistula
            ◊ Exteriorization preferred for cochlear involvement
            ◊ Removal and repair preferred for small fistulae
    - Petrous apicitis—spectrum of disease ranging from asymptomatic effusion to abscess formation
        - Often similar presentation to suppurative otitis media
        - Gradenigo syndrome: (1) otorrhea, (2) retro-orbital pain (irritation of CN V at Meckel cave), (3) diplopia due to CN VI palsy
        - Diagnosis: HRCT temporal bones showing dissolution of bony septae and coalescence; MRI to evaluate intracranial complications as needed
        - Treatment: IV antibiotics first-line therapy; consider myringotomy and ventilation tube; surgical petrosectomy for abscess formation or failure of medical therapy
            ◊ Surgical approach depends on anatomy and air cell tracts (eg, retrolabyrinthine, infralabyrinthine, subarcuate; translabyrinthine in non-hearing ear)
    - Abscess formation
        - Subperiosteal abscess—results from AOM and mastoiditis
        - Bezold abscess—erosion of the mastoid tip with abscess formation deep to the SCM muscle
        - Zygomatic root abscess
- Intracranial complications
    - Meningitis—most common intracranial complication of AOM/COM
        - Increased incidence in inner ear anomalies, temporal bone fractures
        - Etiology: hematogenous spread, direct extension, iatrogenic injury during surgery

  - Pathogens: same as AOM and COM
  - Signs/symptoms: severe headache, photophobia, nausea/vomiting, fever, malaise, and lethargy
    - ◊ Ominous—vision changes, seizures, ataxia, altered mental status
    - ◊ Brudzinski sign—passive neck flexion causes flexion of both legs
    - ◊ Kernig sign—when thigh flexed, pain with passive extension of knee
  - Diagnosis: lumbar puncture
  - Treatment: broad-spectrum IV antibiotics with CSF penetration; 7 to 10 days IV therapy followed by 2 to 3 weeks culture-directed PO therapy
    - ◊ Corticosteroids decrease auditory and neurologic sequelae.
    - ◊ M&T (Myringotomy and Tube) for AOM, mastoidectomy for COM.
    - ◊ Monitor hearing for SNHL; consider urgent CI in cases of bilateral SNHL.
- ○ Lateral sinus thrombosis—17% to 20% of OM intracranial complications
  - Etiology: extension of infection into perisinus space, intimal damage followed by mural thrombosis
  - Signs/symptoms: "picket-fence fevers," headache, malaise and fatigue, edema and tenderness over mastoid and SCM (Griesinger sign)
    - ◊ Complicated cases: septic emboli, intracranial abscess, lower cranial neuropathies
  - Imaging: HRCT with contrast shows sinus wall enhancement with sinus hypodensity ("delta sign"), MRV with sinus flow void
  - Treatment: M&T +/− mastoidectomy
    - ◊ Anticoagulation controversial—no evidence regarding neurological outcomes, recommended for involvement of sagittal, transverse, or cavernous sinus
- ○ Otitic hydrocephalus—increased ICP with normal CSF on LP
  - Etiology: infection and thrombosis of transverse sinus with extension to involve superior sagittal sinus, prevents CSF absorption through arachnoid villi resulting in increased ICP
  - Signs/symptoms: increased ICP (headaches, nausea/vomiting, visual changes, lethargy, papilledema), can mimic meningitis in some cases
  - Diagnosis: MRI/MRV
  - Treatment: Mastoidectomy with M&T
    - ◊ In absence of otologic infection, treatment is medical
    - ◊ Lower ICP (mannitol, fluid restriction, corticosteroids)
    - ◊ Consider anticoagulation for sagittal sinus thrombosis
    - ◊ Lumbar drainage or shunt in recalcitrant cases
- ○ Subdural empyema
  - Signs/symptoms: severe headache, nuchal rigidity, altered mental status with focal neurological deficits, papilledema
  - Diagnosis with imaging (MRI or CT with contrast); LP with normal intracranial pressure
  - Treatment: urgent neurosurgical drainage with IV antibiotics
- ○ Epidural abscess
  - Signs/symptoms: deep mastoid pain, similar to coalescent mastoiditis, often discovered incidentally on imaging or during surgery
  - Diagnosis: CT or MRI shows enhancing fluid-filled cavity
  - Treatment: surgery only recommended treatment, IV antibiotics postoperatively
- ○ Intraparenchymal abscess—second most common intracranial complication of OM after meningitis, typically temporal lobe and cerebellum

- Signs/symptoms: Three stages of disease
  1. Encephalitis: headache, fever, nausea/vomiting, mental status changes, seizures
  2. Quiescent (coalescent): acute symptoms abate
  3. Rupture/expansion: return of acute symptoms, signs of increased ICP, meningeal signs
- Focal deficits in up to 70%
  - ◊ Cerebellum—ataxia, dysmetria, nystagmus, tremor
  - ◊ Temporal lobe—visual deficits, hemiparesis, aphasia
- Diagnosis: imaging with MRI or CT with contrast
- Pathogens: *S. aureus* most common; Gram-negative rods; anaerobic bacteria
- Treatment: broad-spectrum antibiotics with urgent neurosurgical intervention
  - ◊ Urgent neurosurgical intervention when neurologically stable (< 24 hours when possible)
  - ◊ IV steroids and anticonvulsants

- Noninfectious
  - Congenital cholesteatoma—develops from rests of embryonic epithelial cells in middle ear
    - Occurs in anterosuperior quadrant of mesotympanum and TM or adjacent to malleus and posterior mesotympanum
    - Presentation: 2 to 6 years of age—white mass beneath drum, usually adjacent to malleus
    - Imaging: HRCT temporal bone to evaluate extent of disease
    - Treatment: surgical removal
  - Otosclerosis
    - Epidemiology: Caucasians 8% to 12%, clinical disease 0.52%; African American population 1%, clinical disease 0.1%.
    - Female:male ratio 2:1.
    - Genetics: approximately 50% have positive family history; 70% autosomal dominant with 25% to 40% penetrance
    - Pathology:
      - ◊ Early phase—vascular, spongy bone progressing to fibrosis
      - ◊ Late phase—new bone replaced with sclerotic bone
      - ◊ Anterior oval window (fissula ante fenestram): most common location, 70% to 90%. Round window: 30% to 70%; cochlear: 14%; extensive involvement: 10% to 12%
      - ◊ Measles virus associated with otosclerotic foci
    - Symptoms: progressive conductive or mixed hearing loss; typical presentation age of 30 to 50; associated with pregnancy in 30% to 63%; paracusis of Willis (hearing better in noise), 36% to 85%; tinnitus, 75% to 100%; imbalance, 22%; vertigo, 26%; Schwartze's sign (promontory hyperemia), 10%
    - Audiometry: progressive, low frequency, conductive or mixed hearing loss; maximum conductive component, 60 dB; Carhart notch is depressed bone threshold at 2000 Hz; word discrimination often 70% or better
    - Acoustic reflex: No reflex suggests fixed stapes.
      - ◊ *Biphasic reflex (on–off)*: Occurs in 94% with symptoms of less than 5 years and in 9% greater than 10 years. (40% of normals have biphasic acoustic reflexes.)
      - ◊ If normal reflex consider other possible etiologies (superior semicircular canal dehiscence syndrome)
    - Tuning forks: Weber lateralizes to affected ear; Rinne is negative—bone greater than air, masking the opposite ear with unilateral hearing loss. Applying the tuning forks to the teeth rather than the forehead will increase the sensitivity 5 to 10 dB.

Tuning Fork	*Air–Bone Gap*
Negative 256 Hz Rinne	15 dB or more
Negative 512 Hz Rinne	25 dB or more
Negative 1024 Hz Rinne	35 dB or more

- Computed tomography:
  - ◊ HRCT temporal bone (0.5-0.6 mm) of labyrinth, axial and coronal views; areas of reduced bone density, cochlear deformity. Indications for imaging—rapid loss of bone threshold, cochlear otosclerosis, questionable conductive hearing loss, vestibular complaints, third window symptoms
- Surgical indications:
  - ◊ CHL 20 dB or greater; negative Rinne test, 512 Hz (good candidate); if 1024 Hz also negative (excellent candidate); good bone conduction threshold; speech discrimination greater than 70%; stable middle and inner ear
  - ◊ Poorer-hearing ear always operated first
- Other considerations:
  - ◊ Hearing disability; occupation; hobbies (scuba diving); inability to use a hearing aid at air conduction thresholds but aidable bone thresholds
- Surgical contraindications: Only or better-hearing ear; ear with better speech discrimination; perforated TM; active middle ear disease; active Ménière disease; prolapsed facial nerve
- Relative contraindications:
  - ◊ Less than 18 years of age; poor eustachian tube function; air conduction threshold less than 30 dB; air–bone gap less than 15 dB; aidable hearing with bone conduction greater than 40 dB:
  - ◊ *Occupation*: roofer, acrobat, scuba diver; sommelier (chorda)
- Medical treatment
  - ◊ Sodium fluoride, calcium, vitamin D (widely accepted but not FDA approved)
- Surgical Results
  - ◊ Dependent on surgeon's experience more than prosthesis; *Experienced surgeon*: closure of ABG less than 10 dB, 90% to 95%
  - ◊ Revision surgery (lifetime): 5%
  - ◊ Significant sensorineural hearing loss, less than 5%
  - ◊ Mild transient vertigo, 5%; Severe persistent vertigo, less than 5%
  - ◊ Dysgeusia, 5% to 10%
- Intraoperative complications:
  - ◊ Torn tympanomeatal flap; dislocation of incus; fractured incus; perilymph gusher (1/300); vertigo; sensorineural hearing loss; floating footplate
- Revision stapes surgery:
  - ◊ Up to 5% of cases
  - ◊ Displaced prosthesis from incus necrosis is most common
  - ◊ Other causes: displaced prosthesis, perilymph fistula, tympanic membrane perforation or retraction, reparative granuloma

○ Congenital ossicular fixation—stapes fixation is most common followed by malleus fixation
- 35 to 50 dB air–bone gap
- CT is important to evaluate for ossicular deformity or fixation
- X-linked stapes fixation: surgery contraindicated (stapes gusher)
  - ◊ Widened cochlear aperture at internal auditory canal

- Systemic diseases
  - Granulomatosis with polyangiitis(GPA)—ear involvement 30% to 50% of patients
    - Overall, 10% have SNHL.
    - CHL from chronic serous otitis media most common. 30% of patients with middle ear involvement have associated SNHL.
  - Sarcoidosis—associated with facial nerve paralysis and cochlear-vestibular neuropathy
  - Paget disease—*osteitis deformans*
    - male:female ratio 4:1; inherited autosomal dominant
    - Symptoms: thickening of the skull; mixed/conductive hearing loss; thickening of the ossicles with fixation
    - Pathology: vascular, spongy bone, thick or enlarged ossicle, and otic capsule
    - Radiology: CT shows thickening of cortical bone, ossicles, and otic capsule
    - Treatment: consider stapedectomy in patients with CHL versus hearing aid

Inner Ear

- Infectious
  - Serous labyrinthitis
    - Most common in pediatric population due to incidence of AOM
    - Inflammation of labyrinth in the absence of bacteria or virus
    - Etiology: bacteria enter labyrinth through oval window (OW), round window (RW), or labyrinthine fistula
      - ◊ Labyrinthine dysfunction due to changes in ionic potentials rather than neuroepithelial destruction; function can return to normal after inflammatory state subsides
    - Signs/symptoms: typically unilateral, dizziness, hearing loss (mild to severe SNHL)
    - Diagnosis: culture of ME effusion when present, audiogram, vestibular testing when necessary; imaging indicated only with other suspected complications of OM
    - Treatment: oral antibiotics typically effective; steroids (oral and/or IT) may improve hearing outcomes but data are lacking
      - ◊ Myringotomy for unresolving middle ear infection
  - Suppurative labyrinthitis—most commonly associated with COM in the modern era
    - Etiology: bacteria can reach cochlea through different mechanisms
      - ◊ Subarachnoid space (meningitis)—enter scala tympani via patent cochlear aqueduct or via IAC
      - ◊ Temporal bone (osteomyelitis)
      - ◊ Middle ear (otitis media with or without cholesteatoma)
    - Signs/symptoms: vestibular dysfunction, fever, meningeal signs, purulent OM; hearing loss, frequently bilateral in meningitic labyrinthitis
      - ◊ 2% to 20% with deafness following bacterial labyrinthitis
      - ◊ Incidence of hearing loss varies by bacterial strain—*S. pneumoniae* (20%), *H. influenzae* (12%), *Neisseria meningitides* (5%)
    - Diagnosis: cultures via myringotomy or lumbar puncture
      - ◊ Audiogram, vestibular testing
    - Imaging: HRCT temporal bone; if SNHL, MRI + HRCT temporal bone increases sensitivity and specificity of evaluating for cochlear obstruction
    - Treatment
      - ◊ Parenteral antibiotics with CSF penetration
      - ◊ M&T if noncholesteatoma otogenic infection; tympanomastoidectomy if cholesteatoma present

  - ◊ Steroids improve hearing outcomes in meningitic labyrinthitis
  - ◊ Early CI for signs of ossification in bilateral SNHL
- ○ Spirochetes
  - – Syphilitic labyrinthitis (*Treponema pallidum*)—can be congenital or acquired
    - ◊ Congenital syphilis
      - * 30% with SNHL; variable rate of progression
      - * Can present as bilateral sudden SNHL
    - ◊ Acquired syphilis
      - * Deafness usually occurs during secondary or tertiary syphilis
      - * Often with symptoms associated with neurosyphilis (80% with neurosyphilis have hearing loss)
      - * Often abrupt in onset, bilateral, and progressive
      - * Usually with minimal vestibular symptoms
    - ◊ Histopathology: lymphocytic labyrinthitis, obliterative endarteritis, and destruction of neuroepithelium; leads to osteitis of otic capsule and membranous labyrinth
    - ◊ Signs/symptoms: variable pattern of hearing loss (sudden, fluctuating, progressive)
    - ◊ Often mimics Meniere disease (fluctuating SNHL, aural fullness, episodic vertigo)
      - * Tullio phenomenon: vertigo and nystagmus precipitated by loud noise
      - * Hennebert sign: positive fistula test with an intact TM
    - ◊ Diagnosis: VDRL or RPR used for screening; false negatives in early and late stages
      - * If VDRL or RPR—requires confirmatory testing
      - * FTA-ABS (fluorescent treponemal antibody-absorption) test, greater than 95% sensitive for secondary and tertiary syphilis
    - ◊ Treatment:
      - * Early stage: single IM dose of benzathine penicillin G 2.4 million units
      - * Late-stage neurosyphilis: aqueous crystalline penicillin G 18 to 24 million units per day given as 3 to 4 million units IV every 4 hours for 10 to 14 days
      - * High-dose prednisone (1 mg/kg up to 80 mg) for 4 weeks
      - * 30% to 50% will show improvement in hearing and vestibular dysfunction
  - – Mycobacterium (*M. tuberculosis*)—rare cause of labyrinthitis
    - ◊ Associated with tuberculous meningitis, most common in high-risk patients (eg, HIV+)
- ○ Cytomegalovirus (CMV)—herpesvirus, DNA virus
  - – Most common cause of nonsyndromic congenital SNHL in United States.
  - – 7% to 15% of asymptomatic children will develop hearing loss.
  - – Congenital CMV is a spectrum of disease, most severe form called cytomegalic inclusion disease (CID).
  - – 35% to 50% of CID patients have bilateral deafness.
  - – Up to 23% with less severe manifestations may also have SNHL.
  - – Etiology.
    - ◊ Acute changes include viral inclusion cysts in neuroepithelium, stria vascularis, and supporting cells
    - ◊ Macrophage inflammatory proteins thought to play a significant role in CMV-related hearing loss
    - ◊ Late changes include hydrops, extracellular calcifications, strial atrophy, loss of sensory and support cells in organ of Corti

- Signs/symptoms in CID:
  - ◊ Deafness, microcephaly, hepatosplenomegaly, jaundice, intracerebral calcifications
  - ◊ Blueberry muffin rash (blue-gray purpura due to extramedullary hematopoiesis)
  - ◊ Patients with symptomatic infection have worse hearing loss and higher likelihood of progressive pattern
- Diagnosis
  - ◊ Gold standard: detection of CMV DNA via PCR in body fluid or tissue sample (saliva, urine, blood, CSF, placenta) prior to Day 21 of life
  - ◊ Dried blood spots from Guthrie cards can be used retrospectively with variable sensitivity (up to 80%)
- Treatment
  - ◊ Oral valganciclovir and IV ganciclovir equivalent
  - ◊ IV ganciclovir recommended if infant NPO
  - ◊ Dosing:
    - * 6 mg/kg/dose of IV ganciclovir twice daily
    - * 16 mg/kg/dose of oral valganciclovir twice daily
  - ◊ No outcome differences between 6 weeks versus 6 months of treatment
  - ◊ Treated infants followed with audiograms until age 6 and ophthalmology surveillance until age 5

○ Mumps—paramyxovirus, RNA virus
- Hearing loss affects 1 in 20,000 patients with mumps infection
- Introduction of mumps vaccine led to significant decline in cases
- Etiology
  - ◊ Predominantly affects cochlea, atrophy of organ of Corti and stria vascularis
  - ◊ Route of spread hematogenous or through cochlear aqueduct or modiolus
- Signs and symptoms: unilateral or bilateral parotid swelling, salivary adenitis, orchioepididymitis
  - ◊ HL can be mild to profound, usually high frequency and sudden in onset
- Diagnosis: often clinical diagnosis
  - ◊ Serological detection of IgM antibodies can confirm
  - ◊ Viral isolation via oral swab through PCR can confirm
- Treatment
  - ◊ Primary prevention with MMR vaccine (measles, mumps, rubella)
  - ◊ Treatment often supportive
  - ◊ Oral steroids have variable success for sudden HL
  - ◊ No antiviral therapy currently available

○ Measles (rubeola)—paramyxovirus, RNA virus
- Infection of otic capsule has been implicated as cause of otosclerosis
- Etiology
  - ◊ Inflammation, fibrous infiltration, and ossification of basal turn of cochlea
  - ◊ Degeneration of organ of Corti, stria, and vestibular neuroepithelium
- Signs/symptoms: three Cs—cough, coryza, conjunctivitis
  - ◊ Koplik spots—"grain of rice" spots on oral mucosa
  - ◊ Subacute sclerosing panencephalitis—rare progressive neural degeneration occurring months to years after infection
- Diagnosis: typically clinical diagnosis based on symptoms and signs
- Treatment: generally supportive
  - ◊ Vitamin A may decrease morbidity and mortality.

- Herpes simplex virus 1 (HSV-1)—Herpesvirus, DNA Virus
  - Role as causative agent in SSNHL remains controversial
  - Incidence of SNHL in congenital HSV-1 is approximately 10%
  - Signs/symptoms: SSNHL vertigo, flu-like prodrome, encephalitis in advanced cases; often with oral lesions at the time of infection
  - Treatment: acyclovir or valcyclovir
    - ◊ Randomized controlled trials show no added benefit of antivirals for improving hearing outcomes in ISSNHL
- Herpes zoster—Herpesvirus, DNA virus
  - Latent infection within spiral or vestibular ganglion may result in labyrinthine infection
  - Signs/symptoms: often occurs with facial paralysis and/or herpetic skin eruption over auricle or within EAC (herpes zoster oticus)
    - ◊ When associated with facial nerve involvement—Ramsay Hunt Syndrome
    - ◊ Typically severe unilateral SNHL
    - ◊ Vestibular symptoms common
  - Diagnosis: Tzanck smear of ruptured vesicles to identify multinucleated giant cells
  - Treatment
    - ◊ VZV vaccine introduced in 2006 reduced the number of shingles cases, but effect on RHS is yet unknown
    - ◊ High-dose oral steroids and antiviral therapy
    - ◊ No differences in oral versus IV antiviral therapy
    - ◊ Recovery of hearing loss is poor despite recovery of facial nerve function
- Rubella (German measles)—Togavirus, RNA virus
  - Incidence low in developed countries due to MMR vaccine
  - Up to 50% of newborns with congenital rubella have HL
  - Acquired infection generally not associated with HL
  - Etiology
    - ◊ Cochlear and saccular degeneration
    - ◊ Atrophy of stria vascularis
    - ◊ Utricle and semicircular canals generally unaffected
  - Signs/symptoms of congenital rubella:
    - ◊ Cataracts, micro-ophthalmia, cardiac defects, "Blueberry muffin" skin rash, developmental delay, hearing loss
      - * Greater than 50% with profound hearing loss
      - * Usually bilateral
      - * Most often affects mid-frequencies
  - Diagnosis: viral isolation from nasopharyngeal swab or urine during first weeks of life
    - ◊ Serology difficult to interpret due to transplacental transmission of IgG
    - ◊ Identification of IgM in neonatal serum is diagnostic
  - Treatment: no current antiviral medication targets the rubella virus
    - ◊ Supportive care with hearing aids or CI for hearing loss as indicated

- Noninfectious
  - Idiopathic sudden sensorineural hearing loss (ISSNHL)
    - Epidemiology: 5 to 20/100,000 per year, median age 40 to 54 years, male=female
    - 30 dB loss over 3 frequencies within a 3-day period
    - Presentation: may initially present with aural fullness and tinnitus prior to hearing complaints. Typically unilateral
    - Pathophysiology remains unclear

- Treatment: high-dose oral steroid regimen
  - ◊ Intratympanic steroids have been suggested for use as first-line treatment and salvage therapy.
  - ◊ No evidence for antiviral therapy.
- Factors associated with low likelihood of hearing recovery:
  - ◊ Flat and high-frequency hearing loss
  - ◊ More severe hearing loss
  - ◊ Presence of vertigo
  - ◊ Advanced age

- Perilymphatic fistulas
  - Presentation: sudden or progressive hearing loss (SNHL or mixed) associated with roaring tinnitus, dysacusis, disequilibrium
  - May be seen in setting of stapes surgery or trauma (especially barotrauma)
  - Diagnosis:
    - ◊ Hennebert sign (vertigo with pneumatic otoscopy)
    - ◊ Serial audiograms and imaging to rule out retrocochlear pathology
  - Treatment: observation 7 to 10 days with bed rest and minimized straining (stool softeners)
    - ◊ Surgery is considered with progressive hearing loss and persistent symptoms.
      - * In nonoperated patient, perilymph leak around annular ligament of stapes is most common.
- Autoimmune inner ear disease (AIED)
  - Classically defined as rapidly progressive bilateral SNHL that responds to immunosuppressive agents
    - ◊ Primary AIED—symptoms only involving inner ear
    - ◊ Secondary AIED—inner ear and systemic involvement
  - Primary AIED—poorly defined with no gold standard for diagnosis
    - ◊ Pathophysiology: Theorized to occur from localized labyrinthine immune reaction to antigen resulting in physiologic changes leading to symptoms. Response is likely initiated in the endolymphatic sac as it contains the only immunocompetent cells in the labyrinth.
    - ◊ Symptoms: Patients typically develop bilateral SNHL that worsens over weeks to months.
    - ◊ Hearing may fluctuate, but overall trend is toward worse hearing.
    - ◊ 50% of patients have vestibular complaints.
  - Treatment: Corticosteroids are mainstay of treatment but highly variable results.
    - ◊ 60 mg for 4 weeks; if pure-tone thresholds improve 15 dB in a single frequency or 10 dB or more in two or more consecutive frequencies, patients are considered steroid-responders.
    - ◊ Responders continue steroid therapy at full dose until audiometric recovery plateaus, then steroids taper over 8 weeks to maintenance dose (5-20 mg every other day).
    - ◊ No clear understanding of how and when to discontinue maintenance dose. Nonresponders are tapered off steroids.
    - ◊ Alternative and adjuvant therapies include methotrexate, cyclophosphamide, etanercept, and intratympanic steroids
- Secondary AIED
  - Cogan syndrome—classic symptoms include SNHL, vertigo, tinnitus, and interstitial keratitis
    - ◊ Atypical Cogan syndrome includes patients with nonkeratitic ocular inflammation

- GPA—see earlier discussion
- Antiphospholipid antibody syndrome—autoimmune disorder causing coagulopathy, recurrent thrombi, and spontaneous abortions
  - ◊ Have antiphospholipid, antilupus anticoagulant, or anticardiolipin antibody
  - ◊ Can develop SNHL likely due to labyrinthine thrombus formation
- Systemic lupus erythematosus—necrotizing vasculitis with chronic otitis media, SNHL, and/or vestibular symptoms

○ Presbycusis—SNHL related to age without other identifiable cause
- Progressive hearing loss, typically in high frequencies first
- More severe hearing loss in men
- Schuknecht four classifications of presbycusis:
  - ◊ Neural—loss of auditory nerve fibers, worse than expected speech discrimination based on pure tone thresholds
  - ◊ Strial—atrophy of stria vascularis, relatively flat audiograms
  - ◊ Sensory—progressive loss of hair cells beginning in the basal turn of the cochlea, leads to high-frequency loss
  - ◊ Cochlear conductive—increased basilar membrane stiffness results in gradually descending hearing loss
- Treatment: Hearing aids when word recognition scores are good. Cochlear implantation with poor word recognition.

○ Noise-induced hearing loss
- Temporary threshold shift (TTS)—loud noise exposure that causes SNHL that resolves within 24 hours
  - ◊ Level of injury dependent on sound level (dB) and sound frequency (high frequency causing more injury)
  - ◊ Continuous and longer sound exposure causes a greater threshold shift than interrupted noise
- Permanent threshold shift (PTS)—noise exposure that leads to SNHL lasting greater than 24 hours
  - ◊ Can result from single exposure or repeated exposure over time
  - ◊ Like TTS, level of injury is related to sound level and frequency
  - ◊ Controversial whether injury continues after sound insult ceases or stops with sound
- Diagnosis:
  - ◊ Typically hearing loss around 3 to 6 kHz with recovery at higher frequencies
    - * Greatest hearing loss seen at 4 kHz
    - * 3 to 6 kHz notch is often lost over time
  - ◊ Acoustic reflexes (tensor tympani and stapedius muscle) likely play a protective role
    - * Given delay (40-150 msec) between noise and reflex, not entirely protective
    - * Most protective at frequencies less than 2 kHz
- Pathophysiology
  - ◊ Injury occurs initially at outer hair cells (OHC), OHC stereocilia become stiffened by injury and less responsive to noise.
- In TTS, stereocilia likely recover normal mobility, and hearing subsequently recovers. In PTS, repetitive injury or louder noise exposure causes more significant damage leading to loss of stereocilia and OHC and inner hair cell death

- Prevention
  - ◊ Clear susceptibility difference for NIHL between individuals, no genetic or predictive causes identified
  - ◊ Occupational Safety and Health Administration has clear allowances for duration of noise exposure
    - * Exposure to sound greater than 90 dB for 8 h/day requires hearing protection

OSHA Noise Level Standards

dB Level	*Duration (hour)*
90	8
92	6
95	4
97	3
100	2
102	1.5
105	1
110	0.5
115	<0.25

- Ototoxicity
  - Aminoglycosides—individual drugs vary in impact on cochlear and vestibular systems
    - ◊ Kanamycin, amikacin, neomycin, tobramycin are most cochleotoxic.
    - ◊ OHCs in basal turn injured first (high-frequency SNHL), with continued insult, spiral ganglion cells involved.
    - ◊ Hearing loss typically occurs during treatment but may arise 1 to 3 weeks after completion.
    - ◊ Ribosomal mitochondrial 12S mutations increase susceptibility.
  - Cisplatin—dose-dependent SNHL
    - ◊ Advanced age, children less than 5 years old, and noise exposure also increase the likelihood and severity of SNHL.
    - ◊ Hearing loss is permanent and bilateral.
    - ◊ Injury occurs initially at OHC, but may ultimately affect stria vascularis and ganglion cells.
  - Loop diuretics (furosemide)—results in transient SNHL
    - ◊ Stria vascularis is most common site of injury.
  - Salicylates—bilateral flat SNHL
    - ◊ Dose dependent and typically reversible
    - ◊ Injury occurs initially at OHC; spiral ganglion can be affected with prolonged treatment
  - Ototopicals
    - ◊ Both gentamicin and neomycin/polymyxin have reports of ototoxicity when used with perforated TM.
    - ◊ Chlorhexidine has been shown to be ototoxic if enters the middle ear.

Bibliography

1. Kimberlin DW, Jester PM, Sanchez PJ, et al. Valganciclovir for symptomatic congenital cytomegalovirus disease. *N Engl J Med*. 2015;372(10):933-943.
2. Smith JA, Danner CJ. Complications of chronic otitis media and cholesteatoma. *Otolaryngol Clin N Am*. 2006;39:1237-1255.
3. Rosenfeld RM, Shin JJ, Schwartz SR, et al. Clinical practice guideline: otitis media with effusion (Update). *Otolaryngol Head Neck Surg*. 2016;154(1 Suppl):S1-S41.
4. Merchant SN, Durand ML, Adams JC. Sudden deafness: is it viral? *ORL J Otorhinolaryngol Relat Spec*. 2008;70(1):52-60.
5. Little SC, Kesser BW. Radiographic classification of temporal bone fractures: clinical predictability using a new system. *Arch Otolaryngol Head Neck Surg*. 2006;132:1300-1304.

Questions

1. A 30-year-old woman presents to your office after undergoing successful stapedotomy for otosclerosis. She asks about the chances that her children will have otosclerosis. You tell her:
   A. Your children will definitely have hearing loss from otosclerosis.
   B. There is a 50% chance that your children will have hearing loss from otosclerosis.
   C. There is a chance your children will inherit the gene, but their level of hearing loss will vary.
   D. Only females can inherit the otosclerosis gene.
   E. There is no genetic component to otosclerosis.

2. A HIV-positive patient presents with severe aural pain (especially at night) and otorrhea. He has failed multiple courses of topical antibiotics. On physical examination, granulation tissue is visualized at the isthmus of the EAC. What is the most likely diagnosis?
   A. Malignant otitis externa
   B. Granular myringitis
   C. Chronic otitis externa
   D. Coalescent mastoiditis

3. Which patients should be given antibiotics as a first-line treatment for AOM?
   A. Children older than 2 years of age with mild symptoms or uncertain diagnosis
   B. Children older than 6 months with moderate to severe otalgia older than 48 hours or temperature greater than 39°C
   C. Nonsevere, bilateral AOM in children 6 to 23 months
   D. B and C
   E. All of the above

4. A patient presents to the emergency room with vertigo and hearing loss after a toothpick went in his ear. The ear canal is filled with blood, but a small perforation is seen. How would you manage this patient?
   A. Antibiotic drops
   B. Bed rest and labyrinthine sedatives
   C. Emergency surgery—tympanoplasty and ossicular reconstruction
   D. Emergency surgery—tympanoplasty, tissue seal of the oval window, and secondary reconstruction
   E. Re-evaluate in 6 weeks

5. According to OSHA standards, someone who works in a factory regularly exposed to 95 dB noise can work for how long before requiring hearing protection?

   A. 1 hour

   B. 2 hours

   C. 4 hours

   D. 6 hours

Chapter 21
Tumors of the Temporal Bone

Selected Benign Tumors

See Table 21-1.

Glomus Tumor (Paraganglioma)

A. Most common neoplasm of the middle ear and second most common neoplasm of the temporal bone/cerebellopontine angle (CPA)
   a. Glomus tympanicum (GT)
   b. Glomus jugulare (JG)
   c. Glomus vagale (GV)

B. Caucasians more commonly affected

C. Female preponderance (5:1)

D. May be multifocal (10%)

E. Majority are sporadic, 40% are hereditary
   a. Genetic testing recommended for screening and surveillance recommendations for patients and relatives.
   b. Hereditary variants are associated with increased risk for multifocal and metastatic disease.

F. Rarely malignant (2%-4%), highest risk in glomus vagale
   a. Diagnosis requires metastasis to non-neuroendocrine tissue.
   b. Most common sites are lymph nodes, bone, lung, and liver.
   c. Metastases can occur at any time after primary tumor resection.

G. Rarely functional in temporal bone tumors (extra-adrenal locations)
   a. 5% secrete neuroactive peptides.
   b. Symptoms: palpitations, sweating, hypertension, headaches, syncope.
   c. Some patients are asymptomatic.
   d. Can result in catastrophic hypertension upon induction of anesthesia if not identified and treated preoperatively.
      i. Treat hypertension upon anesthesia induction with phentolamine (nonselective alpha blocker).
      ii. To prevent induction hypertension, treat with phenoxybenzamine (nonselective alpha-blocker) or doxazosin (selective alpha blocker) 7 to 14 days preoperatively.

Table 21-1 Tumors of the Temporal Bone

	Benign	*Malignant*
EAC	Osteoma Adenoma	SCCA BCCA Adenocarcinoma (ceruminous) Melanoma Direct extension of tumors from surrounding areas
ME/Mastoid	Lipoma/choristoma Glomus tympanicum Hemangioma Endolymphatic sac tumor Adenomatous neuroendocrine	SCCA Adenoid cystic carcinoma Acinic cell carcinoma Rhabdomyosarcoma
Petrous Apex	Schwannoma (facial/vestibular) Meningioma Hemangioma Glomus jugulare Chondrosarcoma	SCCA Osteosarcoma Chondroma Lymphoma Metastatic carcinoma to the temporal bone (TB) Direct extension of tumors of the surrounding area

BCCA, basal cell carcinoma; SCCA, squamous cell carcinoma.

H. Biology
   a. Arise from chemoreceptor cells of the neuroendocrine system
      i. Derived from parasympathetic paraganglia in the head and neck
      ii. Found in the jugular dome, tympanic promontory along Jacobson and Arnold nerves
   b. Pathology
      i. Type I chief cells that grow in nests (zellballen, "ball of cells")
      ii. Type II sustentacular cells
   c. Genetics (Table 21-2)
      i. Familial tumors are caused by a genetic defect in mitochondrial DNA encoding for succinyl dehydrogenase subunit B, C, or D (SDHB, SDHC, SDHD), involved in the mitochondrial electron transport chain.
         1. This is thought to be the mutation in sporadic tumors too.

Table 21-2 SDH Mutations in Familial Paragangliomas

Gene	*Tumor Syndrome*	*Locus*	*Inheritance*	*Head & Neck*	*Adrenal*	*Risk of Malignancy*	*Unique Features*
SDHD	PGL1	11q23	AD(I)	91%-98%	16%-21%	8%	Multiple tumors
SDHAF2	PGL2	11q13.1	AD(I)	70%-91%	0%	0%	Imprinting
SDHC	PGL3	1q21	AD	88%	< 10%	< 10%	Single tumors
SDHB	PGL4	1p35-p36	AD	27%-31%	18%-28%	13%-23%	Malignancy
SDHA	PGL5	5p15.33	AD	<3%	< 10%	< 10%	

(I): maternal imprinting implies the disease is only expressed when mutation is passed on from the father.

ii. SDH mutations result in pseudohypoxia and upregulation of hypoxia-inducing factor 1-α.
iii. SDHD and SDHC have highest risk of developing head and neck paragangliomas.
iv. SDHB has highest risk of malignancy.
v. Phenotype is maternally imprinted (passed via male carrier).
   1. Why phenotype can skip a generation?
   2. Autosomal dominant.

I. Classification schemes (Table 21-3)
   a. Fisch
   b. Glasscock-Jackson

Table 21-3 Glomus Tumor Classification Schemes

Fisch	
Type A	Limited to the middle ear
Type B	Limited to the tympanomastoid area with no involvement of the infralabyrinthine compartment
Type C	Involves the infralabyrinthine compartment and petrous apex C1—limited involvement of carotid canal C2—invasion of the vertical portion of carotid canal C3—invasion of the horizontal portion of the carotid canal, does not involve the foramen lacerum C4—involves the entire course of the intrapetrous carotid
Type D	Intracranial extension De1—extradural, extension of < 2 cm De2—extradural, extension of > 2 cm Di1—intradural, extension of < 2 cm Di2—intradural, extension of > 2 cm Di3—intradural, unresectable
Glasscock-Jackson	
Glomus tympanicum	
Type I	Limited to the promontory
Type II	Completely filling the middle ear
Type III	Filling middle ear and extending into the mastoid
Type IV	Filling middle ear, into the mastoid, tympanic membrane (TM), and into the external auditory canal (EAC) (may extend anterior to the internal carotid artery)
Glomus jugulare	
Type I	Small tumor involving the jugular bulb, middle ear, and mastoid
Type II	Extending under the internal auditory canal (IAC), may have intracranial extension
Type III	Extending into petrous apex, may have intracranial extension
Type IV	Extending beyond the petrous apex into the clivus or infratemporal fossa, may have intracranial extension

J. Diagnosis
   a. Symptoms
      i. Pulsatile tinnitus (80%)
      ii. Hearing loss, conductive or mixed (60%)
      iii. Aural fullness (32%)
      iv. Otalgia (13%)
      v. Hoarseness/dysphagia (15%)
      vi. Facial weakness (15%)
      vii. Functional tumors: palpitations, unexplained weight loss, uncontrolled hypertension, headaches
   b. Physical examination
      i. Middle ear mass
         1. Brown sign: blanching of purple, pulsatile middle ear mass with pneumatic otoscopy
         2. Ear canal mass
         3. Neck mass or pharyngeal fullness
         4. Cranial nerve deficits
            a. Audiogram
            b. Laryngoscopy
   c. Labs
      i. 24-Hour urine or plasma-free vanillylmandelic acid (VMA), metanephrines
         1. Used to exclude a functional component
   d. Radiography
      i. Computed tomography (CT) temporal bone
         1. Evaluate extent of lesion. Used to classify tumor as GT or GJ.
         2. Evaluate extent of carotid canal involvement.
         3. Differentiate mass from high-riding jugular bulb or aberrant internal carotid artery.
         4. Glomus tumors are infiltrative and erosive into the bone.
      ii. Magnetic resonance imaging (MRI) posterior fossa with contrast
         1. Identify extent of the mass and assess for intracranial extension
         2. Classic "salt and pepper" appearance due to hemorrhage and flow voids within the tumor
      iii. Contrast-enhanced MRA (MR angiogram)
         1. Early intense arterial enhancement
         2. Improved detection of multifocal paragangliomas
      iv. Nuclear medicine functional imaging: ^{68}Ga-DOTATATE (Gallium 68 Somatostatin receptor imaging)
         1. Superior sensitivity
         2. First-line imaging if suspected multifocal and metastatic disease
         3. Determines eligibility for targeted peptide-receptor therapy
         4. Alternative functional imaging studies: ^{111}In-pentetreotide, ^{18}F-FDG PET/CT for metastases, ^{123}I-MIBG to identify candidates for ^{131}I-MIBG therapy

K. Treatment: Goal is to achieve tumor control while preserving critical neurovascular functions.
   a. Observation: active surveillance
      i. For smaller, less than 2 to 3 cm, symptomatic tumors and nonfunctional tumors

ii. Slow growth rate, 0.8 to 2 mm/y; slower growth in patients greater than age 50
iii. Over half of tumors do not grow

b. Radiation
  i. Can be used as primary modality or for residual/recurrent disease
  ii. Stereotactic radiosurgery, intensity-modulated radiation therapy (IMRT), or proton therapy
  iii. Prevents tumor growth via obliterative endarteritis
  iv. Lower doses used for single fraction (15 Gy) and external beam (40-45 Gy)
  v. Stereotactic radiosurgery has reported 90% to 94% rate of tumor control
    1. Risks: Radiation-induced malignancy, osteoradionecrosis of the skull base, temporal lobe necrosis, cranial nerve injury

c. Surgery
  i. For larger, growing, functional, and/or symptomatic tumors
  ii. GT
    1. Small tumors limited to the promontory can be removed via transcanal, endoscopic, or anterior tympanotomy approaches.
    2. Larger tumors require wider exposure via mastoidectomy and posterior tympanotomy.
  iii. GJ
    1. Requires proximal control of the internal jugular vein/external and internal carotid artery in the neck and sigmoid sinus.
    2. Large tumors may require transposition of the facial nerve to expose the tumor anteriorly.
    3. Infratemporal fossa approach (Fisch type A) is method of choice for removal.
    4. Considerable care required to preserve the lower cranial nerves (IX-XII).
      a. Most centers currently remove as much tumor as possible while preserving lower cranial nerve function and treat postoperatively with stereotactic radiosurgery in the case of tumor growth.
    5. For very large tumors, may need to stage the procedure if blood loss greater than 3 L and proceed with intracranial resection later
    6. Preoperative embolization for Fisch C and D tumors
      a. Four-vessel angiography to identify feeding vessels
      b. Main feeding vessels: ascending pharyngeal artery, occipital artery, posterior auricular artery
      c. Embolization should be performed 24 to 48 hours prior to surgery
      d. Significantly improves intraoperative blood loss
    7. Preoperative balloon occlusion testing of the ipsilateral internal carotid artery should be performed if imaging suggests arterial invasion

d. Therapeutic nuclear medicine: Theranostics
  i. Uses peptide receptor-mediated radionucleotides to target specific pathologic tissue with radiation doses
  ii. For locally unresectable or metastatic disease
  iii. Example: MIBG scan-positive tumors: treat with ^{131}I-MIBG

L. Posttreatment surveillance
  a. Local recurrence, metachronous lesions, and distant metastases may occur at any time, but risk is less than 10%.
  b. Annual imaging (MRI) recommended with closer interval follow-up in patients with high risk for multifocal or metastatic disease.

Endolymphatic Sac Tumor

A. Locally aggressive, slow-growing neoplasm originating from the endolymphatic sac or duct
   a. Endolymphatic sac is contiguous with the posterior cranial fossa.
   b. Endolymphatic sac/duct regulates volume and pressure of endolymph, immune responses of inner ear, and elimination of endolymphatic waste.
   c. Tumors disrupt the petrous bone and can expand into the middle ear, otic capsule, middle, and posterior cranial fossa.
B. Histologically described as a destructive papillary cystic adenomatous tumor of the temporal bone
C. Sporadic tumors more common
   a. Diagnosis occurs in fourth and fifth decades
D. Von Hippel-Lindau (VHL) associated tumors less common
   a. VHL caused by loss of function of tumor suppressor gene (chromosome 3p25.5), ubiquitin ligase, autosomal dominant
      i. Controls hypoxia-inducing factors, which regulate angiogenesis and metabolism
      ii. Associated malignant tumors
         1. Clear cell renal carcinoma, pancreatic neuroendocrine tumors, pheochromocytomas, broad ligament cystadenomas
      iii. Associated benign tumors
         1. Retinal hemangioblastoma, cerebellar hemangioblastoma, spinal cord hemangioblastoma, epididymal cystadenoma, endolymphatic sac tumors, renal/pancreatic cysts
      iv. Diagnosis: Genetic testing
   b. More common in females
   c. Can be presenting sign in 30% of patients with VHL
   d. 30% will have bilateral endolymphatic sac tumors
E. Symptoms: Due to disruption of otic capsule
   a. Often mimic endolymphatic hydrops due to obstruction of the normal flow and resorption patterns of endolymph
   b. Sensorineural hearing loss, tinnitus, vertigo, aural fullness
   c. Sudden hearing loss can result from intralabyrinthine hemorrhage
   d. Middle ear extension can mimic Eustachian tube dysfunction and otitis media
   e. Late symptoms include facial paresis, symptoms of brain stem compression, and lower cranial neuropathies
   f. No cases of distant metastases, but several cases of spinal metastases
F. Imaging
   a. CT: bony destruction of posterior fossa plate centered over the operculum with central calcifications
   b. MRI
      i. T1: heterogenous, hypo, iso, or hyperintense. Hyperintensity from intralesional hemorrhage (methemoglobin, hemosiderin, cholesterol crystals), hypointensity from residual bone or calcifications
      ii. T2: heterogeneous (highly vascular)
      iii. T1 with contrast: heterogenous enhancement
G. Staging: Bambakidis-Megerian Staging System
   a. Grade I: confined to temporal bone, middle ear, and/or external auditory canal
      i. Surgery: hearing preservation retrolabyrinthine transdural approach

   b. Grade II: Extension into posterior fossa
      i. Surgery: extended retrolabyrinthine transdural approach versus translabyrinthine approach (for poor hearing)
   c. Grade III: Extension into middle cranial fossa
      i. Surgery: subtemporal craniotomy with petrosectomy
   d. Grade IV: Extension into clivus and/or sphenoid wing
      i. Surgery: staged anterior and posterior fossa techniques
H. Differential diagnosis: paraganglioma, choroid plexus tumor, metastasis, eosinophilic granuloma, meningioma, arachnoid granulation, aneurysmal bone cyst, primary bone tumors
I. Treatment
   a. Surgery with gross total resection is the treatment of choice
      i. Long-term cure is 90% with gross total resection.
      ii. Can be difficult to achieve complete resection.
      iii. Consider preoperative embolization for larger tumors.
   b. Radiation
      i. Sparse data for primary radiotherapy
      ii. Adjuvant radiation with good control rates reported after subtotal resection or for unresectable recurrence
J. Follow up
   a. High rate of recurrence, long-term follow-up necessary
      i. 20% recurrence rate in sporadic disease
      ii. 12% recurrence rate in VHL-associated disease
   b. Disease-free survival 47.6 months in sporadic disease, 49.8 months in VHL-associated disease

Hemangioma

A. Benign tumors that arise from blood vessels account for 0.7% of all temporal bone neoplasms
   a. Occur most frequently in fifth and sixth decades
B. Typically associated with the facial nerve, particularly the geniculate ganglion
   a. Less common locations: internal auditory canal (IAC), cerebellopontine angle (CPA), tympanic and mastoid segments of the facial nerve
C. Symptoms
   a. Most common symptom is progressive facial weakness (sudden paralysis more rare)
      i. Cause facial weakness out of proportion to their size
   b. Sensorineural or conductive hearing loss, vestibular symptoms
   c. Mechanisms for symptoms include local tumor bony destruction, nerve compression, nerve infiltration, or vascular steal
D. Imaging
   a. CT: infiltrative erosive lesion centered at the geniculate ganglion with intralesional stippled calcifications
      i. Can erode cochlear or labyrinth
   b. MRI: hypo- to isointense on T1 imaging, enhances avidly with contrast
E. Treatment
   a. Observation: Natural history data are lacking.
   b. Surgery

i. Early intervention thought to increase likelihood of anatomic and functional facial nerve preservation
ii. Small lesions: can be meticulously dissected free from the facial nerve when centered at the geniculate fossa with preservation of facial function
iii. IAC/CPA lesions
1. For normal preoperative facial function, decompress IAC as tumor resection often involves facial nerve resection and grafting
2. For preoperative facial paralysis at or worse than House Brackmann grade IV, resect tumor with nerve graft. Facial nerve function outcomes are better with shorter duration of preoperative facial weakness.

c. Radiation
i. Stereotactic radiosurgery has been reported, but no current long-term tumor control rates.

F. Follow up
a. Surveillance imaging mandatory with subtotal resection

Middle Ear Adenomatous Neuroendocrine Tumor (MEANT)

A. Rare tumors with uncertain biological behavior and unpredictable clinical course
a. Epithelial-derived adenomatous tumors with neuroendocrine differentiation.
i. Other terminology: middle ear adenoma, carcinoid tumor, adenomatous tumor of the middle ear
b. No reliable histopathological or immunohistochemical predictors of tumor behavior or clinical outcome have been identified.
i. Some tumors behave indolently, confined to the tympanic cavity.
ii. Other tumors are aggressive with malignant characteristics and metastasize.
c. Neuroendocrine tumors in other organs (lungs and GI tract most common) have organ-specific grading schemes to stratify aggressiveness and differentiate neuroendocrine tumor versus carcinoma, but this has not been differentiated in MEANTs.

B. Presenting symptoms
a. Conductive or mixed hearing loss
b. Aural fullness
c. Tinnitus, pulsatile or high frequency
d. Carcinoid syndrome
e. Facial nerve paresis

C. Physical exam
a. Pink middle ear mass with bulging tympanic membrane

D. Imaging
a. CT temporal bone
i. Similar to tympanic paraganglioma, but MEANTs can develop in atypical positions (not centered over promontory or hypotympanum)
b. MRI posterior fossa with contrast
i. 80% of tumors enhance with Gadolinium, T1 hyperintense in most cases, T2 hypointense in most cases
ii. No restricted diffusion on diffusion-weighted imaging
c. Octreotide scintigraphy using 6.3mCi ^{111}In-labeled octreotide

E. Differential diagnosis
   a. Temporal bone paragangliomas (unlike paraganglioma, these can develop in locations other than hypotympanum, nonpulsatile, pink)
   b. Cholesteatoma (MEANTs do show restricted diffusion on MRI)
F. Staging
   a. T1: Tumor confined to middle ear cavity that does not envelop or adhere to ossicles
   b. T2a: Tumor fills middle ear cleft and encases ossicles with/without ossicular erosion
   c. T2b: Tumor extends into mastoid
   d. T2c: Tumor extends through tympanic membrane into ear canal
   e. T3: Tumor adheres to important neurovascular structures such as petrous internal carotid artery, facial nerve, sigmoid sinus, dura
   f. T4: Intradural tumor extension
   g. N0: No regional lymph node metastases
   h. N1: Regional lymph node metastases (parotid and cervical chain most common)
   i. M0: No metastases
   j. M1: Metastatic disease (bone, liver, lung most common)
   k. S0: Tumor is nonsecretory
   l. S1: Hormone-secreting tumor (eg, serotonin)
G. Treatment
   a. Complete surgical resection is treatment of choice.
      i. Most common surgical approach is tympanomastoidectomy.
      ii. For more widespread or aggressive disease, more extensive surgical resection is warranted such as subtotal petrosectomy.
   b. Postoperative radiation and/or chemotherapy, treatment with somatostatin analogues, and peptide radionuclide receptor therapy have been reported.
H. Surveillance
   a. High recurrent rates (71% recurrence rate in report with longest follow-up)
      i. One-third of T2 tumors and two-thirds of T3 tumors developed local recurrence at a median duration of 6 years.
      ii. Some advocate for a second-look procedure 1 year postoperatively.
   b. Need long-term follow-up.

Choristoma (Lipochoristoma, Lipomatous tumor, Lipoma)

A. Rare mass of middle ear or internal auditory canal
   a. Choristoma: histologically normal tissue in abnormal location
B. Symptoms
   a. Conductive hearing loss/middle ear effusion if in the middle ear
   b. SNHL, tinnitus, dizziness if in the internal auditory canal/cerebellopontine angle
C. Imaging
   a. MRI posterior fossa with contrast
      i. Choristoma/lipomas are hyperintense on T1 without contrast and do not enhance with gadolinium.
      ii. Differential diagnoses: vestibular schwannoma, epidermoid cysts, meningioma, arachnoid cysts, dermoid cysts, hemangiomas.
      iii. Depend on imaging characteristics to differentiate lipoma from other tumors.
D. Treatment
   a. Observation with annual audiogram, MRIs every 2 to 3 years.

b. Tumor growth is rare (1.4% incidence of tumor growth and most in younger patients).
c. Lipomas tend to envelop nerves, making removal with nerve preservation difficult. Surgery is not recommended.

Vestibular Schwannoma (VS)

A. Most common tumor of the internal auditory canal (IAC) and cerebellopontine angle (CPA)
   a. Represents 8% to 10% of all intracranial tumors with lifetime prevalence of 1 in 500 persons.
   b. Schwannomas most commonly arise from the vestibular nerve, but may arise from any cranial nerve including the facial, cochlear, trigeminal, or lower cranial nerves.
      i. Tumors arise from somatic mutations of the *NF2* gene.
   c. VS are benign, slow-growing tumors with an average growth of 1 to 2 mm per year.
      i. Some tumors do not show any growth on serial imaging.
   d. Histology shows Antoni A fibers (fibrillary, polar, elongated tissue) and Antoni B fibers (loosely reticulated tissue).
   e. Neurofibromatosis type 2 (NF2) and NF2-related Schwannomatosis (NF2-SWN) characterized by bilateral VS.
      i. Rare, prevalence of 1:60,000
      ii. Autosomal dominant inheritance, *NF2* gene on chromosome 22q 11.2 (loss of function of the tumor suppressor gene encoding Merlin)
      iii. Loss of tumor suppressor function also causes meningiomas, ependymomas, posterior lenticular opacities, and cutaneous schwannomas
B. Symptoms
   a. Asymmetric sensorineural hearing loss (SNHL) (audiogram may show poorer speech discrimination score than expected with louder presentation)
   b. Tinnitus
   c. Dizziness
C. Diagnosis: Imaging
   a. MRI brain and posterior fossa with contrast shows a characteristic T1-enhancing mass within or centered over the IAC.
D. Treatment
   a. Observation: for small tumors, serviceable hearing, older age, medical comorbidities
      i. Some tumors never grow and do not require treatment.
      ii. Annual imaging recommended to detect tumor growth.
      iii. Newer approach: "Size threshold surveillance approach"
         1. Traditionally, treatment has been recommended for linear tumor growth greater than 2 mm, but newer data suggest it is safe to accept some tumor growth up to a size threshold range of approximately 15 mm of CPA extension.
   b. Radiosurgery
      i. Modalities: Gamma knife (single dose, 12-13 Gy), Linear accelerator (LINAC): Novalis or BrainLAB, Cyberknife (20-25 Gy in 5 treatments), proton beam therapy
      ii. Indications: Enlarging tumors, tumors less than 2.5 cm, patients who cannot tolerate surgery

iii. Risks
1. Hearing loss (Rate of serviceable hearing 10 years after radiosurgery is 29%)
2. Facial nerve dysfunction (1% risk)
3. Trigeminal paresthesia or pain
4. Communicating hydrocephalus
5. Malignant transformation (1:1000 risk over 30 years)

iv. Outcomes
1. 90% to 95% long-term tumor control rate
2. Better long-term quality of life for dizziness/imbalance for patients undergoing radiation or observation than surgery

v. Adjuvant treatment after subtotal or near-total surgical resection
1. 95% rate of tumor control with radiosurgery after primary microsurgery

c. Microsurgery
i. Goal of gross total tumor resection, sparing the facial nerve
1. Tumors less than 1.5 cm are eligible for hearing preservation.
2. Subtotal or near-total resection can be necessary to preserve the facial nerve.
a. Tumor remnant can grow and require postoperative treatment with radiation.

ii. Three surgical approaches
1. Translabyrinthine approach
a. For any size tumor, including large tumors
b. Hearing is sacrificed as part of the approach
c. No brain retraction
d. Facial nerve is identified in the fundus before tumor removal begins
2. Retrosigmoid approach
a. Potential for hearing preservation in tumors less than 1.5 cm and more medially located in the IAC
b. Can be used for any size tumor
c. Requires cerebellar retraction
d. High risk of chronic headaches
3. Middle fossa approach
a. Potential for hearing preservation
b. Indicated for tumors less than 1.5 cm in the IAC
c. Requires retraction of the temporal lobe (rare side effects are memory changes, word finding difficulties, or seizures)

d. Pharmacologic therapies
i. No FDA-approved drugs for treatment of sporadic VS or NF2, but there are ongoing clinical trials for multiple drugs.
1. Most studied drug: Bevacizumab (humanized immunoglobulin G1), which is a monoclonal antibody that binds vascular endothelial growth factor (VEGF). Bevacizumab has shown hearing improvement and volumetric reduction of VS.

Facial Nerve Schwannoma

A. Most common facial nerve tumor (Hemangioma is the second most common facial nerve tumor).
B. Geniculate ganglion is the most common site of a facial nerve schwannoma.
C. MRI shows enhancement with gadolinium contrast.
D. On CT, schwannomas show smooth remodeling of the bone, whereas Hemangiomas show bony erosion and ground-glass appearance.

E. Treatment is based on facial nerve function, tumor location, and size.
F. Schwannomas with normal or near-normal function can usually be observed with serial imaging.
G. In schwannomas with a House-Brackmann Grade 3 or poorer facial function, tumor removal and facial reanimation procedures are considered.
H. Tumor decompression can be considered with early and mild paresis.
I. Radiation can be considered in a small growing tumor.
J. Surgical approaches are based on hearing status and tumor location. The middle fossa and/or transmastoid approach are used for tumors with serviceable hearing. The translabyrinthine approach is used for tumors with nonserviceable hearing.

Meningioma

A. Second most common tumor of the CPA.
B. Arises from arachnoid cap cells, which are cells in the arachnoid layer of the meninges covering the brain.
C. Imaging characteristic that differentiate a meningioma from a vestibular schwannoma include: dural tail, eccentric location to the IAC, calcifications, hyperostosis of adjacent bone, less enhancement, and more homogenous with gadolinium contrast.
D. Symptoms based on tumor location and size: may include SNHL, tinnitus, imbalance/vertigo, facial paresthesia or numbness, diplopia, or ataxia.
E. World Health Organization (WHO) classification of meningiomas
    i. Benign (Grade 1)—meningiothelial, fibrous, translational, psammomatous, angiomatous, secretory, lymphoplasmacyte-rich, and microcystic
    ii. Atypical (Grade 2)—chordoid, clear cell, atypical
    iii. Anaplastic/malignant (Grade 3)—papillary, rhabdoid, anaplastic
F. Hearing preservation or even hearing improvement more common with meningiomas compared to vestibular schwannomas.
G. Histology characterized by psammoma bodies, which can be seen in many tumors.

Chondrosarcoma

A. Rare malignant tumors, produce a chondroid (cartilaginous) matrix. Rarely metastasizes
B. Less than 1% of all intracranial neoplasms, 6% of skull base tumors
C. Typically arising from synchondroses (spheno-occipital or petroclival sutures)
D. Imaging
    i. Characteristics similar to chordomas, but tend to be more eccentrically located, with no imaging hallmarks distinguishing low grade from high grade
E. Pathology
    i. WHO Grade 1 (well-differentiated) and 2 (intermediate-differentiated), low-grade and significantly more frequent
    ii. WHO Grade 3 (high grade, poorly differentiated), mesenchymal chordoma subtype
    iii. Nonreactive for keratin and EMA, and more frequently firm with calcifications
F. Treatment
    i. Same as chordomas: surgery followed by radiation
G. Prognosis
    i. Younger age, female gender, and smaller tumor size are associated with increased survival.
    ii. SEER database reports 5- and 10-year mortality rates of 87% and 68% respectively, substantially higher when only considering low-grade chondrosarcomas.

Chordoma

A. Rare low-grade malignant tumor originating from embryonic notochordal tissue.
B. Mainly occur in the axial bone, mostly in the spheno-occipital junction.
C. 0.1% to 0.2% of all intracranial neoplasms.
D. Metastasis is rare.
E. Symptoms
   i. Produce morbidity and mortality through local growth.
   ii. Headache is a frequently presenting symptom.
F. MRI Imaging
   i. Classically hyperintense on T2WI, hypointense on T1WI
   ii. 30% demonstrate calcifications within the tumor
G. Pathology
   i. Three histologic subtypes: classical/conventional (most common), chondroid, and dedifferentiated
   ii. Stain positive for brachyury, S-100, cytokeratin, epithelial membrane antigen (EMA)
   iii. Physaliferous cells are pathognomonic
H. Treatment
   i. Maximal resection with aggressive high-dose postoperative radiation therapy.
   ii. Surgical approach is dependent on size and location; an anterior approach is favored, because most of these tumors arise midline in the clivus.
   iii. Disease lateral to the carotid will require lateral skull base approaches.
   iv. Residual tumor is treated with adjuvant radiation.
   v. Fractionated stereotactic radiosurgery, with a median dose of 67 Gy, yields approximately 50% 5-year local control.
   vi. Proton beam and carbon ion therapy are effective with 5-year local control rates above 70%.
I. Outcome
   i. SEER database notes median overall survival of 7.7 years.
   ii. Patients under 40 years of age have better long-term survival (68%) at 10 years as compared to those patients older than 40 years of age (43%).
   iii. 5-year overall survival is 6 times more likely with gross or near-total resections, compared with subtotal resections.

Squamous Cell Carcinoma

A. Squamous cell carcinoma (SCC) is the most common primary malignancy of the temporal bone (39%).
   i. Followed in decreasing order by basal cell carcinoma, adenocarcinoma, adenoid cystic carcinoma, mucoepidermoid carcinoma, ceruminoma, melanoma, and sarcoma
B. Risk factors include chronic irritation or inflammation.
C. Many possible routes of spread.
D. Symptoms include: otalgia, otorrhea, hearing loss, facial palsy, and parotid mass.
E. Preoperative evaluation
   i. Audiogram
   ii. CT temporal bone and neck with contrast (can metastasize to parotid and cervical lymph nodes)
   iii. MRI with gadolinium to identify local spread to soft tissue, perineural disease, and dural involvement.
   iv. CT chest with IV contrast, CXR, or PET scan to evaluate for distant metastases.

Table 21-4 T-Staging for Squamous Cell Carcinoma of the Temporal Bone

T Stage	*Extent of Disease*
T1	Tumor limited to EAC without evidence of bony erosion or soft tissue involvement
T2	Tumor causes limited bony erosion (not full thickness) or < 0.5 cm of soft tissue involvement
T3	Tumor erodes through the bony EAC with limited (< 0.5 cm) soft tissue involvement; or involves middle ear and/or mastoid
T4	Tumor erodes into the medial wall of the middle ear to involve the cochlea, labyrinth, petrous apex, jugular foramen, carotid canal, or dura; soft tissue involvement of > 0.5 cm (temporomandibular joint [TMJ], styloid or parotid); evidence of facial paresis/paralysis

Reproduced with permission from Moody SA, Hirsch BE, Myers EN. Squamous cell carcinoma of the external auditory canal: an evaluation of a staging system, *Am J Otol*. 2000 Jul;21(4):582-588.

F. Most widely used staging for SCC of the temporal bone is the modified University of Pittsburgh Staging System (Table 21-4).
G. Treatment
   i. Low-grade EAC lesions not involving the bone, sleeve resection (removes the bony EAC skin, cartilaginous EAC portion, and +/− tympanic membrane, leaving the bony EAC intact).
   ii. Lesions involving bone require a lateral temporal bone resection (LTBR) at minimum.
   iii. When disease extends into the middle ear, subtotal temporal bone resection (STBR) is indicated (drill into the petrous temporal bone and otic capsule until obtaining negative margins).
   iv. Total temporal bone resection (TTBR) includes a STBR + sigmoid sinus and possibly petrous carotid artery resection. TTBR has no proven survival benefit to date and is rarely done.
   v. Parotidectomy and neck dissection are performed for local or lymphatic spread of disease. Prophylactic parotidectomy +/− neck dissection in patients with T3 or T4 disease.
   vi. Postoperative radiation (50-60 Gy) is generally offered to all patients with T2, T3, or T4 disease.
   vii. Chemotherapy should be considered for T4 tumors, residual disease after surgery, or metastatic disease.
   viii. Immunotherapy remains under investigation (Table 21-5).
H. Reported survival rates per T staging include for T1 (48%-100%), T2 (28%-100%), T3 (17%-100%), and T4 (14.3%-54.0%).

Rhabdomyosarcoma

A. Most common pediatric temporal bone malignancy.
   i. Most commonly affects the head and neck region, accounting for 35% to 40% of all rhabdomyosarcomas.
   ii. Most frequently encountered in the orbit, paranasal sinuses, and nasopharynx.
   iii. Only 5% present in the temporal bone.
B. Originate from embryologic skeletal muscle cells.
C. Symptoms: otalgia, otorrhea, hearing loss, headache, aural polyp, facial nerve weakness, and regional lymphadenopathy.
D. Imaging: CT temporal bone. MRI of IAC with and without contrast.

Table 21-5 Temporal Bone Resection

Surgery	*Tissues Removed*	*Limits of Dissection*
LTBR	En bloc removal of cartilaginous and bony EAC, TM, malleus, incus Optional: parotidectomy, neck dissection, mandibular condyle	A: capsule of TMJ S: epitympanum, root of zygoma P: mastoid cavity I: facial nerve, hypotympanic bone, infratemporal fossa M: stapes
STBR	LTBR + contents of ME and mastoid, otic capsule, medial wall of ME Optional: facial nerve, dura, infratemporal fossa, sigmoid, brain parenchyma May be piecemeal or en bloc resection	A: anterior capsule of TMJ, mandibular ramus S: middle fossa dura P: dura of posterior fossa I: infratemporal fossa M: IAC, petrous apex with neurovascular structures
TTBR	STBR + petrous apex and neurovascular bundle Piecemeal resection used when carotid and lower CN preserved; en bloc resection requires sacrifice of carotid and lower CN	A: anterior capsule of TMJ, mandibular ramus S: temporal lobe P: cerebellum I: Infratemporal fossa M: +/− carotid, clivus

A: anterior; I: inferior; M: medial; P: posterior; S: superior.

E. Pathology/Histology:
   i. Three classifications: embryonal (most common), alveolar, and pleomorphic.
   ii. Embryonal is subdivided into spindle cell, botryoid, and embryonal (conventional) subtypes.
   iii. Better prognosis for embryonal tumors compared with alveolar.
   iv. Pleomorphic most commonly encountered in adults.
   v. Spindle cell and botryoid tumors are more favorable.

F. Can originate from external auditory canal, middle ear, and mastoid cavity

G. Soft Tissue Sarcoma Committee of the Children's Oncology Group developed current staging grouping system (Table 21-6).
   i. Includes tumor stage at diagnosis, with T2 tumors involving structures outside external ear and tympanomastoid space, and assigning an 'a' or 'b' for tumors smaller or larger than 5 cm in diameter
   ii. Assignment of tumor group after surgery based on resection and then risk classification and histologic subtype
   iii. All temporal bone tumors are considered parameningeal, and thus by definition, unfavorable, at minimum Stage II tumor stage

H. Treatment
   i. Debate as to whether to surgically resect or biopsy, followed by primary chemoradiation.
   ii. Many recommend wide surgical resection with clear margins, since the extent of resection determines prognosis.

Table 21-6 TNM Staging System for Rhabdomyosarcoma

Stage	*Site*	*T*	*N*	*M*
I	Orbit, HN (× parameningeal), genitourinary (GU) nonbladder/nonprostate	T1 or T2a or b	N0 or N1	M0
II	Bladder/prostate, extremity, cranial, parameningeal	T1 or T2a or b	N0	M0
III	Bladder/prostate, extremity, cranial, parameningeal	T1 or T2a or b	N1	M0
IV	All sites	T1 or T2a or b	N0 or N1	M1
Group 1	Localized disease, completely excised, no microscopic residual A. Confined to site of origin, completely resected B. Infiltrating beyond the site of origin, completely resected			
Group 2	Total gross resection A. Gross resection with evidence of microscopic local residual B. Regional disease with involved lymph nodes, completely resected with no microscopic residual C. Microscopic local and/or nodal residual			
Group 3	Incomplete resection or biopsy with gross residual			
Group 4	Distant metastasis			

iii. SRS indications include residual or recurrent disease within the jugular foramen or perineurial invasion into the internal auditory canal, Meckel cave, or cavernous sinus.
iv. Most pediatric high-grade sarcomas are treated with surgical resection followed by 50 to 70 Gy external beam radiation with multidrug chemotherapy.
v. External beam radiation to the skull base in children can lead to eustachian tube dysfunction, osteoradionecrosis, sensorineural hearing loss, cataract development, impaired cranial bone and tooth development, as well as pituitary dysfunction and chronic headache

I. 5-year survival rates by risk classification include 90% for low-risk group, 60% to 80% for intermediate risk group, and 20% to 40% in the high-risk group.

Acknowledgements

The authors would like to acknowledge the previous work of Jacob Hunter MD, Walter Kutz MD, and Brandon Isaacson MD in writing this chapter for the 12th edition, much of which has been used here and updated.

Bibliography

Lin EP, Chin BB, Fishbein L, et al. Head and neck paragangliomas: an update on the molecular classification, state-of-the-art imaging, and management recommendations. *Radiol Imaging Cancer*. 2022 May;4(3):e210088.

Lovin BD, Gidley PW. Squamous cell carcinoma of the temporal bone: a current review. *Laryngoscope Investig Otolaryngol*. 2019 Nov 13;4(6):684-692.

Marinelli, JP, Cass, SP, Mann, SE, et al. Adenomatous neuroendocrine tumors of the middle ear: a multi-institutional investigation of 32 cases and development of a staging system. *Otol Neurotol.* 39(8):e712-e721, Sept 2018.

Moore MG, Netterville JL, Mendenhall WM, Isaacson B, Nussenbaum B. Head and neck paragangliomas: an update on evaluation and management. *Otolaryngol Head Neck Surg.* 2016;154:597-605.

Van der Lans RJL, Engel MSD, Rijken JA, et al. Neuroendocrine neoplasms of the middle ear: Unpredictable tumor behavior and tendency for recurrence. *Head Neck.* 2021 June; 43(6): 1848-1853.

Questions

1. A 39-year-old man presents with 9 months of progressive right facial weakness. The audiogram shows normal hearing bilaterally. The patient is otherwise healthy with a normal birth history. There is no history of cancer or malignancy. On physical examination, the right CN VII is House-Brackmann 3/6. Left CN VII is normal. MRI shows a small enhancing lesion at the geniculate ganglion. CT shows calcifications in the area of the lesion. What is the next step in management?
   A. Decompress via the middle cranial fossa approach (Key)
   B. Repeat imaging in 6 to 12 months (Distractor)
   C. Resect the lesion and perform a nerve graft procedure (Distractor)
   D. Stereotactic radiation (Distractor)

2. A 32-year-old man presents with left pulsatile tinnitus and hearing loss, which has been progressing over the past 7 years. On physical examination, a mass is noted in the left middle ear. Auscultation of the left neck and periauricular area reveals an objective bruit. MRI of the internal auditory canal shows an enhancing mass at the jugular foramen with a salt and pepper appearance. Which additional scan would be appropriate to order in this patient during the workup?
   A. [^{68}Ga]-DOTATATE PET/CT (Key)
   B. Functional MRI (Distractor)
   C. ^{99m}technetium-diphosphonate scan (Distractor)
   D. MRI of the abdomen (Distractor)

3. A 62-year-old man presents with severe left otalgia with otorrhea. He has been to several doctors who have all prescribed antibiotic otologic drops. His pain continues to worsen. On examination, friable tissue is noted. A biopsy is taken and reveals squamous cell carcinoma. CT scan shows bony erosion of the anterior external auditory canal. There is no extension into the middle ear. MRI shows enhancement into the parotid gland. What is the appropriate treatment option?
   A. Sleeve resection (Distractor)
   B. Lateral temporal bone resection (Distractor)
   C. Lateral temporal bone resection with parotidectomy (Key)
   D. Total temporal bone resection (Distractor)

4. State True or False. MRI surveillance in 1 year is an acceptable treatment option for a 65-year-old man with an untreated 1.2 cm vestibular schwannoma, which showed 2 mm of growth over the past year on his annual MRI.

5. A 50-year-old woman presents with unilateral fluctuating hearing loss and vertigo. An MRI shows an enhancing posterior fossa mass. CT scan shows bony destruction of the posterior fossa plate centered over the operculum with central calcifications. All the following are true of this tumor EXCEPT
   A. Genetic testing should be performed to evaluate for Von Hippel-Lindau disease (Distractor).
   B. Treatment is surgical resection (Distractor).
   C. Long-term surveillance after surgical resection is not necessary (Key).
   D. Can be associated with other benign and malignant tumors (Distractor).

Chapter 22
Endoscopic Ear Surgery

Introduction

Endoscopic ear surgery (EES) is a minimally invasive approach similar to standard microscopic techniques. Initially endoscope was used to assist traditional operations to visualize middle ear's hidden areas. Therefore, instrumentals, optics, light, and camera systems improvements allowed endoscope to be a main tool in middle ear surgery.

Anatomy

Middle ear is an irregular cavity filled with air in the center of the temporal bone, in tympanic portion. See Figures 22-1 to 22-7.

Limits

- Superior: called tegmen, a plate of bone below middle cranial fossa dura and temporal lobe.
- Inferior: narrow and thin plate of bone above jugular bulb. Careful approach to middle ear is necessary if the patient has a high or dehiscent jugular bulb.
- Medial: cochlear promontory (cochlear basal turn), tympanic plexus (Jacobson nerve), oval and round windows, tympanic segment of facial nerve, and lateral semicircular canal.
- Lateral: tympanic membrane, annulus fibrosus, and scutum.
- Anterior: formed by petrous bone. From superior to inferior:
  (a) Tensor tympani muscle canal
  (b) Eustachian tube
  (c) Internal carotid artery (vertical segment)
- Posterior: formed by the petrous bone and *aditus ad antrum* that communicates attic and mastoid antrum.

Epitympanum (Attic)

- It is the upper portion of middle ear cavity above tympanic membrane level and an imaginary plane through malleus short process.
- Communicates with mastoid antrum.
- Plays a fundamental role in ventilation routes.

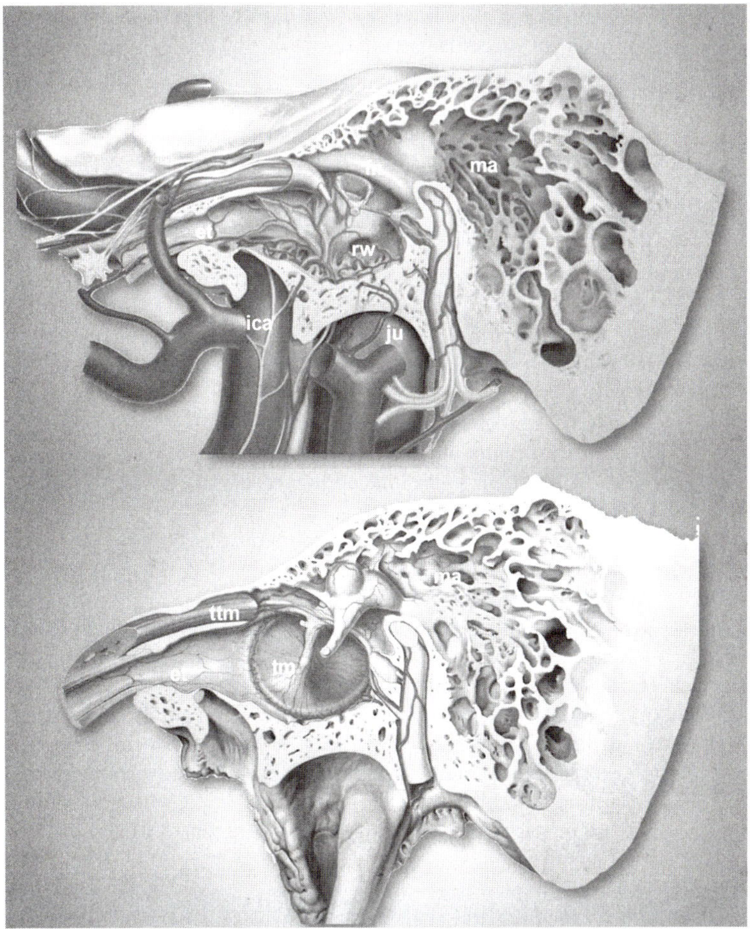

Figure 22-1 Schematic view of the middle ear anatomy and its limits. et: eustachian tube; fn: facial nerve; ica: internal carotid artery; ju: jugular vein; ma: mastoid antrum; rw: round window; tm: tympanic membrane; ttm: tensor tympani muscle.

- Limits:
  (a) Superior: tegmen tympani
  (b) Inferior: tympanic diaphragm and isthmus
  (c) Medial: facial nerve canal and lateral semicircular canal
  (d) Lateral: pars flaccida of tympanic membrane and scutum (Chaussé spur)
  (e) Anterior: zygomatic root
  (f) Posterior: incudal fossa and aditus ad antrum
- Posterior epitympanum compartment is posterior to superior malleal fold
  (a) Posterior part of malleus head
  (b) (Incus body and short process
  (c) Posterior route ventilation: most important pathway to attic
- Anterior epitympanum compartment is anterior to superior malleal fold
  (a) Anterior portion of malleus head
  (b) Anterior route of ventilation: accessory pathway to attic

- Tympanic diaphragm is made of various folds and ligaments:
  (a) Posterior incudal ligament
  (b) Lateral incudomalleal fold
  (c) Lateral malleal fold
  (d) Lateral malleal ligament
  (e) Anterior malleal fold
  (f) Anterior malleal ligament
  (g) Tensor tympani fold (or Posterior malleal fold)
  (h) Tensor tympani muscle tendon
- Tympanic isthmus is a 2.5 mm opening in the tympanic diaphragm that ventilates entire attic.
  (a) (Anterior tympanic isthmus: between incudostapedial joint and tensor tympani tendon. It is the largest and most important ventilation route to attic. Granulation tissue and blockages at this region lead to attic selective dysventilation, chronic edema, exudate, inflammation, infections, retraction pockets, and cholesteatoma.
  (b) Posterior tympanic isthmus: posterior to incudostapedial joint, between stapedial muscle tendon, pyramidal eminence, and incus short process.
- Prussak space:
  (a) Superior: lateral malleal fold (tympanic diaphragm)
  (b) Inferior: malleus neck
  (c) Medial: malleus head
  (d) Lateral: pars flaccida of tympanic membrane (Sharpnell membrane)
  (e) Anterior: anterior malleal fold
  (f) Posterior: posterior malleal fold
  (g) Ventilation route: independent, rough, narrow, through posterior pocket of von Troltsch. Thick and viscous secretions may close posterior pocket and lead to sectorial dysventilation of Prussak Space, pars flaccida membrane retraction, and adhesion to malleus neck. This could happen without any involvement of anterior and posterior epitympanum, aditus, and mastoid cells.

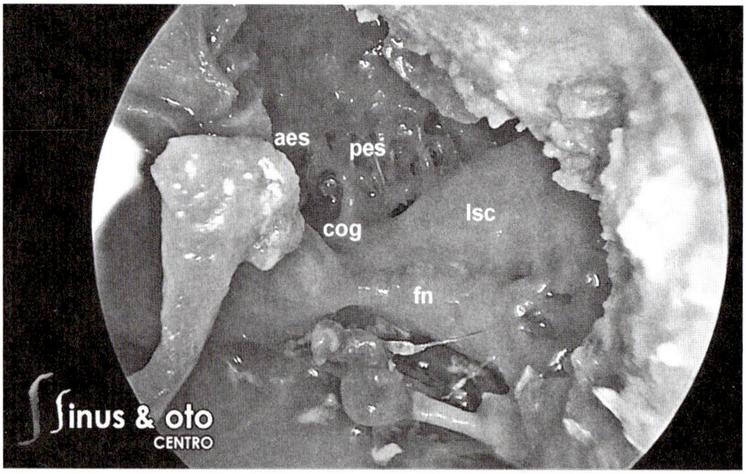

Figure 22-2 Attic: endoscopic view of left ear showing: aes: anterior epitympanic space; pes: posterior epitympanic space (separated in some cases by the COG). The COG can also separate the supratubal recess from the aes.fn: facial nerve; lsc: lateral semicircular canal.

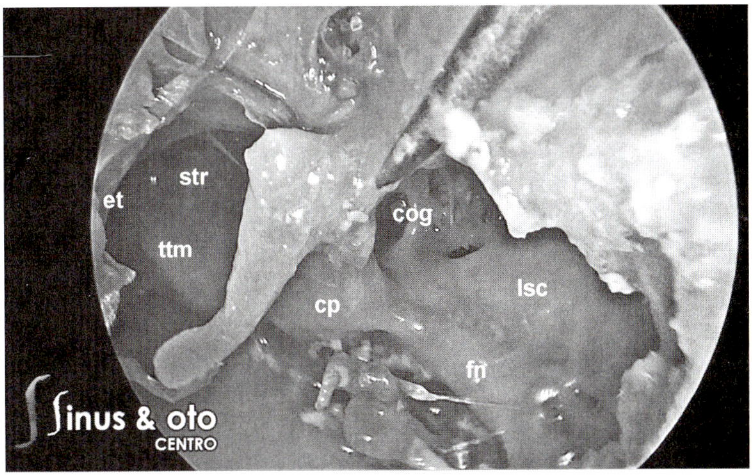

Figure 22-3 Endoscopic view of left ear showing: cp: cochleariform process; et: Eustachian tube; fn: facial nerve; lsc: lateral semicircular canal; str: supratubal recess; ttm: tensor tympani muscle.

Mesotympanum

- It is the central, longest, and narrowest compartment of middle ear.
- Limits:
  (a) Superior: tympanic diaphragm, open to epitympanum (attic)
  (b) Inferior: open to hypotympanum
  (c) Medial: promontory
  (d) Lateral: pars tensa of tympanic membrane
  (e) Anterior: open to protympanum
  (f) Posterior: open to retrotympanum

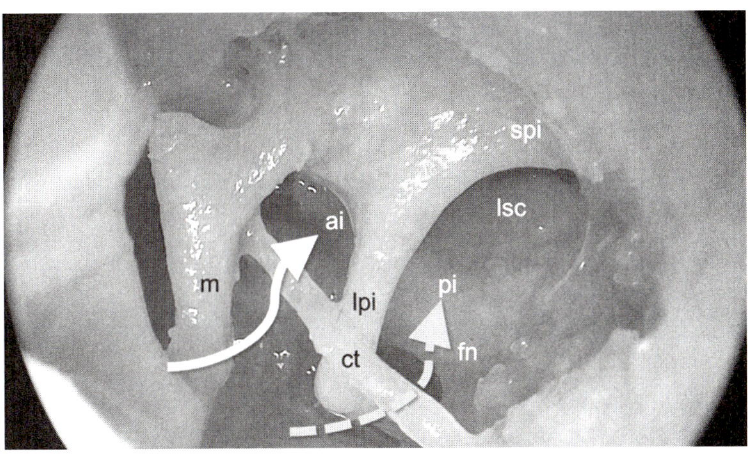

Figure 22-4 Endoscopic view of left ear showing the main ventilation routes between the Eustachian tube and mastoid antrum. ai: anterior isthmus; ct: chorda tympani; fn: facial nerve; lpi: long process of incus; lsc: lateral semicircular canal; m: malleus; pi: posterior isthmus. The tympanic isthmus is a passage, the main ventilation route, between the cochleariform process and the incudostapedial joint.

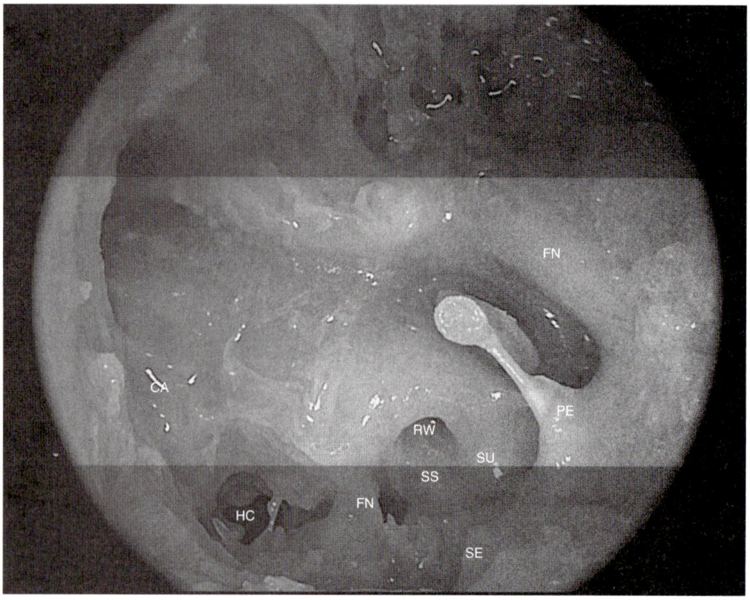

Figure 22-5 Endoscopic view of left ear (without malleus and incus) to demonstrate the divisions between epitympanum, mesotympanum (in the middle), and hypotympanum.

- Structures:
  (a) (Malleus: handle (manubrium)
  (b) Incus: long process and lenticular process
  (c) Stapes: capitulum, anterior and posterior crus, footplate, stapedial tendon
  (d) Cochlear promontory (cochlea basal turn)
  (e) Tympanic plexus (Jacobson nerve) and inferior tympanic artery (branch of the ascending pharyngeal artery)
  (f) Caroticotympanic arteries (branches of the internal carotid artery)

Hypotympanum

- It is the lowest portion of the tympanic cavity, below a horizontal plane passing through inferior margin of the external auditory canal and promontory.
- Walls:
  (a) Inferior: jugular bulb
  (b) Outer: tympanic bone
  (c) Medial: lower portion of the promontory and part of the petrous bone, which is usually pneumatized and air cells may reach petroux apex (subcochlear tunnel)
  (d) Anterior: dense bone of petrous bone and carotid canal
  (e) Posterior: styloid complex and mastoid portion of the facial nerve, frequently has retrofacial air cells

Retrotympanum

- It consists of several spaces in the posterior portion of tympanic cavity.
- Microscopic approaches can't properly visualize this region, where most of middle ear diseases like retraction pockets and cholesteatoma occur.

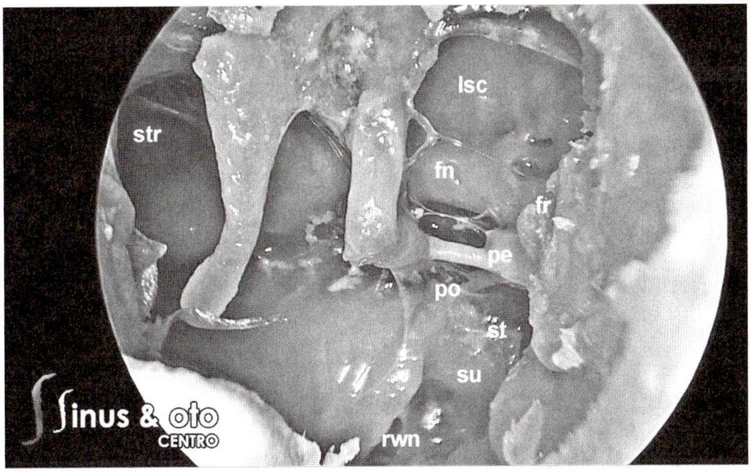

Figure 22-6 Endoscopic view of left ear showing: fn: facial nerve; lsc: lateral semicircular canal; pe: pyramidal eminence; po: ponticulus; rwn: round window niche; su: subiculum; st: sinus tympani; rwn: round window niche; str: supratubal recess.

- Most of posterior tympanotomy and wall down mastoidectomy achieves to reach retrotympanum.
- Angled endoscopes through transcanal techniques permit a better and complete visualization of retrotympanum, preserving mastoid cell system.

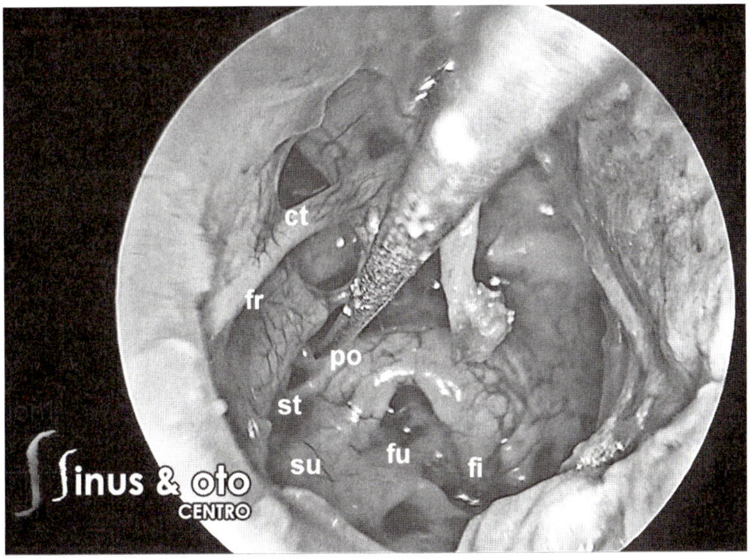

Figure 22-7 Endoscopic view of right ear showing: po: ponticulus (note the variations between the ponticulus. It can be present in a bridge shape, in the multiple shape, and absent). su: subiculum. The space between the ponticulus and subiculum is called sinus tympani. fi: finiculus. The space between the subiculum and finiculus is called sinus sub-tympanicum. fu: fustis, a reliable anatomic landmark for the round window.

- Structures:
  (a) Facial recess: spaces lateral to mastoid portion of the facial nerve and pyramidal ridge (between pyramidal and styloid eminence)
    - Facial sinus: between incudal fossa and chordal ridge (link pyramidal and chordal eminence)
    - Lateral tympanic sinus: inferior to chordal ridge, between pyramidal and styloid ridges
  (b) Facial nerve (tympanic portion)
  (c) Pyramidal eminence, stapedial tendon, stapes, and oval window
  (d) Posterior tympanic sinus
  (e) Ponticulus: bony ridge from promontory to the pyramidal eminence, partial or completely absent in 10% of population
  (f) Sinus tympani: largest space (sinus), variable in size, shape, and depth
    - Superior: ponticulus and pyramidal eminence
    - Inferior: subiculum and the styloid eminence
    - Lateral: pyramidal ridge
    - Anterior: promontory
    - Posterolateral: tympanic and mastoid portions of the facial nerve, lateral semicircular canal, and vestibule
  (g) (Subiculum: bony ridge from posterior tip of round window niche to styloid eminence, is rarely a bridge
  (h) Subtympanic sinus
  (i) Area concomerata: pars media called fustis bone, the floor of round window niche (tegmen, anterior and posterior pillar)
  (j) Finiculus: ridge or bridge between anterior pillar of round window niche and jugular wall, borderline between retrotympanum and protympanum

Protympanum

- Limits:
  (a) Superior: tensor tympani muscle bony semicanal, cochleariform process, tensor tympani fold
  (b) Inferior: finiculus, retrotympanum
  (c) Medial: carotid canal
  (d) Lateral: thin plate of tympanic bone, mandibular fossa
  (e) Anterior: bony portion of the Eustachian tube (1 cm in adults, approximately)
  (f) Posterior: promontory
- Supratubal recess: between tympanic orifice of Eustachian tube and tensor tympani fold; it is small or absent if tensor fold is horizontal.

Indications

Endoscope allows a better visualization and access to tympanic cavity. Therefore, any middle ear disease could be performed by endoscopic transcanal approach.

- Otitis media with effusion: ventilation tube insertion
- Chronic otitis media: myringoplasty
- Dysventilation syndromes, retraction pocket and atelectasis: myringoplasty
- Cholesteatoma:

(a) Transcanal exclusively: attic, Prussak space, or mesotympanic involvement
(b) Combined approach: antral or mastoid cell involvement, lateral semicircular canal or mastoid tegmen dehiscence, relative indication to narrow external ear canal

- Otosclerosis: stapes surgery
- Ossicular reconstruction
- Middle ear benign tumors: glomus tympanicum, adenoma, osteoma
- Assist cochlear implantation

Nowadays, it's possible to perform lateral skull base in an endoscopic-assisted or an exclusive endoscopic approach. Some applications are:

- Cholesteatoma with medial extension to inner ear
- Cholesterol granuloma of petrous apex
- Acoustic neuroma in internal ear canal fundus
- Cochlear or facial nerve schwannomas

EES principles are:

- Use ear canal as a natural corridor to tympanic cavity.
- Restore middle ear ventilation routes to mastoid.
- Preserve normal tissues and structures.
- Reduce bone and soft tissue dissection to achieve tympanic cavity.

Advantages

- Endoscope tip bypasses the narrowest portion and tortuosity of external ear canal, so it is rarely necessary to widen the canal.
- Direct, clear, and wide visualization of entire eardrum, annulus fibrosus, anterior limit of perforation, tympanic cavity, chorda tympani, ossicular chain, tympanic segment of facial nerve, round and oval windows.
- Minimally invasive approach.
- Natural and direct approach to disease site in middle ear cleft.
- No need for periauricular incisions and dissection.
- No need for bone drilling of external ear canal or mastoid.
- Preservation of mastoid cell system (mucosa and transmucosal gas exchange).
- Possible to restore ventilation routes to attic.
- Better control of cholesteatoma in hidden areas.
- Less trauma to chorda tympani, especially in stapes surgery.
- No need to curette or drill external ear canal to visualize and access stapes anterior crus and footplate.
- Direct and better visualization of tympanic segment of facial nerve, avoiding lesions and facial palsy.
- Possibility to better understand middle ear anatomy and teach residents and ENT specialists.

Disadvantages

- One-handed surgery and difficulty in controlling excessive bleeding.
- Excessive heat dissipation in major structures: avoid by using regular light source at lower intensity (approximately 40% to 50%) and continuous cleaning of endoscope tip.
- Direct trauma to major and delicate structures like ossicular chain by endoscope tip.

- Loss of depth perception and binocular vision.
- Fogging and smearing of the tip of the endoscope.
- Technique is more difficult.
- Learning curve is longer and harder: needs more training and laboratory practice.
- Cost of specific equipment.

Instruments

- Hopkins endoscope of 110 to 140 mm length, 3 or 4 mm diameter, 0 degree lent.
- 30 or 45 degree angled lents could be necessary to see "middle ear corners," for example: sinus tympani, facial recess, attic, *aditus ad antrum*.
- Camera system should have triple charge-coupled device (3CCD), to avoid "red-out" images in small fields with bleedings. Also high-definition camera allows better identification of important structures.
- Xenon light and fiber-optic cable of 180 cm length are preferred.
- Microscope should be prepared to use if needed.
- Standard instruments for microscopic surgery: mastoid retractors, microdrill, micromotor handles straight and curved, set of cutting and diamond burs, suction instruments, soft tissue dissectors, scissors, forceps, and periosteal raspatory.
- Microsurgical instruments: microforceps, microcup, microalligator, straight and curved microscissors, set of different angles and lengths microhooks; needles; elevators, round cutting knife (45 degree angle), sickle knives, Rosen elevator, House curette, set of fine suction tips with control hole, and others.
- Special instruments based on International Working Group on Endoscopic Ear Surgery are available for advanced functional EES and skull base surgery. It includes some sets: curved shaft dissectors, sharp hooks, curved suction cannulae, curved curettes, curved microcups forceps of 10 cm working length, suction and shaft instruments, for example: round cutting knife with suction.
- Piezosurgery device performs fine movements to cut bone with 0.3 to 0.6 mm width without necrosis. It is used mostly for lateral endoscopic skull base surgery.
- Vesalius is a special monopolar and bipolar device that enables cutting and also coagulating soft tissue without temperature elevation. It is precise, delicate, and without thermal damage to raise tympanomeatal flap and to dissect cholesteatoma from ossicles and attic compartments.
- Laser has flexible fibers that achieve recesses, oval window, and ossicles webs. Potassium titanyl phosphate (KTP) laser removes granulation tissue, reduces residual disease, and improves hearing by ossicle preservation. Some studies show that stapedotomy with laser has better audiologic outcomes.

Preparation

- It is essential to have a high-resolution CT scan available: axial and coronal views at least.
- Operation room is prepared similar to microscope surgery. Although, endoscope tower is placed facing the surgeon, and monitor stays at the level of surgeon's eyes.
- Surgeon can be seated or in a standing position. Surgeon's arm should be placed above patient or surgical table to stabilize image.
- Patient lies in supine position, with head slightly extended and lateralized. Chest elevation of about 30 degrees reduces bleeding.

- Controlled intraoperative hypotension (mean arterial pressure reduced about 30%) and bradycardia (heart rate about 60 bpm) also avoids bleeding.
- Adhesive tape places hair around ear away from surgical field. Perform antisepsis with povidone-iodine, 5% concentration preferably, to avoid ototoxic effect.
- Place surgical patties soaked in 1:1000 epinephrine solution into ear canal while trimming external ear canal hair to prevent smearing blood or wax on endoscope tip.
- Always use antifog solution.

Tips and Pitfalls

- Tympanomeatal flap elevation is the first step in any EES. It is also the most challenging part for the beginners, inexperienced with one-hand technique.
- How to reduce bleeding and raise flap using only one hand and instrument?
  (a) Injection of local anesthetic with vasoconstrictor into the ear canal skin.
  (b) Abuse of small cottonoid pledgets soaked in 1:1000 epinephrine solution.
  (c) Irrigation with saline at body temperature cleans operation field, vulnerable to "red out" and improves surgeon's view to better understand important structures.
  (d) Increased hemorrhage is controlled by packing ear canal for 5 to 15 minutes.
- Horizontal incisions are made at 5 or 6 o'clock and at 12 or 1 o'clock (right ear) or at 12 or 11 o'clock (left ear). Incision begins next to tympanic membrane and extends laterally before osseocartilaginous junction (about 0.5 to 1 cm or two times the size of round cutting knife). Flap length should not be too short nor too long.
- Raise flap using an aspirator or a round cutting knife. Small surgical patties soaked with epinephrine are placed between flap and bone to absorb blood, to maintain flap integrity, and to broadly elevate skin off the bone.
- Narrow canal is harder to elevate flap. Once tympanic cavity is achieved, enlarge ear canal with curette to improve access.
- Bleeding generally stops after reaching middle ear. It is important to identify and preserve chorda tympani.
- Posterior malleolar ligament is detached from posterior tympanic spine using a hook.
- Tympanic membrane is pushed anteriorly to separate *pars flaccida* from notch of Rivinus with microcup or microalligator forceps.
- Careful dissection of malleolar handle up to the umbo using a hook or a needle, and then, divide final ligament with microscissors to expose and access the ventilation routes by tympanic isthmus.
- Usually oval window can be seen without external ear canal bone removal, which reduces the risk of damage to the chorda tympani.
- Endoscope most of the time remains lateral to the annulus, to avoid damage to middle ear delicate structures.

Outcomes

- EES complications are much the same as for microscopic surgery. Remember, it's to perform traditional transcanal techniques with another tool, the endoscope.
- Cholesteatoma residual disease missed by the microscope, but detected by the endoscope after canal up or canal down mastoidectomy ranges between 16.7% and 37.5%. Most frequent sites are: sinus tympani, facial recess, undersurface of the scutum, and

anterior epitympanic recess. Therefore, endoscope is a valuable tool to improve cholesteatoma surgery results.

- Cholesteatoma residual disease after endoscopic-only and combined technique is 6.2%, with a mean follow-up of 23.4 months. Conversion to microscope approach occurs in 4.3% to 23.8% of procedures.
- Tympanoplasty perforation closure rates of endoscopic technique are 85.1%, comparable to microscopic approach of 86.4%. Also improvement of air-bone gap is similar. However, endoscopic tympanoplasty has a lower canaloplasty rate and more desirable cosmetic result.
- Endoscopic stapes surgery has a median postoperative air-bone gap of 9.0 dB HL, similar to previously published in the literature. Although studies are needed to compare scutum removal, postoperative taste changes, pain score, and other aspects.
- Endoscopic cochlear implantation is a controversial application. Although round window is better visualized by endoscope and several small studies showed complete insertions, patient follow-up duration is limited (6-7 months). Cochlear basal turn trajectory is more aligned by posterior tympanotomy, so traditional mastoidectomy remains favored.
- Endoscopic lateral skull base surgery is a recent application; therefore, outcome studies are ongoing to describe and quantify the endoscope effects.

Bibliography

Hunter JB, Zuniga MG, Leite J, et al. Surgical and audiologic outcomes in endoscopic stapes surgery across 4 institutions. *Otolaryngol Head Neck Surg.* 2016;154(6):1093-1098.

Kiringoda R, Kozin ED, Lee DJ. Outcomes in endoscopic ear surgery. *Otolaryngol Clin North Am.* 2016; 49(5):1271-1290.

Presutti L. Marchioni D. *Endoscopic Ear surgery: principles, indications, and techniques.* 1st ed. Germany: Georg Thieme Verlag KG; 2015.

Tseng CC, Lai MT, Wu CC, Yuan SP, Ding YF. Comparison of the efficacy of endoscopic tympanoplasty and microscopic tympanoplasty: a systematic review and meta-analysis. *Laryngoscope.* 2017;127(8):1890-1896.

Questions

1. The most important characteristic of anterior tympanic isthmus is
   A. Next to the jugular bulb
   B. Communicates with middle cranial fossa dura
   C. Largest ventilation route to attic
   D. Irregular cavity filled with air
   E. Contains tympanic segment of facial nerve

2. Microscopic approach can't properly visualize this region
   A. Epitympanum
   B. Prussak space
   C. Mesotympanum
   D. Hypotympanum
   E. Retrotympanum

3. These are advantages of endoscopic technique, except
   A. Minimally invasive approach
   B. Easier and requires a smaller learning curve
   C. No need of periauricular incisions
   D. Preservation of mastoid cell system
   E. Possible to restore ventilation routes to attic

4. Essential instruments for endoscopic ear surgery are:
   A. Hopkins endoscope of 3 or 4 mm diameter, 0 degree lent
   B. Camera system with triple charge-coupled device (3CCD)
   C. Xenon light and fiber-optic cable
   D. Microsurgical instruments
   E. All items above

5. Cholesteatoma residual disease is most frequent in these sites, except
   A. Long process of incus
   B. Sinus tympani
   C. Facial recess
   D. Undersurface of the scutum
   E. Anterior epitympanic recess

Chapter 23
Lateral Skull Base Surgery Approaches

Anatomy

Temporal Bone/Petrous Apex

- The temporal bone is divided into five parts: squamous, petrous, tympanic, mastoid, and styloid process.
- There are four fissures dividing the main parts of the temporal bone:
  - Petrosquamous fissure
  - Petrotympanic fissure
  - Tympanosquamous fissure
  - Tympanomastoid fissure
- The petrous apex is shaped like a pyramid and is located between the middle fossa and posterior fossa.
  - The anterosuperior surface forms the middle fossa floor.
    - The arcuate eminence is a prominence on the middle fossa floor
      - ◊ The height of the arcuate eminence is variable.
      - ◊ It serves as a marker for superior semicircular canal identification, but this is not a reliable relationship and should be used with caution.[1]
    - The hiatus for the greater superficial petrosal nerve (GSPN) exits anterolaterally to the arcuate eminence.
  - Posterior surface
    - The posterior surface of the temporal bone is the anterolateral wall of the posterior cranial fossa.
    - Extends medially from the posterior semicircular canal and the endolymphatic sac to the petroclinoid ligament and Dorello canal, an intradural space containing the abducens nerve (cranial nerve VI).
    - Bounded superiorly and inferiorly by the superior and inferior petrosal sinuses.
    - The internal auditory (IAC) canal lies midway across the posterior surface.
      - ◊ The medial portion of the IAC is called the porus acousticus.
      - ◊ The lateral portion of the IAC, called the fundus, is divided into a superior and an inferior portion by a horizontal ridge called the transverse or falciform crest. The facial nerve and superior vestibular nerve are in the superior portion while the cochlear nerve and inferior vestibular nerve are in the inferior portion.

            ◊ A vertical ridge of bone called Bill bar separates the superior portion into anterior and posterior divisions. The facial nerve and nervus intermedius are located anteriorly and the superior vestibular nerve is located posteriorly.
            ◊ The cochlear nerve lies anterior to the inferior vestibular nerve in the inferior portion.
        - The endolymphatic sac lies on the posteroinferior face of the temporal bone.
            ◊ The endolymphatic duct passes through the vestibular aqueduct, which enters the temporal bone lateral to the operculum and travels to the inferior surface of the vestibule.
    - Inferior surface
        - Forms the external surface of the cranial base.
        - The carotid canal and jugular foramen are located medial and posterior to the styloid process, with the carotid artery anterior to the jugular vein.
        - The jugular foramen is divided into the pars nervosa and the pars vascularis, which are separated by a fibro-osseous band off of the jugular spine.
            ◊ Anteromedially, the pars nervosa contains the inferior petrosal sinus, CN IX, and Jacobsen nerve (branch of CN IX).
            ◊ Posterolaterally, pars vascularis contains the jugular bulb, CN X, CN XI, and Arnold nerve (branch of CN X).
        - The cochlear aqueduct contains the perilymphatic duct and connects the perilymph of the scala tympani to the cerebrospinal fluid space in the posterior fossa. It opens into the posterior fossa near the pars nervosa of the jugular foramen. The cochlear vein runs parallel with cochlear aqueduct and drains blood from the cochlea to the jugular bulb.
        - The hypoglossal canal is medial and inferior to the jugular foramen.
        - The digastric ridge runs along the medial aspect of the mastoid tip and intersects with the stylomastoid foramen.
        - The styloid process is anterior to the stylomastoid foramen, where the facial nerve (CN VII) exits the mastoid.
        - The spine of the sphenoid is anterior to the vertical segment of the carotid canal.
        - The cartilaginous portion of the Eustachian tube begins medial to the spine of the sphenoid.

The Facial Nerve

The facial nerve is a mixed nerve with a circuitous course through the brain stem, cerebellopontine angle (CPA), and temporal bone.

- Nuclei/Brain stem
    - Facial nucleus: Motor fibers innervate the muscles of facial expression, stapedius muscle, stylohyoid muscle, and the posterior belly of the digastric muscle.
    - Superior salivary nucleus: Parasympathetic innervation to the submandibular, sublingual, and lacrimal glands via the chorda tympani and the GSPN.
    - Solitary nucleus: Special sensory (taste) sensation of the anterior two-thirds of the tongue via the chorda tympani nerve.
    - Spinal nucleus of the trigeminal nerve: Transmits sensory information from the pinna and the external auditory canal (EAC) via the posterior auricular nerve.
- Course of the facial nerve
    - Exits the anterolateral brain stem at the level of the pons.
        - Cranial nerve VII root entry zone is inferior and medial to the root entry zone of cranial nerve VIII.

- Six segments
  - Intracranial or cisternal segment in the CPA: runs in a superior-anterior trajectory from its root entry zone to eventually lie superior to cranial nerve VIII at the medial opening of the IAC (porus acusticus).
  - Meatal or canalicular segment: The facial nerve and nervus intermedius pass through the anterosuperior quadrant of the IAC from the porus acusticus medially to the fundus laterally.
  - Labyrinthine segment: The nerve enters the facial nerve canal (or fallopian canal) after exiting the IAC. At the geniculate ganglion, it gives off the GSPN.
    - ◊ This is the shortest and narrowest portion of the fallopian canal (mean diameter: 0.97 mm + 35 mm; range: 0.44-2.19 mm).
  - Tympanic segment: The nerve passes horizontally in the middle ear from the geniculate ganglion to the second genu at the pyramidal eminence.
  - Mastoid segment: The nerve passes vertically through the mastoid until exiting the temporal bone at the stylomastoid foramen.
  - Extratemporal segment: From the stylomastoid foramen, the nerve branches into superior and inferior portions at the pes anserinus before dividing into its terminal branches (frontal, zygomatic, buccal, marginal mandibular, and cervical).

Clinical Investigation

- Perform a complete history and physical exam with particular attention to subjective hearing changes, tinnitus, vertigo/imbalance, facial numbness, facial twitching, swallowing problems, and voice changes. Document any prior ear surgeries, trauma, ear drainage, or ear infections. Physical exam should include microscopic otoscopy, a full cranial nerve exam, and a tuning fork exam if indicated.
- Audiogram is a required part of the initial evaluation in all diseases of the temporal bone and CPA.
  - Asymmetric hearing loss is an indication for additional imaging, preferably a contrasted magnetic resonance imaging (MRI) to rule out a retrocochlear process.
- Imaging
  - Fine-cut computed tomography (CT) evaluation of the temporal bone is used to identify abnormal bony anatomy, particularly for surgical planning and guidance. CT is also the study of choice for assessment of mucosal disease in the middle ear or mastoid.
  - CT arteriography can be used to investigate vascular anomalies, particularly in the case of pulsatile tinnitus.
  - MRI with gadolinium contrast identifies and delineates intracranial soft tissue, nerves, and tumors of the CPA. It is also useful in defining intracranial extension of various temporal bone pathologies.
- Vestibular testing
  - Physical exam can be used to assess the peripheral vestibular system, vision, and proprioception. Objective vestibular testing can be useful to evaluate undifferentiated dizziness and may include videonystagmography (VNG), video head impulse testing (VHIT), vestibular evoked myogenic potentials (VEMPs), rotary chair, and posturography.
  - VEMPs are an important part of the preoperative workup of superior semicircular canal dehiscence and other third-window phenomenon.

Tumors of the Temporal Bone

- External auditory canal (EAC)
  - Benign
    - Pleomorphic adenoma
    - Ceruminous adenoma
  - Malignant
    - Squamous cell carcinoma (SCC)
    - Basal cell carcinoma
    - Sarcoma
    - Melanoma
    - Lymphoma
    - Adenocarcinoma
    - Adenoid cystic carcinoma
    - Ceruminous adenocarcinoma
- Middle ear and mastoid
  - Benign
    - Paraganglioma (Glomus tumors)
    - Myxoma
    - Lipoma
    - Hemangioma
    - Schwannoma
    - Endolymphatic sac tumor
    - Neurofibroma
    - Osteoma
    - Chondroblastoma
    - Giant cell tumor
    - Meningioma
    - Teratoma
  - Malignant
    - Squamous cell carcinoma (SCC)
    - Basal cell carcinoma
    - Adenocarcinoma
    - Carcinoid tumor
    - Rhabdomyosarcoma
    - Malignant paraganglioma
    - Malignant schwannoma
    - Hemangiopericytoma
    - Osteosarcoma
    - Chondrosarcoma
    - Malignant germ cell tumor

Paraganglioma/Glomus Tumors

- Paragangliomas are the most common tumors of the middle ear.
  - Benign neuroendocrine tumors arising from autonomic paraganglia, which derives from neural crest cells during embryonic development.
  - Common lateral skull base locations:
    - Glomus tympanicum: arise from Jacobson nerve on the promontory of the middle ear; arterial supply is the inferior tympanic artery; can extend to hypotympanum, protympanum, or mastoid

    - Glomus jugulare: arises from Vagus nerve at the jugular bulb; arterial supply is the ascending pharyngeal artery; erode the jugular foramen and jugular spine; can extend through the hypotympanum into the middle ear and mastoid, can also extend intracranially
  - May present with hearing loss, pulsatile tinnitus, vertigo, cranial nerve neuropathies (V, VI, VII, VIII, IX, X, XI, and XII), aural pain, or neck mass.
- 1% of paragangliomas display physiologically significant catecholamine secretion. Presence of tachycardia, arrhythmias, flushing, or labile hypertension should prompt analysis of 24-hour urine specimen for excess catecholamines (dopamine, norepinephrine, and epinephrine) and catecholamine metabolites (metanephrine, normetanephrine, vanillylmandelic acid).
- Two major classifications:
  - Fisch classification:[2]
    - Class A: limited to the middle ear space
    - Class B: limited to the middle ear and mastoid
    - Class C: involvement of infralabyrinthine components and extending to the petrous apex
      - ◊ C1: involving jugular foramen and jugular bulb with limited involvement of carotid canal
      - ◊ C2: involving the vertical portion of the carotid canal
      - ◊ C3: involving the horizontal portion of the carotid canal
    - Class D: Intracranial extension
      - ◊ D1: intradural extension < 2 cm
      - ◊ D2: intradural extension > 2 cm
      - ◊ D3: neurologically unresectable
  - Glasscock-Jackson classification:[3]
    - Glomus tympanicum
      - ◊ Type 1: small mass limited to the promontory
      - ◊ Type 2: completely filling middle ear space
      - ◊ Type 3: filling the middle ear with extension into mastoid
      - ◊ Type 4: extension beyond the mastoid, through the EAC or anteriorly to the carotid artery
    - Glomus jugulare:
      - ◊ Type 1: involving jugular bulb, middle ear, and mastoid
      - ◊ Type 2: extending to the internal auditory canal
      - ◊ Type 3: extending to the petrous apex, may have intracranial extension
      - ◊ Type 4: extending into clivus or infratemporal fossa, may have intracranial extension

Glomus Tympanicum Resection

- Type 1 and 2 tumors often resected via a transcanal approach, with or without use of an endoscope
- Extension to the mastoid, petrous apex, or EAC will require a mastoidectomy with extended facial recess or a subtotal petrosectomy

Transcanal Glomus Tympanicum Resection

- A superiorly based tympanomeatal flap is elevated.
  - Tympanic membrane should elevate off the tumor.
- Inferior canalplasty improves access to the hypotympanum. Anterior canalplasty improves access to the protympanum. Atticotomy improves access to the epitympanum.

- Ideally, the feeding vessel is identified and cauterized with a bipolar or laser. If tumor size does not allow this cauterization, the tumor can be sequentially debulked.
  - Hemostasis during debulking requires temporary packing of the middle ear and use of hemostatic agents.
  - The ossicular chain can often be left intact.
- Drilling in the hypotympanum can clear microscopic disease and provide additional hemostasis.
- If tumor extends into the mastoid or cannot be reached in the hypotympanum, then a mastoidectomy with an extended facial recess can be added.

Subtotal Petrosectomy Glomus Jugulare Resection

- Approach first described by Rambo in 1958 and modified by Fisch in 1965.
- Management of glomus jugulare tumors has moved away from gross total resection and more toward partial debulking with adjuvant radiation. Specific treatment planning depends on tumor size and associated deficits/symptoms.
- Advantages of the subtotal petrosectomy with ear canal closure include improved access to the middle ear, mastoid, hypotympanum, petrous apex, and jugular bulb region. This approach can also be advantageous for advanced chronic ear disease, osteoradionecrosis, or cerebrospinal fluid leaks.
- Ear canal closure creates a maximal conductive hearing loss, but preservation of the cochlea may facilitate future rehabilitation with an osseointegrated implant.
- There are two ways to facilitate ear canal closure:
  - 1. Postauricular incision with transection of the skin at the bony-cartilaginous junction. The tubular skin canal is then inverted out of the ear canal and oversewn.
  - 2. A laterally based flap of tragal skin is elevated with canal incisions at 6- and 12 o'clock positions. The flap is sized in the conchal bowl. Conchal bowl skin is removed or pushed medially for subsequent resection. The tragal flap then gets sewn to the conchal bowl (modified Rambo technique)
    - Any ear canal closure requires diligent removal of epithelium on the canal skin and tympanic membrane to prevent future cholesteatoma development. The malleus and incus are removed, but the stapes should be preserved.
- Postauricular incision and mastoidectomy are performed. The mastoidectomy is thorough with exenteration of all air cells and mucosalized surfaces. The posterior EAC and chorda tympani are removed.
- Based on disease location, additional drilling in the hypotympanum, retrofacial recess, or jugular bulb region can be performed.
  - Debate exists regarding the utility of plugging the Eustachian tube or use of an abdominal fat graft to fill the cavity.
- Fisch described three approaches to the infratemporal fossa:
  - Type A: closure of the EAC and subtotal petrosectomy; originally described with mobilization of the facial nerve but now the nerve is often left its bony canal (fallopian bridge) to protect it; venous system is controlled be decompressing the sigmoid sinus and securing access to the jugular vein in the neck, carotid artery is also dissected in the neck for potential control; good for jugular foramen and infralabyrinthine pathology, classic technique for gross total glomus jugulare resection
  - Type B: Type A approach plus zygomatic osteotomy and glenoid resection to facilitate exposure of the horizontal portion of the petrous carotid artery; may require sacrifice of V3 trigeminal nerve branch, middle meningeal artery, or GSPN
  - Type C: Type B approach plus additional drilling around the petrous carotid to access the pterygopalatine fossa and nasopharynx

Squamous Cell Carcinoma

Staging of SCC of the Temporal Bone Determines Surgical Approach

- T1: limited to EAC without bony erosion
- T2: limited bony erosion or limited soft tissue involvement
- T3: full-thickness EAC erosion with limited (< 5 mm) soft tissue involvement or middle ear involvement
- T4: erosion of cochlea, petrous apex, medial wall of middle ear, carotid canal, jugular foramen, dura, or extensive (> 5 mm) soft tissue involvement; facial nerve involvement
  - Sleeve resection should be used with caution for T1 tumors due to a higher risk of recurrence.
  - T1, T2, and T3 tumors may be managed with lateral temporal bone resection.
  - More extensive surgery (subtotal or total temporal bone resection) may be required in the case of T3 and T4 tumors. However, long-term morbidity is significantly increased with these procedures without a clear improvement in recurrence rate or mortality.
  - Parotidectomy and/or neck dissection may be included with the resection.
  - Lymphatic spread from a temporal bone squamous cell carcinoma is rare, and a single positive node automatically classifies it as advanced disease (N0 or N1)
    - T1N1 = Stage III
    - T2, T3, T4N1 = Stage IV
  - Adjuvant radiation is often recommended for tumors staged > T2

Lateral Temporal Bone Resection

- Incision determined partly by need for neck dissection, parotidectomy, or other oncologic surgery. Auriculectomy or partial auriculectomy may be required.
- A stepped incision is made through the fascia, muscle, and periosteum. Periosteum is elevated anteriorly toward the root of the zygoma and inferiorly to the mastoid tip.
- If the pinna is not involved, the ear canal is sectioned at the bony cartilaginous junction and closed in multiple layers.
  - The temporalis muscle and the temporoparietal fascia can be preserved and reflected forward to be used later in reconstruction.
- Mastoidectomy is performed with skeletonization of the facial nerve, tegmen, sigmoid sinus, and bony ear canal.
- The mastoid tip is removed and the digastric muscle is exposed to facilitate facial nerve exposure at the stylomastoid foramen.
- Inferiorly, an extended facial recess approach is performed, which includes sacrifice of the chorda tympani and exposure of the inferior annulus. This creates an inferior trough around the EAC.
- Superiorly, the zygomatic root is drilled away and the head of malleus is exposed. This creates a superior trough around the EAC.
- The superior and inferior troughs are continued anteriorly until the glenoid fossa is reached.
- The incudostapedial joint is sectioned and the incus is removed. The tensor tympani tendon is transected.
- The specimen is mobilized and separated from the soft tissues anteriorly.
  - Osteotomes are not recommended due to potential for carotid injury.
- A rotational flap or free flap may be required for closure if auriculectomy performed.

Subtotal Temporal Bone Resection

- Dissection extends medially to the petrous apex and otic capsule.
- Includes removal of the cochlea, labyrinth, and often facial nerve.
  - Carotid artery and jugular bulb are exposed but not resected.

Total Temporal Bone Resection

- Medial dissection continues into the infratemporal fossa.
- Resection includes the petrous apex with or without resection of the petrous carotid artery. The Sigmoid-Jugular venous system may also need to be resected. Dura of the middle fossa or posterior fossa may also be resected.

Approaches to the Internal Auditory Canal and Cerebellopontine Angle

Tumors of the Internal Auditory Canal (IAC) and the Cerebellopontine Angle (CPA)

- Majority of tumors in the CPA are benign and slow growing.
  - 75% to 85% are vestibular schwannomas.
  - 10% to 15% are meningiomas.
  - Remaining tumors include: epidermoids, other cranial nerve schwannomas, arachnoid cysts, lipoma, endolymphatic sac tumors, and metastatic lesions.
  - CPA tumors have low risk of malignancy (~1%)
    - Malignancies in the CPA often present with significant cranial nerve dysfunction and/or pain.
- Vestibular schwannomas (acoustic neuromas) are benign tumors, most commonly of the superior or inferior vestibular nerve.
  - Histologically composed of Antoni A (nuclear palisading known as Verocay bodies) and Antoni B (loosely organized, myxoid) regions.
  - Growth rate is typically 1 to 2 mm per year. Growth is saltatory (nonlinear).
  - 95% occur in a sporadic fashion, while 5% are associated with neurofibromatosis type 2 or familial vestibular schwannoma.
  - Asymmetric sensorineural hearing loss with gradual progression is the most common presenting symptom, but 10% to 20% of patients can present with sudden-onset sensorineural hearing loss. Other symptoms include tinnitus, imbalance, facial numbness, Hitselberger sign (numbness of the EAC and conchal bowl).
  - Small to medium-sized tumors may undergo a period of observation to determine growth rate prior to intervention. Treatment options include stereotactic radiosurgery or surgical resection.

Translabyrinthine Approach

- This approach was first introduced in 1904 by Panse but did not become a standard approach until its reintroduction by William House in 1964.
- Advantages
  - Minimized cerebellar retraction
  - Drilling is performed extradurally.
  - Visualize facial nerve prior to tumor dissection
  - Early exposure of the lateral IAC and wide exposure of the CPA.
- Disadvantages
  - Loss of residual acoustic hearing

  - Approach typically takes longer
  - Can be dependent on mastoid and sigmoid sinus anatomy
- Technique
  - A curved postauricular incision is made 3 cm behind the postauricular crease.
  - A complete mastoidectomy is performed with identification of the facial nerve.
  - The sigmoid sinus is decompressed except for a thin wafer of bone that may be left covering the sinus (Bill island).
  - Complete labyrinthectomy is performed.
  - All bone covering the dura from the sigmoid sinus to the porus acousticus is removed as well as the bone covering the middle fossa dura.
  - The IAC is skeletonized 270 degrees with a superior trough between the middle fossa dura and IAC, and an inferior trough between the IAC and jugular bulb.
  - The labyrinthine segment of the facial nerve is identified together with the vertical crest (Bill bar) which separates the facial nerve from the superior vestibular nerve in the lateralmost aspect of the IAC.
  - The dura over the IAC and posterior fossa is incised and reflected away to reveal the tumor and the cerebellum.
  - Facial nerve stimulation is used to confirm that the facial nerve is not draped across the superficial surface of the tumor prior to tumor debulking.
  - Tumor dissection may proceed in a medial to lateral or lateral to medial fashion.
  - Tumor debulking proceeds with bipolar cautery, CO_2 laser, ultrasonic aspiration, and sharp microdissection.
  - The superior vestibular nerve together with the tumor in the lateral IAC is reflected off the facial nerve to develop the facial nerve-tumor interface.
  - A facial recess may be opened to improve visualization when packing the middle ear space.
  - The middle ear space is filled with muscle or fascia, and open air-cell tracts are occluded with bone wax.
  - The craniotomy is packed with abdominal fat. Bone cement or an absorbable or titanium mesh plate may be used to further reinforce the craniotomy closure.
  - The incision is closed in three layers and a tight headwrap or Glasscock dressing is typically used.

Transotic Approach

- The transotic approach, as described by Ugo Fisch, is a modification of the translabyrinthine approach.
- Provides additional exposure anteriorly for tumors extending toward the petrous apex or into the cochlea by drilling out the cochlea and anterior petrous apex.
- In its initial description, the transotic approach required anterior reflection of the facial nerve, but this was later modified to preserve the facial nerve in the fallopian canal.

Transcochlear Approach

- First described by House and Hitselberger in 1975.
- Like the transotic approach, this extension of the translabyrinthine approach improves access for tumors extending anteriorly and into the petrous apex.
- In addition to the translabyrinthine resection, the transcochlear approach includes removal of the EAC with blind sac closure, drilling of the cochlea and petrous apex, and mobilization of the facial nerve.
- Mobilization of the facial nerve results in high rates of facial nerve weakness.

Retrolabyrinthine Approach

- Originally described by Hitselberger and Pulec in 1972 for section of the fifth nerve, use of this approach has been expanded.
- Can be combined with the retrosigmoid approach for improved exposure of the posterior fossa without ablation of the otic capsule.
- Alone is a limited approach to the posterior fossa.
- Technique
  - A postauricular incision is made and a layered flap created.
  - A cortical mastoidectomy is performed.
  - The dura is skeletonized along posterior fossa and superiorly along the middle fossa dura.
  - The facial nerve, labyrinth, and incus are identified.
  - The sigmoid sinus is decorticated, and retrosigmoid air cells are removed to expose the retrosigmoid dura.
  - A dural flap is made parallel to the sigmoid sinus (behind the endolymphatic sac) up to the level of the superior petrosal sinus.
  - The cerebellum is retracted and the arachnoid incised, exposing the seventh to eighth nerve complex.
  - After nerve section or tumor removal, the dura is closed. Abdominal fat may be used to obliterate the surgical defect prior to layered wound closure.

Endoscopic Transcanal Approaches

- Defined by Marchioni in 2015.[5]
- Represent minimally invasive approaches through the EAC.
- Extensions of these approaches enable hybrid endoscopic-microscopic adaptations.
  - Suprageniculate corridor: opening between the floor of the middle fossa and the geniculate ganglion, can extend anteriorly into the petrous apex
  - Transpromontorial corridor: opening the cochlea and vestibule along with drilling the inferior IAC, exposes the IAC and CPA
  - Infracochlear corridor: opening between the cochlea, carotid, and jugular bulb, can extend anteriorly to the petrous apex

Retrosigmoid Craniotomy

- Advantages
  - Faster access to the CPA than translabyrinthine approach
  - Possibility of preserving acoustic hearing in appropriately sized tumors (< 2 cm)
  - Wide exposure of the posterior fossa with an advantage in visualizing tumors with significant inferior extension or extension into Meckel cave
- Disadvantages
  - Increased incidence of postoperative headache
  - Limited access to the lateral IAC
  - Requires intracranial drilling
  - May require cerebellar retraction, particularly in the case of large tumors
- Technique
  - The patient is positioned either supine or in the "park-bench" position, and the head is secured in pins.
  - A curvilinear incision 3 cm posterior to the postauricular sulcus is made down to bone. The cervical muscles are detached from the calvarium to expose the mastoid and suboccipital area.

  - A craniotomy is made with boundaries of the sigmoid sinus anteriorly and the transverse sinus superiorly. The asterion (the junction of the occipital, parietal, and temporal bones) is a useful landmark for the junction of the transverse and sigmoid sinuses.
  - Opened mastoid air cells are sealed with bone wax to prevent CSF leaks ("Wax in, wax out").
  - A dural flap is opened and reflected.
  - CSF is drained from the cisterna magna by piercing the arachnoid of the cistern and retracting the cerebellum superiorly. This allows relaxation of the cerebellum so that it falls away and minimizes the need for retraction which may lead to swelling. A cottonoid is placed over the cerebellum to protect it.
  - Division of additional arachnoid bands and gentle dissection of bridging veins away from the tumor opens the CPA and reveals the tumor.
  - The operculum is an important landmark that identifies the entry point of the endolymphatic duct.
  - The porous acusticus is identified, and a dural incision is made over the IAC with care to preserve the endolymphatic sac. Dural flaps are retracted away from the bone.
  - The bone overlying the IAC is removed medially to laterally, with troughs 180° to 270° around the IAC. In general, up to 7 mm of bone can be removed safely from the medial aspect of the IAC.
  - The lateral extent of the tumor is reflected medially, and the facial nerve-tumor interface is developed.
  - Tumor debulking is performed, and the capsule is gradually folded in on itself with care to identify the root entry zones of VII and VIII. Lower cranial nerves (IX, X, XI) are frequently encountered early in the dissection.
  - The IAC is plugged with fascia, muscle, and/or fat. Care is taken to fill any air cells with bone wax to prevent CSF egress.
  - A watertight dural closure is performed. Any additional air cells at the margins of the craniotomy are sealed with bone wax ("Wax in, wax out").
  - The bone flap is replaced and secured with plates. The wound is closed in layers, and a headwrap may be placed.

Far Lateral Approach

- Introduced by Heros in 1986. The approach is an inferolateral extension of a retrosigmoid craniotomy along with a C1 hemilaminectomy.
- Advantages
  - Increased exposure to lesions lying anterior to dentate ligament and between the foramen magnum, lower third of the clivus, and C2.
  - Drilling the occipital condyle provides additional lateral exposure of the jugular tubercle and posterior jugular foramen.
    - Transcondylar, supracondylar, and paracondylar extensions
  - Consider use in foramen magnum meningiomas, lower cranial nerve schwannomas, aneurysms of the vertebral artery, vertebrobasilar junction, and posterior inferior cerebellar artery (PICA).
- Disadvantages
  - Potential injury to the vertebral artery or PICA
  - Instability of the craniocervical junction
- Technique
  - Similar positioning considerations as those for a retrosigmoid craniotomy

  - Skin incision must allow access to the nuchal muscles which are released from the superior nuchal line and mastoid. The nuchal muscles are reflected in a single block to expose the lateral suboccipital region, lateral condyle of C1, and C1 hemilamina.
    - A cuff of muscle should be left at the superior nuchal line to facilitate closure of the myocutaneous flap.
  - Occipital artery and vertebral arteries are identified in the posterior neck triangle during the approach.
  - Craniotomy is a lateral and posterior extension of the retrosigmoid opening
    - Extends down to the foramen magnum
  - Three intradural triangles defined by the course of the lower cranial nerves provide working corridors:
    - Vagoaccessory triangle
    - Suprahyoglossal triangle
    - Infrahyoglossal triangle

Middle Cranial Fossa Approach

- Advantages
  - Hearing preservation approach to intracanalicular tumors. Approximately 50% to 75% chance of hearing preservation.
  - Lower risk of postoperative CSF leak.
- Disadvantages
  - Slight increased risk to facial nerve due to having to work around the facial nerve.
  - Requires temporal lobe retraction, which has additional risks in patients over the age of 65.
  - Not suitable for tumors with significant CPA extension due to limited exposure of the posterior fossa.
- Technique
  - An incision is made anterior to the auricle and extending into the hairline in either a straight line or reverse question mark.
  - The temporalis muscle is elevated off the bone and protected with a moist raytech during retraction.
  - An anteriorly based 5 × 5 cm craniotomy is performed (two-thirds anterior, one-third posterior to the EAC)
  - The dura is carefully dissected off the middle fossa floor posteriorly to anteriorly to protect the GSPN, which may be dehiscent. The middle meningeal artery may be sacrificed.
  - The temporal lobe is retracted using a House-Urban retractor placed under the lip of the petrous ridge.
  - The IAC bisects the line made by the GSPN anteriorly and the arcuate eminence (superior semicircular canal) posteriorly.
  - The IAC is drilled 270 degrees from medial to lateral. The lateral limit of the dissection is Bill bar.
  - The tumor is removed using microdissection medially to laterally.
  - The IAC is plugged with fascia, muscle, and/or fat and the bone flap is replaced.
  - The incision is closed in layers, and a headwrap may be placed.

Extended Middle Cranial Fossa Approach (Kawase Approach; Anterior Petrosectomy)

- First described by Takeshi Kawase in 1985. Indication was better access for clipping of a basilar artery aneurysm.

- Consider use to approach pathologies like: petroclival meningioma, trigeminal schwannoma, chordoma, chondrosarcoma, pontine cavernoma, or basilar artery aneurysm
- Advantages
  - Increased exposure to the petrous apex, clivus, Meckel cave, and prepontine space
- Disadvantages
  - Sacrifice of the middle meningeal artery
  - Possible need to sacrifice the GSPN
  - Dissection around the petrous segment of the carotid artery
- Technique
  - Similar setup and initial approach as the middle fossa craniotomy.
  - The middle meningeal artery is sacrificed to facilitate more anterior exposure
  - Drilling or dissection of the anterior petrous bone exposes the boundaries of the Kawase triangle: petrous ridge (medial), arcuate eminence (posterior), and GSPN (lateral).
  - The modified Dolenc-Kawase (MDK) rhomboid dissection involves an intradural dissection for better exposure of the trigeminal nerve and Gasserian ganglion. This improves access to Dorello canal, clivus, and the prepontine space.

Complications and Outcomes

- Complications following skull base surgery can be serious. For this reason, the patient is typically kept in the hospital for a period of observation and frequent neuro checks.
- Sensorineural hearing loss and vestibulopathy may result from disturbing the otic capsule, which may be planned or inadvertent.
- Damage to the facial nerve may occur during mastoidectomy or during tumor removal in the IAC and CPA.
- Changes in taste are common due to the risk of injury to the chorda tympani or the nervus intermedius.
- Additional cranial nerve injury can occur with any of the nerves adjacent to the surgical resection, most commonly cranial nerves V, VI, VII, VIII, IX, X, and XI.
- Cerebrospinal fluid leak
  - CSF leaks commonly resolve spontaneously.
  - May resolve with a lumbar drain as conservative management, or re-exploration if lumbar drain fails.
  - May be further complicated by tension pneumocephalus.
- Meningitis.
  - Can occur with or without an accompanying CSF leak.
  - The efficacy of prophylactic antibiotics for CSF leak is controversial.
  - Perioperative antibiotics are generally continued in the setting of active CSF leak following skull base surgery.
- Wound complications include wound dehiscence, infection, craniotomy bone flap loss, and hematoma.
- Intracranial hemorrhage or stroke.
- Mortality after resection of tumors of the skull base is rare.
- Sacrifice of the carotid artery requires preoperative balloon occlusion tests. However, serious complications can still occur if carotid artery sacrifice is required.
- Myocardial infarction, pulmonary embolism, and cerebral edema make up the remainder of the commonest causes of perioperative death and occur mostly in the elderly with multiple medical comorbidities.

Bibliography

1. García-Barrios A, Cisneros AI, Obon J, Crovetto R, Benito J, Whyte J. Anatomical study between the correlation of the arcuate eminence and the superior semicircular canal. *Surg Radiol Anat.* 2021;43(11):1845-1850.
2. Fisch U. Infratemporal fossa approach for glomus tumors of the temporal bone. *Ann Otol Rhinol Laryngol.* 1982;91(5 Pt 1):474-479.
3. Jackson CG, Glasscock ME, Harris PF. Glomus tumors. Diagnosis, classification, and management of large lesions. *Arch Otolaryngol.* 1982;108(7):401-410.
4. Moody SA, Hirsch BE, Myers EN. Squamous cell carcinoma of the external auditory canal: an evaluation of a staging system. *Am J Otol.* 2000;21:582-588.
5. Marchioni D, Alicandri-Ciufelli M, Rubini A, Presutti L. Endoscopic transcanal corridors to the lateral skull base: Initial experiences. *Laryngoscope.* 2015;125:S1-S13.

Questions

1. Which brain stem nucleus is responsible for the special sense of taste?
   A. Facial nucleus
   B. Superior salivary nucleus
   C. Solitary nucleus
   D. Spinal nucleus of the trigeminal nerve

2. The facial nerve lies in which quadrant of the lateral IAC?
   A. Anterior-superior
   B. Posterior-superior
   C. Anterior-inferior
   D. Posterior-inferior

3. A patient presents with a T2N1M0 squamous cell carcinoma. What stage is their cancer?
   A. Stage I
   B. Stage II
   C. Stage III
   D. Stage IV

4. Indication for use of a far lateral approach includes access to which structure?
   A. Petrous carotid artery
   B. Meckel cave
   C. Foramen magnum
   D. Lateral semicircular canal

5. Which structure is not a boundary for the Kawase Triangle?
   A. Arcuate eminence
   B. Petrous ridge
   C. Greater superficial petrosal nerve
   D. Internal auditory canal

Part 3
Rhinology

Chapter 24
Sinonasal Development and Anatomy

Nasal Cavity

1. Nasal embryology
   - The embryologic precursors of the nasal turbinates arise in the eighth week of gestation as ridges along the lateral nasal wall.
   - **Maxilloturbinal**: originates inferiorly from the maxillary process and gives rise to inferior turbinate
   - **Ethmoturbinals**: arise superiorly from ethmoid bone; five arise with only four persisting throughout development
     (a) First ethmoturbinal:
       - Ascending portion gives rise to agger nasi
       - Descending portion gives rise to UP
       - Regresses during development
     (b) Second ethmoturbinal: gives rise to middle turbinate
     (c) Third ethmoturbinal: gives rise to superior turbinate
     (d) Fourth and fifth ethmoturbinals: give rise to supreme turbinate (when present)
   - **Primary furrows**: form the recesses separating the ethmoturbinals and give rise to meati
     - First primary furrow: separates first and second ethmoturbinals; gives rise to middle meatus
     - Second primary furrow: gives rise to superior meatus
     - Third primary furrow: gives rise to supreme meatus

2. External nasal anatomy
   A. Subcutaneous layers of the nose
   Mnemonic = "**S**ubcutaneous **F**at **D**ee**P**"
      - S = **S**uperficial fatty layer (connected to dermis)
      - F = **F**ibromuscular layer (nasal SMAS)
      - D = **D**eep fatty layers (contains neurovascular system)
      - P = **P**eriostium/Perichondrium
         - Optimal plane of dissection is located between D and P as it is avascular and heals with minimal fibrosis
   B. External nasal landmarks
      - **Nasion**: corresponds to nasofrontal suture
      - **Radix**: nasal root; centered at nasion, extends inferiorly to the level of the lateral canthus and superiorly by equivalent distance
      - **Rhinion**: corresponds to bony-cartilaginous junction along nasal dorsum
      - **Supratip break**: a break in the nasal profile separating the nasal dorsum and lobule located immediately superior to the tip defining point
      - **Supratip lobule**: portion of lobule located superior to tip-defining point
      - **Tip defining point**: Two points located at the highest, medial, and cephalic portion of the lateral crus; corresponds to light reflex externally
      - **Infratip lobule**: portion of lobule located inferior to tip-defining point and superior to infratip break
      - **Infratip break**: lobule-columella junction
      - **Nasal sill**: nostril rim located between columella and alar facial attachment
   C. Nasal tip support
      (a) Major tip supports
         1. Medial and lateral crura
         2. Attachment of medial crura to caudal edge of quadrangular cartilage
         3. Attachment of upper lateral cartilage to lower lateral cartilage ("scroll area")
      (b) Minor tip supports
         1. Skin-soft tissue envelope (attachment of lower lateral cartilage to overlying skin and musculature)
         2. Sesamoid complex (located between lateral crura and pyriform aperture)
         3. Interdomal ligament (located between lower lateral cartilages)
         4. Anterior nasal spine
         5. Cartilaginous septal dorsum
         6. Membranous nasal septum
   D. Nasal osteology
      - Two nasal bones fuse in the midline to form a pyramidal shape
      - Nasal bones are thicker superiorly than inferiorly
      - Nasal bone attachments =
         - Superior: nasal process of frontal bone
         - Lateral: frontal process of maxilla
      - Pyriform aperture = bony opening into the nasal cavity bounded by:
         - Superior: caudal margin of nasal bones
         - Inferior: alveolar process of maxilla
         - Lateral: frontal process of maxilla
         - Medial: nasal septum
   E. Nasal cartilages
      - **Upper lateral cartilage (ULC):**
         - Attached superiorly to nasal bones

- Articulates inferiorly with the cephalic margin of the LLC most often forming an interlocking scroll
- Thickens medially where it becomes continuous with the quadrangular cartilage of the septum forming the cartilaginous portion of the nasal dorsum

- **Lower lateral cartilage (LLC)**:
  - Provides the shape of the nasal tip
  - Composed of medial and lateral crura
- **Sesamoid cartilages**:
  - Small cartilages located lateral to the lateral crus

F. Nasal septum

- Comprised of both bony and cartilaginous components, lined by either a mucoperiosteal or mucoperichondrial layer
  - Cartilage = quadrangular cartilage
  - Bone = perpendicular plate of ethmoid, vomer, crest of the maxillary bone, crest of the palatine bone; minor contributions from crest of sphenoid bone and nasal spine of frontal bone
- **Membranous (mobile) septum**:
  - Cartilage-deficient membrane adjoining the columella to the caudal septum
  - Site of hemitransfixion/transfixion incision
- **Keystone area**:
  - Corresponds to convergence of caudal margin of nasal bone, perpendicular plate of ethmoid, cephalic margin of ULC, and cartilaginous septum
  - Failure to preserve this region can result in nasal collapse
- **Vomeronasal organ** (Jacobsen organ):
  - Auxiliary olfactory organ involved in the perception of pheromones in mammals.
  - Function in humans is controversial as it largely regresses in-utero and is thought to be vestigial in nature.
  - Identified as a groove in the anterior-inferior nasal septum.

G. Nasal musculature

- Elevators

  Function = shortens nose and dilates nostrils
  - Procerus
  - Levator labii superioris alaeque nasi
  - Anomalous nasi
- Depressors:

  Function = lengthens nose and dilates nostrils
  - Depressor septi
  - Alar Nasalis
- Compressors:

  Function = lengthens nose and constricts nostrils
  - Compressor narium minor
  - Transverse nasalis

3. Anatomy of the nasal cavity

A. Nasal valves

- Important contributors to nasal airway resistance
- Regions at greatest potential for collapse resulting in nasal airway obstruction
  - **Internal nasal valve**:
    - Bounded by nasal septum, caudal edge of ULC, anterior face of inferior turbinate
    - Normally forms 10 to 15-degree nasal valve angle

- Narrowest cross-sectional area of the nasal cavity and site of greatest nasal airflow resistance
- Does not undergo change in dimension during inspiration

◦ **External nasal valve**:
- Bounded by nasal ala laterally, nasal septum and columella medially
- Situated caudal to internal nasal valve
- Normally dilates during inspiration

B. Nasal vestibule
- Entrance of nasal cavity lined by hair-bearing skin, sebaceous, and sweat glands
- Boundaries:
  - ◦ Medial = nasal septum
  - ◦ Superior and lateral = LLC
  - ◦ Inferior = alveolar process of maxilla
  - ◦ Posterior = Limen nasi (Limen vestibule), formed by the caudal margin of the ULC
    - Posterior boundary coincides with the transition from the skin of the nasal vestibule to the mucosal surface (pseudostratified ciliated columnar epithelium) of the nasal cavity

C. Lateral nasal wall (Figure 24-1 and Figure 24-2)
- **Osteology of the lateral nasal wall** (from anterior to posterior):
  - ◦ Frontal process of maxilla
  - ◦ Lacrimal bone
  - ◦ Medial maxillary wall inferiorly, lamina papyracea (LP) superiorly
  - ◦ Perpendicular plate of the palatine bone
  - ◦ Medial pterygoid plate of the sphenoid bone
    - Latter two structures form the sphenopalatine foramen

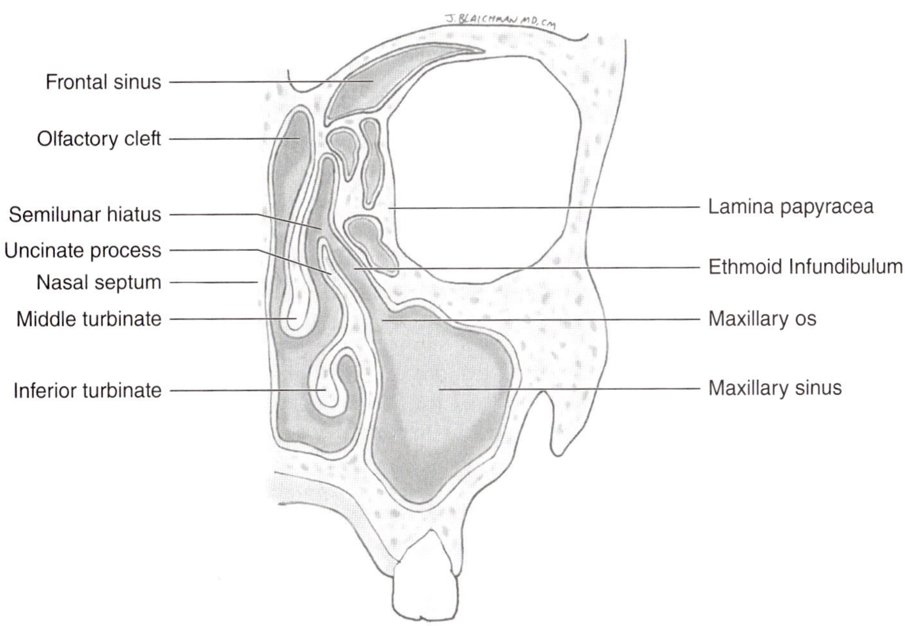

Figure 24-1 Coronal sinus. *(Illustrations by Dr. Jason I. Blaichman MDCM, FRCPC.)*

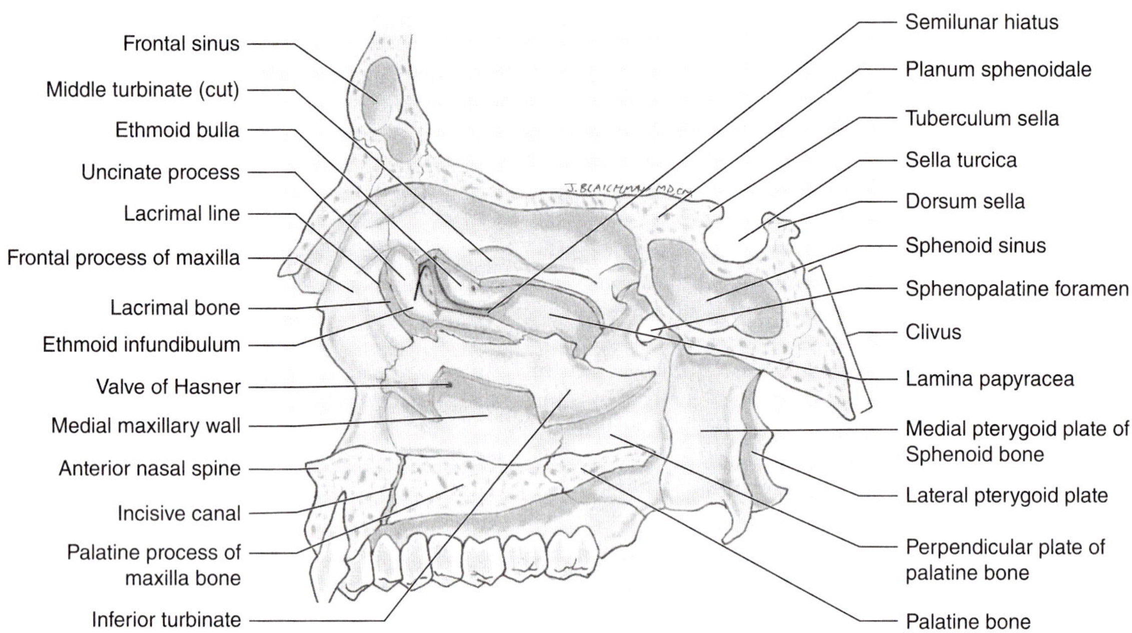

Figure 24-2 Lateral nasal wall bone. *(Illustrations by Dr. Jason I. Blaichman MDCM, FRCPC.)*

- **Lamella of the lateral nasal wall**: five lamella from anterior to posterior
  1. First lamella = uncinate process (UP)
  2. Second lamella = ethmoid bulla (EB)
  3. Third lamella = basal lamella of middle turbinate (MT)
  4. Fourth lamella = basal lamella of superior turbinate
  5. Fifth lamella = basal lamella of supreme turbinate (when present)
- **Meatus**: air space located beneath and lateral to the turbinate of the same name
  - **Inferior meatus**: contains slit-like opening (termed **Hasner valve)** corresponding to site of drainage of the nasolacrimal duct, located ~ 1 cm posterior to anterior face of inferior turbinate
  - **Middle meatus:** site of drainage of frontal, anterior ethmoid and maxillary sinuses
  - **Superior meatus**: site of drainage of posterior ethmoid and sphenoid sinuses; Sphenoethmoidal recess located within posterior aspect of superior meatus
- **Turbinates**:
  - Shelves of bone encased in erectile mucosa capable of altering nasal airway cross-sectional area
  - Covered by ciliated pseudostratified columnar epithelium
  - Assist in maintaining directional and laminar airflow
  - Inferior, middle, superior, and occasionally supreme
  - All originate from ethmoid bone except for inferior turbinate
- **Middle turbinate (MT)**:
  - Anterior end attaches to frontal process of maxilla forming axilla of the MT
  - Has three sites of attachment oriented in three planes

A. **Anterior** portion of MT:
  - Oriented in sagittal plane
  - Attached to junction of cribriform plate and lateral lamella
  - Delimits fovea ethmoidalis (roof of ethmoid sinus) from cribriform plate
B. **Middle** portion of MT (aka basal [ground] lamella):
  - Oriented in coronal plane (vertical)
  - Attached laterally to LP
  - Delimits anterior and posterior ethmoid sinus
C. **Posterior** portion of MT (aka horizontal attachment):
  - Oriented in axial plane (horizontal)
  - Attached to the crista ethmoidalis of the perpendicular process of palatine bone just anterior to sphenopalatine foramen
  - Potential site of postoperative epistaxis when MT is resected
  - Preservation reduces risk of postoperative MT lateralization

- Possible variations of the MT include:
  - **Concha Bullosa**: pneumatized MT; present in one-third of the population
  - **Paradoxical MT**: the lateral surface of the MT is convex rather than concave
- **Lacrimal (maxillary) line**:
  - Endoscopic landmark of suture line along medial orbital wall at the junction of the frontal process of the maxilla and lacrimal bone
  - Site of attachment of the UP to the lateral nasal wall
- **Uncinate process (UP)**:
  - Crescent-shaped, mucosal-lined bone of ethmoid origin which shields natural ostium of the maxillary sinus
  - May narrow ethmoid infundibulum when pneumatized
  - Vertical portion attaches anteriorly to the lacrimal line
  - Horizontal portion attaches inferiorly to the inferior turbinate
  - Site of superior attachment of vertical portion determines frontal sinus drainage pathway
    - Superior attachment to LP:
      - ◊ Frontal sinus drainage occurs medial to the UP, directly into the middle meatus
      - ◊ Results in blind pouch of the superior portion of the ethmoid infundibulum (termed **Recessus Terminalis**)
      - ◊ Most common configuration (80%)
    - Superior attachment to fovea ethmoidalis or MT:
      - ◊ Frontal sinus drainage occurs lateral to the UP and directly into the ethmoid infundibulum
      - ◊ Less common configuration (20%)
- **Ethmoid infundibulum**:
  - Three-dimensional trough bounded by the UP medially, the LP laterally, and the EB posterosuperiorly
  - Opens inferiorly at maxillary sinus ostium
- **Hiatus semilunaris**:
  - Two-dimensional, crescenteric window into the ethmoid infundibulum
  - Bounded by UP anteriorly and EB posteriorly
- **Nasal fontanelles**:
  - Areas of bony dehiscence of the lateral nasal wall typically covered by mucosa of the middle meatus, connective tissue and mucosa of the maxillary sinus
  - Site of accessory ostia when mucosa absent, most commonly located in posterior fontanelle (up to 30% of people)

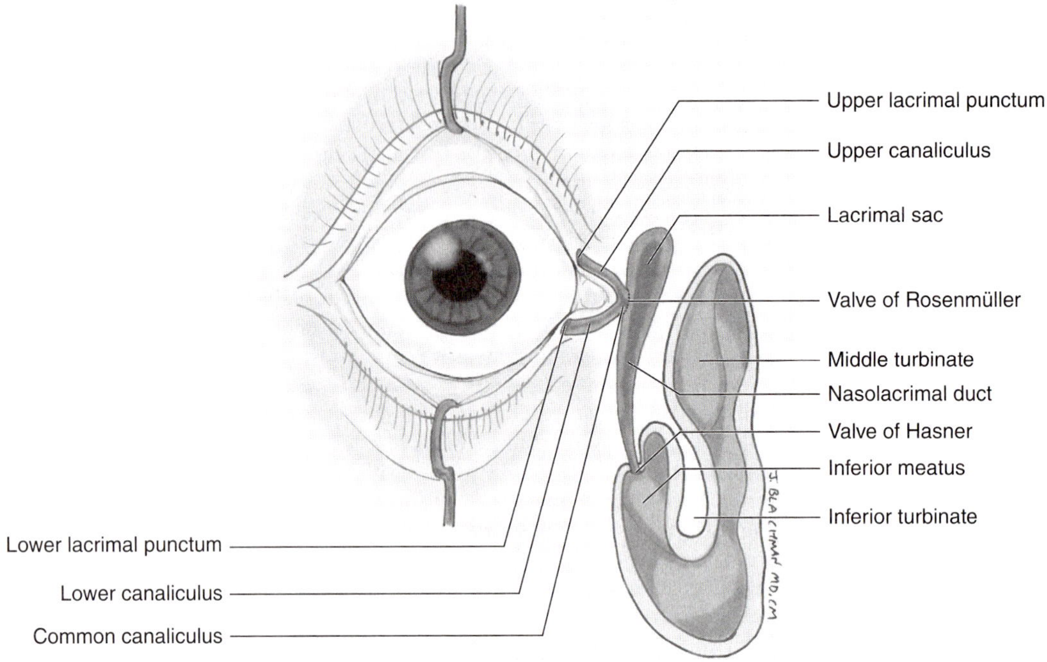

Figure 24-3 Nasolacrimal system. *(Illustrations by Dr. Jason I. Blaichman MDCM, FRCPC.)*

- **Posterior fontanelle**
  - Located posterior to horizontal process of UP
  - Located posterior to natural maxillary os and oriented in sagittal plane (compared to oblique orientation of natural maxillary os)
- **Anterior fontanelle**
  - Located anterior to UP articulation with inferior turbinate
- **Osteomeatal Complex (OMC)**:
  - Region within the middle meatus bounded as follows:
    (a) Posterior: basal lamella of the MT
    (b) Medial: MT
    (c) Lateral: LP
    (d) Superior: fovea ethmoidalis
      - Region of interest in the pathophysiology of acute bacterial rhinosinusitis as it is a regional confluence of drainage pathways of the maxillary, anterior ethmoid and frontal sinuses.
- **Nasolacrimal system**: intimately related to the lateral nasal wall (Figure 24-3)
  - Tear drainage pathway as follows:
    - Upper and lower lacrimal punctum → Upper and lower canaliculus → Common canaliculus (present in 90%) → Valve of Rosenmüller (one-way valve preventing reflux into canaliculi) → Lacrimal sac → Nasolacrimal duct → Valve of Hasner → Inferior meatus
- **Lacrimal fossa**: (Figure 24-4)
  - Bony, oval-shaped recess containing the lacrimal sac
  - Comprised of two parts

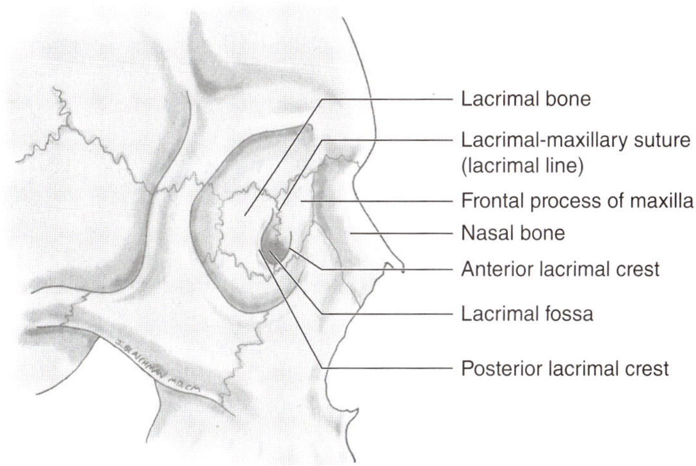

Figure 24-4 Lacrimal bone. *(Illustrations by Dr. Jason I. Blaichman MDCM, FRCPC.)*

- Anterior lacrimal crest: formed by frontal process of maxilla
- Posterior lacrimal crest: formed by lacrimal bone
- The suture line between these two bones corresponds to the lacrimal (maxillary) line, an important endoscopic landmark (see above)

- **Lacrimal sac**:
  - Much of the sac is located above the axilla of the MT (~ 0.9 cm) and above the common canaliculus (~ 0.5 cm)
  - Relevant during dacrocystorhinostomy to ensure adequate lacrimal sac exposure

4. Vascular anatomy
   A. Vascular anatomy of the external nose
      1. Facial artery branches (external carotid artery)
         (a) Angular artery →lateral nasal artery
            - Supplies lateral surface of caudal nose
         (b) Superior labial artery → columellar artery
            - Supplies columella and nasal tip
      2. Ophthalmic artery branches (Internal carotid artery)
         (a) Dorsal nasal artery
            - Supplies nasal dorsum
         (b) External nasal branch of anterior ethmoid artery
            - Supplies nasal dorsum and tip
   B. Vascular anatomy of the nasal cavity
      1. Internal carotid artery branches (both branches of the ophthalmic artery)
         (a) Anterior ethmoid artery (AEA):
            - Larger than posterior ethmoid artery (PEA)
            - Exits orbit between superior oblique and medial rectus muscle via anterior ethmoid foramen (~24 mm posterior to anterior rim of lacrimal fossa) within the frontoethmoid suture
            - Courses anteromedially along the skull base either within a bony canal (dehiscent in 40%) or within a mesentery below skull base

- Delineates posterior limit of frontal recess
- Enters anterior cranial fossa medially by piercing the lateral lamella, rendering it the weakest portion of the skull base (one-tenth as strong as the fovea ethmoidalis)
- Supplies anterior one-third of the nasal cavity

(b) Posterior ethmoid artery (PEA):
- Exits orbit via posterior ethmoid foramen (~ **12** mm posterior to anterior ethmoid foramen, **6** mm anterior to optic ring)
- Supplies posterior nasal cavity

2. External carotid artery branches
   (a) Internal maxillary artery (IMA) branches
      1. Descending palatine artery → greater palatine artery
         - Passes through greater palatine canal located along posterior aspect of the perpendicular plate of the palatine bone
         - Potential for injury with dissection of the posterior medial maxillary wall at its junction with posterior maxillary sinus wall
         - Supplies anteroinferior nasal cavity including nasal septum via incisive foramen
      2. Pharyngeal branch of IMA (aka palatovaginal artery)
         - Courses through pharyngeal (aka palatovaginal) canal which arises from the posterior wall of the Pterygopalatine fossa (PPF), coursing posteriorly within the roof of the nasopharynx
         - Supplies posterosuperior nasal cavity and nasopharynx
      3. Sphenopalatine artery (SPA)
         - Enters nasal cavity via sphenopalatine foramen (SPF), multiple SPA branches and/or accessory foramina may exist
         - SPF located within superior meatus, between basal lamella of MT and superior turbinate
      4. Posterior septal branch
         - Courses along sphenoid rostrum inferior to natural sphenoid os
         - Risk of injury with inferior extension of sphenoidotomy
         - Supplies nasal septum (vascular supply of pedicled nasoseptal flap)
      5. Posterior lateral nasal branch
         - Runs along the middle and inferior turbinates, providing their vascular supply
   (b) Facial artery branches
      - Superior labial artery → alar branch
      - Supplies nasal vestibule and anterior nasal cavity
3. Nasal cavity vascular plexuses
   (a) **Woodruff's plexus**:
      - Aggregation of vessels (posterior lateral nasal + pharyngeal branch of IMA) within the posterior inferior meatus
      - Previously thought to be arterial, now shown to be venous in nature
   (b) **Kiesselbach plexus** (aka Little's area)
      - Located in the anterior nasal septum
      - Most common site of anterior epistaxis
      - Formed by posterior septal branch of SPA, AEA, greater palatine artery, alar branch of superior labial artery

4. Venous drainage of nasal cavity
   - Anterior and posterior ethmoid veins →superior ophthalmic vein → cavernous sinus
   - Sphenopalatine vein →pterygoid plexus
     - As this is a valveless venous system, there is a potential for retrograde spread of infection intracranially (cavernous sinus in particular)
   - **Diploic veins of Breschet**:
     - Provide venous drainage of the frontal sinuses
     - Course through multiple anterior and posterior table foramina (breschet's canals)
     - Communicate with the dural sinuses (cavernous sinus and superior sagittal sinus)
     - Contributes to intracranial spread of infection
5. Sensory innervation
   (a) External nose
      1. Branches of ophthalmic division of cranial nerve V (V1)
         a. Infratrochlear nerve
            - supplies lateral nose above medial canthus
         b. External anterior ethmoidal nerve
            - supplies nasal tip, dorsum and ala
      2. Branches of Maxillary division of cranial nerve V (V2)
         a. Infraorbital nerve
            - supplies lateral nose and ala
         b. Anterior superior alveolar nerve (branch of infraorbital nerve)
            - minor contribution to nasal tip and columella

   (b) Nasal cavity
      1. Branches of ophthalmic division of cranial nerve V (V1)
         a. Internal nasal branch of anterior ethmoidal nerve
            - supplies anterior and superior regions of the nasal cavity
         b. Posterior ethmoidal nerve
            - supplies posterior nasal cavity
      2. Branches of maxillary division of cranial nerve V (V2)
         a. Sphenopalatine (Nasopalatine) nerve (anastomoses with greater palatine nerve)
            - supplies posterior nasal cavity
         b. Anterior superior alveolar nerve
            - supplies anterior nasal cavity and nasal floor
6. Autonomic innervation
   (a) Sympathetic innervation
      Function: Vasoconstriction
      Preganglionic: sympathetic chain
      Ganglion: Superior cervical ganglion
      Postganglionic: Deep petrosal nerve joins with greater superficial petrosal nerve (GSPN) →vidian nerve (passes through sphenopalatine ganglion without synapsing) → distributed to nasal mucosa with sensory nerves

   (b) Parasympathetic innervation
      Function: Vasodilation and mediates nasal secretions
      Preganglionic: Superior salivatory nucleus (CN VII) → nervus intermedius (leaves CN VII at geniculate ganglion with GSPN to form vidian nerve)
      Ganglion: Sphenopalatine ganglion
      Postganglionic: distributed to nasal mucosa with deep branches of V2

Paranasal Sinuses (Figure 24-5)

1. Paranasal sinus embryology (in order of completed development)
   A. Ethmoid sinus:
      - First to develop in utero
      - Most developed at birth (completely developed in number of cells but not in size)
      - Anterior ethmoid originates from middle meatus
      - Posterior ethmoid originates from superior meatus
      - Other structures originating from ethmoid bone include middle, superior and supreme turbinate, cribriform plate and perpendicular plate of ethmoid
   B. Maxillary sinus:
      - In early childhood, floor of sinus is situated above nasal floor due to presence of unerupted dentition
      - Roof of sinus sloped downward from medial to lateral due to disproportionately large orbit relative to midface
   C. Sphenoid sinus:
      - Pneumatization begins postnatally (~ 1 year of age)
      - Conversion of red bone marrow to fatty marrow precedes pneumatization
      - Pneumatization occurs following marrow involution with subsequent epithelialization of the sinus mucosal lining
      - Failure of this conversion process results in arrested pneumatization (see sphenoid sinus section)
      - Pneumatization progresses in an inferior posterolateral direction
      - Adult size reached by age 12 beyond which size remains constant though shape may change

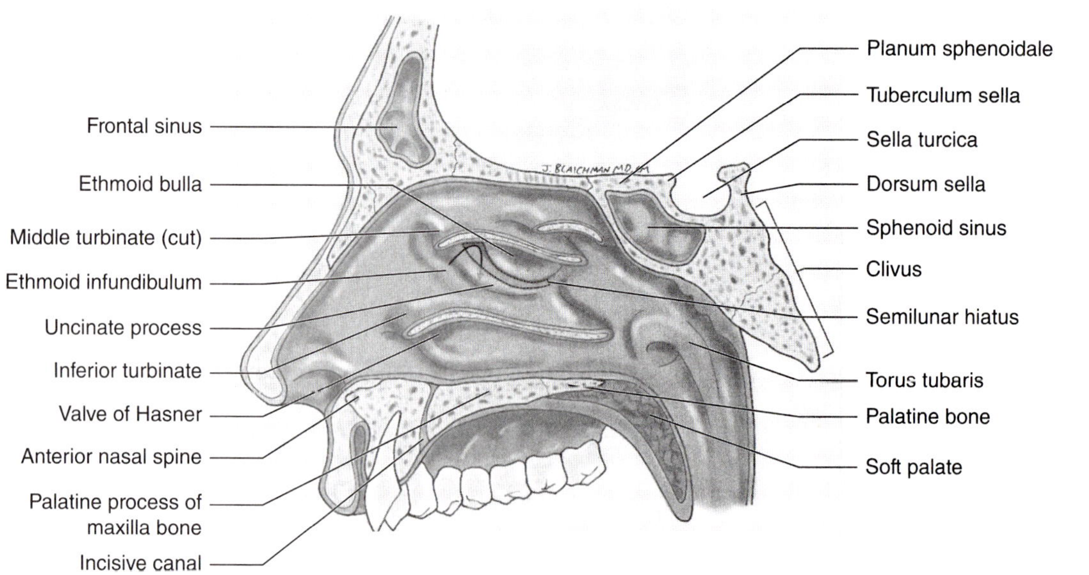

Figure 24-5 Lateral nasal wall mucosa. *(Illustrations by Dr. Jason I. Blaichman MDCM, FRCPC.)*

D. Frontal sinus:
- Last sinus to begin and complete development
- Majority of development occurs postnatally with pneumatization continuing into early adulthood
- Only ethmoid and maxillary sinuses are present at birth

  Order of paranasal sinuses according to size (from largest to smallest)
  - Maxillary sinus
  - Frontal sinus
  - Sphenoid sinus
  - Ethmoid sinus

2. Paranasal sinus anatomy

A. Ethmoid sinus

1. Anterior ethmoid sinus (anterior to MT ground lamella)
- Anterior ethmoid cells are generally smaller but greater in number

(a) **Agger nasi**:
- Most anterior ethmoid cell
- Projects anterior to axilla of the MT creating a bulge in the lateral nasal wall
- Posterior limit forms the anterior border of the frontal recess
- Anteroposterior distance of the frontal recess largely determined by degree of pneumatization of the agger nasi cell
- A large, well pneumatized agger nasi cell confers a small frontal beak which gives rise to a large frontal anteroposterior distance

(b) **Ethmoid bulla**:
- Largest anterior ethmoid cell
- Attached laterally to LP
- Most constant and identifiable ethmoid cell

(c) **Sinus lateralis**:
- Made up of the suprabullar and retrobullar recesses
- Site of suprabullar recess = above EB in the absence of a suprabullar cell
- Site of retrobullar recess = posterior to EB, anterior to MT basal lamella
- Boundaries include EB anteriorly, basal lamella of MT posteriorly, MT medially, LP laterally, and fovea ethmoidalis superiorly

(d) **Suprabullar cell**:
- Ethmoid cell located above EB without pneumatizing into frontal sinus
- Fovea ethmoidalis (ethmoid roof/skull base) forms roof of this cell

(e) **Frontal bulla cell:**
- Suprabullar cell which pneumatizes into frontal sinus along posterior wall of frontal sinus

(f) **Supraorbital ethmoid cell**:
- Ethmoid cell located posterolateral to the frontal sinus ostium with pneumatization lateral to the LP and superolateral to the orbital roof (orbital plate of the frontal bone)
- Anterior ethmoid artery typically located within the posterior wall of the cell along or immediately beneath the skull base

(g) **Haller cell** (Infraorbital ethmoid cell):
- Most common anatomic variation within the maxillary sinus
- Most commonly originates from the anterior ethmoid sinus
- Pneumatizes along the inferomedial orbit and may obstruct the natural drainage pathway of the maxillary sinus

2. Posterior ethmoid sinus (posterior to basal lamella of MT)
   - Posterior ethmoid cells are generally larger but fewer in number
     (a) **Onodi cell** (Sphenoethmoidal cell):
       - Posterior ethmoid cell which pneumatizes posteriorly over the superolateral aspect of the sphenoid sinus
       - When present, the optic nerve and occasionally the internal carotid artery can project along the superolateral wall of the Onodi cell rather than the sphenoid sinus, placing them at increased risk of iatrogenic injury
       - Incidence is ~ 30%
       - Identified on coronal CT scan as a horizontal septation within the sphenoid sinus, posterior to the bony choanal arch
         - Onodi cell located superolateral
         - Sphenoid sinus located inferomedial
3. Fovea ethmoidalis and skull base
   - **Fovea ethmoidalis** (ethmoid roof):
     - Formed by orbital plate of frontal bone
     - Slopes downward (~ 15 degrees) from anterior to posterior and lateral to medial
     - Posteromedial region of fovea ethmoidalis theoretically at greater risk of injury during ESS given its lower height
     - Attaches to lateral lamella medially
   - **Lateral lamella**:
     - Formed by ethmoid bone
     - Forms lateral surface of cribriform fossa
     - Thinnest and weakest bone in the skull base
   - **Cribriform plate**:
     - Forms floor of cribriform fossa
     - Perforated by multiple olfactory nerve fibers
     - Also slopes downward as it passes posteriorly
4. Keros classification
   - Classification system for assessing the depth of the olfactory fossa (corresponds to the length of lateral lamella)
   - Lateral lamella of cribriform plate is the thinnest bone in the skull base
   - Increasing risk of cerebrospinal fluid (CSF) leak during endoscopic sinus surgery (ESS) with increasing Keros type due to low cribriform fossa and increased length of thin lateral lamella (more subject to fracture)
     - Type 1: 1-3 mm (second most common configuration)
     - Type 2: 4-7 mm (majority of cases)
     - Type 3: 8-16 mm (rare)
     - Type 4: asymmetric between two sides

B. Maxillary sinus
1. Boundaries of maxillary sinus
   - Superior: orbital floor
   - Inferior: alveolar and palatine process of maxilla
   - Lateral: zygoma
   - Medial: lateral nasal wall
   - Posterior: pterygopalatine (PPF) and Infratemporal fossa (ITF)
   - Anterior: facial surface of maxilla
2. Endoscopic landmarks associated with the maxillary sinus
   - Roof of maxillary sinus: approximates height of sphenoid sinus floor
   - Posterior wall of maxillary sinus: approximates depth of sphenoid rostrum

- Medial maxillary wall of maxillary sinus:
  - With normal maxillary sinus pneumatization, it is located in line with a vertical line drawn tangential to LP
  - When maxillary sinus is hypoplastic or atelectatic, medial maxillary wall may be lateral to LP

3. Foramen of Maxillary bone
   - **Infraorbital foramen**:
     - Contains infraorbital nerve, artery, and vein
     - Runs along maxillary sinus roof within infraorbital canal
     - Iatrogenic injury possible if canal is dehiscent (incidence of 14%)
   - **Incisive foramen**:
     - Contains greater palatine artery and nerve
   - **Maxillary os**:
     - Located within posterior one-third of ethmoid infundibulum
   - **Superior alveolar foramen**:
     - Contains posterior, middle, and anterior superior nerve, artery, and vein

C. Sphenoid sinus

1. Classification of sphenoid pneumatization
   - **Conchal**:
     - Absent pneumatization, sinus is filled with cancellous bone
     - Rare
   - **Presellar**:
     - Pneumatization anterior to a vertical line drawn through tuberculum sella
     - second most common pattern
   - **Sellar**
     - Pneumatization extends beyond a vertical line drawn through turberculum sella
     - Majority of cases
   - **Postsellar**:
     - Pneumatization extends beyond the dorsum sella
   - **Arrested pneumatization** (arrested development):
     - Developmental variant resulting in persistence of atypical fatty marrow within a nonpneumatized region of the sphenoid sinus
     - Incidental finding on imaging as patients are typically asymptomatic -Distinct from sphenoid hypoplasia wherein a normal bony trabecular pattern is present within the sphenoid sinus
     - Can be mistaken for a skull base lesion
     - Most commonly occurs in sphenoid sinus
2. Walls and recesses of the sphenoid sinus (Figure 24-6)
   - **Planum sphenoidale**:
     - Forms sphenoid roof
     - Contiguous anteriorly with fovea ethmoidalis
   - **Sphenoid rostrum**:
     - Forms sphenoid face and anterior floor
     - Articulates anteriorly with the vomer and perpendicular plate of ethmoid forming a keel
   - **Sella turcica**:
     - Latin for Turkish saddle
     - Rounded projection along posterosuperior wall in a well pneumatized sphenoid sinus
     - Forms floor of hypophyseal fossa (containing pituitary gland; middle cranial fossa)

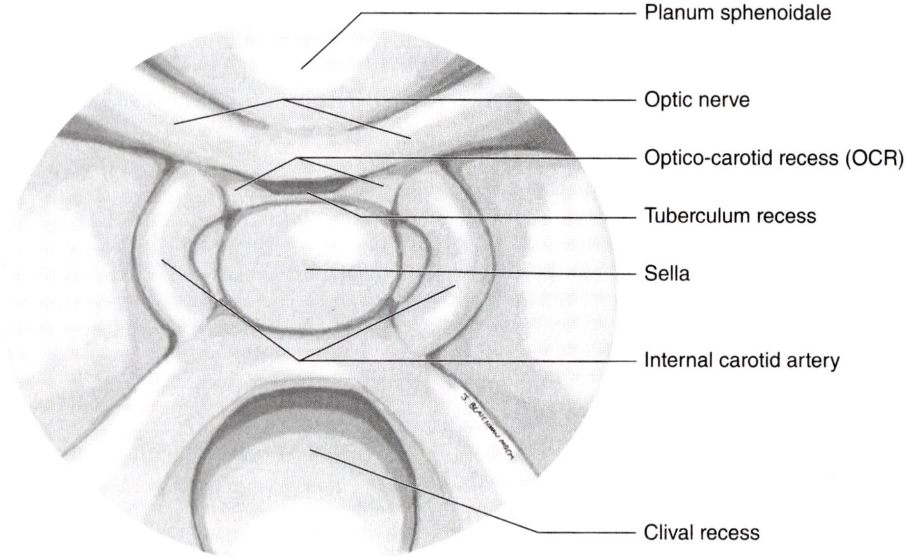

Figure 24-6 Sphenoid. *(Illustrations by Dr. Jason I. Blaichman MDCM, FRCPC.)*

    - May be attenuated or anteriorly displaced in the presence of a pituitary macroadenoma
    - Bounded anterosuperiorly by **tuberculum sella** and posteriorly by **dorsum sella**
- **Lateral pterygoid recess** (lateral recess):
    - Inferolateral pneumatization of the sphenoid sinus
    - Common location for spontaneous CSF leak and encephalocele
- **Lateral wall of sphenoid**:
    - Forms medial wall of cavernous sinus
    - When well pneumatized, bony impressions of the internal carotid artery (partially dehiscent in 25%) and optic nerve (dehiscent in 6%) can be visualized
- **Opticocarotid recess**:
    - Bony depression between the optic nerve superiorly and the cavernous internal carotid artery segment inferiorly
    - Located posterosuperiorly along the lateral wall of a well pneumatized sphenoid sinus
- **Sphenoid intersinus septum**:
    - May asymmetrically divide the sphenoid sinus
    - Must be removed with caution in transnasal endoscopic approaches to the skull base when inserts onto or in the vicinity of the carotid and/or optic canal
- **Clival recess**:
    - Forms posteroinferior wall of the sphenoid sinus if well pneumatized
    - Separates sphenoid sinus from posterior cranial fossa
- **Choanal arch**:
    - Forms the floor of the sphenoid
    - Corresponds to roof of nasopharynx
    - Bordered laterally by the medial pterygoid process

3. Landmarks for sphenoid ostium
   - Most reliable landmark = between the nasal septum and posterior insertion of the superior turbinate at the level of maxillary sinus roof
   - One-third of the way up from choana to skull base
   - 1.5 cm superior to the bony choanal arch
   - 7 cm at a 30-degree angle from the anterior nasal spine
   - Approximately at the level of the maxillary sinus roof

D. Frontal sinus
- Made up of two frontal sinuses, frequently asymmetric, separated by an intersinus septum
- Thick anterior wall, thin posterior wall (anterior wall of anterior cranial fossa)
- **Frontal beak**: thick bone of the frontal process of maxilla, anterior to the agger nasi that projects posteriorly into the frontal recess, thereby limiting its anteroposterior distance
  1. Frontal recess
     - Hourglass space with the narrowest portion corresponding to the frontal os
     - Communicates with the frontal sinus superiorly and anterior ethmoid inferiorly
     - Boundaries
       - Anterior = frontal beak/agger nasi
       - Medial = lateral lamella
       - Lateral = LP
       - Posterior = EB/Suprabullar recess
       - Posterosuperior = fovea ethmoidalis
       - Significant variation accounts for the complexity of frontal sinus dissection
  2. Frontal sinus cells
     - **Frontal ethmoidal cells**:
       - Anterior ethmoidal cells in contact with the anterior wall of the frontal recess (frontal process of maxilla)
       - Three classification schemes exist
         1. Kuhn classification: [1]
            ◊ Type 1: single cell above agger nasi cell
            ◊ Type 2: tier of cells above agger nasi cell
            ◊ Type 3: single cell pneumatizing into the frontal sinus
            ◊ Type 4: isolated cell within the frontal sinus
         2. Modified Kuhn classification (Wormald):[2]
            ◊ Type 1 and 2: no change from previous classification
            ◊ Type 3: cell pneumatizing into the frontal sinus but less than 50% of the vertical height of the sinus
            ◊ Type 4: cell pneumatizing into the frontal sinus greater than 50% of the vertical height of the sinus
               * Change in classification prompted by rarity of initial definition of Type 4 cell
         3. International frontal sinus anatomy classification (IFAC)[3]
            ◊ Supra agger cell: anterior-lateral ethmoidal cell, located above the agger nasi cell (not pneumatizing into the frontal sinus)
            ◊ Supra agger frontal cell: anterior-lateral ethmoidal cell that extends into the frontal sinus

        - ◊ Supra bulla cell: cell above the bulla ethmoidalis that does not enter the frontal sinus
        - ◊ Supra bulla frontal cell: cell that originates in the supra bulla region and pneumatizes along the skull base into the posterior region of the frontal sinus
        - ◊ Supraorbital ethmoid cell: cell that pneumatizes around anterior to, or posterior to the anterior ethmoid artery over the roof of the orbit
        - ◊ Frontal septal cell: medially based cell attached to or located in the interfrontal sinus septum
    - **Intersinus septal cell**:
        - Pneumatization of the interfrontal sinus septum
        - Originates medially, thereby displacing frontal sinus drainage pathway laterally
        - Other relevant frontal recess cells include agger nasi cell, suprabullar cells, frontal bulla cells, and supraorbital ethmoid cells (see description above)

Abbreviations

ULC = upper lateral cartilage
LLC = lower lateral cartilage
MT = middle turbinate
UP = uncinate process
EB = ethmoid bulla
LP = lamina papyracea (medial orbital wall)
GSPN = greater superficial petrosal nerve
ESS = endoscopic sinus surgery
IMA = internal maxillary artery
SPA = sphenopalatine artery
SPF = sphenopalatine foramen
AEA = anterior ethmoid artery

Questions

1. Which of the following anatomical structures does not arise from the ethmoid bone?
   A. Uncinate process
   B. Inferior turbinate
   C. Agger nasi
   D. Middle turbinate

2. Which of the following sites corresponds to the weakest portion of the anterior cranial fossa skull base?
   A. Junction of the posterior fovea ethmoidalis and lateral lamella
   B. Lateral lamella, at the site of insertion of the anterior ethmoid artery
   C. Skull base attachment of the middle turbinate
   D. Superior attachment of the perpendicular plate of the ethmoid bone

3. Which of the following anatomic structures would be encountered first when extending a maxillary antrostomy posteriorly from the natural maxillary os toward the posterior maxillary sinus wall?
   A. Nasolacrimal duct
   B. Sphenopalatine artery
   C. Descending palatine artery
   D. Posterior septal artery

4. Presence of an onodi cell places which of the following structures at greatest risk intraoperatively?
   A. Pituitary gland
   B. Palatovaginal artery
   C. Medial rectus muscle
   D. Optic nerve

5. Which of the following cells would most likely displace the frontal sinus drainage pathway laterally?
   A. Intersinus septal cell
   B. Supraorbital ethmoid cell
   C. Agger nasi
   D. Frontal bulla cell

References

1. Bent JP, Cuilty-Siller C, Kuhn FA. The frontal cell as a cause of frontal sinus obstruction. *Am J Rhinol.* 1994;8(4):185-192.
2. Wormald PJ, Xun Chan SZ. Surgical techniques for the removal of frontal recess cells obstructing the frontal ostium. *Am J Rhinol.* 2003;17(4):221-226.
3. Wormald PJ, Hoseman W, Callejas C, et al. The international frontal sinus anatomy classification (IFAC) and classification of the extent of endoscopic frontal sinus surgery (EFSS). *Int Forum Allergy Rhinol.* 2016;6(7):677-696.

Chapter 25
Nasal Function and Evaluation of Taste and Smell

Nasal Function

A. Warming and humidification
   i. Air is humidified to 98% relative humidity.
   ii. Air is warmed through heat diffusion and convection to an optimal range for ciliary function.
B. Regulation of nasal secretions
   i. Proteins in mucus layer and airway surface liquid (ASL)
      a. Plasma proteins
         1. Albumin
         2. Immunoglobulins (IgG, IgM, IgA)
      b. Serous cell products
         1. Antibacterial defense molecules
            - Lysozymes
            - Lactoferrin
            - Defensins
            - Cathelicidins
            - Secretory component, IgA, and complement
      c. Mucous cell products
         1. Mucoglycoproteins
         2. Mucins
      d. Epithelial goblet cell products
         1. Macromolecules and ions
   ii. ASL thickness modified by epithelial ion pumps
      a. Dysfunction in cystic fibrosis transmembrane conductance regulator (CFTR) results in ASL dehydration
      b. Plasma extravasation controlled by interepithelial tight junctions
         1. Vasodilation increases plasma extravasation
         2. Vasoconstriction reduces plasma extravasation
C. Regulation of airway resistance
   i. Autonomic innervation modulates airway resistance
      a. Vidian nerve
         1. Formed by the greater superficial petrosal (preganglionic parasympathetic fibers) and deep petrosal nerves (postganglionic sympathetic fibers)

2. Postganglionic fibers join sphenopalatine nerve
   - Parasympathetic neurons
     (a) Vasointestinal peptide (cotransmitter to acetylcholine)
       - Vasodilation at arterial and venous sinusoidal vessels
       - Enhanced secretory activity, thickened mucosa, increased airway resistance
       - Mast cell degranulation
         - Release of histamine, bradykinin, arachidonic acid metabolites, ions
   - Sympathetic neurons
     (a) Neuropeptide Y (Co-transmitter to noradrenaline)
       - Vasoconstriction of vessels reduces mucosal blood flow, shrinks mucosa, decreases airway resistance

ii. Nonadrenergic, noncholinergic responses
  a. Trigeminal sensory neurons use peptides as neurotransmitters
    1. Secreted by macrophages, eosinophils, lymphocytes, dendritic cells
    2. Substance P, neurokinin A, calcitonin gene-related peptide (CGRP)
       - Induce vasodilation
       - Increase vascular permeability
       - Increase nasal resistance
       - Stimulate glandular secretion
       - Leukocyte chemotaxis
       - Mast cell degranulation

iii. Nasal cycle
  a. Cyclical vascular phenomenon that occurs in 80% of normal individuals
  b. Alternating congestion/decongestion every 3 to 7 hours
  c. Centrally mediated autonomic tone of capacitance vessels of erectile mucosa

iv. Other influences on nasal resistance
  a. Exercise decreases nasal resistance
  b. Irritants (dust, smoke), cold/dry air, alcohol, pregnancy, hypothyroidism, and medications can cause congestion of capacitance vessels
    1. Medications that can cause nasal congestion
       - Antihypertensives (alpha and beta blockers)
       - Oral contraceptives
       - Antidepressants
       - Nonsteroidal anti-inflammatory medications
       - Decongestants in excess may result in rhinitis medicamentosa
  c. Atrophic rhinitis
    1. Chronic, degenerative disorder characterized by nasal crusting, malodorous discharge, and nasal obstruction
       - Atrophy of serous and mucinous glands
       - Loss of cilia and goblet cells
       - Inflammatory cell infiltrates
    2. Possible causes
       - Underlying chronic inflammatory disease
         (a) Granulomatous disorders
       - Irradiation
       - Bacterial and viral infection
       - Excessive nasal surgery

D. Nasal airflow
   i. At low flow rates, airflow is laminar.
   ii. Maximum velocity occurs in the narrowest segment—the nasal valve.
      a. Bernoulli principle
         1. Increased airflow velocity leads to negative pressure and nasal valve collapse
      b. Poiseuille law
         1. Airflow resistance is inversely proportional to fourth power of the radius.
         2. Small decrease in cross-sectional area produces large increase in airway resistance.
   iii. Relatively slow flow rates found in olfactory region with quiet breathing.
   iv. During inspiration, main flow stream occurs in the lower and middle airway (space between middle meatus and nasal septum).
   v. During expiration, maximum velocity is lower but expiratory air is evenly distributed across inferior, middle, and olfactory regions.
   vi. Diagnostic testing of nasal airflow.
      a. Objective diagnostic measures of nasal airflow often poorly correlate with patient-reported symptoms
      b. Nasal inspiratory peak flow
         1. Objective, physiologic measurement of nasal airflow during maximal forced nasal inspiration
         2. Advantages: portable equipment, easy to use
         3. Disadvantages: test-retest variability, influenced by the lower airway, influenced by nasal valve collapse
      c. Rhinomanometry
         1. Pressure sensors placed with and without decongestion to develop flow-pressure curves
         2. Measurements calculated to determine airflow resistance
         3. Advantages: functional test, may be done on both sides simultaneously
         4. Disadvantages: time, expense, inability to identify site of obstruction
      d. Acoustic rhinometry
         1. Sound waves transmitted into nasal cavity, which is reflected back and converted into digital impulses constructed on a rhinogram
         2. Detects variances in cross-sectional area along predetermined points in the nasal cavity
         3. Advantages: fast test, localizes area of obstruction
         4. Disadvantages: technically challenging, expensive, unable to accurately measure beyond narrow apertures
      e. Computational fluid dynamics
         1. Technique that uses mathematical calculations (Navier–Stokes equations) based on an imaging study (CT or MRI) to predict airflow in the nasal cavity
         2. Advantages: nonintrusive, can be used to simulate effects of surgery
         3. Disadvantages: time consuming, unclear correlation to patient symptoms, requires imaging study

E. Immunology/mucociliary clearance
   i. First line of defense against bacteria/viruses
   ii. Mucociliary transport of microorganisms and noxious particles
      a. Mucus travels along ciliated columnar epithelial cells of nasal mucosa at a rate of 2 to 10 mm/h

iii. Seromucinous glands and goblet cells secrete mucus
iv. Periciliary fluid contains immunomodulating cells/proteins: macrophages, neutrophils, basophils, eosinophils, mast cells, B and T leukocytes, immunoglobulins A, G, M, E, lysozymes, lactoferrin, interferon
v. Particles >12 μm may be filtered
vi. Evaluation of mucociliary function
   a. Saccharin test
      1. 0.5 mm saccharin particle placed approximately 1 cm behind the anterior end of the inferior turbinate
      2. Measure time until the first experience of sweet taste
   b. 99Tc-macroaggregated albumin scintigraphy
      1. Radiolabeled droplet placed in anterior nasal floor
      2. Gamma camera systems obtain dynamic images to measure transport time between a reference point and the nasopharynx
   c. Electron microscopy
      1. Absent or shortened outer dynein arms of ciliary ultrastructure observed in patients with ciliary dyskinesia
   d. Nasal nitric oxide measurements
      1. Reduced in patients with primary ciliary dyskinesia and cystic fibrosis

F. Olfaction
   i. Basic terminology
      a. Smell—the perception of an odor
      b. Taste—the perception of salty, sweet, sour, bitter, umami
      c. Flavor—the complex interaction of smell, taste, and somatic sensation
         1. Mediated by CNs I, V, VII, IX, and X in the nose, oral cavity, pharynx, and larynx
      d. Anosmia—inability to detect all odors
      e. Hyposmia—decreased ability to detect odors
      f. Dysosmia—altered perception of smell
         1. Parosmia—odor stimulus present, but incorrectly identified
            - Often mistaking pleasant or neutral odors for unpleasant ones
         2. Phantosmia—odor stimulus absent, but still perceive smell (olfactory hallucination)
      g. Ageusia—inability to taste
      h. Hypogeusia—decreased ability to taste
      i. Dysgeusia—distorted sense of taste

Anatomy and Physiology of Olfaction and Taste

A. Olfaction plays a primary role in the regulation of food intake, the perception of flavor, and in the detection of irritating and toxic substances.
   i. Humans can discriminate more than 1 trillion olfactory stimuli.
B. In a normal young adult, the olfactory system consists of 6 to 30 million olfactory sensory neurons (OSNs).
C. Olfactory neuroepithelium
   i. Thick, pseudostratified, columnar, nonciliated epithelium
   ii. Present primarily at the olfactory cleft, also found at the superior-posterior septum, superior turbinate, superior and medial aspect of middle turbinate

iii. Contains multiple cell types
    a. Olfactory sensory neurons—bipolar cells, axons form the olfactory nerve
    b. Basal cells—capable of regenerating OSNs throughout life and following injury
    c. Bowman glands—secrete mucus
    d. Sustentacular/supporting cells—secrete mucopolysaccharides into mucus that dissolve hydrophobic odorants, allowing them to bind receptors on OSNs

D. Olfactory mucosa is sheltered during normal respiration, limiting olfaction.
  i. Orthonasal olfaction: Sniffing redistributes airflow to the upper portion of the nasal cavities, leading to the perception of odorant.
  ii. Retronasal olfaction: Retrograde perception of odorants from the oropharynx while eating or drinking.
    • Contributes to perception of flavor
  iii. Orthonasal and retronasal olfaction may be processed differently, thus leading to different perceived smells with the same odorant.

E. Olfactory transduction:
  i. Movement of odors from the air phase of the nasal cavity into the aqueous phase of the olfactory mucus.
  ii. Odorants are transported through aqueous medium to olfactory receptor proteins on OSNs dendritic cilia.
  iii. Odorant recognized by distinct combination of olfactory receptors.
  iv. OSNs are unique in that each cell serves as both a receptor cell and first-order neuron.
    a. Axons are projected directly from the nasal cavity into the brain without an intervening synapse.
  v. Olfactory transduction involves a G-protein-mediated cascade.
    a. Results in membrane depolarization through the influx of calcium and sodium, outflow of chloride.
  vi. Action potential travels down the axon of the olfactory receptor cell.
    a. Meets with axons of other olfactory receptor cells to form the olfactory nerve
    b. Axons traverse the cribriform plate of the ethmoid bone and synapse to second-order neurons in glomeruli of the olfactory bulb
    c. Second-order neurons merge to form olfactory tract
  vii. Olfactory tract travels to the piriform cortex, hippocampus, thalamus, and amygdala.
    a. Encodes representations of odor quality, identity, memory, and the coordination of olfaction, vision, and taste.
    b. Thalamus is involved in the interpretation of odors.
    c. Amygdala responds to the intensity of emotionally significant pleasant or unpleasant odors.
    d. Entorhinal cortex preprocesses information entering the hippocampus, which is involved in learning and memory.
    e. Orbitofrontal cortex provides interpretive processing.
      1. Corresponds to Brodmann areas 10, 11, 25
  viii. While sight and hearing are processed by a relay center in the cerebral hemisphere, smell has a direct route to many parts of the brain.
    a. Sight and hearing are more closely connected with higher functioning.
    b. Smell is associated with emotion.

ix. Trigeminal system (CN V) delivers somatosensory information from within the nasal cavity through branches of the ophthalmic and maxillary divisions.
   a. Stinging, burning, pungent sensations mediated by trigeminal afferents
   b. Cell bodies of trigeminal afferents located in Gasserian ganglion within Meckel cave
   c. Axons project to the trigeminal nucleus in the brain stem, thalamus, and insular and cingulate cortices (both part of the limbic system)

F. Taste
   i. Taste refers to sensations arising from the taste buds
      a. Salty, sweet, sour, bitter, umami
   ii. Flavor is the combination of taste and smell.
      a. Tastants contact the taste buds on the tongue, oropharynx, and larynx.
      b. Retronasal olfaction occurs as food is chewed and swallowed.
         1. Odorants pumped behind the palate into the nasal cavity
   iii. Taste mediated by CN VII, IX, and X
      a. Anterior two-thirds of the tongue
         1. Chorda tympani (CN VII), runs along lingual nerve
      b. Posterior one-third of the tongue and junction of the hard and soft palate
         1. Lingual branch of the glossopharyngeal nerve (CN IX)
      c. Laryngeal surface of the epiglottis
         1. Superior laryngeal nerve branch of the vagus nerve (CN X)

G. Taste map myth
   i. Although studies have shown that thresholds for certain sensations are lower in certain areas of the tongue, the differences are very small.

Olfactory and Taste Disorders

A. 200,000 patient visits a year in the United States for smell and taste disturbances

B. Prevalence: estimates ranging from 1.4% to 23% worldwide
   a. Risk factors: male sex, concurrent sinonasal disorders, smoking, alcohol abuse, obesity, low socioeconomic status, minority status

C. Olfactory dysfunction (OD) is independently associated with increased risk of all-cause mortality

D. Chemosensory loss is age-dependent
   i. Prevalence of olfactory dysfunction is 34.5% for mean age greater than 55 years, versus 7.5% for mean age less than 55 years
   ii. Declining olfaction correlates with increased cognitive decline, frailty, and mortality in older adults

E. Etiology:
   i. Olfactory dysfunction can result from pathologic processes at any level along the olfactory pathway, from the nasal cavity to the brain
      a. Conductive defects interfere with transport and access of odorants to the olfactory neuroepithelium
         1. Acute or chronic inflammation—chronic rhinosinusitis (CRS) with or without polyps, viral/bacterial infections, allergic rhinitis, atrophic rhinitis
         2. Iatrogenic injury (surgery disrupting olfactory epithelium)
         3. Radiation therapy

b. Sensorineural loss results from injury at the receptor region or damage to the central olfactory pathways
   1. Post-viral olfactory dysfunction
      a. Local inflammation, injury to olfactory epithelium, supporting cells, and nerves—exact mechanism unclear
      b. Non-COVID-19 related
         i. Most commonly rhinovirus and coronavirus
c. COVID-19 related
   i. Overall prevalence of OD in early COVID-19 pandemic was 47% to 67%
   ii. Some evidence that supporting cells infected by COVID-19, not OSNs
   iii. Persistent OD in 30% of patients 6 months after initial infection
   iv. Later variants of COVID-19 less likely to cause OD
   2. Head trauma: 7% to 22% occurrence of OD after head injury
      a. Fractures and shearing injury can disrupt the olfactory axons that perforate the cribriform plate
      b. Anosmia more common than hyposmia
      c. Usually permanent (only about 10% improve)
      d. More common when the trauma is associated with loss of consciousness, moderate to severe head injury, and skull fracture
   3. Neoplasms
      a. Meningiomas of inferior frontal region
      b. Olfactory neuroblastoma: rare tumor of the olfactory neuroepithelium
      c. Others: sinonasal tumors, pituitary adenoma, craniopharyngioma, glioma
   4. Toxin exposure: environmental pollutants or work-related
      a. Cadmium and manganese metal exposure in particular
   5. Neurodegenerative disorders
      a. Alzheimer disease, Parkinson disease, multiple sclerosis (MS), amyotrophic lateral sclerosis (ALS)
      b. Olfactory loss may be the first clinical sign of disease
   6. Congenital abnormalities
      a. Kallmann syndrome: X-linked disorder with congenital anosmia and hypogonadotropic hypogonadism
   7. Other possible causes of OD: medications, smoking, vitamin deficiency (B_6, B_{12}), autoimmune disease, hypothyroidism, depression, schizophrenia, epilepsy, anorexia

Evaluation of Olfactory Function

A. History
   i. Identify underlying cause
      a. Timing can help distinguish possible etiologies, such as sudden onset (post-URI, posttraumatic), gradual/fluctuating onset (sinusitis, allergies, neurodegenerative diseases), and congenital (Kallmann syndrome)
   ii. Clarify the taste-smell distinction
      a. Taste dysfunction: diminished or altered basic taste perception (sweet, sour, salty, bitter, umami)
      b. Olfactory dysfunction: flavor complaints, decreased or altered smell and taste

B. Physical examination
   i. Complete head and neck, neurologic examination
   ii. Cognition and mood
   iii. Signs of systemic disease
   iv. Nasal endoscopy
      a. Zero-or 30-degree rigid scope, 4 mm or smaller
      b. Topical decongestant may impair assessment of obstruction; however, it does not affect olfactory function
      c. Topical anesthetic may cause temporary olfactory dysfunction; therefore, avoid if planning to perform olfactory testing
      d. Evaluate color of mucosa, presence of inflamed or hypertrophic mucosa, presence of nasal polyps, masses, or secretions, and anatomic abnormalities

C. Labs
   i. Not typically part of workup; however, can obtain complete blood count (CBC), comprehensive metabolic panel (CMP), thyroid-stimulating hormone (TSH), IgE levels in the appropriate patient

D. Smell threshold and identification tests
   i. Sniffin' sticks: odor-producing pens placed 2 cm from the nose
      a. Reliable, validated assessment for odor threshold, discrimination, and identification
   ii. Alcohol sniff test
      a. Open alcohol packet, wave it in front of the nose, measure the distance from the nostrils at the time of detection
      b. Normally able to detect odor at approximately 30 cm, move 1 cm closer with each expiration until detection
      c. Anosmic patients will not detect odor of alcohol, but may have trigeminal reactivity when very close to the nose
   iii. Smell identification test (SIT-40, previously known as "UPSIT")
      a. Self-administered, standardized 40-item, multiple choice scratch-and-sniff test
      b. High test-retest reliability for smell identification, does not test thresholds
      c. Most widely used clinical test
      d. Adjusts for age and gender
      e. Patient scored as normal (score of 35-40), mild, moderate, or severe microsmia (score of 19-34), anosmia (score of 6-18), or probable malingering (score of 5 or less)
         1. Malingering appears as the reporting of fewer correct responses than expected based on chance
         2. Present strong CN V stimulant (ammonia) to test for malingering

E. Gustatory testing: no convenient standardized tests for taste function
   i. Solutions or edible strips containing sweet, salty, bitter, and sour components may be used; umami is not usually screened as it is poorly detected

F. Imaging
   i. CT scan
      a. Consider if history or exam is suggestive of paranasal sinus disease, iatrogenic injury, or trauma
   ii. MRI
      a. Consider if suspected congenital, neurogenic/sensory etiology, or intracranial tumor
      b. Coronal MRI from frontal sinus to posterior corpus callosum is technique of choice to image the olfactory bulbs, tracts, and cortical parenchyma.
   iii. Obtaining imaging is controversial, particularly if endoscopy is unrevealing

Treatment of Olfactory Dysfunction

A. Address underlying cause
  a. Inflammatory disease with or without polyps addressed with medical or surgical management
  b. Olfactory outcomes following ESS for CRS variable and challenging to predict
  c. Presence of nasal polyposis is predictive of postoperative olfactory improvement
    i. Short-term management of OD in CRSwNP with oral corticosteroids is recommended
    ii. Long-term management with topical corticosteroids
    iii. Biologics effective for severe, refractory CRSwNP shown to improve olfaction
B. Several medical therapies under investigation for postviral, posttraumatic, and idiopathic anosmia
  a. So far, insufficient evidence to recommend use of these treatments
  b. Topical, locally injected, and systemic steroids
  c. Alpha lipoic acid: fatty acid derivative that acts as an antioxidant
  d. Theophylline: phosphodiesterase inhibitor thought to increase olfactory sensitivity
    i. Chronic use associated with need for repeated serum monitoring due to narrow therapeutic range and potential toxicities (seizures, MI)
  e. Oral or intranasal zinc: zinc deficiency previously thought to cause OD
  f. Topical or injected platelet-rich plasma (PRP): releases growth factors and cytokines
  g. Oral or topical high-dose vitamin A: precursor of retinoic acid, a transcription regulator
C. Olfactory training
  i. Unclear evidence if olfactory training is effective
  ii. Repeated exposure to odor stimuli in attempt to improve odor detection and discrimination
  iii. Frequent short-term exposure to odors, typically for several weeks
  iv. Considered in patients with olfactory loss due to URI, head trauma, and neurodegenerative disorders
D. Treatment of phantosmia
  i. No accepted gold standard treatment, limited studies demonstrating benefit with medical therapy selected based on the most likely etiology (antimigraine, antipsychotic, antiepileptic)
  ii. Olfactory mucosa excision has been described, although this only demonstrated short-term improvement and is highly risky

Bibliography

Geurkink N. Nasal anatomy, physiology, and function. *J Allergy Clin Immunol.* 1983;72:123-128.

Papon JF, Coste A. Physiology of the nose. European manual of medicine. *Otolaryngol Head Neck Surg.* 2010;173-175.

Patel ZM, Holbrook EH, Turner JH, et al. International consensus statement on allergy and rhinology: Olfaction. *Int Forum Allergy Rhinol.* 2022;12(4):327-680.

Whitcroft KL, Altundag A, Balungwe P, et al. Position paper on olfactory dysfunction: 2023. *Rhinology.* 2023;61(33):1-108.

Questions

1. Which of the following contributes to the parasympathetic response in the nasal cavity?
   A. Substance P
   B. Vasointestinal peptide
   C. Neuropeptide Y
   D. Neurokinin A
   E. Calcitonin gene-related peptide

2. Which diagnostic test of nasal function allows for the localization of an area of obstruction?
   A. Rhinomanometry
   B. Nasal nitric oxide measurements
   C. Acoustic rhinometry
   D. Nasal inspiratory peak flow
   E. 99Tc-macroaggregated albumin scintigraphy

3. Which of the following decreases nasal resistance?
   A. Exercise
   B. Oral contraceptives
   C. Cold air
   D. Beta-blockers
   E. Nonsteroidal anti-inflammatory medications

4. Which of the following mediates taste on the posterior one-third of the tongue?
   A. CN VII
   B. CN IX
   C. CN V
   D. CN XII

5. What sensory dysfunction is characterized by distortion in the perceived quality of an odor?
   A. Anosmia
   B. Hyposmia
   C. Dysgeusia
   D. Parosmia
   E. Phantosmia

Chapter 26
Acute and Chronic Sinusitis

Classification and Diagnosis

- Sinusitis is an inflammatory disease affecting one or more of the paranasal sinuses and can be subdivided into either acute or chronic sinusitis depending on the length of symptoms:
- **Acute rhinosinusitis (ARS)**: Sinonasal inflammation lasting less than 4 weeks with sudden onset of symptoms
  - Symptoms: nasal obstruction OR nasal discharge (anterior/posterior) AND facial pain/pressure OR reduction/loss of smell
  - Often precipitated by an upper respiratory viral infection
- **Chronic rhinosinusitis (CRS):** Symptomatic inflammation of the paranasal sinuses and nasal cavity for a duration longer than 12 weeks
  - To make a diagnosis of CRS, two or more of the following cardinal symptoms must be present for twelve weeks or longer:
    - Mucopurulent drainage (anterior or posterior)
    - Nasal obstruction/congestion
    - Facial pain or pressure
    - Hyposmia or anosmia
  - In addition to documentation of two or more of the above symptoms, inflammation of the nasal mucosa must be confirmed by one of the following findings:
    - Polyps in the nasal cavity or middle meatus, confirmed with endoscopy or anterior rhinoscopy
    - Purulence or edema in the middle meatus or anterior ethmoid cavity
    - Radiographic (CT) evidence of mucosal thickening, edema, or other findings consistent with inflammation
- CRS can be punctuated by acute exacerbations, sometimes referred to as "acute-on-chronic" rhinosinusitis, in which symptoms worsen secondary to an acute infection or other environmental insult.
- Recurrent acute sinusitis refers to four or more discrete episodes of sinusitis in 1 year, with asymptomatic periods between episodes, and is treated differently from CRS.

Subtypes

- Acute rhinosinusitis
  - Acute viral rhinosinusitis (AVRS): symptoms or signs present for less than 10 days without worsening symptoms
  - Acute bacterial rhinosinusitis (ABRS): persistent symptoms beyond 10 days or worsening of symptoms after 5 days indicate postviral ABRS (double sickening)
  - Recurrent ARS (RARS): four or more episodes of ARS with symptom-free intervals between episodes
- Chronic rhinosinusitis
  - Overall prevalence (all types) ranges from 4.5% to 12.5% in Western populations.
  - There are generally three subtypes of CRS recognized:
    - Chronic rhinosinusitis with nasal polyposis (CRSwNP)—20% to 33%
      - ◊ Excessive TH-2 inflammation, eosinophilic infiltration, histamine, IL-5, IL-13
    - Chronic rhinosinusitis without nasal polyposis (CRSsNP)—60% to 65%
      - ◊ Neutrophilic infiltration, IL-1, IL-16, tumor necrosis factor α (TNF-α)
      - ◊ Can be due to primary/acquired mucociliary failure, immunodeficiency, or anatomic factors
    - Allergic fungal rhinosinusitis (AFS)—8% to 12%
  - In practice, there can be an overlap of several of the above inflammatory markers and etiologies in both CRSwNP and CRSsNP.
  - Ongoing research will further classify CRS based on microscopic, genomic, and microbiomic categorizations.

Pathogenesis

- **Acute Sinusitis:**
  - Viruses: Viral upper respiratory infection inhibits sinonasal mucociliary clearance and can precede ABRS.
  - *Haemophilus influenza, Streptococcus pneumonia, Moraxella catarrhalis* are the most common causative organisms in both adults and children in ABRS.
  - Allergy, environmental irritants, and microbes cause mucosal swelling and sinus ostial obstruction.
  - Anatomic abnormalities block natural drainage pathways: septal deviation/spur, middle turbinate concha bullosa, prominent agger nasi cell or frontal cells, Haller cells.
  - Allergic rhinitis with systemic IgE-mediated response.
  - Odontogenic infections
    - Recent dental procedures (extractions) or periapical disease can result in ABRS, predominately starting in the maxillary sinus.
    - Ongoing odontogenic infections can lead to the development of CRS.
  - Environmental factors (smoking, daycare attendance for children).
- **Chronic Sinusitis:**
  - Whereas ABRS is marked by a suppurative, neutrophil-predominate infectious etiology, CRS is characterized by an inflammatory response where eosinophils are the predominant inflammatory cell in both atopic and nonatopic individuals.

- Contributing factors to CRS include anatomy, local physiological factors, and systemic physiological factors. Many of these can overlap, making a targeted diagnosis and treatment plan difficult to develop.
- Multiple episodes of ABRS may ultimately lead to the development of chronic sinusitis (predominately inflammatory process)
- **Anatomic factors**
  - Blockage of the osteomeatal complex, sphenoethmoidal recess, frontal recess, or other natural drainage pathways by anatomic abnormalities can cause or prolong chronic sinusitis.
    - ◊ Septal deviation, turbinate hypertrophy, middle turbinate concha bullosa, paradoxical turbinates, prominent agger nasi cell, Haller cells, prominent ethmoid bulla, pneumatization and inversion of uncinate process, hypoplastic sinuses, accessory maxillary ostia → recirculation
- **Local physiologic factors**
  - Mucociliary impairment: ciliary function plays an important role in the clearance of sinuses
    - ◊ The ciliary beat of the epithelium removes allergens, bacteria, and pollutants trapped in the mucus or gel layer of the mucociliary blanket through natural drainage pathways (ostia).
    - ◊ Loss of ciliary function may result from infection, inflammation, toxins, or direct mucosal injury:
      - * Occupational exposures, cigarette smoke inhalation, silent sinus syndrome, chronic odontogenic infection
      - * Direct injury from bacterial toxins: eg, Staphylococcus
      - * Postsurgical trauma/mucosal stripping
      - * Genetic abnormalities: eg, primary ciliary dyskinesia
    - ◊ Alterations in the viscosity and production of mucous can also lead to chronic sinusitis.
      - * Decreased hydration
      - * Patients with cystic fibrosis have thick mucous due to alterations in water and electrolyte (Cl^-) transport
- **Bacterial infection:** Chronic bacterial infection results in direct, non-reversible, toxic injury to sinonasal mucosa and can lead to acute exacerbations as well.
  - Inspissated secretions and hypoxia in occluded sinuses result in bacterial growth, which in turn secretes inflammatory mediators and toxins which directly damage the ciliated respiratory epithelium → decreased mucociliary clearance.
  - Sinus microbiome: The paranasal sinuses possess a diverse population of commensal bacteria in normal, healthy individuals.
    - ◊ Decreases in the biodiversity of bacteria in the sinuses have been implicated in the development of some CRS phenotypes.
    - ◊ This is similar to disease processes caused by decreased gut flora diversity, such as inflammatory bowel disease and obesity.
    - ◊ Whether changes in microbiome diversity are a cause or effect of CRS has yet to be firmly established.
  - Direct bacterial infection: Common CRS pathogens include *Pseudomonas aeruginosa, Staphylococcus aureus, Fusobacterium, Peptostreptococcus, Prevotella, Bacteroides, Klebsiella pneumoniae, Corynebacterium genus, Proteus mirabilis, Enterobacter, and Escherichia coli.*

- ◊ *P. aeruginosa* is frequently cultured from immunocompromised patients, patients with cystic fibrosis, and those undergoing revision surgery.
- ◊ Patients with CRS show a decrease in microbiome diversity compared to healthy controls.
- ◊ Patients with CRS have a higher incidence of antibiotic resistance.

- Bacterial biofilms: three-dimensional polysaccharide matrices which adhere to sinonasal mucosa and contain living bacteria colonies
  - ◊ Bacteria such as *S. aureus* and *P. aeruginosa* establish biofilms which allow them to evade host defenses and develop decreased susceptibility to systemic and local antibiotic therapy.
  - ◊ These bacteria demonstrate an altered phenotype with atypical growth and gene transcription.
  - ◊ Biofilms elicit a considerable immunologic reaction and can be difficult to eradicate from the paranasal sinuses.
  - ◊ Their formation may explain the persistence of inflammation in some medically recalcitrant CRS, especially in patients who have undergone prior surgery.
  - ◊ Mechanical debridement with sinonasal irrigations may be effective in disrupting biofilms, especially if a surfactant is added to the irrigation medium.
- Bacterial superantigen: Bacteria possess the ability to secrete pathogenic exotoxins, or superantigens, that can activate large subpopulations of the T-lymphocyte pool. This process has been proposed as a potential unifying theory for the pathogenesis of CRS.
  - ◊ T-cell superantigens bind to MHC-II histocompatibility complexes on antigen-presenting cells and the T-cell receptors of T lymphocytes that are separate from the antigen-binding sites, resulting in activation of up to 30% of the T-lymphocyte pool (normal < 0.01%) and massive TH-2 cytokine release.
  - ◊ Activation of CD4+ and CD8+ cells together → TH-2 cytokine release → eosinophil recruitment, mast cell degranulation, and generation of nasal polyps.

- **Fungal infection:** mycetoma/fungal ball, chronic invasive fungal sinusitis, allergic fungal sinusitis
  - IgE-independent fungal inflammation: Fungus may be a possible inflammatory trigger for CRS independent of a type-IgE allergic mechanism as seen in allergic fungal sinusitis (AFS).
    - ◊ Eosinophils cluster around fungi, and there is evidence that they are recruited and activated as a response to fungi in patients with CRS.
    - ◊ Furthermore, peripheral lymphocytes from CRS patients will produce large quantities of inflammatory cytokines when they are exposed to certain fungal antigens.
    - ◊ The environmental fungi present in the sinonasal cavity may activate and induce inflammation independent of an allergic response.
  - Allergic fungal sinusitis: a form of CRSwNP defined by the Bent and Kuhn criteria for AFS:
    - ◊ Type 1 hypersensitivity
    - ◊ Nasal polyposis
    - ◊ Characteristic CT findings: sinus opacification with areas of increased density/attenuation due to ferromagnetic elements produced by fungi, bony erosion or expansion can be present

      - ◊ Eosinophilic mucin: thick, green, peanut butter-consistency with Charcot-Leyden crystals, fungal hyphae, and eosinophils
      - ◊ Fungal stain or culture
  - **Osteitis:** inflammation of bone commonly found in patients with refractory CRS
    - Characterized by neo-osteogenesis, bony remodeling, and thickening of the mucosa secondary to infection adjacent to the affected bone.
    - Can occur in distal sites via the Haversian canal system within the bone, although histologic studies do not always reveal bacteria within the bone itself.
    - Osteitis is associated with a greater chance of recurrent disease and poor outcomes after surgery.
- Systemic physiologic factors
  - **Pulmonary**
    - Asthma: significant modifying factor for CRS
      - ◊ 84% to 100% of patients with severe asthma have abnormal sinus CTs.
      - ◊ Histologically, CRS can demonstrate the TH-2-type inflammatory response seen in asthmatics where eosinophils are the predominant inflammatory cells in both atopic and nonatopic individuals.
      - ◊ Control of asthma improves CRS symptoms in many patients.
    - Allergy: There is increased prevalence of allergic rhinitis in patients with CRS (25%-75% of cases).
      - ◊ Allergy is thought to be more prevalent in patients with CRSwNP compared to those with CRSsNP, although a direct link establishing causality has not been discovered.
      - ◊ Allergy avoidance and immunotherapy are thought to be potential modulators for patients with CRS.
      - ◊ Perennial allergies may worsen CRS more than seasonal allergies.
    - Aspirin exacerbated respiratory disease (AERD)/Samter Triad: nasal polyposis, aspirin (ASA) sensitivity, and asthma; mediated by production of proinflammatory mediators, mainly leukotrienes
      - ◊ Typically presents in the third or fourth decade. Often starts with rhinitis, followed by asthma, and lastly ASA sensitivity.
      - ◊ Arachidonic acid is normally cleaved from cellular membranes by phospholipase A2 and subsequently shunted to either the leukotriene pathway by the enzyme 5-lipoxygenase or the prostaglandin pathway by the enzyme cyclooxygenase.
      - ◊ Leukotrienes, also known as the slow-reacting substances of anaphylaxis, are a class of inflammatory mediators that increase vascular permeability, inflammatory cell chemotaxis, and smooth muscle constriction.
      - ◊ Prostaglandin E2, a product of the cyclooxygenase pathway, inhibits 5-lipoxygenase in a feedback loop.
      - ◊ Aspirin and other nonsteroidal anti-inflammatory drugs inhibit cyclooxygenase and decrease prostaglandin E2, resulting in a net increase in leukotrienes → this results in acute exacerbations of symptoms (eg, bronchoconstriction, mucous hypersecretion, vasodilation).
      - ◊ Nasal polyps in AERD patients typically have a higher eosinophilic load and are generally more refractory to treatment than other forms of CRS.
      - ◊ Patients with AERD may benefit from aspirin desensitization.

- Rheumatologic/Autoimmune
  - Granulomatosis with polyangiitis (GPA, formerly Wegener granulomatosis), sarcoidosis, eosinophilic granulomatosis with polyangiitis (EGPA, Churg-Strauss Syndrome).
  - Diagnosis of these rheumatologic disorders can be assisted by pathologic tissue sampling from the sinonasal cavity.
- Immunologic
  - The interface between the nasal mucosa and the external environment contains both a mechanical and innate immune protective barrier that helps maintain the integrity and function of the respiratory epithelium.
  - Disorders of the innate immune system (at the level of the sinonasal mucosa) or the adaptive immune system (cell-mediated immunity) can lead to CRS.
  - Inherited or acquired immunodeficiencies can cause or worsen CRS: common-variable immunodeficiency (CVID), HIV, leukemia/hematologic malignancy, IgA/IgG/IgM deficiency, specific antibody deficiency, IgG subclass deficiency, chronic steroid administration, chemotherapy, uncontrolled diabetes mellitus.
  - IgG4-related disease.
  - Nitric oxide is thought to assist the innate immune system, and normal paranasal sinus mucosa is a reservoir for nitric oxide.
    - ◊ Nitric oxide has been shown to be bactericidal against *P. aeruginosa.*
    - ◊ Less exhaled nitric oxide is found in patients with CRS and CF.
    - ◊ The presence or lack of nitric oxide may represent a target for future therapies.
- Genetic
  - Cystic fibrosis, Kartagener syndrome (situs inversus, CRS, and bronchiectasis), primary ciliary dyskinesia (PCD)

Complications of Acute Rhinosinusitis

- Cause of spread:
  - Hematogenous: retrograde thrombophlebitis through valveless veins (veins of Breschet)
  - Direct spread: through lamina papyracea, posterior table of frontal sinus
- Ophthalmologic:
  - Chandler classification
    - Preseptal cellulitis
      - ◊ Infection of orbital contents anterior to orbital septum: eyelid and periorbital soft tissue
      - ◊ Symptoms: fever, pain, conjunctival injection, blurry vision, epiphora, periorbital swelling
      - ◊ Management: systemic broad-spectrum antibiotics and close follow-up
    - Orbital cellulitis
      - ◊ Infection of soft tissues posterior to orbital septum
      - ◊ Symptoms: chemosis, proptosis, ocular pain, restricted/painful movement of extraocular muscles
    - Subperiosteal abscess
      - ◊ Extraconal abscess between periorbita and sinus
      - ◊ Symptoms similar to orbital cellulitis may also have fixed globe/ophthalmoplegia and impaired visual acuity
      - ◊ Displacement of globe laterally or downward

      - Orbital abscess
        - ◊ Intraconal abscess
        - ◊ Symptoms similar to subperiosteal abscess, with high potential for vision loss
      - Cavernous sinus thrombosis
        - ◊ Symptoms: bilateral lid drop, exophthalmos, ophthalmic nerve neuralgia, cranial nerve palsies retroocular headache, complete ophthalmoplegia, papilledema, and/or signs of meningeal irritation associated with spiking fevers
        - ◊ MR venogram is gold standard for diagnosis; shows absence of venous flow in the affected cavernous sinus
    - Management of orbital complications
      - Except for preseptal cellulitis, admission, IV antibiotics (may observe in early stages in pediatric patients on antibiotics for orbital cellulitis) and surgical debridement/drainage of sinuses
      - Canthotomy/cantholysis for emergent orbital decompression
      - Afferent pupillary defect indicates optic nerve compression and requires urgent surgery
      - For cavernous sinus thrombosis, use of anticoagulants is controversial
    - Superior orbital fissure (SOF) syndrome
      - Compression of SOF contents: third, fourth, and sixth CN
      - Symptoms: immobile globe; dilated pupils that are nonreactive to light; ptosis; and hypoesthesia of the eyelids, cornea, and conjunctiva
      - Requires emergency surgery and IV antibiotics
    - Orbital apex syndrome: similar to SOF syndrome, but involves optic foramen, resulting in visual loss
- Intracranial:
    - CT is first step for diagnosis; MRI increases sensitivity
      - Subdural abscess
        - ◊ Abscess that stays on one side of falx cerebri
        - ◊ Most common intracranial complication in adults
        - ◊ Causes increased intracranial pressure, cerebritis, and meningeal irritation
        - ◊ Symptoms: fever, headache, mental status changes, orbital cellulitis
        - ◊ Associated with polymicrobial infections: *Streptococcus*, *Staphylococcus*, anaerobic gram-positive cocci, and anaerobic gram-negative bacilli
        - ◊ Requires immediate surgical intervention and antibiotics
      - Epidural abscess
        - ◊ Abscess that can cross midline/anterior to falx cerebri
        - ◊ Common intracranial complication in pediatrics
        - ◊ Similar symptoms to subdural abscess, but may be less severe
        - ◊ Requires immediate surgical intervention and antibiotics
      - Meningitis
        - ◊ Obtain imaging prior to lumbar drainage if suspected
- Pott puffy tumor::
    - Subperiosteal abscess of osteomyelitis of frontal bone
      - Anterior wall of frontal sinus presents with "doughy" edema of skin over frontal bone
      - Management: broad-spectrum IV antibiotics, surgical debridement of sequestered bone, drainage of frontal sinus (endoscopic or open)
- Mucocele:
    - Collection of sinus secretions trapped due to obstruction of sinus outflow tract; expansile process with bony remodeling on imaging
      - Mucopyocele: infected mucocele
      - Requires endoscopic drainage and marsupialization

Medical Treatment

Goals of Treatment

- Decrease symptomology and return to baseline sinonasal functionality (eg, airway patency, olfaction)
- Prevent or resolve chronic sinusitis
- Decrease exacerbations of co-morbidities (ie, asthma)
- Reestablish patency of ostiomeatal complex and mucociliary clearance
- Reduce inflammation and restore drainage of infected sinuses
- Eradicate bacterial infection and minimize risk of complications

Local/Topical Medical Treatment

- Topical steroids are an effective alternative to oral corticosteroid therapy with a far more limited side-effect profile.
- Commercially available nasal steroids include fluticasone, budesonide, mometasone, and others.
  - Generally dispensed in a spray bottle delivery device.
  - Systemic absorption: Budesonide > Fluticasone > Mometasone.
  - Budesonide is safe for use during pregnancy. (Pregnancy Category B)
  - Combination sprays are also available (fluticasone + azelastine) when indicated.
- Off-label therapy using respules or custom compounded nasal steroids and antibiotics which can be suspended in large-volume nasal saline irrigations.
- Medicated saline irrigations may be more effective than sprays at treating harder to reach sinuses (eg, frontal and sphenoid) and have a mechanical effect by displacing allergens and other particulate matter due to their larger volume.
- Side effects of topical nasal steroids include epistaxis, mucosal thinning, and excessively dry mucosa.

Systemic Medical Treatment

- *Acute sinusitis*
  - For mild or uncomplicated acute sinusitis, offer observation if follow-up is ensured. Otherwise, can offer initial antibiotic therapy
  - With moderate to severe disease (symptoms persistent or worsening; temperature > 38 degrees Celsius), offer antibiotic.
    - First line: amoxicillin with or without clavulanate (has potential for GI upset, bacterial resistance).
    - In penicillin allergic patients: doxycycline or respiratory quinolone (levofloxacin or moxifloxacin).
    - If no improvement on initial antibiotics, prescribe alternate antibiotic and consider complications or other causes of illness.
    - Endoscopically directed cultures can be useful to identify causative organisms.
  - Oral corticosteroids not recommended for acute sinusitis
  - Insufficient evidence for benefit of decongestants and antihistamines
  - Imaging usually not required unless complications suspected
- *Chronic sinusitis*
  - Broad-spectrum antibiotics such as amoxicillin with clavulanate acid, third-generation cephalosporins, respiratory fluoroquinolones, tetracyclines, or macrolides are effective against CRS pathogens.

  - Antibiotic resistance should be expected for patients who have had endoscopic sinus surgery or long-standing disease.
  - Endoscopy-guided, culture-directed antibiotics should be administered whenever possible.
- Macrolides such as clarithromycin and roxithromycin exhibit both an anti-inflammatory and bacteriostatic effect which can be beneficial for patients with CRSsNP.
- Tetracyclines such as doxycycline can downregulate inflammatory factors in addition to bacteriostatic effect in patients with CRSwNP.
- Antibiotics may be prescribed on a long-term basis, greater than 12 weeks
- In rare occasions, IV antibiotics and consultation with an infectious disease specialist may be required for patients infected with multidrug-resistant bacteria.
- Potential side effects of prolonged antibiotic treatment must be discussed with patients prior to initiation of therapy.
  - Fluoroquinolones: tendon rupture
  - Clarithromycin: cardiac disease
  - Doxycycline: sun sensitivity, teeth discoloration
- Oral corticosteroids (prednisone, methylprednisolone, dexamethasone) control eosinophilic disease by downregulating cytokines responsible for inflammation and shrinking polyposis.
- Nasal obstruction, hyposmia, and other sinonasal symptoms can improve significantly with oral steroids.
- Corticosteroids are generally prescribed in a burst dose followed by a taper (eg, 1 mg/kg initially followed by a 10-14 day taper).
- Informed consent is important given the potentially severe side-effects of oral steroid therapy (eg, avascular necrosis of the hip, hyperglycemia, psychosis). Complications can occur with short doses but are more common with prolonged therapy.

- *Allergy and asthma control*
  - CRSwNP is often comorbid with allergic disease and atopy. Allergy testing, allergen avoidance, and immunotherapy (subcutaneous or sublingual) should be pursued in affected patients.
  - Immunomodulators such as omalizumab (anti-IgE monoclonal antibody) can reduce sinonasal symptoms in atopic patients.
  - Leukotriene inhibitors (eg, Montelukast) are effective for asthmatic/atopic patients.
  - Patients with comorbid asthma or allergic disease should be managed with a consulting pulmonologist. Control of comorbid asthma has been shown to improve sinonasal symptoms, and vice-versa.
- *Management of comorbid conditions*
  - Patients with rheumatologic, immunologic, pulmonary, or genetic manifestations of sinonasal disease benefit from consultation with appropriate physician specialists.

Medical Treatment by CRS Phenotype

- *CRSwNP*: oral/topical corticosteroids, immunotherapy, immunomodulators (eg, dupilumab, mepolizumab), oral antibiotics (eg, doxycycline)
- *CRSsNP*: oral/topical culture-directed antibiotics (eg, macrolides), oral/topical antibiotics, saline irrigation
- *AFS*: oral/topical corticosteroids, immunotherapy (no benefit from oral or topical antifungals)
- *AERD*: anti-leukotriene therapy (zileuton), antibiotic therapy, aspirin desensitization, immunomodulators, oral/topical corticosteroids
- *CF*: sinonasal irrigations (with or without corticosteroids), CFTR modulators

Aspirin Desensitization

- A subset of patients with CRS suffers from aspirin (ASA) exacerbated respiratory disease (AERD).
- Desensitizing these patients to ASA may improve their pulmonary and sinonasal disease.
- ASA desensitization has a risk of significant adverse events, including anaphylaxis and gastric bleeding, and therefore should be performed in an appropriately equipped setting.
- ASA desensitization may be considered in patients with AERD who are refractory to both medical and surgical therapies.

Biologics

- Humanized monoclonal antibody therapies have been increasingly used to target type II inflammation in patients with CRSwNP with other comorbid conditions. They are typically reserved for patients with recalcitrant CRSwNP.
- Biologics are associated with high cost and cost effectiveness and utility have yet to be defined.
- **Anti-Immunoglobulin-E Therapy**
    - Immunoglobulin-E (IgE) in an inflammatory mediator responsible for mast cell activation.
    - Many CRSwNP patients with concurrent asthma and allergy have been found to have elevated serum IgE levels.
    - Monoclonal anti-IgE antibodies have been developed and function by binding free serum IgE and decreasing the availability of IgE receptors on.
        - Mast cells, basophils, dendritic cells
    - Omalizumab is an anti-IgE monoclonal antibody approved for maintenance use in CRSwNP patients ≥ 18 years of age with inadequate response to nasal corticosteroids or greater than 6 years of age with moderate to severe uncontrolled allergic asthma.
    - Potential adverse effects of omalizumab include:
        - Headaches
        - Injection site reactions
        - Pulmonary embolism/deep vein thrombosis
        - Cardiovascular (myocardial infarction, angina)
    - Long-term safety profile has been well established in patients with allergic asthma and chronic idiopathic urticaria and has been shown not to increase the rate of tumor.
    - Omalizumab has been shown to improve nasal polyp score (NPS) and nasal congestion score (NCS) with associated improvements in QoL (SNOT-22) and smell (UPSIT score) in patients with CRSwNP.
- **Anti-Interleukin-5 Therapy**
    - Interleukin-5 (IL-5) mediates inflammation by increasing growth, recruitment, and activation of eosinophils. Commonly elevated in CRSwNP.
    - Anti-IL-5, mepolizumab, therapy involves humanized IgG monoclonal antibodies that bind free IL-5.
    - Mepolizumab, reslizumab, benralizumab are commercially available anti-IL-5 therapies for asthma but only mepolizumab is approved for CRSwNP at this time.
        - Mepolizumab is currently approved for use in severe eosinophilic asthma and is shown to reduce OCS usage. It has also been shown to improve eosinophilic granulomatosis with polyangiitis.
        - Mepolizumab has been shown to reduce the occurrence of repeat ESS, usage of OCS, and improved symptomology, such as smell, in patients with CRSwNP especially in patients with high blood eosinophil count.

- Anti-IL-5 receptor monoclonal antibody, benralizumab, has been shown to induce eosinophil apoptosis and reduce blood and tissue eosinophilia.
- Mepolizumab has demonstrated consistent safety profile.
- Potential adverse effects of anti-IL-5 therapy includes:
  - Headache
  - Opportunistic infection
  - Injection site reactions

- **Anti-Interleukin-4R Therapy**
  - Interleukin-4 (IL-4) and Interleukin-13 (IL-13) are mediators of Type 2 inflammation.
  - IL-4 has also been shown to potentiate the immune response of fibroblasts in CRS.
  - CRSwNP who have comorbid asthma have high levels of IL-4/IL-13 driving type 2 inflammation.
  - Dupilumab is a monoclonal antibody that targets the α subunit of the IL-4 receptor (Rα). This leads to inhibition of IL4 and IL13 which then targets downstream cytokines.
  - Potential adverse effects of dupilumab include:
    - Headache
    - URI
    - Local injection reactions
    - Rash
    - Conjunctivitis
  - In large phase III trials, dupilumab in addition to intranasal steroids has been shown to improve symptom scores, reduce polyp size, improve smell, reduce OCS usage and need for ESS when compared to placebo.
  - These benefits were found throughout many subpopulations including patients with AERD, recalcitrant CRSwNP, and comorbid asthma patients.

Surgical Treatment

Patient Selection

- Surgical treatment for acute rhinosinusitis is reserved for patients with acute complications (orbital/intracranial).
- Surgical treatment for chronic rhinosinusitis is an option after a trial of "maximal medical therapy," which consists of an extended course of antibiotics, oral and/or topical steroids, and other symptomatic treatments.
- The presence of diffuse nasal polyposis unresponsive to medical therapy, suspected fungal sinusitis, or mucocele are generally straightforward indications for surgery.
- With minor mucosal disease, or when the primary complaint is recurrent sinusitis or headache, a decision to proceed with surgery is more equivocal.
  - Headache correlates poorly with sinus disease, and severe pain is unusual in CRS.
- In the absence of complicated sinusitis (orbital or intracranial extension), fungal sinusitis, neoplasm, or other urgent indications, a decision to pursue surgery is driven by the patient's quality of life.
- General guidelines:
  - The patient should meet the diagnostic requirements for CRS.
  - The patient should have had a trial of maximal medical therapy.

  - There should be persistent evidence of mucosal disease (radiographic or endoscopic).
  - Preoperative CT should be performed at least 4 weeks following the onset of medical therapy.
  - Performing elective sinus surgery on patients who continue to smoke may result in increased scarring and worsening of symptoms. Smoking cessation should be encouraged.
  - Alternative diagnoses should be explored prior to surgery, and treatment should be initiated if possible (rheumatologic/immunologic diseases, neoplasm, etc.).
  - Patients should be advised that disease recurrence and need for revision surgery are possible.

Surgical Techniques

- Oral steroid therapy 5 to 7 days prior to surgery may improve the operative field and reduce polyp burden.
- Raising the head of bed, using total-intravenous anesthesia, controlling blood pressure, and irrigating with warm saline can reduce intraoperative blood loss.
- The general goals of surgery for CRS are removal of disease (polyps, osteitic bone), re-establishment of sinus aeration/drainage, and improvement of postoperative topical drug delivery.
  - Polyp resection should be as complete as possible while preserving the mucoperiosteum, limiting mucosal stripping, and limiting exposed bone.
  - Osteitic bone should be removed as completely as possible.
  - Frozen-section and/or permanent pathologic analysis can be utilized if there is suspicion for underlying neoplasm or systemic disorder (eg, sarcoidosis).
  - The middle turbinate should be preserved whenever possible, but removal of extensive polyposis may destabilize its bony attachments, prompting the surgeon to remove the middle turbinate to prevent lateralization and to decrease inflammatory load.
  - Removal of bony partitions within the ethmoid sinuses and widening openings to the maxillary, sphenoid, and frontal sinus should be performed to facilitate delivery of postoperative medications via sinonasal irrigation.
  - Severe frontal sinus disease, particularly in revision cases, may require more extensive techniques such as a modified Lothrop (Draf 3) procedure.
  - Thick, tenacious debris may be encountered in patients with allergic fungal sinusitis, requiring serial saline flushes and curved instrumentation to completely clear debris and allergic mucin from impacted sinuses.
  - Postoperative packing is based on surgeon preference and is available in a variety of materials and formulations.
  - Placement of steroid-eluting stents, particularly in the frontal recess, may decrease polypoid recurrence.
- Intraoperative CT-guided navigation is generally indicated for revision surgery, difficult anatomy, or for teaching purposes.

Post-Surgical Therapy and Surveillance

- Antibiotic coverage is started in the operating room and can be continued postoperatively based on intraoperative culture.
- Saline irrigations and topical steroid irrigations are instituted in the early postoperative period and continued until the cavity is endoscopically normal.

- Oral steroids (CRSwNP) are tapered during the postoperative period based on the endoscopic appearance of the mucosa.
- Postoperative debridements are necessary to remove packing and ensure proper healing of sinonasal tissues (eg, prevent middle turbinate lateralization, synechiae).
- Postoperatively, patients may require short courses of antibiotics and/or oral steroids to avoid recurrent mucosal disease and bacterial sinusitis following a viral upper respiratory infection.
- Polyp recurrence postsurgery can be detected on in-office endoscopy and treated with oral/topical corticosteroids, in-office polypectomy, in-office placement of steroid-eluting stents/materials, or revision surgery.

Pediatric Rhinosinusitis

Pediatric Acute Rhinosinusitis

- Strong relation between viral URI and ARS
- Similar symptoms to adults (purulent nasal discharge, nasal obstruction, facial pain/pressure)
- Pediatric patients more likely to present with behavioral problems (ie, irritability) or cough, and less likely headache or fatigue
- Definition:
    - Sudden onset of two or more of the following symptoms: nasal blockage/obstruction/congestion or discolored nasal discharge or cough (daytime and nighttime) for less than 12 weeks
    - Subdivisions:
        - Acute viral rhinosinusitis
        - Acute postviral rhinosinusitis
            - ◊ Increase of symptoms after 5 days or persistent symptoms after 10 days with less than 12 weeks duration
    - Acute bacterial rhinosinusitis
            - ◊ Presence of at least three symptoms/signs including: discolored discharge (with unilateral predominance) and purulent secretions; severe local pain (with unilateral predominance); fever (> 38°C); elevated ESR/CRP; and double sickening
- Contributing factors
    - Rhinitis, coexisting medical conditions (CF, immune deficiency, ciliary dyskinesia), and environmental factors (smoking, daycare)
- Diagnosis and management
    - Diagnosis based on history and physical (anterior rhinoscopy)
    - Can be difficult to differentiate between adenoiditis and ARS
    - Imaging not indicated unless complications suspected
    - Antibiotics (Amoxicillin or amoxicillin-clavulanate) indicated for children with complications, comorbid diseases, severe onset of disease or worsening course
    - No efficacy of decongestants, antihistamines, or nasal irrigations

Pediatric Chronic Rhinosinusitis (PCRS)

- Defined as at least 90 continuous days of two or more symptoms of purulent rhinorrhea, nasal obstruction, facial pressure/pain, or cough and either endoscopic signs of mucosal edema, purulent discharge, or nasal polyposis and/or CT scan changes showing mucosal changes within the OMC and/or sinuses in pediatric patients aged 18 or younger

- Predisposing factors may include any of the following:
  - Viral URTIs
  - Day care attendance
  - Allergic rhinitis
  - Anatomic abnormalities
  - Gastroesophageal reflux
  - Immunodeficiency
  - Second-hand smoke
  - Ciliary dysfunction (PCD, Kartagener syndrome)
  - Adenoiditis/tonsillitis
  - Otitis media
  - Cystic fibrosis
- Twenty consecutive days of antibiotic therapy may produce a superior clinical response in PCRS patients. Culture-directed antibiotics are preferable but can be more difficult to obtain in children.
- Topical nasal steroids and saline irrigations are a beneficial adjunctive medication to antibiotics.
- Adenoidectomy is an effective first-line surgical treatment for children up to age 12 with chronic rhinosinusitis and may have a benefit independent of ESS.
- Endoscopic sinus surgery can be performed after medical therapy, adenoidectomy, or both have failed.
  - A CT scan of the sinuses should be obtained prior to surgery.
- Surgery may be indicated more urgently in cases of mucocele, nasal polyposis, fungal rhinosinusitis, or orbital/intracranial extension of disease.
- Postoperative debridement is difficult in children and efforts to minimize packing and/or need for return trips to the operating room should be made.

Bibliography

Batra PS, Tong L, Citardi MJ. Analysis of comorbidities and objective parameters in refractory chronic rhinosinusitis. *Laryngoscope*. 2013;123:S1-S11.

Brietzke SE, Shin JJ, Choi S, et al. Clinical consensus statement: pediatric chronic rhinosinusitis. *Otolaryngol Head Neck Surg*. 2014;151(4):542-553.

Fokkens WJ, Lund VJ, Mullol J, et al. EPOS 2012: European position paper on rhinosinusitis and nasal polyps 2012. A summary for otorhinolaryngologists. *Rhinology*. 2012 Mar;50(1):1-12.

Rosenfeld RM, Piccirillo JF, Chandrasekhar SS, et al. Clinical Practice Guideline (Update): Adult sinusitis. *Otolaryngol Head Neck Surg*. 2015;152(2S):S1-S39.

Tabaee A, McCoul ED, et al. Refractory chronic rhinosinusitis. *Otolaryngol Clin N Am*. 2017;50(1).

Questions

1. What is the direct end-effect of aspirin in patients with Samter's triad?
   A. Promotion of cyclooxygenase
   B. Inhibition of cyclooxygenase
   C. Promotion of phospholipase A2
   D. Inhibition of phospholipase A2

2. Which of the following is not one of the cardinal symptoms of chronic rhinosinusitis?
   A. Epistaxis
   B. Mucopurulent drainage
   C. Facial pain/pressure
   D. Hyposmia or anosmia

3. What is considered first-line therapy for ARS?
   A. Antihistamines
   B. Intranasal corticosteroids
   C. Decongestants
   D. Oral corticosteroids

4. What is NOT a presenting symptom of preseptal cellulitis?
   A. Periorbital edema
   B. Conjunctival injection
   C. Restricted extraocular movements
   D. Fever

5. Which of the following classes of antibiotics is particularly useful for treating sinonasal inflammation in patients with CRSsNP?
   A. Fluoroquinolones
   B. Tetracyclines
   C. Cephalosporins
   D. Macrolides

Chapter 27
Fungal Rhinosinusitis

Introduction

- With increased recognition over the past 30 years, fungal rhinosinusitis (FRS) represents a heterogeneous group of disorders whose manifestation depends on host immunologic function and fungus-specific factors.
- The first known case of fungal sinusitis by Plaignaud in 1791 reported a 22-year-old soldier with maxillary pain and "fungal tumor."
- Initial diagnostic focus on the causative organism led to widely used terms: "aspergillosis," "mucormycosis," or "zygomycosis." Modern classification schema relies more on disease characteristics than fungal speciation.
- Detailed understanding of mycology remains important in the diagnosis and treatment of FRS.
- Modern endoscopy and imaging modalities have allowed for the development of contemporary diagnostic criteria and targeted surgical treatment.

Classification

- FRS is best characterized as invasive or noninvasive—defined by the histopathological presence of fungal invasion into sinonasal soft tissue, more specifically angioinvasion.
- Three noninvasive forms of FRS
  (a) Fungal ball (ie, mycetoma)
  (b) Allergic fungal rhinosinusitis (AFRS)
  (c) Saprophytic fungal infestation
- Three invasive forms of FRS
  (a) Acute invasive fungal rhinosinusitis (AIFS)
  (b) Chronic invasive fungal rhinosinusitis
  (c) Granulomatous invasive fungal sinusitis
- Refinement of this classification will evolve with our understanding of the pathophysiologic role of fungi in rhinosinusitis.

Principles of Mycology

- With millions of species, fungus is a large, ubiquitous eukaryotic group of organisms that are subclassified into yeasts and molds.
- Characteristics of molds:
  (a) Mold is a type of fungus that grows and branches in multicellular filaments called hyphae. Mold colony comprises interwoven hyphae.
  (b) Molds reproduce by producing spores, which can be sexual or asexual.
  (c) Branching patterns (ie, 45 vs 90 degrees) and presence of septations (ie, septate, pauci-septate, or aseptate/coenocytic) of the hyphae are useful for further classification.
- Characteristics of yeasts:
  (a) In contrast, yeasts are unicellular and round fungal organisms.
  (b) They most commonly reproduce asexually by fission or budding, and less commonly via sexual spores in unfavorable growth conditions.
  (c) Multiple attached buds form a pseudohyphae, which appear structurally similar but are distinct from true hyphae.
- Both molds and yeasts have sexual or asexual reproductive cycles and may undergo sporulation. Fungal spores are ubiquitous in the environment and immunologically inert until their germination into yeast or hyphae.
- Molds are responsible for most noninvasive and invasive forms of FRS and are further classified into septate, pauci-septate, or aseptate as well as dematiaceous or hyaline.
- Pauci-septate or aseptate molds—largely responsible for invasive disease
  (a) **Class *Zygomycetes***
    - Order *Mucorales*
      - Genera *Rhizopus, Mucor, Rhizomucor, Absidia, Cunninghamella*
- Septate molds—largely responsible for non-invasive disease
  (a) **Dematiaceous** molds (dark-colored)
    - *Bipolaris, Curvularia, Penicillum, Alternaria, Cladosporium*
  (b) **Hyaline** molds (light-colored)
    - *Aspergillus, Pseudallescheria, Fusarium*
- "Mucormycosis" should not be used interchangeably with AIFS as other molds within the class Zygomycetes as well as *Aspergillus* are common etiologic organisms.
- Fungi are universally found within normal healthy human nose and paranasal sinuses, likely via inhalational spores.
- The pathogenicity of sinonasal fungus depends on the host's immune system; in immunocompetent hosts, the relationship is most commonly commensal.

Noninvasive Fungal Sinusitis

Fungal Ball (Mycetoma, Aspergilloma)

- Presents largely in immunocompetent patients.
- Dense amalgamation of fungal hyphae can be identified in the involved sinus.
- This entity usually affects a single sinus, but may also affect multiple sinuses in ipsilateral or bilateral disease.
  (a) Maxillary sinus (most common)
  (b) Sphenoid sinus (second most common)
  (c) Ethmoid sinus > frontal sinus

- Many fungal balls are asymptomatic and incidentally found on radiologic exams performed for other reasons (ie, head computed tomography [CT], dental X-rays).
- However, fungal balls may be associated with chronic rhinosinusitis (CRS) or recurrent acute rhinosinusitis (RARS) of the involved sinus. Nonspecific symptoms may include:
  (a) Pressure and fullness of the cheek or forehead (maxillary sinus, frontal sinus)
  (b) Retro-orbital pressure (sphenoid sinus)
  (c) Nasal drainage (purulent if secondary bacterial infection)

Diagnosis

- Endoscopy:
  (a) Endoscopy may vary from normal to mild mucosal edema to frank polyposis with mucopurulence.
  (b) Grossly, fungal balls have been described as gritty, dirt-like, clay-like, chalky, or cheesy debris. The underlying mucosa appears edematous and inflamed. These findings confirm the preoperative diagnosis (Figure 27-1).
- CT:
  (a) Nonenhanced sinus CT is the study of choice.
  (b) CT often demonstrates a partially or completely opacified sinus.
  (c) It most commonly affects the maxillary sinus followed by the sphenoid sinus.
  (d) Areas of differential densities within the opacified sinus are more specific and provide evidence for the diagnosis (Figure 27-2).
  (e) Bony confines of the affected sinus are often thickened and hyperostotic. CT may also reveal bony remodeling or erosion.

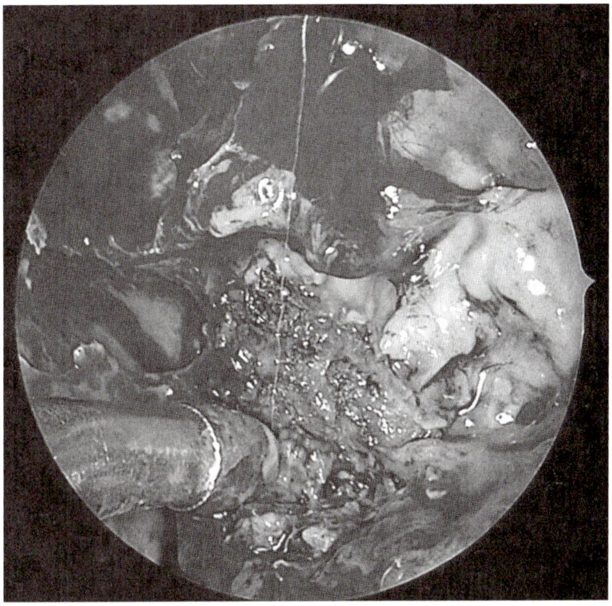

Figure 27-1 Intraoperative endoscopy into the left maxillary sinus reveals dense, chalky, discrete balls of fungal elements and associated purulent debris.

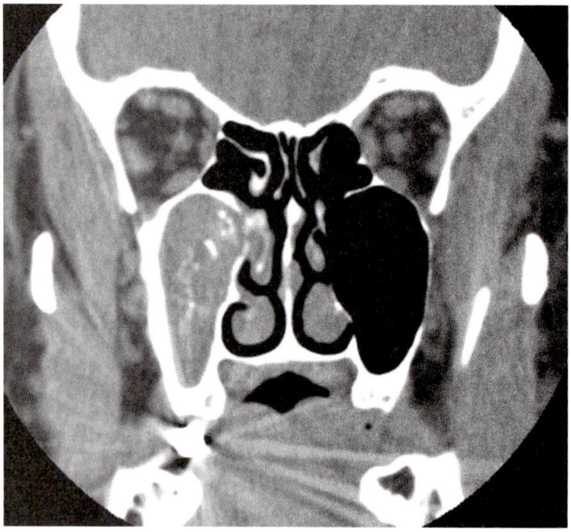

Figure 27-2 Coronal CT in soft tissue window of a patient with isolated right maxillary fungal ball demonstrates multifocal hyperdensities, sinus opacification, and sinus wall thickening.

- Magnetic resonance imaging (MRI):
  (a) MRI is less specific than CT in diagnosis.
  (b) Dehydration of the fungal content produces variable low signal intensities in T1/T2 weighted MR images. Calcification and paramagnetic substances in the fungal ball may contribute to areas of low T2 signal.
  (c) Longstanding disease may produce loss of signals in T1 and T2 MRI, mimicking aerated sinuses.
  (d) Fungal content will not enhance with administration of gadolinium; however, inflamed peripheral mucosa will demonstrate enhancement.
- Culture and pathology
  (a) A*spergillus species* are most commonly implicated by histology as cultures are often unrevealing and may be negative in as many as 70% of cases.
  (b) Microscopic examination of the sinus mucosa demonstrates the following: (Figure 27-3)
    - Densely packed conglomeration of septate fungal hyphae (dematiaceous or hyaline molds)
    - Nonspecific chronic inflammatory changes without evidence of fungal invasion

Treatment

- Surgery is the mainstay of treatment.
  (a) Oral and topical antifungal therapy is ineffective against fungal balls.
  (b) Postoperative medical treatment is frequently deployed but should not be considered necessary.
- Goals of surgery
  (a) Confirm diagnosis
  (b) Complete extirpation of fungal debris
  (c) Wide ostial patency for postoperative irrigation, debridement, and surveillance

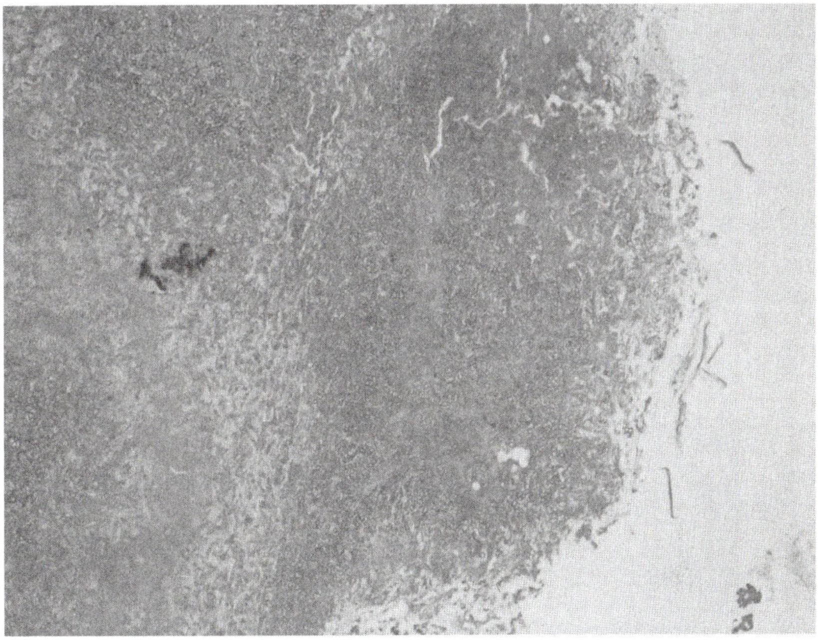

Figure 27-3 A large fungal ball under intermediate powered microscopy reveals tightly packed hyphae with inflammatory exudates and cell debris. Fungal invasion is not seen.

- Recurrence is uncommon after thorough endoscopic surgery.
- Rare progression of fungal ball to invasive FRS has been documented in immunocompromised patients. Risk for progression or secondary infection and the unlikelihood of spontaneous disease resolution suggest that surgical treatment is indicated even in asymptomatic individuals.
- Surveillance may be offered in clinically quiescent fungal balls in elderly patients or those with significant medical comorbidities and anesthetic risks.

Allergic Fungal Rhinosinusitis (AFRS)

- This noninvasive form of FRS commonly presents with nasal polyposis, of which hypersensitivity to extramucosal fungi is the basis.
- AFRS is considered a subtype of chronic rhinosinusitis—accounting for 5% to 10% of CRS cases.
- It commonly affects young, immunocompetent individuals with fungal atopy.
- Highest incidence occurs in the south along the Mississippi basin, the southeast, and the southwest secondary to the climatic exposure (ie, warm temperatures, high humidity) to fungi which facilitate their proliferation.
- First recognized by Safirstein et al. in 1976, AFRS shares clinical similarity with allergic bronchopulmonary aspergillosis (ABPA). Thick, inspissated mucus were found in the paranasal sinuses as well as the bronchial passages of ABPA patients.
- The thick, viscous green/brown mucous found in the paranasal sinuses of AFRS patients is known as allergic mucin, or more accurately, eosinophilic mucin (EM) (Figure 27-4).

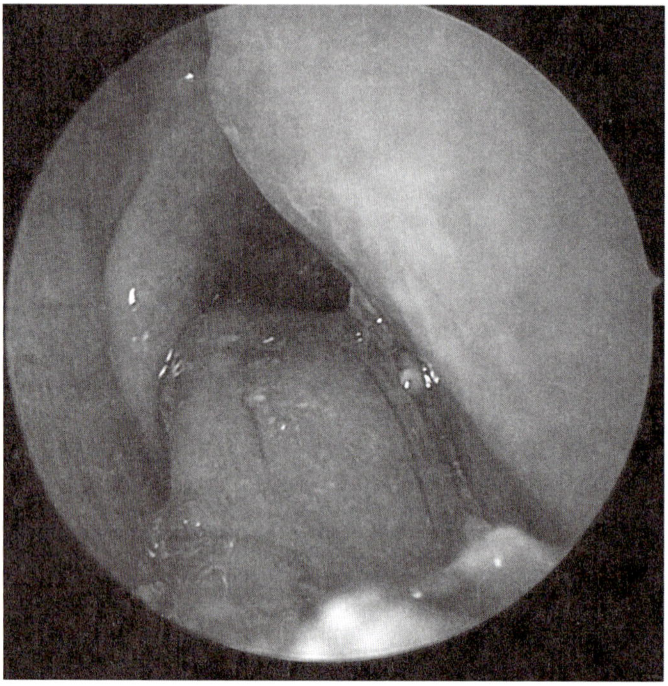

Figure 27-4 Allergic fungal rhinosinusitis is characterized by the presence of thick, inspissated eosinophilic mucin demonstrated in this endoscopic image.

(a) EM is characterized by necrotic inflammatory cells, eosinophils, and Charcot-Leyden crystals (byproduct of eosinophil breakdown), and commonly contains elements of fungal hyphae that are readily visualized with fungal stains.

- AFRS is known for its high recidivism and resistance to conventional therapy with antifungals, steroids, and surgical extirpation.

Pathophysiology

- Abnormal IgE-mediated immune response to fungal antigen incites an influx of eosinophils and mast cells via inflammatory pathways leading to mucus stasis, mucosal edema, ostial obstruction, build-up of tenacious fungal debris, and polyp formation.
  (a) This fungal-driven locally destructive immune response may then expand to adjacent sinuses and incite sinus expansion and bone erosion.
  (b) In addition to IgE, recent evidence suggests a robust, epithelial cell-driven Th2 immune response (ie, IL-25, IL-33, TSLP) in both AFRS and CRSwNP.
- *Aspergillus* and the dematiaceous fungi (*Alternaria, Bipolaris, Curvularia, Exophilia, Fusarium*) have been implicated. Classically, a large, predominant fungal load is identified within the eosinophilic mucin of the affected sinuses, suggesting its etiologic role.
- Controversy
  (a) Despite the classic, well-known Bent and Kuhn diagnostic criteria (see below), its clinical application is not universally accepted, given the incomplete understanding of the pathogenesis of AFRS.
  (b) As fungus could be cultured from the majority of healthy controls and CRS patients, the distinction between AFRS and AFS-like CRS remains in contention.

(c) Eosinophilic inflammation remains the central theme in what appears to be a spectrum of disease.
(d) **Eosinophilic mucin rhinosinusitis (EMRS)**
- Clinical (ie, gross) features of AFRS.
- The driving pathological mechanism is not a hypersensitivity to fungal antigen, but rather a systemic dysregulation associated with upper and lower airway eosinophilia.
  1. Absence of fungus (ie, lack of identifiable fungal elements in cultures or histologically on smears)
  2. Absence of IgE-mediated fungal hypersensitivity
- Peripheral total IgE is elevated, albeit significantly less so than that of AFRS.
- Driving pathological mechanism is not hypersensitivity to fungal antigen but systemic immunologic dysregulation of upper and lower airway and mucosal barrier disruption.
- As a systemic disease, EMRS presents uniformly with bilateral involvement and is more commonly associated with aspirin-sensitive asthma, and IgG1 immunodeficiency than does classic AFRS.

(e) **Non-allergic eosinophilic fungal rhinosinusitis (EFRS)**
- Clinical features of AFRS
  1. Presence of fungus (ie, positive cultures or visualized in eosinophilic mucin)
  2. Absence of IgE-mediated fungal hypersensitivity on skin-prick and intradermal testing
- There is also a lack of significant peripheral total or fungal-specific IgE elevation; however, local sinonasal IgE levels remain elevated.
- It was therefore postulated that certain fungi could elicit eosinophilic inflammation and mucosal epithelial barrier disruption with major basic protein (MBP) in the absence of type I hypersensitivity.

(f) More than fungal antigens, other possible contributors to the process of eosinophilic inflammation include staphylococcal-derived superantigens.
- Superantigen has the ability to incite massive immune reaction through nonspecific polyclonal activation of T cells.
- Specific IgE to staphylococcal enterotoxin (SE-IgE) is an independent risk for asthma and total IgE elevation, and is found in high percentage of AFRS patients in some study cohorts.
- Both fungi and *Staphylococcus aureus* have been detected on electron microscopy of biofilm in AFRS patients.

Diagnosis

- Clinical Presentation
  (a) Insidious onset and slow progression lasting months to years are typical.
  (b) CRS symptomatology (mucous drainage, nasal obstruction, facial pressure, smell loss) with allergic component (ie, sneezing, watery eyes).
  (c) Advanced cases may present with bony dehiscence and/or orbital deformities such as proptosis from bony expansion.
- Diagnostic criteria
  (a) Bent and Kuhn (1994)
  - Major criteria
    1. Type I hypersensitivity to common fungi
    2. Nasal polyposis
    3. Characteristic CT findings (see below)

4. Eosinophilic mucin without fungal invasion
5. Positive fungal stain/smear

- Minor criteria
  1. Asthma
  2. Unilateral disease
  3. Bone erosion on CT
  4. Fungal culture
  5. Charcot-Leyden crystals
  6. Serum eosinophilia
- According to Bent and Kuhn, formal diagnosis of AFRS requires meeting all five major criteria, while the minor criteria act to support the diagnosis.

- CT
  (a) Ethmoid sinuses are most commonly involved, followed by maxillary, sphenoid, and frontal sinuses.
  (b) Sinus expansion may be present with bony demineralization, remodeling, or erosion, which in severe cases may lead to telecanthus or other facial deformities.
  (c) Partial to full opacification of involved sinuses may be unilateral or bilateral; eosinophilic mucin causes increased attenuation on noncontrast CT (Figure 27-5).
  (d) Differential density is related to heavy metals or calcium salt precipitate within the mucin. Heterogeneous attenuation may be punctate foci or diffuse, ground glass in pattern.

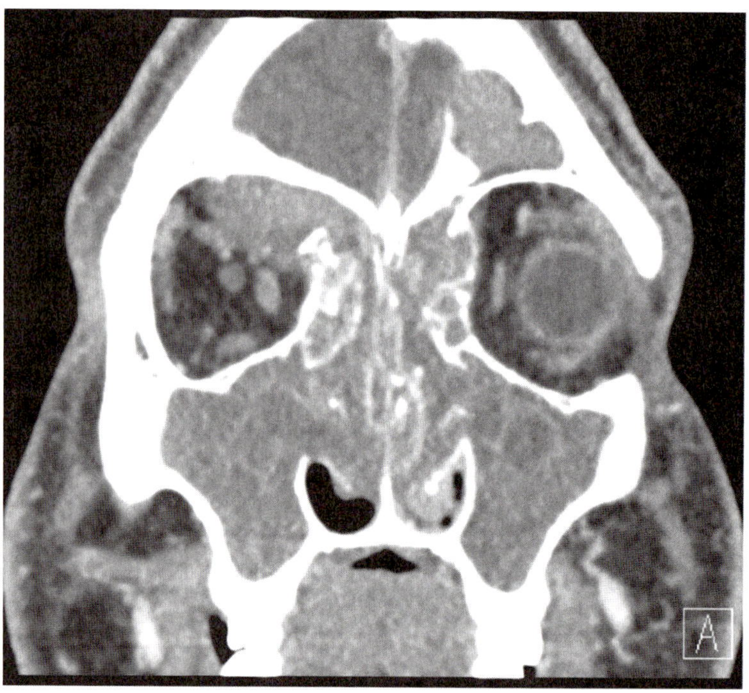

Figure 27-5 Coronal CT at the level of the posterior ethmoid sinuses demonstrating diffuse and extensive bilateral maxillary and ethmoid sinuses opacification and heterogeneous attenuation suggesting allergic fungal rhinosinusitis. There is also evidence of bony erosion along the medial orbital wall.

- MRI
  (a) High-protein concentration and dehydration of mucin causes isointense to hypointense T1 signal and hypointense to signal void on T2-weighted imaging.
  (b) Sinus mucosa demonstrates peripheral enhancement with contrast, while eosinophilic mucin does not enhance.
- Culture and pathology
  (a) Culture may help confirm diagnosis or assist in treatment of associated bacterial infection.
  (b) Tissue histology demonstrates polypoid mucosa with prominent eosinophilic infiltrates.
  (c) Eosinophilic mucin aspirate (most sensitive)
    - Branching, noninvasive fungal hyphae (may be absent)
    - Typical lamellated sheets of eosinophils
    - Elongated eosinophilic breakdown products known as Charcot-Leyden crystals

Treatment

- Surgery combined with topical and oral corticosteroids is the standard of care.
- Goals of surgery are the same in all forms of noninvasive fungal disease (see earlier discussion). Surgery should be performed in a meticulous, thorough manner to allow for complete surgical extirpation of fungal disease and patency of involved sinuses for topical delivery of medication.
- Prolonged postoperative surveillance is indicated for its high recidivism.
- Corticosteroids
  - Retrospective evidence has demonstrated improved outcomes with use of topical and systemic corticosteroids (ie, improved symptom scores, fewer revision surgeries, and disease recurrences)
    - In general, prednisone should be administered in the immediate postoperative period. Some clinicians utilize prednisone 0.5 mg/kg/day for 2 to 3 weeks with tapered perioperative steroids to reduce intraoperative inflammatory burden and bleeding.
    - Topical steroids as nasal sprays or irrigations may be used concomitantly in a prolonged setting. This can be tapered off following the stabilization of mucosal health.
  - No rigorous analysis has confirmed the utility of one treatment protocol over the other. However, in recent years, as the long-term effects of systemic corticosteroids are more readily recognized, the focus has shifted toward enhancing delivery of topical corticosteroids which remain a mainstay.
  - Traditional methods of topical steroid delivery have been shown to have limited deposition in upper and posterior parts of the nasal cavity and sinuses (frontal and sphenoid sinuses in particular). In recent years, to address this challenge, exhalation delivery systems using fluticasone (EDS-FLU) have demonstrated significant promise in improving drug deposition in these areas.
- Immunotherapy (IT)
  (a) Immunotherapy with fungal antigens to dematiaceous species has been shown in limited retrospective studies to decrease polyp recurrence, nasal crusting, quality of life, decreased systemic corticosteroid use, and quality of life.
  (b) Postoperative IT may also reduce rates of recurrence and revision surgery.
  (c) Fear of the theoretical risk of iatrogenic type III (immune-complex mediated) reaction from fungal allergen-specific IgG has limited immunotherapy research. However, thus far, no study has reported any type III reactions or other severe local or delayed reactions.

- Biologic agents
  - (a) Available agents being approved for CRSwNP target type II inflammatory mediators; IgE, IL-4, IL-5, and IL-13. Their role in AFRS has been focused on recalcitrant disease.
  - (b) Dupilumab, a blocker of IL-4 and IL-13 signaling, is currently undergoing phase III clinical trials for AFRS. At present, the published literature on its effectiveness is limited to case reports and case series, some of which have demonstrated improvement.
  - (c) In a study of patients with AFRS and concurrent asthma, monthly mepolizumab, an IL-5 inhibitor, demonstrated improvements in objective modified Lund-Kennedy scores and eosinophil counts.
  - (d) IgE blocker, Omalizumab may also have a role in AFRS management given the elevated, often exaggerated serum IgE associated with the disease.
- Culture-directed antibiotics should be administered for any evidence of frank mucopurulence. AFRS exacerbations are often heralded by secondary acute bacterial sinus infections. Of note, patients with AFRS exhibit significantly higher levels of *S. aureus* compared to those without AFRS, although its exact role in the disease's pathogenesis remains unclear.
  - (a) Empirical use of antistaphylococcal agents in postoperative regimen is used by some otolaryngologists.
  - (b) Mupirocin irrigation—with its effectiveness against planktonic and biofilm forms of *S. aureus*—also has theoretical benefits.
- Antifungals
  - (a) Sparse, uncontrolled case series have not demonstrated support for use of topical or oral antifungals in AFS.
  - (b) Cochrane reviews of both topical and oral antifungals in the broader CRS population do not show any benefit.
  - (c) Oral or topical antifungals are not recommended.

Saprophytic Fungal Infestation

- Fungal colonization of mucous crusts occurs within the nasal and paranasal cavities.
- Ubiquitous environmental fungal spores germinate over moist crusting.
- This affects patients who have undergone previous nasal or sinus surgeries with disrupted mucociliary clearance.
- Patients are usually asymptomatic or complain of foul odor.
- Diagnosis is clinical and based on endoscopic surveillance examination.
- Treatment is endoscopic debridement of spore-encrusted mucous secretions; recurrence is rare after thorough debridement.
- Potential progression of untreated infestation into fungal ball has been predicted.

Invasive Fungal Sinusitis

Acute Invasive Fungal Sinusitis

- Hallmark of invasive fungal sinusitis is perineural invasion or angioinvasion by fungi.
- AIFS affects immunocompromised individuals, specifically with neutropenia or neutrophil dysfunction.
  - (a) Hematologic malignancies (ic, bone marrow transplantation)
  - (b) Chemotherapy-induced neutropenia
  - (c) Chronic immunosuppression (ie, solid organ transplantation)

(d) Diabetes with ketoacidosis
(e) Advanced HIV infection (eg, AIDS) with concomitant neutrophil dysfunction
(f) Dialysis patients administered deferoxamine

- Early diagnosis is crucial as the infection is rapidly progressive and fatal if not properly identified and promptly treated.
- Tissue biopsy is paramount for rapid diagnosis and treatment in patients with comorbid risk factors.
- Mortality rate remains high despite treatment; largest systematic review demonstrates 50% mortality for all-cause acute invasive fungal sinusitis (AIFS).
  (a) Negative prognosticators: advanced age, palatal or facial involvement, severe neutropenia ($\leq$ 500 neutrophils/μL blood), CRP elevation ($\geq$ 5.50 mg/dL), altered mental status, renal/liver failure, intracranial extension
  (b) Positive prognosticators: reversible immunosuppression (ie, diabetes with ketoacidosis), surgical resection, treatment with liposomal amphotericin B

Mycology

- Causative fungal species are widely distributed within the environment; normally functioning as saprophytes.
- Fungal spores may inhabit the aerodigestive tract and become pathogenic under optimized conditions.
- The most common causative fungi are the Zygomycetes class/Mucorales order of fungi (ie, Mucor, Rhizopus), followed by the *Aspergillus* species.
- "Mucormycosis" refers to a specific fungal infection and should not be used interchangeably as "AIFS" unless confirmed by culture speciation.
- Although Mucor species are suggested to be more aggressive, often associated with increased neurovascular and orbital invasion, multiple studies have shown that the type of fungus does not predict survival outcomes.
- Zygomycetes (class)
  (a) Fast-growing, coenocytic molds, with irregular nonseptate or pauci-septate hyphae branching at wide angles (typically 90°).
  (b) *Mucorales* (order)
    - *Rhizopus—most common in AIFS, Mucor, Rhizomucor, Absidia, Cunninghamella* (genera)
  (c) Growth of Mucorales fungi is facilitated by acidotic conditions by its enzyme, ketone reductase; as such, patients with diabetic ketoacidosis are uniquely at risk for AIFS.
  (d) Abnormal transferrin binding in diabetic or dialysis patients, leading to iron overload, has been implicated in enhancing fungal growth and pathogenicity, particularly at risk are those receiving iron-chelating agents such as deferoxamine. Deferoxamine acts as a siderophore for Rhizopus species, increasing iron uptake and thereby promoting fungal proliferation and invasion.
- *Aspergillus* (genus)
  (a) Ubiquitous hyaline mold with regular septate hyphae branching at acute angles (45°)
    - *Fumigatus*—most common Aspergillus AIFS, *flavus, niger, terreus* (species)

Diagnosis

- Clinical Presentation
  (a) Variable presentation of rhinosinusitis which can make diagnosis highly challenging—insidious to rapid onset and progression over days to weeks
    - Mucous drainage, nasal obstruction, facial pressure, smell loss, fever, epistaxis, foul smell; there is no pathognomonic symptom.

   (b) Vision changes and neurological deficits (ie, mental status changes, cranial nerve deficits, esp. numbness) need to be explicitly sought on history and exam as extrasinus extension are common and indicative of advanced, progressive disease. The infraorbital nerve and associated premaxillary numbness is frequently present.
- Physical exam
   (a) Nasal cavity: Commonly with mucosal edema and mucous drainage that is indistinguishable from other causes of rhinosinusitis; edema alone may be the indicative of early AIFS. Rarely, more worrisome signs of white necrotic debris or black eschar (typically mucor) may present and involve the turbinate and septum.
   (b) Orbit: proptosis, ecchymosis, ophthalmoplegia, blindness.
   (c) Oral cavity: hard or soft palate ischemia or necrosis (Figure 27-6).
   (d) Nasal endoscopy: pale, ischemic mucosa (early), thick crusting and mucous, mucopurulence, anesthesia to manipulation, minimal to absent bleeding on biopsy, frank necrosis and ulceration (late).
- Laboratory workup
   (a) Basal metabolic panel to assess for hyperglycemia/ketoacidosis and CBC with differential to assess the absolute neutrophil count should be checked.
   (b) No absolute plasma glucose level has been definitively linked with AIFS.
   (c) Patients with ANC less than 500/μL are at highest risk.
- Tissue biopsy
   (a) Gold standard for diagnosis: operative endoscopy and biopsy may be more sensitive than bedside evaluation. Areas most commonly involved include the middle turbinate, nasal septum or nasal floor.

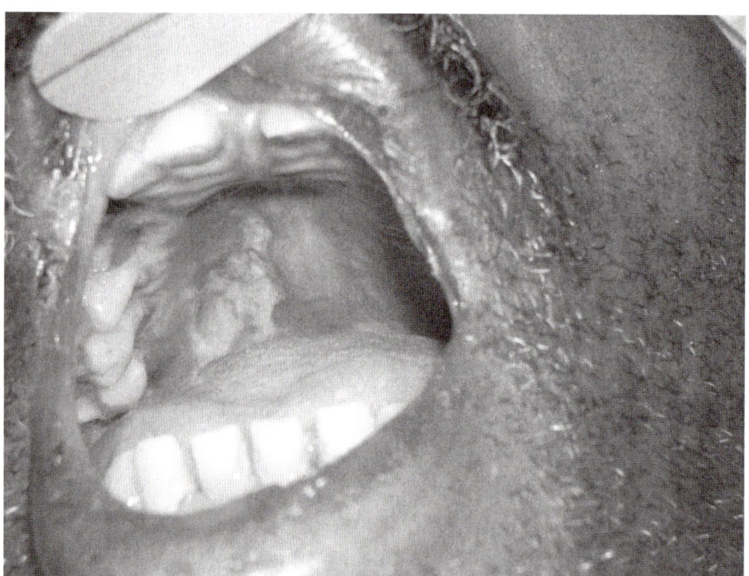

Figure 27-6 Clinical photograph showing ulcer with necrosis in the anterior palate in a patient with palatal mucormycosis.

(b) Angioinvasion or perineural invasion of fungal elements are pathognomonic for AIFS.
  - Absence of fungal hyphae on initial biopsy does not rule out AIFS when high clinical suspicion exists and may warrant further workup including imaging or formal surgical exploration.

(c) Frozen section biopsies remain key in early diagnosis with high sensitivity and specificity.
  - Antero-inferior portion of middle turbinate best site for biopsy
  - 85% sensitivity, 100% specificity
  - Multiple biopsies of suspicious nasal sites may enhance sensitivity.

(d) Definitive histologic stains to identify fungus must include the silver stain; calcofluor white stain may also be used.
  - Silver is deposited into the fungal cell wall readily and therefore is very sensitive to fungal cells.
  - Gram and H&E stains highlight fungal cytoplasm which may be sparse due to rapid cytoplasmic transference to growing fungal tips; high false negatives.

- Culture
  (a) Due to the time required for fungal growth, awaiting culture results is ill-advised, and the absence of growth does not rule out invasive disease.
  (b) However, positive fungal culture may guide antifungal therapy and support the diagnosis in the appropriate clinical setting.
- PCR
  (a) Broad-range PCR is an effective tool for diagnosing invasive fungal infections and identifying fungal species. Studies support it as a complement to traditional methods.
  (b) Preliminary and final results are obtained faster than with culture, with an improved ability to identify fungal species, including rare ones that are difficult to identify morphologically.
- Fungal culture, direct examination, PCR, and antifungal susceptibility testing are collectively recommended for AIFS cases, as they can identify cases that other assays might miss.
- Imaging is nonspecific for AIFS.
- CT
  (a) Noncontrast CT of the sinuses is the modality of choice to assess bony changes and mucoperiosteal thickening.
  (b) Unilateral soft tissue mucosal thickening along turbinates, septum, nasal walls are consistent early CT findings.
    - Mucosal irregularities are often consistent with endoscopic findings of mucosal edema, inflammation, or necrosis.
    - Sinus opacification is also a nonspecific finding.

  a) Worrisome CT findings include soft tissue emphysema and bony erosion—the latter suggesting late-phase changes.

  (c) Extrasinus fat stranding or infiltration needs to be evaluated closely for potential involvement.
    - Periantral soft tissue infiltration (ie, obliteration of fat, nasal floor, or palatal defect)
    - Intraorbital extension from ethmoid disease (may occur without lamina papyracea dehiscence)
    - Masticator space
    - Pterygopalatine and infratemporal fossae

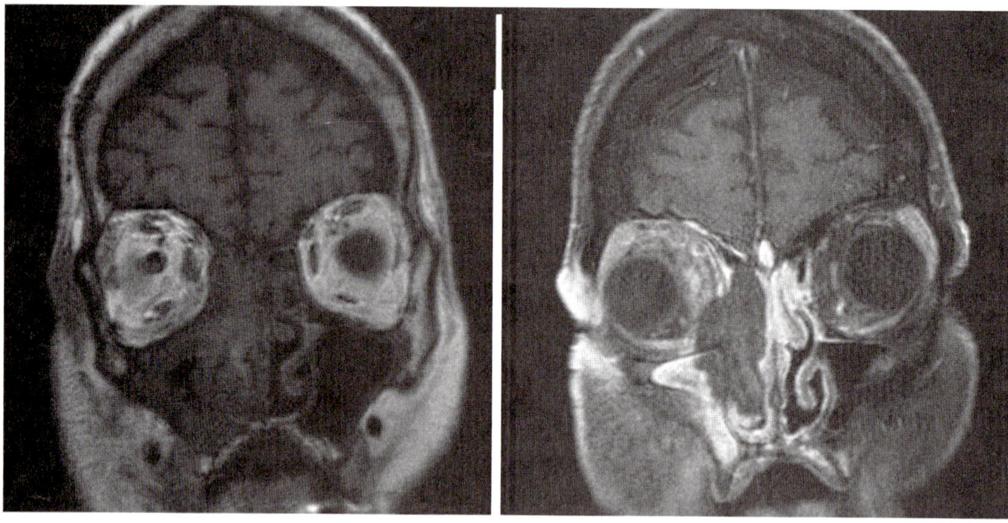

Figure 27-7 Angioinvasion of acute invasive fungal sinusitis causes devascularization of sinonasal mucosa, in particular the middle turbinate, which does not enhance on post-contrast enhanced T1-weighted MRI (right pane). This is referred to as the *black turbinate sign* and is important for the early detection of AIFS.

- MRI
  (a) MRI with contrast (gadolinium, Gd) is the modality of choice to evaluate soft tissue extension.
  (b) T1 and T2 demonstrate low to intermediate signaling in affected regions.
  (c) "Black turbinate sign" or the lack of enhancement with Gd in the sinonasal mucosa on T1/T2 signal is highly suggestive of mucosal necrosis from fungal angioinvasion (Figure 27-7). On the other hand, extra-sinus invasion would typically be enhanced with Gd.
  (d) Particular attention should be paid to orbit or cranial invasion.
    - Leptomingeal involvement
    - Cavernous sinus thrombosis (ie, engorgement of superior ophthalmic vein)
    - Intracranial extension

Treatment

- Three pillars of treatment include surgical eradication of disease, reversal of immunosuppression, and prolonged intravenous antifungal therapy. Currently, there are no evidence-based recommendations for the diagnosis, prognosis, and treatment of AIFS. Previous documents have outlined these aspects, but most recommendations remain based on expert opinion.
- Several studies have shown that early surgery, within 7 days of diagnosis, (improving survival rates from 57.1% to 83.5%). In contrast, delays of over 14 days from disease onset significantly worsen outcomes, increasing death rates from 30.9% to 33.3%.
- Surgical debridement
  (a) There is a lack of literature and guidelines on the necessary extent of resection, the role of extended surgical approaches, the choice between open, endoscopic, or combined techniques, and the considerations for repeat resections following initial treatment.

(b) Endoscopic surgery may be preferred for disease limited to the sinonasal cavity. At times, extensive endoscopic techniques such as Denker's or Caldwell-Luc antrostomy and medial maxillectomy for maxillary sinus disease, transmaxillary approaches for pterygopalatine or infratemporal involvement, and Draf III for frontal disease may be necessary.
(c) Open approaches (ie, maxillectomy, orbital exenteration) reserved for the presence of intraorbital extension, palatal, and/or intracerebral involvement.
(d) Unfortunately, aggressive open-approach resection including orbital exenteration has not been shown to improve outcomes.
   - In large systematic review, patients who underwent endoscopic resection had improved survival (64%) compared to those with open resection (54%).
   - No statistically significant improvement in survival outcome in patients undergoing orbital exenteration.
   - These findings may be secondary to higher fungal burden in those who received open surgical approaches. In effort to reduce the fungal load, patients and caregivers must be counseled accordingly prior to disfiguring debridement.
(e) In general, extent of debridement includes nonviable tissue until normal bleeding mucosal surfaces or noneroded bony confines are reached. Despite loss of surgical landmarks in advanced disease, meticulous dissection and maintenance of the skull base is important in preventing intracranial extension of disease.
(f) Intraoperative frozen section analysis has been used to guide surgical debridement. While frozen sections have a 100% positive predictive value for AIFRS, the negative predictive value is only 70%, meaning a negative result does not guarantee clear margins.
(g) "Second-look" endoscopic evaluation of residual disease should be performed at regular intervals following initial surgery until stabilization of sinonasal mucosa.

- Reversal of immunosuppression
  (a) Consultation with appropriate specialties
     - Endocrinology: reversal of hyperglycemia in diabetic, ketoacidotic patients
     - Rheumatology, nephrology, hepatology: autoimmune disorders and solid organ transplantations
  (b) Survival outcomes are improved in patients whose immunosuppression can be rapidly reversed (ie, diabetes).
- Hyperbaric oxygen has been utilized adjunctively in small case series; however, evidence of its usefulness in AIFS is still lacking.
- Immune enhancement therapies in AIFS are investigational and lack evidence for wider application; strategies have been employed in intractable disease in small case series with mixed results.
  (a) Cytokine therapy: GM-CSF, G-CSF (widely used to reduce neutropenic days and neutropenia-related hospitalization), M-CSF, IFN-gamma
  (b) Granulocyte transfusion
- Prolonged antifungal therapy
  (a) Depending on the suspected fungal organism, amphotericin B, azoles, and caspofungin have all been effective in reducing mortality.
  (b) Evidence on the optimal duration of treatment is limited, but factors such as disease extent, hematologic status, timing of surgery, and smoking status may influence treatment length.

(c) Amphotericin B
- Antifungal of choice for empirical treatment of AIFS when culture results are unavailable or if speciation reveals zygomycosis.
- The basis of empiric amphotericin is based on expert opinion and is principled on its broad-spectrum coverage of Mucorales and aspergillus.
  1. 1 mg/kg/day for conventional formulation (significantly less costly)
  2. 5 mg/kg/day for liposomal formulation (eg, Ambisome → or Abelcet → are preferred for reduced nephrotoxicity and increased CNS penetration)
  3. Lipid formulations are as effective as conventional deoxycholate formulation.
  4. Some retrospective studies have found that patients who received liposomal formulations of amphotericin B had an overall improved survival compared to those receiving conventional amphotericin B.
- Poor side effect profile: nephrotoxicity from acute tubular necrosis, anaphylaxis
- *Aspergillus terreus* is inherently resistant to amphotericin.

(d) Voriconazole
- Antifungal of choice for AIFS by *Aspergillus* spp. and *Pseudallescheria boydii*
  1. In multicenter randomized trial for invasive aspergillosis, voriconazole was found to have improved partial or complete response, lower mortality, regimen change, and side effect profile than amphotericin B deoxycholate.
- Trough measurements are needed to keep serum concentration between 1 and 5.5 μg/mL due to variable metabolism in patients.
- Mucorales species are intrinsically resistant to voriconazole.
- Typically, treatment begins with IV administration and then transitions to oral therapy based on clinical, biochemical, and radiologic assessments.

(e) Isavuconazole
- Approved by US Food and Drug Administration (FDA) in 2015 for treatment of invasive aspergillosis based on noninferiority trial against voriconazole.
- Used as an alternative to voriconazole in AIFS caused by *Aspergillus* spp.

(f) Posaconazole
- Approved by FDA in 2013 for treatment of invasive aspergillosis and candidiasis.
- In vitro potency against *Aspergillus* and *Zygomycetes* is similar to that of amphotericin and greater than voriconazole.
- Used as an alternative to voriconazole or amphotericin B in AIFS.

(g) Itraconazole is not proven to be effective against invasive fungal disease in immunocompromised patients.

(h) Oral antifungal agents may be initiated for long-term administration (ie, 3-6 months) after control of disease—or indefinitely in those who require lifelong immunosuppression.
- Oral posaconazole and isavuconazole have been used.

(i) Current data does not support a recommendation for the use of topical antifungals in AIFS.

(j) Intraorbital antifungal therapy has limited evidence, studies have lacked standardized protocols, and offers no clear benefit for orbital preservation. However, it may be considered for patients with complete vision loss and ophthalmoplegia, as it poses minimal harm.

An infectious disease consult is warranted for antifungal management.

- Surveillance

(a) No consensus; a few studies have varied between weekly or bi-weekly nasal endoscopy after initiating antifungal therapy and surgical debridement until reversal of neutropenia and immune function recovery.

(b) A study has advocated for extended follow-up until normal sinus function and re-mucosalization are fully restored. Survivors may develop significant scarring and sinus obstruction. Some may experience other sinonasal infectious complications or recurrences over a year after the initial surgery.

Chronic Invasive Fungal Sinusitis

- Chronic, indolent form (lasting > 4 weeks) of fungal rhinosinusitis with tissue invasion.
- Likely a less fulminant form of AIFS.
- Affects older patients who are immunocompetent or mildly immunocompromised (ie, diabetes mellitus or low-dose glucocorticoids).
- Hyaline mold (*Aspergillus* spp.) and dematiaceous molds are more commonly implicated than mucorales spp.
- Commonly presents with months of symptoms typical of chronic rhinosinusitis (ie, maxillary pressure) prior to development of a complication.
  - Proptosis or visual changes from orbital invasion
  - Neurologic changes or cranial neuropathies
  - Pre-antral cellulitis

Diagnosis

- Similar to that AIFS; however, time course and immune status distinguishes chronic invasive fungal sinusitis from AIFS.
- Tissue biopsy is vital for diagnosis.
  (a) Dense hyphae similar to that of fungal ball
  (b) Tissue invasion with necrosis
- CT
  (a) Affected sinus(es) with mass lesion and mucosal thickening
  (b) Bony erosion and extra-sinus involvement are common
- MRI
  (a) Similar to AIFS. T1 and T2 with iso-or hypointense signals relative to muscle in affected regions

Treatment

- Similar to that of AIFS
  (a) Reversal of immunosuppression
  (b) Surgical debridement
  (c) Prolonged antifungal treatment
- Long-term surveillance is indicated.

Granulomatous Invasive Fungal Sinusitis

- Rare form of chronic invasive fungal rhinosinusitis characterized by granuloma formation.
- Mainly reported in Middle East, South Asia, and African countries (ie, Sudan, India, Pakistan, Saudi Arabia); more rarely in the United States.
- Largely affects healthy, immunocompetent patients.
- *Aspergillus flavus* and *Aspergillus fumigatus* most common causative pathogens.
- Most common symptom is unilateral proptosis rather than CRS symptoms.
- Often mistaken for a suspected tumor until intraoperative evaluation and pathology confirmation.
- Disease is often advanced due to its indolent nature.

Diagnosis

- Biopsy
  (a) Noncaseating granuloma formation with foreign body reaction
  (b) Multinucleated giant cells
  (c) Dense background fibrosis and vasculitis
- CT
  (a) Large expansive, hyperdense mass with homogenous contrast enhancement
    - Lack dual-density secretion commonly seen in fungal balls
  (b) Bony erosion and extra-sinus involvement are common
- MRI
  (a) T1/T2 hypointensity
  (b) Intense, homogenous enhancement
  (c) Cerebritis—foci of parenchymal enhancement—are commonly found adjacent to solid lesion

Treatment

- Limited experience due to rarity
- Surgical resection and prolonged antifungal therapy.
  (a) Surgery is crucial due to the poor penetration of antifungal drugs into fibrotic lesions.
- Most studies note complete regression or clinical improvement in the majority of patients who undergo treatment
- Case reports support conservative, orbit-sparing surgical approaches given their responsiveness to therapy.

Conclusion

- Fungal rhinosinusitis encompasses a wide range of fungal-related inflammatory disorders from colonization, hypersensitivity, to infection.
- Current classification scheme subdivides FRS into noninvasive and invasive forms; invasive forms may be rapidly deteriorating and fatal if expeditious diagnosis and treatment is not accomplished.
- Endoscopic evaluation and surgery provide a powerful tool for diagnosis confirmation and treatment in all forms of FRS.
- The role of fungi in AFRS, EFRS, and EMRS remains controversial and unclear; however, eosinophilic inflammation plays a common role.

Bibliography

Chakrabarti A, Denning DW, Ferguson BJ, et al. Fungal rhinosinusitis: a categorization and definitional schema addressing current controversies. *Laryngoscope*. 2009;119:1809-1818.

Ferguson BJ. Eosinophilic mucin rhinosinusitis: a distinct clinicopathological entity. *Laryngoscope*. 2000;110:799-813.

Mabry RL, Mabry CS. Allergic fungal sinusitis: the role of immunotherapy. *Otolaryngol Clin North Am*. 2000;33:433-440.

Safirstein BH. Allergic bronchopulmonary aspergillosis with obstruction of the upper respiratory tract. *Chest*. 1976; 70:788-790.

Turner JH, Soudry E, Nayak JV, et al. Survival outcomes in acute invasive fungal sinusitis: a systematic review and quantitative synthesis of published evidence. *Laryngoscope*. 2013;123:1112-1118.

Questions

1. Which of the following portends a better prognosis in acute invasive fungal sinusitis?
   A. Lack of visual or neurological symptoms
   B. *Aspergillus* as causative fungus
   C. Aggressive open-approach resection
   D. Diabetic patient in ketoacidosis

2. Which of the following is true regarding allergic fungal rhinosinusitis?
   A. Oral antifungals may reduce postoperative mucosal inflammation and recurrence of disease.
   B. Positive fungal cultures are required for diagnosis and directed antifungal therapy.
   C. Surgery is usually not necessary as polyps and mucin respond readily to appropriate medical management.
   D. More than IgE-mediated hypersensitivity, robust T helper 2-driven adaptive immune response to fungal antigen drive the AFS inflammatory cascade.

3. Which is the best treatment for invasive sinusitis of hyaline mold with regular septate hyphae branching at acute angles?
   A. IV isavuconazole
   B. Liposomal amphotericin B
   C. IV voriconazole
   D. IV piperacillin-tazobactam

4. How is chronic invasive sinusitis clinically differentiated from acute invasive fungal sinusitis?
   A. Tissue biopsy
   B. Time course of symptoms
   C. Degree of extra-sinus invasion
   D. Fungal stain and culture

5. Which of the following is false in acute invasive fungal sinusitis?
   A. Oral antifungals have no role in the treatment of invasive fungal sinusitis.
   B. *Mucor* growth is optimized in acidotic conditions due to an increased availability of serum iron.
   C. Infection with *Mucorales* spp. is more destructive and fatal than *Aspergillus* spp.
   D. Invasive disease by *Pseudoallescheria boydii* is resistant to amphotericin B, and requires voriconazole.

Chapter 28
Diseases of the Nasal Cavity

Congenital Midline Masses

Background

- Incidence is 1:20,000 to 1:40,000
- Includes nasal dermoid, glioma, and encephalocele

Embryology

- Formation due to the failure of closure of the anterior neuropore
- Transient opening between frontal and nasal bones known as fonticulus frontalis at eighth week of gestation
  - *Prenasal space* forms between frontal and nasal bones and the cartilaginous nasal capsule.
  - *Foramen cecum*, an opening between the skull base and frontal bone, into the prenasal space. A projection of dura (diverticulum) passes through this foramen.
  - Dural diverticulum typically regresses with fusion of skull base and frontal bone. Failure results in neuroglial or ectodermal elements to remain in prenasal space with potential intracranial connection.

Nasal Dermoid

- Pathophysiology
  - Retained ectodermal and mesodermal elements from incomplete regression of dura from prenasal space or fonticulus frontalis. Form cysts filled with squamous epithelium, keratin debris, and connective tissue.
- Epidemiology
  - Most common midline nasal mass
  - 1% to 3% of all dermoid cysts, 11% to 12% of head and neck dermoids
- Presentation
  - Most commonly on nasal dorsum, may occur from nasal tip to glabella
  - Can be intranasal, intracranial, or extranasal masses
  - Nasal pit present in 45% to 84%, may contain hair
  - Firm, nontender, nonpulsatile, noncompressible mass without transillumination
  - Tendency for repeated infections, ranging from cellulitis to abscess
- Diagnosis
  - CT and MRI, the latter is important to determine intracranial extension

- Complications
  - Repeat infection, nasal skin necrosis, cartilage and bony destruction, CSF leak, meningitis
- Treatment
  - Early excision with removal of cyst, tract, and involved bone, cartilage, and septum
  - Open rhinoplasty approach optimal with wide exposure and superior cosmesis

Nasal Glioma

- Pathophysiology
  - Unencapsulated, ectopic glial tissue
  - Mass covered with nasal mucosa or skin containing heterotopic glial cells
- Presentation
  - 20% with intracranial connection through stalk
  - 60% external, 30% internal, 10% combined
  - Firm, nontender, nonpulsatile, noncompressible mass without transillumination
  - External are typically red with telangiectasias, internal glistening gray or purple
- Diagnosis
  - CT and/or MRI
- Complications
  - Cosmetic deformity, nasal obstruction, meningitis
- Treatment
  - Complete surgical excision
  - External nasal approach or lateral rhinotomy for extracranial lesions
  - Intracranial extension may warrant craniotomy to anterior cranial fossa

Encephalocele

- Pathophysiology
  - Herniation of CNS tissue through defect at the skull base, meningeal sac containing glial tissue
    - Failed closure of anterior neuropore or poor migration of neural crest cells, communicates with the subarachnoid space
  - Terminology differs based on CNS contents
    - Meningocele (meninges only)
    - Meningoencephalocele (meninges and brain)
    - Meningoencephalocystocele (meninges, brain, and ventricular system)
  - Varies by location
    - Posterior most common (occipital, non-nasal type)
    - Anterior
      - ◊ Sincipital (frontoethmoid): defect at foramen cecum between frontal and ethmoid bones
        - * Nasofrontal—glabellar
        - * Nasoethmoid—lateral nose
        - * Nasoorbital—medial orbital wall
      - ◊ Basal
        - * Transethmoidal
        - * Sphenoethmoidal
        - * Transphenoidal
        - * Sphenomaxillary
- Epidemiology
  - 1:4000 live births

- Presentation
  - External lesions are soft, compressible masses
  - Intranasal lesions are bluish, high in nasal cavity, compressible, and pulsatile
- Diagnosis
  - CT and/or MRI (look for bony defects and intracranial communication)
  - Positive Furstenberg sign (expansion of mass with crying or compression of internal jugular vein)
- Complications
  - Cosmetic deformity (large external lesions can be deforming), CSF leak, meningitis, hydrocephalus
- Treatment
  - Repair skull base defect, prevent further herniation and CSF leak, reduce chances of above complications
  - Open approach/craniotomy for external lesions
  - Endoscopic repair
    - Transnasal
    - Encephalocele identified and fulgurated
    - Repaired in multilayer fashion
    - Options include fat or fascia underlay, +/– bone graft with free mucosal graft or pedicled nasoseptal flap overlay

Teratoma

- Pathophysiology
  - Tumors with all three embryonic germ layers
  - Often contain connective tissue and hair, sometimes teeth
  - Rapid growth
- Epidemiology
  - 1 in 4000 live births
  - Head and neck comprise 2% to 9% of all teratomas
    - Nasopharynx and cervical neck most common
  - Presentation
    - Dyspnea at birth due to intermittent airway obstruction
    - Dysphagia
    - Firm tumors, noncompressible
  - Diagnosis
    - CT and/or MRI
      - ◊ CT reveals calcifications and intracranial extension
      - ◊ Exclude other masses (ie, encephalocele)
    - Negative Furstenberg test
  - Treatment
    - Secure airway
    - Complete surgical excision (small risk of malignancy)

Cysts

Nasopalatine Duct Cyst

- Pathophysiology
  - Originally thought to be trapped epithelium between embryological processes
  - Develops from the oronasal duct in incisive canal

- Cystic mass lined by nasal epithelium superiorly, then cuboidal and then squamous epithelium as it approaches the oral cavity
- Epidemiology
  - Most common non-odontogenic cyst
  - Fourth to sixth decade of life
- Presentation
  - Typically asymptomatic
  - Hard palate swelling, pain, nasal obstruction
- Diagnosis
  - CT
    - Well-circumscribed, round, ovoid, or heart-shaped lesions of the maxilla
- Treatment
  - Surgical enucleation
    - Recurrence in 0% to 11%

Nasoalveolar Cyst (Nasolabial Cyst)

- Pathophysiology
  - Non-odontogenic cyst
  - Nasal epithelium trapped between maxillary, median, and lateral nasal processes.
  - Sometimes from displaced nasolacrimal duct tissue
  - Cyst-like structure with connective tissue lined by pseudostratified columnar nasal epithelium
- Epidemiology
  - More common in women
  - 10% bilateral
- Presentation
  - May present with nasal obstruction or pain, facial asymmetry, effacement of nasolabial fold
  - Gingivobuccal sulcus obliterated
  - Firm, nontender, cyst-like mass
- Diagnosis
  - CT
    - Homogenous, hypodense, cystic structure
    - Non-rim enhancing
- Treatment
  - Surgical excision
    - Sublabial excision
    - Endoscopic marsupialization

Nasolacrimal Duct Cyst (Dacryocystocele)

- Pathophysiology
  - Failure of opening of distal nasolacrimal duct leading to accumulation of secretions and expansion of the nasolacrimal duct
- Presentation
  - Located anterior to the nasolacrimal duct in the inferior meatus, crust near opening in Hasner valve
  - Commonly asymptomatic
  - Symptoms include epiphora, nasal obstruction, dacryocystitis
  - Respiratory distress in infants if large (obligate nasal breathers)

- Diagnosis
  - Physical exam and CT
    - Cystic mass within the nasolacrimal duct
- Treatment
  - Endoscopic marsupialization with concurrent probing of the nasolacrimal duct

Thornwaldt Cyst

- Pathogenesis
  - Sixth week of development.
  - Notochord begins to regress from its most cephalic extent. If a communication develops between the notochord and the primitive foregut, respiratory epithelium and formation of a potential space in the midline can occur. If the nasopharyngeal opening of this communication becomes obstructed, a cyst may form.
  - Cyst forms in midline nasopharynx.
- Epidemiology
  - Uncommon
- Presentation
  - Usually asymptomatic
  - Postnasal drainage, ear fullness, serous otitis media, headache, cervical myalgia
  - Midline smooth submucosal mass in the midline nasopharynx
- Diagnosis
  - Nasal endoscopy, CT, or MRI
    - Midline cystic mass between longus capitis muscles
    - High T_1 and T_2 signal
- Treatment
  - Observation
  - Endoscopic marsupialization if symptomatic

Rathke Pouch Cyst

- Pathogenesis
  - Failure of obliteration of Rathke pouch (diverticulum of ectoderm that forms the anterior lobe of the pituitary and pars intermedius)
    - Leave persistent craniopharyngeal canal
  - Single layer of epithelium with goblet cells
- Epidemiology
  - Commonly found incidentally on CT or MRI
  - Incidence varies
  - Female predominance
- Presentation
  - Asymptomatic
  - Can cause mass effect and compress adjacent structures, including pituitary gland, optic chiasm, or hypothalamus with enlargement
  - May cause headaches, visual impairment, and endocrine abnormalities
- Diagnosis
  - MRI
    - Well-circumscribed, cystic mass within the sella turcica
    - May have suprasellar component and generally displaces the pituitary gland and stalk posteriorly
    - T_1 hypointense, T_2 hyperintense
- Treatment
  - Endoscopic transsphenoidal marsupialization and drainage

Intra-adenoidal Cyst

- Pathogenesis
  - Caused by occlusion of the embryonic groove on the pharyngeal tonsil prior to the lymphoid tissue appears causing a cyst
  - Crypts of lymphoid tissue, with some columnar and squamous epithelium
- Presentation
  - Midline cystic structure with groove
  - Sometimes asymptomatic but could cause snoring, serous otitis media with effusion
- Diagnosis
  - Nasal endoscopy, CT, MRI
- Treatment
  - Observation
  - Adenoidectomy, endoscopic marsupialization

Rhinitides

Allergic Rhinitis

- Background
  - IgE-mediated nasal condition resulting from allergen exposure in a sensitized individual
  - Nasal symptoms
    - Nasal congestion, rhinorrhea (anterior and posterior), nasal pruritus, palatal pruritus, postnasal drainage, smell disturbance
  - Ocular symptoms
    - Ocular pruritus, watery eyes
- Pathophysiology:
  - Gel and Coombs type I hypersensitivity
  - Sensitization
    - After initial exposure to an antigen, antigen-processing cells (macrophages, dendritic cells) present the processed peptides to T-helper cells
    - Upon subsequent exposure to the same antigen, these cells are stimulated to differentiate into either more T-helper or B cells
    - B cells further differentiate into plasma cells and produce IgE specific to that antigen
    - Allergen-specific IgE molecules then bind to the surface of mast cells, sensitizing them
  - Early phase response starts within 5 to 15 minutes
    - Mast cells degranulate releasing histamine, heparin, and tryptase producing sneezing, rhinorrhea, congestion, and pruritus
    - Degranulation also triggers formation of prostaglandin PGD2, leukotrienes LTC4, LTD4, LTE4, and platelet-activating factor (PAF)
    - Symptoms include nasal itching, nasal congestion, and rhinorrhea
  - Late-phase response begins 4 to 8 hours later
    - Caused by newly arrived inflammatory cells recruited by cytokines
    - Eosinophils, neutrophils, and basophils prolong the earlier reactions and lead to chronic inflammation
    - Symptoms include nasal blockage, increased mucus secretion, and nasal hyperresponsiveness

- Seasonal allergies present at particular time of the year according to seasonal allergens (grass, trees, pollen, ragweed)
- Perennial allergies are present all year round (dust mites, dogs, cats)

Non-allergic Rhinitis

- Chronic symptoms of nasal congestion, rhinorrhea, and posterior nasal drainage
- May be distinguished from allergic rhinitis by consistent presence of symptoms, lack of nasal or ocular pruritus
- Possible triggers include strong fragrances, tobacco smoke, changes in temperature, and cleaning products
- *Infectious rhinitis*: most common is viral (rhinovirus, respiratory syncytial virus, parainfluenza virus, adenovirus, influenza virus, enterovirus)
- *Vasomotor rhinitis (Nonallergic rhinopathy [NAR])*: Most common type of nonallergic rhinitis.
    - Heterogeneous group of patients with chronic nasal symptoms that are not immunologic or infectious in origin and are usually not associated with nasal eosinophilia.
    - Postulated to be an imbalance in the autonomic system where the parasympathetic system predominates leading to vasodilation and mucosal edema.
    - Changes in climate (temperature, humidity, barometric pressure), strong odors (perfume, cooking smells, flowers, chemicals), environmental tobacco smoke, pollutants, exercise, and alcohol ingestion exacerbate symptoms.
    - Primarily in adults with female predominance (2:1 to 3:1 female-to-male ratio).
    - Diagnosis of exclusion.
- *Hormone-induced rhinitis*: associated with hormonal imbalance
    - Hypothyroidism, acromegaly, menopause, puberty, or menstruation
    - Physiologic changes in pregnancy (expanded blood volume, vascular pooling, plasma leakage, and smooth muscle relaxation) exacerbate preexisting rhinitis
        - Rhinitis occurs in one-fifth of pregnancies and peaks in the second trimester.
- *Occupational rhinitis*: rhinitis at the workplace; usually due to inhaled irritants and frequently associated with concurrent occupational asthma
- *Chemical rhinitis*: nasal irritation due to some chemicals; chlorine-induced rhinitis, water-soluble agents (ammonia, formaldehyde, sulfur dioxide)
- *Smoke-induced rhinitis:* rhinorrhea and congestion due to smoke exposure
    - Does not appear to be driven by IgE-mediated hypersensitivity
    - Mechanism: likely multifactorial with neurogenic (substance P, neurokinin A) and irritant (altered mucociliary flow) etiologies leading to rhinitis
- *Drug-induced rhinitis:* can be classified into local inflammatory, neurogenic and idiopathic types
    - *Local inflammatory:* NSAIDs, aspirin
    - *Neurogenic:* α and β-adrenergic receptor modulators (prazosin, metoprolol, clonidine); phosphodiesterase inhibitors (sildenafil, tadalafil); ACE inhibitors (ramipril, captopril, lisinopril)
    - *Idiopathic:* psychotropics (amitriptyline, alprazolam), immunomodulators (cyclosporine), hormones (estrogen, oral contraceptives), antihypertensives (hydralazine, hydrochlorothiazide), other (gabapentin, gingko biloba)
- *Rhinitis medicamentosa*: tachyphylaxis associated with prolonged use of nasal sympathomimetics
    - Exact duration unknown, but recommendations not to exceed 3 days of continued use to avoid rebound phenomenon

  - Alpha receptors in the nose are desensitized; rebound congestion due to overuse of decongestants
  - Treatment includes discontinuation of decongestants and intranasal corticosteroids
  - During the withdrawal process, a short course of systemic steroids is sometimes required
  - Underlying rhinitis or anatomic issues that initiated the decongestant use should be addressed
- *Gustatory rhinitis*: watery rhinorrhea due to vasodilation after eating, especially with spicy or hot foods
  - Vagally mediated phenomenon
  - Pre-prandial treatment with topical ipratropium is often effective
- *Food-induced rhinitis*: rhinitis as part of systemic IgE-mediated food allergy reaction
  - Pollen-food allergy syndrome, also known as oral allergy syndrome, experience oropharyngeal itching, tingling, swelling, and symptoms of allergic rhinitis after ingestion of certain raw fruits and vegetables
  - Affects up to one-half of pollen-allergic patients due to ingestion of cross-reactive, heat-labile food proteins of plant origin
  - Patients do not have reactions if food is cooked due to heat-labile food proteins
- *Age-related rhinorrhea:* rhinitis of the older adult
  - Clear rhinorrhea increases with age, likely due to less sensitive autonomic function leading to imbalance between sympathetic and parasympathetic tone
- *Nonallergic rhinitis with eosinophilia syndrome (NARES):* perennial disorder usually in middle-aged adults
  - Most common type of inflammatory nonallergic rhinitis
  - Rhinitis with approximately 10% to 20% eosinophils on nasal smears in the setting of negative assessment for aeroallergen-specific IgE
  - Symptoms of nasal congestion, rhinorrhea, sneezing, pruritus, and hyposmia (hyposmia more pronounced than in allergic rhinitis)
  - Usually responds well to topical nasal corticosteroids
  - Associated with aspirin-exacerbated respiratory disease

Atrophic Rhinitis

- Also called rhinitis sicca or ozena
- Mucosal colonization with *Klebsiella ozaenae* and other pathogenic organisms
- Nasal mucosa degenerates and loses mucociliary function
- Histology demonstrates squamous metaplasia, glandular atrophy, diffuse endarteritis obliterans
- Presents with foul smell, yellow or green nasal crusting, anosmia with atrophy and fibrosis of mucosa
- Primary atrophic rhinitis
  - Most prevalent in developing countries in subtropical and temperate climate zones
  - Etiology is unknown, but bacterial infection is thought to be involved from *Klebsiella ozaenae*, *Staphylococcus aureus*, *Proteus mirabilis*, and *Escherichia coli.*
- Secondary atrophic rhinitis
  - More prevalent in developed countries, less severe and less progressive
  - Usually secondary to trauma, sinonasal surgery, irradiation, or underlying granulomatous disease
- Management: nasal saline irrigation, antibiotics

Viral Rhinitis

- Viral infection of the sinonasal mucosa, "common cold"
- Risk factors include families with multiple children, daycare, healthcare workers, stress, allergic rhinitis, humidity
- Rhinovirus and coronavirus account for 50%
- Others include parainfluenza, RSV, adenovirus, coxsackievirus, echovirus, influenza, and enterovirus
- Transmission occurs through contact or aerosolization of infectious secretions
- *Symptoms:* watery rhinorrhea of acute onset, sneezing, congestion, pharyngitis, cough, olfactory loss, headache, malaise, conjunctivitis, lymphadenopathy
- Potential transition to bacterial infection (0.5%-2%)
- Diagnostic tests typically not necessary; serologic, tissue culture, PCR assays available
- Treatment is supportive with rest, hydration, topical and systemic decongestants, mucolytics, and nasal irrigations

Bacterial Rhinitis

- Often due to secondarily infected viral rhinitis and may be part of bacterial rhinosinusitis.
- Organisms commonly include *Streptococcus, Haemophilus influenzae, S. aureus, Bordetella pertussis,* chlamydia, diphtheria.
- Symptoms are similar to viral rhinitis with more prominent yellow to green purulent discharge.
- Treatment includes antibiotics and supportive therapy.

Granulomatous Diseases

Granulomatosis with Polyangiitis (GPA) (formerly Wegener Granulomatosis)

- Idiopathic disease characterized by a triad of necrotizing granulomas of respiratory tract (85%), glomerulonephritis (75%), and systemic vasculitis
- Sinonasal symptoms usually manifest early with severe nasal crusting, epistaxis, rhinorrhea, and secondary rhinosinusitis.
- Nasal biopsy is often nondiagnostic.
- Cytoplasmic pattern (+c-ANCA) strongly associated with 60% to 90% positive testing.
- Consultation with rheumatology for systemic treatment.
- Nasal treatment includes saline irrigations, nasal moisturization, and topical antibiotic irrigations.

Eosinophilic granulomatosis with polyangiitis (EGPA) (formerly Churg-Strauss syndrome)

- Small-sized vessel vasculitis in patients aged 30 to 50 years
- Rhinitis, CRS with nasal polyposis, anosmia
- Suspected in patients with asthma, increased peripheral blood eosinophil count (> 10%) and pulmonary manifestations
- Associated with p-ANCA
- Treatment includes high doses of corticosteroids and immunosuppressants
- New anti-IL-5 therapy with clinical benefit
- Nasal management includes irrigations, culture-directed antibiotics, nasal steroids, and surgery (select cases)

Sarcoidosis

- Multisystem inflammatory disease with noncaseating granulomas.
- Symptoms include nasal obstruction, epistaxis, nasal pain, epiphora, and anosmia.
- Nasal exam may show erythematous, edematous, friable, and hypertrophied mucosa. Submucosal yellow nodules may be seen. Nasal polyps, lupus pernio, and septal perforation have been reported.
- More common in young, female, and African Americans.
- Serum ACE levels may be elevated.
- Treatment includes systemic steroids and immunosuppressants including newer biologic therapy (anti-TNF agents).
- Nasal management includes irrigations, nasal steroids, and surgery (select cases).

Rhinoscleroma

- Chronic granulomatous disease due to *Klebsiella rhinoscleromatis*
- Endemic to Central America, Chile, Central Africa, India, Indonesia, Middle East
- More common in females (13:1 female-male ratio); second to third decade of life in crowded, rural areas with poor hygienic and nutritional conditions
- Usually affects nasal cavity, but may also affect the larynx, nasopharynx, or paranasal sinuses
- Contracted by direct inhalation of droplets or contaminated material beginning in areas of epithelial transition (nasal vestibule, larynx, etc.)
- Symptoms include nasal obstruction, rhinorrhea, anosmia, epistaxis, nasal deformity; may also involve laryngeal, tracheal and bronchial airway, oropharynx (absent uvula)
- Three stages of disease progression
    - Catarrhal/rhinitic: persistent purulent rhinorrhea, nasal honeycomb-color crusting
    - Granulomatous/florid: painless granulomatous masses in nose and upper respiratory tract, septal destruction, thickened soft palate
    - Sclerotic/cicatricial: lesions heal with extensive dense fibrotic scarring with narrowing of the nasal passages, anosmia, dysphonia, stridor
- Key pathologic findings:
    - *Mikulicz cells*: large macrophages with clear cytoplasm containing bacilli
    - *Russell bodies:* bloated plasma cells with birefringent inclusions
    - Pseudoepitheliomatous hyperplasia is present
- Treatment includes long-term antibiotics (tetracycline, fluoroquinolones), biopsy, and debridement

Rhinosporidiosis

- Chronic granulomatous infection of the nose and external eye caused by *Rhinosporidium seeberi.*
- Endemic to Africa, Pakistan, Sri Lanka, and India.
- Transepithelial transmission by exposure to spores in contaminated dust, soil, or stagnant water (public bathing).
- Eyes and nasal cavity most common affected sites with symptoms of nasal obstruction, epistaxis, rhinorrhea, or foreign body sensation.
- Exam demonstrates friable, polypoid, exophytic mass lesion with submucosal studding of the erythematous surface with white spores ("strawberry" appearance); infection of palpebral conjunctivae.
- *Histopathology*: pseudoepitheliomatous hyperplasia, presence of *R. seeberi.*
- Treatment requires surgical excision and dapsone.

Nasal Infections

Septal Abscess

- Septal abscess can occur as a result of septal hematoma.
  - Septal hematoma occurs in 0.8% to 1.6% cases of nasal trauma in which mechanical force ruptures perichondrial blood vessels leading to accumulation of blood in the submucoperichondrial space and stripping of cartilage of its blood supply
  - Can result in avascular necrosis of the cartilage and act a potential nidus for infection leading to septal abscess
- More common in males and children.
- Mucoperichondrium is less adherent in children leading to additional risk.
- Other potential causes of septal abscess include injury of septum via nasogastric tube, furunculosis, sinusitis (direct extension from sphenoiditis), dental infection, iatrogenic (septoplasty).
- Symptoms include widened septum, severe pain, fever, erythema in nasal vestibule, nasal obstruction.
- May appear as bilateral purple/dusky nasal septal swellings obstructing airway
- Causative organisms include *S. aureus* (70%), *H. influenzae, group A beta-hemolytic strep, S. pneumoniae, Klebsiella pneumoniae, enterobacteriaceae.*
- Complications can be severe and may include dissolution of septal cartilage, saddle nose deformity, nasal valve collapse, facial cellulitis, sepsis, orbital extension, cavernous sinus thrombosis, intracranial extension including epidural abscess, meningitis, and intracranial abscess.
- Treatment entails prompt operative incision and drainage, followed by culture-directed antibiotic therapy.

Nasal Cellulitis

- External nasal infection of the deep dermis and subcutaneous fat
- Symptoms include induration, nasal erythema, edema, tenderness
- Predisposing factors to nasal cellulitis include direct trauma, contiguous spread from dental infections, sinusitis, immunodeficiency including diabetes and chronic steroid use
- Common causative organisms include
  - Group A beta-hemolytic streptococcus and *S. aureus.*
  - *H. influenza* may be causative in pediatric cellulitis.
  - Cryptococcus in immunocompromised patients.
- Prompt aggressive antibiotic therapy is indicated as disease may spread to the cavernous sinus via the superior ophthalmic vein and pterygoid plexus through the valveless facial vein.
- Mild cases can be treated with a first-generation cephalosporin (cephalexin), amoxicillin-clavulanate, or erythromycin (PCN allergic). Prior history of MRSA requires treatment with trimethoprim-sulfamethoxazole, clindamycin, doxycycline, or minocycline.
- Severe cellulitis requires hospitalization with parenteral antibiotics with coverage of MRSA.

Erysipelas

- Erysipelas is an infection of upper dermis and superficial lymphatics of the face.
- Lesions are raised above the level of the surrounding skin with clear demarcation between involved and uninvolved tissue.
- Symptoms include acute-onset "butterfly" involvement of face associated with fevers and chills.

- Primarily affects the young, elderly, and immunocompromised.
- *Streptococcus pyogenes* is the causative organism.
- Treatment includes oral penicillin therapy with macrolides for PCN allergy. First-and second-generation cephalosporins as well as fluoroquinolones may be used in complicated cases.

Nasal Vestibulitis (Folliculitis)

- Infection of the nasal vestibule commonly attributed to *S. aureus*.
- Risk factors include digital trauma, excessive nose blowing, trimming vibrissae.
- No association has been confirmed with nasal steroid use.
- Symptoms include anterior nasal pain, swelling, and tenderness to palpation or movement of the nose. Nasal crusting or pustules may be present. The nasal septum is often spared as disease is limited to the vestibular skin hair follicles.
- Treatment includes the use of warm compresses and topical antimicrobials (polymyxin, bacitracin, neomycin, mupirocin, retapamulin).
- *Furunculosis* is a deep variety of vestibulitis associated with perifollicular erythema and edema with possible abscess formation. Untreated infections can lead to facial cellulitis and complications such as cavernous sinus thrombosis. Treatment includes topical antimicrobials, oral anti-staphylococcals, warm compresses, and prompt incision and drainage if necessary.
- *Carbuncle* is a term used to describe a group of furuncles.

Rhinophyma

- Rhinophyma is a form of end-stage acne rosacea in which there is massive hypertrophy and hyperplasia of the sebaceous glands of the nose.
- Presents primarily in middle-aged to elderly white males, associated with facial flushing.
- Symptoms: begins with acne rosacea in adolescence; oily, cystic, thick nasal skin which progresses to large pits, fissures, and lobulations deforming the nose. May progress to nasal obstruction when advanced.
- Possible association with vitamin deficiencies, stress, androgenic hormone influences, chronic infections with *Demodex folliculorum*; no association with alcohol.
- Rhinophyma has been described in association with squamous cell carcinoma and basal cell carcinoma; however, no direct cause proven.
- Medical therapy includes topical antibiotics (metronidazole, clindamycin), topical anti-inflammatory (azelaic acid, benzoyl peroxide), topical retinoids, isotretinoin, oral antibiotics (metronidazole, macrolides, tetracyclines).
- Surgical treatment of nasal deformity treated with decortication (partial or full-thickness excision), laser excision (Er:YAG, CO2 laser), or dermabrasion followed by skin grafting.

Epistaxis

Background

- 16% of US population suffers from epistaxis annually.
- Accounts for about 500,000 emergency room visits per year.
- Most are self-limited and do not require medical attention.
- Almost 90% of nose bleeds arise anteriorly.

Vascular Anatomy

- Terminal branches from internal and external carotid arteries with numerous anastomoses.
- External carotid sends two major branches to the nasal cavity.
  - Internal maxillary artery (IMA)
    - Sphenopalatine artery (SPA) is the terminal branch that gains access to the nasal cavity through the sphenopalatine foramen. Divides into lateral nasal artery, supplying the lateral nasal wall, and posterior septal artery, supplying the posterior nasal septum.
    - Descending palatine branch of IMA supplies the anterior nasal septum and floor of the nose.
  - Facial artery
    - Courses superiorly within the nasofacial crease as the angular artery supplying the nose
    - Superior labial artery sends small branches to supply the nasal vestibule and anterior nasal septum
- The internal carotid artery supplies two terminal branches arising in the orbit from the ophthalmic artery.
  - Anterior ethmoid artery (AEA) supplies the lateral and anterior one-third of the nasal cavity.
  - Posterior ethmoid artery (PEA) supplies small portion of the superior turbinate and adjacent posterior septum.
- Kiesselbach plexus is a confluence of vessels along the anterior nasal septum located within Little's area
  - Receives vascular supply from septal branches of SPA, greater palatine artery, anterior ethmoid artery, and superior labial artery
  - Anastomotic highway between internal and external carotid systems
- Woodruff plexus, known as nasopharyngeal plexus is located at the posterior 1 cm of the nasal floor, inferior meatus, and middle meatus

Pathophysiology

- Local and iatrogenic factors
  - Digital trauma
  - Dry air
  - Nasal sprays (decongestants, topical steroids)
  - Drugs (cocaine, heroin)
  - Tobacco (cigarette smoke, snuff)
  - Pollution (chemical and environmental irritants)
  - Inflammatory diseases (rhinitis, sinusitis)
  - Granulomatous diseases (granulomatosis with polyangiitis, sarcoidosis)
  - Structural deformity (septal deviation/spur and perforation)
  - Nasal instrumentation (oxygen cannula, intubation, airway, nasogastric tube)
  - Facial trauma (maxillofacial, nasal)
  - Surgery (rhinoplasty, septoplasty, sinus surgery, skull base surgery)
  - Neoplasms (nasopharyngeal angiofibroma, sinonasal papilloma, squamous cell carcinoma)
- Systemic factors
  - Medications (aspirin, NSAIDS, warfarin, heparin, vitamin E)
  - OTC supplements (garlic, gingko, ginseng, fish oil)

- Blood dyscrasias (acquired or hereditary)
- Hematologic malignancies
- Platelet dysfunction and thrombocytopenia
- Cardiovascular diseases (coronary artery disease, hypertension)
- Vitamin A, D, C, E, or K deficiency
- Alcohol use
- Liver failure
- Chronic renal failure and uremia

Management

- Anterior epistaxis, mild
  - Inspect nasal cavity with headlight and speculum
  - Formal diagnostic endoscopy may be warranted to confirm the absence of other bleeding sources
  - Remove any clots obscuring site of bleeding
  - Apply topical decongestant and anesthesia with atomizer, cottonoids, wisps of cotton
  - Chemical cautery with silver nitrate generally suffices
  - Absorbable hemostatic agents like Gelfoam or Surgicel applied over cauterization site to minimize risk of rebleeding
  - Refrain from anticoagulants for 7 to 10 days (if not medically contraindicated)
  - Avoid strenuous activity and nasal blowing
  - Humidity, saline sprays, and emollients
- Anterior epistaxis, moderate to severe
  - Office treatment in most cases.
  - Formal diagnostic nasal endoscopy to identify and control sources of bleeding.
  - Topical decongestant and anesthesia as above.
  - Transoral greater palatine foramen block may be considered to reduce bleeding.
  - Inject bleeding area with lidocaine with epinephrine.
  - Bipolar electrical cautery for definitive control of bleeding.
  - If unable to tolerate office treatment or medically unstable, perform in operating room under general or monitored care anesthesia.
  - Absorbable (Gelfoam or Surgicel) or nonabsorbable (Merocel, Vaseline gauze) nasal packing can be used as an alternative.
  - Tranexamic acid (topical, po or IV).
- Posterior epistaxis
  - Patient stabilization (airway, breathing, circulation)
  - Posterior nasal packing
    - Anteroposterior (AP) pack
    - Tamponade vessels of anterior and posterior nasal cavity
    - Foley catheter with 30-cc balloon or gauze (2×2s or tonsil balls) to pack the nasopharynx
    - Both nasal cavities packed with Vaseline gauze or absorbable packing
    - Alternate options include dual balloon epistaxis devices
    - Antibiotic therapy to prevent toxic shock syndrome from *S. aureus*
    - Observation in stepdown or ICU with cardiac monitoring and supplemental oxygen
    - High failure rate of 38% from posterior packing

  - Associated with multiple complications (mucosal trauma, alar necrosis, oroantral fistula, otitis media, respiratory obstruction, local infection, aspiration, significant pain, cardiopulmonary compromise)
  - Typically not required in the endoscopic era
  - Tranexamic acid (topical, po or IV)
- Internal maxillary artery ligation
  - Rarely needed with the advent of endoscopic techniques
  - Gingivobuccal approach to pterygomaxillary fossa
  - IMA isolated and vascular clips applied to the main trunk and branches
  - 10% to 15% failure rate
  - Complications include facial numbness or hypoesthesia, cranial nerve palsies, epiphora, damage to tooth roots, oroantral fistula, sinusitis, orbital penetration, and blindness
- Transnasal endoscopic SPA ligation (TESPAL) or cautery
  - Preferred method for intractable, posterior epistaxis
  - Definitive control of the terminal blood supply
  - Performed under general anesthesia
  - Mucosal incision anterior to the crista ethmoidalis of palatine bone
  - Medially based mucosal flap raised from lateral nasal wall
  - SPA and associated terminal branches cauterized with bipolar cautery
  - Vascular clips may be applied but are generally unnecessary
  - Patient discharged home the next day
  - 95% to 98% success rate with shorter hospital stay
  - Complications include crusting, synechiae, palatal/nasal paresthesia, orbital injury
- Anterior and posterior ethmoid artery ligation
  - Adjunct to TESPAL or IMA ligation, especially in cases of rebleeding
  - May be required in cases of nasal or maxillofacial trauma
  - Approached through standard Lynch incision
  - Anterior ethmoid artery arises from the fronto-ethmoid suture line 22 to 24 mm posterior to anterior lacrimal crest
  - Vascular clips and/or bipolar cautery applied prior to AEA division
  - PEA is approximately 12 mm posterior to AEA
  - Clipping or cautery of PEA performed with extreme caution given proximity to optic nerve (3-7 mm)
  - Complications include scarring, telecanthus, lacrimal system injury, hypoesthesia, enophthalmos, orbital hematoma, and blindness
- Embolization
  - Utilized for epistaxis intractable to previous measures as above
  - Useful in medically unstable patients, vascular malformations, large sinonasal malignancies requiring preoperative or palliative vascular control, and after craniofacial trauma with severe distortion of normal anatomy
  - Performed under local anesthesia via transfemoral catheterization
  - Bilateral external and internal carotid angiography performed to identify the bleeding source or other vascular abnormalities
  - Bilateral IMA embolization performed if single, clear source of bleeding is not identified
  - Multiple embolic materials may be used including polyvinyl alcohol particles, platinum coils, or Gelfoam particles
  - Average success rate reported at 88% with 12% complication rate

   - Complications include groin and/or retroperitoneal hematoma, groin numbness, femoral artery pseudoaneurysm, crusting, sinusitis, facial pain, paresthesia, stroke, and ophthalmic artery occlusion with blindness

Hereditary Hemorrhagic Telangiectasia (HHT)

- Background
  - Also known as Osler-Weber-Rendu syndrome
  - Occurs mainly in whites (1:5,000-10,000)
  - Autosomal dominant inheritance pattern
  - Characterized by telangiectasias of the skin/mucosal membranes and AVMs of internal organs
- Pathophysiology
  - Defect in signaling of TGF-β1
  - Adversely affects connective tissue and matrix production required to support and guide proliferating blood vessels during angiogenesis
  - HHT type 1 is caused by a mutation in the endoglin gene (chromosomal locus 9q34)
  - HHT type 2 is caused by a mutation in the *ALK1* gene (chromosomal locus 12q1)
- Curacao criteria for clinical diagnosis
  - Spontaneous or recurrent epistaxis
  - Telangiectasia of multiple mucosal or skin sites
  - Telangiectasia of multiple visceral sites (GI, pulmonary, hepatic, cerebral, spinal AVMs)
  - Family history of first-degree relative with HHT
  - Diagnosis definite if three or more criteria met
  - Diagnosis possible if two criteria met
- Clinical features
  - 80% to 90% develop epistaxis by age 21
  - 80% to 90% develop skin/oral cavity lesions by 30s/40s
  - GI AVMs 20% to 25%
  - Pulmonary AVMs 30%
  - Cerebral AVMs 5% to 15%
  - Hepatic AVMs 40% to 70% (usually asymptomatic)
  - Spinals AVMs rare
- Diagnostic workup
  - Comprehensive head and neck examination
  - Diagnostic nasal endoscopy
  - MRI brain with contrast for cerebral AVMs
  - Transthoracic contrast echocardiography for pulmonary AVMs
  - Endoscopy for GI AVMs (symptomatic in 25%)
  - Doppler ultrasound or CT scan for hepatic AVMs (symptomatic in 8%)
  - Genetic counseling
- Treatment options for HHT-related epistaxis
  - Humidification
  - Saline sprays/rinses
  - Topical emollients (Sesame/Rose Geranium oil)
  - Hormonal therapies (estrogen, tamoxifen)
  - Tranexamic acid (TA)
  - Bevacizumab (VEGF inhibitor) via topical or intravenous route to reduce epistaxis
  - Photocoagulation (bipolar cautery, lasers, coblation)

- Septodermoplasty
  - Mucosa replaced by full-or split-thickness skin graft
  - Reduce need for multiple laser procedures by 50%
- Young's procedure
  - Unilateral or bilateral nasal valve closure
  - Effective in 83% cases
  - Rebleeding can be very problematic after nasal closure

Nasal Hemangioma

- Background
  - Benign tumor of vascular origin
  - Based on histopathology, they can be classified as capillary, cavernous, and mixed types
- Clinical features
  - Nasal obstruction, epistaxis, and in children can result in poor feeding
  - Can spontaneously regress in children and in pregnancy
- Diagnostic workup
  - CT for more extensive lesions
- Treatment
  - Endoscopic excision

Respiratory Epithelial Adenomatoid Hamartoma (REAH)

- Background
  - Rare benign tumors of the upper airway and can be misdiagnosed as polyp or malignant tumor
  - Pathophysiology: Non-neoplastic hamartomatous overgrowth of respiratory epithelium often found at the olfactory cleft and posterior nasal septum
  - Higher incidence in patients with long-standing sinonasal inflammation
- Clinical features
  - Most commonly seen in men between the third and ninth decades of life
  - Majority are asymptomatic but can present with nasal obstruction, hyposmia, facial pain, and headache while symptomatic
- Diagnosis
  - Imaging which shows bilateral widening masses in the olfactory cleft without bone erosion should raise the suspicion for REAH.
- Management
  - Correctly identifying REAH can avoid unnecessary treatment.
  - Surgical excision is an option for symptomatic lesions.

Empty Nose Syndrome

- Background
  - Described in 1990 as a postsurgical disorder characterized by paradoxical symptomatic nasal obstruction in patients with a patent nasal airway

- Pathogenesis
  - Poorly understood.
  - Aggregate knowledge regarding empty nose syndrome (ENS) is limited, as the entity is quite rare.
  - Levels of evidence in the literature regarding ENS are quite low, with most of the literature being case series or expert opinion
- Clinical features
  - Nasal obstruction, nasal dryness, burning sensation in the nose, and a sense of suffocation.
  - Reduced sleep, anxiety, and depression are often accompanying symptoms.
  - Patients frequently become preoccupied with maintaining sensation of breathing.
  - Difficult due to lack of reliable physical signs.
  - Validated assessment tools such as Empty Nose Syndrome-6-Item questionnaire (ENS6Q) and cotton test can help to assess symptom severity and possible candidacy for surgical intervention.
- Management
  - ENS symptoms can be managed through moisturization, counselling, and in selected cases, tissue expansion.

Bibliography

Alobid I, Guilemany JM, Mullol J. Nasal manifestations of systemic illnesses. *Curr Allergy Asthma Rep*. 2004;4:208-216.

American Academy of Otolaryngology—Head and Neck Surgery position statement on empty nose syndrome, December 9, 2024.

Fitzhugh VA, Mirani N. Respiratory epithelial adenomatoid hamartoma: a review. *Head Neck Pathol.* 2008;2(3):203-208.

Kanowitz SJ, Citardi MJ, Batra PS. Contemporary management strategies for epistaxis. In Stucker FJ, De Souza C, Kenyon GS, Lian TS, Draf W, Schick B, eds. Rhinology and Facial Plastic Surgery. New York, NY: Springer-Verlag; 2009. Chapter 12. 139-148.

Rodriguez DP, Orscheln ES, Koch BL. Masses of the nose, nasal cavity, and nasopharynx in children. *Radiographics*. 2017;37:1704-1730.

Wise SK, Lin SY, Toskala E, et al. International Consensus Statement on Allergy and Rhinology: Allergic Rhinitis. *Int Forum Allergy Rhinol.* 2018;8:108-352.

Witkowski JA, Parish LC. Bacterial skin infections: management of the common streptococcal and staphylococcal lesions. *Postgrad Med*. 1982;72:166-178.

Questions

1. Of the neurogenic tumors, congenital encephaloceles may demonstrate which of the following characteristics during physical exam?
   A. Positive Furstenberg test
   B. Nasal pit that may contain hair
   C. Mass covered by nasal mucosa or skin
   D. Noncompressible, nonpulsatile midline mass

2. Rathke pouch cyst forms due to which of the following embryologic pathways?
   A. Failed closure of anterior neuropore or poor migration of neural crest cells
   B. Failure of obliteration of diverticulum of ectoderm that forms the anterior lobe of the pituitary and pars intermedius
   C. Failure of opening of distal nasolacrimal duct leading to accumulation of secretions and expansion of the nasolacrimal duct
   D. Nasal epithelium trapped between maxillary, median, and lateral nasal processes

3. Granulomatosis with polyangiitis (GPA) presents with severe nasal crusting and epistaxis. Which of the following would be most likely to be elevated in GPA patients?
   A. IgA
   B. p-ANCA
   C. c-ANCA
   D. Serum ACE

4. Rhinophyma is associated with all of the following except
   A. Demodex folliculorum
   B. Acne rosacea
   C. Squamous cell carcinoma
   D. *Klebsiella ozaenae*

5. Diagnosis of hereditary hemorrhagic telangiectasia (HHT) using Curacao criteria includes all of the following except
   A. Spontaneous or recurrent epistaxis
   B. Telangiectasia of multiple visceral sites including GI, pulmonary, hepatic, cerebral, and spinal AVMs
   C. Telangiectasia of multiple mucosal or skin sites
   D. Autosomal recessive pattern of inheritance

Chapter 29
Tumors of the Paranasal Sinuses

General Principles

Overview

- Sinonasal tumors exhibit remarkable variety both in histopathology and tumor behavior, ranging from benign lesions to high-grade, highly fatal malignancies.
- Sinonasal malignancy is very rare (incidence 0.56 per 100,000 per year), representing less than 1% of all malignancies and less than 5% of head and neck cancers.
- Approximately 60% of malignancies begin in the maxillary sinus, 25% in the nasal cavity, and 15% in the ethmoid labyrinth; less than 1% occur in the sphenoid or frontal sinus.
- Most common in middle-aged and older adults (80% in age $\geq$ 55 years) but may occur across the age spectrum.
- Twice as common in men than in women.

History and Presentation

- Presentation depends on which anatomic subsites of the sinonasal cavity are involved.
- Presence of unilateral symptoms are common and should raise concern.
- Symptoms of sinonasal tumors are often quite nonspecific, which may lead to delay in diagnosis:
  - Nasal obstruction (typically unilateral)
  - Epistaxis
  - Rhinorrhea
  - Chronic rhinosinusitis (obstruction of sinus drainage pathways by tumor)
  - Hyposmia/anosmia
  - Headache
  - Proptosis
  - Ophthalmoplegia
  - Diplopia
  - Facial pain
  - Facial paresthesia/hypoesthesia
  - Trismus
  - Neck mass (regional metastasis)

Risk Factors

- Squamous cell carcinoma (SCC): wood dust, leather dust, nickel, glue, chromium, aflatoxin, mustard gas, volatile hydrocarbons, formaldehyde, arsenic, tobacco smoke, presence of inverted papilloma (IP)
- Adenocarcinoma: wood dust (eg, woodworking, furniture-making); leather work
- Human papillomavirus (HPV) has been identified in some tumors, but unclear whether this is a causative agent versus merely an associated finding
  - Recent studies in sinonasal SCC suggest possible causative relationship in approximately 31% of cases, with epidemiologic and prognostic implications (HPV-positive patients are younger and have better 5-year overall survival).
  - High-risk HPV (eg, HPV 16 and 18) may cause dysplastic IP and development of SCC.

Evaluation and Workup

In-Office Examination

- Comprehensive head and neck examination
- In-office rigid nasal endoscopy to appreciate site(s) involved and extent of tumor
- Valsalva maneuver under direct visualization—expansion suggests intracranial extension of mass such as in an encephalocele (ie, positive Furstenberg sign)
- Assess for ease and safety of in-office biopsy, if considered, facilitated by nasal endoscopy

Differential Diagnosis

- Non-neoplastic lesions
  - Encephalocele/meningoencephalocele
  - Inflammatory polyp
  - Fungal ball (mycetoma)
  - Mucocele/mucous retention cyst
  - Fibrous dysplasia
  - Nasal foreign body
  - Granulomatous diseases (eg, granulomatosis with polyangiitis [GPA], sarcoidosis, syphilis, tuberculosis)
- Benign neoplasms—exhibit varying degrees of growth/locally destructive behavior, and in some cases may cause significant morbidity (eg, severe or recurrent epistaxis, sinus outflow obstruction, etc.); detailed discussions to follow for select pathologies
  - Antrochoanal polyp
  - Sinonasal papilloma—exophytic, oncocytic, inverted
    - Oncocytic and inverted papillomas have malignant potential
    - Exophytic and inverted papillomas have association with HPV
  - Respiratory epithelial adenomatoid hamartoma (REAH)
  - Osteoma
  - Ossifying fibroma
  - Chondroma
  - Schwannoma
  - Fibroma/neurofibroma
  - Odontogenic tumors (may present in maxillary sinus)

- Vascular tumors
    - Hemangioma
    - Lobular capillary hemangioma (ie, pyogenic granuloma)
    - Juvenile nasopharyngeal angiofibroma
- Malignant neoplasms
  - Squamous cell carcinoma
  - Adenocarcinoma
  - Esthesioneuroblastoma
  - Sinonasal neuroendocrine carcinoma (SNEC)
  - Sinonasal undifferentiated carcinoma (SNUC) and associated subtypes
    - SMARCB1-deficient sinonasal carcinoma
    - SMARCA4-deficient sinonasal carcinoma
    - NUT carcinoma
  - Adenoid cystic carcinoma
  - Sarcomas
    - Rhabdomyosarcoma
    - Osteosarcoma
    - Chondrosarcoma
  - Lymphoma
    - NK T-cell lymphoma
    - Other non-Hodgkin lymphomas
  - Sinonasal glomangiopericytoma (formerly hemangiopericytoma)
  - Mucosal melanoma
  - Clival chordoma
  - Primary nasopharyngeal carcinoma

Imaging

- Typically, both computed tomography (CT) and magnetic resonance imaging (MRI) with contrast will be obtained for any lesion that appears malignant.
- CT is most helpful for delineating bony anatomy and assessing for erosion/invasion of structures such as orbit, cribriform plate/skull base.
  - Certain lesions such as juvenile nasopharyngeal angiofibroma (JNA), fibrous dysplasia, osteomas, and inverting papilloma (IP) can be diagnosed with high degrees of certainty on CT imaging alone
    - Site of attachment of IP often demonstrates area of hyperostosis
  - CT angiography (CTA) is helpful to evaluate vascular lesions and may be performed with preoperative embolization of such tumors.
- **MRI** is most helpful for providing information on surrounding soft tissue (eg, periorbita, dura, cavernous sinus) as well as differentiating tumor from trapped secretions.
  - Tumor will often enhance on postcontrast T1-weighted MRI.
  - Trapped secretions will typically be hyperintense on T2 due to water content (unless they have become significantly inspissated and dehydrated).
- **Positron emission tomography (PET)** scan is used for staging biopsy-proven malignancies—assesses for regional (ie, cervical node) and distant metastatic disease.
- For maxillary sinus tumors, can assess tumor relationship to **Ohngren's line**
  - Imaginary line from angle of mandible to medial canthus, dividing maxillary sinus into anterior-inferior and posterior-superior parts
  - Tumors arising in posterior-superior portion (above Ohngren line) associated with poorer prognosis due to earlier invasion of orbit, skull base/pterygopalatine fossa

Biopsy Considerations

- In-office biopsy may be pursued in certain cases if imaging has already been obtained and is not suggestive of a lesion with intracranial connection (meningoencephalocele) or extension and/or an extensive vascular composition.
- Theoretical benefit of in-office biopsy is accelerating diagnosis and therefore time to treatment, as well as sparing patient a trip to the operating room/general anesthetic.
- Possible pitfalls of in-office biopsy include:
  - Greater difficulty controlling epistaxis in the office setting
  - May be difficult to get a sample of sufficient size and cellular viability (and failure to obtain definitive diagnosis will ultimately slow diagnostic process down)
  - Cannot safely biopsy certain lesions (eg, significant vascular component)
  - Don't have access to intraoperative frozen section pathology
- If any concern as to the safety or likelihood of success of in-office biopsy, it is best to proceed to the operating room for a more thorough procedure under controlled conditions and with access to intraoperative frozen section pathology to ensure successful diagnosis.
- Discovery of cervical adenopathy on physical exam and/or imaging warrants fine-needle aspiration biopsy.

Staging of Sinonasal Malignancy

- Tumor/Node/Metastasis (TNM) staging system for sinonasal malignancies is divided by subsite (nasal cavity/ethmoid sinus versus maxillary sinus)
- N and M staging similar to that used for other head and neck malignancies
- Other disease entities have their own staging system (eg, Kadish system for esthesioneuroblastoma)
- Maxillary sinus T staging
  - T1: tumor limited to maxillary sinus mucosa (no bone involvement)
  - T2: bone involvement, can include hard palate and/or middle meatus
  - T3: tumor invades any of the following—medial/inferior orbit, posterior maxillary sinus wall, pterygopalatine fossa, ethmoid sinuses, or cheek subcutaneous tissue
  - T4a: tumor invades any of the following—anterior orbit, cheek skin, pterygoid plates, infratemporal fossa, cribriform plate, sphenoid sinus, or frontal sinus
  - T4b: tumor invades any of the following—orbital apex, dura, brain, middle cranial fossa, cranial nerves (other than V2), nasopharynx, or clivus
- Nasal cavity/ethmoid sinus T staging
  - T1: tumor limited to one sinonasal subsite (septum, floor, lateral wall, vestibule, left/right ethmoid sinus)
  - T2: tumor involves two subsites, or otherwise extends to involve adjacent region
  - T3: tumor invades any of the following—medial/inferior orbit, maxillary sinus, palate, cribriform plate
  - T4a: tumor invades any of the following—anterior orbit, nose/cheek skin, pterygoid plates, sphenoid sinus, frontal sinus, minimal extension to anterior cranial fossa
  - T4b: tumor invades any of the following—orbital apex, dura, brain, middle cranial fossa, cranial nerves (other than V2), nasopharynx, or clivus
- Nodal staging of sinonasal malignancies
  - N0: no evidence of nodal metastasis
  - N1: metastasis in single ipsilateral lymph node ≤ 3 cm

- N2a: metastasis in single ipsilateral lymph node 3 to 6 cm
- N2b: metastasis in multiple ipsilateral lymph nodes < 6 cm
- N2c: metastasis in bilateral/contralateral lymph nodes < 6 cm
- N3a: metastasis in any lymph node > 6 cm
- N3b: any lymph node metastasis with extranodal extension

- Metastasis staging of sinonasal malignancies
  - M0: no distant metastasis
  - M1: distant metastasis present

Benign Neoplasms

Antrochoanal Polyp

- Smooth polypoid mass extending from maxillary sinus into nasal cavity and nasopharynx
- Thought to develop because of negative pressure generated with swallowing
- **Management:** endoscopic sinus surgery with complete removal

Sinonasal (Schneiderian) Papilloma

- Derived from the sinonasal Schneiderian membrane, which consists of pseudostratified ciliated columnar epithelium and underlying periosteum
- Divided into three subtypes: exophytic, oncocytic, and inverted
  - Frequency: inverted (62%-78%) > exophytic (10%-33%) > oncocytic (~6%)
- **Exophytic:**
  - Associated with low-risk HPV (subtypes 6 and 11)
  - Do not undergo malignant transformation
  - Most commonly arise from nasal septum
- **Oncocytic:**
  - 4% to 17% of cases develop malignant transformation (typically SCC)
  - *KRAS* mutations
  - No HPV association
  - Most commonly arise from lateral nasal wall or maxillary sinus
- **Inverted:**
  - Second most common benign sinonasal tumor
  - 5% to 15% of cases develop malignant transformation (typically SCC)
  - *EGFR* mutations
  - HPV appears to be a factor for tumorigenesis, though role of higher risk subtypes for malignant transformation remains unclear (in contrast to *de novo* sinonasal SCC where the causative association has been made more clearly)
  - Most commonly arise from lateral nasal wall or maxillary sinus (especially medial maxillary wall)
  - Classically on CT may see a focal area of osteitis or hyperostosis representing the attachment site
- **Management:** Complete surgical resection, most commonly through a purely endoscopic approach, with focused attention to managing site of attachment
  - Complete surgical resection for inverted and oncocytic papillomas includes addressing the attachment site—removal of mucosa with drilling and/or cauterization of bone at the site—to avoid unacceptably high recurrence rates

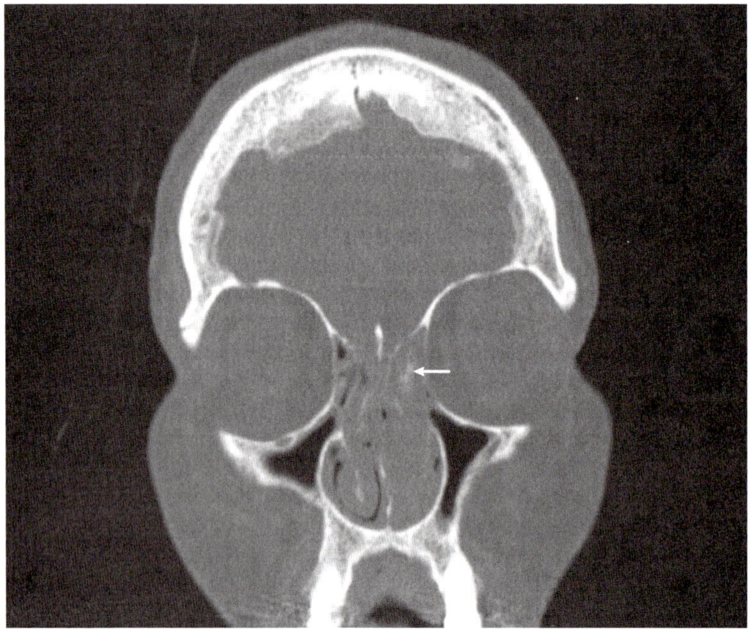

Figure 29-1 This CT scan demonstrates hyperostosis in the left ethmoid labyrinth which represents the site of attachment of an inverted papilloma in this patient.

- Often require expanded endoscopic approaches such as endoscopic medial maxillectomy or Denker approach
- Occasionally open approaches are needed as well (such as Caldwell-Luc) often in conjunction with endoscopic surgery (Figure 29-1)

Respiratory Epithelial Adenomatoid Hamartoma (REAH)

- Controversy exists as to whether REAH represents a true non-neoplastic entity versus actual neoplasm
- Commonly associated with chronic rhinosinusitis with nasal polyposis (CRSwNP)—recent data suggest 50.1% of REAH occurs with concurrent CRSwNP
- Presents as a polypoid mass, usually darker and more opaque than inflammatory polyps, most commonly arising in the olfactory cleft, and may be unilateral or bilateral
- May mimic more sinister pathology (eg, esthesioneuroblastoma) due to location/appearance
- Histologically demonstrates glandular proliferation, thickened hyalinized basement membrane, often with background of inflamed stroma
- **Management:** endoscopic resection; endoscopic sinus surgery if associated with CRS

Osteoma

- Most common benign sinonasal tumor
- Most commonly found in frontal sinus, followed by ethmoid and maxillary sinuses
- Diagnosed on CT—similar density to surrounding bone
- Associated with Gardner syndrome

  - Subtype of familial adenomatous polyposis (FAP), presenting with innumerable colonic polyps, osteomas, fibromas, epidermoid cysts, and dental anomalies (eg, supernumerary teeth)
- **Management:** observation for asymptomatic lesions; excision (typically endoscopic) for lesions obstructing sinus outflow or that are otherwise causing significant mass effect

Ossifying Fibroma

- True benign neoplasm characterized by fibrous tissue and bone with a true capsule, in contrast to fibrous dysplasia (see following discussion).
- Sinonasal ossifying fibroma is rare, typically (but not exclusively) occurring in the second and third decades, and disproportionately affects black women.
- CT appearance: well-defined, multiloculated lesion, bordered by a peripheral eggshell-like dense rim.
- **Management:** resection (endoscopic where feasible)—can be challenging due to possible adherence to dura and periorbita, and recurrence rates in such cases are higher.

Fibrous Dysplasia versus Ossifying Fibroma

	Fibrous Dysplasia	*Ossifying Fibroma*
Pathophysiology	Genetic defect in osteoblastic differentiation and maturation leading to replacement of bone with immature woven bone and fibrous tissue	True neoplasm composed of fibrous and bony tissue with a true capsule
CT imaging findings	Early phases (high-density fibrous tissue), radiolucent or lytic appearance similar to simple bone cyst Later phases (bony tissue increases), ground glass or sclerotic appearance	Well-defined, multiloculated lesion bordered by peripheral eggshell-like dense rim
Symptoms and complications	May obstruct sinus outflow, compress the orbit or optic nerve (visual disturbance and diplopia), or cause aesthetic deformities	Usually presents as a discrete nasal mass causing nasal obstruction which can cause mass effect/sinus outflow obstruction when large
Management	Partial or complete resection depending on location, symptoms, goals of surgery, aesthetic factors	Resection (endoscopic if feasible)
Other notes	Associated with McCune-Albright syndrome, which also manifests with café-au-lait spots and precocious puberty, due to defects in G_s alpha subunit	

Schwannoma

- Arise from Schwann cells in myelin sheath, in sinonasal cavity most commonly from trigeminal nerve branches (V_1 or V_2)
- Most commonly arises in ethmoid sinus, followed by maxillary sinus and nasal cavity
- May be found in pterygopalatine fossa
- Intracranial extension in 8.5%
- Well-delineated, firm to rubbery, with favorable dissection plane between tumor and surrounding tissue

- Histopathologically demonstrate Antoni A (cellular areas with Verocay bodies—palisading areas) mixed with hypocellular Antoni B areas
- **MRI** is most helpful imaging study
  - **T1:** Iso-or hypointense
  - **T1 postcontrast:** intensely enhances
  - **T2:** hyperintense with heterogeneity, sometimes areas of cystic degeneration
- **Management:** surgical resection

Lobular Capillary Hemangioma (Pyogenic Granuloma)

- Benign proliferation of capillaries most commonly on the anterior nasal septum that may be associated with local trauma (eg, digital trauma), pregnancy, other hormonal influences
- Usually presents with recurrent epistaxis
- **Management:** complete resection (usually endoscopic)

Juvenile Nasopharyngeal Angiofibroma (JNA)

- Highly vascular tumor arising from region of sphenopalatine foramen (SPF) and pterygopalatine fossa (PPF)
- Presents most commonly with recurrent epistaxis (may be severe) and nasal obstruction
- Almost exclusively seen in adolescent males which would suggest a role for androgenic hormones in tumorigenesis/tumor growth
- May see **Holman-Miller sign** on CT—anterior bowing of the posterior wall of maxillary sinus as tumor expands PPF
- Blood supply from branches of internal maxillary artery (external carotid system) most commonly, but as tumor grows there can be contributions from internal carotid system
- Benign but expansile and locally aggressive—may expand into sinuses, skull base, orbit, infratemporal fossa due to relationship of SPF/PPF with surrounding structures
- Histologically, JNAs demonstrate vessels of varying caliber, large fibroblast component with dense stroma
- **Management:**
  - Preoperative angiography and embolization of feeder vessels from external carotid system is performed 24 to 72 hours before surgery to reduce intraoperative blood loss.
  - Endoscopic resection has been shown to be superior to pure open approaches in terms of recurrence rates.
  - For massive tumors, combined endoscopic and open approaches may be needed.
- Variety of staging systems have been created, but University of Pittsburgh Medical Center (UPMC) system incorporates residual vascularity of tumor after preoperative embolization, allowing for more accurate prediction of intraoperative blood loss (Figure 29-2).

UPMC Staging System for JNA

Stage I	Tumor limited to nasal cavity and medial PPF
Stage II	Tumor extends to sinuses, lateral PPF
Stage III	Tumor extends to orbit, skull base, infratemporal fossa without residual vascularity
Stage IV	Tumor extends to orbit, skull base, infratemporal fossa with residual vascularity
Stage V	Intracranial extension with residual vascularity M: medial intracranial extension L: lateral intracranial extension

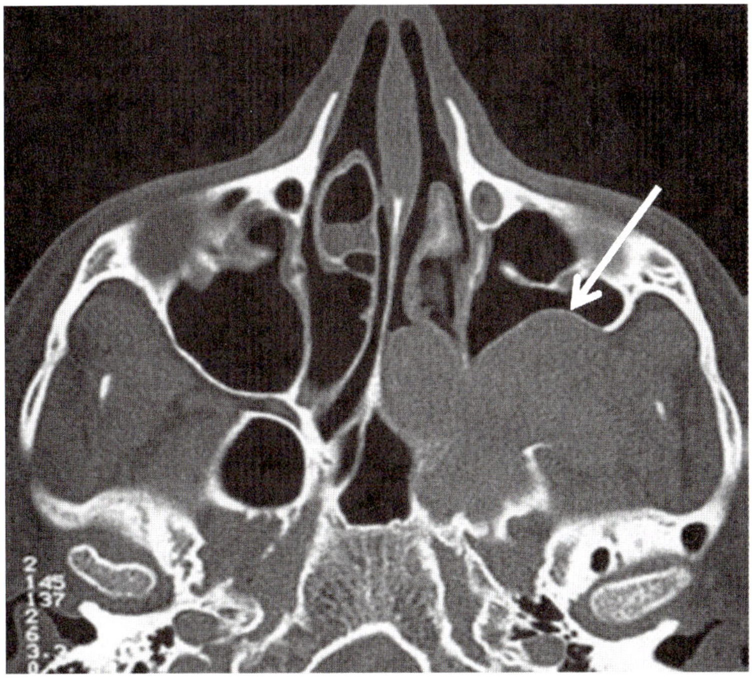

Figure 29-2 Anterior bowing of the posterior maxillary sinus wall—the Holman-Miller sign—is a classic finding on CT in JNA.

Malignant Neoplasms

Squamous Cell Carcinoma

- Most common sinonasal cancer, representing 41.9% to 51.6% of sinonasal malignancies
  - May arise *de novo* or in context of IP (5%-15% of cases of IP become malignant)
- Most commonly arises maxillary sinus (60%), followed by nasal cavity (25%) and ethmoid sinus (15%).
- Histologically may be described as keratinizing or nonkeratinizing (characterized by a "blue cell tumor" appearance without keratin formation).
  - Stains positively for cytokeratin
- Recent studies have elucidated the role of HPV, which appears to play an etiologic role in 25% of sinonasal SCC, and has similar prognostic implications to oropharyngeal squamous cell carcinoma—patients with HPV+ sinonasal SCC tend to be younger and have a better prognosis.
  - HPV-related multiphenotypic sinonasal carcinoma is a subtype of nonkeratinizing SCC first described in 2013, which has a favorable clinical outcome despite aggressive histomorphology.
- Five-year overall survival 56% for *de novo* SCC, 65% for SCC arising from IP.
- **Management:** negative margin surgical resection with adjuvant radiation therapy
  - Management of N0 neck: higher risk of occult neck metastasis in advanced T stage and maxillary sinus primary tumors, therefore need to consider elective neck dissection or elective neck irradiation in these patients

- Adjuvant chemotherapy may be added to radiation for positive margins or extranodal extension if neck dissection performed
- Consideration for immunotherapy (eg, nivolumab or pembrolizumab) for unresectable recurrent or metastatic SCC

- Expanding role for neoadjuvant chemotherapy: for certain patients with locally advanced tumors, neoadjuvant chemotherapy may be able to downstage tumor making negative-margin resection and orbital preservation more likely, as well as potentially improving overall survival

Adenocarcinoma

- Second most common sinonasal cancer—21% of all sinonasal malignancies
- More than one-half of cases occur in the nasal cavity and ethmoid sinuses
- Histopathologically divided into intestinal type and nonintestinal type (which is further characterized as low grade and high grade)
  - Intestinal type has association with wood dust exposure
  - May stain positively for CK20, CDX2, villin, MUC2
- Five-year survival 63%
- **Management:** surgical resection, often followed by radiation (especially in advanced T-stage tumors, high grade, or positive surgical margins)
  - Adjuvant chemotherapy may be considered in certain cases (eg, for positive margins) especially for intestinal type.

Esthesioneuroblastoma (Olfactory Neuroblastoma)

- Rare sinonasal malignancy arising from olfactory neuroepithelium (in olfactory cleft)
  - Comprises 2% to 6% of all sinonasal malignancies
- Bimodal age distribution, peaking in second and sixth decades
- Small round blue cell tumor whose histopathological stage is described by **Hyams grading system** with significant prognostic importance
  - Lower Hyams grades (I and II) characterized by less mitosis, absent necrosis, and presence of Homer-Wright pseudorosettes
  - Higher Hyams grades (III and IV) characterized by higher levels of mitosis and necrosis and presence of Flexner-Wintersteiner rosettes
  - Often stains positively for chromogranin, synaptophysin, and S-100
- **Kadish system** is a unique staging for esthesioneuroblastoma
  - **Kadish A:** tumor confined to nasal cavity
  - **Kadish B:** extension into paranasal sinuses
  - **Kadish C:** extension to skull base, dura/intracranial space, and/or orbit
  - **Kadish D:** regional (neck node) or distant metastasis
  - Note that Kadish C lesions with dural involvement have a worse prognosis than those without direct dural involvement; invasion of dura predicts recurrence and metastasis with worse overall survival
- 5-year overall survival 56% to 80% for lower Hyams grade lesions compared with 20% to 40% for high-grade lesions
- **Management:** surgical resection followed by adjuvant radiotherapy
  - N0 neck is typically not electively treated, though in some centers this may be considered in cases of dural invasion or high-grade tumors
  - Chemotherapy typically reserved for palliation in distant metastatic disease (Figure 29-3)

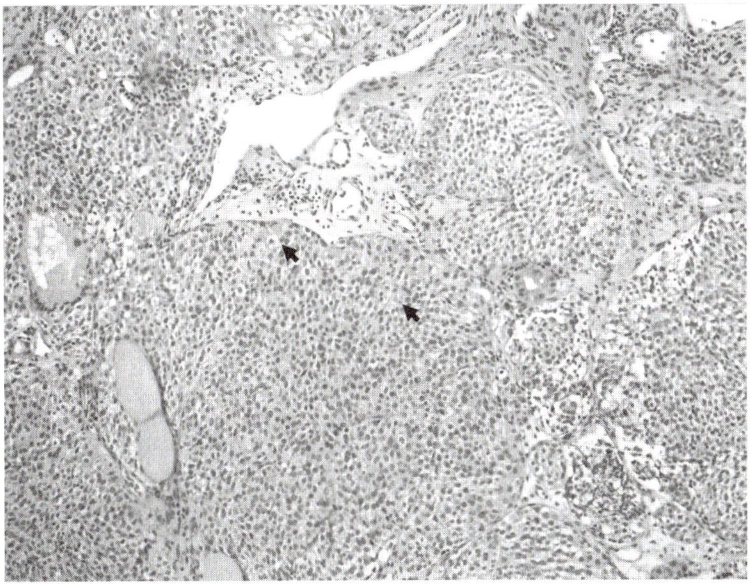

Figure 29-3 Histopathologic appearance of a Hyams grade II esthesioneuroblastoma—small round blue cells with poorly formed pseudorosettes, indicated by arrows.

Sinonasal Neuroendocrine Carcinoma (SNEC)

- Rare and aggressive cancer comprising 2% of all sinonasal malignancies
- Five-year disease-specific survival ranges from 50% to 70% but is considerably lower for higher grade pathology (eg, small-cell variant)
- Has a propensity for distant metastasis and can be associated with paraneoplastic syndromes, such as syndrome of inappropriate antidiuretic hormone secretion and Lambert-Eaton myasthenic syndrome
- Histopathology demonstrates small round blue cells that form nests, glands, rosettes with markers of neuroendocrine differentiation (eg, may be positive for chromogranin, synaptophysin, CD56, N-CAM, cytokeratin)
- **Management:** in many centers, induction chemotherapy most commonly cisplatin and etoposide (a common neuroendocrine tumor regimen) is used
  - Greater than 50% response → consolidation chemoradiation
  - Less than 50% response but surgically resectable → surgery followed by radiation
  - Less than 50% response and not surgically resectable → chemoradiation (this group has a poor prognosis)

Sinonasal Undifferentiated Carcinoma (SNUC)

- Rare and highly aggressive—5% of all sinonasal malignancies
- Strong tendency for distant metastasis
- Five-year survival 34.9%
- Histopathology demonstrates a small round blue cell tumor frequently with necrosis
  - Stains positively for cytokeratins, but negative for neuroendocrine markers like chromogranin and synaptophysin

- **Management:**
  - Traditionally, surgery followed by radiation often with chemotherapy.
  - Like in SNEC, induction chemotherapy (commonly cisplatin and etoposide) is now being used in many centers with the decision to move forward with consolidation chemoradiation versus surgery followed by (chemo)radiation based on tumor response.
- **SNUC variants:** with more sophisticated immunohistochemistry, several subtypes of poorly differentiated sinonasal malignancies which all previously fell under the SNUC umbrella have been described
  - **SMARCB1-deficient carcinoma:** tumor cells with loss of expression of tumor suppressor SMARCB1 (INI-1) leading to dysregulation of SWI/SNF pathway
    - Highly aggressive with regional and distant metastasis
  - **SMARCA4-deficient carcinoma**: also leads to derangement in SWI/SNF pathway due to tumor suppressor loss
  - **NUT carcinoma:** 5q14 rearrangement in *NUT* (nuclear protein in testis) gene
    - Highly aggressive and tends to present in younger patients
    - 50% of NUT carcinomas present in the lung, 40% in sinonasal tract, 10% other sites (eg, bladder, pancreas, retroperitoneum)

Sinonasal Adenoid Cystic Carcinoma (ACC)

- Represents 10% to 25% of cases of adenoid cystic carcinoma
- Most commonly occurs in maxillary sinus followed by nasal cavity
- Very strong propensity for perineural invasion and late distant metastasis, sometimes occurring many years after treatment of the primary tumor
- Sinonasal ACC also has a tendency toward local recurrence and invasion of nearby critical structures such as orbit and skull base
- Three histologic variants: cribriform (best prognosis), tubular, and solid (worst prognosis)
- **Management:** negative margin resection whenever possible (often difficult to achieve) followed by adjuvant radiation; chemotherapy usually reserved for palliation

Lymphomas

- A variety of lymphomas may present in the sinonasal cavity, including B-cell (more common in the western world) and T-cell lymphomas (more common in Asia and South America).
- Role of the surgeon is primarily obtaining an adequate biopsy for identification of the tumor type, which requires immunohistochemical analysis.
- Sinonasal B-cell lymphomas are typically treated with some combination of chemotherapy, radiation, and immunotherapy (eg, rituximab).
  - Most common type: diffuse large B-cell lymphoma
- **Sinonasal NK/T cell lymphoma (ENKTL):**
  - A rare but aggressive tumor associated with Epstein-Barr virus (EBV)
  - Symptoms and signs are often nonspecific and include nasal obstruction, epistaxis, rhinorrhea, mucosal ulceration, and a rapidly enlarging nasal mass
  - **Management:** chemotherapy and radiation (combination superior to either alone)

Sinonasal Sarcomas

- Overall represent a very rare group of sinonasal tumors—only 1% to 3% of head and neck tumors are sarcomas, and among sinonasal tumors, epithelial-derived tumors are far more common.

- Rhabdomyosarcoma
  - Embryonal subtype more common in children.
  - Alveolar subtype more common in adolescents and adults, more aggressive.
  - Treatment is typically chemotherapy with radiation (role of surgeon is usually in obtaining a biopsy and salvage surgery when needed).
- Sinonasal osteosarcoma and chondrosarcoma are exceedingly rare but often treated in a multimodality fashion (surgery with adjuvant radiation and/or chemotherapy).

Glomangiopericytoma

- A vascular tumor of the sinonasal tract that behaves as a low-grade malignancy with low distant metastatic potential but propensity for recurrence with incomplete resection
  - When it does occur, distant metastasis usually follows a long period of time with the disease and multiple recurrences
- **Management:** negative margin surgical resection provides an excellent prognosis both in terms of survival and prevention of recurrence

Sinonasal Mucosal Melanoma (SNMM)

- A rare but highly aggressive disease usually affecting older adults and, unlike cutaneous melanoma, unrelated to sun exposure
  - **All** mucosal melanomas are at minimum T3 lesions
  - 5-year survival 22%
  - Early and repeated recurrences; distant metastasis ultimately affects about one-half of patients
- The nasal cavity is the most common site for SNMM and presents with more localized disease, whereas a paranasal sinus primary site (especially maxillary and ethmoid) portends a worse prognosis.
- Classically appears as a pigmented tumor affecting the sinonasal mucosa, but in some cases, malignant cells do not produce melanin (amelanotic melanoma)
  - Small round blue cell tumor +/− melanin production
  - Tumor cells express S-100, Melan-A, HMB-45, and MITF
  - Unlike cutaneous melanoma, SNMM does not have frequent BRAF mutations, but does have c-KIT mutations more often than cutaneous disease
- **Management:**
  - Negative-margin surgical resection with adjuvant radiotherapy.
  - Usually, no elective neck dissection is performed for the clinically N0 neck in sinonasal mucosal melanoma.
  - Immunotherapy:
    - BRAF inhibitors (eg, vemurafenib) are not usually effective.
    - Imatinib has been used with good effect in patients whose tumor cells harbor c-KIT mutations.
    - Checkpoint inhibitors such as pembrolizumab, nivolumab, and ipilimumab have also been used.
    - Neoadjuvant immunotherapy is being investigated due to very high risk of distant metastasis over time.

Clival Chordoma

- Chordomas are rare tumors derived from a **notochord** remnant that can arise anywhere along the path of the embryonic notochord, from skull base to sacrum.
  - Notochord is the precursor to vertebral disc material
  - **Clival chordoma** can involve the nasopharynx and/or sinonasal cavity by extension from the clivus

- Tend to be slow growing but locally aggressive
- Histopathology shows characteristic **physaliphorous cells** with a "soap bubble" appearance
  - These cells uniquely stain positive for **brachyury**
- **Management:** aggressive surgical resection followed by adjuvant radiotherapy
- Prognosis better for younger patients—10-year survival 68% in patients less than 40 years old versus 43% in patients greater than 40 years old

Surgical Approaches for Sinonasal Malignancy

Open Approaches

- Historically, open craniofacial resection was the gold standard for treating sinonasal malignancy, but with significant morbidity (36.3% of cases) and a 4.7% mortality rate.
  - Morbidity includes wound (infection, dehiscence, flap necrosis); central nervous system (meningitis, pneumocephalus, cerebrospinal fluid [CSF] leak); orbital (nasolacrimal duct obstruction, diplopia, blindness); and systemic (myocardial infarction, renal, pulmonary, urinary tract infection) complications
- Open craniofacial resection involves combining transfacial incisions with a bicoronal craniotomy to address tumor affecting the anterior cranial base.
- Several other open procedures are also used depending on the location and extent of the pathology including the Caldwell-Luc approach to the maxillary sinus, partial and total maxillectomy, and orbital exenteration for extensive orbital invasion.
- There was historically an emphasis on en bloc resection of the entire tumor, but over time as the endoscopic endonasal approach gained popularity, piecemeal resection/debulking followed by addressing the tumor attachment site in an en bloc fashion has been shown to have similar or in some cases superior survival outcomes.
- There is still a role for open approaches depending on extent of disease, or for combined approaches in which some components of the procedure are performed in an open approach, whereas others are done endoscopically.

Endoscopic Endonasal Approach

- Has become the gold standard for most sinonasal malignancies and benign tumors given development of more advanced techniques and excellent visualization/magnification with endoscopic technology.
- Can be used as the sole approach for many pathologies.
- Outcomes are typically as good or superior to open approaches with less morbidity, shorter length of hospital stay, and no external incisions, though it should be noted that the previously mentioned complications for open approaches are still possible with endoscopic approaches.
- Typically, technique involves debulking the tumor and following it back to its attachment site where an en bloc resection can then take place in the case of malignancy.
- Contraindications to a purely endoscopic approach for resection of sinonasal malignancy:
  - Invasion of nasal bone, palate, skin/subcutaneous tissueExtensive invasion/involvement of:

  - Frontal sinus (especially laterally and anterior table)
  - Orbit (ie, significant invasion beyond periorbita and fat which suggests need for possible exenteration)
  - Lateral, anterior, or inferior aspects of maxillary sinus
  - Lateral supraorbital dura
  - Infratemporal fossa
  - Intracranial space with massive involvement of dura/brain parenchyma

Overview of Skull Base Reconstruction

General Principles

- Considerations include size of the dural defect as well as presence/absence of a CSF leak (and if present whether high flow or low flow)
  - Size of the dural defect has been classified into small (< 1 cm), intermediate (1-3 cm), and large (> 3 cm) defects
  - High-flow leak: defect in connection with a CSF cistern or ventricle
  - Low-flow leak: leak present but no connection to a CSF cistern or ventricle
- When there is no CSF leak present and the defect is small, a simple subdural or extradural inlay of a synthetic material is often sufficient (eg, bovine collagen dural substitute).
- A low-flow leak can typically be successfully repaired with a free mucosal graft onlay harvested from a variety of sites (eg, nasal floor, septum, inferior/middle turbinate) and may be combined with an inlay of synthetic or other autologous material.
- For large dural defects (which often have an accompanying high flow leak), free mucosal grafts have an unacceptably high rate of postoperative CSF leak (> 15%), but vascularized pedicled flaps (most commonly a nasoseptal flap) are used to lower this rate considerably (< 5%), usually as part of a multilayered closure with an inlay material.
  - Inlay materials for high-flow leaks may include synthetic materials or autologous tissue—fascia lata is a commonly used, robust tissue that is often used.
- Subarachnoid drains have historically been and continue to be used (institution-and surgeon-dependent), but evidence suggests that with good reconstruction, even high flow leaks can be safely repaired without CSF diversion.
  - Maintain consideration for lumbar drainage in "high flow, high risk" leaks—patients with morbid obesity, previously operated or irradiated field, recurrent high-flow leak

Vascularized Pedicled Flaps

- Detailed discussion of vascularized pedicled flaps is provided elsewhere in this book, but an overview is provided here.
- **Nasoseptal flap (NSF)**
  - Mucoperichondrium/mucoperiosteum harvested from the nasal septum (can be extended onto the nasal floor and even onto the lateral nasal wall); workhorse flap for skull base reconstruction.
  - Pedicle is based on posterior septal branch of sphenopalatine artery (SPA) and is located between the natural ostium of the sphenoid sinus and the choanal arch.

- Useful for defects of many sizes and locations, including anterior cranial fossa, sella/tuberculum/planum, and posterior fossa.
- Generally will use NSF for most endoscopic approaches unless it is directly invaded by tumor.

- **Pericranial flap**
  - Robust flap that can be used for very large defects, especially anterior fossa
  - Based on supratrochlear and supraorbital arteries
  - Can be harvested via an open approach or endoscopic assisted
  - Needs to be passed through a nasionectomy into the nasal cavity
- **Inferior turbinate/lateral nasal wall flap**
  - Another flap that can be used when NSF is unavailable
  - Based on two SPA branches to the inferior turbinate—a larger one which travels toward the inferior meatus and a smaller branch on the medial surface of the turbinate
  - Arc of rotation is somewhat limited; most suited for clival defects
- **Temporoparietal fascia flap**
  - Based on superficial temporal artery
  - A laterally based flap that needs to be tunneled through the infratemporal fossa into the PPF and nasal cavity (technically challenging)
  - Rarely used but most suited for posterior fossa defects

Microvascular Free Flaps

- Typically reserved for when all other reconstructive options are unavailable
- Examples include radial forearm free flap and anterolateral thigh flap
- Additional details provided in chapter on free-flap reconstruction

Bibliography

Cerebrospinal Fluid Rhinorrhea: Guide to Comprehensive Management. Sindwani R, Roxbury C. eds. Elsevier, St Louis, MO; 2023.

Johncilla M, Vickie YJ. Soft tissue tumors of the sinonasal tract. *Semin Diagn Pathol*. 2016;33(2):81-90.

Kuan EC, Wang EC, Adappa ND, et al. International Consensus Statement on Allergy and Rhinology: Sinonasal Tumors. *Int Forum Allergy Rhinol*. 2024;14(2):149-608.

Sindwani R, Woodard TD, Recinos PF. Endoscopic cranial base and pituitary surgery. *Otolaryngol Clin North Am*. Feb 2016;49:1-263.

Thawani R, Kim MS, Arastu A, et al. The contemporary management of cancers of the sinonasal tract in adults. *CA Cancer J Clin*. 2023;73(1):72-112.

Questions

1. The nasoseptal flap is a vascularized, pedicled flap used in skull base reconstruction based on which of the following arteries?
   A. Palatovaginal artery
   B. Main trunk of sphenopalatine artery
   C. Posterior septal branch of sphenopalatine artery
   D. Septal branch of posterior ethmoidal artery
   E. Septal branch of superior labial artery

2. The Holman-Miller sign refers to which of the following?
   A. Anterior bowing of the posterior wall of the maxillary sinus seen on CT sinus
   B. Posterior bowing of the posterior wall of the maxillary sinus seen on CT sinus
   C. Focal point of hyperostosis/osteitis seen on CT sinus
   D. T2 hyperintensity seen on MRI in association with sinonasal malignancy
   E. T2 hypointensity seen on MRI in association with sinonasal malignancy

3. Physaliphorous cells are associated with which of the following tumors?
   A. Esthesioneuroblastoma
   B. Sinonasal undifferentiated carcinoma
   C. Sinonasal neuroendocrine carcinoma
   D. Squamous cell carcinoma
   E. Chordoma

4. Small round blue cells with neuroendocrine marker differentiation and the presence of pseudorosettes and/or rosettes describes which of the following?
   A. Squamous cell carcinoma
   B. Sinonasal neuroendocrine carcinoma
   C. Sinonasal undifferentiated carcinoma
   D. Esthesioneuroblastoma
   E. Juvenile nasopharyngeal angiofibroma

5. Which of the following is true about sinonasal mucosal melanoma?
   A. It carries a better prognosis than cutaneous mucosal melanoma.
   B. The minimum T stage is T3.
   C. It has a high rate of BRAF mutations.
   D. Chemotherapy is the mainstay of treatment.
   E. It always produces melanin pigment.

Chapter 30
Endoscopic Sinus Surgery

Introduction

- There has been an evolution in the theories of pathogenesis and clinical management of sinonasal inflammatory disease that has revolutionized the practice of otolaryngologists.
- Diseases previously managed with open procedures are now widely managed with endoscopic approaches as the technology too has greatly improved.
- Further, the advancement of topical therapies and in-office procedures has created opportunities to manage disease, while creating cost-saving techniques and possibly improving patient safety.
- However, the variability of the anatomy and their critical relationship with the sinonasal cavities, still remain true and a detailed knowledge of the embryology and anatomy of the paranasal sinuses is necessary to avoid potentially disastrous surgical complications.

Embryology of Paranasal Sinuses

Ethmoturbinals (Figure 30-1)

- Development heralded by the appearance of a series of ridges or folds on the lateral nasal wall at approximately the eighth week.
- 6 to 7 folds emerge initially, but eventually only 3 to 4 ridges persist.
- Persistent ridges are referred to as ethmoturbinals from an ethmoid origin:
    - First ethmoturbinal—rudimentary and incomplete in humans
        - Ascending portion forms the agger nasi
        - Descending portion forms the uncinate process
    - Second ethmoturbinal—forms the middle turbinate
    - Third ethmoturbinal—forms the superior turbinate
    - Fourth and fifth ethmoturbinals—fuse to form the supreme turbinate
- Furrows form between the ethmoturbinals and ultimately establish the primordial nasal meati and recesses.
    - First furrow (between the first and second ethmoturbinals)
        - Descending aspect forms the ethmoidal infundibulum, hiatus semilunaris, and middle meatus.
            - ◊ The primordial maxillary sinus develops from the inferior aspect of the ethmoid infundibulum.
        - Ascending aspect contributes to the frontal recess.

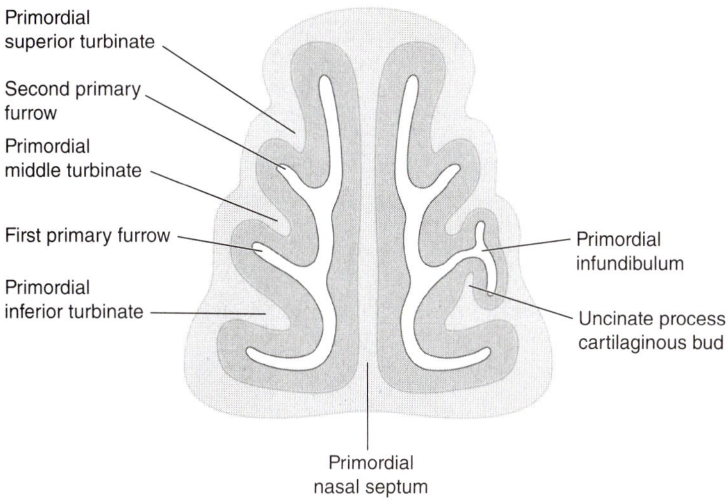

Figure 30-1 Fetal cartilaginous capsule at 9-12 weeks.

- Second furrow (between the second and third ethmoturbinals) forms the superior meatus.
- Third furrow (between the third and fourth ethmoturbinals) forms the supreme meatus.

Contemporary Sinus Embryology Theory

- In addition to the traditional ridge and furrow concept of development, a cartilaginous capsule surrounds the developing nasal cavity and plays a role in sinonasal development.
- At 8 weeks, three soft-tissue elevations or preturbinates are seen that correlate to the future inferior, middle, and superior turbinates.
- At 9 to 10 weeks, a soft-tissue elevation and underlying cartilaginous bud emerge that correspond to the future uncinate process.
- By 13 to 14 weeks, a space develops lateral to the uncinate anlagen that corresponds to the ethmoidal infundibulum.
- By 16 weeks, the future maxillary sinus begins to develop from the inferior aspect of the infundibulum.
- All three turbinates and each paranasal sinus arise from the cartilaginous nasal capsule which resorb or ossify over time.

Anatomic Considerations in Endoscopic Sinus Surgery (ESS)

The Lamellae

- The basal or ground lamella of the middle turbinate divides the anterior and posterior ethmoid air cells.
- The frontal, maxillary, and anterior ethmoid cells arise from the region of the anterior ethmoid and therefore drain into the middle meatus.

- The posterior ethmoid cells lie posterior to the basal lamella and therefore drain into the superior and supreme meati.
- The sphenoid sinus drains into the sphenoethmoid recess medial to the superior turbinate.

Agger Nasi

- The agger nasi is a region, rather than a particular air cell, bordered by the following:
  - Anteriorly: frontal process of the maxilla
  - Superiorly: frontal recess or sinus
  - Anterolaterally: nasal bones
  - Inferolaterally: lacrimal bone
  - Inferomedially: uncinate process of the ethmoid bone

Uncinate Process

- A hook-like, sagittally oriented structure measuring 3 to 4 mm wide and 1.5 to 2 cm in length.
- The posterior margin is free and forms the anterior boundary of the hiatus semilunaris while forming the medial wall of the ethmoidal infundibulum.
- It attaches anteriorly and superiorly to the ethmoidal crest of the maxilla and just inferiorly fuses with the posterior aspect of the lacrimal bone.
- Posteriorly, it attaches to the ethmoidal process of the inferior turbinate and palatine bones.
- Superior aspect most commonly bends laterally to insert on the lamina papyracea creating the *recessus terminalis*, a blind pouch, which drives the frontal recess superior and medial to this portion of the uncinate.
- Alternatively, the uncinate process may occasionally attach superiorly to the ethmoid roof or even bend medially to attach to the middle turbinate which guides the frontal recess lateral to the uncinate.
- The inferior aspect forms part of the medial wall of the maxillary sinus. The maxillary sinus natural ostium lies lateral and superior to this part, and thus, this portion of the uncinate must be removed to widen the natural ostium.

Nasal Fontanelles

- The attachment of the uncinate process to the inferior turbinate divides the medial wall of the maxillary sinus into anterior and posterior regions of periosteum covered by mucosa. These are called the anterior and posterior fontanelles.
- An accessory ostium represents a perforated fontanelle (20%-25% of patients), typically the posterior fontanelle, and perhaps indicates prior sinus disease.

Ethmoid Bulla

- Superiorly, the anterior wall of the ethmoid bulla can extend to the skull base and form the posterior limit of the frontal recess.
- Posteriorly, the bulla may blend with the basal lamella or have a space between it and the basal lamella labeled the retrobullar recess. A space above the bulla is termed the suprabullar recess, while collectively, these spaces are referred to as the *sinus lateralis*.

Hiatus Semilunaris

- Defined as a two-dimensional, crescent-shaped gap between the posterior free margin of the uncinate process and the anterior wall of the ethmoid bulla for which the middle meatus communicates with the ethmoid infundibulum.

Ethmoidal Infundibulum

- Described as a funnel-shaped passage which channels secretions into the middle meatus from the anterior ethmoid cells and the maxillary sinus and, in some cases, the frontal recess.
- It has the following borders:
  - Medial: uncinate process
  - Lateral: lamina papyracea
  - Posterior: anterior wall of ethmoid bulla
  - Anterior and superior: frontal process of the maxilla
  - Superior and lateral: lacrimal bone

Osteomeatal Unit

- The osteomeatal unit is not a discrete anatomic structure but rather is a functional designation that describes the drainage pathway of the maxillary, frontal, and anterior ethmoid sinuses.
- Collectively, it also encompasses the middle meatus, uncinate process, and ethmoid infundibulum.

Frontal Recess and Sinus

- The frontal recess is the most anterior and superior aspect of the anterior ethmoid sinus that forms the connection with the frontal sinus.
- The boundaries of the frontal recess are as follows:
  - Lateral: lamina papyracea
  - Medial: middle turbinate
  - Anterior: the posterior superior wall of the agger nasi cell (when present)
  - Posterior: anterior wall of the ethmoid bulla (if it extends to the skull base)
- The frontal recess tapers as it approaches the superiorly located internal ostium of the frontal sinus.
- Above the ostium, it again widens as the anterior and posterior tables diverge to their respective positions giving an hourglass appearance, with the narrowest portion being the frontal ostium.
- Most commonly the recess opens just medial to the posterior aspect of the uncinate process.

Anterior Ethmoid Artery (AEA)

- The AEA is highly variable with regard to the skull base. It may lie within the skull base, be dehiscent, or sit up to 4 mm below the skull base in a mesentery.
- The AEA traverses from the orbit (lateral) to the lateral lamella of the cribriform plate (medial) along the ethmoid roof in a posterior-to-anterior direction.
- From an anterior-to-posterior direction, the artery lies just behind the bulla ethmoidalis or any stacked air cells above the bulla. The one exception is a supraorbital ethmoid cell, whereby the artery may sit anterior, within, or posterior to this cell.
- Radiographically, the artery can be seen piercing the medial orbit, commonly referred to as the "nipple sign," just posterior to the globe in the area where the superior oblique and medial rectus are closely adjacent to one another.

Middle Turbinate

- Originating from the ethmoid bone, the anterior middle turbinate attaches laterally at the agger nasi region, specifically at the crista ethmoidalis maxillae.

- It courses superiorly and medially to attach vertically to the lateral aspect of the cribriform plate, where anterior cranial fossa dura may invaginate the turbinate with olfactory filaments.
- This segment is in a near coronal plane anteriorly and near axial plane posteriorly and represents the basal lamella dividing the ethmoid labyrinth into anterior and posterior components.
- The most posterior aspect is the inferior attachment of the turbinate at the crista ethmoidalis of the perpendicular process of the palatine bone, just anterior to the sphenopalatine foramen. Cauterization of the root of the middle turbinate at this location should be considered when resecting the middle turbinate due to the close proximity of vessels arising from the sphenopalatine foramen.
- Pneumatization of the vertical portion of the middle turbinate is described as intralamellar while pneumatization of the head of the middle turbinate is referred to as a concha bullosa.

Ethmoid Roof and Cribriform Plate

- Typically, the ethmoid roof slopes inferiorly and medially, and is thinner medially than laterally.
- Medially, the roof is formed by the lateral lamella of the cribriform, which is variable in its vertical height.
- A low-lying or asymmetric skull base must be recognized prior to surgery to avoid the potential complication of a cerebrospinal fluid (CSF) leak.
- Keros described three ethmoid roof variations based on the lateral lamella vertical height:
  - Keros Type I: 1-to 3-mm depth to the olfactory fossa
  - Keros Type II: 4-to 7-mm depth to the olfactory fossa
  - Keros Type III: 8-to 16-mm depth to the olfactory fossa
- The third Keros group is considered the highest-risk configuration for inadvertent intracranial injury because of the long, thin lateral lamella adjacent to the ethmoid sinuses, but it does not consider the skull base height posteriorly which is evaluated by comparing the ratio of the ethmoid height to that of the maxillary sinus.

Sphenoethmoidal (Onodi) Cell

- A posterior ethmoid cell that pneumatizes over the superolateral aspect of the sphenoid sinus is called an Onodi cell.
- If present, the optic nerve and the internal carotid artery become intimately related to this cell, thus putting these structures at risk if this anatomic variation is not identified.

Sphenoid Sinus

- The sphenoid ostium is near the height of the maxillary sinus roof and the face of the sphenoid is at the same depth as the posterior wall of the maxillary sinus.
- Located centrally within the skull, the sinus has highly variable pneumatization. Laterally, the sinus may pneumatize for a variable distance under the middle cranial fossa (lateral recess); inferiorly, it may pneumatize to a variable extent into the pterygoid processes, and posteriorly, it may pneumatize for a variable distance inferior to the sella turcica creating the clival recess.
- This inter-sinus septum is highly variable and may attach laterally to one side in the region of the carotid artery, an important consideration if it is being surgically manipulated.

- Critical midline structures that border the sinus include the sella turcica, superior intercavernous sinus, and the planum sphenoidale.
- In well-pneumatized sphenoid sinuses, the vidian canal may be identified inferolaterally.
- Lateral to the sinus lie the carotid artery, the optic nerve, the cavernous sinus, and the third through sixth cranial nerves (excluding V3).
- The optic nerve and internal carotid artery are covered by a thin layer of bone and can indent the sphenoid sinus lateral and posteriorly. The optico-carotid recess represents pneumatization between these structures.
- The carotid canal may be dehiscent in up to 22% of specimens, while dehiscence of the optic canal occurs in 5% of cases.

Surgical Management of Sinonasal Disease

Objective of Endoscopic Sinus Surgery (ESS)

- The goal of ESS is to promote physiologic sinus drainage, sinus ventilation, improve mucosal health for restoration of healthy sinus function, and also provide access for medication delivery in some cases.
- ESS debrides inflamed tissue and removes the obstructive nature of disease, but surgery alone is only one step in restoring healthy sinus function. Medical management is also key for improving overall sinonasal health and may be augmented by topical treatment for long-term management of inflammation.
- In select cases, surgery alone is adequate in managing the disease. Such conditions include fungus balls and silent sinus syndrome.

Evaluation, Diagnosis, and Preoperative Management

Patient Selection

- Deciding to proceed with surgery in the presence of severe disease is relatively easy. Large mucoceles, inflammatory complications, or diffuse nasal polyposis unresponsive to medical therapy require surgery for appropriate outcomes.
- Minor disease, recurrent sinusitis, or headaches are more challenging indications for surgery.
- Differential diagnoses and underlying systemic conditions should also be considered due to the requisite ancillary treatments needed. Without identifying immunodeficiencies, cystic fibrosis, ciliary dysmotility, or systemic conditions (such as vasculitis), adequate outcomes cannot be accomplished.
- One should also consider the patient's response to previous medical treatments and surgical procedures. Those with poor medical responsiveness are more likely to have poor symptom control compared to responsive patients. Prior to revision surgery, the surgeon should identify the cause of surgical failure.
- Patient expectations should be tempered. Symptoms with poor objective endoscopic and radiographic correlation may not be ideal surgical candidates.
- General guidelines before ESS:
    - The patient should have a trial of appropriate medical therapy (see below).
    - Realistic expectations of surgical results should be set. Severe pain is unusual in chronic rhinosinusitis (CRS), and headaches correlate poorly with sinus disease;

- therefore, patients should understand that these conditions are not likely to improve with surgery.
  - Smoking cessation should be pursued, as tobacco smoke may result in increased scarring and worsening of symptoms.

Recurrent Acute Rhinosinusitis (RARS)

- Four or more episodes per year of acute bacterial rhinosinusitis (ABRS) with distinct symptom-free intervals between episodes.
- Contributing factors may include anatomic anomalies, viral infections, allergy, and immunodeficiency, but each lacks clear evidence of causality.
- Medical management should be managed the same as ABRS.
- Surgical management may be helpful in a select population but ESS has not been shown to reduce antibiotic usage.

Appropriate Medical Therapy (AMT)

- Maximal medical therapy has been replaced by the term AMT, which more accurately describes appropriate nonsurgical options without negatively impacting surgical outcomes.
- For CRS without nasal polyposis (CRSsNP), a trial of intranasal corticosteroids (INCS), saline irrigations, and oral antibiotics are recommended.
- For CRS with nasal polyposis (CRSwNP), a trial of INCS, saline irrigations, and a single short course of oral corticosteroids is recommended.
- The recommended duration of antibiotics is 3 weeks at a minimum.
- Success is defined as symptomatic relief, and failure is defined as insufficient symptomatic response with persistent endoscopic or radiologic evidence of CRS.

Diagnostic Nasal Endoscopy

- The development of the modern rigid nasal endoscope represents a major advance in rhinologic diagnostic capability.
- Nasal endoscopy is more sensitive for the diagnosis of accessible disease than computed tomography (CT) and provides essential complementary information for patient diagnosis.
- Endoscopy permits detailed evaluation of the middle meatus and sphenoethmoidal recess for mucosal edema, polyps, or purulence.
- The 30° 2.7-mm (pediatric) endoscope is the most useful endoscope as it provides an ample viewing field and is well tolerated by most patients. A 45° or 70° telescope may be helpful in some patients.
- The patient remains in a sitting or supine position.
- The nasal cavities are sprayed with a topical decongestant and local anesthetic.
- The endoscope lens is treated with a thin film of antifog solution and introduced slowly under direct vision.
- A complete examination can be successfully accomplished in a step-wise manner:
  - First, pass the endoscope along the nasal floor while inspecting the overall anatomy, identifying any septal obstructions, the presence of pathologic secretions or polyps, and the condition of nasal mucosa. Further inspection allows a complete evaluation of the nasopharynx, including both eustachian tube orifices.
  - Next, pass the scope between the middle and inferior turbinates allowing for inspection of the inferior portion of the middle meatus, fontanelles, and the presence of accessory maxillary ostia. The scope is then passed medial to the middle turbinate

and advanced posteriorly to examine the sphenoethmoidal recess. Rotating the scope superiorly and slightly laterally allows for visualization of the superior turbinate and meatus as well as the slit-like or oval ostia of the sphenoid sinus.

- Finally, the examination is completed as the telescope is withdrawn. As the scope is brought back anteriorly, it can frequently be rotated laterally under the middle turbinate into the posterior aspect of the middle meatus. The bulla ethmoidalis, hiatus semilunaris, and infundibular entrance are inspected. Withdrawing the telescope further can provide an excellent view of the middle turbinate, uncinate process, and surrounding mucosa.

Imaging

- High-resolution CT scans should be performed at least 4 weeks after initiating medical therapy for the most recent episode of CRS and at least 2 weeks following the most recent upper respiratory infection.
- Radiographic (or endoscopic) evidence of mucosal disease should be present to diagnose CRS.
- Preoperative imaging evaluation is key in identifying possible anatomic variants that can lead to adverse outcomes (see below for imaging checklist).
- Opacification adjacent to skull base dehiscence is an indication for magnetic resonance imaging (MRI) to rule out a meningoencephalocele prior to surgery.

Surgical Indications (Inflammatory Disease)

- CRSwNP and CRSsNP recalcitrant to medical treatment
- Fungal rhinosinusitis (invasive and noninvasive forms)
- Recurrent acute rhinosinusitis (may be helpful in a select population)
- Complications of rhinosinusitis (mucoceles, orbital/subperiosteal infections, intracranial complications)
- Antrochoanal polyp

Surgical Indications (Non-inflammatory Disease)

- Benign and malignant sinonasal neoplasms
- Silent sinus syndrome and chronic maxillary atelectasis
- CSF leak and meningoencephalocele
- Endoscopic access to skull base tumors
- Endoscopic orbital decompression for thyroid eye disease
- Choanal atresia repair
- Recurrent epistaxis
- Sinus foreign body removal

Surgical Concepts

Extent of Surgery

- Relief of ostial obstruction is paramount.
- Remove inflammatory mucosa, bony partitions, and osteitic bone in the area of disease as completely as possible.
- Extend the dissection one step beyond the extent of disease (if possible).
- Septoplasty is used for surgical access and postoperative surveillance (see below).

- Complete ESS addressing all the sinuses is recommended in patients with diffuse disease to facilitate the delivery of postoperative topical therapy and reduce the inflammatory burden.

Mucosal Preservation

- Mucosal preservation, and thereby preserving the mucoperiosteum and avoiding exposed bone, is essential in modern ESS.
- Preservation of mucosa reduces osteitis, crust formation, stenosis, pain, and undesirable scarring while facilitating healing.
- Native mucosal lining is vital to maintaining mucociliary clearance.

Surgical Exposure

- Wide exposure is optimal, thus limiting the risk of disorientation and facilitating instrument movement.
- Narrow surgical fields often result out of fear of orbital or skull base injury, at times a result of a lack of understanding the surgical anatomy.
- Early identification of key landmarks, like the lamina papyracea or skull base, allow for avoidance of such injuries.

Natural Ostia Inclusion

- Natural mucociliary clearance patterns mobilize mucus toward the natural ostium of a sinus.
- Connecting surgical ostia with the natural ostia ensures normal mucus outflow.
- Discontinuity between a surgical and natural ostium can result in recirculation and potentially recalcitrant CRS.

Management of Nasal Septum

- Septoplasty is indicated when a deviated septum otherwise obstructs surgical access to the sinuses or inhibits adequate postsurgical aeration, postoperative surveillance or debridement, and postoperative topical medication delivery.
- Goal of septoplasty is visualization of the anterior superior attachment of the middle turbinate with the 0° telescope.
- ESS is started on the contralateral side to the deviation to allow for better visualization and to reduce the risk of septal trauma.
- The septoplasty is then performed prior to completing the second surgical side.
- Endoscopic approach to septoplasty allows improved visualization of the septum without changing instrumentation or the need for a headlight.

Management of the Middle Turbinate

- Preservation of the middle turbinate is ideal, but resection may be required if marked disease is present or concern for lateralization is high.
  - Middle turbinate lateralization may compromise patency of the middle meatus, which is essential in maintaining long-term ventilation and drainage of the maxillary, ethmoid, and frontal sinuses.
- Techniques to prevent lateralization include suture techniques, Bolgerization, partial resection of the middle turbinate, and various forms of stents.
- Middle turbinate resection may be useful in cases with heavy disease burden and to improve access. Overly aggressive resection comes with potential risks for CSF leaks and olfactory disturbance.

Image Guidance

- Allows for real-time localization of surgical instruments and critical structures within the surgical field.
- Image guidance is not a substitute for a thorough understanding of the patient's anatomy.
- Appropriate indications for use include:
  - Revision sinus surgery
  - Distorted sinus anatomy of developmental, postoperative, or traumatic origin
  - Extensive sinonasal polyposis
  - Pathology that involves the frontal, posterior ethmoid, and sphenoid sinuses
  - Disease abutting the skull base, orbit, optic nerve, or internal carotid artery
  - CSF rhinorrhea or conditions in which there is a skull base defect
  - Benign and malignant sinonasal neoplasms

Powered Instrumentation

- Powered microdebriders are useful in debulking hypertrophic sinonasal mucosal lining, sinonasal polyps, or tumors.
  - Microdebriders cut the desired mucosa sharply and minimize mucosal stripping.
  - Multiple angulated blades exist. The 60° blade is commonly used for the frontal sinuses.
- Drills are useful in complex sinus surgery and skull base tumors.

Balloon Sinus Dilation

- Balloon dilation is advocated when the goal is atraumatic dilation of sinus ostia to restore sinus ventilation and normal drainage.
- An expert panel reached consensus about the following statements regarding balloon sinus dilation:
  - It is not appropriate for those without both sinonasal symptoms and positive findings of disease on CT scans.
  - It is not appropriate for the management of headaches or obstructive sleep apnea in patients who do not meet criteria for CRS or recurrent ARS.
  - CT scanning is required before balloon dilation is performed.
  - It is not appropriate for patients with sinonasal symptoms that lack CT evidence of sinonasal disease.
  - It can be appropriate as an adjunct procedure to ESS in patients with CRSsNP.
  - It can have a role in persistent sinus disease after previous ESS.
  - It can have a role in recurrent ARS based on symptoms and CT evidence of ostial occlusion and mucosal thickening.
  - It can improve short-term QOL outcomes in patients with limited CRSsNP.
  - It can be effective in frontal sinusitis.

Avoiding and Managing Intraoperative Complications

- Critical to avoiding operative complications is a thorough understanding of anatomical concepts and how they apply to the particular patient.

Intraoperative Bleeding

- Deliver topical and/or infiltrative vasoconstriction at the beginning of the case.
- Avoid unnecessary mucosal trauma, particularly along the nasal septum.
- The anterior ethmoid artery is dehiscent in approximately 40% of patients as it travels in a bony mesentery along the ethmoid roof. Early identification is imperative to risk reduction.
- Careful resection of tissue in the area of the sphenopalatine foramen and the associated arterial branches. Enlargement of the middle meatal antrostomy posteriorly and resection of the sphenoid face inferiorly place arterial branches at risk for injury.
- Suction electrocautery and topical vasoconstrictors often are adequate for immediate hemostasis.
- Elevating the head of the bed 17° improves blood loss without interfering in instrument management, particularly the frontal sinus.
- Repeated warm saline irrigations (104°-114°F) have been shown to be effective in reducing blood loss intraoperatively.
- Persistent bleeding, in some cases, may require ending the surgery prior to completion of the procedure.

Orbital Injury

- Early identification of the lamina papyracea is crucial.
- Avoiding dissection along the orbit can often times lead to spatial disorientation when removing ethmoidal cells. Upon positively identifying the lamina papyracea, deliberate dissection along this structure allows for safe removal of air cells while also maintaining the lateral dissection limits.
- Care should be taken in the posterior ethmoid cells, particularly when sphenoethmoidal (Onodi) cells are present, as the optic nerve and carotid artery are present along the superior and lateral walls of this structure.
- Identify and preserve the anterior ethmoid artery.
  - Inadvertent arterial ligation can result in vessel retraction within the orbit and a subsequent orbital hematoma.
  - If bony resection is needed adjacent to the vessel, resection should first occur medially (toward the lateral lamella), because it reduces the risk of arterial retraction into the orbit and facilitates operative control of the vessel.
- Management of orbital complications
  - Upon intraoperative violation of the lamina papyracea with orbital fat exposure, further dissection should be terminated in the immediate region. Orbital fat should not be removed or resected.
  - Avoid nasal packing when orbital contents have been violated to avoid elevated intraorbital pressure.
  - Early signs of an orbital hematoma include chemosis and proptosis suggesting an orbital compartment syndrome may be imminent.
    - Immediate lateral canthotomy and cantholysis are required for pressure reduction. Endoscopic orbital decompression may also be performed, and ophthalmology consult obtained.
    - Medical management of orbital hematoma includes topical timolol and intravenous acetazolamide, mannitol, and high-dose steroids.

Skull Base Injury

- The skull base is consistent anatomically at the roof of the sphenoid sinus. By first identifying the skull base posteriorly at the sphenoid sinus and then dissecting anteriorly, one can maintain consistent visualization of the skull base.

- Medial dissection should be performed carefully as there is variable height anatomically between patients around the lateral lamella and cribriform plate, which are easily penetrated with instruments.
- Thru-cutting instruments should be used to remove partitions attached to the skull base.
- To avoid disorientation, a 0° telescope should be used until the skull base is identified. Then a 30° scope is appropriate for the remaining dissection.

CSF Rhinorrhea

- Intraoperative identification of CSF rhinorrhea should be managed at the time of surgery.
- Remove any residual bony partitions around the defect to create a flat surface for graft placement.
- Adjacent sinus mucosa should be removed to create an area of denuded bone for the graft.
- Place a free overlay nasal mucosal graft over the leak site. The middle turbinate and nasal floor mucosa offer reliable free mucosal grafts.
- Secure the graft with several layers of absorbable collagen-based packing with or without a nonabsorbable sponge layer.
- Consider a postoperative head CT and MRI to rule out the possibility of intracranial bleeding and injury.
- Consider neurosurgical and infectious disease consultations.

Endoscopic Sinus Surgery

Historical Surgical Approaches

Messerklinger

- Anterior-to-posterior dissection in the following manner:
  - Removal of the uncinate process exposes the ethmoidal infundibulum permitting visualization of the ethmoid bulla.
  - The ethmoid bulla is removed, which exposes the frontal sinus outflow tract and the ethmoid roof.
  - Resection of the remaining anterior ethmoid cells is followed by removal of the basal lamella of the middle turbinate and the posterior ethmoidectomy.
  - The sphenoidotomy is performed by identifying and enlarging the sphenoid ostium.
  - A 30° endoscope is then used to identify the natural ostium of the maxillary sinus and to perform the middle meatal antrostomy.

Wigand

- Posterior-to-anterior approach along the skull base in the following manner:
  - Removal of the low posterior ethmoid cells until the face of the sphenoid is identified.
  - Sphenoidotomy is then performed, which permits identification of the skull base at the face of the sphenoid sinus.
  - With the skull base identified, the dissection of remnant ethmoid partitions is continued in a posterior to anterior fashion along the ethmoid roof.

Surgical Steps

Surgeon Review of Imaging

- Accurate knowledge of the patient's surgical anatomy is essential to safe and effective surgery.
- Anatomical landmarks should be reviewed the day of surgery with the aid of imaging.
- Key landmarks include:
  - Height, slope, shape, symmetry, and integrity of the skull base
  - Position of the anterior ethmoid artery relative to the skull base
  - Shape and integrity of the lamina papyracea (ie, orbital content in sinus)
  - Relative height of the posterior ethmoid sinuses to the posteromedial roof of the maxillary sinus
  - Rotation and position of the uncinate process
  - Presence of named cells: Onodi or Haller cells
  - Frontal recess anatomy: frontal recess diameter and relationship of ethmoid cells in the outflow tract
  - Sphenoid sinus: dehiscence of carotid artery or optic nerve; also note any attachment of intersphenoid sinus septum to carotid canal
  - CLOSE mnemonic also helps identify key landmarks to review on CT:
    - C = Cribriform plate
    - L = Lamina papyracea
    - O = Onodi cell
    - S = Sphenoid sinus pneumatization
    - E = (Anterior) Ethmoid artery

Surgical Team Safety Check

- All members of the surgical team should ensure the following:
  - Topical epinephrine/oxymetazoline is stained and labeled appropriately.
  - Injectable anesthetic is labeled and left unstained.
  - Suction cautery/bipolar cautery is immediately available in the room.
  - Hemostatic materials are immediately available in the room.
  - Culture swabs or suction traps are available in the room.
  - Method of specimen collection is reviewed (sidedness, microdebrider trap, fresh/formalin).

Preparation of Nasal Cavity

- Under local or general anesthesia, the nose is decongested prior to surgery with oxymetazoline or topical epinephrine (1:1000) on nasal pledgets.
- Endoscopic injection with 1% Xylocaine with 1:100,000 epinephrine is an option:
  - Anterior to the attachment of the middle turbinate
  - Anterior to the inferior portion of the uncinate process
  - Inferior aspect of middle turbinate
  - Transnasal or transoral sphenopalatine block for posterior ethmoid or sphenoid sinus dissections
  - Perform slowly as temporary diplopia can occur and visual loss has been reported

Uncinectomy

- The first and one of the most important steps in ESS is identification and complete removal of the uncinate process.
- Care must be taken to avoid violation of the lamina papyracea due to its close proximity to the uncinate.

- Uncinectomy is performed in the following manner:
  - Visualization of the posterior (free) edge of the uncinate process.
  - Pediatric backbiter placed behind the posterior free margin of the uncinate at the transition zone of the vertical (superior two-thirds) and horizontal (inferior one-third) segments of the uncinate.
  - Cut anteriorly to the level of the maxillary line, which is the junction of the anterior uncinate border and the medial vertical buttress of the maxilla housing the nasolacrimal duct.
  - A J-curette is then used to reflect the superior segment of the uncinate process medially and 90° angled graspers are used to remove the vertical segment (push-pull motion).
  - Side biting and back-biting instruments are used to remove the horizontal segment of the uncinate.

Middle Meatal Antrostomy

- The natural ostium of the maxillary sinus lies anteriorly and opens at a 45° angle in the floor of the infundibulum.
- Mucociliary clearance patterns are directed toward the natural maxillary ostium.
  - An accessory ostium should not be confused with the natural ostium.
  - Failure to connect the natural and accessory ostia may result in recirculation.
- Angled endoscopes (30°, 45°, or 70°) are critical to ensuring visualization of the natural ostium of the maxillary sinus.
- A double-ball probe positioned in an inferior-lateral direction is used to probe the natural ostium.
  - Directing the double-ball probe directly lateral may result in orbital injury.
- The natural ostium is then opened using a combination of back biting and 90° angled graspers.
- Through-cutting instruments may be used to expand the antrostomy posteriorly.
- Side-biting antrum punches are useful to expand the antrostomy inferiorly and/or superiorly.
- The appropriate size of the middle meatal antrostomy should be tailored to the patient's disease.

Extended Maxillary Sinus Procedures

- Endoscopic maxillary mega-antrostomy includes partial inferior turbinectomy and widening of the maxillary antrostomy to the level of the nasal cavity floor.
- This procedure is indicated when mucociliary clearance is ineffective.
- Endoscopic modified medial maxillectomy is used for the management of benign sinonasal neoplasms and requires complete inferior turbinectomy and widening of the antrostomy to its anatomic limits.
- Denker operation is an extension of the medial maxillectomy beyond the nasolacrimal duct anteriorly to the level of the pyriform aperture which allows access and visualization of far lateral and anterior disease.
- Endoscopic-assisted sublabial anterior maxillotomy (Caldwell-Luc approach) is rarely indicated for inflammatory disease but may be beneficial in disease which is difficult to access through endonasal routes.
- Inferior meatal antrostomy is rarely indicated and could lead to recirculation of mucus, but it may be used in mucociliary dysfunction conditions.

Ethmoidectomy

- Appropriate dissection requires early identification of several landmarks from anterior to posterior as each successive step is performed: ethmoid bulla, lamina papyracea, basal lamella of the middle turbinate, superior turbinate and its basal lamella, anterior face of the sphenoid sinus.
- The ethmoidectomy should begin with a 0° telescope. Transition to an angled telescope does not occur until the skull base has been defined in the posterior ethmoid cavity and the surgeon has reached the limits of nonangulated instruments.
- The bulla ethmoidalis is resected first. This step begins with placing a J-curette into the retrobullar space. In a posterior-to-anterior direction the bulla is resected with the curette followed by resection of bone and soft tissue with grasping devices and a microdebrider. If the retrobullar space is not well-defined, blunt dissection of the bulla ethmoidalis is initiated medially and inferiorly.
- Upon dissection, attention should then be turned toward defining the lamina papyracea, which is a constant landmark through the entire ethmoidectomy. Cutting and grasping instruments are used for this portion.
- Next, management of the basal lamella occurs.
  - If the surgery is to be limited to the anterior ethmoidectomy, attention should then turn toward any agger nasi cells and supra-bullar cells (see below).
  - If a posterior ethmoidectomy is to be performed, the horizontal and vertical segments of the basal lamella are to be identified. The optimal location for penetrating the basal lamella is medially and inferiorly which protects against skull base and orbital injury. One should be careful to protect the horizontal segment of the basal lamella so as not to destabilize the middle turbinate.
- A J-curette in the inverted position (pointing down) perforates the basal lamella. Biting and grasping forceps are then used for dissection in a medial-to-lateral direction until the lamina papyracea is defined.
- The posterior ethmoidectomy is continued with the use of biting and grasping instruments and the aid of the microdebrider. A complete ethmoidectomy should include removal of all partitions until the sphenoid face is visualized and the following structures are defined: the superior turbinate medially, the basal lamella of the superior turbinate inferiorly, the skull base superiorly, and the lamina papyracea laterally. Collectively, this parallelogram of structures is referred to as "Bolger box."
  - The surgeon should be cognizant of the existence of any sphenoethmoidal (Onodi) cells, which can be mistaken for the sphenoid sinus. The optico-carotid recess may form the posterior apex of the Onodi cell.
- If a superior ethmoid or frontal recess dissection is planned, the skull base should be identified when possible within the posterior ethmoid sinus. However, this is most safely performed after the sphenoidotomy has been completed and the skull base has been defined within the sphenoid sinus (see sphenoidotomy below).
- Once the skull base has been identified and the limits of straight instruments have been reached, transition to an angled endoscope occurs. Most commonly, 30° or 45° endoscopes are used.
- Removal of partitions along the skull base should be performed with a J-curette and small, angled thru-cutting instruments.
- Dissection of the agger nasi region is required for a complete ethmoidectomy.

Sphenoidotomy

- The most posterior ethmoid cell characteristically has a pyramidal shape with the apex pointing posteriorly, laterally, and superiorly toward the optic nerve. The sphenoid sinus lies inferiorly, medially, and posterior to this cell. In some cases, a sphenoethmoidal (Onodi) cell aerates beyond the anterior face of the sphenoid sinus.

Surgical Approaches to the Sphenoid Sinus

- Transseptal approach: historically utilized in pituitary or midline skull base tumor approaches. A submucosal dissection along the nasal septum anterior-to-posterior until the sphenoid rostrum (midline) is identified. Bilateral sphenoid ostia are identified and enlarged followed by removal of the sphenoid rostrum and intersinus septum. The goal of this approach is to create a common sphenoid cavity.
- Transnasal approach: indicated for isolated sphenoid sinus disease or when approaching tumors within the sphenoid skull base.
  - The middle turbinate is carefully medialized with a Freer elevator to not destabilize the basal lamella.
  - The superior turbinate is identified and cut sharply as it transitions from the vertical to the horizontal segment.
  - The natural sphenoid ostium is invariably located medial to the superior turbinate attachment, approximately 1.5 cm above the choana. A stapes curette, J curette, or freer elevator may be used to bluntly palpate the ostium and curette/enlarge the bony edges.
  - The ostium is further enlarged with a 2-mm Kerrison rongeur or a sphenoid mushroom punch. Any use of a microdebrider should be limited to the ostium itself, and the blades of the debrider should be directed medially and inferiorly with the purpose of defining the ostium. Lateral dissection with a microdebrider may inadvertently injure the optic nerve or carotid artery, which are dehiscent in 5% and 20% of cases, respectively.
  - Lowering the anterior face of the sphenoid sinus is required in certain cases. This can be safely performed with the same instruments. However, it should be noted that the posterior septal branch of the sphenopalatine artery courses in the mucosa overlying the inferior sphenoid face. Injury to this branch can be controlled utilizing a bipolar or suction cautery.
- Transethmoidal approach: indicated when a sphenoethmoidectomy is to be performed and often prior to the ethmoid skull base dissection.
  - The safest method of entering the sphenoid from within the ethmoid sinus is via the natural ostium of the sphenoid sinus.
  - First, the superior turbinate is cut sharply at the transition of the vertical and horizontal segment of the lamella allowing for direct visualization of the sphenoid ostium, which invariably lies medial to the superior turbinate attachment. This permits improved access to the sphenoid sinus for debridement and surveillance. Resection of the inferior half or one-third of the superior turbinate does not appear to disrupt olfactory function.
  - A stapes curette, J curette, or a freer elevator may be used to bluntly palpate the ostium and curette the bony edges. The ostium is further enlarged as described above utilizing Kerrison rongeurs and sphenoid mushroom punches.

Extended Sphenoid Sinus Procedures

- Extended dissection is indicated for access to extensive disease or previous surgical failure.

- Classification of sphenoid surgery:
  - Type I – identification of ostium without further intervention
  - Type II—enlargement of ostium to the level of the cranial base and inferiorly to one-half of the sinus height
  - Type III—widening the ostium to the floor of the sinus and to its most lateral extent
- Bilateral extended sphenoidotomy includes bilateral sphenoidotomies, posterior nasal septectomy, sphenoid rostrum resection, and intersinus septectomy to create a common cavity with a broad drainage pathway ("Sphenoid rescue").
  - This may be indicated in large mucoceles, fungus balls, extensive nasal polyposis, or in revision cases.

Frontal Sinus Surgery

- The key to a successful frontal sinus dissection is a thorough understanding of the patient's anatomy (see above "Anatomic considerations in ESS") and complete resection of ethmoid partitions anterior and posterior to the frontal recess.
- Upon completion of the dissection, the frontal recess forms a funnel shape and is bounded by:
  - Anterior—frontal beak and agger nasi region
  - Medial—variable depending on the degree of dissection (see below)
  - Lateral—orbit
  - Posterior—posterior table of the frontal sinus and skull base
- Essential instruments include angled endoscopes (30°, 45°, or 70°), a frontal sinus curette, frontal sinus recess forceps, and angled Thru-cut instruments, a 60° or 90° microdebrider, and a 60° angled mushroom punch, a Hoseman punch, or a Cobra punch. A high-speed angled (65° or 70°) drill may be needed for extended frontal sinus dissections.

Classification of Extended Endoscopic Frontal Sinus Dissection

Draf Classification (Historical)

- Draf type 1 frontal recess surgery: all superior ethmoid partitions within the inferior portion of the frontal recess are removed while the infundibulum remains un-dissected.
- Draf type 2 frontal sinusotomy
  - Draf type 2a: the infundibulum of the frontal recess is enlarged from the lamina papyracea laterally to the middle turbinate medially.
  - Draf type 2b: resection of the floor of the frontal sinus is extended further medially to the nasal septum by removing the anterior attachment of the middle turbinate, exposing the ventral margin of the olfactory fossa. This is utilized in cases where the ostium is stenotic, and the middle turbinate root has become osteitic further narrowing the frontal sinus recess.
- Draf type 3 (Modified Lothrop) frontal sinusotomy: the Draf 2b is further extended medially on both sides through resection of the superior nasal septum and frontal sinus septum creating one common frontal sinus cavity. The result is resection of the frontal sinus floor from orbit to orbit.

International Classification of the Extent of Endoscopic Frontal Sinus Surgery:

- Grades 0 through 3 relate to surgery of the frontal recess below the frontal sinus ostium, or the narrowest point between the sinus and recess:
  - Grade 0—balloon sinus dilation without tissue removal
  - Grade 1—removal of cells in the frontal recess not obstructing the ostium
  - Grade 2—removal of cells directly obstructing the ostium
  - Grade 3—removal of cells pneumatizing through the frontal ostium into the frontal sinus without enlargement of the frontal ostium

- Grades 4 through 6 require bone removal which enlarges the ostium:
  - Grade 4—removal of cells that pneumatize through the ostium with enlargement of the ostium itself
  - Grade 5—ostium enlargement from the lamina papyracea to the nasal septum
  - Grade 6—resection of the floor of the frontal sinus creating a common ostium between the right and left sides; formerly known as a Draf 3 procedure
- Frontal sinus trephination is indicated for complicated acute or chronic frontal sinusitis, frontal osteomyelitis, far lateral sinus disease, and difficult to access supra-agger frontal cells.
- Frontal sinus osteoplastic flap with or without obliteration is indicated for recalcitrant frontal sinus disease after failure of ESS, mucoceles, tumors, and osteomyelitis.
  - The procedure frequently involves a bicoronal incision across the vertex of the head with an inferiorly based bone flap hinged on pericranium with eradication of frontal sinus mucosa.
  - Obliteration with fat, muscle, or nonautologous materials and occlusion of the frontal recess are necessary to prevent future disease, although mucoceles many years later are common.

Frontal Sinusotomy Approach and Dissection

- The anterior ethmoid artery is highly variable in relation to the skull base. In some cases, it may extend as much as 4 mm below the level of the skull base in a bony mesentery. This artery defines the posterior limit of the frontal recess dissection; therefore, early identification is essential to performing a safe and effective dissection.
- Once the anterior ethmoid artery has been positively identified, a frontal sinus curette is used to remove any ethmoid partitions in a posterior-to-anterior direction. The dissection should be performed laterally along the medial orbital wall to avoid inadvertent injury to the lateral lamella or cribriform plate.
- After removing ethmoid partitions posterior to the recess, the agger nasi region should be cleared of any remaining partitions through the use of a curette.
- Next, careful inspection should reveal the opening to the frontal recess. Typically, the outflow tract is displaced medially by agger nasi and suprabullar cells. However, in the presence of a frontal septal cell, the entrance to the frontal sinus will be displaced laterally.
- A frontal sinus probe or image guidance probe may be used to confirm access to the frontal recess.
- Depending on the intended degree of frontal ostium expansion, further dissection may be performed.
- When expanding the frontal sinus ostium, care must be taken to avoid stripping mucosa whenever possible. This is particularly important in maintaining normal mucociliary outflow and preventing stenosis of the sinusotomy.
- The ostium is bounded anteriorly and medially by the frontal sinus beak. Posteriorly lies the skull base and laterally sits the orbit. When expanding the ostium, attention should be paid toward expanding the areas of the beak. This permits safe expansion of the ostium, functional mucosal preservation, and limits risk to the orbit or skull base.

Use of Packing

- Perioperative use of absorbable and nonabsorbable materials is highly variable in technique and use.
- For the purpose of hemostasis, evidence suggests packing is not essential in most cases and will not necessarily reduce the risk of epistaxis.

- Some studies, though, have shown an advantage to packing with regard to wound healing. However, evidence is limited and it has not been shown to necessarily be more advantageous to early debridement.

Steroid Eluting Stents

- Propel and SINUVA are FDA-approved corticosteroid-releasing implants.
- These are biodegradable stents that provide sustained localized medication (mometasone furoate) release over 30 to 90 days.
- Propel is the only device shown to reduce interventions, lysis of adhesions, and nasal polyposis in the postoperative period.
- Patient-specific factors should dictate when use is appropriate.

Postoperative Management

Sinus Cavity Debridement

- Research has suggested that early and frequent postoperative debridements have been associated with improved postoperative cavity appearance and a reduction in synechiae formation.
- Impaired mucociliary function continues 3 to 12 weeks after surgery. Retained blood and mucus can promote a persistent inflammatory response and microbe colonization.
- Typically, the first endoscopic debridement occurs 5 to 7 days after surgery, at which time any packing is removed. Subsequent debridements occur 2 to 4 weeks later depending on the status of the sinonasal cavity.
- Particular focus is on the removal of any blood, crusting, or retained bone fragments. Visible scars should be divided, in particular in the area of the frontal recess.

Medical Therapy Following Surgery

Hypertonic or Isotonic Saline Irrigations

- Initiation of irrigations is recommended beginning 24 to 48 hours after surgery and should be continued throughout the postoperative period.

Topical Corticosteroids

- INCS use is supported by the literature. Evidence has suggested that INCS significantly improve endoscopic appearance, symptom control, and recurrence rate of nasal polyps.
- Steroid irrigations, if appropriate, have been shown to reduce edema and may eliminate the necessity for oral steroids.

Systemic Corticosteroids

- Current evidence is lacking for the routine use of systemic corticosteroids in the postoperative period.
- Current guidelines suggest that systemic administration has benefits in patients with CRSwNP. This philosophy can be applied to postoperative management.
- With regard to patients with CRSsNP, systemic steroids lack evidence of being beneficial, but may be an option.

Antibiotics

- The benefits of routine antibiotics in the postoperative period have not been demonstrated in the literature.

- The application of such medication is patient-specific, especially if purulence is encountered intra-operatively, and further consideration should be given when packing is placed perioperatively.

Management of Postoperative Complications

- Historically, rates of CSF leak, orbital hematoma, or significant bleeding are 1%.
- Overall complication rates of ESS are less than 3%.

Management of Postoperative Epistaxis

- Application of topical hemostatic vasoconstrictive agents or absorbable packing may be beneficial.
- Endoscopic localization of the bleeding site with treatment via electrocautery or non-absorbable packing of the bleeding site may be required.
- Consider arterial ligation or embolization for refractory cases.

Postoperative CSF Rhinorrhea

- Early repair of CSF leaks identified postoperatively should be performed.
- Unlike most closed-head injury CSF leaks, which often times close spontaneously and have a 5% rate of meningitis, iatrogenic CSF leaks have a 20% incidence of meningitis with long-term follow-up if managed nonsurgically.

Long-Term Management of ESS Patients

- Since CRS is typically a multifactorial disease, surgery is only a part of the overall management of patients.
- Scheduled visits with endoscopic evaluation are critical to the evaluation of persistent or recurrent disease. Regular visits can identify advancing disease that is amenable to medical management long before the return of patient symptoms. Thus, the need for revision surgery may be avoided.
- Although updated imaging is indicated in revision surgery when image guidance is utilized, endoscopic surveillance of the sinonasal cavity is often sufficient when deciding if revision surgery is indicated.
- Sinonasal irrigations continue to be a part of the patient's long-term management in most cases, and INCS have been shown to benefit patients as well.
- Further medical management should adhere to well-established clinical guidelines for CRS.

Reasons for Failure of Primary FESS

- Middle turbinate lateralization, incomplete air cell removal, and unidentified Haller or Onodi cells may lead to obstruction of natural drainage pathways.
- Synechiae and scarring can lead to stenosis of outflow tracts.
- Incomplete communication between the surgical and natural ostium can lead to recirculation of mucus.
- Neo-osteogenesis and recurrent nasal polyposis are common causes of revision sinus surgery.
- Common patient conditions that show higher rates of revision surgery include CRSwNP, allergic fungal sinusitis, disorders of mucociliary clearance, immunodeficiencies, and aspirin-exacerbated respiratory disease (AERD), all of which may be less responsive to standard medical or surgical treatment.

Pediatric Chronic Rhinosinusitis

- The development is thought to be multifactorial, much like adult CRS; however, the adenoids distinguish the pediatric disease from adults.
- Evidence suggests the adenoids act as a reservoir of bacteria, have a high degree of biofilm formation, and correlate with lateral nasal wall cultures.
- Common microbes include alpha hemolytic streptococci, *Streptococcus pneumoniae*, *Haemophilus influenza*, and *Moraxella catarrhalis* with an increase in *Staphylococcus aureus* and anaerobic bacterial cultures.
- At least two of the following are required for diagnosis: nasal congestion, colored nasal discharge, facial pressure or pain, or cough beyond 12 weeks in association with visualized purulence or mucosal edema on examination.
- First-line medical therapy begins with nasal saline irrigations and INCS, while antibiotics and systemic steroids are reserved for exacerbations.
- Empiric antibiotics with a transition to culture-guided therapy for 3 to 12 weeks is recommended.
- Surgery is reserved for recalcitrant disease and often begins with an adenoidectomy, which is effective in removing obstructions and reducing reservoir loads.
- ESS may be used in conjunction with adenoidectomy or for persistent disease depending on the etiology of CRS.

Bibliography

Orlandi RR, Kingdom TT, Smith TL, et al. International consensus statement on allergy and rhinology: rhinosinusitis 2021. *Int Forum Allergy Rhinol.* 2021;11(3):213-739.

Palmer JN, Chiu AG. *Atlas of Endoscopic Sinus and Skull Base Surgery.* Philadelphia, PA: Elsevier Saunders; 2013:3-168.

Piccirillo JF, Payne SC, Rosenfeld RM, et al. Clinical consensus statement: balloon dilation of the sinuses. *Otolaryngol Head Neck Surg.* 2018;158(2):203-214.

McCoul ED, Tabaee A. A practical approach to refractory chronic rhinosinusitis. *Otolaryngol Clin North Am.* 2017;50(1):183-198.

Wise SK, Orlandi RR, DelGaudio JM. Sinonasal development and anatomy. In: Kennedy DW, Hwang PH. *Rhinology: Diseases of the Nose, Sinuses, and Skull Base.* New York, NY: Thieme Medical Publishers, Inc.; 2012:1-21.

Questions

1. The uncinate process originates from which of the following ethmoturbinal portions?
   A. Ascending portion of the first ethmoturbinal
   B. Descending portion of the first ethmoturbinal
   C. Second ethmoturbinal
   D. Third ethmoturbinal

2. Appropriate medical therapy recommendations for chronic rhinosinusitis with nasal polyposis include
   A. A single short course of systemic steroids
   B. A trial of topical antibiotics for 3-4 weeks
   C. A trial of oral antibiotics for 3-4 weeks
   D. Anti-leukotriene therapy

3. Which antibiotic would best treat a patient with 4 months of rhinosinusitis with nasal polyps and elevated IgE levels?
   A. Doxycycline
   B. Azithromycin
   C. Amoxicillin/Clavulanate
   D. Culture-directed antibiotic

4. In relation to structures along the anterior skull base, which answer best describes the relative position of the anterior ethmoid artery?
   A. The artery lies anterior to or within a frontal bullar cell.
   B. The artery lies directly posterior to a supra-agger cell.
   C. The artery lies anterior, within, or posterior to a supraorbital ethmoid cell.
   D. The artery may be directly anterior or posterior to the frontal recess.

5. With regard to iatrogenic skull base injury with CSF rhinorrhea, which is true?
   A. Postoperative identification requires immediate surgical repair.
   B. Intraoperative recognition of CSF leaks may be watched conservatively as the majority of cases will heal spontaneously.
   C. A trial of conservative management is appropriate in all cases.
   D. 20% of iatrogenic CSF leaks result in meningitis.

Chapter 31
Endoscopic Skull Base Surgery

Principles and Concepts

- Effective management of skull base lesions requires a collaborative team effort involving a broad range of specialties, including neurosurgery, otolaryngology, neuroradiology, radiation oncology, medical oncology, endocrinology, and pathology.
  - Cases should be discussed at tumor boards to decide the best therapeutic strategy.
- Substantial progress in anatomic understanding, surgical techniques, and instrumentation has allowed exposing and resecting skull base lesions via endoscopic endonasal approaches.
- Endoscopic approaches are now considered the standard for certain skull base lesions, while open approaches remain crucial for managing others. Rather than being opposing philosophies, open and endoscopic techniques are complementary.
  - The skull base team must be proficient in both.
  - The selected approach should provide proper exposure for resection with the least morbidity. Crossing the plane of cranial nerves or major vessels (eg, internal carotid artery) should be avoided.
  - Some lesions have a clear indication for an open or an endoscopic approach, but often there is no single universally accepted approach for a lesion. The decision to use an endoscopic, open, combined, or staged approach will depend on the team's preference according to their expertise and experience.
  - Whether open or endoscopic, the intradural neurosurgical microdissection principles remain the same.

Assessment

Symptoms and Signs

1. Intracranial mass effect
   a. Compression of structures (malignant neoplasms will also invade structures)
      Cranial nerves (CN)
      - Anterior fossa skull base tumors
        - CN I (olfaction) by compression (eg, olfactory groove meningioma) or invasion (eg, olfactory neuroblastoma)

- Middle fossa skull base tumors
  - Optic chiasm compression (bitemporal hemianopia). Several midline middle cranial fossa tumors (eg, pituitary macroadenoma, craniopharyngioma, tuberculum sella meningioma)
  - CN II: Tuberculum sella meningioma can extend into the optic canals, causing vision loss and a relative afferent pupillary defect due to nerve compression.
  - Cavernous sinus (CS) compression/invasion (eg, pituitary macroadenomas) can involve CN III, IV, and/or VI, with subsequent diplopia
    - CN VI runs within the CS, lateral to the internal carotid artery (ICA), unlike the other cranial nerves, which run within the lateral wall of the cavernous sinus. Since CN VI is the most medial cranial nerve in the CS, it is more vulnerable to being affected by tumors invading it or by surgical resection within this area.
    - The ophthalmic branch of CN V also runs within the lateral wall of the CS and can be affected by tumors invading it.
  - Branches of CN V can be involved in perineural invasion (PNI) from skin cancer of the face (eg, SCC or melanoma), with tumor tracking back along the nerve to the trigeminal (Gasserian) ganglion or even the brain stem. In some cases, cranial neuropathies from tumoral PNI may occur in the absence of a clinically obvious cutaneous lesion and may be the presenting symptom. CN VII can also be similarly affected.
- Posterior fossa skull base tumors
  - CN VI: Has the longest intracranial course of all CN running from its origin in the brain stem to its exit in the posterior fossa. It is particularly vulnerable to being affected by tumors located in the ventral posterior fossa (eg, chordoma, chondrosarcoma), but can also be false localizing sign of any intracranial tumor.
  - Tumors located or extending to the cerebellopontine angle can affect CN VII and VIII.
  - Tumors located or extending to jugular foramen may affect CN IX, X, and XI.
  - Tumors extending to hypoglossal canal can affect CN XII.
- Anterior fossa skull base tumors
  - Personality changes: alterations in mood, irritability, apathy, or emotional flatness as well as disinhibition
  - Loss of executive function: Difficulty with tasks requiring planning, organizing, and problem-solving
- Middle fossa skull base tumors
  - Hypothalamic syndrome (eg, craniopharyngioma)
- Posterior fossa skull base tumors
  - Cerebellum: cerebellar syndrome
  - Brainstem:
    - Altered consciousness: ranging from confusion to complete loss of consciousness (coma)
    - Respiratory and cardiovascular abnormalities
    - Focal neurological deficits (sensory or motor)

b. Increased intracranial pressure
- Headaches: typically, worse in the morning or when lying down
- Vomiting: often without nausea (projectile vomiting)
- Altered mental status: ranging from confusion to coma
- Papilledema
- Seizures
- Cushing triad: hypertension, bradycardia, and irregular respiration

c. Obstructive hydrocephalus: usually relatively rapid onset of increased intracranial pressure
   - Symptoms of increased intracranial pressure
   - Gait disturbances and urinary incontinence can be present

2. Sinonasal symptoms
   - Tumors arising from or extending to the sinonasal region produce nonspecific symptoms: nasal obstruction, rhinorrhea, facial pain/pressure or headaches, and hyposmia/anosmia
   - Red flags to suspect a sinonasal tumor:
     - Unilateral symptoms
     - Recurrent epistaxis
3. Pituitary function abnormalities
   - Hypopituitarism (involving one or more hormone axes) due to compression of the normal gland by tumors. Typically caused by pituitary macroadenomas (other causes include craniopharyngiomas and tuberculum Sella meningiomas).
   - Hypersecretion of hormone (functioning pituitary adenomas). Most common are:
     - Prolactin: oligo/amenorrhea, galactorrhea, altered libido, infertility
     - GH: Acromegaly (adults): facial changes, hands and feet enlargement, hypertension and cardiomegaly, sleep apnea, diabetes, impotence. Gigantism (before puberty)
     - ACTH (Cushing disease): central obesity, buffalo hump, moon face, purple striae, acne and facial redness, osteoporosis, hypertension, diabetes, hirsutism, fatigue
   - Workup: blood tests to determine the functional status of the hypothalamic-pituitary axis include prolactin, morning cortisol, ACTH, GH, IGF-1, TSH, free T4, LH, FSH, testosterone, and serum sodium
     - Bilateral inferior petrosal sinus sampling (BIPSS): Invasive test consisting of catheterization of the inferior petrosal sinuses. Useful in patients with Cushing syndrome and no evident pituitary adenoma on MRI. Allows to confirm pituitary origin of excess ACTH (Cushing disease) and the location of the adenoma (right vs left side of the gland) to guide surgery.

Imaging

- Computer tomography (CT) and magnetic resonance (MR) are complementary, and in most tumors, both should be performed.
- Enable determination of the location and extension of skull base tumors, as well as regional and distant dissemination in case of malignant disease.
- Frequently allow to infer the diagnosis when lesions exhibit characteristic radiological features (eg, pituitary adenoma, Rathke cyst, meningioma, craniopharyngioma, chordoma, chondrosarcoma).
- Allow the use of intraoperative navigation when acquired with appropriate protocols.

CT: Ideal to assess bone involvement. It allows:

- Differentiating a lesion that causes bone remodeling (suggestive of a benign lesion) from one that causes bone destruction (suggestive of a malignant lesion)
  - Exceptions to this behavior in skull base pathology include prolactinomas and meningiomas, which are benign lesions that may not respect bone.
- Determining the sinonasal and critical neurovascular anatomy to plan endoscopic approach

MR: Ideal to assess soft tissue. It allows:

A. Differentiating soft tissue lesions from inflammatory changes and secretions.
B. Detecting perineural invasion.

C. Assessing periorbital, orbital, dural, and intracranial involvement, key structures that require close review because invasion of either of these structures may warrant more extensive resection and reconstruction.
  - Reliable signs of periorbital involvement include:
    - Enhancement or enlargement of extraocular muscles
    - Stranding of periorbital fat
    - Loss or nodularity of plane between the orbital tissue and the mass
  - Dural invasion is likely present when nodular or smooth thickening of the dura is more than 5 mm in length.

D. Measurement of the diffusion of water molecules within tissues helps to differentiate between benign and malignant lesions.
  - Diffusion-weighted imaging (DWI): Malignant tumors often exhibit restricted diffusion due to their higher cellularity, appearing bright or hyperintense, whereas benign lesions typically show low signal intensity or appear darker.
  - Apparent diffusion coefficient (ADC): Is a quantitative measure derived from DWI that provides numerical values representing the degree of water diffusion within tissue. Malignant tumors generally have lower ADC values, indicating restricted diffusion, which is commonly seen in areas of high cellularity. These tumors appear dark or hypointense on ADC maps (opposite to their appearance on DWI).
    - One exception to this rule is chondrosarcoma that is composed largely of cartilaginous matrix, which allows relatively free diffusion of water molecules and hence shows low restriction and higher ADC values (bright). Higher-grade chondrosarcomas typically have lower ADC values due to their higher cellularity.

E. Postoperative surveillance. Imaging modality of choice to assess the degree of resection (ideally performed within 24 hours of resection or after 3 months to avoid postoperative artifacts) and for posttreatment surveillance of skull base neoplastic disease.
  - DWI and ADC are also useful for posttreatment surveillance (eg, in chordoma surveillance, low ADC values are helpful in distinguishing remnant/recurrence from fluid, inflammation, or postoperative changes)
  - Depending on the tumor pathology, 6 monthly or annual surveillance scans may be indicated for long-term follow-up.

PET CT: Useful for detecting distant metastasis (for staging or surveillance purposes)

- FDG (18F-fluorodeoxyglucose): most frequently used radiotracer. Detects areas of increased metabolic activity
- DOTATATE (gallium-68-labeled DOTATATE): is a somatostatin analog. More sensitive and specific than FDG PET when tumor expresses somatostatin receptors (certain neuroendocrine tumors, meningiomas, and paragangliomas)

Biopsy

- Histological diagnosis must be obtained to plan treatment for sinonasal tumors. Diagnosis may be complex and requires a trained experienced pathologist.
  - Treatment modality of different sinonasal malignancies differs and is mainly driven by histology. Nononcological resection of sinonasal masses without a histological diagnosis must be avoided and may affect prognosis.

- Intracranial lesions without sinonasal extension may be difficult to biopsy prior to definitive surgery. Tumors like meningiomas, chordomas, and chondrosarcomas typically have distinctive radiological features that allow for fairly accurate inference of the diagnosis. Surgery is usually planned and tailored to the presumed pathology. However, it is recommended to send intraoperative fresh frozen samples to confirm the suspected diagnosis.

Pathologies

Neoplastic Disease

Benign

i. Pituitary neuroendocrine tumors (PitNET or formally called adenoma)

Origin/etiology:

- benign neoplasm of the pituitary gland

Features:

- 90% of all sellar tumors
- 10% to 15% of all intracranial tumors

Epidemiology:

- They can occur at any age but are most frequently diagnosed in adults aged 30 to 50 years.
- 10% prevalence.

Classification:

- Size: macroadenoma (1 cm or greater) versus microadenoma (< 1 cm)
- Functional status: Nonfunctioning (15%-54% of pituitary adenomas) versus functioning (secretory adenomas):
  - Prolactin-secreting pituitary adenomas
  - GH-secreting tumors 8% to 16% of pituitary adenomas
  - ACTH-secreting tumors 2% to 6% of pituitary adenomas
  - TSH-secreting tumors 1% of pituitary adenomas
  - Gonadotropin-secreting tumors 1% of pituitary adenomas

Clinical Presentation:
Two main factors determine symptoms associated with pituitary adenomas:

- Mass effect: bitemporal hemianopia (peripheral vision should be tested to determine impingement on the optic chiasm), headache, and/or hypopituitarism
- Endocrine disorder: depends on the hormone produced in excess or compression of stalk causing diabetes insipidus

Imaging:

- CT: Although benign, they can be locally aggressive tumors and not respect the bone on imaging (eg, prolactinoma).
- MR: gold standard to evaluate the pituitary gland

    - Allows evaluation of optic nerve and optic chiasm compression and cavernous invasion by macroadenomas
    - Most microadenomas enhance less intensely than the normal portion of the pituitary gland after gadolinium contrast

Treatment:

- Prolactinomas:
    - First-line therapy consists of dopamine agonists (bromocriptine or cabergoline). These medications may not be tolerated due to a high incidence of side effects (nausea, dizziness, headaches, drowsiness).
    - Surgery is reserved for patients who fail or don't tolerate medical therapy.
    - Radiotherapy and radiosurgery are options to consider when medical therapy fails or is not tolerated, and surgery is not a suitable option (eg, advanced age and unfit for general anesthesia) or cannot achieve gross total resection (eg, cavernous sinus invasion).
- All other pituitary adenomas:
    - Transsphenoidal pituitary surgery is the first-line therapy for other pituitary adenomas requiring treatment.
    - Small, nonfunctioning adenomas do not need surgery and can be observed.
- Medical therapy is reserved for those not cured by surgery
    - GH-secreting tumors: somatostatin analogues, cabergoline, and pegvisomant
    - ACTH-secreting tumors: ketoconazole, mifepristone, and pasireotide
    - TSH-secreting tumors: somatostatin analogues

ii. Rathke cyst

- Benign, nonneoplastic cyst that originates from remnants of Rathke pouch, typically found in the sella and suprasellar region (included in this section to group it with pituitary adenomas)
- Very common incidence of approximately 15%; however, most are small and asymptomatic
- Rarely do these lesions ultimately become symptomatic, approximately 2%
- Female preponderance (2:1), with a peak in incidence between 40 and 50 years of age
- Symptoms due to compression of suprasellar structures, pituitary gland
- Endoscopic surgical drainage with marsupialization of the cyst into the sphenoid sinus is reserved for symptomatic cysts

iii. Meningioma

Origin/etiology:

- Extra-axial tumor arising from the arachnoid cap cells within the arachnoid mater

Features:

- Most common benign intracranial tumor, accounting for 15% to 25% of primary intracranial tumors
- Risk factors include exposure to ionizing radiation (previous radiotherapy) and exogenous hormones
- Meningiomas can occur anywhere along the meninges, including any part of the skull base (eg, olfactory groove, planum, tuberculum, petroclival region, foramen magnum)

Epidemiology:

- Female preponderance
- Incidence increases with age, most common between 30 and 70 years of age

Classification: The World Health Organization (WHO) classification (based on histological features) remains widely used:

- Grade I (benign):
  - Most common type (80%-90%)
  - Slow growing and with low risk of recurrence if completely resected
- Grade II (atypical):
  - Represent 15% to 20%
  - More aggressive than grade I. Higher recurrence rate (even after complete resection) and tendency to invade brain
- Grade III (anaplastic/malignant meningiomas):
  - Represent 1% to 3%
  - Highly aggressive (high recurrence rate, rapid growth, and brain invasion)
  - Often metastasizes outside the central nervous system

Clinical Presentation:

- Depends on the location. Symptoms mainly due to mass effect

Imaging:

- CT:
  - Usually hyperdense relative to brain, but can be isointense.
  - Homogeneous contrast enhancement (grade II or III may show heterogeneous enhancement because of necrosis and cystic areas).
  - Often demonstrate a "dural tail."
  - Calcifications within the tumor are common.
  - Hyperostosis at the attachment site is frequent.
    - However, they can be locally aggressive tumors and may not respect the bone causing osteolysis
- MR:
  - T1: isointense or slightly hypointense compared to brain tissue. Strong, uniform enhancement with gadolinium
    - Dural tail sign: enhancement extends along the dura beyond the tumor appearing as a "tail." Characteristic of meningiomas
  - T2: typically, isointense or hyperintense. Allows to visualize cerebral edema associated with meningiomas
  - FLAIR: offers better contrast near CSF-filled spaces to assess cerebral edema
  - DWI/ADC: may suggest atypical or malignant meningiomas when there is restricted diffusion (bright DWI and dark ADC)
- 68Ga DOTATATE PET: more specific and sensitive than FDG in detecting both typical and atypical meningiomas. Helps to assess recurrent or residual meningioma, especially in difficult-to-image locations like the skull base

Treatment:

- Observation: small, asymptomatic, stable meningiomas
- Surgery: presence of neurologic deficit or progressive growth with threat of deficit
  - Anterior skull base: endoscopic transcribiform approach is a valid option when olfaction has been lost

    - Avoids brain retraction
    - Enables early tumor devascularization (bipolar cautery of the ethmoidal arteries)
    - Allows comfortable drilling of the hyperostotic bone
    - When olfaction is preserved, open approaches are often favored
  - Tuberculum sella: Endoscopic approach is an excellent alternative.
    - Provides direct access without brain retraction.
    - Allows comfortable drilling of the hyperostotic bone.
    - Enables removal of tumor extension into the optic canals.
    - Lateral extension of the tumor (eg, above the anterior clinoid process) may limit exposure through an endoscopic approach. A combined open/endoscopic or open approach may be more suitable in this scenario.
  - Posterior fossa: Endoscopic transclival approach provides direct access, but lateral extension of the tumor may warrant a combined or alternative approach.
- Radiotherapy: often used as adjuvant treatment after resecting grade II and III meningiomas, or when complete resection is not possible in grade I

iv. Craniopharyngioma

Origin/etiology:

- Two different histopathological subtypes have been described. It has long been hypothesized that, although they share common histological features, both entities have different pathogenesis.
  - Adamantinomatous subtype: neoplastic transformation of embryonic epithelial remnants of the Rathke pouch or primitive craniopharyngeal duct and typically originate in the region of the pituitary infundibulum
  - Papillary subtype: is thought to form from metaplasia or somatic mutations of differentiated cells

Features:

- Adamantinomatous: high prevalence of CTNNB1 mutations affecting the Wnt/beta-catenin pathway
- Papillary: high prevalence of BRAF V600E (Val 600 Glu) mutation has been identified and appears to be exclusive to this subtype

Epidemiology:

- Adamantinomatous: is the most common subtype overall, accounting for 90% and can occur at any age
  - Childhood craniopharyngiomas are almost exclusively the adamantinomatous subtype
- Papillary: almost exclusively seen in adults and accounts for 10% of tumors
  - Frequently presents as a solid tumor with little mineralization

Classification: according to their suprasellar extension relative to the infundibulum (useful to plan the appropriate endoscopic approach)

- Type I: preinfundibular (anterior to the pituitary infundibulum)
  - A transplanum transtuberculum approach to the prechiasmatic cistern is required
- Type II: transinfundibular (extending into the stalk)
  - A transplanum transtuberculum approach and vertical incision of the pituitary stalk are necessary to gain access to the tumor

- Type III: retroinfundibular, extending behind the gland and stalk
    - A transplanum transtuberculum approach augmented by mobilization of the pituitary gland (eg, hemi transposition) to get access to the retroinfundibular space is required.
        - IIIa: extending into the third ventricle
        - IIIb: extending into the interpeduncular cistern
- Type IV: isolated to the third ventricle and/or optic recess. It is not accessible via an endonasal approach.

Clinical Presentation:

- Compressive symptoms related to its location (headaches, visual field alterations, pituitary gland dysfunction, and/or hypothalamic dysfunction)
- Hydrocephalus due to CSF flow obstruction

Imaging: They have mixed cystic and solid components (cysts are not a significant feature of papillary subtype). Calcifications are frequently observed in the adamantinomatous subtype

- CT: highly sensitive to calcifications (hyperdense areas).
- MR:
    - T1:
        - Cysts. Adamantinomatous: iso to hyperintense to grey matter (due to high protein content "motor oil cysts"). Papillary: usually hypointense
        - Solid areas enhance with gadolinium contrast
    - T2: cystic areas appear hyperintense
    - Flair: helps differentiate the cystic components from surrounding brain tissue and CSF

Treatment:

- Surgery: Maximal resection without compromise of nearby structures (hypothalamus, optic nerves, pituitary stalk) is the preferred approach to optimize both quality of life and disease control.
- Radiotherapy: As adjuvant therapy when gross total resection (GTR) is deemed unsafe, and subtotal resection is preferred in an attempt to preserve as much pituitary and cranial nerve function as possible.
    - Radiotherapy after subtotal resection (STR) has shown to decrease tumor recurrence from 55%-85% to 0%-20%.
    - This has led some surgeons preferring to perform STR with planned radiation therapy in an attempt to preserve as much pituitary and cranial nerve function as possible.
- BRAF/MEK inhibitor dual therapy is currently being explored as an adjuvant/neoadjuvant systemic therapy for papillomatous subtype.
- Malignant: Please see Chapter 29

Meningoencephalocele/Idiopathic Cerebrospinal Fluid (CSF) Leak

a. They develop in the context of idiopathic intracranial hypertension (IIH).
    - Risk factors: obesity, medications (eg, tetracyclines, Vitamin A derivatives), hormonal changes
    - Epidemiology: typically affects young overweight women of childbearing age, though it can occur in anyone

- Symptoms and signs: headaches, visual disturbances, pulsatile tinnitus, dizziness, papilledema
- Imaging
  - CT: thinned skull base, dilated foramina (eg, foramen rotundum, jugular foramen)
  - MR: More sensitive than CT scan
    - Empty sella and flattened pituitary gland
    - Optic nerve sheath dilation
    - Flattening of the posterior globe
    - Transverse sinus stenosis (seen on MR venography)
    - Absence of hydrocephalus (small or slit-like lateral ventricles)
    - Enlarged Meckel's cave
      - ◊ Diagnosis of IIH: Lumbar puncture to confirm elevated intracranial pressure.
    - Should be performed once the leak has been closed (active leaking may falsely decrease opening pressure)
    - Normal intracranial opening pressure is between 10 and 15 cm H_2O

b. Diagnosis of CSF leak

Symptoms & signs:

- Unilateral clear watery nasal discharge
  - Positional
  - It increases with Valsalva
  - Salty or metallic taste
- Headaches associated with CSF leak are typically positional, worsening when standing or sitting upright (due to traction on pain-sensitive structures caused by brain sagging), and improving when lying down

Confirmation of CSF:

- Beta-2 transferrin protein detection: considered the gold standard (found exclusively in the CSF, aqueous humor of the eye, and perilymph)
- Beta-trace protein detection: found in much higher concentrations in CSF compared to other body fluids. Faster, but not as widely available as beta-2 transferrin in many clinical settings

Imaging

- Signs of IIH
- Enable to detect the site of leaking (thin cut coronal reconstruction)
  - If CSF leak is confirmed and no evident anterior skull base or sphenoid defect is detected on imaging, assessment of tegmen timpani is warranted. Rarely, middle ear CSF leaks can manifest as CSF rhinorrhea through the eustachian tube.

c. Common locations
- Cribriform plate
- Lateral sphenoid recess (lateral to V2)
- Temporal bone (tegmen tympani)

d. Treatment

Surgical repair

- Off-label intrathecal fluorescein may be useful to confirm the leaking site or coexistent leaks which can be present in up to 40%.

- Bipolar cautery of the meningoencephalocele is required to reduce it and expose the skull base defect.
- Repair options include fat, free mucosal grafts or pedicles flaps depending on size and location of leak. Multilayered closures often preferred.

Management of IIH

- Weight loss
- Acetazolamide: It reduces the production of CSF. Effective in treating moderate increases in intracranial pressure.
- Shunt surgery: necessary to treat severe increases in intracranial pressure (eg, above 35cm H2O). Lumbo-peritoneal shunt is the most frequently used. Ventriculoperitoneal is an alternative in selected cases.

Inflammatory Disease

Panus: granulation tissue that forms in response to chronic inflammation, typically seen in joints affected by rheumatoid arthritis. Around the odontoid process can cause:

- Erosion of the odontoid process or surrounding bone structures
- Atlantoaxial instability
- Compression of the spinal cord or brain stem
  - Treatment: endoscopic odontoidectomy

Approaches

Table 31-1 provides an overview of the preferred endoscopic approaches for treating the most common skull base pathologies.

Reconstruction

- Multilayer reconstruction is the preferred method for closing defects after endoscopic skull base surgery.
- There is no one standard way of closing skull base defects.
  - The reconstruction technique should be tailored to the defect.
  - Different experienced teams will close the same defect in different ways.
- Technique selection depends on many factors including size and location of the dural defect, magnitude of the CSF leak (low flow vs high flow), available tissue for reconstruction, and the preference of the surgical team.
- Commonly used alternatives for reconstruction include:
  - Dural closure:
    - Synthetic dural substitute and/or autologous graft (fat and/or fascia lata).
    - They can be placed intradural (inlay), extradural (onlay), or as gasket seal.
  - Extracranial closure (overlay):
    a. Free mucoperiosteal grafts:
       - Typically obtained from middle turbinate, inferior turbinate, or nasal cavity floor
       - Usually used for reconstruction of small to moderate size (eg, < 2 cm^2), low-flow skull base defects

Table 31-1 Most Frequent Histologies According to Location and Typical Endoscopic Approaches. Combination of These Approaches Can Be Tailored to the Extent of the Lesion

SB location	*Pathology*	*Endoscopic Approaches*	*Potential Risks to Avoid*
Sagittal Plane			
Anterior SB	Olfactory Neuroblastoma[a] Meningioma (olfactory groove) Sinonasal malignancy[a]	Transcribiform	Injury to AEA with retraction and retrobulbar hematoma formation
	Meningoencephalocele/CSF leak	Endoscopic sinus surgery	
Middle SB	Sellar tumors	Transsellar +/− Cavernous sinus[b]	Avulsion of Inferior hypophyseal artery from ICA (major bleeding)
	Meningioma (tuberculum sella)	Transtuberculum/transplanum	Injury to superior hypophyseal artery causing vision loss
		+/− Optic nerve decompression	Injury to ophthalmic artery causing vision loss
	Craniopharyngioma	Transtuberculum/transplanum (grade I, II, III) + Pituitary gland hemitransposition (grade III)	Injury to superior hypophyseal artery causing vision loss
	Meningoencephalocele/CSF leak	Transpterygoid approach to sphenoid lateral recess	Scarifies vascularization of ipsilateral nasoseptal flap
Posterior SB	Chordoma (clival)	Transclival[c] +/− Posterior clinoidectomy	Injury to CN VI causing diplopia
	Meningioma	Transclival[c]	Injury to perforating vessels supplying the brain stem causes catastrophic sequelae
CC junction	Rheumatoid arthritis (panus)	Odontoidectomy[d]	
Coronal Plane			
	Chondrosarcoma	Petrous apex + Transpterygoid	Injury to CN VI causing diplopia
	JNA[a]	Transpterygoid +/− Infratemporal[e]	Scarifies vascularization of ipsilateral nasoseptal flap

AEA: anterior ethmoidal artery; CC: craniocervical; CSF: cerebrospinal fluid; ICA: internal carotid artery; JNA: juvenile nasopharyngeal angiofibroma; SB: skull base.

[a]Large lesions often benefit from a combined open and endoscopic approach.

[b]Extension into the cavernous sinus may be necessary for tumors invading it.

[c]A transpterygoid approach can be added to extend lateral access or improve surgical maneuverability.

[d]Spinal stabilization (eg, posterior occipitocervical fusion) is typically necessary to prevent instability created by ligament sectioning and bone removal.

[e]Additional endoscopic approaches (eg, transorbital) may be required depending on the extension of the tumor.

b. Vascularized flaps: Evidence strongly suggests that they reduce the rates of postoperative CSF leakage in cases of large dural defects or high-flow intraoperative CSF leaks.
   (a) Local flaps. Most used options include:
      – Nasoseptal: workhorse for reconstruction with local vascularized flap. Supplied by the nasoseptal artery, a branch of the posterior septal artery (a terminal branch of the internal maxillary artery). Can incorporate the mucoperiosteum of the floor of the nasal cavity to increase its size.

- Lateral wall: can be fashioned posteriorly based (supplied by the posterolateral nasal artery, branch of the sphenopalatine artery) or anteriorly based (supplied by the angular and lateral nasal branches of the facial artery and anterior ethmoidal artery). Can incorporate the mucoperiosteum of the floor of the nasal cavity to increase its size.
- Middle turbinate: difficult to harvest and not very long reach. Valid alternative for small to medium-sized anterior skull base defects. Supplied from branches of the sphenopalatine artery.

(b) Regional flaps:
- Pericranial or galeopericranial. Supplied by the supraorbital and supratrochlear vessels. Very good option to reconstruct big anterior skull base defects (eg, transcribiform resection).
- Temporoparietal fascia. Supplied by the superficial temporal artery. Very good option to reconstruct posterior defects (eg, transclival approaches).

c. Free microvascular tissue transfer (widely known as "free flaps"): Last resource when there are no suitable local or regional flaps available.
- Common alternatives used for skull base reconstruction include free radial forearm flap and vastus lateralis free flap.
- Other options include latissimus dorsi and rectus abdominis.

Complications

Intraoperative

i. Bleeding
- Adequate management of venous and arterial bleeding is key to a successful surgery. A poor field of vision is often the starting point leading to complications.

ii. Internal carotid artery injury
- Rare but potentially life-threatening complication
- Estimated incidence in endoscopic skull base surgery: 0.4% (0.001%-2.5%)
- Most ICA injuries occur during pituitary surgery (by far the most common endoscopic skull base surgery performed worldwide)
  - According to pathology, chondroid neoplasms (chordoma, chondrosarcoma) have the highest incidence (estimated in 2% risk) compared to endoscopic resection of pituitary tumor (estimated in 0.3%)
- Treatment:
  - Obtaining adequate visualization of the defect with a large-bore suction and two surgeons' technique is vital to control the bleeding.
  - A piece of crushed muscle taken from the neck or thigh can be placed to patch the injury.
  - This area is then covered by a nasoseptal flap and supported by gentle cavity packing.
  - Immediately after control of bleeding, the patient should be taken to interventional radiology for angiogram assessment.

iii. Orbital Injury

Unintentional orbital fat exposure:
- Does not present a significant problem if promptly identified and the injury is limited to just fat herniation

Extraocular muscle injury:

- Can result in permanent diplopia, especially if the muscle is transected.
- The medial rectus muscle is at particular risk during endoscopic approaches.
- Surgical options to repair damage to these muscles usually have modest results.

Retrobulbar hematoma:

- Secondary to injury to an ethmoidal artery (usually the anterior) resulting in retraction into the orbit with subsequent retrobulbar hematoma formation. Increase intraocular pressure can lead to permanent vision loss if not timely identified and decompressed.
  - Clinical diagnosis: development of proptosis, ecchymosis, and edema of the eyelids. Palpation of a rock-hard eyeball suggests a significant increase in pressure in the retrobulbar space. If available, a tonometer will give an objective measure of the eye globe pressure.
  - Treatment: immediate orbital decompression. Options include lateral canthotomy and inferior cantholysis, and endoscopic medial orbital decompression (removing the lamina papyracea and incising the periorbita).

iv. Neural injury
- Can result from direct trauma or secondary to vascular injury (eg, superior hypophyseal artery, perforating vessels supplying the brainstem).
- Selecting an appropriate approach to avoid crossing the plane of a given CN helps to prevent an injury.
- During endoscopic approaches to the skull base, practically every CN can be at risk, depending on the size and location of the tumor, and the selected approach. However, the most common cranial neuropathy encountered is CN VI palsy.
- Aggressive resection of craniopharyngioma may result in injury to the hypothalamus causing hypothalamic syndrome.
- When an unexpected paralysis or decrease in vision is noted postoperatively, imaging studies may assist in distinguishing etiologies, such as infarcts or compression from hematoma.
  - Additionally, other sources of compression should be addressed, such as nasal packing compressing the optic nerves resulting in postoperative visual loss.

Postoperative

i. Bleeding

Epistaxis

- In case of massive bleeding, first ensure that the patient is protecting the airway. If in respiratory distress, especially in the setting of high-volume bleeding, securing the airway takes priority.
  - Of note, generally rapid sequence intubation is recommended to avoid positive pressure mask ventilation and potential pneumocephalus.
- If the patient is stable, an attempt should be made with a rigid nasal endoscope to inspect the nasal cavity for any potential sources of bleeding.
  - According to these findings, one can consider conservative management, medical management with topical decongestants or hemostatic agents, absorbable and/or nonabsorbable packing, and/or operative evaluation and control.
  - Treatment must consider the specifics of the surgical approach previously performed to avoid damaging the repair.

Intracranial

- May manifest as sudden headache or development of new neurological deficits.
- Usually, bleeding occurs within the surgical bed, but it can also take place in different locations as subdural hematoma or distant site bleeding.
- Urgent assessment with imaging will confirm the bleeding and determine the site and magnitude of it.
- Surgery for evacuation will be required if significant compression of neural structures develops or if there is increase in the size of the hematoma, suggesting recurrent or persistent bleeding.

ii. CSF leak
- Postoperative CSF leak rate depends on multiple factors, including the team's experience, location, and extent of the surgical resection, size of the dural defect, and type of reconstruction.
- Sellar defects have the lowest rate of postoperative CSF leak (4.8%) followed by parasellar defects (9.0%) and anterior fossa defects (13.0%). Posterior fossa/clival defects are associated with the highest rate of reconstructive failure at 19%.
- Postoperative CSF leaks typically manifest in the first few days after surgery (approximately two-thirds). Delayed CSF leaks, presenting after 1 week of surgery, are less common.
- Risk factors for postoperative CSF leaks include elevated BMI (> 25) or high intraventricular pressure, poor healing due to Cushing disease or diabetes mellitus, and prior radiotherapy to the surgical site.
- Clinical presentation includes rhinorrhea, headache, and meningitis.
- Imaging: ascertain the presence of pneumocephalus on CT may help to confirm the diagnosis.
- Diagnosis: clinical by detecting CSF leakage on tilt test or in nasal endoscopy combined with a provoking maneuver. Beta-2 transferrin testing is usually not practical because it takes considerable time to process, and the protein can remain detectable in sinonasal secretions for several days after surgery.
- Treatment: immediate surgical exploration and repair to avoid the associated risk of meningitis or tension pneumocephalus is usually favored; however, placement of a lumbar drain may successfully resolve low-flow postoperative CSF leaks, especially if reconstructed with a vascularized flap.

iii. Tension pneumocephalus
- Rare but potentially life-threatening complication.
- Continued ingress of air results in increased intracranial pressure and compression of the brain.
- It usually develops progressively over days, but it can manifest as early as in the immediate postoperative period.
- Clinical manifestations include headaches, seizures, and reduced level of consciousness.
- Imaging: characteristic finding of "Mount Fuji sign" on CT imaging confirms the diagnosis.
- Treatment: emergently releasing the trapped air and repairing the skull base defect.

iv. Central nervous system infections
- Rare but potentially devastating.
- Overall risk of postoperative meningitis after endonasal skull base surgery is estimated around 1% to 2%.
- Others include subdural empyema and intraparenchymal abscess.

v. Neurological: They have a delayed presentation and arise as the result of other complications (eg, vascular injury, bleeding, hypotension, tension pneumocephalus)
   - Seizure
   - Others include visual deficits, motor deficits, ataxia, altered mental status, hydrocephalus

References

Hardesty DA, Montaser A, Kreatsoulas D, et al. Complications after 1002 endoscopic endonasal approach procedures at a single center: lessons learned, 2010-2018. *J Neurosurg*. 2021 Aug 6;136(2):393-404.

Hwang PH, Kennedy DW, Orlandi RR, Wormald PJ. *Rhinology: Diseases of the Nose, Sinuses, and Skull Base*. 2nd ed. New York, NY: Thieme; 2024.

Kuan EC, Wang EW, Adappa ND, et al. International consensus statement on allergy and rhinology: sinonasal tumors. *Int Forum Allergy Rhinol*. 2024 Feb;14(2):149-608.

Wang EW, Zanation AM, Gardner PA, et al. ICAR: endoscopic skull-base surgery. *Int Forum Allergy Rhinol*. 2019 Jul;9(S3):S145-S365.

Questions

1. Which of the following is not an MR finding of IIH?
   A. Empty sella
   B. Flattening of the posterior globe
   C. Hydrocephalus
   D. Transverse sinus stenosis

2. Which protein typically tests positive in cerebrospinal fluid (CSF) analysis?
   A. Hemoglobin
   B. Beta-2 transferrin
   C. Tau protein
   D. Albumin

3. Which of the following statements correctly describes the adamantinomatous and papillary subtypes of craniopharyngioma?
   A. The adamantinomatous subtype is most common in adults and has a high prevalence of BRAF V600E mutations.
   B. The papillary subtype originates from embryonic epithelial remnants of Rathke pouch and is the most common subtype in children.
   C. The adamantinomatous subtype is the most common overall, frequently occurs in children, and is associated with CTNNB1 mutations affecting the WNT/beta-catenin pathway.
   D. The papillary subtype is exclusively seen in children, frequently presents with cystic components, and is associated with CTNNB1 mutations.

4. Which of the following is true regarding complications of endoscopic skull base surgery?
   A. Most reported internal carotid artery injuries have occurred during chordoma and chondrosarcoma surgery.
   B. Most reported internal carotid artery injuries have occurred during pituitary surgery.
   C. Anterior fossa defects have the highest rate of postoperative CSF leaks.
   D. The most frequent cause of retrobulbar hematoma is breach of the periorbita with the microdebrider.
   E. The most common cause of diplopia after endoscopic skull base surgery is inferior rectus muscle injury.

5. Which of the following is true regarding skull base reconstruction?
   A. Vascularized flaps decrease the rate of postoperative CSF leaks after closure of small, low-flow defects.
   B. Vascularized flaps decrease the rate of postoperative CSF leaks after closure of large or high-flow defects.
   C. Allografts are superior to autologous grafts to repair the dura.
   D. Autologous grafts are superior to Allografts to repair the dura.

Chapter 32
Transorbital Approaches

Introduction

- The orbit continues to be considered a danger zone for many otolaryngology centers around the world.
- The division of expertise between otolaryngology, ophthalmology, and neurosurgery has traditionally caused surgeons to avoid complex approaches within this area.
- New technologies and understanding have now opened possibilities to address orbital pathology while minimizing tissue disruption.
- More recently, the orbit is increasingly being utilized (either alone or in multiportal surgery) as an effective means of accessing difficult areas of the sinuses and skull base.
- The advent of the endoscope allows for increased vision, illumination, and precision when operating within the orbit.
- Transorbital corridors can effectively address orbital and skull base pathology with reduced operative morbidity.
- New concepts of anatomic compartmentalization of the orbit have facilitated endoscopic intraconal approaches and classification systems.

Endoscopic Endonasal Management of Orbital Tumors

- Whilst a multiplicity of options exists for the external approach to orbital tumors, challenges remain regarding accessing the medial and inferior orbit.
- Poor illumination, bleeding, orbital fat obstruction, and considerable globe retraction restrict adequate access.
- The endoscope and transnasal corridors now offer an excellent access strategy for these tumors, with minimal associated morbidity.

Orbital Tumors

- Represent approximately 25% of all orbital disease.
- Occur at a rate of 3 to 5 tumors per million population per year.
- No obvious differences between races and genders.
- Benign lesions are more common than malignant ones.
  - (a) Most common lesions are vasculogenic (17% of all orbital masses).
  - (b) Orbital pseudotumor (8%), non-Hodgkin lymphoma (8%), and optic nerve gliomas (4%) are also common.

Pathology

- Vasculogenic
  - (a) Infantile hemangioma
  - (b) Venous malformations
  - (c) Lymphangioma
  - (d) Orbital varix
- Lymphocytic
  - (a) Orbital pseudotumor
  - (b) Lymphoma (ocular adnexal lymphoma; OAL)
  - (c) Leukemia
- Neurogenic and nerve sheath
  - (a) Optic nerve glioma
  - (b) Optic nerve meningioma
  - (c) Schwannoma
  - (d) Neurofibroma
- Osseous and fibro-osseous lesions
  - (a) Osteoma
  - (b) Ewing sarcoma
  - (c) Aneurysmal bone cysts
- Mesenchymal tumors
  - (a) Solitary fibrous tumor
  - (b) Histiocytoma and hemangiopericytoma
  - (c) Fibrous dysplasia
  - (d) Fibrosarcoma
  - (e) Juvenile xanthogranuloma
  - (f) Rhabdomyosarcoma
- Lacrimal gland
  - (a) Adenocarcinoma
  - (b) Adenoid cystic carcinoma
  - (c) Pleomorphic adenoma

Signs and Symptoms of Orbital Neoplasms

- Proptosis
- Globe dystopia
- Pain, especially in relation to eye movement
- Decreased vision or visual fields
- Periocular oedema, erythema
- Epiphora
- Trigeminal nerve numbness

Diagnostic Evaluation

- Otolaryngologist assessment
- Ophthalmologist assessment
  - (a) Visual field testing
  - (b) Visual acuity (VA) testing
  - (c) Complete eye exam with extraocular muscle (EOM) testing
- Neurosurgical assessment
  - (a) If any adjunct craniotomy is required

- Imaging
  (a) High-resolution CT
    - Delineates bony anatomy and landmarks
    - Assess for any concurrent sinonasal disease or extension
    - Can be used for intra-op image guidance, but may not always be reliable as orbital tumors can mobilize during operative manipulation of orbital fat
  (b) MRI with contrast
    - Characterize the lesion
    - Delineates neurovascular anatomy
    - Course of the ophthalmic artery in relation to the optic nerve is particularly pertinent
- Angiography may be indicated in certain cases only, particularly with optic canal involvement.

The ORBIT Classification of Intra-Orbital Tumors

- Orbital resection by intranasal technique (ORBIT).
- Classification system that provides a framework for standardized tumor localization and reporting of outcomes (Figure 32-1).
- Anterior and posterior intraconal compartments are delineated by the takeoff of the inferomedial trunk of the ophthalmic artery which may be approximated radiologically by the intersection of the ophthalmic artery and optic nerve.
- All tumors are classified into five classes:
  (a) Class I—Extraconal
  (b) Class II—Intraconal and anterior to intersection of ophthalmic artery and optic nerve
  (c) Class III—Intraconal and posterior to intersection of ophthalmic artery and optic nerve
  (d) Class IV—Orbital tumor with extension into the pterygopalatine or infratemporal fossae through inferior orbital fissure
  (e) Class V—Orbital tumor with intracranial extension via the superior orbital fissure

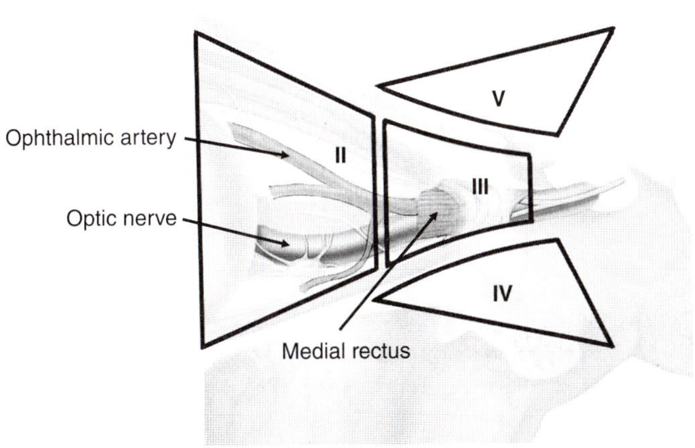

Figure 32-1 The ORBIT classification by class. ORBIT, orbital resection by intranasal technique. Image adapted from original by Patrick J. Lynch, medical illustrator, licensed under CC BY 2.5.

Surgical Technique

- Approach
  (a) An endonasal endoscopic approach can often be used for tumors whose epicenters occur within the orbit with the exception of the superotemporal quadrant.
  (b) A single nostril can be utilized for extraconal tumors.
  (c) For intraconal access, a binarial, four-handed technique can be employed via a trans-septal approach to enable cooperative visualization, suction, dissection, and retraction.
- Sinonasal work and preparation
  (a) Wide exposure of the lamina is required.
  (b) This is achieved by performing a maxillary antrostomy and then taking down the cells of the ethmoid and sphenoid sinuses.
  (c) The frontal recess and sinus cells can be spared to protect this area from secondary fat obstruction.
  (d) Once exposed, the lamina is completely removed.
  (e) The orbital process of the palatine bone may be drilled to enhance inferolateral dissection and retraction.
- Incision into periorbita
  (a) The periorbita assists in containing orbital fat and preventing it from prolapsing into the field.
  (b) Therefore, the periorbital incision must be chosen carefully.
  (c) Typically, a reverse hockey-stick incision is made just anterior to the site of the lesion.
  (d) This allows adequate access, whilst ensuring fat anterior to the lesion does not obscure the field.
- Medial rectus retraction
  (a) The medial rectus muscle represents both the landmark and barrier to the medial intraconal space.
  (b) Effective and atraumatic retraction is necessary to access the intraconal space, whilst minimizing morbidity.
  (c) Multiple methods have been reported to retract this muscle endoscopically.
    - Transchoanal vessel loop placement
    - Trans-septal suture or vessel loop placement
    - Trans-septal retraction using an angled instrument
  (d) Dynamic retraction with angled instruments is preferred to reduce the risk of tonic traction injury to the medial rectus neurovascular bundle and ophthalmic artery
    - Downsides include requirement of a septal window and occupation of an extra-surgical hand for retraction.
- Management of orbital fat and bleeding
  (a) Orbital fat needs to be handled with care and retracted to visualize the tumor and progress with dissection.
  (b) Cottonoid pledgets can be utilized to separate and retract fat to provide adequate access.
  (c) Whilst bipolar cautery can be performed judiciously and on low setting for extraconal fat, no diathermy technique should be used for intraconal fat.
    - Electric and thermal cautery disperses easily within the orbit, and can be the source of injury to critical structures
  (d) To navigate the orbital fat, saline-soaked cottonoids are utilized to retract the fat as required, as well as absorb any bleeding.
  (e) Warm saline washes can also be utilized to promote hemostasis and reduce bleeding within the orbit.

- Tumor dissection
  - (a) Blunt dissection is utilized through the orbital fat to isolate the tumor.
  - (b) An extracapsular dissection of the tumor is often possible.
  - (c) The tumor is dissected circumferentially, with approximately 270 degrees being freed from surrounding tissue.
  - (d) Once relatively free, the tumor is tractioned anteriorly along the plane of the optic nerve to allow for final dissection of lateral attachments.
  - (e) Dissection between the tumor capsule and optic nerve should be avoided to prevent nervous injury or ophthalmic artery vasospasm.
- Reconstruction
  - (a) Reconstruction of the medial orbital wall should be considered in cases of intraconal tumor removal.
    - Preserves orbital volume
    - Reduces diplopia
    - Prevents enophthalmos
  - (b) Multiple options exist for reconstruction.
  - (c) Immediate rigid reconstruction can result in orbital compartment syndrome and should be avoided.
  - (d) Pedicled nasoseptal flap reconstruction is favorable.
    - Can cover both medial and inferior orbital walls.
    - The flap permits swelling and fluid extravasation within the orbit without allowing intraocular pressures to elevate.
    - Contracts over time to result in a semi-rigid construct.

Postoperative Considerations

(a) Check the patient's visual acuity and range of motion when awake.
(b) Nasal packing should be avoided, as it may place pressure on the orbit and contribute to orbital compartment syndrome.
(c) Gelfoam or similar soft packs may be placed alongside the flap to provide support to the area.
(d) Gentle saline sprays may be initiated within 24 to 48 hours; however, high-volume irrigations should be delayed until 1 week to prevent accumulation within the orbit.
(e) Post-op antibiotics are typically not required.
(f) If any concerns over vision decrement or new diplopia, close follow-up with ophthalmology is recommended for serial examinations.

Transorbital Ethmoid Artery Ligation

- Anterior ethmoid artery ligation continues to be one of the most common transorbital procedures performed by otolaryngologists.
- Is a useful technique in the setting of refractory epistaxis (general management of epistaxis discussed elsewhere).
- Is often the third line of management after nasal packing and sphenopalatine artery (SPA) ligation/embolization has failed.

General Considerations

- The anterior and posterior ethmoid arteries, as branches of the ophthalmic artery, are a part of the internal carotid artery system.

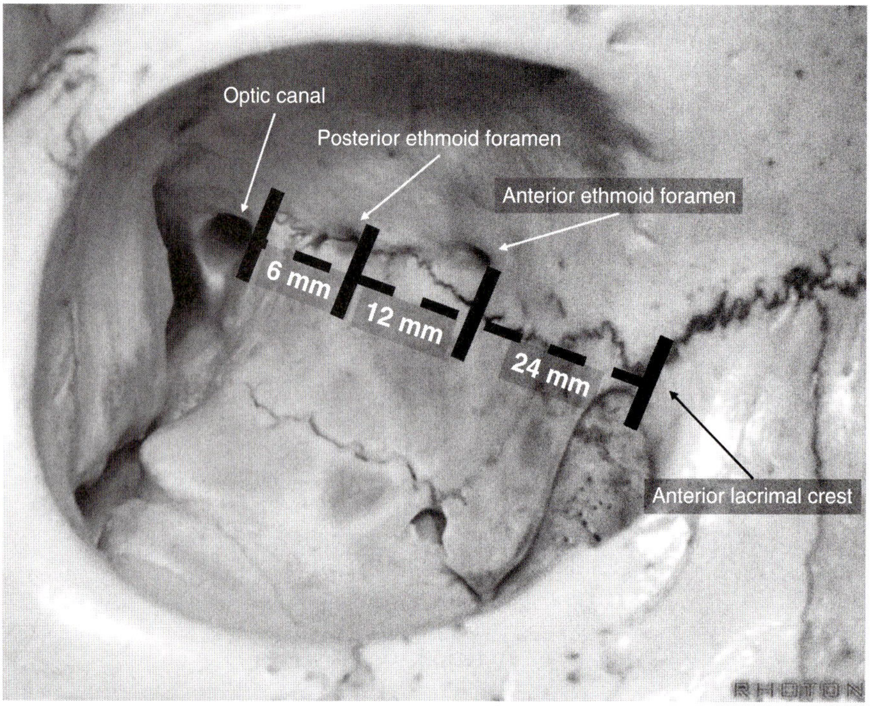

Figure 32-2 Right orbital bony anatomy demonstrating the relationship between the anterior lacrimal crest and significant neurovascular structures.
Image adapted from the Rhoton Collection. Courtesy of the Rhoton Collection, American Association of Neurological Surgeons (AANS)/Neurosurgical Research and Education Foundation (NREF).

- This results in a contraindication to radiologic embolization of these vessels (due to high stroke/vision loss risk).
  (a) Any ligation must therefore be performed surgically.
- Traditionally, a lynch incision would have been the standard approach, but this results in unnecessary scarring and cosmetic deformity.
  (a) A transcaruncular approach is now often preferred.
- Whilst this approach can be performed with a headlight, the endoscope now allows for markedly increased visibility and precision.
- The rule of halves can be remembered to guide surgeons during their approach to critical neurovascular structures of the medial orbital wall (Figure 32-2). That is:
  (a) 24 mm from the anterior lacrimal crest is the anterior ethmoidal foramen (AEF).
  (b) 12 mm from the AEF is the posterior ethmoidal foramen (PEF).
  (c) 6 mm from the PEF is the optic canal.

Surgical Technique

- Incision
  (a) A transcaruncular incision is made, and the incision carried down to the periosteum of the orbit.
  (b) Bipolar cautery may be required to cauterize the diploic veins that exit in this region; however, an avascular plane can be identified and utilized.

- Dissection
  (a) Once the periosteum is identified, a Cottle elevator can be used to elevate the periosteum from the maxilla and lamina papyracea.
  (b) The orbital contents are gently retracted using a malleable retractor.
  (c) The frontoethmoidal suture line is followed posteriorly, as this identifies the level at which the arterial canals enter the orbit.
  (d) From the anterior lacrimal crest, the AEA can be found approximately 24 mm posteriorly, at the level of the frontoethmoidal suture line.
- Ligation
  (a) Once this is identified, it can be cauterized and clipped. Arterial transection is at the discretion of the surgeon but is often not required.
  If the posterior ethmoid artery ligation is required, it can then be found by continuing to elevate the periorbita posteriorly along the frontoethmoidal suture line another 12 mm.
- Once the procedure is completed, instruments are retracted out of the orbit and the incision is left to heal.

Postoperative Considerations

- Check the patient's visual acuity and range of motion once awake.
- The optic nerve and superior oblique muscle are at risk of thermal injury if bipolar cautery is utilized.
- Minor periorbital bruising can be expected in the immediate postoperative period.

Transorbital Access to the Lateral Frontal Sinus (Periorbital Suspension Technique)

Introduction

- The frontal sinus continues to be a challenging region, even for rhinologists.
- Management of the frontal sinus has advanced significantly over the past few decades.
- Improved minimally invasive techniques have resulted in a significant decrease in the use of more traditional, invasive, and open approaches.
- The far lateral frontal sinus is perhaps the most inaccessible region in modern endoscopic sinus surgery, given the limitations in both visualization and instrumentation.
- Some pathologies (such as tumors, encephaloceles, and mucoceles) can center in this lateral region and thus require novel approaches to address in a purely endoscopic fashion.
- These pathologies can now be accessed either via a TONES approach (see following discussion) or a purely transnasal periorbital suspension approach.

Common Pathology of the Far Lateral Frontal Sinus

- Tumors
  (a) Inverting papilloma (most common)
  (b) Meningioma
  (c) Melanoma
- Obstructive/inflammatory
  (a) Mucocele
- Osseous and fibro-osseous disease
  (a) Osteoma
  (b) Ossifying fibroma
  (c) Fibrous dysplasia

- CSF leak
  (a) Meningoencephalocele
  (b) Idiopathic intracranial Hypertension and spontaneous CSF leak
  (c) Iatrogenic or traumatic CSF leak

Preoperative Evaluation

- Otolaryngologist assessment with endoscopic assessment
- Biopsy of lesion as indicated
  (a) To prevent CSF leak, avoid biopsy if meningoencephalocele is suspected
    - In this instance, obtain imaging first before proceeding
- Pre-operative ophthalmologist assessment
  (a) Baseline vision and EOM testing if concern for orbital extension of the pathology
- Imaging
  (a) High-resolution CT in all patients
    - Standard imaging for sinonasal pathology
    - Allows assessment of bony landmarks and extent of disease
    - Provides intraoperative image guidance
  (b) MRI with contrast in all patients
    - Allows assessment of any intracranial extension of disease
    - Allows for assessment of intraorbital extension of disease
    - Can characterize pathologies

Surgical Technique (Figure 32-3)

- Preparation of the nasal cavity
  (a) Extensive functional endoscopic sinus surgery needs to be performed (either unilaterally or bilaterally).
  (b) This must include either a Draf IIb or Draf III (Modified Lothrop; frontal drill-out) procedure.

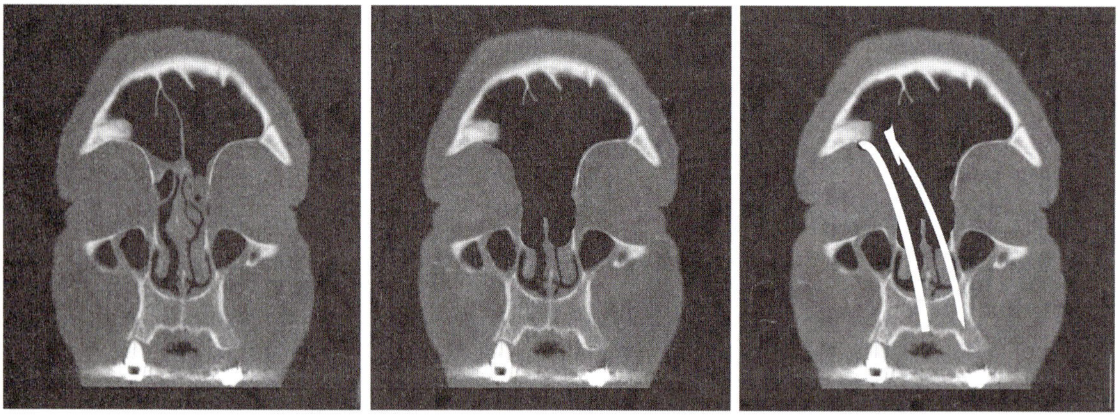

A B C

Figure 32-3 Adapted CT image demonstrating the periorbital suspension technique. **(A)** Patient CT revealing a heterogenous tumor in the right lateral frontal sinus, normally inaccessible via standard endoscopic techniques. **(B)** Adapted CT with Draf III performed and right orbital roof removed. **(C)** The periorbital suspension technique. A malleable retractor (curved line) displacing the right orbital contents. Operative instruments (curved arrow) can access the lateral frontal sinus and pathology via the contralateral nasal passage in a transeptal approach.

- Draf III and associated superior septectomy allow for more lateral pathology to be accessed by utilizing the contralateral nares and creating a greater working angle for instruments
- Exposure of the lamina and orbital roof
  (a) The medial wall and lamina papyracea are removed from the lacrimal sac anteriorly to the anterior ethmoid artery posteriorly.
    - Whilst the entirety of these structures may be removed, they need only be removed in the upper one-third to half to allow adequate access
  (b) The anterior ethmoid artery is then isolated, cauterized, and divided.
  (c) The periorbita is left intact to contain orbital contents and prevent prolapse of fat into the field.
- Removal of superior orbital wall
  (a) With a curved, malleable retractor, the exposed periorbita and orbit contents are displaced gently in an inferior and lateral direction.
    - This maneuver elevates the periorbita from the superior orbital roof, protecting the orbit.
  (b) The superior orbital wall is then removed using a diamond burr drill or cutting instruments to fully expose the lateral frontal sinus.
  (c) Anteriorly, the trochlea-periorbit complex must be identified and preserved.
    - Damage to this will cause EOM imbalance and diplopia.
- Access
  (a) Access to the lateral frontal sinus can now be achieved.
  (b) For maximum exposure, a Draf III, use of the contralateral nasal passage/nares, and curved instruments are required.
    - This allows for maximum angle and reach into the ipsilateral frontal sinus.
  (c) Depending on the extent of pathology, the above steps can be modified to reduce the extent of exposure and risks of morbidity.
- Reconstruction
  (a) Generally, no reconstruction of the orbital wall is required.
  (b) The intact periorbita will contain the orbital contents and prevent frontal sinus occlusion.
  (c) Maintaining the lower half to two-thirds of the lamina and medial orbital wall will ensure the orbital contents do not herniate into the sinuses over time.

Postoperative Considerations

- Nasal packing may be performed inferiorly, taking care not to place direct pressure on the exposed periorbita.
- Nasal saline rinses can commence gently on day 1 post-op, then per usual from the end of week 1.
- Patients may wish to avoid use of CPAP in the immediate postoperative period to avoid any undue pressure on the exposed orbit.
- Prophylactic antibiotics are given as per usual sinus surgery.

Transorbital Neuroendoscopic Surgery (TONES)

Introduction

- Complete transorbital surgery was traditionally considered far too unsafe to attempt until recently.
- New techniques developed since the 2010s have now opened the possibility of accessing the skull base via the orbit.

- These techniques involve following surgical planes along the orbital wall, whilst simultaneously retracting the orbital contents gently to open a working space within the orbit itself.
- Combined with hidden incisions into the eyelid, conjunctivae and caruncle allows for a truly minimally invasive approach.
- These approaches, used in the correct context, can avoid large craniotomy incisions and approaches of the past.
- TONES should be performed in conjunction with a neurosurgeon.
  (a) The otolaryngologist provides and opens a corridor of work.
  (b) The neurosurgeon performs the intracranial component.

The Routes of Transorbital Neuroendoscopic Surgery (TONES)

- There are four planes available in transorbital neuroendoscopic surgery (Figure 32-4):
  (a) Superior
  (b) Medial
  (c) Inferior
  (d) Lateral
- Each gives access to different aspects of the skull base and sinuses.
- Each plane has different considerations in regard to pathology accessible, incision and dissection pathways (described in the following discussion).

Pathology Addressed with TONES:

- Superior approach:
  (a) Superior orbital tumors/cysts
  (b) Anterior cranial fossa CSF leaks/meningoceles

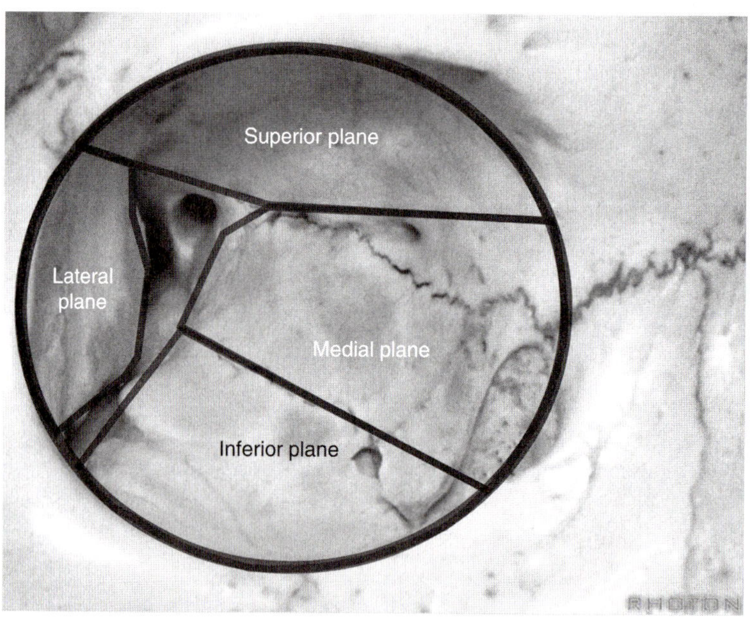

Figure 32-4 Right bony orbit demonstrating the access available from the four planes of transorbital neuroendoscopic surgery. Image adapted from the Rhoton Collection. Courtesy of the Rhoton Collection, American Association of Neurological Surgeons (AANS)/Neurosurgical Research and Education Foundation (NREF).

(c) Anterior cranial fossa meningiomas/tumors
(d) Lateral frontal sinus (tumors, mucoceles, CSF leaks)

- Medial approach:
  (a) Ethmoid arteries (for ligation)
  (b) Medial orbital tumors
  (c) Optic nerve decompression
  (d) Lateral sphenoid recess pathology (via transseptal approach)
  (e) Medial cavernous sinus
  (f) CSF leaks/ meningoceles
- Inferior approach:
  (a) Infraorbital nerve pathology to foramen rotundum
  (b) Inferior orbital fractures
  (c) Inferior orbital tumors/cysts
  (d) Maxillary sinus tumors with orbital floor invasion
- Lateral approach:
  (a) Sphenoid wing meningiomas
  (b) Infratemporal fossa lesions
  (c) Middle cranial fossa lesions
  (d) Lateral cavernous sinus lesions
  (e) Superior orbital fissure lesions
  (f) Lateral orbit or optic nerve lesions
  (g) Optic nerve decompression (lateral)

Preoperative Evaluation

- Otolaryngologist assessment with endoscopic assessment
  (a) Full cranial nerve assessment and documentation
- Neurosurgeon assessment
- Preoperative ophthalmologist assessment in all patients
  (a) Baseline vision and EOM testing
  (b) Intraocular pressure assessment
  (c) Especially required if pre-existing orbital disease exists
- Imaging
  (a) High-resolution CT and MRI scan in all patients
    - Allows for fusion navigation
    - Allows for complete characterization of pathology
    - Allows for planning for possible surgical approaches

Choice of Approach

- The advent of TONES highlights the myriad of choices that are now available to the surgeon when considering their approach to specific pathology.
- Ultimately, several factors should be considered when deciding on the appropriate surgical approach:
  (a) Morbidity to patient
  (b) Nearby critical structures (especially neurovascular)
  (c) Ease of access for instrumentation
  (d) Working window and working distance
  (e) Reconstruction requirements
  (f) Surgical experience
  (g) Patient preferences

Superior Plane Surgical Approach

- Incision:
  (a) Superior eyelid crease incision is typically chosen to allow adequate access whilst ensuring the levator palpebrae muscle is not transected.
    - 6 mm above the superior eyelid margin
  (b) A preseptal dissection plane is carried out to the orbital rim.
    - This allows for avoidance of the levator palpebrae muscle
    - Will also prevent orbital fat from entering field and obscuring view
- Dissection
  (a) Orbital periosteum incised at the superior orbital rim.
  (b) Anteromedially, the supratrochlear and supraorbital nerves can be identified as they exit the periosteum.
    - Drilling of the foreman they enter allows further retraction and preservation of the nerves.
  (c) Freer elevator can then be used to elevate periosteum from rim all the way back to the orbital apex.
  (d) Bone is resected as required to achieve desired surgical outcome.
- Surgical access:
  (a) Frontal sinuses (anteriorly)
    - Lateral aspect of the ipsilateral sinus
    - Medial aspect of the contralateral sinus
  (b) Anterior cranial fossa (posteriorly)
  (c) Greater and lesser wings of the sphenoid
- Postoperative considerations:
  (a) Bony defects in the orbital roof do not typically require reconstruction.
  (b) Any cerebrospinal fluid (CSF) leaks encountered can be repaired using standard techniques.
  (c) Dura pulsation against orbital contents usually subsides 2 weeks postoperatively.

Medial Plane Surgical Approach

- Incision:
  (a) Access gained through a precaruncular
    - Caruncle gently lateralized; incision made between caruncle and medial canthus using Wescott scissors
  (b) Transcaruncular incision may also be utilized, but will invariably breech the orbital septum and allow fat to prolapse into the field
  (c) Incision extended superiorly and inferiorly
- Dissection:
  (a) Enter preseptal plane and follow the posterior limb of the medial canthal tendon to the posterior lacrimal crest.
  (b) Incise periosteum of the lamina papyracea and dissect the plane between it and medial orbital bone.
  (c) Dissection extends from the floor to the skull base; ethmoid arteries cauterized/divided as needed.
- Surgical access:
  (a) Medial orbital wall
  (b) Anterior and posterior ethmoid arteries
  (c) Frontal, ethmoid, and sphenoid sinuses (contralateral lateral recess)
  (d) Optic nerve

- Postoperative considerations:
  (a) Bone defect reconstruction only if significant, to preserve orbital volume and prevent herniation of orbital contents into sinuses.
    - Keeping periorbita intact will often negate the need for this.

Inferior Plane Surgical Approach

- Incision:
  (a) Transconjunctival incision, directed toward the inferior orbital rim
    - This incision can be extended medially into a transcaruncular incision or laterally into a canthotomy/cantholysis incision.

  (b) Care is taken to avoid injury to the lacrimal system.
- Dissection:
  (a) Dissect through orbital fat to the orbital rim; incise periosteum.
  (b) Elevate periosteum, exposing the origin of the inferior oblique muscle.
  (c) Continue dissection posteriorly to the orbital apex, along the floor to the inferior orbital fissure.
  (d) Infraorbital nerve typically left undisturbed unless intentionally dissected.
  (e) Dissection can be extended medially or laterally to the anterior aspect of the inferior fissure.
  (f) Bone is resected as required to achieve desired surgical outcome.
- Surgical access:
  (a) Inferior orbit
  (b) Infraorbital nerve to foramen rotundum and trigeminal ganglion
  (c) Superior maxillary sinus tumors
- Reconstruction and postoperative care:
  (a) Orbital floor reconstruction is more common than medial wall reconstruction.
  (b) Incision typically left open.
  (c) If extended approach results in conjunctival edema, a temporary tarsorrhaphy suture is placed to prevent prolapse and exposure damage.

Lateral Plane Surgical Approach

- Incision:
  (a) Retrocanthal or lateral canthotomy/cantholysis
  (b) May also use extended upper lid crease incision above the lateral canthus
  (c) Allows greatest exposure for superolateral pathology such as with the sphenoid wing
- Dissection:
  (a) Dissection through the preaponeurotic space toward orbital rim and the periosteum is subsequently incised and elevated.
  (b) Periosteum is then elevated posteriorly off the lateral orbital wall until the superior orbital fissure is encountered.
  (c) Bipolar cautery applied to the recurrent branch of the middle meningeal artery just anterior to the superior orbital fissure.
  (d) Lateral orbital bone can be drilled away as required, leaving a 5 mm anterior bony rim to provide structure and avoid postoperative reconstruction.
  (e) Exposure of the temporalis muscle and dura of the temporal fossa achieved by drilling the lesser wing of the sphenoid bone.
- Surgical access
  (a) Wide lateral portal provides access to the intracranial component of sphenoid wing meningiomas and the superior orbital fissure
  (b) Infratemporal fossa

  (c) Superior orbital fissure
  (d) Middle cranial fossa
  (e) Cavernous sinus
- Reconstruction and postoperative considerations:
  (a) Reconstruction is not required if the anterior bony orbital rim is left intact as this provides adequate structural support.

Multiportal Surgery

- The above dissection planes and pathways can be utilized with traditional endonasal endoscopic techniques to allow for access to previously inaccessible areas.
- Examples of this would include:
  (a) Using the superior transorbital plane in addition to an endonasal Draf III to access pathology of the lateral frontal sinus.
  (b) Using a medial approach alongside an endonasal approach with a posterior septectomy can allow access into the lateral sphenoid sinus to address CSF leaks and meningoceles.
  (c) For maxillary sinus malignancies, the inferior plane can be utilized alongside the endonasal extended maxillary approaches to assess for pathology extension into the orbit/infraorbital nerve and assist with tumor manipulation.

Postoperative Considerations

- Wound care:
  (a) No dressings required
  (b) Topical ocular lubricant used regularly for 7 days
  (c) Topical antibiotic ointment used on cutaneous incision site for 7 days
- Orbit checks
  (a) Observe VA and EOM when awake and then as needed.
  (b) Ophthalmology review within 2 to 4 weeks post-op.
- Obtain postoperative CT scan in all patients with intracranial component on the evening of surgery.
- Prophylactic oral antibiotics for 5 to 7 days.

Conclusion

- Transorbital endoscopic surgery continues to be in its infancy, but is rapidly developing and being adopted across the world.
- The orbit is no longer considered a "no go" zone for the endoscopic rhinologist.
- In many cases, an endoscopic transorbital approach can be utilized effectively to address pathology of the orbit, sinuses, and skull base.
- The use of endoscopic transorbital techniques is reducing the utilization and reliance on large craniotomies and open approaches.
- These new ports can be effectively used alone or in combination with established endonasal routes to tailor the surgery to both the patient and the anatomical access required.
- Ongoing collaboration between otolaryngology, ophthalmology, and neurosurgery is essential for these approaches and will continue to open new possibilities and corridors for addressing previously difficult areas.

Bibliography

Jafari A, Adappa ND, Anagnos VJ, et al. Orbital resection by intranasal technique (ORBIT): A new classification system for reporting endoscopically resectable primary benign orbital tumors. *IFAR*. 2023;13(10):152-863.

Tilak A, Purvis J, Pena-Garcia A, et al. Above and beyond: periorbital suspension for endoscopic access to difficult frontal sinus pathology. *Laryngoscope*. 2022;132:538-544.

Moe KS, Bergeron CM, Ellenbogen RG. Transorbital neuroendoscopic surgery. *Neurosurgery*. 2010;67(3 Suppl Operative): ons16-28.

Questions

1. How far from the anterior lacrimal crest can the anterior ethmoid artery be found?
   A. 10-15 mm
   B. 20-25 mm
   C. 30-35 mm
   D. 40 mm

2. What are the most common types of tumors in the orbit?
   A. Lymphocytic tumors, such as lymphoma
   B. Neurogenic tumors such as optic gliomas
   C. Vascular tumors such as cavernous hemangioma
   D. Fibro-osseous lesions such as fibrous dysplasia

3. In classifying tumors of the orbit, those that enter the pterygopalatine fossa would be considered ORBIT
   A. Class II
   B. Class III
   C. Class IV
   D. Class V

4. Damage to which structure may lead to postoperative orbital mobility issues?
   A. Superior orbital roof
   B. The periorbita-trochlea complex
   C. The anterior ethmoid artery
   D. The posterior ethmoid artery

5. TONES can provide access to
   A. Aspects of the anterior cranial fossa
   B. Aspects of the middle cranial fossa
   C. Aspects of the infratemporal fossa
   D. All of the above

Part 4
Head and Neck

Chapter 33
Salivary Gland Diseases

I. Anatomy

A. Parotid gland
  1. Anatomic boundaries
    (a) Anterior: masseter muscle
    (b) Posterior: tragal cartilage, sternocleidomastoid muscle (SCM)
    (c) Deep: parapharyngeal space (prestyloid)
    (d) Superior: zygomatic arch
    (e) Superficial: platysma muscle
    (f) Inferomedial: posterior digastric muscle
    (g) Lateral: parotidomasseteric fascia
  2. Superficial and deep lobes defined by the plane of the facial nerve. Most of the gland parenchyma (~80%) lies within the superficial lobe.
  3. Parotid tail: inferior 2 cm of superficial parotid gland, lateral to digastric, and anterior to sternocleidomastoid muscle
  4. Encased by superficial layer of deep cervical fascia (parotid fascia)
    (a) Deep to the superficial musculoaponeurotic system (SMAS)
    (b) Contiguous with masseter fascia anteriorly, SCM fascia posteriorly

5. Arterial anatomy
   (a) Terminal external carotid artery (ECA) courses medial to the digastric muscle and the deep parotid gland.
   (b) Deeply, the ECA divides into the internal maxillary artery and superficial temporal artery (STA).
   (c) ECA course can be torturous at the inferior parotid gland and can infrequently be encountered during superficial parotidectomy or require ligation with deep lobe/parapharyngeal space (PPS) surgery.
   (d) STA is typically identified superficially during superior gland dissection, posterior to the frontal branch of facial nerve.
6. Venous anatomy
   (a) Retromandibular vein (RMV) runs within the gland parenchyma, formed by the maxillary and superficial temporal veins.
   (b) Retromandibular vein drains to external jugular vein or posterior facial vein.
   (c) Variably, branches from RMV to facial vein or internal jugular vein will exist.
   (d) RMV is often used as a radiographic proxy for the depth of the facial nerve, although the nerve can sometimes run deep or within two branches of the RMV.
7. Lymphatics
   (a) Majority of lymph nodes are located within superficial lobe of the parotid gland
   (b) Primarily drains facial skin, eyelids, scalp, and ear
8. Stensen duct
   (a) Traverses superficial to the masseter muscle then pierces through the buccinator to the oral mucosa.
   (b) The duct punctum is adjacent to the maxillary second molar.
9. The great auricular nerve
   (a) Arises from C2 and C3 nerve branches of the cervical plexus.
   (b) Provides sensation to the skin overlying the parotid and mastoid, as well as the external ear.
   (c) A posterior branch can be saved variably during parotidectomy to spare some auricular sensation, depending on the nature and location of parotid pathology.
10. Facial nerve
    (a) Exits the temporal bone at the stylomastoid foramen along the tympanomastoid suture line (the gap between the tympanic plate and mastoid process).
    (b) Stylomastoid foramen lies *posterolateral* to the styloid process and *anteromedial* to the mastoid process.
    (c) The main trunk branches within the parotid into the upper and lower divisions at the *pes anserinus* ("goose's foot").
    (d) Traditionally, five main branches are described (temporal, zygomatic, buccal, marginal mandibular, and cervical). However, branching patterns are variable, and more numerous branches often exist.
    (e) Facial nerve trunk course is typically more superficial in children younger than 2 years.
11. Anatomic landmarks of main trunk of facial nerve
    (a) Tympanomastoid suture line is the most dependable landmark with palpation of junction of styloid and mastoid bones.
    (b) Just superior to, and at the level of, the posterior belly of the digastric muscle.
    (c) 1 cm deep and inferior to the tragal pointer. This can be variable depending on parotid pathology.

(d) Retrograde dissection along one of the distal facial nerve branches.
(e) Mastoid segment identification via mastoidectomy.

12. Autonomic nerve supply
    (a) Parasympathetic: fibers of CN IX (glossopharyngeal nerve) synapse in otic ganglion, then postganglionic fibers travel with auriculotemporal nerve → secrete acetylcholine → secretion of saliva
    (b) Sympathetic: superior cervical ganglion → secrete norepinephrine (NE) → gland vasoconstriction, thickened saliva
13. Parapharyngeal space
    (a) Inverted pyramid, boundaries include:
        i. Superior: skull base, petrous temporal bone
        ii. Inferior: hyoid bone
        iii. Medial: pharyngeal constrictors
        iv. Lateral: pterygoid musculature
        v. Posterior: carotid sheath/vertebral bodies
        vi. Anterior: pterygomandibular raphe
    (b) *Prestyloid* compartment: deep lobe of parotid, adipose tissue
    (c) *Poststyloid* compartment: carotid sheath, CNs IX-XII, sympathetic chain

B. Submandibular gland
1. Gland anatomy
    (a) Bounded by the inferior mandible and anterior and posterior belly of the digastric muscle (submandibular triangle)
    (b) Superficial and deep lobes divided by mylohyoid muscle
2. Vascular anatomy
    (a) The facial artery courses deep to the posterior belly of the digastric muscle but has a tortuous course to the superficial aspect of the gland superiorly. Small branches from the facial and submental arteries (variable in number) supply the gland.
    (b) The facial vein lies lateral to the gland and drains into the internal jugular vein or, rarely, the external jugular vein.
    (c) Wharton's duct travels around the posterior mylohyoid muscle to drain to the floor of the mouth. The lingual nerve travels from lateral to medial under the duct.
3. Nerve anatomy
    (a) Parasympathetic: facial nerve → chorda tympani (travels within lingual nerve) → submandibular ganglion → salivary secretion (acetylcholine)
    (b) Sympathetic: superior cervical ganglion → postganglionic fibers run along the external carotid artery to the gland to stimulate secretion
    (c) The lingual nerve (sensory) traverses the floor of the mouth and attaches to the deep surface of the submandibular gland via the submandibular ganglion (parasympathetic).
    (d) The hypoglossal nerve (motor to the tongue) runs medial to the submandibular gland and can quickly be found deep at the junction of the mylohyoid muscle and anterior belly of the digastric.
4. Relevant lymph nodes are periglandular (outside of gland capsule); typically, there are 3 to 6 nodes below the mandible around the gland.
5. When glands are *unstimulated*, the submandibular gland produces roughly 70% of resting state saliva (more is produced by parotid when glands are stimulated).

C. Sublingual and minor salivary glands
   i. The sublingual glands, the smallest of the major salivary glands, are paired glands in the floor of the mouth, bounded inferiorly by the mylohyoid muscle, medially by genioglossus muscle, and laterally by the mandible.
   ii. Sublingual glands drain via ducts of Rivinus; the largest duct (duct of Bartholin) drains into Wharton's duct.
   iii. Mucoceles of the sublingual glands are called ranulas. A "plunging" ranula is defined by herniation through the mylohyoid muscle into the neck.
   iv. Minor salivary glands are located throughout the upper airway but are concentrated in the oral cavity (esp. the palate and lip), numbering from 600 to 1000 unnamed glands.

II. Imaging

A. Neoplasms

Imaging modality should be chosen according to the radiographic question at hand, institutional availability, and individual surgeon experience.

1. Ultrasound
   (a) No ionizing radiation, real-time clinical or intraoperative information, and high sensitivity for salivary pathology.
   (b) Loss of fatty hilum, rounded lymph node shape, and abnormal peripheral vascularity can suggest malignancy.
   (c) The deep aspect of lesions in PPS can be difficult to visualize.
   (d) A bimanual exam with a finger in the floor of the mouth can help with the visualization of sublingual/FOM lesions.
   (e) Sialolithiasis (stones) can also be reliably identified on ultrasound
   (f) Image-guided fine/core needle biopsies can be obtained quickly and easily.
2. Magnetic resonance imaging (MRI) provides excellent soft tissue detail of neoplastic salivary lesions.
   (a) A normal gland is hyperintense (bright) on unenhanced T1-weighted images due to high fat content.
   (b) All neoplasms are generally hypointense (dark) on T1 images.
   (c) Low-density differentiated masses (benign and low-grade malignancy) tend to be hyperintense on T2 images (more water content).
   (d) Salivary malignancies tend to be T2 hypointense (denser) but more reliably identified by irregular/infiltrative borders.
   (e) Warthin tumors are isointense/hyperintense on T1 (cysts containing cholesterol) and variable/heterogeneous intensity on T2.
   (f) Diffusion-weighted imaging can be helpful as hypercellular neoplasms demonstrate restricted water motion.
   (g) Postcontrast T1 sequences are helpful for identifying perineural invasion in malignancy.
3. Computerized tomography (CT) scans are widely available and commonly used for salivary tumor imaging.
   (a) Inferior soft tissue detail relative to MRI, but often sufficient.
   (b) Early cortical erosion of the mandible or skull base is better determined by CT, relative to MR, which is better at determining bone marrow and intracranial involvement.

(c) Excellent for delineation of potential malignant adenopathy.
(d) CT-guided FNA can be diagnostic in nonpalpable lesions that are not amenable to ultrasound (US)-guided biopsy.
(e) Sialoliths or other calcifications readily identified.

4. Nuclear scintigraphy
   (a) Tc-99m pertechnetate is rarely utilized but may help in diagnosing Warthin tumor (concentrates the radiocontrast agent).
5. PET-CT fluorodeoxyglucose (PET-FDG) is generally used to identify regional and distant metastases in known malignancies. Warthin tumors are FDG-avid, while some low-grade salivary carcinomas can show low PET-avidity, so PET cannot necessarily distinguish between malignant and benign lesions.
6. Inflammatory lesions
   (a) Ultrasound and CT (contrast not needed) have high sensitivity for sialoliths. Plain radiographs can also be used, but FOM stones can be obscured by the mandible.
   (b) Sialography (sialogram) utilizes injected contrast into a cannulated salivary duct and can be useful in identifying and localizing stones, ductal strictures, and penetrating trauma. Technically difficult and contraindicated in acute sialadenitis.
   (c) MR sialography can image the salivary ducts without duct cannulation (T2-weighted sequences can highlight duct).
7. Systemic diseases
   (a) Calcifications in Sjögren disease or sarcoidosis: US or CT
   (b) Sialography or MRI sialography may help stage Sjögren disease.
   (c) Multiple modalities (CT, US, MRI) can be used to identify mucosa-associated lymphoid tissue (MALT) lymphoma in Sjögren patients.
   (d) Radiographic bilateral parotid cysts should prompt workup for HIV/AIDS.
8. Parapharyngeal space (PPS) mass imaging
   (a) MRI definition outstanding, and should be standardly obtained for any PPS mass.
   (b) *Prestyloid* masses tend to displace the carotid posterolaterally.
   (c) *Poststyloid* masses tend to put carotid anteromedially and/or splay vessels.
   (d) Pleomorphic adenomas emanating from deep lobe of parotid are characteristically bright on T2-weighted MRI.
   (e) Dotatate PET/CT (Ga-68) can be used to define poststyloid PPS mass as paraganglioma.

III. Physiology, Embryology, and Related Topics

A. Embryology
   1. Glands first develop around 6 to 8 weeks of gestation.
   2. Develop via branching morphogenesis.
   3. Glands are functional at birth.
   4. Lymph nodes form within the pseudocapsule of the parotid gland, but they do not form within the capsule of other salivary glands.

B. Salivary physiology and function
   1. Between 0.5 and 1.5 L of human saliva is produced daily.
   2. Parotid gland secretion is the least viscous and most dependent on salivary stimulation.

3. Submandibular gland secretion tends to be more viscous (higher mucin content) and predominates as unstimulated saliva.
4. Involved in the early digestion of starches and triglycerides with secreted amylases (alpha-amylase most abundant) and lipases.
5. Lubricates a food bolus with mucous glycoproteins, assisting with speech, mastication, swallowing, and taste.
6. Provides dental protection by buffering oral pH, diluting sugars, and aiding enamel remineralization.
7. Saliva also plays an immunologic role: secretory component/IgA, lysozymes, autolysin, and lactoferrin protect against viral and bacterial infection.

C. Neurophysiology
1. Salivary flow is under autonomic nervous system control
2. Parasympathetic cholinergic stimulation: increased salivary flow triggered by acetylcholine release → downstream Ca^{2+} release, stimulating transport activity in acinar and ductal cells.
3. Sympathetic beta-adrenergic stimulation: thickens saliva via neurotransmitter norepinephrine using G-protein–activated second messenger, cyclic adenosine monophosphate (cAMP).

D. Pathologic flow states
1. Cystic fibrosis results in abnormal chloride regulation with failure of reabsorption of NaCl in the ductal cells, resulting in more viscous and less voluminous saliva.
2. Drugs are the most common source of xerostomia: anticholinergics, antidepressants/antipsychotics (eg, haloperidol), opioids, and antihistamines, among others.
3. Xerostomia in elderly individuals is often the product of medical comorbidities and polypharmacy, as well as changes in the chemical composition of saliva (increased mucin creating viscous saliva).
4. Radioactive iodine given for thyroid cancer accumulates in salivary tissue and can cause chronic xerostomia (especially with doses > 150 mCi).
5. External beam radiation for head and neck malignancies/lymphoma causes both acute and chronic xerostomia.
6. Salivary flow can be quantified with sialometry, which typically involves unstimulated salivary collection for 5 to 10 minutes (various techniques exist). Sialometry specimens can also be used for sialochemistry analysis.

E. Salivary histology
1. Secretory (acinar) cells are organized into discrete secretory units called acini.
2. Acini can be serous, mucous, or mixed serous/mucous.
3. Acini converge into intercalated ducts → striated ducts → interlobular (excretory) ducts
4. Myoepithelial cells surround intercalated ducts to regulate salivary flow.
5. The parotid gland is primarily composed of serous acini and watery saliva.
6. The submandibular gland has mixed serous and mucous acini.
7. Sublingual gland with predominantly mucous acini: most viscous saliva.

F. Benign non-neoplastic pathology
1. Adenomatoid hyperplasia
   (a) Asymptomatic submucosal nodule generally over the hard palate.
   (b) Hyperplasia of mucinous acini
   (c) If symptomatic, surgical excision can be offered for cure

2. Sialadenosis (a.k.a. sialosis)
   (a) Painless enlargement of the salivary glands.
   (b) Histologically characterized by enlarged acinar cells.
   (c) Myoepithelial atrophy and neural degeneration are also seen.
3. Necrotizing sialometaplasia
   (a) Presents as a painless ulcer on the posterior hard palate.
   (b) Can be preceded by trauma or local anesthetic infiltration in the palate.
   (c) While clinically often misinterpreted as malignancy, it is benign and self-limited. Most lesions recede within several weeks to several months.
4. Accessory/heterotopic salivary gland tissue (SGT)
   (a) Accessory SGT: salivary tissue remote from the salivary gland occurring along major salivary ducts. Accessory parotid tissue is common along Stensen duct.
   (b) Heterotopic SGT: rest of salivary tissue in an abnormal location without associated duct; examples include cervical lymph nodes, middle ear, thyroid, and pituitary.
5. Amyloidosis
   (a) Salivary amyloidosis can present as painless gland enlargement with xerostomia.
   (b) Histology: positive Congo red staining (apple-green birefringence on polarized view)
   (c) Localized salivary involvement is very rare and can be associated with Sjögren syndrome or lymphoma.
6. Lipomatosis
   (a) Diffuse parenchymal deposition of adipose tissue in the salivary gland (parotid most common)
   (b) Gland enlarges without discrete mass
   (c) Associated with aging, diabetes, cirrhosis, alcoholism, and malnutrition
7. Cheilitis glandularis
   (a) Nodular, swollen lower lip with clear mucous secretions, typically seen in adult males.
   (b) Etiology unknown
   (c) Treatments include topical antibiotics and steroids, rarely surgical excision.

IV. Sialadenitis

A. Acute suppurative sialadenitis
   1. Elderly, debilitated, dehydrated, and postsurgical patients are most affected by nonsialolith acute sialadenitis.
   2. Parotid is the most common site of acute infection; saliva is less mucinous with poor antimicrobial activity (cf. submandibular gland).
   3. Sialolith-related sialadenitis more commonly involves the submandibular gland.
   4. Regardless of etiology, *Staphylococcus aureus* is the most common pathogen cultured. MRSA should be a consideration, especially for hospitalized patients.
   5. Ultrasound or CT may identify stone or abscess; sialography and sialendoscopy are contraindicated during acute infection.

6. Treatment: Beta-lactamase and anaerobic sensitive antibiotics, hydration, gland massage, and sialagogues. In mild cases, antibiotics may be excluded.
7. In cases of salivary abscess, ultrasound-guided aspiration can be attempted to drain and obtain cultures. Rarely are surgical incision and drainage needed in recalcitrant cases.

B. Chronic obstructive sialadenitis
1. Sialolithiasis may result in scarred, stenotic ducts and sialectasia, leading to diminished secretory function of the gland.
2. Other causes can include RAI-induced external beam radiation and systemic diseases (see below) that cause chronic inflammation and scarring of ducts.
3. Conservative treatment with antibiotics, hydration, and gland massage can improve many cases.
4. Removal of sialolith or interventional sialendoscopy can return gland function and obviate gland removal.

C. Mumps
1. Caused by the mumps virus of the *Paramyxoviridae* family of viruses.
2. United States cases have dropped drastically since the introduction of the MMR vaccine in 1971.
3. Peak age 4 to 6 years. In addition to parotitis, symptoms include fevers, malaise, orchitis, encephalitis, and even sensorineural hearing loss.
4. Bilateral parotitis usually begins 2 to 3 weeks after viral exposure. Unilateral is rare.
5. Self-limited clinical course; treatment is supportive with hydration, warm packs, etc.

D. HIV-related salivary gland disease
1. Diffuse parotid enlargement from lymphoid hyperplasia can be a presenting symptom of HIV infection.
2. Bilateral lymphoepithelial cysts often develop in parotid.
3. Can develop sicca syndrome like Sjögren syndrome—diffuse infiltrative lymphocytosis syndrome (DILS) due to infiltration with CD8+ lymphocytes.
4. Dx: HIV+ serology, associated cervical adenopathy, and nasopharyngeal lymphoid hypertrophy.
5. Cysts often involute with appropriate antiretroviral treatment; surgery is rarely recommended/required for the parotid deformity.
6. Intraparotid lymphoma can develop in HIV+ patients, presenting as a solid (noncystic) mass.

E. Infectious granulomatous diseases
1. Tuberculous sialadenitis: Extrapulmonary tuberculosis typically caused by *Mycobacterium tuberculosis.*
2. Atypical mycobacterial infection
   (a) Most often a pediatric infection, 16 to 36 months old
   (b) Characteristic violaceous hue of skin, sinus tracts
   (c) Chest X-ray (CXR) negative, PPD nonreactive
   (d) High cure rates with surgical excision +/− antimycobacterial antibiotics (referral to Infectious Disease often helpful)
3. Actinomycosis
   (a) Gram-positive anaerobic *Actinomyces* species, microscopically characterized by branched, filamentous rods with sulfur granules.
   (b) Risk factors include poor oral hygiene, dental/mandibular infections, alcoholism, and immunosuppression (HIV, lymphoma, chemotherapy, etc.)
   (c) Treatment involves a prolonged antibiotic course (typically over 6 weeks of penicillin G, beta-lactam, or cephalosporin)

4. Cat scratch disease
   (a) Caused by *Bartonella henselae*, inoculated from cat scratch or cat flea bite.
   (b) Sialadenitis can be secondary to parotid lymph node lymphadenitis.
   (c) Diagnosed on serology and polymerase chain reaction (PCR), microscopic Warthin-Starry stain reaction, and histologic necrotizing stellate abscesses.
   (d) Typically self-limited, resolving over 2 to 6 months; antibiotics used in severe cases.
5. Toxoplasmosis
   (a) Caused by *Toxoplasmosis gondii* protozoan parasite
   (b) Can present as an isolated parotid mass
   (c) Associated with raw meat, contact with animal feces, unpasteurized milk
   (d) Diagnosis: tissue culture, IgM/IgG serology
   (e) Treated with pyrimethamine and sulfadiazine. Mild cases can be observed for resolution.

F. Noninfectious granulomatous diseases
1. Sarcoidosis
   (a) Systemic disease of unknown etiology, characterized by noncaseating granulomas.
   (b) Can present as a painless swelling of the parotid gland.
   (c) Alternative salivary presentation is Heerfordt syndrome (parotitis, fever, facial nerve palsy, and anterior uveitis).
   (d) Corticosteroids are standard treatment.
2. Granulomatosis with polyangiitis (GPA, formerly Wegener granulomatosis)
   (a) ANCA-associated vasculitis: systemic necrotizing granulomatous inflammatory lesions
   (b) May involve major salivary glands; parotid abscesses reported
   (c) Treatment: steroids, other immunosuppressants
3. Xanthogranulomatous sialadenitis
   (a) Rare inflammatory lesion that presents as a persistent salivary mass
   (b) Associated with Warthin tumor
   (c) Most are surgically excised, given the propensity to mimic malignancy
4. Sjögren syndrome
   (a) Chronic autoimmune disease characterized by xerostomia and xeropthalmia
   (b) Parotid hypertrophy is also common with xerostomia
   (c) Diagnosis: anti-Ro (SS-A) and anti-La (SS-B) serologies, minor salivary gland biopsy
   (d) Associated with the development of non-Hodgkin lymphoma (20x risk of unaffected individual)
   (e) Supportive treatment: salivary substitutes, pilocarpine, NSAIDs, artificial tears.

G. Sialolithiasis
1. Not associated with higher rates of nephrolithiasis or cholelithiasis.
2. CT is the standard imaging technique to identify and characterize stones. However, ultrasound has excellent sensitivity for sialoliths and can be utilized intraoperatively to identify stones and confirm removal.
3. Improvements in sialendoscopy technology have greatly improved minimally invasive approaches to sialolith removal. Stones 3 to 5 mm can usually be extracted endoscopically, while a combined endoscopic/open approach can be used for larger stone extraction.

4. Hilar or intraparenchymal stones are not amenable to transoral extraction, and either a transfacial approach (parotid) or gland excision (submandibular) should be utilized.
5. Intracorporeal versus extracorporeal shock wave therapy is not currently FDA-approved in the United States.

V. Pediatric Salivary Gland Disease

A. Parotitis
   1. Neonatal suppurative parotitis can develop in preterm, male neonates. *S. aureus* is the most common pathogen.
   2. Recurrent parotitis of childhood: more common in males aged 3 to 10, presents with recurrent bacterial infections several times per month. Treatment includes antibiotics and interventional sialendoscopy.
   3. Viral infections include mumps (as above), HIV, cytomegalovirus.

B. Congenital cysts
   1. Parotid dermoid: very rare, soft cystic mass, treated with surgery if cosmetic concerns.
   2. Branchial cleft cysts: Type I can be associated with the parotid gland and facial nerve, with a tract to the membranous external auditory canal.
   3. Polycystic parotid disease: surgery can be offered for cosmetic reasons.

C. Acquired cysts
   1. Ranula: extravasation of saliva, not a true cyst, most often from the sublingual gland. "Plunging" ranula extends beyond the mylohyoid muscle into the neck. Adequate treatment requires sublingual gland resection.
   2. Mucocele: trauma-induced pseudocyst of minor salivary gland; lower lip most common location.

D. Neoplasms
   1. Infantile hemangiomas
      (a) Most common salivary gland neoplasm in children; most spontaneously involute (50% by 5 years, 70% by 7 years).
      (b) Without spontaneous involution, the primary treatment is with a beta-blocker (propranolol).
      (c) Primary surgery is rarely utilized, given success with beta-blockers, but cosmetic procedures can be offered for postinvolutional scarring.
   2. Lymphangiomas, however, rarely involute, and surgery or sclerotherapy (OK-432) is offered.
   3. Based on more recent series, malignancy rate in pediatric salivary tumors is less than 25%.
   4. Mucoepidermoid carcinoma is the most common pediatric salivary malignancy.

E. Sialorrhea/ptyalism
   1. Common in children with cerebral palsy or other neurologic disorders.
   2. Treatment includes salivary Botox injections and anticholinergic medications. Generally, Botox is preferred given its effectiveness and better side effect profile than anticholinergics.
   3. Surgery can be utilized in refractory cases. Bilateral parotid duct ligation and submandibular gland excision are considered the most effective; however, high success rates are also reported for four-duct ligation.

VI. Benign Tumors and Cysts

A. Pleomorphic adenoma (also known as benign mixed tumor)
   1. Most common salivary gland neoplasm, roughly two-thirds of all salivary tumors.
   2. About 85% present in the parotid gland.
   3. Can be within prestyloid PPS emanating from the deep lobe of the parotid, presenting as a submucosal oropharyngeal mass. Small PPS tumors medial to the carotid artery can be removed transorally (with or without robotic assistance).
   4. Histologically characterized by the proliferation of a mixed population of epithelial and myoepithelial cells. Three subtypes: 1) myxoid (hypocellular, most common), 2) cellular, and 3) classic.
   5. There is a low but real risk of malignant transformation of a benign pleomorphic adenoma (1-2% based on large European series).
   6. Enucleation results in an unacceptably high recurrence rate due to a thin, delicate pseudocapsule prone to rupture (particularly hypocellular tumors).
   7. Extracapsular dissection without facial nerve dissection can be utilized by surgeons who are experienced in this technique.
   8. The definitive treatment for tumor recurrence involves resection of all gross tumor. Often this is not achievable without significant morbidity, and clinical judgement must be used. Postoperative radiation may be utilized on a case-by-case basis depending on the location and nature of recurrence.

B. Myoepitheliomas (a.k.a. myoepithelial adenoma) consist entirely of myoepithelial cells, which are much less common than pleomorphic adenoma.

C. Basal cell adenoma
   1. Monomorphic basaloid cell tumors are typically slow-growing and in the parotid gland.
   2. Can be indistinguishable from adenoid cystic carcinoma on FNA cytology.

D. Warthin tumor (papillary cystadenoma lymphomatosum)
   1. The second most common benign neoplasm of the parotid.
   2. Occasionally becomes inflammatory/painful.
   3. Characteristically PET-avid.
   4. Can be multifocal (20%) or bilateral (5%).
   5. Associated with smoking, but etiology unknown.
   6. Histology: oncocytic epithelium, papillary architecture, lymphoid stroma, and cystic spaces.
   7. Can be resected if symptomatic; otherwise, it can be observed after needle biopsy confirmation.
   8. Malignant transformation is exceedingly rare.

E. Canalicular adenoma
   1. Slow-growing, rare variant of basal cell adenoma.
   2. Typically, in minor salivary glands, the mucosal upper lip.
   3. Surgical resection is the mainstay of treatment.

F. Oncocytoma
   1. Rare (< 1%) epithelial tumors, often of the parotid gland in elderly patients.
   2. Like Warthin tumor, it can rarely be multifocal or bilateral.
   3. Malignant transformation is also exceedingly rare.

G. Lipoma
   1. Characteristic appearance on imaging and typically can be observed unless symptomatic or a significant cosmetic issue.

H. Acquired cystic lesions
   1. Sialocele—not a true epithelial-lined cyst. It can be postobstructive, iatrogenic (surgery), or traumatic in origin.
   2. Pseudocysts (mucoceles) are common in minor salivary glands and are typically traumatic in origin.
   3. Benign lymphoepithelial cysts: can be HIV-related or non-HIV-related (epithelial ductal inclusions in lymph nodes).

I. Sialadenosis
   1. Benign noninflammatory swelling of salivary glands.
   2. Etiology is typically metabolic; these causes can include (but are not limited to) bulimia nervosa, diabetes, hypothyroidism, cirrhosis, obesity, and Sjögren syndrome.
   3. Parenchymal atrophy with an increase in adipose deposition, without inflammatory infiltrate.
   4. FNA or gland biopsy is typically performed to rule out underlying neoplasm.
   5. Treatment involves correction of underlying medical condition.

VII. Malignancies

A. Primary salivary malignancies
   1. Heterogenous histology, with 24 salivary gland malignancies identified by the World Health Organization.
   2. Etiology unknown, although not known to be related to smoking or alcohol consumption. Proposed (but not proven) mechanisms include genetics, radiation exposure, viral infection, and environmental exposures.
   3. Presentation
      (a) Often painless, but painful mass can be indicative of perineural invasion.
      (b) Variable growth rate can involve overlying skin, sternocleidomastoid muscle invasion (clinical fixation), masseter or pterygoid muscle (trismus), facial nerve weakness.
      (c) For any presenting salivary mass, the likelihood of malignancy increases according to location: sublingual (most likely malignancy) > minor > submandibular > parotid (least likely malignant
   4. Treatment general principles
      (a) Surgical resection is the primary treatment for epithelial salivary malignancies with adjuvant radiation used for higher grade and stage.
      (b) For clinically N0 disease, elective neck dissection should be performed for high-grade or high-stage (cT3 or cT4) cancers. Levels II and III are typically included but can vary according to surgeon.
      (c) For clinically apparent disease, more extensive dissection typically is performed (Levels I-IV +/− V).
      (d) Postoperative radiotherapy is often applied with close surgical margins, extension beyond the gland capsule, perineural invasion, metastatic lymphadenopathy, high-grade tumors, or recurrent low-grade tumors but is highly dependent upon underlying tumor histology and institutional preference.
      (e) Intensity-modulated radiation therapy (IMRT) is the most utilized type of radiation in salivary gland cancer; this distributes high doses to the intended target, limiting doses to critical normal structures.

(f) Targeted molecular therapy is useful in specific situations, typically in the setting of recurrent/metastatic disease. Targeted mutations can include HER2 (trastuzumab/Herceptin), androgen receptor (anti-androgen receptor therapies), and PDL1 positivity (immunotherapy).

5. Parotid Carcinoma
   (a) A preoperatively functional facial nerve can be preserved in many salivary cancer cases with meticulous nerve dissection.
   (b) If the facial nerve sacrifice is considered due to tumor involvement, malignancy should be histologically confirmed.
   (c) If facial nerve is sacrificed, immediate nerve grafting should be performed. Volitional facial movement can be obtained even with adjuvant radiation. Surgical rehabilitation of affected regions can be selectively undertaken simultaneously.
   (d) Donor nerves for grafting can include great auricular nerve (typically, a distal frozen margin should be taken to ensure this nerve graft is cancer-free), ansa cervicalis, sural nerve, lateral antebrachial cutaneous nerve (if radial forearm flap is harvested), nerve to vastus lateralis (excellent branching pattern; harvested with anterolateral thigh free flap).
   (e) Mastoidectomy may be required if the proximal facial nerve and/or bone of the skull base are involved with the tumor.
6. Submandibular gland carcinoma
   (a) Adequate surgery may include resection of platysma and/or mylohyoid/digastric muscle.
   (b) Marginal mandibular nerve, if involved, may need to be resected and immediately reconstructed.
   (c) Hypoglossal and lingual nerves may also be affected.
7. Sublingual gland carcinoma
   (a) Complete resection is recommended, typically with the floor of the mouth mucosa and possibly the lingual nerve. Lingual nerve should be reconstructed immediately if feasible.
   (b) Floor-of-mouth reconstruction may be necessary to prevent tongue tethering.
8. Minor salivary gland carcinoma
   (a) Resection depends on anatomic location.
   (b) The most common location is on the hard palate, which requires resection with palate reconstruction versus prosthetic placement.

B. Mucoepidermoid carcinoma (MEC)
   1. Most common malignant salivary tumor.
   2. Varying grades from low to intermediate and high grade.
   3. Clear correlation of tumor grade with survival.
   4. Targetable molecular mutations are rare, with poor response rates to immunotherapy even with PDL-1 positivity.

C. Adenoid cystic carcinoma
   1. Comprises roughly 10% of malignant salivary gland neoplasms.
   2. Most common epithelial malignancy of minor salivary, submandibular, and sublingual salivary glands.
   3. Propensity for perineural invasion and distant metastases (lung most common).
   4. Margin control is notoriously difficult despite gross tumor resection.
   5. Lymphatic metastasis is uncommon. Elective neck dissection is less commonly recommended.

6. Histologically divided into three subtypes:
   (a) Cribriform type: "Swiss cheese" pattern, most common, intermediate grade
   (b) Tubular pattern: low grade
   (c) Solid pattern: highest grade, poor prognosis
7. Recurrence can present years if not decades after initial treatment.
8. Adjuvant radiation is recommended in nearly all cases regardless of final surgical pathology.
9. Most common site of failure after surgery and radiation is distant (lung) metastasis or perineural invasion at the skull base.

D. Acinic cell carcinoma
   1. Low-grade epithelial malignancy
   1. Most common in parotid
   2. Multiple subtypes (solid, microcystic, papillary cystic, follicular) are not known to have prognostic significance
   3. Local recurrences more likely than regional or distant

E. Epithelial-myoepithelial carcinoma
   1. 75% in parotid, locally aggressive
   2. Biphasic histology of epithelial and myoepithelial cells
   3. Prognosis overall good

F. Salivary duct carcinoma (SDC)
   1. Rare (4%-6% of salivary cancers), high-grade tumor with high rates of regional and distant metastasis.
   2. Often found within a benign pleomorphic adenoma (SDC ex-pleomorphic adenoma).
   3. Elective neck dissection is almost always performed, given the high rates (> 50%) of regional metastases.
   4. In the setting of recurrent/metastatic disease, HER2-targeted therapy (trastuzumab) or androgen deprivation therapy can be given when HER2/androgen receptor immunohistochemistry is positive.

G. Polymorphous adenocarcinoma (formerly polymorphous low-grade adenocarcinoma)
   1. 95% present in minor salivary glands, most commonly in hard palate. Major salivary gland presentation is rare.
   2. Often slow-growing, with low propensity for neck metastasis.
   3. High-grade transformation is possible but rare.

H. Adenocarcinoma, not otherwise specified (NOS)
   1. "Catch all" category of histologically diverse salivary malignancies that cannot be otherwise classified. This is a small and shrinking category of tumors.

I. Clear cell carcinoma
   1. Rare malignancy of minor salivary glands
   2. Indolent clinical course with rare metastases
   3. Molecularly defined by *EWSR1:ATF1* fusion oncogene

J. Carcinoma ex-pleomorphic adenoma
   1. Arises within a benign mixed tumor, presenting as rapid growth.
   2. Most common histology is salivary duct carcinoma, although any salivary malignancy is possible.
   3. May present as spectrum of transformation from in situ (low grade) to poorly differentiated aggressive (high grade).
   4. Often clinically aggressive, with high metastatic rates, but this depends on the histology of the underlying malignancy.

K. Secretory carcinoma
  1. Previously referred to as mammary analog secretory carcinoma due to its resemblance to secretory carcinoma of the breast due to its association with the tyrosine receptor kinase fusion gene.
  2. Histologically, it is often confused with acinic cell carcinoma (AciCC), but generally is clinically more aggressive with higher rates of cervical metastases than AciCC.
  3. Diagnosis is established by the presence of the *ETV6-NTRK3* gene translocation, which distinguishes this diagnosis from AciCC.

L. Lymphoma
  1. Often misdiagnosed as an epithelial salivary tumor.
  2. Parotid is the most common salivary gland involved. Autoimmune disease (eg, Sjögren syndrome), immunosuppression, HIV/Epstein-Barr Virus, and hepatitis C virus infection are risk factors for development of lymphoma.
  3. Extranodal (primary salivary) lymphoma arises from lymphocytes within the parotid parenchyma, not within the lymph nodes. These salivary gland lymphomas (SGL) are a non-Hodgkin lymphoma originating from B cells.
  4. Most common extranodal lymphoma in salivary glands is mucosa-associated lymphoid tissue (MALT) lymphoma, a marginal-zone B-cell lymphoma
     (a) Marginal zone B-cell lymphoma.
     (b) Often localized disease with favorable prognosis.
     (c) Chronic gastritis from *Helicobacter pylori* infection confers an increased risk of SGL.
     (d) Treatment of MALT lymphoma typically involves low-dose radiation; surgery can also be offered in early cases where complete resection is feasible.
  5. Nodal (a.k.a. secondary) lymphoma can be seen with systemic non-Hodgkin lymphoma.
  6. Surgery may be required for adequate tissue biopsy.

M. Cutaneous cancer metastases to major salivary glands
  1. Squamous cell carcinoma (most common) and melanoma are the most common skin cancers to metastasize to the parotid gland. Others, more rarely, can include Merkel cell carcinoma, eccrine carcinoma (many types including eccrine porocarcinoma and hidradenocarcinoma), and sebaceous carcinoma.
  2. Basal cell carcinoma.
     (a) Very rare metastatic disease
     (b) Occasional direct extension to parotid fascia/gland from the primary tumor
  3. Cutaneous squamous cell carcinoma.
     (a) Typically, parotid metastases are to the superficial intraparotid lymph nodes.
     (b) Usually present within 1 year of the index primary skin cancer in the face/eyelid, scalp, or ear.
     (c) Risk factors of primary tumor for metastasis include diameter greater than 2 cm, thickness greater than 4 mm, locally recurrent disease, perineural invasion, or location in preauricular/ear skin.
     (d) Parotid metastasis from skin primary is associated with a 25% rate of clinically apparent neck metastasis and 35% of occult neck metastasis.
     (e) Adjuvant radiation is recommended following surgical resection of regional metastases.
     (f) In cases with an anticipated need for facial nerve sacrifice due to tumor extent, induction immunotherapy can be considered prior to surgery to improve the likelihood of facial nerve preservation.

4. Melanoma
   (a) Most parotid melanoma arises from a head and neck cutaneous primary. Roughly 4% are of unknown primary origin (determined only after dermatology full body exam, endoscopic evaluation of aerodigestive tract, and full imaging workup have been completed).
   (b) Regional metastatic rates correlate with tumor thickness, the primary determinant of the primary tumor stage.
   (c) Sentinel lymph node biopsy (SLNB) is indicated for cN0 cases with tumor thickness greater than 1mm; it can be "discussed and considered" for tumor thickness 0.8 to 1.0 mm per National Comprehensive Cancer Network (NCCN) guidelines.
   (d) Based on the Multicenter Selective Lymphadenopathy trials, complete neck dissection when SLNB is positive can provide benefits in regional control but does not improve overall or disease-specific survival. Most centers now offer adjuvant immunotherapy without neck dissection when SLNB is positive.

VIII. Xerostomia

A. Radiation-induced xerostomia
   1. Xerostomia syndrome (XS): dry mouth, sore throat, dysgeusia, dental caries/decay, worse speech/swallow function.
   2. Irreversible damage secondary to radiation therapy can begin at 25 Gy. With IMRT techniques, salivary gland dosing can be reduced.
   3. XS can occur with radioactive iodine (RAI) treatment in a dose-dependent fashion (> 100 mCi). RAI can also induce chronic sialadenitis, for which sialendoscopy can be helpful in addressing ductal strictures and mucous plugs.

B. Xerostomia treatment/palliation
   1. Frequent water drinking, sialagogues, dry mouth oral rinse, salivary substitutes (many gels, rinses, sprays, etc. available).
   2. Systemic sialagogues: pilocarpine, cevimeline, bethanechol; many systemic side effects, generally poorly tolerated.
   3. Amifostine: radioprotectant that scavenges and binds oxygen-free radicals; Some studies of IV administration during radiation may decrease acute mucositis and long-term xerostomia.
   4. Palifermin: derivative of keratinocyte growth factor, also used to mitigate mucositis and xerostomia for radiation.
   5. Submandibular salivary gland transfer is utilized prior to radiation at some centers. The gland is surgically released and repositioned in the submental space to allow radiation shielding by the mandible.

IX. Surgery

A. Parotid gland surgery
   1. Parotidectomy
      (a) Careful review of cross-sectional imaging with attention to possible deep lobe involvement, metastatic disease to cervical lymph nodes, relationship to skull base, perineural invasion of facial nerve (MRI).

(b) Fine-needle or core-needle biopsy to determine epithelial tumor versus lymphocyte-related tumor and risk of carcinoma. Generally, this should be performed under ultrasound guidance to improve diagnostic accuracy.
(c) Plan incision: Modified Blair is standard, but facelift incision can be utilized for benign posterior tumors. Neck dissection extension can be incorporated into the incision as needed for lymphadenectomy or PPS dissection.
(d) Informed consent: careful discussion of risks of transient versus permanent facial nerve weakness, numbness of ear and neck, gustatory sweating (Frey syndrome), cosmetic changes (hollowing), hematoma, infection (rare), and recurrence.
(e) Depending on the pathology/tumor, the posterior branch of the great auricular nerve can sometimes be spared.
(f) Facial nerve identification landmarks: tympanomastoid suture line, styloid-mastoid interface, posterior belly of the digastric muscle, tragal pointer (see "Parotid Gland" section P above).
(g) Once the main trunk of the facial nerve is identified, dissection can proceed distally with care to protect all nerve branches.
(h) Retrograde facial nerve dissection can be used to facilitate facial nerve dissection in select cases such as scarring or dense tumors at the main trunk/skull base. Some surgeons utilize retrograde dissection routinely.
(i) Soft-tissue reconstruction: Some surgeons utilize abdominal fat graft or alloderm to help with contour defects. Nonvascularized grafts are generally avoided when adjuvant radiation is anticipated due to the risk of infection/necrosis of the graft.
(j) When larger soft tissue contouring is needed (ie, total parotidectomy with neck dissection), vascularized grafts can be utilized, including submental artery island rotational flap, radial forearm, or anterolateral thigh free flap.
(k) Frey syndrome (FS): gustatory sweating caused by abnormal reinnervation between severed parasympathetic cholinergic nerve fibers of the parotid with sympathetic receptors innervating skin sweat glands.
(l) FS treatment: topical antiperspirants/anticholinergics, botulinum injections. Some surgeons place an acellular dermal matrix between the defect and skin flap at the time of surgery to help prevent FS.
(m) Sialocele: localized collection of saliva that can collect after surgery or trauma and typically resolves spontaneously within 1 month. Botox injections of remnant salivary tissue can be used in refractory cases.
(n) Accessory parotid tumors can be accessed transcervically with an extended skin flap. Rarely small, anterior, benign tumors can be accessed transorally through the buccal mucosa. Accessory parotid tumors are often near the zygomatic and buccal branches of the facial nerve.
(o) Experience is evolving using extracapsular dissection, which does not routinely utilize facial nerve dissection, for the management of select benign tumors in experienced hands.

B. Deep lobe parotid/parapharyngeal space tumors
   1. Roughly 20% of parotid salivary tissue is in the "deep lobe" deep to the facial nerve, and tumors here often extend into the PPS.
   2. Deep lobe and PPS tumors can be removed by a transcervical approach with transparotid extension as needed. Techniques to improve access include nasal intubation (able to close jaw), division of digastric muscle, and division of external carotid artery. Mandibulotomy is rarely necessary.

3. Tumors medial to the carotid artery and not abutting the skull base can be considered for removal via transoral approach, with or without a surgical robot. Size limitations of tumors that can be removed are dictated by the size of mouth opening, the quality of oropharyngeal exposure, and the degree of lateral extension.
4. Complications include facial nerve paresis, lower cranial nerve injury, first-bite syndrome, tumor spillage, and recurrence.

C. Submandibular/sublingual tumors
1. For submandibular tumors, the incision is designed along a skin crease at least two finger breadths below the inferior mandible.
2. The marginal mandibular nerve runs in the superficial aspect of the submandibular gland fascia and can be preserved with the release of the fascia and/or Hayes Martin maneuver (ligation and upwards reflection of the facial vein). This nerve may require resection and reconstruction in select malignant cases.
3. In level I, the hypoglossal nerve lies deep at the junction of the mylohyoid muscle and the digastric tendon.
4. Caudal retraction of the submandibular gland and anterior retraction of the mylohyoid muscle expose the lingual nerve superiorly. The gland is divided from the lingual nerve at the submandibular ganglion.
5. Small sublingual tumors may be removed via a transoral approach, transposing Wharton's duct and avoiding the lingual nerve. The high incidence of malignancy in these tumors must be considered when undertaking resection.
6. Larger or malignant sublingual tumors may require en bloc resection of the floor of mouth and level I, including lingual nerve resection and reconstruction.

X. Approach to Evaluation for Salivary Gland Disease

A. History
1. Age and gender
2. Anatomic location (ie, which gland is involved)
   (a) Risk of malignancy increases with a decrease in size of gland
   (b) Parotid < submandibular < sublingual < minor salivary gland
3. Character and location of pain
4. Neurological symptoms (numbness, weakness)
5. Associated symptoms
   (a) Xerostomia/xerophthalmia
   (b) Malocclusion, dental caries, trismus
   (c) Otalgia
   (d) Fever, unintentional weight loss
   (e) Neck swelling/lymphadenopathy
   (f) Weight loss, loss of appetite
6. Social history: Smoking/alcohol exposure, ionizing radiation exposure, international travel, infectious exposure, and sexual history
7. Family history
   (a) Autoimmune disorders
   (b) Head and neck cancer
   (c) Leukemia/lymphoma
   (d) Genetic disorders/syndromes

B. Physical examination
   1. Vital signs (systemic signs of disease)
   2. Complete head and neck examination
      (a) Single versus multigland involvement
      (b) Intraoral examination of salivary ducts and orifices
      (c) Examination of eyes, lacrimal glands, and ducts
      (d) Cranial nerve examination, including flexible laryngoscopy as appropriate
      (e) Neck examination for lymphadenopathy (unilateral versus bilateral)

C. Imaging studies
   1. Ultrasound: rapid, in-office evaluation, no radiation exposure
   2. CT: quick and widely available, cross-sectional imaging is simple to interpret and generally inexpensive. Excellent for associated bony anatomy and lymph node assessment. It can also be used to evaluate the chest for possible concomitant metastatic/granulomatous disease.
   3. MRI: no radiation, excellent soft tissue detail if the patient can lie still, but time-consuming and often expensive. Superior assessment of perineural spread.
   4. Sialendoscopy: directly evaluate the ductal system with immediate intervention as appropriate.

D. Laboratory studies
   1. Selective utilization of laboratory tests can help support or refute some salivary diagnoses, especially as they pertain to systemic or infectious diseases.
      (a) Complete blood count +/− differential (nonspecific, can indicate hematologic dx)
      (b) Erythrocyte sedimentation rate (ESR) and C-reactive protein (CRP)
      (c) Serum calcium and angiotensin-converting enzyme elevation (sarcoidosis)
      (d) Autoantibodies: rheumatoid factor (RF), antinuclear antibodies (ANA), anti-SSA and anti-SSB (Sjögren syndrome)
      (e) Thyroid-stimulating hormone (hypothyroidism)
      (f) Complete metabolic panel (hepatic or renal dysfunction)
      (g) Human immunodeficiency virus testing (antibody, antigen/antibody, and nucleic acid tests available)
      (h) Nutritional or vitamin deficiencies (eg, protein, iron, vitamins A/B/C deficiency)

E. Sialendoscopy
   1. Diagnostic and therapeutic sialendoscopy may be utilized for direct visualization of major ductal systems and immediate intervention.
   2. Treatable conditions identified on sialendoscopy include:
      (a) Stricture/stenosis
      (b) Sialolithiasis
      (c) Inflammatory debris/mucous plugs

F. Fine-needle aspiration biopsy (FNAB)
   1. Can be quickly collected in a clinic for rapid diagnosis of both benign and malignant palpable lesions. Ultrasound guidance can improve accuracy and is essential in nonpalpable lesions.
   2. Helps clarify the difference between lymphocytic and epithelial tumors.
   3. Diagnostic accuracy influenced by cellular yield and cytopathologist experience.
   4. Stains and cultures of aspirates can also be performed in the setting of suspected infection.

G. Core needle biopsy
   1. Typically collected with larger, commercially available core biopsy devices which obtain larger tissue specimens.
   2. Histologic ultrastructure and higher cellular yield can improve diagnostic accuracy over FNAB.
   3. Molecular testing can also be more easily sent from a core biopsy specimen.

H. Diagnostic gland biopsy
   1. A lower lip biopsy of minor salivary glands is a simple and valuable method of tissue sampling for inflammatory disorders (Sjögren syndrome); typically, these can be performed in a clinic with local anesthesia.
   2. Rarely, an incisional biopsy of a major salivary gland is needed to render a definitive diagnosis. This should only be pursued after adequate image-guided core biopsy has been performed and is nondiagnostic. Difficult entities to diagnose can include:
      (a) Amyloidosis
      (b) Sarcoidosis
      (c) Sjögren syndrome
      (d) Lymphoma
      (e) IgG4 disease

XI. Classification of Salivary Gland Disorders

A. Non-neoplastic salivary gland disorders and dysfunction
   1. Inflammatory disorders and dysfunction
      (a) Acute sialadenitis
         i. Viral: paramyxovirus (mumps), cytomegalovirus, coxsackievirus A and B, influenza, echovirus, COVID-19 (rare)
         ii. Bacterial (suppurative): typically preceded by salivary stasis, for example, stones or dehydration. *S. aureus* is the most common pathogen cultured.
         iii. Radiation-induced (both acute and chronic forms)
         iv. Necrotizing sialometaplasia
      (b) Chronic sialadenitis
         i. Obstructive: persistent/recurrent inflammation from stones, duct strictures, external tumor compression, foreign body, etc.
         ii. Granulomatous disease
            a. Sarcoidosis
            b. Granulomatosis with polyangiitis (GPA, formerly Wegener granulomatosis)
            c. Infectious: tuberculosis, actinomycosis, bartonella (cat-scratch disease)
            d. Xanthogranulomatous sialadenitis (associated with Warthin tumor)
         iii. Autoimmune: Sjögren syndrome, GPA, IgG4-related sialadenitis
         iv. Chronic sclerosing sialadenitis (a.k.a. Küttner tumor)
         v. HIV-associated salivary gland disease, with or without lymphoepithelial cysts
   2. Noninflammatory disorders and dysfunction
      (a) Acute
         i. Trauma (penetrating or blunt to gland or duct)
         ii. Pneumoparotid (playing a wind instrument, dental procedure, etc.)

(b) Chronic
  i. Age-related xerostomia
  ii. Sialadenosis (a.k.a. sialosis): chronic gland enlargement
    a. Endocrine disorders
    b. Diabetes mellitus
    c. Hypothyroidism
    d. Pregnancy and lactation
  iii. Nutritional/metabolic disorders
    a. Alcoholism
    b. Cirrhosis
    c. Obesity
    d. Nutritional/vitamin deficiency states
    e. Bulimia nervosa
  iv. Medications
    a. Iodine
    b. Valproic acid
    c. Thiourea

(c) Amyloidosis

(d) Idiopathic

B. Neoplastic salivary gland disease
  1. Benign
    (a) Pleomorphic adenoma
    (b) Warthin tumor
    (c) Oncocytoma
    (d) Basal cell adenoma
    (e) Myoepithelioma
  2. Malignant
    (a) Mucoepidermoid carcinoma
    (b) Adenoid cystic carcinoma
    (c) Adenocarcinoma
    (d) Acinic cell carcinoma
    (e) Salivary duct carcinoma
    (f) Clear cell carcinoma
    (g) Lymphoma
    (h) Carcinoma ex pleomorphic carcinoma
    (i) Metastatic cutaneous malignancy (squamous cell carcinoma, basal cell carcinoma [rare], melanoma, Merkel cell carcinoma)
    (j) Primary squamous cell carcinoma (rare)

Questions

1. What is the most common pathogen cultured from acute suppurative sialadenitis?
   A. *Streptococcus pyogenes*
   B. *Staphylococcus aureus*
   C. Mixed anaerobic flora
   D. *Escherichia coli*
   E. *Actinomyces* spp.

2. Which benign salivary tumor is characteristically avid on PET-CT scan?
   A. Pleomorphic adenoma
   B. Myoepithelioma
   C. Warthin tumor (papillary cystadenoma lymphomatosum)
   D. Lipoma
   E. none of the above

3. From which nerve(s) does the great auricular nerve arise?
   A. C2 and C3 nerve branches of cervical plexus
   B. C4 and C5 nerve branches of cervical plexus
   C. C6 and C7 nerve branches of cervical plexus
   D. Auriculotemporal nerve
   E. Sensory branches of the vagus nerve

4. Which salivary gland tumor is defined by the *ETV6:NTRK3* gene translocation?
   A. Adenocarcinoma, NOS
   B. Adenoid cystic carcinoma
   C. Pleomorphic adenoma
   D. Carcinoma ex-pleomorphic adenoma
   E. Secretory carcinoma

5. If treatment is required, pediatric head and neck/salivary hemangiomas are typically treated first with
   A. Sclerotherapy
   B. Brachytherapy
   C. Surgery
   D. External beam radiation
   E. Propranolol

Bibliography

Andreasen S, Therkildsen MH, Bjørndal K, Homøe P. Pleomorphic adenoma of the parotid gland 1985-2010: a Danish nationwide study of incidence, recurrence rate, and malignant transformation. *Head Neck*. 2016;38 Suppl 1:E1364-E1369.

Astor FC, Hanft KL, Ciocon JO. Xerostomia: a prevalent condition in the elderly. *Ear, Nose Throat J*. 1999;78(7):476-479.

Barrett AW. Wegener's granulomatosis of the major salivary glands. *J Oral Pathol Med*. 2012;41(10): 721-727.

Bittmann S, Luchter E, Bittmann L, Moschüring-Alieva E, Villalon G. Current aspects of treatment options of chronic sialorrhea in children. *J Clin Med Res*. 2022;14(6):246-249.

Chason H, Downs B. Anatomy, Head and Neck, Parotid Gland. europepmc.org. Published 2024. https://europepmc.org/article/NBK/nbk534225. Accessed 2024.

Derbel A, Frikha F, Guermazi M, et al. Localized amyloidosis involving parotid and submandibular glands associated to Sjogren syndrome: rare association. *La Revue De Médecine Interne*. 2021;42:A353-A354.

Deschler DG. Extracapsular dissection of benign parotid tumors. *JAMA Otolaryngol Head Neck Surg*. 2014;140(8):770-771.

Deschler DG, Eisele DW. Surgery for primary malignant parotid neoplasms. *Adv Otorhinolaryngol.* 2016;78:83-94.

Geiger JL, Ismaila N, Beadle B, et al. Management of salivary gland malignancy: ASCO Guideline. *J Clin Oncol.* 2021;39(17):1909-1941.

Ghannam M, Singh P. Anatomy, Head and Neck, Salivary Glands. europepmc.org. Published 2019. https://europepmc.org/article/nbk/nbk538325. Accessed 2019.

Grewal JS, Bordoni B, Ryan J. Anatomy, Head and Neck, Sublingual Gland. Europepmc.org. Published 2016. Available at: https://europepmc.org/article/nbk/nbk535426. Accessed 16/11/2024.

Huoh KC, Eisele DW. Etiologic factors in sialolithiasis. *Otolaryngology–Head and Neck Surgery.* 2011;145(6):935-939.

Jesberg P, Monzon A, Gitomer SA, Herrmann BW. Pediatric primary salivary gland tumors. *Am J Otolaryngol.* 2023;44(5):103948.

Kapourani A, Kontogiannopoulos KN, Barmpalexis P. A review on the role of pilocarpine on the management of xerostomia and the importance of the topical administration systems development. *Pharmaceuticals.* 2022;15(6):762.

Larson AR, Annick Aubin-Pouliot, Delagnes E, Zheng M, Chang JL, Ryan WR. Surgeon-performed ultrasound for chronic obstructive sialadenitis helps predict sialendoscopic findings and outcomes. *Otolaryngology.* 2017;157(6):973-980.

Larson AR, Ryan WR. Transoral excision of parapharyngeal space tumors. *Otolaryngol Clin North Am.* 2021;54(3):531-541.

Mydlarz W, Schmitt N, Eisele D. Salivary Gland Diseases. In: Chan Y, Goddard JC, eds. *K. J. Lee's Essential Otolaryngology.* McGraw Hill Professional; 2019.

Ogawa M, Yokoo S, Yamaguchi T, et al. Diagnosis and treatment of secretory carcinoma arising from the oral minor salivary gland. *Medicine.* 2021;100(51):e28390.

Prendes BL, Orloff L, Eisele D. Therapeutic sialendoscopy for the management of radioiodine sialadenitis. *Archives of Otolaryngology–Head & Neck Surgery.* 2012;138(1):15.

Rao V, Curran J, Blair EA, Sweiss NJ. Salivary glands sarcoidosis. *Operative Techniques in Otolaryngology-Head and Neck Surgery.* 2008;19(4):234-236.

Seethala RR. An update on grading of salivary gland carcinomas. *Head Neck Pathol.* 2009;3(1):69-77.

Seikaly H, Jha N, Harris JR, et al. Long-term outcomes of submandibular gland transfer for prevention of postradiation xerostomia. *Archives of Otolaryngology–Head & Neck Surgery.* 2004;130(8):956.

Senthilnathan N, Rajaram Mohan K, Fenn SM, Pethagounder Thangavelu R. Necrotizing sialometaplasia: a diagnostic challenge to oral physicians. *Cureus.* 2022;14(12).

Skalova A, Ilmo Leivo, Henrik Hellquist, et al. Clear cell neoplasms of salivary glands: a diagnostic challenge. *Adv Anatomic Pathol.* 2022;29(4):217-226.

Sunavala-Dossabhoy G. Radioactive iodine: an unappreciated threat to salivary gland function. *Oral Diseases.* 2018;24(1-2):198-201.

Swetter SM, Thompson JA, Albertini MR, et al. NCCN Guidelines® Insights: Melanoma: Cutaneous, Version 2.2021. *J Natl Compr Canc Netw.* 2021;19(4):364-376.

Thoeny HC. Imaging of salivary gland tumours. *Cancer Imaging.* 2007;7(1):52-62.

Thackray A, Lucas R. *Tumors of the Major Salivary Glands. Atlas of Tumor Pathology, Series 2, Fascicle 10.* Armed Forces Institute of Pathology; 1974:107-117.

Urquhart A, Hutchins LG, Berg RL. Preoperative computed tomography scans for parotid tumor evaluation. *Laryngoscope.* 2001;111(11):1984-1988.

Valstar MH, de Ridder M, van den Broek EC, et al. Salivary gland pleomorphic adenoma in the Netherlands: a nationwide observational study of primary tumor incidence, malignant transformation, recurrence, and risk factors for recurrence. *Oral Oncol.* 2017;66:93-99.

Chapter 34
Anatomy and Physiology of the Upper Aerodigestive Tract

Anatomy and Physiology of the Oral Cavity

Overview

Boundaries of the Oral Cavity

- Anterior: vermillion border of the lips
- Posterior: junction of hard and soft palate (superiorly), circumvallate papillae or linea terminalis (inferiorly), and the retromolar trigones (laterally)

Subunits

- Lips, buccal mucosa, upper (maxillary) and lower (mandibular) alveolar ridges, retromolar trigone, hard palate, floor of mouth, and oral tongue (anterior two-thirds)
- Function
- Intake and mastication, oral phase of deglutition, speech, and protection from noxious substances

Anatomy of the Lip

Surface Anatomy

- Vermillion: nonkeratinized squamous epithelium, capillaries give its characteristic color
- Vermillion border: transition point from external skin to internal mucous membrane
- Philtrum ridges and Cupid bow (on upper lip)
- Oral commissure: lateral junction between upper and lower lip

Perioral Musculature

- Innervation: facial nerve (CN VII)
- *Modiolus*: tendinous thickening at oral commissure that serves as an attachment site for several upper and lower lip muscles
- Muscles that insert on modiolus: orbicularis oris (forms a sphincter around the mouth, purses the lips, presses lips against teeth), buccinator (presses the lips and cheek against the teeth), levator anguli oris (elevates the commissure), depressor anguli oris (depresses and laterally moves commissure), zygomaticus major (elevates and laterally moves commissure), risorius (laterally moves the commissure)
- Muscles that insert on upper lip: levator labii superioris (elevates), levator superioris alaeque nasi (dilates nostril and elevates), zygomaticus minor (elevates and laterally moves commissure)
- Muscles that insert on lower lip: depressor labii inferioris (depresses and pulls it laterally), mentalis (elevates), platysma (depressor)

Sensory Innervation

- Upper lip: infraorbital nerve (CN V2)
- Lower lip: mental nerve (CN V3)

Vascular Supply

- Inferior and superior labial arteries from facial artery

Lymphatic Drainage

- Primarily to submandibular lymph nodes
- Midline lower lip also to submental lymph nodes
- Upper lip also to preauricular, infraparotid, and perifacial lymph nodes

Teeth

Layers of the Teeth (Four Major Components)

- Enamel: hardest, calcium phosphate white outer part, formed by ameloblasts (amelogenesis)
- Dentin: layer under the enamel, formed by odontoblasts (dentinogenesis)
  - Unlike enamel, dentin continues to form throughout life and sensate
- Pulp: inner structure with blood vessels and nerves
- Cementum: surface layer of the tooth root composed of connective tissue that binds tooth roots to gingiva and alveolar bone, formed by cementoblasts

Periodontal Ligament

- Connects teeth to alveolar bone through cementum, formed by fibroblasts

Alveolar Bone

- Surrounds the tooth roots, formed by osteoblasts

Nomenclature

- Incisors (8): central and lateral
- Canines (4): between incisors and premolars
- Premolars (8): first and second
- Molars (8 children, 12 adults): first, second, third (wisdom teeth)
- Deciduous teeth (20): no premolars, named superiorly right to left (A-J), inferiorly left to right (K–T)
- Adult teeth (32): numbered superiorly right to left (1-16), inferiorly left to right (17-32)

Muscles of Mastication

Masseter Muscle

- Origin: zygomatic arch
- Insertion: angle and lateral surface of ramus of mandible, coronoid process
- Action: elevation and protrusion of the mandible
- Innervation: masseteric nerve (branch of mandibular nerve, CN V3)

Temporalis Muscle

- Origin: temporal lines (parietal and frontal bone), superior temporal surface of sphenoid bone
- Insertion: coronoid process of mandible
- Action: elevation and retraction of mandible
- Innervation: deep temporal nerve (branch of mandibular nerve, CN V3)

Lateral Pterygoid Muscle

- Origin: greater wing of the sphenoid bone (superior head), lateral pterygoid plate (inferior head)
- Insertion: anterior condyle (superior head) and pterygoid fovea at medial side of the ramus (inferior head)
- Action: depression and protrusion of the mandible, side-to-side movement of mandible
- Innervation: lateral pterygoid nerve (branch of mandibular nerve, CN V3)

Medial Pterygoid Muscle

- Origin: medial lateral pterygoid plate (deep head), pyramidal process of palatine bone, and maxillary tuberosity (superficial head)
- Insertion: medial angle of the mandible
- Action: elevation and side-to-side movements of mandible
- Innervation: medial pterygoid nerve (branch of mandibular nerve, CN V3)

Anatomy of the Tongue

Surface Anatomy

- Papillae: cover the anterior two-thirds of the tongue
  - Filiform: majority; trigeminal nerve endings transmit temperature, texture, and pain; no taste function
  - Fungiform: mushroom shaped with taste buds on superior surface, majority are in anterior 2 cm
  - Foliate: taste buds on lateral surface, located in lateral tongue
  - Circumvallate: large with taste buds on lateral surface, located in V shape at junction of the anterior and posterior tongue
- Sulcus terminalis: groove at the anterior margin of the circumvallate papillae
- Foramen cecum (caecum linguae): pit at the sulcus terminalis where embryologic thyroid begins its descent (etiology of lingual thyroid and thyroglossal duct cyst)
- Frenulum: anterior fold of mucous membrane attaches the anterior inferior aspect of the tongue to the floor mouth and gingiva, may be congenitally short (tongue tied)
- Wharton ducts (submandibular gland ducts) open on either side of the frenulum
- Lingual tonsil: lymphoid tissue extending over the base of the tongue (oropharynx)
- Valleculae: depressions on either side of the midline glossoepiglottic fold extending to pharyngoepiglottic fold laterally (oropharynx)

Muscles of the Tongue

- Genioglossus (extrinsic muscle)
  - Origin: mental spine of the mandible
  - Insertion: hyoid bone and bottom of the tongue
  - Function: provides bulk, depresses, and protrudes the tongue
  - Innervation: hypoglossal nerve (CN XII)
- Hyoglossus (extrinsic muscle)
  - Origin: body and greater cornu of the hyoid bone
  - Insertion: side of the tongue
  - Function: depress and retract the tongue
  - Innervation: hypoglossal nerve (CN XII)
- Styloglossus (extrinsic muscle)
  - Origin: styloid process of temporal bone
  - Insertion: tip and side of tongue

  - Function: retract and elevate the tongue
  - Innervation: hypoglossal nerve (CN XII)
- Palatoglossus (extrinsic muscle)
  - Origin: palatine aponeurosis of the soft palate
  - Insertion: side and dorsum of the tongue
  - Function: elevates the posterior tongue, closes the oropharyngeal isthmus, initiation of swallow, and prevents spillage of saliva into oropharynx
  - Innervation: pharyngeal branch of vagus nerve (CN X)
- Intrinsic muscles of the tongue: include superior and inferior longitudinal, vertical, and transverse
  - Innervation: hypoglossal nerve (CN XII)
  - Function: alter shape of the tongue
- *Fibrous septae* (*septum linguae*): defines midline with triangular fat pad that is visualized on axial CT scan

Vascular Supply

- Arterial supply: lingual artery (second branch of the external carotid artery)
- Venous drainage: lingual vein and vena comitans of the hypoglossal nerve (Ranine vein)

Lymphatic Drainage

- Anterior tongue: tip drains to submental nodes; central tongue drains to ipsilateral and contralateral nodes; lateral tongue drains to ipsilateral nodes (level I-III) or may have skip drainage to nodes in level IV
- Posterior tongue: drains to both ipsilateral and contralateral deep cervical nodes (jugulodigastric)

Sensory Innervation

- Anterior two-thirds (oral tongue): sensation of touch, pain, temperature via lingual nerve (CN V3)
- Posterior one-third (tongue base): touch and gag (visceral afferent) sensation via glossopharyngeal nerve (CN IX) to nucleus solitarius

Taste (Special Sensory Innervation)

- Taste bud: specialized epithelial cells including taste cells (type 1, 2, 3), supportive or basal cells, and neuronal processes
  - Receptors within microvilli of taste cells are within the taste pore at the surface of the epithelium
  - Five basic tastes: sweet, sour, bitter, salty, and umami (savory)
  - Sensation of flavor is from combination of taste, olfactory, and trigeminal sensory inputs and modulated by emotion, physiological and metabolic state, as well as learning (acquired taste)
- Anterior two-thirds (oral tongue): taste receptors in fungiform and foliate papillae → afferent fibers (via lingual nerve) → chorda tympani (CN VII) → geniculate ganglion → intermediary nerve → nucleus solitarius
- Posterior one-third (tongue base): taste receptors in foliate and circumvallate papillae, posterior oropharynx, vallecula, and base of tongue → glossopharyngeal (CN IX) → inferior petrosal ganglion → nucleus solitarius
- Taste receptors on laryngeal surface of epiglottis → superior laryngeal nerve → vagus nerve (CN X) → nucleus solitarius

Anatomy of the Hard Palate

Surface Anatomy

- Forms the anterior two-thirds of the palate
- Bony framework: palatine process of the maxilla (anteriorly), horizontal plates of palatine bones (posteriorly)
- Covered with stratified squamous epithelium attached firmly to underlying bone

Foramina

- Incisive foramen: midline of anterior palate, contains nasopalatine nerve and branch of sphenopalatine artery (from floor of nasal cavity)
- Greater palatine foramen: depression palpable 1 cm medial to second molar, contains greater palatine nerve and descending palatine vessels
- Lesser palatine foramen: posterior to greater palatine foramen, contains lesser palatine nerve and artery (to soft palate)

Sensory Innervation

- Nasopalatine and greater palatine nerves (CN V2)

Vascular Supply

- Arterial supply: maxillary artery →descending palatine artery → greater palatine artery
- Venous drainage: hard palate veins → pterygoid plexus → internal jugular vein

Lymphatic Drainage

- Upper cervical lymphatics or lateral retropharyngeal nodes

Anatomy and Physiology of the Pharynx

Overview

Boundaries

- Nasopharynx: from base of skull to soft palate
- Oropharynx: from junction of hard and soft palate (superiorly) and line of circumvallate papillae (inferiorly) to valleculae (plane of hyoid bone)
- Hypopharynx: from level of hyoid bone (pharyngoepiglottic folds) to inferior border of cricoid cartilage

Subunits

- Nasopharynx: lateral walls (fossa of Rosenmuller, Eustachian tube orifice), vault/roof, posterior wall
- Oropharynx: soft palate and uvula, base of tongue, pharyngoepiglottic and glosso-epiglottic folds, palatine arch (including tonsillar fossae, palatine tonsils, and pillars), lateral and posterior oropharyngeal walls, and valleculae
- Hypopharynx: pyriform sinus (or laryngopharyngeal sulcus, bordered by aryepiglottic folds medially, thyroid cartilage anteriorly, apex is at level of cricoid cartilage), posterior and lateral pharyngeal walls (lateral merges with lateral wall of pyriform sinus), and postcricoid region (inferior to arytenoids, extends to inferior margin of cricoid cartilage, contiguous with medial walls of pyriform sinuses)

Function

- Common pathway for air and food, swallowing, speech, airway protection

Anatomy of the Soft Palate

Function

- Attaches to the posterior margin of the hard palate and acts as a "flutter valve"
- Elevation: closes pharyngeal isthmus and seals off nasopharynx from oropharynx (prevents reflux of food)
- Depression: closes oropharyngeal isthmus and seals off oral cavity from oropharynx (allows you to chew and breathe at the same time)

Muscles

- Palatoglossus (anterior pillar): approximates palate to tongue and narrows oropharyngeal opening, involved in swallowing
- Palatopharyngeus (posterior pillar): raises larynx and pharynx, closing oropharyngeal aperture, involved in breathing
- Musculus uvulae: shortens uvula
- Levator veli palatini: raises soft palate to contact posterior pharyngeal wall, involved in swallowing
- Tensor veli palatini: pulls soft palate laterally to give rigidity and firmness to palate, involved in swallowing
  - Originates in part on the eustachian tube cartilage, so contraction opens tube

Motor Innervation

- Trigeminal nerve → branch of mandibular nerve (CN V3 motor division) → tensor veli palatini
- Vagus nerve (CN X) → pharyngeal plexus → remainder of palatal muscles

Sensory Innervation

- Glossopharyngeal (CN IX) and lesser palatine nerve (CN V2)

Vascular Supply

- Arterial supply:
  - Maxillary artery → descending palatine artery → lesser palatine artery
  - Facial artery → ascending palatine artery
- Venous drainage:
  - Soft palate veins → pharyngeal plexus → internal jugular vein
  - Soft palate veins → external palatine vein → tonsillar fossa → facial vein

Lymphatic Drainage

- Deep cervical lymph nodes

Anatomy of Tonsillar Tissues

Components of Waldeyer Ring

- Adenoids—midline pharynx
- Palatine tonsils—between palatoglossal and palatopharyngeal arches
- Lingual tonsils—posterior third of tongue
- Gerlach tonsils (Tubal tonsils)—small lymphoid nodules within lip of fossa of Rosenmuller, posterior to torus tubarius of Eustachian tube opening in nasopharynx
- Lateral pharyngeal bands—lymphoid tissue behind posterior pillars

Immunology

- B lymphocytes proliferate in germinal centers
- Immunoglobulins (IgG, A, M, D), complement component, interferon, lysozymes, and cytokines accumulate in tonsil tissue

- Tonsils and adenoids: first line of immune defense, especially in children (no proven negative immunologic impact of adenoidectomy and tonsillectomy)

Microbiologic Environment of the Adult Mouth

- Bacteria: Staphylococci (first oral microbe in neonate from skin contamination), nonhemolytic streptococci, lactobacilli, *Actinomyces*, *Leptothrix*, *Neisseria*, *Bacteroides*, Spirochetes, micrococci
- Viruses: myxovirus, adenovirus, picornavirus, coronavirus, human papillomavirus (HPV)

Arterial Supply to the Palatine Tonsils (five)

- Facial → Tonsillar branch → tonsil (main branch)
- Facial → Ascending palatine → tonsil
- Lingual → Dorsal lingual → tonsil
- Ascending pharyngeal → tonsil
- Maxillary → descending palatine → lesser palatine → tonsil

Lymphatic Drainage

- Through pharyngeal wall into jugulodigastric nodes

Anatomy of Pharyngeal Walls

Pharyngeal Constrictor Muscles

- Function: narrow the pharyngeal cavity sequentially from top to bottom to move a bolus of food through the pharynx into the esophagus
- Innervation: vagus nerve (CN X)
- **Superior constrictor muscle**
  - Origin: pterygomandibular raphe and adjacent bone on the mandible and pterygoid Hamulus
  - Insertion: median raphe
- **Middle constrictor muscle**
  - Origin: hyoid bone and stylohyoid ligaments
  - Insertion: median raphe
- **Inferior constrictor muscle**
  - Origin: cricoid cartilage and oblique line of thyroid cartilage
  - Insertion: median raphe
  - **Cricopharyngeus**: most inferior portion of the inferior constrictor, acts as the upper esophageal sphincter (UES)
  - Narrowest portion of pharyngeal cavity: inferior constrictor attachment to cricoid cartilage
  - Killian dehiscence: triangular dehiscence between inferior constrictor and cricopharyngeus, through which a Zenker diverticulum can form
  - Laimer-Hackerman space: between posterior cricopharyngeus and esophageal musculature
  - Killian-Jamieson space: lateral dehiscence inferior to cricopharyngeus where branches of the inferior thyroid artery pass

Pharyngeal Longitudinal Muscles

- **Stylopharyngeus**
  - Origin: styloid process of temporal bone
  - Insertion: pharyngeal wall
  - Action: elevate the pharynx
  - Innervation: glossopharyngeal nerve (CN IX)

- **Salpingopharyngeus**
  - Origin: cartilaginous part of the pharyngotympanic tube
  - Insertion: pharyngeal wall
  - Action: elevate the pharynx
  - Innervation: vagus nerve (CN X)
- **Palatopharyngeus**
  - Origin: upper surface of palatine aponeurosis (soft palate)
  - Insertion: circles the inner aspect of the pharyngeal wall and interdigitates with inner aspect of superior constrictor to create ***Passavant ridge*** (a prominent ridge of the deep aspect of the pharyngeal wall)
  - Action: elevates the pharynx, seals off nasopharynx from oropharynx
  - Innervation: vagus nerve (CN X)

Gaps in Oropharyngeal Walls

- Oropharyngeal triangle: gap between superior and middle constrictor and posterior border of mylohyoid (floor of mouth)
  - Allows stylopharyngeus to slip into the pharyngeal wall
  - Allows passage of structures associated with the tongue—muscles (styloglossus, hyoglossus), vessels (lingual artery and vein), nerves (lingual, hypoglossal CN XII, glossopharyngeal CN XI), and lymphatics
- Between middle and inferior constrictor: passage of internal laryngeal vessels and nerves through thyrohyoid membrane and into the larynx
- Below inferior constrictor: recurrent laryngeal nerves and inferior laryngeal vessels enter the larynx posterior to the inferior horn of the thyroid cartilage and deep to this margin

Motor Innervation

- Pharyngeal branch of the vagus nerve (CN X) through the pharyngeal plexus → all muscles of the pharynx except stylopharyngeus
- Pharyngeal branch of the glossopharyngeal nerve (CN IX) → stylopharyngeus

Sensory Innervation

- Nasopharynx: pharyngeal branch of maxillary nerve (CN V_2)
- Oropharynx: glossopharyngeal nerve (CN IX) via pharyngeal plexus (afferent limb of the gag reflex)
- Laryngopharynx: vagus nerve (CN X) via the internal laryngeal branch of the superior laryngeal nerve

Arterial Supply to the Pharynx

- Upper pharynx—from branches of external carotid
  - Ascending pharyngeal artery
  - Ascending palatine and tonsillar branches of facial artery
  - Numerous branches of maxillary and lingual arteries
- Lower pharynx
  - Pharyngeal branches from inferior thyroid artery (branch from thyrocervical trunk from subclavian artery)

Venous Drainage of the Pharynx

- Pharyngeal plexus → pterygoid plexus (infratemporal fossa) → facial and internal jugular veins

Lymphatic Drainage of the Pharynx

- Deep cervical nodes (retropharyngeal, paratracheal, infrahyoid)

Anatomy and Physiology of the Esophagus

Overview

Boundaries

- From cricoid cartilage to the cardia of the stomach

Subunits

- UES, body (cervical, thoracic, intra-abdominal), and lower esophageal sphincter (LES)

Dimensions

- Incisors to cricopharyngeal sphincter is ~16 cm, to stomach 38 to 40 cm (in adults)
- Lumen 20 mm

Anatomy of the Esophagus

Layers of the Esophagus (from innermost to outermost)

- Mucosa: stratified squamous epithelium with minimal secretory function and poor absorption, lamina propria, muscularis mucosa
- Submucosa: connective tissue, blood and lymphatic vessels, and parasympathetic ganglion cells and fibers (Meissner plexus) that control secretions and blood flow
- Muscularis propria
  - Inner circular muscle
  - Auerbach (myenteric) plexus: controls motility, regulates peristalsis
  - Outer longitudinal muscle

Musculature

- Upper third (cervical esophagus): mainly striated muscle
- Lower two-thirds (thoracic esophagus): smooth muscle

Innervation

- Vagus nerves rotate clockwise when viewed from above (left moves to anterior surface, right moves to posterior surface)

Blood Supply

- Upper third: inferior thyroid artery
- Middle third: thoracic aorta
- Inferior third: left gastric and inferior phrenic arteries

Function of the Esophagus

Upper esophageal sphincter (UES)

- Under tonic contraction at rest, relaxes with swallowing, actively dilated by laryngeal elevation during deglutition

Bolus Transit

- Upper one-third is striated voluntary muscle and has most rapid peristalsis (less than 1 second transit)
- Lower two-thirds is involuntary smooth muscle (approximately 3-second transit)
- Gravity plays only minor role in normal swallowing (position changes minimal)
- Over-distension of esophagus leads to spasm

Peristalsis

- Primary: physiologic propulsive wave of sequential constriction and shortening
- Secondary: nonphysiologic retrograde peristalsis
- Tertiary: nonphysiologic segmental constriction without propulsion

Lower Esophageal Sphincter (LES)

- Closure prevents reflux of gastric contents into esophagus
- Function controlled by parasympathetic tone (acetylcholine) and gastrin
- Not a true anatomic structure, but an active zone of high pressure extending 1 to 2 cm above and below diaphragm that relaxes during passage of the peristaltic wave
- Angle of His: oblique angle of entry of the esophagus into the stomach, absent in infants predisposing them to reflux
- Diaphragmatic crura surrounding hiatus create a sling which assists in sphincteric function (this effect is lost with a hiatal hernia)

Physiology of Normal and Abnormal Swallowing

Overview of Normal Swallowing

- Laryngopharynx functions as a "time-share" for respiration and deglutition.
  - Most basic function of the larynx is airway protection.
  - During deglutition, the formed bolus must move completely through the pharynx while the glottis is closed (adults must interrupt respiration to swallow).
- Normal swallow has three phases: oral, pharyngeal, and esophageal.

Oral Phase

Function

- Prepares the food for delivery to the pharynx
- Under voluntary control

Components

- Mastication
- Addition and mixing of saliva
- Control of bolus: lips, tongue, buccinator, palate
- Selection and verification of safety of bolus (volume, taste, fish bones, etc.)
- Ends when the bolus is pressed against the faucial arches (pressure-sensitive receptors on anterior tonsillar pillar mediated by CN IX and X) to trigger the next involuntary phase

Pharyngeal Phase

Function

- Moves the bolus quickly (less than 1 second) over the closed glottis and through UES into the esophagus
- Under involuntary control

Components

- Nasopharyngeal closure with soft palate elevation (levator and tensor veli palatini) and contraction of superior constrictor (Passavant ridge)—prevents regurgitation
- Cessation of respiration (usually during expiration)
- Glottic closure: approximation of true vocal folds, false vocal folds, arytenoids followed by epiglottis
- Bolus propulsion: via tongue base protrusion ("tongue driving force") and contraction of the pharyngeal constrictor muscles (from top to bottom)

- Laryngeal elevation: contraction of suprahyoid muscles and thyrohyoid muscle results in protection of laryngeal vestibule, epiglottic rotation, and active dilation of cricopharyngeal sphincter
- Epiglottic rotation: active due to laryngeal elevation, pharyngeal constriction, and tongue base retraction; passive due to pressure of bolus
- UES dilation: three important factors contribute to UES opening
  - Relaxation of cricopharyngeus muscle
  - Active dilation from contraction of suprahyoid and thyrohyoid muscles pulls hyolaryngeal complex forward (most important component)
  - Pressure of descending bolus

Esophageal Phase

Function

- Conveys bolus to stomach in average of 3 to 6 seconds with primary peristalsis and relaxation of lower esophageal sphincter (LES)

Components

- Initial peristaltic wave of relaxation to accommodate the bolus
- Followed by wave of contraction to propel the bolus
- Relaxation of lower esophageal sphincter

Innervation of Swallowing

Sensory Receptors

- Found on soft palate, tongue base, tonsillar pillars, posterior pharyngeal wall

Central Ganglions

- CN V—Gasserian ganglion
- CN IX—inferior (Andersch) ganglion and superior/smaller (Ehrenritter) ganglion
- CN X—inferior (jugular) ganglion and superior (nodose) ganglion

Efferent Pathways

- CN V: teeth, jaw, masticators, mylohyoid, tensor veli palatini, anterior belly of digastrics
- CN VII: lips, facial musculature including buccinator, stylohyoid, posterior belly of digastrics
- CN IX: pharynx (stylopharyngeus)
- CN X: pharynx, larynx, esophagus (levator veli palatini, palatopharyngeus, salpingopharyngeus, intrinsic laryngeal muscles, cricopharyngeus, pharyngeal constrictors)
- CN XII: tongue muscles

Overview of Abnormal Swallowing

- Defective deglutition results in inadequate nutrition and/or aspiration due to failure to protect the airway
- Dysphagia may be oral, pharyngeal, or esophageal

Diagnostic Studies

- Bedside swallow evaluation
- Modified barium swallow (MBS): fluoroscopic exam evaluates all three phases

- Esophagram: evaluates esophagus
- Fiberoptic endoscopic examination of swallowing (FEES) with or without sensory testing
- Esophagoscopy: sedated transoral or unsedated transnasal route (TNE)

Clinical Manifestations and Treatment of Dysphagia by Subsite

Oral Dysfunction

- Associated with tumor, surgery, stroke (brain stem), facial paralysis, other neuromuscular disorders
- Clinical features: poor oral control, oral incompetence, oral residue, or failure to initiate swallow
- Treatment: tongue strengthening and articulation exercises

Tongue Base Weakness

- Associated with inanition, neuromuscular disease, stroke, brain stem disorder
- Clinical features: poor bolus propulsion with residue in valleculae or tongue base on MBS or FEES
- Treatment: chin tuck to close vallecula, tongue base strengthening exercises, liquid rinse during meals

Pharyngeal Sensory Loss

- Associated with stroke, gastroesophageal reflux, aging, or surgical injury (superior laryngeal nerve)
- Clinical features: retained pharyngeal secretions on MBS or FEES, decreased sensation on sensory testing, silent (without coughing) penetration of laryngeal vestibule, aspiration (typically worse with thin liquids)
- Treatment: thickening of liquids (provides more time for pharyngeal response), swallowing with chin tucked and rotated to the affected side (to route the bolus to the contralateral pyriform sinus)

Vocal Cord Weakness or Paralysis

- Associated with aging, debilitation, Parkinson disease, or sensory deficit caused by vagal nerve injury
- Clinical features: failure of glottic closure, vocal cord bowing, breathy voice, aspiration of thin liquids
- Treatment: vocal cord adduction exercises, vocal cord augmentation/medialization

Failure of Laryngeal Elevation

- Associated with neuromuscular disorders, debilitation, stroke (brain stem)
- Clinical features: residue over tongue base and pyriform sinus and failure of cricopharyngeal opening on MBS and FEES
- Treatment: laryngeal elevation exercises, Mendelsohn maneuver (hold larynx as high as possible for as long as possible with each swallow), electromyography (EMG) biofeedback, transcutaneous electric stimulation of suprahyoid muscles

Generalized Pharyngeal Weakness

- Associated with stroke and a variety of general and neuromuscular diseases
- Clinical features: moderate to severe residue with failure to clear on subsequent swallows, secondary penetration/aspiration, worse with solids than with liquids
- Treatment: multiple consecutive swallows, small bites, liquid wash between bites

Failure of UES Opening

- Associated with failure of laryngeal elevation, gastroesophageal reflux, neuromuscular disease, and Zenker diverticulum
- Clinical features: cricopharyngeal "bar" or a pharyngeal diverticulum seen on radiographic exam, pharyngeal residue, or regurgitation following a swallow
  - Pharyngeal bar may be present in up to 30% of asymptomatic elderly
- Treatment: strengthening of active UES opening or reduction of sphincteric closure (chemodenervation or cricopharyngeal myotomy)

Disorders of Peristalsis

- Reduced (atony), excessive (spasm), or disordered (secondary or tertiary)

Chapter 35
Disorders of the Upper Aerodigestive Tract

Disorders of the Oral Cavity

Common Childhood Diseases With Oral Cavity Manifestations

- Measles (rubeola): Koplik spots (pale round spots on erythematous base) seen on buccal and lingual mucosa
- Chicken pox (varicella): vesicles
- Scarlet fever: strawberry tongue
- Kawasaki disease: strawberry tongue
- Congenital heart disease: gingivitis, cyanotic gums

Dental and Periodontal Diseases

Dental Developmental Abnormalities

- Hypodontia and anodontia (partial or complete): hereditary absence of teeth
- Dilaceration: abnormal development of the tooth root resulting in angular malformation of the root, caused by trauma or developmental disturbances
- Supernumerary teeth: extra tooth in addition to the normal series, can be found in any region of the dental arch (anterior maxilla is most common), associated with Gardner syndrome
- Enamel hypoplasia: can appear as pits in teeth due to localized areas of defective or absent enamel, associated with low calcium
- Enamel discoloration: may be due to antibiotics (tetracycline given prior to tooth eruption, around age 8), food, porphyria, severe neonatal jaundice, too much fluoride, or genetic defects (dentinogenesis, amelogenesis)
- Single central upper incisor: associated with pyriform aperture stenosis, nasal stenosis, choanal atresia

Infectious and Inflammatory Diseases

- Dental caries: formed by bacteria breaking down enamel and entering deeper structures
  - *Streptococcus mutans* and *Lactobacillus*
- Gingivitis: inflammation around and between teeth
  - Hormonal changes in women
  - Medications: anticonvulsants, antiangina
  - Smoking, cancer, HIV, diabetes

- **Acute necrotizing ulcerative gingivitis (ANUG, Vincent angina, trench mouth)**
  - Due to synergistic mixed anaerobic infection including *Borrelia vincentii* (fusiform bacillus)
  - **Noma:** acute necrotizing gingivitis that rapidly spreads into adjacent soft tissue, most commonly seen in third-world countries, with the highest incidence in children
  - Clinical features: fetid odor to breath, excessive salivation, bleeding gingiva
  - Treatment: oral hygiene and penicillin
- Periodontitis: inflammation of periodontal ligament, cementum, alveolar bone
  - *Prophyromonas gingivalis* and *Treponema denticola*
  - **Papillon-Lefevre syndrome**—periodontitis, hyperkeratosis of soles of feet and palms of hand, calcification of the dura
- Alveolar abscess: due to caries involving root canal
  - May lead to sinusitis, osteomyelitis, Ludwig angina, bacteremia
- Actinomyces: gram-positive bacteria, forms abscesses with masses of bacteria that resemble "sulfur granules"
- See Chapter 34 for cysts and tumors of the jaw

Normal Variants Mimicking Pathology

Torus Palatinus and Torus Mandibularis

- Benign bony exostoses, common on lingual or buccal aspect of anterior mandible or midline hard palate, usually appear in the second decade of life and slowly grow
- Developmental anomaly, broad-based, smooth bony masses covered in mucosa, consists of dense lamellar bone
- Treatment: none unless they interfere with denture placement

Developmental Cysts

- Dermoid cysts: contain elements of epidermal appendages such as hair follicles, sweat glands, and connective tissue, can be seen in the floor of mouth
- Enteric duplication cysts (choristomas): contain elements of GI mucosa, appear at birth as swelling of the tongue or floor of mouth
- Nasoalveolar cysts: usually present in adolescence with swelling in the nasolabial area with unilateral elevation of the nasal ala

Leukoedema

- Diffuse mild surface milky opacification, usually of the buccal mucosa
- Normal variant, associated with smoking, cannabis, alcohol, and bacterial infections
- Clinical features: asymptomatic, stretching the mucosa will cause the altered area to disappear (allows differentiation from leukoplakia or hyperkeratotic conditions)

Other Normal Variants Mimicking Pathology

- Geographic tongue (benign migratory glossitis): erythema with surrounding raised yellow-white margins, characterized by wandering pattern in time
- Amalgam tattoo: from dental fillings, can be confused with melanoma

Infectious Mucosal Diseases

Candidiasis

- Opportunistic infection most commonly caused by *Candida albicans* (less commonly *C. tropicalis*, *C. krusei*, *C. glabrata*), multiple clinical forms below
- Risk factors: immunosuppression such as HIV, poorly controlled diabetes, heavy smoking, denture use, radiation, inhaled or topical steroids, xerostomia, and antibiotic use

- Symptoms: range from asymptomatic to burning, dysgeusia, generalized discomfort, and odynophagia (usually in association with pharyngeal or hypopharyngeal involvement)
- *Acute pseudomembranous candidiasis (thrush)*: characteristic soft, white, superficial plaques with inflammatory base (plaques represent colonies of organisms that can be easily mobilized with a tongue depressor)
- *Acute erythematous/atrophic*: atrophic red patches
- *Chronic hyperplastic candidiasis* (leukoplakic-type hyperkeratosis): asymptomatic plaques that cannot be rubbed off, most commonly on buccal mucosa; biopsy to rule out dysplasia
- *Denture-related*: chronic erythematous/atrophic, in distribution of dentures, usually asymptomatic
- *Angular cheilitis*: scaly, fissured, macerated, or erythematous appearance to labial commissures and may extend onto adjacent skin; may be associated with staphylococcus coinfection
- *Median rhomboid glossitis*: smooth reddish area on midline of tongue devoid of papillae, sometimes corresponding lesion on hard palate
- Diagnosis: usually clinical; confirmation can be done with KOH smear, Periodic acid-Schiff (PAS) or methenamine silver stain, or culture on Sabouraud dextrose agar medium
- Treatment: topical nystatin or clotrimazole for mild-to-moderate disease; fluconazole, itraconazole, or ketoconazole for severe disease

Viral (Herpetic) Infections

- *Primary herpes simplex infection*: 48-hour prodrome of fever, malaise, focal mucosal tenderness, and erythema, followed by group of small vesicles with surrounding inflammation, then shallow, painful superficial ulcerations; can involve oral mucosa (usually no vesicles on the gingiva) and oropharynx; self-limiting after 7 to 14 days
- *Recurrent herpes simplex infection*: due to release of latent virus from dermatome-associated ganglion cells
    - **Herpes labialis**: most common form involving the mucocutaneous junction of the lip, similar prodrome of painful tingling followed by vesicles that coalesce, rupture, ulcerate, and then crust
    - **Recurrent intraoral form**: along the greater palatine nerve distribution on hard palate and attached gingiva in the first molar and premolar areas
- *Intraoral varicelliform eruptions*: acute, painful, orofacial lesions in unilateral distribution along trigeminal sensory nerves
- Histopathology: enlarged keratinocytes with multilobulated viral inclusions (Tzanck cells)
- Treatment: symptomatic management, topical and/or systemic antivirals can be used for recurrent infections

Bacterial Stomatitis

- Common pathogens: Streptococci, Staphylococci, Gonococci

Infectious Granulomatous Disease

- Blastomycosis
- Histoplasmosis
- Tuberculosis: painful, deep, irregular ulcer on dorsum of tongue (other sites include palate, lips, buccal mucosa, gingiva)

Noninfectious Mucosal Diseases

Oral Hairy Leukoplakia

- Asymptomatic white lesion caused by Epstein-Barr virus (EBV) in patients with HIV or immunosuppression
- Clinical features: ranges from subtle white keratotic vertical streaks to thick corrugated and shaggy surface on bilateral lateral tongue margins
- Diagnosis: biopsy and testing for presence of EBV (EBV DNA seen on immunohistochemistry within koilocytic epithelial cells of biopsy specimen)
- Histopathology: hyperkeratosis (thickening of stratum corneum) and irregular surface projections, acanthosis (thickening of stratum basale/spinosum), fungal hyphae may be present but do not contribute to the pathology
- Treatment: none necessary, the lesion will disappear with antiretroviral therapy in patients with HIV/AIDS

Premalignant Lesions

- Includes leukoplakia, erythroplakia, oral submucous fibrosis, and lichen planus (see Dermatologic Diseases)

Oral Leukoplakia

- Descriptive term for a white hyperkeratotic lesion that may or may not be associated with dysplasia; most common premalignant oral mucosal lesion (however, most cases are benign)
- Etiology: associated with smoking, chewing tobacco, betel/areca nut, chronic sun exposure (lip)
- Clinical features: most common in middle-age and older men; can be homogeneous and smooth, focal, or diffuse, heterogeneous and multifocal, ulcerative, erosive, speckled, nodular, or verrucous; occurs most frequently on the lip (vermilion) followed by buccal mucosa, mandibular gingiva, tongue, floor of mouth, hard palate, maxillary gingiva, lip mucosa, and soft palate
- Histopathology: ranges from hyperkeratosis and acanthosis to variable degrees of dysplasia, carcinoma in situ, and invasive squamous cell carcinoma (SCC)
- Risk of malignant transformation: up to 10%, greater risk in heterogeneous, speckled, or nodular forms
- Treatment: if benign or minimal dysplasia → periodic observation or elective excision; if moderate dysplasia or worse → removal with excision or ablation

Proliferative Verrucous Leukoplakia

- Uncommon variant of leukoplakia
- Occurs in patients without usual risk factors and in areas less commonly affected by oral SCC, more common in women
- Strong potential for malignant transformation
- Clinical features: multifocal, persistent lesions that evolve over time from thin, flat white patch to leathery, thickened lesion to papillary and then verrucous lesion

Erythroplakia

- A red lesion that cannot be characterized clinically or pathologically as any other definable lesion
- Clinical features: fiery red, granular, sharply demarcated lesion situated at a slightly lower level than surrounding mucosa
- Risk of malignant transformation: ranges up to 50%

Oral Submucous Fibrosis

- Multifactorial disorder caused by habitual use of areca/betel nut (either by chewing, placing in buccal or labial sulcus, or powdered forms) which results in failure of collagen remodeling
- Most common in India
- Clinical features: begins as erythema followed by progressive pallor and scar bands, which may limit jaw opening and tongue mobility
- Histopathology: juxtaposition of atrophic epithelium to subadjacent fibrosis
- Risk of malignant transformation: ranges from 7% to 30%
- Treatment: cessation of areca use; surgical scar release is moderately successful

Dermatologic Diseases

Oral Lichen Planus

- Mucocutaneous autoimmune disorder mediated by CD8+ T-cells, reaction to antigenic components of the epithelium or exogenous antigens
  - Associated conditions: primary sclerosing cholangitis, lupus erythematosus, primary biliary cirrhosis, Sjögren syndrome, hepatitis C
- Clinical features: multifocal and bilateral lesions; six variants including papular, plaquelike, bullous, atrophic, reticular (lacy white lines known as Wickham striae), or erosive (ulcerative lesions with peripheral striae); most commonly occurs on buccal mucosa, tongue, and gingiva
- Histopathology: dense subepithelial band of chronic inflammatory cells (usually T lymphocytes), Civatte bodies (necrotic keratinocytes); direct immunofluorescence (DIF) shows fibrinogen deposition in basement membrane zone
- Risk of malignant transformation: up to 5%, most commonly in erosive or atrophic forms
- Treatment: symptomatic with topical steroids (oral paste or solution), routine monitoring due to risk of dysplasia

Pemphigus Vulgaris

- Autoimmune mucocutaneous disease caused by autoantibodies against keratinocyte adhesion protein, desmoglein 3 (Dsg3), of the epidermis
  - *Paraneoplastic pemphigus*: usually associated with lymphoproliferative malignancies
- Clinical features: usually fifth decade or beyond, vesiculobullous lesions which then rupture and produce pain and ulceration
- Histopathology: separation of the suprabasal layer from basal layer of the epithelium creating a "tombstone" effect; DIF shows intercellular deposition of IgG and complement 3 (C3) between epithelial cells ("chicken-wire" appearance)
- Treatment: topical and systemic immunosuppression

Mucous Membrane (Cicatricial) Pemphigoid

- Autoimmune *subepithelial* mucocutaneous disease with linear deposition of IgG and C3 at the mucosal basement membrane zone
- Clinical features: patchy distribution of erythematous vesicles and bullae, ocular involvement may occur
- Histopathology: separation of mucosal epithelium from underlying lamina propria; DIF shows continuous linear deposition of IgG, IgA, and/or C3 in basement membrane zone
- Treatment: topical steroid if only oral mucosa is involved; dapsone for mild disease; systemic immunosuppression (prednisone, azathioprine, mycophenolate, cyclophosphamide) for severe or rapidly progressive disease

Erythema Multiforme

- Acute mucocutaneous hypersensitivity reaction ranging from self-limited, mild, exanthematous process to fulminant epithelial necrosis of skin and mucosa, as in Stevens-Johnson syndrome (SJS) and toxic epidermal necrolysis (TEN)
  - Triggers: photosensitivity, medications (carbamazepine and phenytoin, antifungals, quinolones, sulfonamides), and viral infections (recurrent HHV-1 most common; also EBV, chronic hepatitis C, parvovirus B19)
- Clinical features: classic target lesions on skin and aphthous-like ulcers and erosions with occasional vesicles and bullae on oral and oropharyngeal mucosa; usually symmetrical distribution, irregular size and shape, covered with fibrinous plaque; extreme tenderness can lead to sialorrhea, dysarthric-type speech, and inability to take oral intake
- Histopathology: spongiosis, apoptotic basal and parabasal cells, intense lymphohistiocytic infiltration and edema within submucosa and superficial lamina propria; keratinocyte necrosis, edema, and vacuolar degeneration in basement membrane zone
- Treatment: symptomatic treatment, steroids for more severe cases

Recurrent Aphthous Stomatitis (Sutton Disease)

- Most common nontraumatic oral ulceration; unknown etiology but many associated conditions including:
  - Crohn disease, Behcet disease (oral ulcerations, conjunctivitis, iritis, and urethritis), celiac disease, food hypersensitivity, Sweet syndrome (acute febrile neutrophilic dermatosis), PFAPA syndrome (periodic fever, aphthous ulcers, pharyngitis, adenitis)
  - Associated medications: NSAIDs, beta-blockers, potassium channel blockers
- *Minor aphthous ulceration*: most common form, less than 1 cm, usually involves anterior oral cavity, heals within 2 weeks
- *Major aphthous ulcers*: greater than 1 cm, usually in posterior aspect of oral cavity and oropharynx, deeply cratered, sharply marginated, and painful, may last for up to 6 weeks or longer if immunocompromised
- *Herpetiform-type aphthous ulcers*: least common, multiple tiny (< 2 mm) shallow ulcers with widespread distribution
- Treatment: symptomatic management and chlorhexidine rinses for mild cases, may give topical steroids and topical analgesics if needed, severe cases may necessitate systemic corticosteroids

Menopausavostomatitis (Senile Atrophy)

- Unknown pathophysiology
- Clinical features: dry oral mucosa with a burning sensation, diffuse erythema, shiny mucosa, and occasionally fissuring in the melobuccal fold
- Treatment: symptomatic management

Mucositis

- Commonly encountered as a result of chemotherapy and radiation (usually appears after second week of treatment)
- Clinical features: painful inflammation and ulceration, dysguesia
- Treatment: symptomatic management

Pigmented Oral Lesions

Mucosal Melanotic Macule

- Pigmented lesion resulting from excess melanin production, may be idiopathic (ephelis), postinflammatory, syndrome-associated (Peutz-Jeghers syndrome), or related to systemic disease (ie, Addison disease)

- Clinical features: small (< 10 mm) pigmented lesion with well-defined borders, most commonly in white females on the vermilion portion of the lower lip
- Treatment: conservative excision during diagnostic phase to rule out melanoma

Mucosal Melanotic Nevus

- Develops from nevus cell (altered melanocytes) proliferation, can appear in the young or at birth as a focal macular or papular pigmented lesion; palate is the most common site

Other Benign Lesions of the Oral Cavity

Papilloma

- Benign solitary growth associated with human papilloma virus 6 and 11 (HPV 6 and 11)
- Clinical features: single, asymptomatic, soft, pedunculated mass with finger-like projections on the lingual, buccal, and labial mucosa and tongue
- Histopathology: projections with fibrovascular core and narrow base
- Treatment: surgical excision or CO_2 laser ablation, recurrence is unlikely

Granular Cell Tumor

- Neural origin
- Congenital epulis: neonatal form, evident at birth, characteristically involves maxillary gingiva
- Clinical features: small (< 1.5 cm), firm, painless, sessile, nodular-appearing lesion most commonly on dorsum of tongue, also may involve soft palate, uvula, and labial mucosa
- Histopathology: large polygonal, oval, or bipolar cells with abundant granular eosinophilic cytoplasm; cells appear in ribbon pattern, extend to surface of epithelium, and demonstrate pseudoepitheliomatous hyperplasia
- Malignant form seen in about 1% of cases
- Treatment: surgical excision; recurrence is rare

Neurofibroma

- Most common peripheral nerve neoplasm derived from Schwann cells and perineural fibroblasts
    - Associated condition: von Recklinghausen neurofibromatosis (NF type 1)
- Clinical features: adolescent or young adult with solitary, soft, painless, slow-growing mass usually on tongue or buccal or labial mucosa
- Rare malignant transformation to sarcoma
- Treatment: surgical excision

Lipoma

- Uncommon growth seen in third decade of life presenting as a soft, slowly growing, mucosa-covered, smooth, painless mass in the buccal or lingual areas or floor of mouth
- Histopathology: mature encapsulated adipocytes
- Treatment: surgical excision

Fibroma

- Solitary sessile or pedunculated lesion that results from trauma or irritation, usually involving the buccal mucosa
- Treatment: surgical excision

Hemangioma

- Soft, painless red or blue mass, most commonly on the lip, that typically presents at birth in a rapid proliferative phase and then spontaneously regresses over the years
    - Associated conditions: Sturge-Weber syndrome, von Hippel-Lindau syndrome
- Treatment: medical therapies including propranolol and steroids (local and systemic), intralesional sclerosing agents, interferons, laser, radiation, or surgical excision if causing deformity or functional problems

Verruciform Xanthoma

- Uncommon, benign oral lesion with cutaneous counterpart, usually on the genitalia; unknown cause
- Clinical features: presents in fifth decade, well-circumscribed lesion ranging from 0.2 to 2 cm with either depressed, flat, or elevated surface that may have varying degrees of granular texture
- Histopathology: numerous xanthoma (macrophage) cells with lipoid droplets and characteristic foamy or flocculent cytoplasm and Periodic acid-Schiff (PAS)-positive and diastase-resistant granules
- Treatment: surgical excision

Pyogenic Granuloma

- Arise in the setting of trauma, pregnancy (epulis gravidarum), or in response to recent tooth extraction (epulis granulomatosa)
- Clinical features: raised or pedunculated lesion, usually less than 2.5 cm, most commonly on gingiva but also seen on labial mucosa or tongue (may look like a hemangioma)
- Histopathology: rich profusion of anastomosing vascular channels in an edematous, inflammatory, and fibrotic stromal background
- Treatment: usually persists indefinitely except for those associated with pregnancy, surgical excision, and removal of traumatic or infective factors

Traumatic (Eosinophilic) Granuloma

- Uncommon benign and self-limiting chronic oral ulcer of unknown cause
- Clinical features: rapid onset of painful, large (1-2 cm) ulcer on lateral or ventral tongue with crateriform center, sharply demarcated margins, firm, indurated qualities
- Histopathology: inflammatory infiltrate with scattered eosinophils between skeletal muscle bundles
- Treatment: observation, topical steroids, excision if diagnosis is in question

Fordyce Granules

- Painless, pinpoint yellow nodules that occur bilaterally on the posterior buccal mucosa
- Represent enlarged ectopic sebaceous glands

Minor Salivary Gland Tumors

- Most common benign salivary gland tumor of minor salivary glands is pleomorphic adenoma, typically presenting as a smooth, slow-growing mass on the hard palate
- Other benign minor salivary gland tumors: papillary cystadenoma, oncocytoma, myoepithelioma

Ranula

- Mucocele of the sublingual gland that presents in the floor of mouth
- Plunging ranula penetrates mylohyoid muscle and presents as a soft submental neck mass
- Treatment: excision should include the entire sublingual gland to prevent recurrence, with care taken to protect submandibular duct and lingual nerve

Necrotizing Sialometaplasia

- Self-healing, ulcerative, inflammatory reaction of unknown cause; typically arise from minor salivary glands in the palate
- Clinical features: painful ulceration and swelling, may mimic malignancy
- Histopathology: lobar necrosis, sialadenitis mixed with submucous metaplasia of excretory ducts and acini, pseudoepitheliomatous hyperplasia
- Treatment: biopsy to confirm diagnosis, close follow-up

Amyloidosis

- Abnormal deposition of extracellular fibril proteins into tissues
  - Dialysis-related amyloid: beta-2-microglobulin
  - Plasma cell disorders: immunoglobulin light chains
  - Familial amyloidosis: transthyretin
- Clinical features: macroglossia
- Histopathology: apple green birefringence with use of polarized light after Congo red staining
- Treatment: treat underlying cause, tongue reduction if symptomatic dysarthria or dysphagia

Other Causes of Macroglossia

- Hemangioma
- Lymphangioma
- Myxedema
- Acromegaly
- Benign cysts
- Pierre Robin (relative macroglossia due to micrognathia)
- Tertiary syphilis
- Von Gierke disease (glycogen storage disease Type I)
- Hurler syndrome (mucopolysaccharidosis)
- Down syndrome
- Actinomycosis

Neoplasms

Squamous Cell Carcinoma (SCC)

- See Chapter 39

Salivary Gland Malignancies

- Includes: mucoepidermoid carcinoma, adenoid cystic carcinoma, acinic cell carcinoma, epithelial-myoepithelial carcinoma, salivary duct carcinoma, adenocarcinoma, carcinoma ex-pleomorphic adenoma

Melanoma

- Rare neoplasm, more common in Asians and blacks
- Most occur on hard or soft palate
- Aggregates of atypical melanocytes with wide variety of morphology, stains positive for S-100, human melanoma black 45 (HMB-45), and melan-A
- Surgery is the main treatment modality; however, poor prognosis for any mucosal melanoma
- Staging starts at T3 for mucosal melanoma

Kaposi Sarcoma

- Violaceous macules on oral mucosa
- Uncommon, except in association with AIDS, considered an AIDS-defining condition

Others

- Lymphoma
- Metastasis (eg, lung, breast)

Systemic Diseases with Oral Mucosal Manifestations

Hematologic Diseases

- Pernicious anemia: lack of vitamin B12; tongue with lobulations on surface or may be shiny, smooth, and red (in advanced cases); oral mucosa may have irregular erythema
- Iron deficiency anemia: oral mucosa is ash gray (may be associated with Plummer-Vinson syndrome), tongue is smooth and devoid of papillae
- Thalassemia (Mediterranean anemia): oral mucosa has diffuse pallor and cyanosis
- Polycythemia: oral mucosa is bright blue-red with gingival bleeding
- Thrombocytopenic purpura: purpura due to a marked decrease in platelets from a variety of causes, initial manifestations are often oral petechiae and ecchymosis
- Acute myeloid leukemia: gingival hyperplasia

Inherited Syndromes

- Osler-Weber-Rendu disease (hereditary hemorrhagic telangiectasia): forms spider-like blood vessels or angiomatous-appearing lesions on the oral mucosa, tongue, and nasal mucosa; associated with recurrent epistaxis; GI tract may be involved and transfusion may be required
- Sturge-Weber syndrome: port-wine stain of the face, oral cavity, or tongue associated with vascular malformations of the meninges and cerebral cortex

Nutritional Deficiencies

- Vitamin A: dyskeratotic changes of skin and mucous membranes, angular cheilitis, defects in dentin and enamel of developing teeth
- Vitamin B2 (riboflavin): angular cheilitis, burning lips, mouth, and tongue
- Vitamin B12 and folate: recurrent aphthous ulcers
- Niacin deficiency (pellagra): swollen tongue
- Vitamin C deficiency (scurvy): perifollicular hemorrhages and petechiae in mouth, gingival hyperplasia, stomatitis
- Vitamin D (results in calcium deficiency): mandibular osteopenia or osteoporosis, enamel hypoplasia
- Vitamin K: oral hemorrhagic bullae
- Folate and iron: atrophic glossitis (atrophy of filiform papillae), angular cheilitis, hyperkeratotic oral mucosal lesions
- Zinc deficiency: taste changes

Conditions Causing Hyperpigmentation

- Melanosis: physiologic pigmentation, dark patches of the oral mucosa
- Amalgam tattoo: well-defined, grayish-black, focal, macular mucosal discoloration or inadvertent tattoo of gingiva from dental amalgam introduced through a mucosal laceration
- Peutz-Jeghers syndrome: melanotic macules periorally
- Kaposi sarcoma: violaceous macules

- Addison disease: brown macules
- Hemochromatosis: bronze
- Xanthomatous disease: yellow/gray
- Hepatitis: yellow/brown hue to oral mucosa
- Lead: blue-gray line that follows margin of gingiva (Burton line)
- Mercury: gray/violet
- Bismuth: a cause of "Black hairy tongue" from lack of papillae desquamation
- Silver: violet/blue/gray
- Hyperparathyroidism: benign bony mass ("brown tumor")

Disorders of the Pharynx

Congenital Disorders

- Cleft palate: due to failure of fusion; associated with a characteristic voice change and nasal regurgitation of liquids; submucous cleft may be present; eustachian tube disorder due to failure of tensor veli palatini to open eustachian tube on swallowing (see Chapter 46)
- Congenital elongation of uvula

Normal Variants Mimicking Disease

- Tonsillolith
- Lingual tonsil hypertrophy
- Lingual thyroid: represents a lack of descent of thyroid tissue during development in the midline dorsal tongue in the area of the foramen cecum; may be associated with obstructive symptoms due to mass effect and with hypothyroidism
- Persistent foramen cecum
- Aberrant carotid artery: tortuous, kinked, or coiled carotid artery may present as a pharyngeal mass; usually asymptomatic, or can cause abnormal sensation in throat; at risk for injury during procedures in the pharynx

Infectious Diseases of the Pharynx

Acute Pharyngitis

- Viral: most common cause
  - Rhinovirus: most common cause of common cold
  - Coronavirus: common cold
  - Parainfluenza: common cold, croup
  - Influenza: types A and B cause widespread outbreaks
  - Adenovirus: pharyngoconjunctival fever (pharyngitis and conjunctivitis)
  - Coxsackie A: herpangina (vesicular eruption on soft palate or anterior pillar with fever), hand-foot-mouth disease
  - Epstein-Barr virus (EBV): infectious mononucleosis
  - Cytomegalovirus (CMV): CMV mononucleosis
  - Herpes simplex type 1 and 2: pharyngitis, gingivostomatitis
  - Human immunodeficiency virus (HIV): acute retroviral syndrome (primary HIV infection)
- Bacterial:
  - Group A beta-hemolytic *Streptococcus pyogenes* (GABHS): pharyngitis, tonsillitis, scarlet fever
  - Non-group A beta-hemolytic streptococcus (groups B, C, G): pharyngitis, tonsillitis
  - Mixed anaerobes: Vincent angina

    - *Neisseria gonorrhoeae*: pharyngitis, tonsillitis
    - *Corynebacterium diphtheriae*: diphtheria (greyish pseudomembrane, if removed can precipitate cardiac toxicity)
    - *Arcanobacterium haemolyticum*: pharyngitis, scarlatiniform rash
    - *Yersinia enterocolitica*: pharyngitis, enterocolitis
    - *Yersinia pestis*: plague
    - *Francisella tularensis*: tularemia, oropharyngeal form
    - *Treponema pallidum*: secondary syphilis
    - *Chlamydia pneumoniae*: pneumonia, pharyngitis
    - *Mycoplasma pneumoniae*: pneumonia, bronchitis, pharyngitis
- Fungal: *Candida spp.*

Acute Tonsillitis

- Etiology: most common is viral, bacterial causes: Group A beta-hemolytic streptococci (GABHS), *Haemophilus influenzae*, *Streptococcus pneumoniae*, *Staphylococcus aureus*, Tuberculosis (immunocompromised)

Quincke Disease

- Swelling of the uvula, often in association with acute bacterial tonsillitis; can also occur with trauma (heroic snoring, burn from hot food or beverage, inhalation of drugs)

Peritonsillar Abscess

- Pus located deep to tonsil capsule between tonsil and superior constrictor muscle
- Clinical presentation: deviation of the tonsil and uvula toward midline, swelling of the soft palate, trismus, hot potato voice, dysphagia
- Complications: dehydration, airway obstruction, parapharyngeal abscess (due to rupture through superior constrictor), venous involvement (thrombosis, phlebitis, bacteremia, endocarditis), arterial involvement (thrombosis, hemorrhage, pseudoaneurysms), mediastinitis, brain abscess, aspiration pneumonia, nephritis (due to streptococcal antigen), peritonitis
- Treatment: surgical drainage, empiric antibiotics

Indications for Tonsillectomy

- Recurrent infections: 3 per year for 3 years, 5 per year for 2 years, 7 or more in 1 year (Paradise criteria), or greater than 2 weeks of school or work missed in 1 year
- Hypertrophy causing upper airway obstruction (sleep disordered breathing or frank sleep apnea) or causing deglutition problems
- Greater than 1 peritonsillar abscess, multiple antibiotic allergies/intolerance, PFAPA
- Diphtheria carrier
- Treatment of early-stage cancer or search for unknown primary (often performed via TORS), suspicion for malignancy with asymmetric enlargement
- *Morbidity of tonsillectomy*: postoperative hemorrhage 2% to 4%, mortality 1 in 25,000 (hemorrhage, airway obstruction, anesthesia)

Noninfectious Inflammatory Diseases of the Pharynx

Noninfectious Pharyngitis

- Sinonasal disease (post-nasal drip, chronic rhinosinusitis)
- Caustic injury (see esophageal section)
- Chronic allergy or irritants (dust, smoking, alcohol)
- Laryngopharyngeal reflux
- Chronic mouth breathing

- Trauma (endotracheal intubation)
- Vocal abuse
- Granulomatous and connective tissue disorders
- Cobblestoning of posterior wall (inflammation of lymphoid rests)

Mucosal Diseases (mostly on soft palate, see above in oral cavity section)

- Aphthous ulcers
- Leukoplakia, erythroplakia
- Squamous papillomas

Eagle Syndrome

- Pain due to elongated styloid process or calcification of stylohyoid ligament often following tonsillectomy or trauma

Angioedema

- Etiology: mediated by excess bradykinin in familial (C1 esterase deficiency) and ACE inhibitor (ACEI)-induced angioedema and by histamine in allergic angioedema
- ACEI-induced angioedema: increased risk in blacks, women, and smokers; can occur at any time following initiation of therapy and even after cessation of therapy
- Clinical features: watery edema, severe swelling may be preceded by sentinel swelling
- Management: antihistamines, glucocorticoids, and epinephrine; awake fiberoptic intubation or tracheostomy may be required

Neoplasms

- Squamous cell carcinoma (SCC, see Chapter 39)
  - Oropharyngeal: may be either standard variant (found in smokers/drinkers) or HPV-related (HPV 16 and 18, high levels of p16, often found in nonsmokers, different biological behavior and response to treatment)
- Lymphoma (base of tongue, tonsil)
- Minor salivary gland tumors (usually malignant)
- Lingual thyroid cancer (base of tongue): due to failure of descent
- Parapharyngeal space masses (benign or malignant)

Disorders of the Nasopharynx

Benign Diseases

- **Adenoid hypertrophy**
- **Thornwaldt (or Tornwaldt) cyst**
  - Benign epithelial growth that originates from Rathke pouch (cleavage line between nasal and pharyngeal embryological processes)
  - Usually incidental finding of a smooth, centrally located mass with a yellow hue
- **Squamous papilloma**
  - Benign epithelial tumor with inverting epithelial changes at the basal membrane (schneiderian or inverting papilloma)
  - Usually incidental finding in the nasopharynx
  - Treatment: surgical excision (base of the lesion must be completely removed with cuff of normal tissue)
- **Craniopharyngioma**
  - Benign tumor that arises from Rathke pouch
  - May present with endocrine or visual disturbances (similar to pituitary tumors), or nasal obstruction (may mimic presentation of adenoid hypertrophy in children)
  - Treatment: surgical excision with or without radiation

- **Angiofibroma (or Juvenile Nasal Angiofibroma, JNA)**
  - Locally infiltrative slow-growing vascular tumor that arises in sphenopalatine foramen and extends laterally via pterygopalatine fossa and into nasopharynx and choanal space (path of least resistance)
  - Treatment: surgical excision (preoperative embolization may reduce risk of intraoperative bleeding) or radiation
- *Other benign lesions*: hairy polyp, teratoma, adenomatous polyps, fibromyxomatous polyps, choanal polyps, osteomas, fibrous dysplasia, solitary fibrous tumors, desmoid fibromatosis, schwannoma

Malignant Diseases

- **Chordoma**: locally aggressive malignancy from notochord remnants that arises from bone of the basisphenoid and erodes through the bony skull base into the sphenoid and nasopharynx
- **Nasopharyngeal carcinoma**: common in Asia; associated with Epstein-Barr Virus (EBV) and diets high in preservatives (salted fish, eggs, vegetables); most common presentation is palpable neck mass; treated with radiation (stage I or II) or chemoradiation (stage III and IV)
- *Other malignant tumors*: undifferentiated carcinoma, squamous cell carcinoma, lymphoma, hemangiopericytoma, malignant fibrous histiocytoma, rhabdomyosarcoma, malignant salivary gland tumors (adenoid cystic carcinoma, mucoepidermoid carcinoma, acinic cell carcinoma, adenocarcinoma), metastatic tumors (adenocarcinoma, papillary carcinoma)

Disorders of the Esophagus

Motility Disorders

Diagnosis of motility disorders:

- Manometry is diagnostic.
- Barium esophagram can be used as initial test due to some characteristic findings.

Achalasia

- Caused by degeneration of Auerbach (myenteric) plexus resulting in aperistalsis, esophageal dilatation, and failure of LES relaxation
  - May be primary (idiopathic) or secondary (such as **Chagas disease**: caused by the parasite *Trypanosoma cruzi,* which infects ganglion cells)
- Clinical features: progressive dysphagia for solids and liquids, regurgitation, chest pain
- Barium esophagram: failure of peristalsis, dilatation, and air-fluid level in the upright position with smooth tapering of the lower esophagus to a closed LES (bird's beak appearance), presence of epiphrenic diverticulum suggests achalasia
- Manometry: simultaneous, low-contraction amplitudes in body (aperistalsis), high or normal baseline LES pressure with abnormal relaxation
- Rule out ***pseudoachalasia*** with upper endoscopy (tumor at gastroesophageal junction)
- Treatment: symptomatic management with pneumatic dilation or surgical myotomy if surgical candidate, or endoscopic injection of LES with botulinum toxin if poor surgical candidate

Diffuse Esophageal Spasm

- Clinical features: intermittent chest pain (if strong contractions) or dysphagia (if weak contractions)

- Barium esophagram: may be normal, spasms may be described as "curling," "tertiary contractions," "corkscrew esophagus," or "rosary bead esophagus"
- Manometry: simultaneous and repetitive contractions of the distal two-thirds of esophagus with normal LES relaxation and some normal peristalsis may be seen
- Treatment: nitrates, calcium channel blockers

Nutcracker Esophagus

- High-amplitude peristalsis causing chest pain (not a true motility disorder)

Presbyesophagus

  - Associated with age and manifested by incoordination of sphincter function, reduced peristalsis, and frequent tertiary contractions

Systemic Causes of Esophageal Motility Disorders

- **Scleroderma (progressive systemic sclerosis)**
  - Small vessel vasculitis resulting in fibrosis of *smooth* muscle and motility abnormalities
  - Manometry: aperistalsis in distal two-thirds of esophagus and very low LES pressure
  - Barium esophagram: dilated esophagus, patulous GEJ, reflux into esophagus
  - At high risk for severe complications of GERD (eg, Barrett esophagus, esophagitis, strictures)
- **Polymyositis**
  - Muscle weakness secondary to inflammatory and degenerative changes in *striated* muscle of the hypopharynx and upper esophagus
  - Manometry: diminished and poorly coordinated peristaltic waves, decreased UES pressure
  - Barium esophagram: esophagus may be dilated
  - Other clinical features: proximal muscle weakness (hip and shoulder) is most common presenting symptom (termed *dermatomyositis* when associated with skin rashes)
- Neuromuscular disorders: **amyotrophic lateral sclerosis** (ALS), neurogenic dysfunction from **amyloidosis**, other dysautonomia
- Endocrine: **diabetes** (decreased peristalsis and esophageal emptying), **hypothyroidism** (decreased amplitude and velocity of peristalsis)
- Irritants: **gastroesophageal reflux** (hypocontraction and LES hypotension), corrosive injury, alcoholism

Inflammatory and Infectious Diseases of the Esophagus

Gastroesophageal Reflux Disease (GERD)

- Abnormal reflux of gastric contents into esophagus; spectrum includes nonerosive reflux disease (most common), reflux esophagitis, and Barrett esophagus
- Clinical features: symptoms may be typical (heartburn, acid regurgitation) or atypical (asthma, laryngitis, cough, chest pain, dental erosions)
- Diagnosis: often made by history, laryngeal examination, and response to empiric therapy if typical symptoms (24-hour pH monitoring was previously the gold standard)
- Barium esophagram: erosions, ulcerations, strictures in reflux esophagitis
- Endoscopy to evaluate mucosa if concerns for esophagitis or Barrett esophagus
- Treatment: lifestyle modifications (head of bed elevation, dietary changes, avoidance of caffeine and nicotine) and antacids (H2 blockers, proton pump inhibitor)

Barrett Esophagus

- Serious complication of chronic GERD resulting in intestinal columnar metaplasia of distal esophagus (instead of normal stratified squamous epithelium) and increased risk of adenocarcinoma
- Endoscopy: salmon-pink columnar mucosa in distal esophagus (instead of normal appearing pale pink squamous mucosa)
- Diagnosis: biopsy showing intestinal metaplasia (characterized by mucin-containing goblet cells)
- Treatment: close surveillance with endoscopy to detect the development of dysplasia and adenocarcinoma

Infectious Esophagitis

- Predominantly in immunosuppressed patients (AIDS, cancer, diabetes, organ transplants)
- Usually involves long segments of esophagus and presents with odynophagia
- **Candida albicans**: most frequent organism
    - Esophagogram: abnormal motility and longitudinal mucosal plaques in early disease and a shaggy appearance in late disease due to coalescence of plaques
    - Endoscopy: white or pale yellow plaques
    - Treatment: antifungals (topical clotrimazole or nystatin if only mild immunosuppression, fluconazole for most patients, amphotericin B if granulocytopenic or severely immunocompromised to prevent disseminated disease)
- **Herpes simplex virus**: second most common organism
    - Esophagogram: discrete ulcers in the mid esophagus
    - Endoscopy: vesicles and ulcers with raised edges, obtain viral culture, biopsy ulcer margins (multinucleated giant cells and ground-glass intranuclear inclusion bodies)
    - Treatment: acyclovir
- **Cytomegalovirus (CMV)**
    - Infects submucosal fibroblasts and endothelial cells
    - Endoscopy: serpiginous erosions and ulcers, biopsy at base of ulcer for diagnosis (intranuclear and cytoplasmic inclusions, halo surrounding nucleus)
    - Treatment: ganciclovir or foscarnet
- Other viral causes: HIV (aphthous ulceration), VZV, EBV, HPV
- **Tuberculous esophagitis**: caused by direct extension from adjacent lymph nodes
- **Histoplasmosis**: granulomatous infection that may cause ulcers or fistulae

Eosinophilic Esophagitis (EoE)

- Associated with other atopic diseases and food allergies
- Presents with dysphagia and food impaction in young adults
- Endoscopy: multiple esophageal rings, biopsy to measure eosinophil density for diagnosis (> 15/hpf)
- PPI trial no longer required for diagnosis
- Treatment: six-food elimination diet, corticosteroid inhaler, esophageal dilation for rings

Other Systemic Causes of Esophagitis

- Radiation esophagitis: superficial ulcerations or granular-appearing mucosa progressing to dysmotility, strictures, and long-standing ulcers
- Crohn disease: aphthous ulcers, cobblestoning, fistulae, strictures
- Behcet's disease: ulcerations
- Epidermolysis bullosa dystrophica: recessive form of epidermolysis bullosa, hereditary skin disorder with recurrent blisters and esophageal involvement

- Pemphigoid
- Alcohol-induced esophagitis
- Graft-versus-host disease

Pill-Induced Esophagitis

- Common offenders include antibiotics (tetracycline, doxycycline), quinidine, potassium chloride, iron sulfate, bisphosphonates, vitamin C; increased risk with bedtime dosing, tortuous esophagus, and not taking water with medications
- Presents with chest pain and odynophagia
- Esophagram or endoscopy: single ulcer (or small cluster of ulcers), plaque, or stricture at areas of physiologic narrowing (mid esophagus/level of aortic arch or distal esophagus)
- Treatment: avoidance of offending agent, dilation for stricture

Esophageal Burns (Caustic Esophagitis)

- Bimodal distribution: 1 to 5 years old (usually accidental and less severe), adolescent/young adult (intentional suicide attempt, usually more severe damage)
- Pathophysiology: mucosal injury occurs within minutes of ingestion and progresses over weeks to months (esophageal wall weakened within first 3 weeks due to mucosal sloughing and bacterial invasion, then scar retraction and stricture formation develop over the following few months)
    - Alkalis (lye, common in drain and household cleaners): cause liquefaction necrosis and are more likely to cause deep burns
    - Acids: cause coagulation necrosis which limits their penetration; however, may be associated with gastric rupture
- Symptoms are variable and may not correlate with severity of burn, oropharyngeal involvement may not be present
- Endoscopy: used to evaluate mucosa and grade the extent of injury within first 12 to 48 hours
- Grading of caustic esophageal injury: almost all grade 0 to IIA will heal without long-term sequelae, majority of grade IIB and III will develop strictures
    - Grade 0: normal mucosa
    - Grade I: edema and erythema of mucosa
    - Grade IIA: hemorrhage, erosions, blisters, superficial ulcers
    - Grade IIB: circumferential lesions
    - Grade IIIA: focal deep gray or brownish-black ulcers (necrosis)
    - Grade IIIB: extensive deep gray or brownish-black ulcers (necrosis)
    - Grade IV: perforation
- Treatment: supportive care, monitor for signs of perforation, intubation may be needed if epiglottis or larynx are involved, management of late sequela (dilation of strictures, monitor for development of squamous cell carcinoma)

Esophageal Trauma

Foreign Bodies

- Most common location is at site of physiologic narrowing (70% UES, 20% level of aortic arch, 10% LES) or pathologic narrowing (scar from prior burn or surgery, or site of peptic stricture)
    - Button batteries cause particularly severe injury due to leakage of alkaline contents and generation of electrical current with surrounding tissues

- Diagnosis: assess for free air and localization of bones or button batteries on plain radiograph or CT scan; esophagram can be used to confirm food disimpaction (no role in initial diagnosis)
- Treatment: prompt removal to avoid pressure necrosis and resultant perforation

Iatrogenic Perforation

- Most commonly occur at sites of narrowing
- Clinical features: sore throat, neck and chest pain following procedure, often with tachycardia out of proportion to fever; fever and subcutaneous emphysema develop later
- Diagnosis: CXR and CT if clinical suspicion present
- Treatment: antibiotics, fluid resuscitation, and early surgical exploration with repair

Mallory-Weiss Syndrome

- Tear of gastroesophageal junction or cardia of stomach due to forceful vomiting, most commonly in alcoholics (usually men > 40)
- Clinical features: massive hematemesis
- Endoscopy for diagnosis and management

Boerhaave Syndrome

- Linear tear 1 to 4 cm in length through all three layers of esophagus due to sudden increase in esophageal pressure, usually due to vomiting
- Rare, 90% occur on left, males more than females (5:1)
- Clinical features: severe knife-like epigastric pain radiating to left shoulder, may not have significant hematemesis; may develop respiratory difficulty, subcutaneous emphysema, and shock (may be difficult to differentiate from myocardial infarction, pulmonary embolus, or perforated ulcer)
- Diagnosis: initial CXR—widened mediastinum, then left pleural effusion or hydro-pneumothorax
- Treatment: thoracotomy and repair

Neoplasms

Malignant Tumors of the Esophagus (see Chapter 39)

- Squamous cell carcinoma: African American men, associated with alcohol, tobacco use, and caustic esophageal injuries, most commonly in mid esophagus
- Adenocarcinoma: white men, association with GERD and Barrett esophagus, most commonly in distal esophagus
- Other malignant neoplasms: sarcomas (leiomyosarcoma, fibrosarcoma)

Benign Tumors of the Esophagus

- Rare
- Include leiomyoma, fibroma, lipoma

Structural Abnormalities

Zenker Diverticulum

- Occurs in Killian dehiscence inferior to fibers of inferior constrictor and superior to cricopharyngeus
- Associated with incomplete relaxation of UES (cricopharyngeal muscle), muscle fibrosis, or failure of active dilatation due to inadequate laryngeal elevation
- Clinical features: oropharyngeal dysphagia, halitosis, regurgitation of undigested food, aspiration, cough

- Diagnosis: barium esophagogram in the lateral projection shows contrast filling the diverticulum during swallowing
- Treatment: cricopharyngeal myotomy with or without excision, suspension, or inversion of sac, or endoscopic diverticulotomy (laser or stapler)

Traction Diverticulum

- Usually midesophageal, typically on left, often due to traction of adjacent inflammatory process (usually tuberculosis)

Epiphrenic Diverticulum

- Occurs just superior to cardioesophageal junction, usually on right side, often from motility disorder

Esophageal Strictures

- Usually symptomatic when lumen is less than 15 mm (normal lumen = 20 mm)
- Treatment: dilation and address underlying cause
- *Intrinsic causes*: acid peptic induced (most common), pill-induced, caustic, infectious, radiation induced, surgical anastomosis, congenital, systemic inflammatory
- *Extrinsic causes*: mediastinal masses (enlarged thyroid, pulmonary or metastatic malignancies), anomalous vessels or aneurysms, cardiomegaly
    - **Dysphagia lusoria (Bayford syndrome or Bayford-Autenrieth dysphagia):** symptomatic compression of the esophagus by aberrant right subclavian artery that originates from descending aorta distal to left subclavian and passes posterior to esophagus to reach the arm; associated with right nonrecurrent recurrent laryngeal nerve and aortic aneurysms. CT is diagnostic. Treatment involves ligation and division with anastomosis of distal subclavian artery to carotid.

Schatzki Ring

- Concentric ring at the distal margin of LES at esophagogastric junction, may be congenital or possible link with GERD
- Clinical features: intermittent solid food dysphagia (if lumen is < 13 mm)
- Barium esophagram is most sensitive test, can also be seen on endoscopy
- Treatment: dilation if symptomatic

Esophageal Webs

- Barium esophagram is best diagnostic test, usually seen on anterior wall and appear asymmetric
- Often associated with **Plummer-Vinson syndrome** (Patterson-Kelly syndrome, sideropenic dysphagia)
    - Etiology unclear, possible relationship to GERD
    - Females > males 10:1, typically of Scandinavian descent
    - Triad: 1) proximal esophageal webs, 2) iron-deficiency anemia, 3) dysphagia
    - May also be associated with hypothyroidism, glossitis, cheilitis, gastritis; increased risk of postcricoid carcinoma
    - Diagnosis: barium esophagram; check CBC, serum iron, ferritin levels
    - Treatment: iron replacement, dilation of web

Hiatal Hernia (HH)

- A portion of stomach passing up through the esophageal hiatus of the diaphragm
- Two types: sliding (most common) in which the esophagogastric junction (EGJ) herniates into the thorax, or paraesophageal in which the EGJ is below the diaphragm while the fundus of the stomach bulges around it and through the diaphragm into the chest cavity
- Associated condition: **Sandifer syndrome**—abnormal contortions of the neck and back associated with unrecognized hiatus hernia in children

Congenital Diaphragmatic Hernia

- Pleuroperitoneal (Bochdalek): defect in posterolateral diaphragm
- Retrosternal (Morgagni): defect is anterior and retrosternal

Congenital Tracheoesophageal Fistula (TEF)

- Abnormal connection between esophagus and trachea.
- Various types: distal TEF with upper esophageal atresia (most common, 85%), blind upper and lower esophageal pouches without a connection to the trachea (8%), true H-type fistula (4%), proximal esophagus opens into trachea (< 1%).
- Clinical features: Infants present with drooling and feeding difficulties, coughing, abdominal distention, vomiting, and cyanosis.
- Diagnosis: Radiographs demonstrate marked air filling the stomach and proximal intestine and often right upper lobe pneumonia (aspiration). Passage of NG tube that meets obstruction 9 to 13 cm from nares suggests diagnosis. CXR with the catheter in place can demonstrate position of pouch as well as air in stomach and intestine. Barium study is diagnostic.
- Prognosis: 60% to 80% survival except if cardiac or genitourinary abnormalities present (then drops to 22%).

Bibliography

Alcaide ML, Bisno AL. Pharyngitis and epiglottitis. *Infect Dis Clin North Am*. 2007 Jun;21(2):449-69, vii.

Amagasa T, Yamashiro M, Uzawa N. Oral premalignant lesions: from a clinical perspective. *Int J Clin Oncol*. 2011 Feb;16(1):5-14.

Gravina SA, Yep GL, Khan M. Human biology of taste. *Ann Saudi Med*. 2013 May-Jun;33(3):217-222.

Kurowski JA, Kay M. Caustic ingestions and foreign bodies ingestions in pediatric patients. *Pediatr Clin North Am*. 2017 Jun;64(3):507-524.

Yardimci G, Kutlubay Z, Engin B, Tuzun Y. Precancerous lesions of oral mucosa. *World J Clin Cases*. 2014 Dec 16;2(12):866-872.

Questions

1. An 88-year-old woman complains of burning mouth. Examination reveals "shiny" tongue. The most likely diagnosis is
   A. Xerostomia due to medications
   B. Senile atrophy
   C. Malabsorption syndrome with essential nutrient deficiency
   D. Congenital absence of filiform papillae

2. A 46-year-old woman is found to have anesthesia of her left hard palate. Sensation in her cheek and upper lip are normal. A CT scan demonstrates a mass in her ipsilateral posterior nasal cavity. Of the following, which is the most likely site of nerve involvement?
   A. Incisural foramen
   B. Foramen rotundum
   C. Greater palatine foramen
   D. Glossopharyngeal nerve

3. A 65-year-old woman complains of dysphagia and skin changes. Manometry shows no peristalsis of the lower third of her esophagus and a dilated lower esophageal sphincter. What is the most likely diagnosis?
   A. Achalasia
   B. Dermatomyositis
   C. Scleroderma
   D. Presbyesophagus

4. A 2-year-old boy presents to the emergency room in the middle of the night after unwitnessed ingestion of a foreign body. He appears to be breathing comfortably with no stridor or evidence of drooling. Radiograph of the neck and chest reveals a thin 2 cm wide round object at the level of C6, with a subtle halo of radiolucency around the circumference. What is the next best step in management?
   A. Discharge home with collection cup since the foreign body is likely a coin and will pass on its own
   B. Schedule for elective foreign body removal in the morning
   C. Observe overnight and take him to the OR if he develops respiratory distress or becomes symptomatic
   D. Take emergently to the OR for removal of foreign body

5. A 38-year-old asymptomatic woman is undergoing right thyroid lobectomy. During the procedure, the right recurrent laryngeal nerve cannot be identified. Review of the CT scan is likely to demonstrate
   A. Aberrant take-off of right subclavian artery, which passes behind the esophagus
   B. Anterior displacement of the nerve by an unexpectedly enlarged parathyroid gland
   C. Congenital laryngeal rotation with hypertrophy of Galen anastomosis
   D. Right-sided porencephaly with congenital absence of right vagus nerve

Chapter 36
Neck Spaces and Fascial Planes

Advances in imaging technology and the development of potent antimicrobial therapies have made it possible to manage many deep neck space infections with medical treatment alone. Nonetheless, a thorough understanding of the neck's anatomical spaces and fascial planes remains essential for predicting patterns of disease spread and assessing potential impacts on surrounding structures. Such knowledge is equally critical if surgical intervention becomes necessary. The primary objective of surgery in these cases is to halt disease progression while preserving vital structures. With the growing prevalence of resistant organisms, such as methicillin-resistant *Staphylococcus aureus* (MRSA), surgery will continue to play a vital role in the management of deep neck space infections.

Anatomy

Triangles of the Neck (Figure 36-1)

Anterior Cervical Triangle

A. Boundaries:
   - i. Superior: mandible
   - ii. Anterior: midline
   - iii. Posterior: sternocleidomastoid

B. Subordinate triangles:
   - i. Submaxillary (digastric) triangle
     - a. Superior: mandible
     - b. Anterior: anterior belly of digastric
     - c. Posterior: posterior belly of digastric
   - ii. Carotid triangle
     - a. Superior: posterior belly of digastric
     - b. Anterior: superior belly of omohyoid
     - c. Posterior: sternocleidomastoid
   - iii. Muscular triangle
     - a. Superior: superior belly of omohyoid
     - b. Anterior: midline
     - c. Posterior: sternocleidomastoid
   - iv. Submental (suprahyoid) triangle
     - a. Superior: symphysis of mandible
     - b. Inferior: hyoid bone
     - c. Lateral: anterior belly of digastric

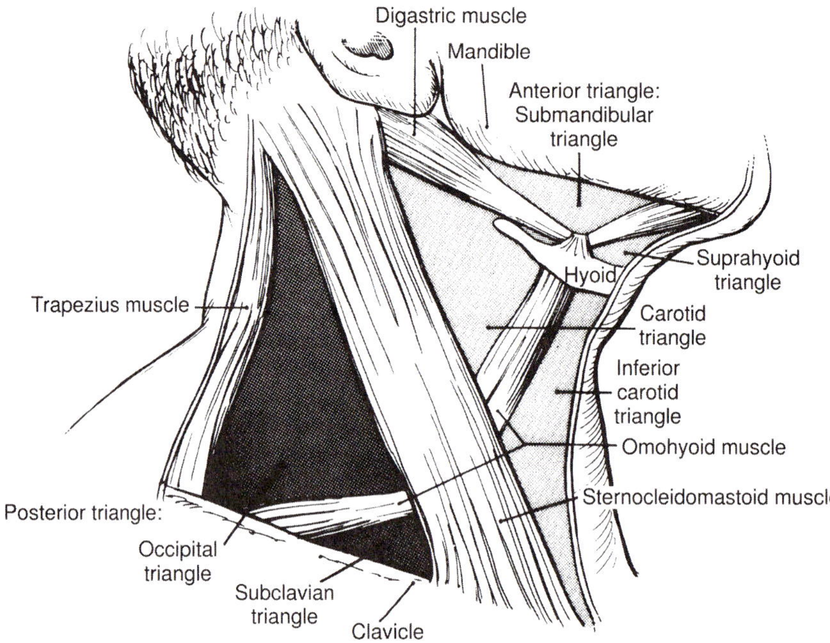

Figure 36-1 Triangles of the neck.

Posterior Cervical Triangle

A. Boundaries:
   i. Anterior: sternocleidomastoid
   ii. Posterior: trapezius
   iii. Inferior: clavicle
B. Subordinate triangles:
   i. Occipital triangle:
      a. Anterior: sternocleidomastoid
      b. Posterior: trapezius
      c. Inferior: omohyoid
   ii. Subclavian triangle:
      a. Superior: omohyoid
      b. Inferior: clavicle
      c. Anterior: sternocleidomastoid

Fascial Planes of the Neck (Figure 36-2)

Superficial Cervical Fascia

A. Envelopes:
   i. Platysma
   ii. Muscles of facial expression
B. Boundaries:
   i. Superior: zygomatic process
   ii. Inferior: clavicle

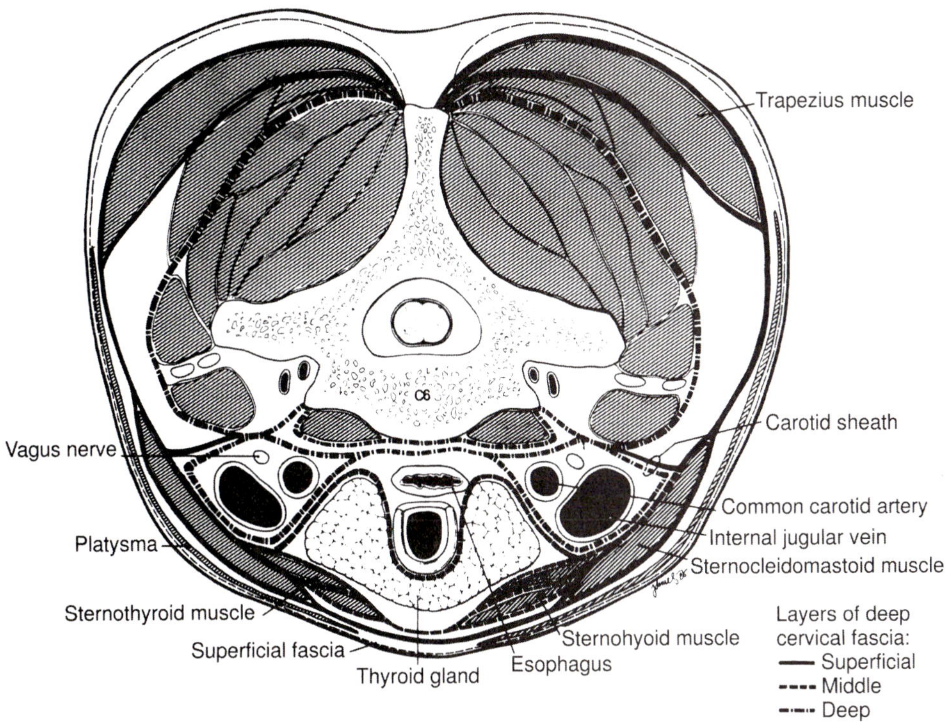

Figure 36-2 Fascial planes of the neck. (*Adapted with permission from Paonessa DF, Goldstein JC: Anatomy and physiology of head and neck infections (with emphasis on the fascia of the face and neck)*, Otolaryngol Clin North Am. *1976 Oct;9(3):561-580.*)

C. Significance:
   i. Main plane of resistance to deep neck spread of cellulitis
   ii. Allows mobility of skin over deep neck structures
   iii. Easily separated when raising neck flaps from deep cervical fascia in the subplatysmal potential space (adipose, sensory nerves, blood vessels)

Deep Cervical Fascia

A. **Superficial layer (investing fascia)**
   i. Envelopes:
      a. Trapezius, sternocleidomastoid, strap muscles
      b. Submandibular and parotid glands
      c. Muscles of mastication: masseter, pterygoids, temporalis
   ii. Boundaries:
      a. Superior: mandible and zygoma
      b. Inferior: clavicle, acromion, spine of scapula
      c. Anterior: hyoid bone
      d. Posterior: mastoid process, superior nuchal line of cervical vertebrae
   iii. Significance:
      a. Outlines masticator space superiorly
      b. Forms stylomandibular ligament posteriorly (separates parapharyngeal and submandibular spaces)
      c. Splits anteroinferiorly to form suprasternal space of Burns

B. **Middle Layer (visceral fascia)**
   i. Envelopes:
      a. Muscular division: strap muscles (sternohyoid, sternothyroid, thyrohyoid, omohyoid)
      b. Visceral division: pharynx, larynx, trachea, esophagus, thyroid, parathyroid, buccinators, constrictor muscles of pharynx
   ii. Boundaries:
      a. Superior: base of skull
      b. Inferior: mediastinum
   iii. Significance:
      a. Forms pretracheal fascia over the trachea
      b. Forms buccopharyngeal fascia which overlies pharyngeal wall (anterior border of retropharyngeal space)
      c. Buccopharyngeal fascia forms midline raphe (posterior midline) and pterygomandibular raphe (lateral pharynx)

C. **Deep Layer (prevertebral fascia)**
   i. Envelopes:
      a. Paraspinous muscles
      b. Cervical vertebrae
   ii. Boundaries:
      a. Superior: base of skull
      b. Inferior: chest
   iii. Significance:
      a. The deep layer of the deep cervical fascia comprises two layers.
      b. The *prevertebral layer* attaches to the transverse processes laterally and covers the vertebral bodies, paraspinous and scalene muscles. Extends from the base of skull to the coccyx.
      c. The *alar layer* lies between the prevertebral layer and the visceral layer of the middle fascia and covers the cervical sympathetic trunk. Extends from the base of skull to the mediastinum.
      d. The *danger space* is the space between the alar and prevertebral layers of the deep cervical fascia.

D. **Carotid Sheath Fascia (Figure 36-3)**
   i. Envelopes:
      a. Common carotid artery
      b. Internal jugular vein
      c. Vagus nerve
   ii. Boundaries:
      a. Superior: base of skull
      b. Inferior: mediastinum
   iii. Significance:
      a. Comprised of all three layers of the deep cervical fascia.
      b. In deep neck space infections, the carotid sheath can act as a barrier to infection spread, but once breached, it can serve as a conduit for rapid extension to the mediastinum (via the "danger space" or retropharyngeal space).
      c. Infections involving the sheath may cause life-threatening complications such as septic thrombophlebitis of the internal jugular vein (Lemierre syndrome).

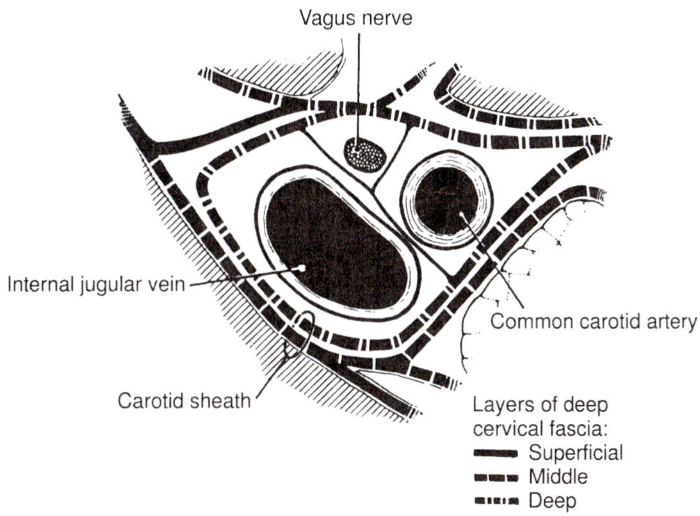

Figure 36-3 Fascial layers of the carotid sheath.

Neck Spaces (Table 36-1)

Parapharyngeal Space

A. Boundaries:
   - i. Superior: base of skull (middle cranial fossa)
   - ii. Inferior: hyoid bone
   - iii. Anterior: pterygomandibular raphe
   - iv. Posterior: prevertebral fascia
   - v. Medial: pharyngobasilar fascia (superiorly), buccopharyngeal fascia covering the superior constrictor
   - vi. Lateral: deep lobe of parotid gland, mandible, medial pterygoid

B. Contents: styloid process divides into a prestyloid and poststyloid compartment. The poststyloid compartment is where the major vessels and cranial nerves reside.
   - i. Prestyloid compartment: muscular (anterior to styloid process)
     - a. Fat
     - b. Lymph nodes
     - c. Internal maxillary artery
     - d. Branches of mandibular nerve V3 (lingual, inferior alveolar, auriculotemporal)
     - e. Medial and lateral pterygoid muscles
     - f. Deep lobe parotid tissue
   - ii. Poststyloid compartment
     - a. Carotid artery
     - b. Internal jugular vein
     - c. Sympathetic chain
     - d. Cranial nerves IX, X, XI, XII

Pterygopalatine (Pterygomaxillary) Fossa

A. Boundaries:
   - i. Superior: sphenoid body, palatine bone (orbital process)
   - ii. Anterior: posterior wall of maxillary antrum

Table 36-1 Major Deep Neck Spaces and Contents

Neck Space	*Boundaries*	*Contents*	*Communicating Spaces*
Peritonsillar	• Medial: palatine tonsil • Lateral: superior constrictor muscle • Anterior: palatoglossus muscle • Posterior: palatopharyngeus muscle	• Loose connective tissue • Tonsillar branches of the lingual, facial, ascending pharyngeal vessels	• Parapharyngeal
Parapharyngeal	• Superior: base of middle fossa • Inferior: hyoid bone • Anterior: pterygomandibular raphe • Posterior: prevertebral fascia • Medial: buccopharyngeal fascia covering the superior constrictor • Lateral: deep lobe parotid, medial pterygoid	Prestyloid • Fat • Lymph nodes • Int. max. artery • Branches of Mandibular Nerve V3 (lingual, inferior alveolar, auriculotemporal) • Pterygoid muscles • Deep lobe parotid Poststyloid • Carotid • Internal jugular • Superior sympathetic • CN IX, X, X, XII	• Peritonsillar • Submandibular • Visceral • Retropharyngeal • Carotid • Masticator • Parotid
Infratemporal fossa	• Superior: sphenoid and temporal skull, fossa medial to zygomatic arch • Anterior: infraorbital fissure, maxilla • Lateral: ramus and coronoid of mandible • Medial: lateral pterygoid plate with tensor and levator palatine muscles	• Pterygoid muscles • Temporalis tendon • Int. max. artery • Pterygoid venous plexus • Mandibular nerve (V3) with otic ganglion	• Temporal fossa • Pterygomaxillary fossa
Pterygomaxillary fossa	• Superior: sphenoid body, palatine bone • Anterior: posterior wall or maxillary antrum • Posterior: pterygoid process, greater wing of sphenoid • Medial: palatine bone • Lateral: temporalis muscle via pterygomaxillary fossa	• Maxillary nerve (V2) • Sphenopalatine ganglion • Int. max. artery	• Infratemporal fossa • Parapharyngeal space • Masticator space • Temporal fossa
Temporal fossa	• Superior: temporal line of skull • Inferior: zygomatic arch • Lateral: temporalis fascia • Medial: pterion skull	• Temporalis muscle • Temporal fat pad	• Infratemporal fossa • Pterygomaxillary fossa
Parotid	• Medial: parapharyngeal space • Lateral: parotid fascia • Superiorly: external auditory canal • Inferiorly: submandibular space	• Parotid gland • Facial nerve • External carotid artery • Posterior facial vein	• Parapharyngeal • Temporal fossa • Masticator

(*Continued*)

Table 36-1 Major Deep Neck Spaces and Contents (*Continued*)

Neck Space	*Boundaries*	*Contents*	*Communicating Spaces*
Masticator	• Medial: fascia medial to pterygoid muscles • Lateral: fascia overlying masseter	• Masseter muscle • Pterygoid muscles • Ramus and posterior body of mandible • Inferior alveolar nerve • Int. max. artery	• Parotid • Pterygomaxillary • Parapharyngeal
Submandibular	• Superior: floor of mouth • Inferior: digastric muscle • Anterior: mylohyoid and anterior belly of the digastric muscle • Posterior: posterior belly of digastric and stylomandibular ligament • Medial: hyoglossus and mylohyoid • Lateral: skin, platysma, mandible	• Sublingual and submandibular glands • Wharton duct • Lingual nerve • Lymph nodes • Facial artery and vein • Marginal branch of VII	• Parapharyngeal • Visceral space
Visceral	• Superior: hyoid bone • Inferior: mediastinum • Anterior: superficial layer of deep cervical fascia • Posterior: retropharyngeal space; prevertebral fascia • Lateral: parapharyngeal space	• Pharynx • Esophagus • Larynx • Trachea • Thyroid gland	• Submandibular • Parapharyngeal • Retropharyngeal
Carotid sheath	• Anterior: sternocleidomastoid muscle • Posterior: prevertebral space • Medial: visceral space • Lateral: sternocleidomastoid muscle	• Carotid artery • Int. jugular vein • Vagus nerve • Ansa cervicalis nerve	• Visceral space • Prevertebral • Parapharyngeal
Retropharyngeal	• Superior: base of skull • Inferior: superior mediastinum • Anterior: pharynx, esophagus • Posterior: alar fascia • Medial: midline raphe of superior constrictor • Lateral: carotid sheath	• Lymph nodes • Connective tissue	• Carotid sheath • Superior mediastinum • Parapharyngeal space • Danger space
Danger	• Superior: Base of skull • Inferior: diaphragm • Anterior: alar fascia of deep layer of deep cervical fascia • Posterior: prevertebral fascia of the deep layer of the deep cervical fascia.	• Loose areolar tissue	• Retropharyngeal • Prevertebral • Mediastinum
Prevertebral	• Superior: base of skull • Inferior: coccyx • Anterior: prevertebral fascia • Posterior: vertebral bodies • Lateral: transverse process of vertebrae	• Dense areolar tissue • Paraspinous, prevertebral, scalene muscles • Vertebral artery and vein • Brachial plexus • Phrenic nerve	• Danger space

   iii. Posterior: pterygoid process, greater wing of sphenoid
   iv. Medial: perpendicular plate of Palatine bone
   v. Lateral: pterygomaxillary fissure
- B. Contents:
   i. Maxillary nerve (V2)
   ii. Sphenopalatine ganglion
   iii. Internal maxillary artery

Masticator Space

- A. Boundaries:
   i. Lateral: fascia over masseter muscle (superficial layer of deep cervical fascia)
   ii. Medial: fascia medial to pterygoid muscles (superficial layer of deep cervical fascia)
- B. Contents:
   i. Masseter muscle
   ii. Lateral and medial pterygoid muscles
   iii. Ramus and posterior body of mandible
   iv. Temporalis muscle tendon
   v. Inferior alveolar nerve (V3)
   vi. Internal maxillary artery

Temporal Fossa

- A. Boundaries:
   i. Superior: temporal line on lateral surface of skull (attachment of temporalis muscle)
   ii. Inferior: zygomatic arch
   iii. Lateral: temporalis fascia
   iv. Medial: skull including pterion
- B. Contents:
   i. Temporalis muscle
   ii. Temporal fat pad

Infratemporal Fossa

- A. Boundaries
   i. Medial: lateral pterygoid plate with tensor and levator palatini muscles, superior constrictor
   ii. Lateral: mandibular ramus, coronoid process
   iii. Anterior: infratemporal surface of maxilla; inferior orbital fissure
   iv. Superior: greater wing of the sphenoid bone, foramen ovale, and spinosum
   v. Inferior: alveolar border of the maxilla
- B. Contents:
   i. Medial and lateral pterygoid muscles
   ii. Insertion of temporalis on coronoid process
   iii. Internal maxillary artery and branches
   iv. Pterygoid venous plexus
   v. V3 with otic ganglion and chorda tympani
   vi. Posterior superior branch of V3

Parotid Space

- A. Boundaries:
   i. Medial: parapharyngeal space
   ii. Lateral: parotid fascia (superficial layer of deep cervical fascia)

iii. Superiorly: external auditory canal
iv. Inferiorly: submandibular space

B. Contents:
i. Parotid gland
ii. Facial nerve
iii. External carotid artery and branches
iv. Retromandibular vein

Peritonsillar Space

A. Boundaries:
i. Medial: Palatine tonsil
ii. Lateral: Superior constrictor muscle
iii. Anterior: palatoglossus muscle
iv. Posterior: palatopharyngeus muscle

B. Contents:
i. Loose connective tissue
ii. Tonsillar branches of lingual, facial, ascending pharyngeal vessels

Submandibular (Submaxillary) Space (Figure 36-4)

A. Boundaries:
i. Superior: floor of mouth mucosa
ii. Inferior: digastric
iii. Anterior: mylohyoid and anterior belly of digastric
iv. Posterior: posterior belly of digastric and stylomandibular ligament
v. Medial: hyoglossus and mylohyoid
vi. Lateral: skin, platysma, mandible

B. The mylohyoid muscle divides the submandibular region into:
a. Sublingual space—above the mylohyoid muscle (between it and the oral mucosa).
b. Submylohyoid (submandibular) space—below the mylohyoid muscle (between it and the skin/subcutaneous tissue of the neck).

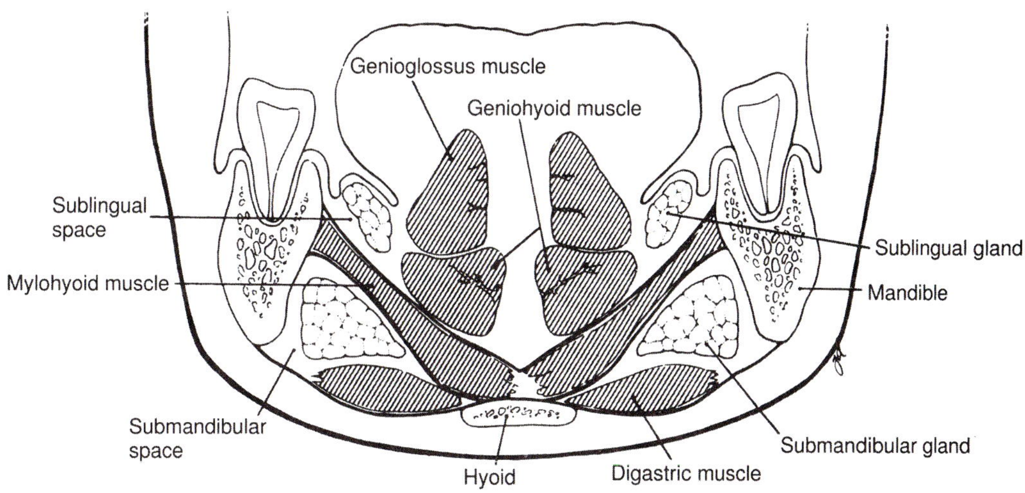

Figure 36-4 Division of the submandibular space into supramylohyoid and inframylohyoid spaces by mylohyoid muscle. (*Adapted with permission from Hollinshead WH, ed:* Anatomy for Surgeons, Head and Neck. *3rd ed. Philadelphia, PA: Harper & Row; 1982.*)

- i. Dental infections and spread:
  - a. The position of a tooth root relative to the mylohyoid line determines where an odontogenic infection spreads:
    1. If the root apex of a mandibular molar is above the mylohyoid line → infection tends to spread into the sublingual space.
    2. If the root apex is below the mylohyoid line → infection tends to spread into the submandibular space.
- i. Sublingual (supramylohyoid) space:
  - a. Sublingual gland
  - b. Wharton duct
  - c. Lingual nerve
- ii. Submandibular (submylohyoid) space:
  - a. Submandibular gland
  - b. Lymph nodes
  - c. Hypoglossal nerve (anterior)
  - d. Facial vein and artery
  - e. Marginal branch of facial nerve

Carotid Sheath Space (See Figure 36-3)

- A. Boundaries:
  - i. Anterior: sternocleidomastoid
  - ii. Posterior: prevertebral space
  - iii. Medial: visceral space
  - iv. Lateral: sternocleidomastoid
- B. Contents:
  - i. Carotid artery
  - ii. Internal jugular vein
  - iii. X nerve
  - iv. Ansa cervicalis

Visceral Space (Pretracheal Space) (Figure 36-5)

- A. Boundaries:
  - i. Superior: hyoid bone
  - ii. Inferior: mediastinum (T4 level/arch of aorta)
  - iii. Anterior: superficial layer of deep cervical fascia
  - iv. Posterior: retropharyngeal space; prevertebral fascia
  - v. Lateral: carotid sheath
- B. Contents:
  - i. Pharynx
  - ii. Esophagus
  - iii. Larynx
  - iv. Trachea
  - v. Thyroid gland

Retropharyngeal (Retrovisceral) Space (Figure 36-6)

- A. Boundaries:
  - i. Superior: base of skull
  - ii. Inferior: the level where the alar fascia fuses with the visceral fascia, which can be anywhere between the T1 and T6 vertebral levels
  - iii. Anterior: pharynx and esophagus (middle layer of deep cervical fascia-buccopharyngeal fascia).

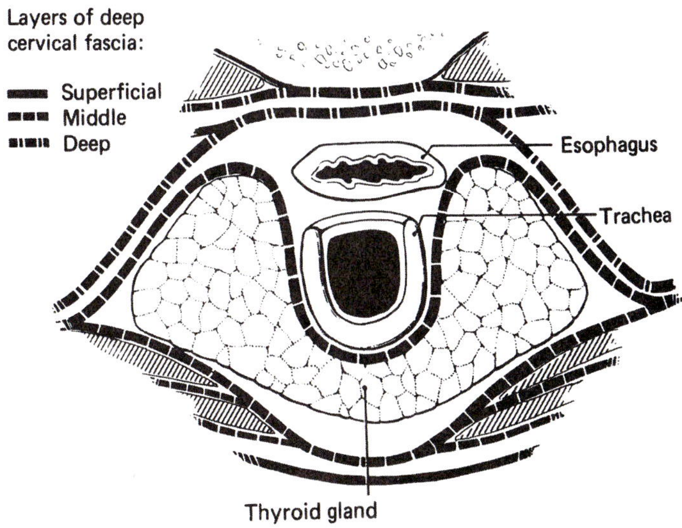

Figure 36-5 Fascial layers surrounding the visceral space.

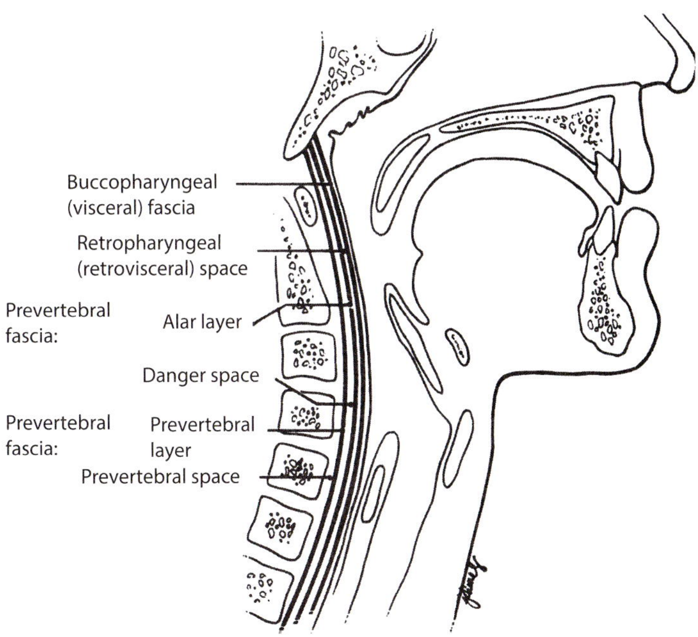

Figure 36-6 Fascial layers of the retrovisceral space. (*Adapted with permission from Hollinshead WH, ed:* Anatomy for Surgeons, Head and Neck. *3rd ed. Philadelphia, PA: Harper & Row; 1982.*)

iv. Posterior: alar fascia
v. Medial: Midline raphe of superior constrictor muscle (results in unilateral abscess in this space)
vi. Lateral: carotid sheath

B. Contents:
i. Retropharyngeal lymph nodes (pediatric infections of sinuses or nasopharynx)
ii. Connective tissue

Danger Space (See Figure 36-6)

A. Boundaries:
i. Superior: base of skull
ii. Inferior: diaphragm
iii. Anterior: alar fascia of deep layer of deep cervical fascia
iv. Posterior: prevertebral fascia of deep layer of deep cervical fascia

B. Contents:
i. Loose areolar tissue
a. Potential for rapid spread of infection through this space resulting in mediastinitis

Prevertebral Space (See Figure 36-6)

A. Boundaries
i. Superior: base of skull
ii. Inferior: coccyx
iii. Anterior: prevertebral fascia (results in midline abscess in this space)
iv. Posterior: vertebral bodies
v. Lateral: transverse process of vertebrae

B. Contents
i. Dense areolar tissue
ii. Muscle: paraspinous, prevertebral, scalene
iii. Vertebral artery and vein
iv. Brachial plexus and phrenic nerve

Deep Neck Space Infections

A. **Etiology (Figure 36-7)**
i. Dental infections (most common in adults)
ii. Acute pharyngitis of Waldeyer ring (most common pediatric)
iii. Cervical lymphadenitis (must rule out associated cancer in adults)
iv. Acute rhinosinusitis (retropharyngeal lymphadenitis)
v. Acute mastoiditis (Bezold abscess)
vi. Iatrogenic (oral surgery; intubation or endoscopic trauma)
vii. Sialadenitis
viii. Foreign body
ix. Penetrating cervicofacial trauma (includes IV drug injection)
x. Cellulitis
xi. Congenital cysts (thyroglossal duct; branchial cleft)
xii. Acquired cysts (laryngoceles; saccular cysts)

B. Microbiology
i. Mixed aerobic and anaerobic polymicrobial oropharyngeal flora (most common)
ii. Streptococcus viridians
iii. *Streptococcus pyogenes* (group A beta-hemolytic strep)
iv. Peptostreptococcus
v. *Staphylococcus epidermidis*

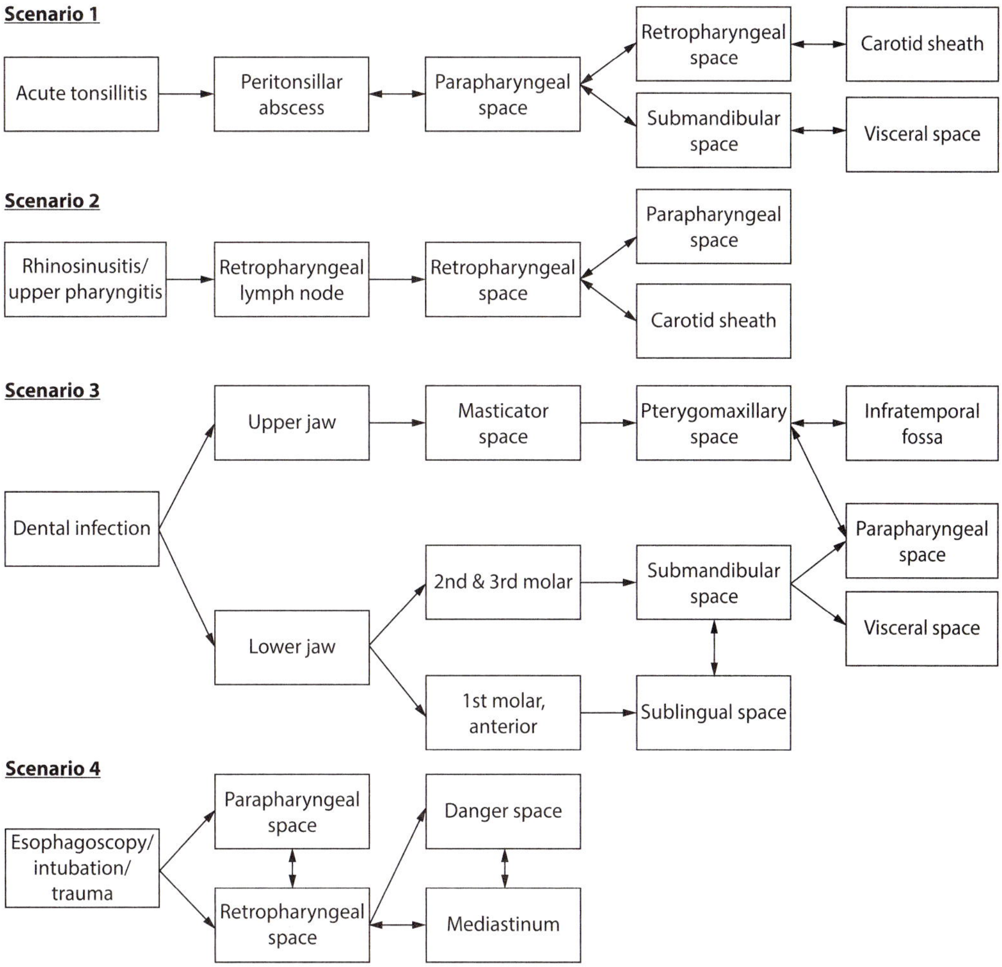

Figure 36-7 Common etiologies and pathways of spread of deep neck infections.

vi. *Staphylococcus aureus*
vii. Methicillin-resistant *Staphylococcus aureus* (MRSA) (the most common isolate in community-acquired deep neck infections in children younger than 2 years)
viii. Bacteroides
ix. Fusobacterium
x. *Neisseria, Pseudomonas, Escherichia, Haemophilus* (occasional)
xi. Actinomyces (gram-positive oropharyngeal saprophyte; necrotic granulomas with "sulfur granules")
xii. Mycobacteria (tuberculous and nontuberculous; necrotizing cervical caseating granulomas; Pott abscess of vertebral body with spread to prevertebral space; acid-fast bacterium; cough, fever, sweats, weight loss).
xiii. *Bartonella henselae* (cat scratch disease; large tender cervical lymph nodes, fever, fatigue)

C. **Clinical evaluation**
   i. **History**
      a. Inflammatory symptoms: pain, fever, swelling, redness.
      b. Localizing symptoms: dysphagia/ odynophagia/drooling (retropharyngeal abscess), "hot potato voice," trismus (peritonsillar abscess), hoarseness, dyspnea, ear pain, neck swelling, otalgia.
      c. Recent infection: dental, sinusitis, otitis.
      d. Recent trauma: IV drug use.
      e. Recent surgery: dental, intubation, endoscopy.
      f. Past medical history: antibiotic allergies.
      g. Immunodeficiency (diabetes; HIV; autoimmune disorder; collagen-vascular disease; hematologic malignancy; recent chemotherapy or steroid) causes increased risk of atypical pathogens and rapidly progressive symptoms.
   ii. **Physical examination**
      a. Palpation:
         1. Localizing tenderness
         2. Crepitus (gas-forming organism)
      b. Otoscopy:
         1. Otitis
         2. Rhinosinusitis
         3. Foreign body
      c. Oral cavity and pharynx
         1. Poor dentition (tooth infection; possible anaerobic organisms)
         2. Trismus (parapharyngeal, pterygomaxillary, masticator spaces)
         3. Floor of mouth edema/tongue swelling (sublingual and submandibular spaces causing Ludwig angina and potential airway emergency)
         4. Purulent discharge from Wharton or Stenson duct (parotid and sublingual/ submandibular spaces; bimanual palpation for stones)
         5. Unilateral tonsil swelling with deviation of uvula (peritonsillar abscess if inflammation present; think tonsillar cancer or parapharyngeal space tumor if no inflammation)
      d. Cranial nerve examination
         1. CN II, III, IV, V, VI can cause reduced vision and eye mobility via retrograde flow of infection through valveless ophthalmic veins.
      e. Awake flexible fiberoptic airway evaluation
         1. Mandatory if hoarseness, dyspnea, stridor, dysphagia/odynophagia without obvious cause.
         2. Normal oximetry common even with critical airway.
         3. Stable airway needs verification prior to transportation to radiology suite.
         4. Identifies patients who may need intubation.
         5. Critical for any floor of mouth swelling
   iii. **Diagnostic testing**
      a. Blood tests
         1. Leukocytosis common
         2. Lack of leukocytosis (virus; immunodeficiency; tumor; congenital cyst)
         3. Basic electrolyte panel (glucose; renal function prior to imaging)
      b. Plain film radiography
         1. Inexpensive, rapid, widely available
         2. Jaw films (Panorex): lucency at dental root (odontogenic abscess); salivary stones

3. Lateral neck films: air-fluid level; greater than 5 mm thickening (child) or greater than 7 mm thickening (adult) at C2 (retropharyngeal infection); arytenoid or epiglottic thickening (thumbprint sign) (supraglottitis)
4. Chest films (dyspnea; tachycardia; cough): lower lobe infiltrate (aspiration pneumonia)

c. Computed tomography with IV contrast
   1. Best overall visualization of neck spaces and structures.
   2. Determines neck spaces requiring drainage, which can be misidentified in 70% of cases based on physical examination alone.
   3. Difficult to differentiate between abscess (pus) or phlegmon (edema). No pus is found on 25% of neck explorations.
   4. Can identify sequelae of infections such as Lemierre syndrome (internal jugular thrombophlebitis).
   5. Metastatic adenopathy (from oropharyngeal primary) needs to be ruled out since this can mimic neck abscess on CT in adult patient.
   6. IV contrast contraindications: allergy, renal failure.

d. Magnetic resonance imaging
   1. Helpful in select cases (intracranial communication or complication; infection of vertebral bodies).
   2. Not recommended if airway or swallowing issues.
   3. MR angiography helpful if thrombi or pseudoaneurysm of major vessel suspected.

e. Ultrasonography
   1. Advantages: noninvasive; no radiation; allows fine needle aspiration; pediatric patients
   2. Limitations: deeper abscesses; obese patients

D. **Treatment**

i. **Airway management**

a. Loss of airway main source of mortality from deep neck infection.

b. Airway most at risk with infection of:
   1. Submandibular space
   2. Parapharyngeal space
   3. Retropharyngeal space

c. Fiberoptic exam evaluates at-risk airway

d. First-line therapy:
   1. Oxygenated face tent with cool humidity
   2. Intravenous steroids
   3. Epinephrine nebulizers
   4. ICU observation if stable and airway greater than 50% normal caliber

e. Intubation
   1. Awake fiberoptic by individual with most expertise
      (a) Awake flexible intubation possible if glottis large enough to pass adult flexible bronchoscope (6 mm)
   2. Surgical airway as a back-up

f. Tracheotomy
   1. Worsening stridor, dyspnea, or obstruction with less than 50% of normal airway diameter.
   2. Awake tracheotomy if patient not easily intubated.
   3. Elective tracheotomy if prolonged (> 48 h) airway edema anticipated. Elective tracheotomy is associated with reduced hospital days and costs compared to prolonged intubation.

ii. **Fluid resuscitation**
   a. Dehydration common due to dysphagia (peritonsillar, retropharyngeal).
   b. Dehydration may be cause of sialadenitis.
   c. Signs of dehydration:
      1. Tachycardia
      2. Dry mucous membranes
      3. Decreased skin turgor
   d. Initial resuscitation: 1 to 2 L of isotonic IV fluids.

iii. **Intravenous antibiotic therapy (Table 36-2)**
   a. Broad-spectrum empiric therapy indicated at diagnosis (should not be delayed for culture).
   b. Clindamycin first-line therapy of choice for children less than 2 years due to increasing rates of MRSA.
   c. Fluids from aspiration/drainage should be sent for culture and sensitivity monitoring.
   d. May delay need for surgical drainage in stable patient:
      1. Contained abscess (intranodal) or phlegmon.
      2. Most pediatric cases.
      3. Abscess size less than 2.5 cm contained within single neck space.
      4. Repeat imaging and/or surgical intervention indicated if no improvement after 48 to 72 hours of therapy.
      5. If improved, continue IV 24 hours beyond symptom resolution followed by 2 weeks of PO therapy.

iv. **Surgical management**
   a. Indications for surgical exploration:
      1. Air-fluid level in neck or gas-forming organism
      2. Abscess present in fascial spaces of neck

Table 36-2 Recommended Antibiotic Therapy for Deep Neck Infections

Community-acquired infection (gram-positive cocci; gram-negative rods; anaerobes)
- Ampicillin-sulbactam 1.5-3.0 g IV every 6 h *or*
- Clindamycin (*if PCN allergy*) 600-900 mg IV every 8 h
- Moxifloxacin (*if Eikenella suspected*) 400 mg QD

Immunocompromised/Nosocomial infection
- **Pseudomonal and gram negatives**
- Ticarcillin-clavulanate 3g IV every 6 h *or*
- Piperacillin-tazobactam 3 g IV every 6 h *or*
- Imipenem-cilastin 500 mg IV every 6 h *or*
- Ciprofloxacin (*if PCN allergy*) 400 mg IV every 12 h
- Levafloxacin (*if PCN allergy*) 750 mg IV every 24 h

Methicillin-resistant *Staphylococcus aureus* (MRSA)
- Clindamycin 600-900 mg every 8 h *and* vancomycin 1 g IV every 12 h
- Trimethoprim-Sulfamethoxazole 10 mg/kg/day divided every 8 h (*if clindamycin resistant*), *and* vancomycin 1 g IV every 12 h

***Necrotizing fasciitis* (mixed gram-positive and expanded anaerobes)**
- Ceftriaxone 2 g IV every 8 h *and* clindamycin 600-900 mg every 8 h *and* metronidazole 500 mg IV every 6 h

Actinomycoses
- Penicillin G 10-20 million units divided every 6 h per day for 4 weeks *then*
- Penicillin V oral 2-4 g divided every 6 h per day for 4-6 mo *or*
- Clindamycin IV and PO if PCN allergy

3. Threatened airway compromise from abscess or phlegmon
4. Failure to respond to 48 to 72 hours of IV antibiotics

b. Goals of surgical exploration:
1. Drainage of abscess for local source control
2. Fluid sampling for culture and sensitivity
3. Irrigation of involved neck space
4. Establishment of external drainage pathway to prevent recurrence
5. Removal of infectious source (dental extraction; foreign body removal)

c. Needle aspiration
1. Lymph nodes containing small abscesses
2. Congenital cysts (with delayed excision after infection subsides)
3. Peritonsillar abscess (adolescent/adult)
4. CT image-guided techniques possible for deep neck spaces

d. Transoral incision and drainage
1. Peritonsillar abscess
   - Performed if not adequately drained by needle aspiration.
   - Premedicate with IV fluids, antibiotics, steroids, and pain medication.
   - Topical anesthetic spray followed by 2 to 3 cc of lidocaine injection over lateral soft palate.
   - Incision on lateral soft palate 5 to 10 mm behind anterior tonsillar pillar, then blunt dissection is used.
   - Irrigation of incision with sterile saline.
   - Oral antibiotics for 10 days.
   - Recurrent abscess possible in 16% adults and 7% of children.
2. Alveolus
   - Remove infected tooth (teeth)
3. Buccal space
   - Incision of buccal mucosa
   - Blunt spreading of buccinator muscle parallel to facial nerve
4. Masticator space
   - Incision through mucosa lateral to retromolar trigone
   - Blunt dissection to masseter
5. Pterygomaxillary space
   - Gingivobuccal sulcus above third maxillary molar with tunnel dissected posteriorly, superiorly, and medially around maxillary tuberosity into pterygomaxillary fossa
   - Alternative route: through posterior wall of maxillary sinus through Caldwell-Luc or transnasal endoscopic approach)
6. Retropharyngeal space
   - Can be accessed transorally or transcervically
   - Incision made over abscess with blunt dissection into pocket

e. Tonsillectomy (peritonsillar abscess)
1. Indications for delayed tonsillectomy:
   - Recurrent peritonsillar abscess
   - Recurrent/chronic tonsillitis
   - Tonsillar hypertrophy with obstructive symptoms
2. Indications for acute "quinsy" tonsillectomy:
   - Recurrent peritonsillar abscess.
   - Massive tonsils causing acute airway obstruction.
   - Patient already under general anesthesia due to comfort issues or poor exposure.

f. Transcervical incision and drainage
   1. Three surgical approaches (choice depends on involved spaces)
      - Modified Blair (parotid) incision
        (a) Parotid space
        (b) Temporal and infratemporal fossa
        (c) Submandibular and parapharyngeal spaces (with extension of neck incision)
      - Horizontal lateral neck incision upper neck (2 cm below mandible body)
        (a) Masticator space (lower border of mandible and staying along lateral surface)
        (b) Submandibular space (between posterior belly of digastric and mandible body)
        (c) Sublingual space (lateral to anterior digastric belly with blunt spreads through mylohyoid muscle)
        (d) Parapharyngeal space/pterygomaxillary space (anterior traction of submandibular gland with blunt dissection superior and medial to posterior belly of digastrics along medial surface of mandible angle)
      - Horizontal lateral neck incision mid-neck (level 3 at cricoid cartilage)
        (a) Retropharyngeal/danger/prevertebral spaces.
        (b) Dissection medial to carotid sheath (retracted laterally) and lateral to strap muscles (retracted medially).
        (c) Deep cervical fascia and paraspinous muscles identified.
        (d) Blunt dissection superior (skull base) to inferior (mediastinum).
   2. Surgical technique
      - Divide superficial cervical fascia and superficial layer of deep fascia.
      - Blunt dissection into involved space.
      - Overdissection puts normal structures at risk and provides path for infection to spread.
      - Avoid finger dissection if suspect IV drug use (broken needles).
      - Culture inflammatory drainage or pus.
      - Copious irrigation of wound.
      - External drainage with Penrose or rubber band drain.
      - Loose closure of wound.

E. **Selected complications of deep neck infections**
   i. **Ludwig angina**
      a. Severe infection of the sublingual and submental spaces.
      b. High mortality from consequent airway compromise.
      c. Most commonly dental origin.
      d. Rapid spread through fascial planes.
      e. Swelling causes posterior tongue displacement and airway obstruction.
      f. Erect, drooling patient, with edema of tongue and floor of mouth; woody, indurated neck.
      g. Airway management is first priority (tracheotomy versus awake fiberoptic intubation).
      h. Wide drainage of bilateral submandibular and sublingual spaces.
      i. IV antibiotic therapy with anaerobic coverage.
   ii. **Cavernous sinus thrombosis**
      a. Life-threatening condition with mortality rate of 30% to 40%
      b. Upper dentition common source of infection

c. Retrograde spread via valveless ophthalmic veins to cavernous sinus
d. Symptoms: fever, lethargy, orbital pain
e. Signs: proptosis, reduced extraocular mobility, dilated pupil, reduced pupillary light reflex

iii. **Lemierre syndrome**
a. Potentially fatal if not recognized.
b. Thrombophlebitis of the internal jugular vein.
c. Most common organism: Fusobacterium necrophorum (anaerobic, gram-negative bacillus).
d. Endotoxin causes platelet aggregation.
e. Associated with pharyngitis, spiking "picket fence" fevers, lethargy, lateral neck tenderness, septic emboli (nodular chest infiltrates and/or septic arthritis).
f. Tobey-Ayer/Queckenstadt test: Compression of internal jugular vein has no effect on CSF pressure in presence of ipsilateral lateral sinus thrombosis when monitoring CSF pressure during a lumbar puncture.
g. CT with IV contrast can demonstrate filling defect in IJ vein.
h. Intravenous beta-lactamase-resistant antibiotics indicated for 2 to 3 weeks.
i. Heparin anticoagulation can be considered.
j. Vein ligation and excision indicated if clinical deterioration occurs.

iv. **Carotid artery pseudoaneurysm or rupture**
a. Associated with infection of retropharyngeal or parapharyngeal space
b. Mortality rate of 20% to 40%
c. Frequency of bleed: internal carotid artery (49%); common carotid artery (9%); external carotid artery (4%); miscellaneous (14%)
d. Possible signs: pulsatile neck mass, Horner syndrome, palsies of CN IX-XII, expanding hematoma, neck ecchymosis, sentinel bright red bleed from nose or mouth, hemorrhagic shock
e. Diagnosis: clinical, MRA, or angiography
f. Treatment: Urgent ligation or stenting of carotid artery

v. **Mediastinitis**
a. Associated with infections of the retropharyngeal (most common; superior mediastinum) and danger spaces (posterior mediastinum to diaphragm).
b. Mortality rate as high as 30% to 40%
c. Possible signs: diffuse neck edema, dyspnea, pleuritic chest pain, tachycardia, hypoxia.
d. Improved survival with combined cervical and thoracic drainage (81%) versus cervical drainage alone (53%)

vi. **Necrotizing fasciitis**
a. Mortality of 20% to 30% (highest with mediastinal extension).
b. More common in older or immunocompromised patients.
c. Dental infection most common cause; mixed aerobic and anaerobic flora.
d. Signs: diffuse spreading erythematous pitting edema of neck with peau-d'orange "orange-peel" appearance; subcutaneous crepitus.
e. Neck CT shows tissue gas in 50% of cases.
f. Treatment: critical care support; broad-spectrum antibiotics, surgical exploration; hyperbaric oxygen.
g. Surgery: debridement to bleeding tissue.

Bibliography

Alexander D, Leonard J, Trail M. Vascular complications of deep neck abscesses. *Laryngoscope*. 1968;78:361.

Brook I. Microbiology and management of peritonsillar, retropharyngeal, and parapharyngeal abscesses. *J Oral Maxillofac Surg*. 2004;62:1545-1550.

Brook I. The increased risk of community-acquired methicillin-resistant *Staphylococcus aureus* in neck infections in young children. *Curr Infect Dis Rep*. 2012;14:119-120.

Cheng J, Elden L. Children with deep space neck infections: our experience with 178 children. *Otolaryngol Head Neck Surg*. 2013;148:1037-1042.

Corsten MJ, Shamji FM, Odell PF, et al. Optimal treatment of descending necrotizing mediastinitis. *Thorax*. 1997;52:702-708.

Crespo AN, Chone CT, Fonseca AS, et al. Clinical versus computed tomography evaluation in the diagnosis and management of deep neck infection. *Sao Paulo Med J*. 2004;122:259-263.

Elliott M, Yong S, Beckenham T. Carotid artery occlusion in association with a retropharyngeal abscess. *Int J Pediatr Otorhinolaryngol*. 2005;70:359-363.

Golpe R, Marin B, Alonso M. Lemierre's syndrome (necrobacillosis). *Postgrad Med J*. 1999;75:141-144.

Kluka EA. Emerging dilemmas with methicillin-resistant *Staphylococcus aureus* infections in children. *Curr Opin Otolaryngol Head Neck Surg*. 2011;19:462-466.

Plaza Mayor G, Martinez-San Millan J, Martinez-Vidal A. Is conservative treatment of deep neck space infections appropriate? *Head Neck*. 2001;23:126-133.

Potter JK, Herford AS, Ellis 3rd E. Tracheotomy versus endotracheal intubation for airway management in deep neck space infections. *J Oral Maxillofac Surg*. 2002;60:349-354.

Smith 2nd JL, Hsu JM, Chang J. Predicting deep neck space abscess using computed tomography. *Am J Otolaryngol*. 2006;27:244-247.

Tung-Yiu W, Jehn-Shyun H, Ching-Hung C, et al. Cervical necrotizing fasciitis of odontogenic origin: a report of 11 cases. *J Oral Maxillofac Surg*. 2000;58:1347-1352.

Questions

1. The prestyloid parapharyngeal space contains all of the following *except*
   A. Fat
   B. Lymph nodes
   C. Glossopharyngeal nerve
   D. Deep lobe of parotid
   E. Medial and lateral pterygoid muscles

2. Masticator space infections can spread directly to all the following spaces *except*
   A. Parotid space
   B. Parapharyngeal space
   C. Pterygomaxillary space
   D. Retropharyngeal space
   E. Buccal space

3. An 18-month-old child presents with fever, dysphagia, drooling, and neck tenderness. The most likely organism is
   A. Pneumococcus
   B. MRSA
   C. *Moraxella catarrhalis*
   D. *Haemophilus influenzae*
   E. Peptostreptococcus

4. A patient presents with fever, dysphagia, and odynophagia. Transoral examination is within normal limits. Pulse oximetry is 100%. The most appropriate next step in management is
   A. Modified barium swallow
   B. PO antibiotic therapy
   C. Antifungal therapy for likely esophageal thrush
   D. Fiberoptic laryngoscopy
   E. Reflux management

5. An emergency room physician calls you concerning a 48-year-old man with poor dentition, unilateral neck swelling, sore throat, odynophagia, and asymmetric tonsils. The neck CT shows a large level II lymph node with rim enhancement just deep to the skin. The next most appropriate step includes
   A. Surgical I&D of the neck abscess
   B. Transoral I&D of presumed peritonsillar abscess
   C. Repeat oral antibiotics with follow-up in 2 to 3 weeks
   D. Dental referral for likely odontogenic infection
   E. Full head and neck examination with FRNA of neck mass for cytopathology

Chapter 37
Thyroid and Parathyroid Glands

"The extirpation of the thyroid gland for goiter typifies perhaps better than any operation the supreme triumph of the surgeon's art."

—Halsted, 1920

Embryology and Anatomy

Embryology

A. The thyroid's medial anlage arises as a ventral diverticulum from the endoderm of the first and second pharyngeal pouches at the foramen cecum.
B. This diverticulum forms at 4 weeks gestation and descends from the base of the tongue to its adult pretracheal position in the root of the neck through a midline anterior path, the thyroglossal duct tract, assuming its final adult position by 7 weeks gestation.
C. If thyroid migration is completely arrested, a lingual thyroid results without normal tissue in the orthotopic location.
D. If the inferior-most portion of the thyroglossal duct tract is maintained, a pyramidal lobe is formed. Persistence of a remnant of thyroid tissue at any point along the rest of the thyroglossal duct tract can develop into a thyroglossal duct cyst that may present as a midline neck mass, frequently in close association with the hyoid bone.
E. The lateral thyroid primordia develop from the fourth and fifth pharyngeal pouches and join the medial anlage as it descends in the neck.
F. Parafollicular C cells arising as ultimobranchial bodies from the neural crest of the fourth pharyngeal pouch migrate and infiltrate the forming lateral thyroid lobes.

Anatomy

A. General
   i. The thyroid gland is composed of two lateral lobes connected by an isthmus, which rests at the level of the second to fourth tracheal cartilages.
   ii. Each thyroid lobe measures approximately 4.5 cm high × 1.5 cm wide × 2 cm deep.
   iii. The pyramidal lobe, a remnant of descent of the thyroid, is present in up to 40% of patients.

B. Fascia
   i. The cervical viscera—including trachea, larynx, and thyroid—are ensheathed by the middle (visceral) layer of the deep cervical fascia.
   ii. It is important to distinguish between the true thyroid capsule and the loose areolar tissue between the true thyroid capsule and strap muscles (ie, the perithyroidal sheath).
      a. True thyroid capsule: tightly adherent to the thyroid parenchyma and continuous with fibrous septa that divide the gland's parenchyma into lobules.
      b. Perithyroidal sheath: thin cobweb-like tissue encountered as the strap muscles are elevated from the ventral surface of the thyroid; typically easily lysed but associated with small bridging vessels extending from the undersurface of the strap muscles to the true thyroid capsule.

C. Ligament of Berry
   i. The thyroid is attached to the laryngotracheal complex through anterior and posterior suspensory ligaments, causing the thyroid to elevate with the larynx and trachea during deglutition.
   ii. The anterior suspensory ligament arises from the anterior aspect of the first several tracheal rings and inserts on the undersurface of the thyroid isthmus.
   iii. The posterior suspensory ligament (ligament of Berry) is a condensation of the middle layer of deep cervical fascia and connects the posterior thyroid to the cricoid cartilage as well as first two tracheal rings. This ligament is well vascularized by a branch of the inferior thyroid artery.
   iv. The recurrent laryngeal nerve (RLN) can actually penetrate the thyroid gland within the ligament of Berry in a significant percentage of patients, placing the RLN at risk of injury in this location during thyroid surgery.

D. Lymphatics
   i. An extensive regional intra- and periglandular lymphatic network exists. The isthmus and medial thyroid lobes drain initially to Delphian, pretracheal, and superior mediastinal nodes, while the lateral thyroid drains initially to the internal jugular chain. The inferior pole drains initially to paratracheal, peri-RLN nodes.

E. Vasculature
   i. The arterial supply to the thyroid is from the superior thyroid artery, a branch of the external carotid artery, and the inferior thyroid artery, a branch of the thyrocervical trunk.
   ii. The thyroid ima artery is a separate, unpaired inferior vessel that may rise from the innominate artery, carotid artery, or aortic arch directly and is present in 1.5% to 12% of cases.
   iii. The thyroid veins include the superior, middle, and inferior thyroid veins (Figure 37-1). The superior thyroid vein is a branch of the internal jugular vein and travels with the superior thyroid artery in the superior pole vascular pedicle. The middle thyroid vein travels without arterial complement and drains into the internal jugular vein. The inferior thyroid vein also travels without arterial complement, extending from the inferior pole to the internal jugular or brachiocephalic vein.

F. Recurrent and superior laryngeal nerves
   i. The cervical branches of the vagus nerve that are of concern during thyroid surgery include both the internal and external branches of the superior laryngeal nerve (SLN), as well as the RLN (Figure 37-2).
   ii. SLN
      a. The SLN's internal branch supplies sensation (general visceral afferents) to the lower pharynx, supraglottic larynx, and base of tongue as well as special visceral afferents to epiglottic taste buds.

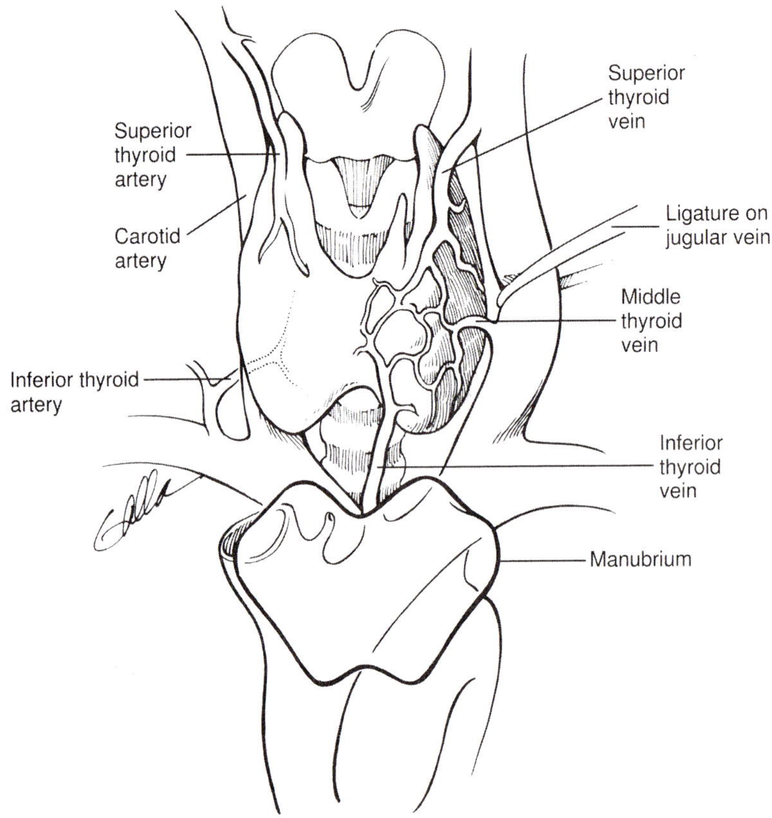

Figure 37-1 Superior thyroid and inferior thyroid arteries (left figure) and superior, middle, and inferior thyroid veins (right figure).

b. The SLN's external branch provides motor innervation (branchial efferents) to the inferior constrictor and cricothyroid muscle. Contraction of the cricothyroid muscle is important for increasing vocal fold length and tension, allowing for the production of high-frequency sounds during phonation.
c. The SLN arises from the upper vagus nerve and descends medial to the carotid sheath. It divides into internal and external branches about 2 to 3 cm above the superior pole of the thyroid.
d. The internal branch travels medially to enter the posterior aspect of the thyrohyoid membrane, providing sensation to the ipsilateral supraglottis.
e. The external branch descends to the region of the superior pole and traverses medially along the inferior constrictor muscle to enter the cricothyroid muscle. In approximately 20% of cases, the external branch travels subfascially on the inferior constrictor as it descends, making it difficult to visualize, though still identifiable through neural stimulation.
f. As the external branch slopes downward on the inferior constrictor musculature, it has a close association with the superior thyroid pole pedicle. Typically, the external branch diverges from the superior pole vascular pedicle 1 cm or more above the superior aspect of the superior thyroid pole. However, in up to

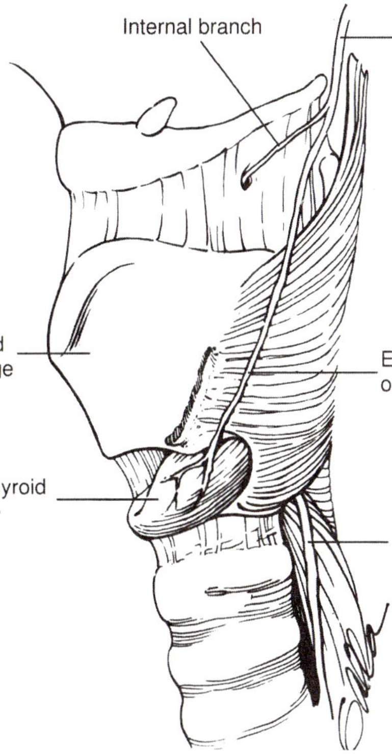

Figure 37-2 Recurrent and superior laryngeal nerves.

20% of cases, the external branch crosses the vessels within 1 cm of the superior thyroid pole, and in 15% of cases (up to 50% in large goiters) the external branch crosses over the actual thyroid parenchyma, placing this nerve at risk during ligation of the superior pole vessels.

iii. RLN
   a. The RLN provides motor innervation (branchial efferents) to the inferior constrictor and all intrinsic laryngeal muscles except the cricothyroid muscle.
   b. The RLN supplies sensation (general visceral afferents) to the larynx (vocal cords and below), upper esophagus, and trachea as well as parasympathetic innervation to the lower pharynx, larynx, trachea, and upper esophagus.
   c. The left RLN emerges from underneath the aortic arch and enters the thoracic inlet on the left in a more paratracheal position and extends upward in a craniocaudal orientation near or within the tracheoesophageal groove, ultimately crossing the distal branches of the inferior thyroid artery. Typically, for the last centimeter or so, the RLN travels close to the lateral border of the trachea prior to laryngeal entry near the ligament of Berry.
   d. The right RLN branches from the vagus nerve and wraps behind the subclavian artery before ascending into the neck base more laterally than does the left RLN. The right RLN ascends the neck in a more oblique fashion, traveling from lateral to medial, crossing the inferior thyroid artery prior to laryngeal nerve entry near the ligament of Berry.

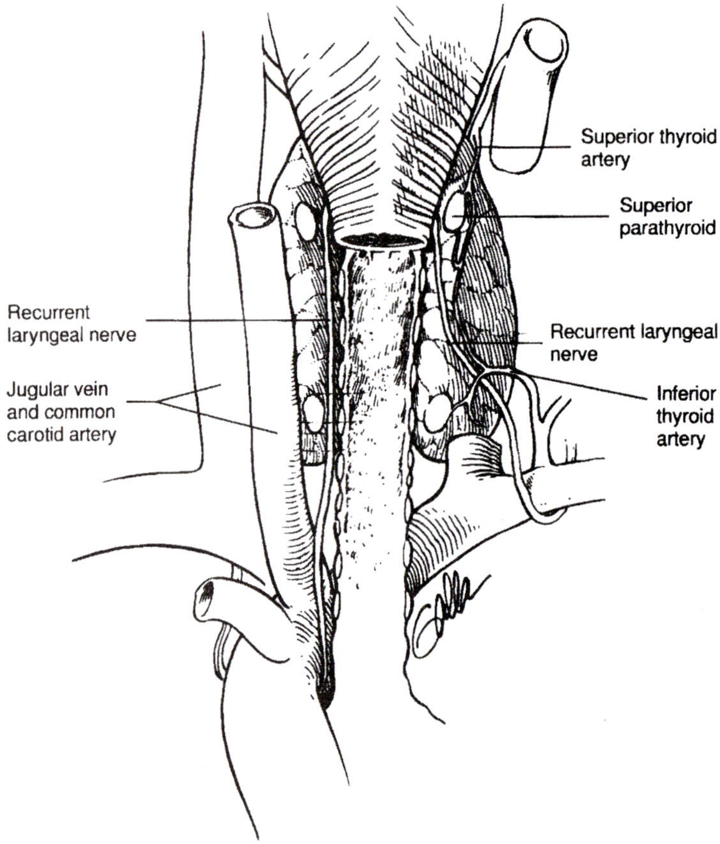

Figure 37-3 Posterior view of thyroid showing superior and inferior thyroid arteries and their relationship to the RLNs.

e. A right nonrecurrent RLN occurs in approximately 0.5% to 1% of cases and is caused by an aberrant right subclavian artery originating from the aortic arch. A left nonrecurrent RLN is extremely rare, with an estimated incidence of 0.04 %, and is associated with major vascular anomalies such as a right-sided aortic arch with aberrant left subclavian artery (often occurring in cases of situs inversus).
f. In approximately one-third of cases, the RLN branches prior to its laryngeal entry point (Figure 37-3).

Physiology

Hormones

The thyroid is composed of follicles that selectively absorb and store iodine from the blood for production of thyroid hormone (TH). The follicles are composed of a single layer of thyroid epithelial cells, which secrete the thyroid hormones triiodothyronine (T_3) and thyroxine (T_4).

Thyroid hormone production and secretion is regulated by thyroid-stimulating hormone (TSH), which is released from the anterior pituitary. As TH decreases, TSH increases in an effort to stimulate the thyroid to maintain the preexisting set point. Increased TSH levels stimulate gland size and vascularity. As TH increases, TSH release is suppressed.

A. T_3
   i. Several times more physiologically potent than T_4.
   ii. 10% of the thyroid gland's production of TH.
   iii. Half-life is 1 day, so reassessment of thyroid function tests after dose change of exogenous T_3 is performed after 1 to 2 weeks.
   iv. 80% of circulating T_3 is created from conversion of T_4 in the periphery.
   v. Exogenous T_3 (levotriiodothyronine) is available as liothyronine.
B. T_4
   i. Strongly correlates with thyroid-stimulating hormone (TSH) level and is believed to play a predominant role in TSH negative feedback.
   ii. About 90% of the thyroid gland's production of TH.
   iii. Half-life is 6 to 7 days; therefore, with a change in exogenous T_4 dose, thyroid function tests are reassessed after 5 to 6 weeks.
   iv. Exogenous T_4 is available as levothyroxine and is the predominant method of thyroid hormone replacement for patients.
C. Both T_4 and T_3
   i. Stimulate calorigenesis, potentiate epinephrine, lower cholesterol levels, and have roles in normal growth and development.
   ii. Iodine is actively transported into the thyroid follicular cell and is oxidized to thyroglobulin-bound tyrosine residues. Four such iodinizations result in the formation of T_4; removal of one residue results in the formation of T_3.
   iii. Subsequently stored bound to thyroglobulin in colloid. The stored hormone is, upon release, taken up from colloid, cleaved off thyroglobulin, and released into the circulation.
   iv. Predominately protein bound (mainly to thyroid-binding globulin), with less than 1% representing free (ie, unbound) hormone.

Pathophysiology

Benign Thyroid Disease

Thyroid Function Tests (Table 37-1)

A. TSH assays (third-generation ultra-sensitivity assays capable of detecting 0.01 mU/L) are often the sole test necessary to sensitively diagnose hypo- or hyperthyroidism.
B. TSH measurements are used not only to monitor replacement therapy but also to measure suppressive therapy postoperatively for thyroid carcinoma.
C. If TSH is high and T_4 is normal, subclinical hypothyroidism is diagnosed. Such a pattern is typically seen in early Hashimoto thyroiditis (also termed chronic lymphocytic thyroiditis).
D. If TSH is low and T_4 and T_3 are normal, subclinical hyperthyroidism is diagnosed. Such a pattern can be seen in multinodular goiter, as the patient develops progressive hyperfunctional regions within the thyroid and moves toward frank hyperthyroidism.
E. Total T_4 and total T_3 laboratory tests measure the total amount of protein-bound and free hormone. There can be significant fluctuation in these total measures depending upon changes in thyroid-binding globulin level.

Table 37-1 Patterns of Thyroid Function Tests

	Euthyroid	*Hyperthyroid*	*Hypothyroid*	*States of High TBG*	*States of Low TBG*
TSH	Normal	↓	↑	Normal	Normal
Total T_4	Normal	↑	↓	↑	↓
T_3 resin uptake (or THBR)	Normal	↑	↓	↓	↑
Free T_4 index	Normal	↑	↓	Normal	Normal

TBG, thyroid-binding globulin; TSH, thyroid-stimulating hormone; T_4, thyroxine; T_3, triiodothyronine.

i. **T_3 resin uptake test:** Allows for correction of total T_4 level for fluctuation in thyroid-binding globulin. T_3 resin uptake measures the binding capacity of existing thyroid-binding globulin. The more available binding sites on native thyroid-binding globulin, the less resin uptake of radio-tagged T_3. Thus, in states of thyroid-binding globulin excess, T3 resin uptake is *low*.
   a. High levels of thyroid-binding globulin occur in pregnancy or with use of birth control pills.
   b. Low thyroid-binding globulin levels can occur in hypoproteinemic states, acromegaly, Cushing syndrome, and with certain drugs such as androgens and anabolic steroids.

Hypothyroidism

- Hypothyroidism is the functional state characterized by decreased TH. In primary gland failure, decreased TH results in increased TSH. In central hypothyroidism (rare), TSH is decreased with resultant decreased TH.
- Hypothyroidism has a variety of causes and can present with a multitude of symptoms. (Table 37-2).
- Treatment for hypothyroidism is typically started at a low dose to avoid abrupt correction, especially in elderly patients or in patients with coronary artery disease.
- Typically, T_4 is started at 0.05 mg PO per day and is slowly increased, titrated to thyroid function levels.
- *Myxedema* refers to nonpitting edema secondary to increased glycosaminoglycan in tissue in severe hypothyroidism.

Table 37-2 Hypothyroidism

Differential Diagnosis	*Clinical Manifestations*
1. Primary gland failure (common) A. Hashimoto thyroiditis B. Iodine deficiency C. Associated with thyroiditis (lymphocytic/postpartum, subacute) D. Radiation-induced (I^{131} or external beam) E. Postsurgical F. Drugs (lithium, iodine) G. Hereditary metabolic defects in hormonogenesis 2. Central hypothyroidism (rare)	Fatigue, slow mentation, change in memory, depression, cold intolerance, hoarseness, brittle hair, dry skin, thick tongue, weight gain, constipation/ileus, menstrual disturbance, bradycardia, nonpitting edema, hyporeflexia, psychosis, hyponatremia, hypoglycemia, coma. In infants, intellectual disability /cretinism.

Table 37-3 Hyperthyroidism

Differential Diagnosis	*Clinical Manifestations*
1. Graves' disease 2. Toxic nodule/multinodular goiter 3. Thyroiditis 4. Exogenous hyperthyroidism/struma ovarii/ functional thyroid cancer 5. Thyrotropin, thyrotropin-like secreting tumor (pituitary, trophoblastic, other)	Weight loss, fatigue, nervousness, tremor, palpitations, increased appetite, heat intolerance, muscle weakness, diarrhea, sweating, menstrual disturbance

Hyperthyroidism

- *Hyperthyroidism* refers to the physiologic state of increased TH biosynthesis and secretion. In primary hyperthyroidism, this leads to TSH suppression.
- Hyperthyroidism can occur as a result of several pathologic entities and presents with characteristic symptoms (Table 37-3).
- By far, Graves' disease and toxic nodular goiter account for most cases of hyperthyroidism. Hyperthyroidism caused by thyroiditis is typically self-limiting.
- *Thyrotoxicosis* refers to the clinical syndrome of TH excess.

Graves' Disease

A. An autoimmune disease that accounts for 60% of clinical hyperthyroidism.
B. Results from activating autoantibodies binding to the TSH receptor, which results in TSH-like activity.
C. More common in females and often presents in the third to fourth decades.
D. Physical examination shows a diffusely enlarged thyroid with increased metabolic activity that is reflected by increased blood flow; thus, a thyroid bruit can often be heard.
E. Thyroid histology shows scattered lymphocytic infiltration.
F. Patients may have an infiltrative ophthalmopathy with exophthalmos. Although considered a part of Graves' disease, the ophthalmopathy typically follows an independent course relative to the thyroid.
G. Patients may also exhibit an infiltrative dermopathy, resulting in localized myxedema (eg, pretibial) and rarely thyroid acropachy, characterized by digital clubbing and edema of the hands and feet.
H. Iodine-123 (I^{123}) scanning shows a diffuse increased gland uptake.
I. Treatments include radioactive iodine ablation, antithyroid drugs, or surgery. Treatment in the United States often involves antithyroid drugs with more definitive treatment with radioactive iodine (RAI) or surgery in refractory or recurrent cases. Treatment with RAI can worsen Graves'-related ophthalmopathy, with surgery usually preferred in these cases.

Toxic Nodular Goiter: Hyperthyroidism can also arise from one or more toxic nodules. In these cases, unlike Graves' disease, the hyperfunctional tissue is restricted to one or more regions within the thyroid gland, which is enlarged in a nodular pattern. Toxic nodular goiter accounts for 5% to 15% of cases of hyperthyroidism but is the most frequent cause of thyrotoxicosis in the elderly.

Toxic Multinodular Goiter

A. Develops from a preexisting nontoxic nodular goiter.
B. Occurs more frequently in endemic goiter, occurring in iodine-deficient regions, and presents more commonly in females.
C. No eye or skin findings that characterize Graves' disease.
D. Progressive nodule formation and evolution of hyperfunctional regions, which elaborate excess TH, resulting in suppression of TSH. This TSH suppression results in the adjacent normal gland becoming less active on I^{123} scans, with hyperfunctional areas lighting up "hot."
E. In early stages, the hyperfunctional region is not autonomous, and a suppression I^{123} shows no uptake. This prehyperthyroid pattern of suppressed TSH but normal T_4 and T_3 is referred to as subclinical hyperthyroidism.
F. The development of overt hyperthyroidism in such patients with exogenous iodine administration (eg, iodine CT contrast) is referred to as the Jod-Basedow phenomenon.
G. With time, the hyperfunctional regions become truly autonomous, continuing to secrete TH despite significant TSH suppression. When true autonomy occurs, I^{123} scanning shows focal hot regions with complete absence of adjacent normal gland. Suppression scanning at this time shows ongoing focal uptake, demonstrating autonomy despite TSH suppression.

Uninodular Toxic Goiter

A. Hyperthyroidism typically does not occur until the nodule is larger than 2.5 cm.
B. Such nodules are usually characterized by enhanced T_3 production relative to T_4.
C. Unlike Graves' disease, there is a low rate of spontaneous remission after antithyroid drug therapy is withdrawn.
D. Treatment is either surgery or radioactive iodine; antithyroid medications are considered only as pretreatment prior to more definitive surgical or radioablative treatment.
E. Surgery quickly and definitively corrects hyperthyroidism and is associated with low morbidity.

Treatment of Hyperthyroidism

Medical Treatment of Hyperthyroidism

When medical treatment is initially offered for hyperthyroidism, treatment is usually initiated with antithyroid drugs to render the patient euthyroid. Radioiodine ablation represents a more definitive treatment modality and involves the oral administration of I^{131}. Areas of increased uptake are preferentially injured through beta-radiation. It is contraindicated in women who are pregnant or lactating.

Antithyroid Medication

A. Propylthiouracil (PTU) and methimazole (thionamides):
   i. Block iodine organification and TH synthesis. PTU also blocks peripheral conversion of T_4 to T_3.
   ii. PTU is given every 8 hours, and methimazole is given daily.
   iii. Typically takes 6 to 8 weeks to render a patient euthyroid.
   iv. Side effects include rash, fever, a lupus-like reaction, and bone marrow suppression (0.3%-0.4% of cases), which is reversible if detected early. PTU has recently been associated with liver failure, especially in children, so methimazole is typically considered the first-line therapy for hyperthyroidism except during pregnancy and lactation.
   v. While both methimazole and PTU cross the placenta equally, there have been rare reports of birth defects with methimazole and so PTU is preferred. PTU also shows less concentration in breast milk than methimazole.

B. Iodides:
   i. Potassium iodide and Lugol solution inhibit organification and prevent TH release.
   ii. Given preoperatively to decrease thyroid gland vascularity.
   iii. Antithyroid effect is transient, with escape within 2 weeks, and is termed the Wolff-Chaikoff effect.
   iv. Prolonged high-dose iodides, especially in the setting of toxic nodular goiter, can result in hyperthyroidism.

C. Beta-adrenergic blockers
   i. Examples include propranolol or nadolol
   ii. Block peripheral TH effects (do not alter TH production)
   iii. Useful in symptomatic control (while other treatments are initiated) and also in transient forms of hyperthyroidism associated with thyroiditis
   iv. Contraindicated in patients with asthma, chronic obstructive pulmonary disease (COPD), cardiac failure, insulin-dependent diabetes, bradyarrhythmias, and those taking monoamine oxidase inhibitors

D. *Advantages* of thionamide treatment of hyperthyroidism:
   i. Quick onset of action
   ii. May facilitate remission with ongoing euthyroid status after discontinuation of the medicine

E. *Disadvantages* of thionamide treatment of hyperthyroidism:
   i. Risk of agranulocytosis
   ii. High rate of hyperthyroid relapse (74% of patients relapsed if followed over a period of 5 years), although newer data suggest improved relapse rates with longer-term use of antithyroid medication, particularly for hyperthyroidism due to Graves' disease.
   iii. Liver failure with PTU

Radioactive Iodine Ablation

A. *Advantages:* Represents an effective, relatively inexpensive, safe, and definitive treatment option.

B. *Disadvantages*:
   i. Up to 80% of patients with Graves' disease and up to 50% of those with toxic nodules treated with radioactive iodine ultimately become hypothyroid.
   ii. Risk of developing malignancy
      a. Some reluctance to treat young patients with radioablation given the potential for long-term development of second malignancies
   iii. Teratogenic effects (conception must be delayed more than 6 months after radioactive iodine treatment)
   iv. Can worsen Graves' ophthalmopathy (especially in smokers)
   v. Less rapid normalization of TH levels than surgery (typically 6-8 weeks)

Surgical Treatment of Hyperthyroidism

A. *Advantages:*
   i. Correction of the hyperthyroid state faster than radioactive iodine and without the risks of antithyroid drugs.
   ii. Especially suited for toxic nodules, where one discrete region of the thyroid may be resected with preservation of contralateral normal tissue.
   iii. Many studies show that when properly done, partial thyroid surgery poses a lower risk of hypothyroidism than radioactive iodine ablation.

B. Surgery for Graves' is considered when there is: (1) failure or significant side effects after medical treatment, (2) need for rapid return to euthyroidism, (3) massive goiter, (4) a wish to avoid radioactive iodine, (5) concern regarding RAI and eye disease or, (6) Graves' with nodules.
C. Thyroid storm, or thyrotoxic crisis, is a rare but acute life-threatening hypermetabolic state induced by the excessive release of thyroid hormones. Preoperative endocrinologic management is essential to return the patient to the euthyroid state to lower the risk of perioperative thyroid storm. Euthyroidism is typically obtained by antithyroid drugs used for 6 weeks prior to surgery with or without beta-adrenergic blockers.
D. When the patient is euthyroid, some consider a 2-week course of preoperative iodide (super saturated potassium iodide [SSKI] or Lugol solution), which is believed to decrease vascularity and gland friability, although the efficacy of such treatment is controversial.
E. Calcium and 25-hydroxy vitamin D should be checked preoperatively and repleted if necessary given the risk of postoperative hypoparathyroidism.
F. The goal of surgery for hyperthyroidism is to remove the hyperfunctional tissue, which typically means total thyroidectomy for Graves' disease. Implicit in this surgical philosophy is that it is preferable to render the patient hypothyroid rather than to provide inadequate resection with recurrent hyperthyroidism.
G. Surgical treatment for Graves' disease:
    i. Total thyroidectomy (or near-total thyroidectomy) is the preferred surgical approach to Graves' disease according to the American Thyroid Association (ATA).
    ii. Alternatives include total lobectomy on one side and contralateral subtotal resection or bilateral subtotal thyroidectomy (decreased risk of hypothyroidism but increased risk of recurrent hyperthyroidism).
    iii. The risk of postoperative hypocalcemia is thought to be higher in Graves' patients due to their underlying hypermetabolic state and increased risk of "hungry bone syndrome."
    iv. Complication rates for total thyroidectomy for Graves' disease in expert hands have been shown to be less than 2% risk of permanent hypoparathyroidism and less than 1% risk of permanent vocal cord paralysis. Mortality is between 1 in 10,000 and 5 in 1,000,000.
H. Surgical treatment for toxic nodule(s):
    i. Resection of the involved portion of the gland (lobectomy).
    ii. In toxic multinodular goiter, it is best to consider both scintillographic and sonographic information in constructing a rational surgical plan, as hot regions of the gland may not correspond to the areas of gross nodularity.
I. Treatment of thyroid storm:
    i. Thyroid storm can happen in the preoperative, intraoperative, or postoperative setting, with signs and symptoms including tachycardia, nausea, tremor, altered mental status, tachycardic hyperthermia, and/or cardiac arrhythmia.
    ii. If thyroid storm occurs during thyroidectomy, the procedure should be stopped.
    iii. Management of thyroid storm includes IV beta blockade, steroids, propylthiouracil, and sodium iodine.

Thyroiditis

Hashimoto Thyroiditis (Chronic lymphocytic thyroiditis)

A. Most common form of thyroiditis and most common single thyroid disease in iodine-sufficient countries.
B. Autoimmune disease with increased thyroid peroxidase antibodies in 70% to 90% of patients.

C. More common in females and often presents in third to fifth decades.
D. Patients presenting with the disease are typically euthyroid but can show symptoms of hypothyroidism in up to 20% of cases. Hypothyroidism often develops with time and results from progressive loss of follicular cells.
E. Presents as painless, firm, symmetric goiter, although regional pain has been reported; typically, both lobes are enlarged.
F. Histologically, there is lymphocytic infiltration with germinal center formation, follicular acinar atrophy, Hürthle cell metaplasia, and fibrosis.
G. $Iodine^{123}$ scanning typically contributes little information to the workup.
H. If patient is hypothyroid, treatment with TH resolves symptoms and usually decreases the size of the goiter.
I. Surgery is considered in cases of large symptomatic goiter refractory to TH and in certain cases of refractory generalized symptoms or rare systemic complications of Hashimoto's.
J. Development of any discrete palpable abnormality not part of the diffuse goiter process (ie, a discrete nodule) should be evaluated with fine-needle aspiration (FNA) despite a preexisting diagnosis of thyroiditis.
K. Rarer fibrous variants of Hashimoto form a massive, firm goiter.
L. A rare complication of Hashimoto is thyroid lymphoma. A rapidly enlarging mass within a Hashimoto gland should raise concern for lymphoma and warrants biopsy.

Subacute Granulomatous Thyroiditis

A. Also known as De Quervain thyroiditis—most common cause of painful thyroid
B. Viral in etiology and presents with enlarged, painful thyroid often seen after upper respiratory tract infection—fever and malaise are common.
C. Pain in the perithyroid region typically radiates up the neck to the angle of the jaw and ear. The pain and enlargement may only involve a portion of the gland and later migrate to the opposite side.
D. About 50% of patients with subacute granulomatous thyroiditis (SGT) present with hyperthyroidism with an elevated TH and sedimentation rate. Pain in the hyperthyroid phase typically resolves in 3 to 6 weeks.
E. I^{123} scanning typically shows less than 2% uptake—this low uptake distinguishes the transient hyperthyroidism of SGT from that of Graves' disease or toxic multinodular goiter.
F. About 50% of patients will enter a hypothyroid phase lasting several months. Most patients ultimately revert to euthyroidism with only 5% developing permanent hypothyroidism.
G. Self-limiting—treat as needed with nonsteroidal anti-inflammatory drugs (NSAIDs) and rarely steroids.

Subacute Lymphocytic Thyroiditis

A. Also termed silent, painless, or postpartum thyroiditis.
B. Etiology unknown but believed to be an autoimmune process.
C. Painless with course similar to subacute thyroiditis.
D. Occurs sporadically but is common in postpartum females (up to 5%).
E. Presents as painless, symmetric thyroid enlargement and reversible hyperthyroidism.
F. Thyrotoxicosis is generally self-limiting with no treatment needed, although permanent hypothyroidism can result in 20% of patients (or more).

Acute Suppurative Thyroiditis

A. Rare thyroid infection often with abscess formation.
B. Most often bacterial (commonly due to *Staphylococcus*, *Streptococcus*, or *Enterobacter*) but can be fungal or even parasitic.

C. Typically presents in the setting of an upper respiratory tract infection (URTI).
D. Treatment is with antibiotics and often incision and drainage in the case of abscess.
E. A left pyriform sinus fistula has been found to be one cause of the spread of infection, especially in children. After acute treatment, especially with recurrent episodes, evaluation for this condition is reasonable with barium swallow, CT, or endoscopy.

Riedel Struma (Invasive Fibrous Thyroiditis)

A. Rare inflammatory process of unknown etiology—the thyroid equivalent to sclerosing cholangitis or retroperitoneal fibrosis.
B. Large, nontender goiter with a woody consistency fixed to surrounding structures.
C. Clinical course characterized by progressive regional symptoms including dysphagia, tracheal compression, and possibly RLN paralysis.
D. Typically euthyroid at presentation but can progress to hypothyroidism.
E. Thyroid histology: extensive fibrosis, the hallmark of which is extrathyroidal extension of fibrosis into surrounding neck structures.
F. Can be confused with malignancy and requires biopsy, often in the form of isthmusectomy, which may be sufficient to relieve symptoms of tracheal and esophageal pressure. Aggressive surgery is usually avoided because of the loss of surgical planes due to extensive extrathyroidal fibrosis. Treatment with steroids can be helpful.

Drug-Induced Thyroiditis

A. Common drugs: amiodarone, interferon-alpha, interleukin-2, lithium, minocycline.
B. Thyroid abnormalities usually resolve when the offending drug is stopped.
C. Amiodarone: can produce thyrotoxicosis through either iodine-induced hyperthyroidism or destructive thyroiditis.

Euthyroid Goiter (Nontoxic Diffuse and Multinodular Goiter)

A. Thyroid enlargement without significant functional derangement may occur with diffuse enlargement (nontoxic diffuse goiter) or through multinodular formation (multinodular goiter).
B. Goiter development can be sporadic or associated with iodine deficiency, inherited metabolic defects, or exposure to goitrogenic agents.
C. Thyroid function tests are normal for nontoxic diffuse goiter. For multinodular goiter, thyroid function tests may show a normal T_4 and T_3, with TSH low normal (subclinical hyperthyroidism) as some of the nodules slowly grow toward autonomy.
D. Goiter may be stable over a period of years or can slowly grow. Nodules within multinodular goiter may also undergo rapid, painful enlargement secondary to hemorrhage. Such a rapid increase in size may be associated with pain and an increase in regional symptoms, including neck pressure, positional shortness of breath, and, rarely more concerning airway distress.
E. 15% to 45% of patients with large cervical goiters or substernal goiters may be asymptomatic. Of note, patients may be asymptomatic and yet have radiographic evidence of substernal extension or tracheal compression and evidence of airway obstruction on flow volume studies.
F. When patients with goiter are symptomatic, they may present with chronic cough, nocturnal dyspnea, choking, dysphagia, and difficulty breathing in different neck positions or in recumbent position. Up to 20% of patients with large cervical and retrosternal goiters may present with acute airway distress, rarely requiring intubation.

G. Surgical consideration should be given to all symptomatic patients, have significant radiographic evidence of airway obstruction or show evidence of substernal goiter (with substernal tissue representing abnormal thyroid tissue that is unavailable for physical exam, monitoring, or FNA). Consideration can be given for significant cosmetic defect as well.
H. The physical examination of such patients should include evaluation of respiratory status, tracheal deviation, and substernal extension. The development of venous engorgement or subjective respiratory discomfort with the arms extended over the head (Pemberton sign) can suggest obstruction of the thoracic inlet from a large or substernal goiter.
I. All patients should have vocal cord mobility assessed.
J. All patients should have a TSH test to rule out subclinical hyperthyroidism.
K. Ultrasound (US) should be performed to evaluate for nodules. Decision for fine-needle aspiration (FNA) biopsy of the nodules should be based on size and ultrasonographic pattern (see thyroid nodule work-up in the following section).
L. If there is significant concern regarding tracheal deviation, compression or substernal extension, an axial CT scan should be performed.
M. Thyroxin suppression can reduce goiter size and has been found to be more helpful in diffuse than in multinodular goiter. The reduction in goiter size is, however, unpredictable. Goiter growth typically resumes after T_4 discontinuation.
N. During surgery for goiter, nerve identification is necessary as in all cases of thyroidectomy. It may be necessary to use a superior approach with identification of the nerve at the laryngeal entry point after superior pole dissection and then retrograde dissection of the nerve.
O. Multiple surgical series suggest that sternotomy for large cervical and substernal goiters is rarely needed. The surgery necessary for cervical and substernal goiter ranges from lobectomy to total thyroidectomy. Subtotal thyroidectomy may rarely be appropriate to preserve parathyroid tissue and avoid permanent hypoparathyroidism when there is concern for injury to multiple parathyroid glands. The incidence of carcinoma (usually small intrathyroidal papillary carcinomas) in such multinodular goiters is approximately 7.5%.

Thyroid Nodules

Background

A. Thyroid nodules are discrete lesions radiographically distinct from surrounding thyroid parenchyma. They are common and increase with age, with the overall prevalence of *palpable* nodules about 5% in women and 1% in men. Detection rates increase to up to 19% to 68% with use of high-resolution ultrasound (with higher rates in women and elderly). Some studies suggest a 50% detection rate of thyroid nodules on high-resolution ultrasound by the time patients reach 60 years old.
B. Though most often asymptomatic, thyroid nodules require evaluation largely because of the risk of malignancy, which is about 10% in thyroid nodules greater than 1 cm. Just over 62,000 new cases of thyroid cancer were estimated in 2023. Until recently, the incidence of thyroid cancer was increasing both throughout the world and in the United States, from 4.9 cases per 100,000 in 1975 to 14.2 per 100,000 in 2014. Much of this increase is attributed primarily to increased detection and evaluation of thyroid nodules. However, with the use of stricter diagnostic criteria for thyroid cancer, the incidence is now decreasing by about 2% per year since 2014.

Table 37-4 Differential Diagnosis of the Thyroid Nodule

95%	Colloid nodule—MNG
	Adenoma
	Cyst
	Focal thyroiditis
	Carcinoma
	S/P hemithyroidectomy
	Hemiagenesis
	Metastasis to thyroid
	Thyroglossal duct cyst
	Nonthyroid:
	Lymph node
	Parathyroid cyst
	Cystic hygroma, dermoid, teratoma
	Laryngocele

MNG, multinodular goiter; S/P, status post.

C. Ninety-five percent of thyroid nodules are benign colloid nodules, adenomas, thyroid cysts, focal thyroiditis, or cancer. However, less likely entities are possible (see Table 37-4).

D. A colloid or adenomatous nodule is a nodule within a gland affected by multinodular goiter. It represents a focal hyperplastic disturbance in thyroid architecture and is generally not a true clonal neoplasm. The umbrella term for these nodules is "follicular nodular disease."

E. True follicular adenomas are monoclonal tumors arising from follicular epithelium and can be autonomous or nonautonomous. It is unknown whether some follicular adenomas have the capability of evolving into follicular carcinoma.

Evaluation and Management of Thyroid Nodules

History The history and physical examination provide the first steps in thyroid cancer risk assessment and provide a clinical context for interpretation of further diagnostic studies including ultrasound and fine-needle aspiration (Table 37-5).

A. Age: Patients less than 30 years of age have a higher risk of carcinoma. In patients older than 60 years of age, follicular nodular disease is more common, and malignant disease, if found, is thought to have a worse prognosis.

B. Gender: Males have an increased risk of a thyroid nodule being malignant, up to double that of females in some studies.

C. Radiation exposure: Childhood exposure to ionizing radiation (such as with the Chernobyl incident) has been shown to significantly increase the risk of papillary thyroid cancer as well as result in more aggressive malignant behavior. Low-dose radiation therapy (eg, 200-500 rads) has been given in the past for adenoidal and tonsillar hypertrophy, thymic enlargement, facial acne, and tinea of the head and neck. Such treatment has been stopped in the United States since 1955. Approximately 1.8% to 10% of patients exposed to low-dose radiation may eventually develop thyroid carcinoma.

Table 37-5 Degree of Clinical Concern for Carcinoma in a Thyroid Nodule Based on History and Physical Examination

Less Concern	*More Concern*
Chronic stable examination	Age < 30 > 60 years
Evidence of a functional disorder (eg, Hashimoto, toxic nodule)	Males
Multinodular gland without dominant nodule	Rapid growth, pain
	History of radiation exposure
	Family history of thyroid carcinoma
	Hard, fixed lesion
	Lymphadenopathy
	Vocal cord paralysis
	Size > 4 cm
	Aerodigestive tract compromise (eg, stridor, dysphagia)

Nodules may develop with a latency of up to 20 to 30 years, requiring ongoing vigilance. Exposure to nuclear fallout, high-dose therapeutic radiation for Hodgkin disease, or scatter exposure from breast radiation also seems to increase the risk of thyroid nodular disease and thyroid cancer.

D. Significant family history of thyroid cancer, especially medullary carcinoma or multiple endocrine neoplasia Type 2 (MEN 2), increases the risk of carcinoma.

Physical Examination

A. Technique: It is best to orient toward the thyroid gland through adjacent cartilaginous laryngeal reference points. Once the thyroid cartilage notch is identified, the anterior ring of the cricoid can be easily found. One thumb-breadth below the cricoid, the isthmus can be palpated on the underlying upper cervical trachea. When identifying the isthmus in the midline or the bilateral thyroid lobes laterally, it is useful to have the patient swallow to have the thyroid roll upward underneath the thumb. With such an examination, nodules of 1 cm or greater can often be detected.

B. Risk of malignancy:
   i. Size of nodule: The risk of follicular malignancy is higher in larger nodules. Larger nodules, particularly greater than 4 cm, are also more difficult to assess, given a higher false negative rate with FNA. Generally, nodules less than 1 cm are not further evaluated as the risk of malignancy is low and even if cancerous, the likelihood of harm is low.
   ii. Other nodule characteristics: Generally, the firmer the nodule, the more is the concern for carcinoma. Fixation to the adjacent laryngotracheal complex also raises concern for malignancy. Rapid growth, pain, or aerodigestive tract compromise are concerning for advanced malignancy but can commonly be associated with benign disease.
   iii. Associated palpable lymphadenopathy and vocal cord paralysis are strong correlates of malignancy. Patients with suspicious thyroid lesions should have a vocal cord examination to assess vocal cord motion. It should be strongly emphasized that voice and swallowing can be normal even when vocal cord paralysis is present.

Laboratory Evaluation

A. Sensitive TSH assay: Excellent screening test to definitively diagnose euthyroidism, hyperthyroidism, or hypothyroidism and is recommended in the initial evaluation of patients with a thyroid nodule.
B. Thyroid peroxidase (TPO) antibodies: helpful if the diagnosis of Hashimoto thyroiditis is suspected.
C. Thyroglobulin
    i. Not helpful in the initial workup of thyroid nodules.
    ii. Secreted by both normal and malignant thyroid tissue.
    iii. The assay is interfered with by antithyroglobulin antibodies that occur in approximately 15% to 25% of patients.
    iv. Extensive overlap in thyroglobulin levels exists between benign thyroid conditions and thyroid carcinoma, rendering this test unhelpful in the initial assessment of malignancy but helpful for cancer surveillance after surgery.
D. Calcitonin: elevated in medullary thyroid cancer but because of the rarity of medullary carcinoma of the thyroid, not thought to be a reasonable routine screening test in patients with a solitary nodule.

Radionuclide Scanning (With Technetium 99m or I^{123})

A. Often used for the workup of thyroid nodularity in the setting of hyperthyroidism to evaluate for hot (hyperactive) nodules. The risk of malignancy in hot nodules is thought to be very low, and fine-needle aspiration is not recommended.
B. 95% of all nodules are found to be cold, with a risk of malignancy of 10% to 15%.

Ultrasonography Thyroid ultrasound is recommended for all patients with one or more suspected thyroid nodules.

A. Evaluation of thyroid nodules: The pattern of sonographic features associated with a nodule on ultrasound confers a risk of malignancy, and when taken into account with the size of a nodule, determines which nodules should undergo fine-needle aspiration. *High suspicion features* include microcalcifications, irregular margins, taller-than-wide status, and extrathyroidal extension. *Intermediate suspicion features* include hypoechogenicity of a solid nodule, and *low suspicion features* include hyper- or isoechogenicity, solid nodule with regular margins, and mixed solid/cystic. *Very low suspicion features* include spongiform appearance and purely cystic (anechoic) appearance, which are felt to be markers of benignity and would not require biopsy.
B. Evaluation of lymph nodes: sensitive technique to identify number, size, and shape of cervical nodes surrounding and distant from the thyroid. Concerning ultrasound features of lymph nodes suggestive of malignancy include microcalcifications, irregular borders, hypervascularity, and loss of the lymph node hilum.
C. Useful in screening for small lesions in patients presenting with metastatic thyroid cancer and for the evaluation of the thyroid in patients with a history of head and neck radiation.
D. Elastography: U/S elastography (USE) has been applied to study the stiffness/elasticity of nodules as a means to help identify risk of malignancy. USE is a relatively new diagnostic tool that evaluates the degree of distortion of US beam under the application of an external force and is based on the principle that the softer parts of tissues deform easier than the harder parts under compression, thus allowing a semiquantitative determination of tissue elasticity. While USE may prove to be a useful noninvasive risk assessment tool, its performance is highly variable and operator dependent and is not yet recommended for widespread use in thyroid nodule work-up.

Fine-Needle Aspiration

A. Fine-needle aspiration (FNA) is the diagnostic procedure of choice for further evaluation of thyroid nodules (Table 37-6). *Ultrasound guidance is strongly recommended because of the improvement in overall sensitivity, specificity, and accuracy of FNA compared to palpation-guided FNA.* Effectiveness of FNA is, in turn, related to the skill of both aspirator and cytopathologist. FNA has significantly decreased the number of patients being sent to surgery by 20% to 50% and has significantly increased the yield of carcinoma in surgical specimens by 10% to 15%.

B. FNA is recommended for nodules suspicious for malignancy. In general, this risk increases for larger nodules and for nodules with more suspicious sonographic features (as discussed above). While different guidelines exist, one of the accepted guidelines for FNA of thyroid nodules is the Thyroid Imaging Reporting and Data System (TI-RADS), which is a point-based scoring system with recommendation for FNA of a nodule if:

≥ *1 cm* with high suspicion features (7+ points, TI-RADS 5)
≥ *1.5 cm* with intermediate suspicion features (4-6 points, TI-RADS 4)
≥ *2.5 cm* with low suspicion features (3 points, TI-RADS 3)
No biopsy for very low suspicion features (0-2 points, TI-RADS 1 and 2)

Table 37-6 Algorithm for the Evaluation of Thyroid Nodules

1. All patients with suspected thyroid nodule(s) should undergo thyroid ultrasound.
2. Patients found to have thyroid nodules ≥ 1 cm should undergo a complete history, physical examination, and measurement of serum TSH.
3. If low TSH, then consider I^{123} or Tc^{99} scanning—if uniform increased uptake or "hot" nodule, then evaluate and treat for hyperthyroidism.
4. If no nodule is seen sonographically and TSH is high, then evaluate and treat for hypothyroidism. If TSH is normal, then no further workup is needed.
5. Based on the combination of nodule size and sonographic characteristics, US-guided FNA should be considered. For high-suspicion features, nodules ≥ 1 cm should be biopsied (TI-RADS 5). For intermediate-suspicion features, nodules ≥ 1.5 cm should be biopsied (TI-RADS 4). For low-suspicion features, nodules ≥ 2.5 cm should be biopsied (TI-RADS 3). In general, very low-suspicion nodules should not be biopsied (TI-RADS 1 or 2).
6. FNA results:
   A. Nondiagnostic/inadequate: Repeat US-guided FNA. If nondiagnostic again, then either close follow-up or surgery based on ultrasonographic features and clinical risk.
   B. Benign: Follow clinically with ultrasound surveillance starting at 12-month intervals. If concerning changes are identified (higher suspicion features or significant growth), then repeat FNA is recommended.
   C. Indeterminate: Consider repeat FNA with molecular testing for supplemental information regarding risk of malignancy. If suspicious for carcinoma, then surgery. If low suspicion for carcinoma, consider surveillance.
   D. Malignant: Surgery is the gold standard for treatment. Active surveillance *may* be considered for select patients with small, low-risk papillary thyroid carcinomas.
7. For purely cystic nodules (TI-RADS 1), aspiration may be considered as a therapeutic option for decompression, and if performed, cytology should be sent. Surgery or ETOH ablation is sometimes recommended for large or recurrent cysts.

Data from Haugen DS, Alexander EK, Bible KC, et al. 2015 American Thyroid Association management guidelines for adult patients with thyroid nodules and differentiated thyroid cancer: the American Thyroid Association task force on thyroid nodules and differentiated thyroid cancer. *Thyroid.* 2016 Jan;26(1):1-133.
Tessler FN, Middleton WD, Grant EG, et al. ACR thyroid imaging, reporting and data system (TI-RADS): white paper of the ACR TI-RADS Committee. *J Am Coll Radiol.* 2017 May;14(5):587-595.

Table 37-7 The 2023 Bethesda System for Reporting Thyroid Cytopathology: Implied Risk of Malignancy and Recommended Clinical Management

Diagnostic Category	*Risk of Malignancy[a] Mean % (range)*	*Risk of Malignancy if excluding NIFTP Mean %*	*Usual Management[b]*
I. Nondiagnostic	13 (5-20)[c]	12	Repeat FNA[d] with ultrasound guidance
II. Benign	4 (2-7)[e]	2	Clinical and ultrasound follow-up
III. Atypia of undetermined significance[f]	22 (13-30)	16	Repeat FNA,[d] molecular testing, diagnostic lobectomy, or surveillance
IV. Follicular neoplasm[g]	30 (23-34)	23	Molecular testing,[h] diagnostic lobectomy
V. Suspicious for malignancy	74 (67-83)	65	Molecular testing,[h] lobectomy or near-total thyroidectomy[i]
VI. Malignant	97 (97-100)	94	Lobectomy or near-total thyroidectomy[i]

[a]These ROM estimates are skewed by selection bias because many thyroid nodules (especially those diagnosed as benign or atypia of undetermined significance) might not undergo surgical excision.
[b]Actual management could depend on other factors (eg, clinical, ultrasound findings), in addition to the FNA interpretation.
[c]The ROM varies with the type and structure of the nodule (ie, solid vs complex vs > 50% cystic); nondiagnostic aspirates from solid nodules are associated with a higher ROM compared with those showing > 50% cystic changes and low-risk ultrasound features.
[d]Studies have shown diagnostic resolution with repeat FNA.
[e]This ROM estimate is based on follow-up of surgically resected nodules, which is skewed by selection bias because most thyroid nodules classified as benign do not undergo surgical excision; using long-term follow-up studies, the best overall ROM estimate for a benign FNA is ~1% to 2%.
[f]This category can be further subclassified into specimens with nuclear versus non-nuclear atypia, the ROM appears to be higher for cases with nuclear atypia.
[g]Includes cases of follicular neoplasm with oncocytic features (formerly Hürthle cell neoplasm).
[h]Molecular analysis can be performed to assess the type of surgical procedure (lobectomy vs total thyroidectomy).
[i]In the case of "suspicious for metastatic tumor" or a "malignant" interpretation indicating a metastatic tumor rather than a primary thyroid malignancy, surgery might not be indicated.
FNA, fine-needle aspiration; ROM, risk of malignancy.
Data from Ali SZ, Baloch ZW, Cochand-Priollet B, et al. The 2023 Bethesda System for Reporting Thyroid Cytopathology. *Thyroid.* 2023 Sep;33(9):1039-1044.

C. The Bethesda classification system is the recommended standardized diagnostic terminology/classification system for reporting thyroid FNA results. This is a six-tiered system for separating FNA results based on risk of malignancy (Table 37-7). While risk of malignancy is estimated for each of the six categories, variability in institution-specific estimated risk is recognized and should be understood by practitioners. The 2017 and more recent 2023 updates additionally account for "non-invasive follicular thyroid neoplasm with papillary-like nuclear features" (or NIFTP), an entity that is no longer considered a cancer, with change in nomenclature to reflect its very low-risk neoplastic status in terms of risk of recurrence or spread. NIFTP is diagnosed and adequately treated with surgical excision and cannot be diagnosed on cytopathology, although the cytologic features of this neoplasm tend to lead to classification on FNA in the indeterminate Bethesda categories (III-V), impacting resultant ROM calculations.
   i. *Nondiagnostic (Bethesda I):* Accounts for about 10% of cases, with risk of malignancy 5% to 20 %. Such aspirates should be repeated under ultrasound guidance. In the event of two nondiagnostic results, patients should be considered for

surgical excision if the nodule demonstrates a suspicious sonographic pattern or there are clinical risk factors for malignancy. Low-risk nodules may be monitored with surveillance.

ii. *Benign (Bethesda II):*
   a. Because the risk of malignancy is very low (2%-7%), no additional immediate work-up is recommended. Management of asymptomatic nodules reported "benign" is usually observation with repetitive examinations and sonograms. Significant growth (≥ 50% increase in volume or ≥ 20% increase in diameter with at least 2 mm increase in 2 or more dimensions) or worrisome change in ultrasound features warrants consideration for repeat FNA. Larger nodules have a higher risk of false negative results, and the risk of malignancy may be higher.
   b. Symptomatic nodules or large nodules greater than 4 cm often warrant additional management:
      1. Purely cystic nodules (anechoic on ultrasound, TI-RADS 1) may be aspirated for decompression if symptomatic. If aspirated, cytology should be sent.
      2. ETOH ablation may be considered for cystic or largely cystic nodules to lower the risk of recurrence after aspiration.
      3. Additional ablative technologies are now available for more solid nodules that are symptomatic and felt to be benign (often with two prior benign biopsies). Microwave ablation (MWA) and radiofrequency ablation (RFA) are newer procedures utilizing heat delivery from a needle inserted under ultrasound guidance for the destruction of the center of a thyroid nodule with resultant decreased nodule volume for symptomatic relief. These therapies do not definitively remove thyroid nodules and do have potential side effects and limitations that must be kept in mind.
      4. Thyroid surgery, with hemithyroidectomy or total thyroidectomy, is the only definitive management for symptomatic benign nodules. However, this comes with the additional risks of surgery and possible need for lifelong thyroid hormone replacement therapy.

iii. *Indeterminate (Bethesda III-V):*
   a. *Atypia of undetermined significance (AUS, Bethesda III):* shows architectural and/or nuclear atypia precluding a "benign" categorization but not sufficient for higher risk category. Risk of malignancy is estimated at 13% to 30% but is variable across centers and influenced by NIFTP. Nuclear atypia is more worrisome than architectural atypia in terms of risk of malignancy. Management options include (1) repeat FNA with possible molecular testing to help further supplement cancer risk assessment, (2) diagnostic/therapeutic surgical excision with lobectomy, or (3) close clinical surveillance.
   b. *Follicular neoplasm (FN, Bethesda IV):*
   One of the main difficulties with FNA in the identification of malignancy is the differentiation of follicular adenoma from follicular carcinoma. This diagnosis hinges on a histologic finding of pericapsular vascular invasion. To definitively differentiate follicular adenoma from follicular carcinoma, histologic evaluation of the entire capsule is necessary—this cannot be achieved with FNA. FNA for follicular lesions is categorized or graded based on several cytopathologic features. The least worrisome pattern on FNA of a follicular lesion would be described as a macrofollicular lesion or colloid adenomatous nodule (benign). A microfollicular lesion with little colloid and with follicular sheets has an increased risk of carcinoma. The overall estimated risk of malignancy in the

FN category is 23% to 34% and is influenced by NIFTP. Management options for this category include most commonly (1) molecular testing to help further supplement cancer risk assessment or (2) diagnostic/therapeutic surgical excision with lobectomy.

1. *Oncocytic neoplasm (previously Hürthle cell neoplasm)* is a subset of this category with presence of oncocytic (Hürthle) cells—large polygonal follicular cells with granular cytoplasm. An oncocytic cell-predominant aspirate may indicate an underlying oncocytic adenoma or oncocytic carcinoma. Oncocytic cells can also be present as metaplastic cells in a variety of thyroid disorders, including multinodular goiter and Hashimoto thyroiditis. Because of the risk of an underlying oncocytic carcinoma, patients with FNA described as oncocytic cell-predominant may undergo repeat biopsy with molecular testing versus diagnostic surgical excision.

c. *Suspicious for malignancy (Bethesda V):* Specimens with cytologic features strongly suspicious for malignancy but not conclusive; confers a 67% to 83% risk of malignancy and is generally managed with molecular testing, thyroid lobectomy, or possible total (or near total) thyroidectomy. This estimated risk of malignancy in this category is also influenced by NIFTP.

iv. *Malignant (Bethesda VI):* When FNA is read as malignant, the chance of malignancy is very high (97%-100%). Well-differentiated thyroid carcinomas are the most common primary thyroid malignancies diagnosed. Otherwise, medullary carcinoma of the thyroid can have a variety of histologic and cytologic forms. Once medullary carcinoma is suspected, calcitonin immunohistochemistry can confirm the FNA diagnosis. Anaplastic carcinoma is often easily identified based on the degree of anaplasia. Lymphoma can be suggested by FNA, but additional tissue with open or core biopsy is often required to confirm the diagnosis. Aspirates read as primary thyroid malignancy are usually treated first-line with surgery.

D. FNA false-negative rate ranges from 1% to 6%. False negatives occur with greater frequency in small lesions less than 1 cm or large lesions greater than 3 to 4 cm.

Molecular Testing

A. Testing for molecular alterations in FNA specimens is primarily proposed for the diagnostic purpose of ruling in or ruling out thyroid malignancy. However, testing may also be used for prognostic purposes and for evaluation of efficacy of certain treatment modalities. The use of molecular testing for diagnostic purposes is primarily reserved for the indeterminate FNA categories of *atypia of undetermined significance, follicular neoplasm*, and less often *suspicious for malignancy*.

B. Genetic drivers for the molecular pathogenesis of thyroid cancer have been identified through ongoing research over the past two decades. As molecular alterations in thyroid cancer continue to be defined, new technologies enabling molecular profiling in individual tumors have made way for the burgeoning development of molecular diagnostic testing. Many molecular markers have been proposed, but only a small minority have been robust enough to modify clinical decision-making and impact care. Long-term outcomes data are still evolving, highlighting the need for appropriate informed consent and acknowledgement of patient preference, pretest probability, and feasibility when considering sending an FNA sample for molecular testing.

C. Molecular testing relies on different next-generation sequencing and gene expression technologies to help "rule in" or "rule out" a cancer. Currently, three genetic testing tools are commercially available in the US—ThyroSeq, Afirma, and ThyGeNEXT/ThyraMIR. These tools vary in technique related to testing substrate (DNA vs RNA) and whether they utilize gene sequencing and/or expression methodologies. Each test has its own published sensitivity, specificity, negative predictive value (NPV), and positive predictive value (PPV).

D. In general, the reported NPV of available molecular testing platforms for cytologically indeterminate nodules has ranged from 94% to 97%, allowing clinicians to use results to "rule out" cancer and prevent unnecessary surgery. It is important to remember, however, that local prevalence of malignancy in each FNA category affects the NPV as well as the PPV of a given test and should be understood.

E. While published overall PPVs are lower for each of the molecular testing platforms (ranging from 47% to 74%), making these tests more difficult to use to "rule in" cancer, certain identified genetic alterations or mutations confer a relatively high risk of malignancy and may be used for clinical decision-making. For example, the BRAF V600E mutation is the most common genetic mutation in papillary thyroid carcinoma, and if identified, confers a 99% risk of malignancy.

F. While there is yet to be one single definitive test to both rule in and rule out malignancy, next-generation testing continues to evolve.

Well-Differentiated Thyroid Cancer (WDTC)

Papillary Carcinoma of the Thyroid

A. *Histopathology*: Papillary thyroid carcinoma (PTC) is characterized histologically by the formation of papillae and unique nuclear features such as nuclear grooves and intranuclear inclusions. The nuclei of the neoplastic epithelium are large, with prominent nucleoli giving an "Orphan Annie eye" appearance. Lesions with any papillary component, even if follicular features predominate, are believed to follow a course consistent with PTC. Unfavorable histologic variants of PTC include diffuse sclerosing, tall-cell, and columnar cell variants.

B. *Clinical behavior and spread*: PTC is strongly lymphotropic, with early spread through intrathyroidal lymphatics as well as to regional cervical lymphatic beds. Nodal metastases from PTC can often undergo cystic formation and may be black in color.

C. PTC has a tendency for multifocality within the thyroid gland.

D. At presentation, approximately 30% of patients with PTC harbor clinically evident cervical nodal disease with a rate of distant metastasis of approximately 3%. In the pediatric population, the nodal metastatic rate can be as high as 60%.

E. The presence of cervical lymph node metastasis may increase the risk of nodal recurrence, particularly with macroscopic nodal disease. Most studies suggest that the presence of microscopic cervical lymph node metastasis does not have significant prognostic implications.

F. *Demographics*: PTC is the most common type of thyroid cancer (80%-85%). It affects all ages (children and adults) and occurs three times more frequently in women. The peak incidence occurs at 40 to 50 years of age in women, while in men, it peaks 10 to 20 years later. Until recently, the incidence of PTC was increasing, although mortality levels remain stable (with most of this increase thought to be secondary to increased detection rates). The majority of PTCs arise spontaneously. Ionizing radiation exposure is a widely studied causative factor of PTC, and the incidence of PTC was increased after the Chernobyl accident. A very small subset of thyroid cancers is associated with syndromes such as Familial Adenomatous Polyposis, Cowden syndrome, and Gardner syndrome.

G. *Etiology and molecular alterations*: The mitogen-activated protein kinase (MAPK) pathway is central to malignant transformation in PTC. In 70% of all cases, alteration in this pathway is found. Specific genetic alterations known to be associated with PTC include RET/PTC, NTRK1, RAS, and BRAF. The BRAF mutation is the most common genetic event in PTC, accounting for approximately 50% of all cases. The presence of a BRAF mutation appears to be a negative prognosticator, associated with a higher frequency of extrathyroidal invasion, cervical lymph node, and distant metastasis, as well as a higher recurrence rate.

H. *Prognosis*: The ten-year survival rates of PTC are over 90%, but age greater than 55 is associated with increased recurrence and mortality rates. Children are more likely to have an advanced stage at the time of diagnosis but overall have an excellent prognosis due to age. Risk stratification is important for prognosis (discussed later).

Follicular Carcinoma

A. *Histopathology*: Follicular carcinoma is a well-differentiated thyroid malignancy, with follicular differentiation lacking features typical of PTC. Follicular lesions are differentiated into benign follicular adenomas, minimally invasive carcinomas, or widely invasive follicular carcinomas by examination of the tumor capsule. Capsular or vascular invasion is the most reliable indication of malignancy. The degree of invasiveness is variable but correlates with the prognosis.

B. *Clinical behavior and spread*: Follicular carcinoma is less likely to present with nodal metastasis compared to papillary carcinoma, as its spread is typically hematologic. However, the rates of distant metastasis at presentation are higher and are estimated at 16% overall. Follicular carcinoma is typically a unifocal lesion, with the incidence of contralateral disease approaching zero.

C. *Demographics*: Follicular carcinoma occurs more commonly in females than in males and in an older age group than PTC, with the median age in the sixth decade.

D. *Etiology and molecular alterations:* The molecular pathogenesis of follicular carcinoma often involves mutations in RAS, PTEN, PIK3CA, and the PAX-PPARG rearrangement. (RAS mutations are also commonly seen in the follicular variant of PTC, however.)

E. *Prognosis*: Follicular carcinomas tend to present in an older age group with a higher rate of distant metastatic disease and, therefore, have a worse prognosis than PTC. The tumor size and degree of invasiveness are key factors in the prognosis.

Oncocytic Carcinoma

A. Previously termed "Hurthle cell carcinoma" and considered a subtype of follicular carcinoma. However, because of an improved understanding of its unique genomic signature and clinical behavior, oncocytic carcinoma (OTC) has been re-classified as a distinct entity of WDTC.

B. *Histopathology:* Oncocytic cells have abundant granular cytoplasm with a round nucleus and prominent nucleolus. Hemosiderin-laden histiocytes may be present.

C. *Clinical behavior and spread:* OTC is more likely to have locoregional (lymph node) metastases than follicular thyroid carcinoma and is more likely to develop distant metastases than papillary thyroid carcinoma.

D. *Demographics:* Accounts for 5% of all thyroid cancers. More commonly found in older patients, although OTC-specific data are limited.

E. *Etiology and molecular alterations:* Often involve chromosomal copy number alterations and novel mutations in mitochondrial DNA.

F. *Prognosis:* Presentation is usually at a higher stage, with worse overall and disease-specific survival compared to other WDTCs. Radioactive iodine uptake is typically poor, with greater reliance being placed on surgery. The overall 10-year DSS for patients with oncocytic carcinoma with low-risk features (minimal capsular/vascular invasion) remains high at near 100%. However, for patients with more widely invasive disease or metastases, the 10-year DSS decreases to 70%.

Prognostic Risk Grouping for Well-Differentiated Thyroid Carcinoma (WDTC)

A. The identification of key prognostic variables makes it possible to segregate patients with WDTC into a large low-risk group and a small high-risk group. Mortality in the low-risk group is approximately 1% to 2%, while in the high-risk group it is approximately 40% to 50%. Segregation of patients into high- and low-risk groups permits appropriately aggressive treatment in the high-risk group with avoidance of excess treatment and its complications in patients in the low-risk category.
B. The key elements of existing prognostic schema for WDTC include:
   i. *Age*: An age threshold of 55 years old is currently used by the American Joint Cancer Committee (AJCC)—TNM staging system for risk stratification of WDTC, with younger patients doing better overall.
      a. Patients younger than 55 years old can only be Stage I or Stage II (based on presence of distant metastatic disease) due to the overall excellent 10-year disease-specific survival (DSS) rates (98%-100% for Stage I and 85%-95% for Stage II).
      b. Patients ≥ 55 years old are grouped based on TNM status into Stage I, II, III, IVA/B (with 10-year DSS rates of 98%-100%, 85%-95%, 60%-70% and < 50%, respectively).
   ii. *Degree of invasiveness/extrathyroidal extension*: Increased invasiveness increases the risk of local, regional, and distant recurrence and decreases survival.
   iii. *Metastasis*: The presence of distant metastasis increases mortality.
   iv. *Sex*: Males generally have a poorer prognosis than females.
   v. *Size*: Lesions greater than 5 cm have a worse prognosis, while lesions less than 1.5 cm have a better prognosis. There is controversy as to the exact tumor size cutoff, with some studies reporting decreased prognosis with lesions greater than 4 cm and better prognosis with lesions less than 1 cm.
C. *The two best-known prognostic schema*: Hay scheme for papillary carcinoma is summarized by the mnemonic AGES—for age, gender, extent, and size. Cady prognostic schema is for PTC and follicular carcinoma and is summarized by the mnemonic AMES—for age, metastasis, extent, and size.

Guidelines for Preoperative Staging of WDTC

A. All patients undergoing thyroid surgery for the treatment of a malignant cytologic finding on FNA should undergo preoperative neck ultrasound for evaluation of the contralateral lobe and cervical lymph nodes. CT scanning of the neck with contrast can be considered.

Specific Guidelines for Appropriate Operative Management of WDTC

A. Recommendations for extent of thyroidectomy:
   i. Total thyroidectomy is indicated in patients with large thyroid cancers (> 4 cm), tumors with extrathyroidal extension, and in patients with metastases. In addition,

those with suspicious cytology with bilateral nodules may prefer total thyroidectomy to avoid the possibility of requiring a future surgery on the contralateral lobe.

ii. A total thyroidectomy should be performed if radioactive iodine therapy is planned.

iii. Lobectomy alone may be sufficient for tumors 1 to 4 cm that are considered low-risk, isolated, and intrathyroidal without cervical nodal disease.

iv. Lobectomy alone should be considered for low-risk tumors less than 1 cm.

B. Central neck dissection should be performed in patients with known lymphatic involvement and in patients with advanced-stage PTC.

i. Systematic evaluation of the central neck nodal beds should be performed (including Delphian, perithyroid, pretracheal, RLN, upper mediastinal, and perithymic regions), with resection of grossly enlarged lymph nodes.

ii. Prophylactic central neck dissection without evidence of clinical disease by either radiologic means or physical examination is controversial. A higher rate of hypoparathyroidism occurs with central neck dissection, and there is a potential to upstage patients due to micrometastatic lymph node disease. Proponents of central neck dissection believe the routine removal of the central nodal beds will remove a potential recurrence source and the potential reoperative morbidity associated with it, permit accurate long-term surveillance, and improve staging accuracy to intensify treatment with radioactive iodine.

C. Total thyroidectomy without central node dissection is usually appropriate for follicular cancer.

D. In patients with biopsy-proven metastatic cervical lymphadenopathy, a lateral neck compartmental lymph node dissection should be performed. If nodal disease is evident in the lateral neck, a selective neck dissection encompassing levels 2 to 4 ± 5 depending on imaging findings, rather than "berry picking," is recommended. Such a systematic neck dissection decreases subsequent nodal recurrence and the need for complicated reoperation but has an unclear impact on survival.

Invasive Disease

A. RLN: When disease is focally adherent to a functioning RLN, it should be dissected off, removing gross disease and preserving the functioning nerve. Even if vocal cord paralysis is noted preoperatively, attempts should be made to preserve the RLN, given the potential for better voice outcomes. An infiltrated RLN may need to be resected if gross disease cannot be removed from the nerve.

B. Strap muscles: Extracapsular disease involving the strap muscles is usually easily managed with resection of the involved musculature.

C. Laryngotracheal complex: Disease invasive to the larynx and trachea is managed with resection of gross disease, with preservation of vital structures when possible. Near-total excision with postoperative adjuvant treatment is equivalent with respect to survival to more radical resection.

D. Neoadjuvant therapy: Systemic tyrosine kinase inhibitor (TKI) therapy is emerging as an important systemic medical treatment offered for symptomatic and progressive advanced thyroid cancer (see discussion below). New studies are not only showing benefit in the post-surgical adjuvant setting, but in the neoadjuvant setting as well to improve rates of surgical resectability and decrease surgical morbidity (with some studies even showing return of RLN function prior to surgery).

Postoperative Management for WDTC

A. Thyroid hormone, usually T_4, is given to suppress TSH to 0.1 to 0.3 mU/L in high-risk patients and 0.5 to 2.0 mU/L in low-risk patients.

B. I^{131} can be given post-thyroidectomy based on the patient's risk stratification and likelihood of harboring metastatic disease. Typically, high-risk patients with PTC and most patients with follicular carcinoma are considered for treatment. There is no good data to suggest radioactive iodine is effective for oncocytic carcinoma.
   i. I^{131} is given in ablative doses ranging from 30 to 100 mCi if patients have undergone less than total thyroidectomy and have greater than 2% uptake on regional neck scanning.
   ii. If adjuvant treatment is necessary or disease is identified on whole body scans, or in high-risk patients, doses of I^{131} (100-200 mCi) are given.

C. External beam radiation (typically 50-60 Gy) has been employed to palliate extensive laryngotracheal disease, prolong local control, and improve quality of life in inoperable cases or where gross disease persists postoperatively. It has also been used to palliate bony and central nervous system (CNS) metastases.

D. Systemic therapy:
   i. Oral small molecule inhibitors targeting different oncogenic pathways important in thyroid cancer have been developed over the past one to two decades. Tyrosine kinase inhibitor (TKI) therapy is now often considered in cases of advanced thyroid cancer, particularly in cases of widespread metastatic disease and especially when there is evidence of disease progression. TKI therapy is not generally considered curative and usually must be continued to maintain disease response. Multiple toxicities are associated with any TKI therapy and must be monitored closely.
   ii. Lenvatinib and sorafenib are multikinase inhibitors that are FDA-approved therapies for RAI-refractory progressive differentiated thyroid carcinoma. Other more targeted therapies include vemurafenib and dabrafenib, examples of BRAF inhibitors, and trametinib, a MEK inhibitor (a component in the same signaling pathway as BRAF). Combination therapy with dabrafenib and trametinib has been studied in combination therapy with dabrafenib for RAI-refractory PTC. Some BRAF and MEK inhibitors have been further shown to restore expression of the sodium iodide symporter and uptake of iodine in thyroid cancer cells in preclinical studies, leading to clinical trials studying their use in possible redifferentiation therapy to reverse RAI resistance.
   iii. Immunotherapy is also an emerging systemic treatment modality, either in isolation or in combination therapy, for advanced thyroid cancer. Pembrolizumab is a monoclonal antibody that blocks the programmed death-1 (PD-1) receptor on cytotoxic T cells and is currently being studied in clinical trials for advanced thyroid cancer.

E. Thyroglobulin is produced by normal and malignant thyroid tissue and can serve as a marker of well-differentiated thyroid cancer after thyroidectomy. If thyroglobulin is low (< 2 ng/mL on T_4 suppression), or unmeasurable after total thyroid ablation, and whole body scanning is negative, patients rarely harbor clinically significant metastatic disease.

F. Cervical ultrasound (US) at 6 and 12 months and then annually for at least 3 to 5 years is recommended to evaluate the thyroid bed as well as central and lateral cervical nodal compartments for disease recurrence or metastasis.

G. PET/CT scanning may be performed and useful on patients with WDTC who have a negative I^{131} scan but with thyroglobulin greater than 10 ng/mL.

Medullary Thyroid Carcinoma (MTC)

A. *Histopathology*: This lesion arises from parafollicular C cells (not thyroid follicular cells). Calcitonin is secreted by normal parafollicular C cells, and calcitonin elevation occurs in C-cell hyperplasia and all forms of medullary thyroid carcinoma (MTC). This tumor marker has proven extremely useful in establishing a diagnosis in asymptomatic relatives of hereditary cases and in postoperative surveillance. Carcinoembryonic antigen (CEA) is another biomarker that can be elevated in MTC, although it is not specific and can be elevated in other conditions such as GI tumors or tobacco use.

B. *Clinical behavior and spread*: MTC has a strong tendency toward paratracheal and lateral neck nodal involvement. MTC tends to recur locally and may metastasize hematogenously to lung, liver, or bone. MTC does not take up iodine.

C. *Etiology and demographics*: MTC represents approximately 5% to 10% of all thyroid cancers. Approximately 75% of MTC occurs as a sporadic neoplasm, typically presenting in the fourth decade as a unifocal lesion. Hereditary MTC accounts for the remaining 25%, occurring in a younger age group with multifocal lesions (Table 37-8). All three forms of hereditary MTC are inherited in an autosomal dominant fashion and are preceded by C-cell hyperplasia.

D. *Molecular alterations:* Germline mutations in the RET protooncogene cause progression from C-cell hyperplasia to MTC in inherited MTC. Over 100 RET mutations have been identified in inherited MTC, representing variable degrees of associated aggressiveness, with the M918T mutation considered the highest risk. Almost half of all sporadic MTC cases will demonstrate somatic RET mutations. Genetic testing is recommended for all new cases of MTC.

E. *Prognosis:* The eighth edition AJCC-TNM staging system estimates 10-year DSS for stage I, II, III, and IV MTC as 100%, 93%, 71%, and 21%, respectively. Large primary tumors, nodal metastases, and distant metastatic disease portend a worse prognosis. Metastatic disease is often suspected when baseline calcitonin levels are greater than 500 pg/mL, warranting additional imaging to standard preoperative neck imaging, including CT Chest, abdominal CT or MRI, and bone scintigraphy or MRI to evaluate for lung, liver, and bone metastases, respectively.

F. *Management*:

i. Surgery is the only curative treatment for MTC and is often more extensive up front compared to WDTC as MTC does not take up radioactive iodine.

a. The standard surgical treatment for MTC is a total thyroidectomy with central neck dissection because of the high rate of central neck lymph node metastases.

b. All patients with clinical lateral neck disease should undergo lateral neck dissection. Given the high incidence of microscopic lateral neck disease, patients with large palpable primary tumors and those with higher calcitonin levels (> 200 pg/mL) can be considered for an ipsilateral prophylactic lateral neck dissection (typically levels II-V). Those with calcitonin levels greater than 500 pg/mL may be considered for prophylactic contralateral lateral neck dissection as well.

c. In patients with known distant metastatic disease, surgery is palliative in nature, and less aggressive surgery may be warranted to minimize complications.

ii. Follow Up

Patients are followed after surgery for evidence of disease recurrence or progression in cases of unresectable disease. Serum calcitonin and CEA "doubling times" are followed, with shorter doubling times corresponding to more aggressive disease. Regular surveillance imaging with neck ultrasound is recommended in the setting of localized disease, with more extensive whole-body imaging for metastatic disease.

Table 37-8 2022 Updated WHO Classification scheme of thyroid neoplasms, 5th edition

Developmental Abnormalities	*Follicular Cell-Derived Neoplasms*	*Other*
Thyroglossal duct cyst Other congenital thyroid abnormalities	Benign tumors a. Thyroid follicular nodular disease[a] b. Follicular adenoma c. Follicular adenoma with papillary architecture d. Oncocytic adenoma of the thyroid Low-risk neoplasms a. Noninvasive follicular thyroid neoplasm with papillary-like nuclear features b. Thyroid tumors of uncertain malignant potential c. Hyalinizing trabecular tumor Malignant neoplasms a. Follicular thyroid carcinoma b. Invasive encapsulated follicular variant papillary carcinoma c. Papillary thyroid carcinoma d. Oncocytic carcinoma of the thyroid e. Follicular-derived carcinomas, high-grade i. Differentiated high-grade thyroid carcinoma ii. Poorly differentiated thyroid carcinoma f. Anaplastic follicular cell-derived thyroid carcinoma	Thyroid C-cell-derived carcinoma a. Medullary thyroid carcinoma Mixed medullary and follicular cell-derived carcinomas Salivary gland-type carcinomas of the thyroid a. Mucoepidermoid carcinoma of the thyroid b. Secretory carcinoma of salivary gland type Thyroid tumors of uncertain histogenesis a. Sclerosing mucoepidermoid carcinoma with eosinophilia b. Cribriform morular thyroid carcinoma Thymic tumors within the thyroid a. Thymoma family b. Spindle epithelial tumor with thymus-like elements c. Thymic carcinoma family Embryonal thyroid neoplasm a. Thyroblastoma

[a]Not considered a true neoplastic condition.

Summarized from the WHO classification of thyroid neoplasms within the 5th edition of the WHO Classification of Endocrine and Neuroendocrine Tumors, 5th Edition, 2022. https://whobluebooks.iarc.who.int/

iii. Systemic therapy:

a. Two multikinase inhibitors have been approved in the treatment of symptomatic, unresectable, locally advanced, or metastatic MTC based on clinical trials showing improvement in progression-free survival compared to placebo. Vandetanib is a multikinase inhibitor against VEGFRs, RET, KIT, and EGFR. Cabozantinib is a multikinase inhibitor against VEGFR2, MET, and RET.

b. Two selective tyrosine inhibitors have been approved for RET-mutated advanced thyroid cancers, including MTC. Selpercatinib and pralsetinib both specifically target RET alterations and have a lower overall toxicity profile than the multikinase inhibitors, making them the treatment of choice when a targetable RET-activating mutation is identified. New studies are emerging showing promise in the neoadjuvant setting with improved surgical resectability and durable effect.

Lymphoma

A. *Histopathology*: Primary thyroid lymphomas are typically of the non-Hodgkin type. Primary thyroid Hodgkin disease is extremely rare. A core biopsy is usually necessary for adequate diagnosis of thyroid lymphoma.
B. *Clinical behavior and spread*: Lymphoma of the thyroid is often rapidly progressive but is a highly curable malignancy if diagnosed promptly and managed correctly at an early stage. Presentation is often of a rapidly enlarging firm painless anterior neck mass and may include hoarseness with evidence of vocal cord paralysis, dysphagia, and regional adenopathy. Treatment is based on the lymphoma subtype and the extent of disease and is similar to the treatment of non-Hodgkin lymphoma (NHL) at other sites. Radiation therapy and chemotherapy are the main treatment modalities, with surgery largely restricted to biopsy or tracheostomy in the setting of airway compromise.
C. *Etiology and demographics*: Thyroid lymphomas constitute only 3% of all NHLs and approximately 1% to 5% of all thyroid malignancies. Thyroid lymphoma often occurs in the sixth to seventh decade of life and is more common in women. Often, there is a history of preexisting hypothyroidism (30%-40% of cases). The incidence of primary thyroid lymphomas in patients with Hashimoto thyroiditis is markedly increased.
D. *Prognosis:* The median all-cause survival for primary thyroid lymphoma is 9.3 to 11.6 years. Prognosis depends on subtype, with advanced stage, older age, tumor size greater than 10 cm, and elevated LDH negatively impacting prognosis.

Anaplastic Carcinoma

A. *Histopathology*: Variable with lack of differentiation of cells and with evidence of chronic inflammation, necrosis, high cellular proliferation, and atypical mitoses. Different morphologic subtypes may include spindle cell or sarcomatoid, giant cell, and squamoid.
B. *Clinical behavior and spread*: Patients often present with a rapidly growing neck mass that is fixed to the laryngotracheal complex, vocal cord paralysis, cervical adenopathy, and distant metastases. Symptoms may include hoarseness, weight loss, bone pain, weakness, and cough. Imaging usually shows a large, widely invasive thyroid cancer with invasion into the laryngotracheal complex and surrounding structures that is usually deemed surgically unresectable at presentation. Anaplastic thyroid cancer (ATC) does not concentrate iodine. Full-body PET/CT imaging and access to expeditious multidisciplinary care are warranted in all newly diagnosed ATC patients.
C. *Demographics:* ATC represents less than 5% of thyroid cancers and occurs in an older age group with a mean age at diagnosis of 65 years. Women are more commonly impacted than men.
D. *Etiology and molecular alterations:* ATC arises from follicular thyroid cells and is believed to occur from a terminal dedifferentiation of previously undetected long-standing differentiated thyroid carcinoma. Immunohistochemistry is essential for diagnosing ATC, with notable loss of thyroid-specific proteins. Common molecular alterations include mutations in BRAF and RAS (thought to be early mutations given presence in WDTC), TERT, as well as p53, beta-catenin, and PIK3CA (likely later mutations).
E. *Prognosis:* The most aggressive thyroid cancer, with a poor prognosis. Median survival is 5 months and 1-year overall survival is 20%. All ATC is considered Stage IV at presentation.

F. *Management:*
   i. Surgery:
      a. In patients without evidence of metastatic disease (50%), surgical resectability of the tumor should be assessed, with the goal of removing all visible disease.
      b. If the tumor is resectable, a total thyroidectomy with cervical lymph node dissection is performed. More aggressive surgery with laryngopharyngectomy, etc., is usually not warranted, given the added morbidity in the setting of an advanced thyroid cancer with an overall poor prognosis.
      c. In patients deemed unresectable, a detailed history, physical exam, and airway evaluation with laryngoscopy can identify those with impending airway compromise who may need consideration for a surgical airway (tracheostomy), such as in the setting of bilateral vocal fold paralysis or significant airway invasion.
   ii. External beam radiation (XRT) and chemotherapy: Postoperative XRT in combination with traditional chemotherapy has shown improved local control rates and survival benefit. For unresectable disease, XRT has traditionally been offered for locoregional palliation. In a minority of patients, XRT, when given alone or in combination with chemotherapy in the neoadjuvant setting, has allowed for delayed primary resection. Chemotherapy regimens have typically been recommended to include a taxane, with or without anthracyclines or platins.
   iii. Tyrosine kinase inhibitors (targeted therapy):
      a. Neoadjuvant therapy: In patients with ATC with a known BRAF-V600E mutation, neoadjuvant TKI combination therapy with dabrafenib (BRAF inhibitor) and trametinib (MEK inhibitor) has been shown to increase the resectability of the primary tumor, as well as improve overall and progression-free survival compared to upfront surgery or no surgery.
      b. Unresectable disease: In addition to BRAF-directed therapy, various other targeted TKI therapies, including RET, ALK, and NTRK inhibitors, are currently under investigation for ATC.
   iv. Immunotherapy: Checkpoint inhibitors such as spartalizumab, a monoclonal antibody against the PD-1 receptor, are being recommended for study in clinical trials in patients with ATC with high PD-L1 expression and no other targetable mutations.

Thyroidectomy: Surgical Anatomy

A. A horizontal neck incision is made within or parallel to a natural skin crease, typically two finger breadths above the sternal notch. A subplatysmal skin flap may be raised.
B. The midline raphe between the strap muscles is divided, and the sternohyoid (more ventral, medial) and sternothyroid (deeper, more lateral) are elevated in one layer off the ventral surface of the thyroid lobe.
C. Through primarily blunt dissection, the lobe is dissected and mobilized. As this is done, the thyroid gland is retracted ventro-medially, and the strap muscles are retracted laterally. The middle thyroid vein should be ligated, providing lateral exposure of the midlobe (Figure 37-4).
D. The inferior pole is dissected with attention toward identifying and preserving the inferior parathyroid, which is typically located within 1 cm inferior or posterior to the thyroid's inferior pole.

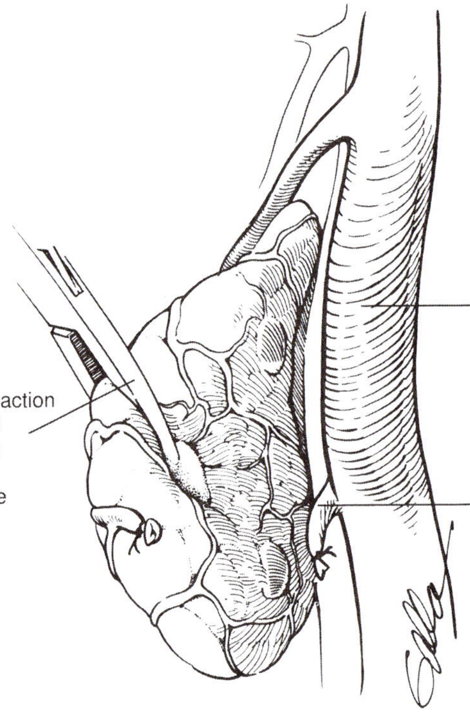

Figure 37-4 Middle thyroid vein division provides for greater lateral exposure.

E. The RLN can be identified through the lateral approach at the mid-polar level, just below the ligament of Berry and its laryngeal entry point, or medial to the tubercle of Zuckerkandl. The RLN is identified as a white, wave-like structure with a characteristic vascular stripe. Extra-laryngeal branching can occur in about one-third of patients above the crossing point of the RLN and inferior thyroid artery. On the right, the RLN traverses a more oblique course than on the left as it courses upwards toward the laryngeal nerve entry site. Intraoperative nerve monitoring (IONM) is often used to facilitate nerve identification, nerve mapping, and prognostication of neural function. The laryngeal entry point is indicated by the inferior cornu of the thyroid cartilage. The possibility of a nonrecurrent RLN on the right should be kept in mind.
F. The RLN should be identified visually in all cases and confirmed electrically through neural monitoring. The vagus nerve should be stimulated at the beginning of surgery before significant dissection to ensure the nerve monitoring circuit is intact (allowing for trust that a negative stimulation is a "true negative"). The vagus nerve should then be stimulated at the end of surgery to ensure the entire length of the RLN is intact (preventing a possible false negative scenario from stimulation of a damaged RLN distal to the site of injury).
G. The distal branches of the inferior and superior thyroid arteries should always be ligated as close to the thyroid as possible to optimize parathyroid preservation (Figure 37-5). If the parathyroid has turned black as a result of its dissection or has a

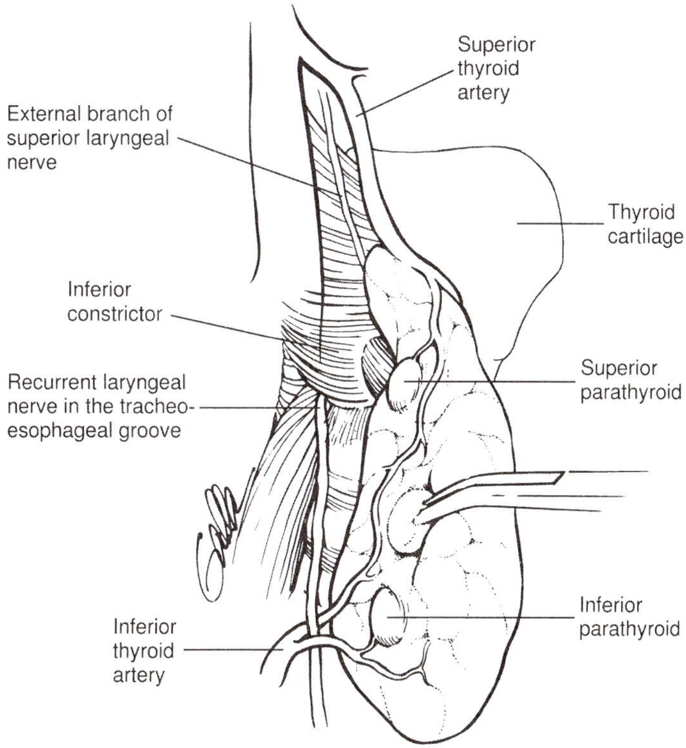

Figure 37-5 Laterally, the inferior thyroid artery and superiorly, the superior thyroid artery are followed to identify inferior and superior parathyroid glands.

questionable vascular pedicle, it can be biopsied, confirmed as parathyroid, and then minced and placed into several muscular pockets in the sternocleidomastoid muscle (SCM).

H. Downward and lateral retraction of the superior pole allows dissection in the interval between the thyroid cartilage medially and the superior pole laterally (cricothyroid space). The superior polar vessels are then ligated at the level of the thyroid capsule. The external branch of the SLN can be, in approximately 20% of cases, closely related to the superior pole vessels at the level of the thyroid capsule and is, therefore, vulnerable to injury. The external branch of the SLN can be electrically identified with a neural monitor.

Surgical Complications

A. *RLN injury and resultant vocal cord paralysis* rates vary because many surgeons do not perform postoperative laryngeal examination, which is essential for determination of accurate postoperative paralysis rates. Many reports reveal rates of 6% to 7%, while some report as high as 23%. The incidence of RLN paralysis increases with bilateral surgery, revision surgery, surgery for malignancy, surgery for substernal goiter, and in patients brought back to surgery for bleeding. RLN injury and resultant vocal cord paralysis can cause hoarseness, dysphagia, and aspiration. Bilateral RLN injury may result in a nearly normal voice but respiratory insufficiency with postoperative stridor. Temporary RLN injury generally resolves within 6 months.

B. *External branch of the superior laryngeal nerve (EBSLN) injury* rates vary widely in the literature (0%-25%), likely secondary to lack of widespread use of intraoperative neural monitoring and difficulty with identification on postoperative exam and laryngoscopy. EBSLN injury results in the reduction of cricothyroid vocal cord tensing with loss of high vocal registers. This leads to loss of projection and high-pitched tones while singing. The affected cord will be lower and bowed, with laryngeal rotation.

C. *Hypoparathyroidism* can result in postoperative hypocalcemia, often most notable on postoperative day two. Early symptoms may include perioral and digital paresthesias, with progressive neuromuscular irritability resulting in spontaneous carpopedal spasm, abdominal cramps, laryngeal stridor, mental status changes, QT prolongation on electrocardiogram, and ultimately tetanic contractions. Chvostek sign is the development of facial twitching with light tapping over the facial nerve. This sign must be assessed preoperatively, as approximately 5% of the normal population has a positive Chvostek sign in the setting of eucalcemia. Trousseau sign is induced by carpal spasm through tourniquet-induced ischemia. Temporary hypoparathyroidism, defined as being of less than 6 months duration, occurs in up to a third of patients after total thyroidectomy. Permanent hypoparathyroidism after total thyroidectomy occurs in approximately 5% to 10% of patients.

D. *Postoperative hematoma* occurs in less than 2% of thyroid surgeries and can occur immediately or several days postoperatively. A hematoma may cause airway obstruction through laryngeal edema and should be treated as a surgical emergency. Endotracheal intubation is difficult in these patients due to edema and compression of the glottis. The use of a postoperative drain has not been shown to decrease hematoma rates.

Parathyroid Glands

A. Parathyroid glands secret parathyroid hormone (PTH), which maintains calcium levels through increased calcium absorption in the gut, mobilization of calcium in bone, inhibition of renal calcium excretion, and stimulation of renal hydroxylase to maintain vitamin D levels.

B. Total calcium levels vary with protein fluctuation, but ionized calcium is maintained within strict ranges. In patients with normal albumin, total serum calcium can be used for monitoring calcium levels. If the albumin level is abnormal, total serum calcium levels can be corrected (total serum calcium levels fall by 0.8 mg/dL for every 1 g/dL fall in albumin), or the ionized calcium can be used for surveillance.

C. Adenomatous or hyperplastic change to the parathyroid glands can cause increased parathyroid hormone secretion which leads to primary hyperparathyroidism. Primary hyperparathyroidism (HPT), which occurs in approximately 1 out of 500 females and 1 out of 2000 males, can be spontaneous, familial, or associated with multiple endocrine neoplasia (MEN) syndromes.

D. Elevated calcium levels (with or without elevated PTH) can be caused by many entities. Elevated calcium combined with elevated PTH helps establish the diagnosis of HPT (provided 24-hour urine calcium is normal to elevated).

E. *Adenoma* implies a single enlarged gland, typically in the context of three other normal glands. Adenomas are benign clonal neoplasms and are hypercellular, consisting of chief and oncocytic cells, with decreased intra- and intercellular fat. A single adenoma occurs in 80% of patients, while double adenomas occur in 2% to 4% of patients and are more common in the elderly.

F. *Hyperplasia,* found in up to 15% of patients, implies that all four glands are involved in the neoplastic change, although the gross enlargement of the glands may be minimal and may be quite asymmetric. Histologically, in hyperplasia there is an increased number of chief and oncocytic cells in multiple parathyroid glands. Four-gland hyperplasia can be sporadic or can occur in familial HPT or in multiple endocrine neoplasia (MEN) syndromes.

G. Parathyroid carcinoma is rare and accounts for approximately 1% of cases of HPT. One should suspect parathyroid carcinoma if serum calcium and PTH levels are *significantly* elevated. In cases of parathyroid carcinoma, preoperative examination may be notable for a palpable perithyroidal firm mass. Intraoperatively and on histopathologic review, the parathyroid is found to be invasive to the thyroid or surrounding tissue. On a molecular level, there is a loss of parafibromin nuclear immunoreactivity in parathyroid carcinoma.

H. Secondary HPT represents a hyperplastic response of parathyroid tissue, typically to renal failure. PTH is significantly elevated with a normal to low calcium level. Secondary HPT is often managed medically (with calcimimetic agents) but may require surgical correction with subtotal parathyroidectomy in advanced cases.

I. Tertiary HPT occurs when the parathyroid response becomes autonomous, persisting after correction of the primary metabolic derangement (typically renal transplant).

J. *Benign familial hypocalciuric hypercalcemia (BFHH)* is associated with mildly elevated calcium and PTH levels; however, unlike HPT, urine calcium levels are low (< 100 mg/24 h and a calcium to creatine clearance ratio < 0.01). BFHH is an autosomal dominant inherited disease, characterized by excess renal calcium reabsorption due to a mutation in the calcium-sensing receptor on the parathyroid gland chief cells. The resulting mild hypercalcemia and PTH, however, do not result in end-organ damage. Given the benign nature of BFHH, treatment including surgery is not indicated. Misdiagnosis of BFHH, which can result in surgical failure, can be avoided by checking a 24-hour urine calcium and creatinine preoperatively.

K. While chronically elevated calcium levels in the past have been detected through "painful bones, kidney stones, abdominal groans, psychic moans, and fatigue overtones," the majority of primary HPT today is detected in asymptomatic or mildly symptomatic patients on routine laboratory screening panels.

L. Symptomatic hypercalcemia or those with an episode of life-threatening hypercalcemia warrants surgical treatment. In addition, surgery is offered to patients with any of the following:
   i. Serum calcium levels greater than 1 mg/dL above the upper limit of normal
   ii. Age less than 50 years
   iii. Creatinine clearance less than 60 cc/min or kidney stones
   iv. Bone density less than two standard deviations below the mean corrected for age, gender, and race

Localization Studies

A. Localization studies should be considered if unilateral, guided, or minimal access surgery is planned, in revision cases and because of the possible ectopic location of the parathyroid glands. Imaging accuracy can vary greatly. Negative imaging repeated at high-volume centers yields a sensitivity of up to 92%. (Figure 37-6).

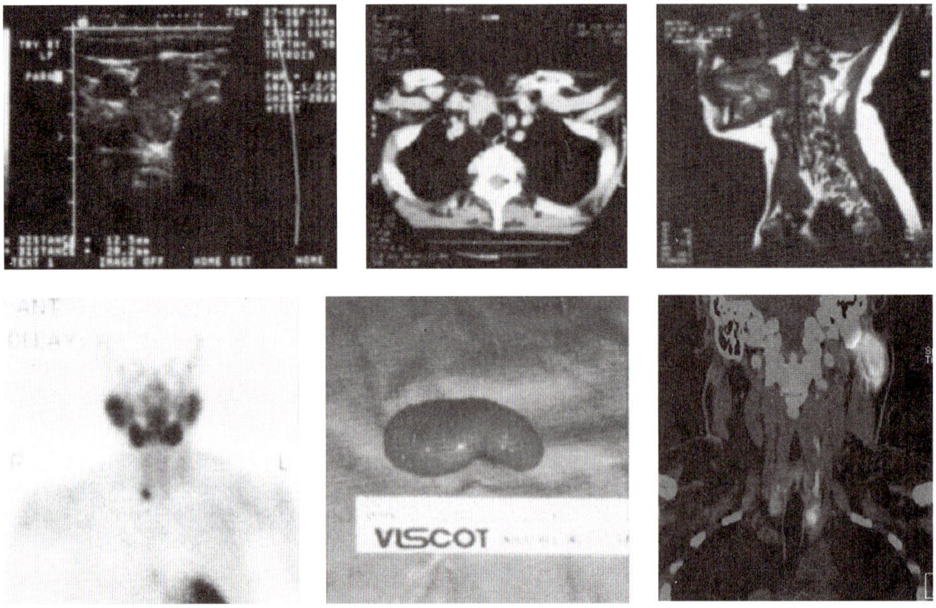

Figure 37-6 Parathyroid localization tests: parathyroid adenoma seen on sonogram, CT, MRI (top), and planar sestamibi scanning, fuset SPECT/CT, and gross pathology of parathyroid adenoma (bottom).

i. Sonography is relatively inexpensive, with sensitivities in the literature ranging from 22% to 89%. Sonography is, however, extremely operator dependent and is poor in evaluating lesions deep in the neck, behind the larynx and trachea, or in the mediastinum.

ii. Sestamibi scanning, with a sensitivity of 89%, can be a useful tool for detecting single adenomas and/or ectopic parathyroid glands. The sensitivity is decreased for small adenomas (typically < 1cm), double adenomas, hyperplasia, and/or concomitant thyroid disease. Technetium 99m methoxyisobutyl isonitrile (Tc^{99}MIBI) is initially taken up by both thyroid and parathyroids. The thyroid uptake is, over time, washed out, yet sestamibi is retained by adenomatous parathyroid glands. The uptake and retention of sestamibi is thought to be related to cellular mitochondrial content. Two-hour washout scans, therefore, reveal any enlarged parathyroids. Single proton emission computerized tomography (SPECT) scanning for primary hyperparathyroidism increases the accuracy of routine sestamibi scanning by about 2% to 3% by providing a three-dimensional picture.

iii. Hybrid SPECT/CT combines the three-dimensional functional information of SPECT with the anatomic information of CT, further improving preoperative localization.

iv. Dynamic-enhanced CT, known as 4D CT scanning was first used in 2006 and has since been shown to be helpful by identifying typical contrast perfusion characteristics of abnormal parathyroid glands. The benefits of high spatial resolution to identify small and/or ectopic glands as well as shorter imaging time, however, must be balanced with the increased radiation exposure to the thyroid (approximately 50-57 times more radiation compared to 99m-Tc-sestamibi). Sensitivity for single gland disease is as high as 94%; however, the sensitivity for MGD ranges from 32% to 60%.

Surgical Theory for Hyperparathyroidism

A. Although a single adenoma is most common, multigland disease and hyperplasia must always be kept in mind when creating the surgical plan. Unilateral exploration guided by preoperative localization studies may allow shorter operative times, a decrease in postsurgical complications, and resultant cost savings.
B. The trend is toward unilateral surgery and minimally invasive approaches with increased reliance on preoperative localization testing and rapid PTH assays for intraoperative PTH assessment. Given the short half-life of PTH (3-5 minutes), approximately 10 to 15 minutes after successful resection of an adenoma the PTH should fall to within normal limits. If PTH drops appropriately, surgery can be concluded with an expected 97% to 99% cure rate.
C. In cases of four-gland hyperplasia, surgical strategies include three-and-a-half-gland subtotal resection or four-gland resection with autotransplantation. In general, the aggressiveness of the surgical approach should relate to the clinical severity of the subtype of four-gland hyperplasia, balanced with the risk of permanent postoperative hypoparathyroidism.

Parathyroid: Surgical Anatomy

A. Parathyroid glands are described as flat-bean or leaf-like in shape and yellow-tan, caramel, or mahogany in color, and thus distinguishable from the brighter, less distinct yellow fat with which the parathyroids are typically closely associated. With age and degree of obesity affecting the degree of intraglandular fat and thus appearance parathyroid glands. They can be observed as discrete bodies gliding within the more amorphous fat surrounding them as this fat is gently manipulated (the gliding sign).
B. The vast majority of humans have four parathyroid glands, but approximately 5% of patients will have more than four glands (supernumerary).
C. Mirror-image symmetry typically occurs for the superior parathyroids as well as for the inferior parathyroids, and this symmetry may assist in finding a contralateral parathyroid.

Superior Parathyroid: Surgical Anatomy

A. The superior parathyroid derives from the fourth branchial pouch and is associated with the lateral thyroid anlage/C-cell complex. Due to the shorter embryologic migratory path, the position of the superior parathyroid glands is more consistent.
B. The superior parathyroid typically occurs at the level of the cricothyroid articulation of the larynx, approximately 1 cm above the intersection of the RLN and inferior thyroid artery. It is closely related to the posterolateral aspect of the superior thyroid pole, often resting on the thyroid capsule in this location and lies *deep or posterior* to the RLN.

Inferior Parathyroid: Surgical Anatomy

A. The inferior parathyroid glands derive from the third branchial pouch and migrate with the thymus anlage. Their position is more variable compared to superior parathyroid glands.

B. The inferior parathyroid is found in close association with the inferior pole of the thyroid, often on the posterolateral aspect of the capsule of the inferior pole or within 1 to 2 cm, and lies *superficial (ventral)* to the RLN. It is often closely associated with the thyrothymic ligament.

C. Parathyroid glands can be found anywhere along the embryologic migratory path. The most common ectopic locations for parathyroid adenomas include retroesophageal, retrotracheal, anterior mediastinal, intrathyroidal, and in the carotid sheath.

Parathyroid Surgery

A. Patients should be positioned supine with slight neck extension.

B. A small midline incision is made in a natural skin crease through skin, subcutaneous tissue, and the platysma. Subplatysmal flaps may be elevated.

C. The strap muscles are separated in the median raphe and then taken off the ventral surface of the thyroid gland. The thyroid gland is then mobilized and retracted medially.

D. The enlarged parathyroid is identified, circumferentially dissected without violation of the thin capsule, and the vascular pedicle is controlled with care not to damage the RLN.

Complications of Parathyroid Surgery

A. Reasons for surgical failure (ie, persistent or recurrent hypercalcemia) in the treatment of HPT include failure to find the adenomatous gland, failure to find a second adenoma, failure to recognize four-gland hyperplasia, failure to identify a supernumerary gland (ie, fifth gland), regrowth of adenoma from the unresected stump of an adenoma, unrecognized parathyroid carcinoma, or incorrect preoperative diagnosis (eg, BFHH).

B. Permanent hypoparathyroidism occurs after surgery in approximately 5% of adenoma cases overall and in 10% to 30% cases of hyperplasia or secondary HPT. Any derangements in PTH postoperatively are followed to assess for normalization. Preoperative vitamin D insufficiency or deficiency may contribute to postoperative hypocalcemia (temporary and permanent).

C. RLN paralysis rates are low, ranging from 0.4% to 4%.

Bibliography

Ali SZ, Baloch ZW, Cochand-Priollet B, et al. The 2023 Bethesda System for reporting thyroid cytopathology. *Thyroid*. 2023 Sept;33(9):1039-1044.

Baloch Z, Asa S, Barletta J, et al. Overview of the 2022 WHO classification of thyroid neoplasms. *Endocrine Pathology*. 2022;33:27-63.

Bischoff L, Ganly I, Fugazzola L, et al. Molecular alterations and comprehensive clinical management of oncocytic thyroid carcinoma – a review and multidisciplinary 2023 update. *JAMA Otolaryngol Head Neck Surg*. 2024 Jan;150(3):265-272.

Haugen DS, Alexander EK, Bible KC, et al. 2015 American Thyroid Association management guidelines for adult patients with thyroid nodules and differentiated thyroid cancer: the American Thyroid Association task force on thyroid nodules and differentiated thyroid cancer. *Thyroid*. 2016 Jan;26(1):1-133.

Karcioglu AS, Ahmed AA, Feng Z, et al. Return of vocal fold motion and surgical preservation of invaded recurrent laryngeal nerves after the use of neoadjuvant therapy in patients presenting with advanced thyroid cancer and vocal fold paralysis: the Lazarus effect. *Thyroid*. 2023 Oct;33(10):1259-1263.

Randolph G. *Surgery of the Thyroid and Parathyroid Glands.* 3rd ed. Philadelphia, PA: Elsevier Saunders; 2021.

Randolph GW, Dralle H, International Intraoperative Monitoring Study Group, et al. International Intraoperative Monitoring Study Group. Electrophysiologic recurrent laryngeal nerve monitoring during thyroid and parathyroid surgery: international standards guideline statement. *Laryngoscope.* 2011 Jan;121 Suppl 1:S1-16.

Shifrin AS, Fahey TJ. *Lange Endocrine Surgery Clinical Diagnosis and Management.* 1st ed. Hong Kong: McGraw Hill; 2025.

Shonka DC Jr, Ho A, Chintakuntlawar AV, et al. American Head and Neck Society Endocrine Surgery Section and International Thyroid Oncology Group consensus statement on mutational testing in thyroid cancer: Defining advanced thyroid cancer and its targeted treatment. *Head Neck.* 2022 Jun;44(6):1277-1300.

Zhao X, Wang J, Dadu R, et al. Surgery after BRAF-directed therapy is associated with improved survival in $BRAF^{V600E}$ mutant anaplastic thyroid cancer: a single-center retrospective cohort study. *Thyroid.* 2023 Apr;33(4):484-491.

Questions

1. A high suspicion feature of a thyroid nodule on ultrasound would include
   A. Spongiform appearance
   B. Solid
   C. Microcalcifications
   D. Cystic appearance
   E. Hypoechogenicity

2. Most parathyroid glands
   A. Are vascularized by the superior thyroid artery
   B. Are in the mediastinum
   C. Are close to or on the thyroid gland
   D. Are often found to be adenomatous at thyroid surgery
   E. Are removed and autotransplanted at surgery

3. Papillary thyroid cancer
   A. Prognosis is worse in the young adult
   B. Is associated with frequent nodal metastasis at presentation
   C. Is associated with capsular invasion
   D. Is typically associated with C-cell hyperplasia
   E. Cannot occur in the pyramidal lobe

4. Medullary cancers
   A. May be associated with RET oncogene mutation
   B. Are always inherited
   C. Result in decrease of calcitonin and carcinoembryonic antigen (CEA)
   D. Never spread to liver or lungs
   E. Are always associated with parathyroid disease

5. Graves' disease
   A. Is associated with focal increased uptake in the thyroid
   B. Can be managed with surgery
   C. Cannot usually be treated with radioactive iodine
   D. Is always associated with eye disease
   E. Generally can be operated on without preoperative medical management

Chapter 38
Cysts and Tumors of the Jaw

Introduction

- Cysts and tumors are rare entities and include a wide differential diagnosis.
- Odontogenic origin pertains to lesions from tooth-related structures, whereas nonodontogenic lesions arise from bone and soft tissue cells.
- Jaw cysts are classified as inflammatory odontogenic, developmental odontogenic, or nonodontogenic.
- Cysts and tumors of odontogenic origin may involve vital and nonvital teeth; therefore, dental exams are essential in the diagnostic phase.
- Clinical features, physical exam, imaging are critical for a differential diagnosis.
- Incisional biopsy versus final treatment will depend on the differential diagnosis.
- Majority of jaw cysts and tumors have good prognosis after complete surgical removal.

Odontogenic Cysts: Inflammatory

A. **Periapical cyst**
   1. **Clinical features**
      - Overall, the most common, accounting for 60% of all odontogenic cysts.
      - Associated with *nonvital* tooth or trauma, not always symptomatic.
      - Necrotic dental pulp creates inflammatory response at root apex creating a fibrous connective tissue wall containing fluid and cellular debris.
   2. **Radiographical features**
      - Radiolucent, single lesion, well-demarcated, unilocular
      - Surrounding the apex of the affected tooth
   3. **Histopathological features**
      - Polymorphonuclear leukocytes (PMNs) intermixed with inflammatory exudate, cellular debris, necrotic material, bacterial colonies.
   4. **Treatment**
      - Removal of underlying inflammatory process through endodontic treatment (root canal) or tooth extraction with enucleation and curettage.
      - Antibiotics and drainage of any soft tissue abscess (if occurs).
   5. **Prognosis**
      - Excellent

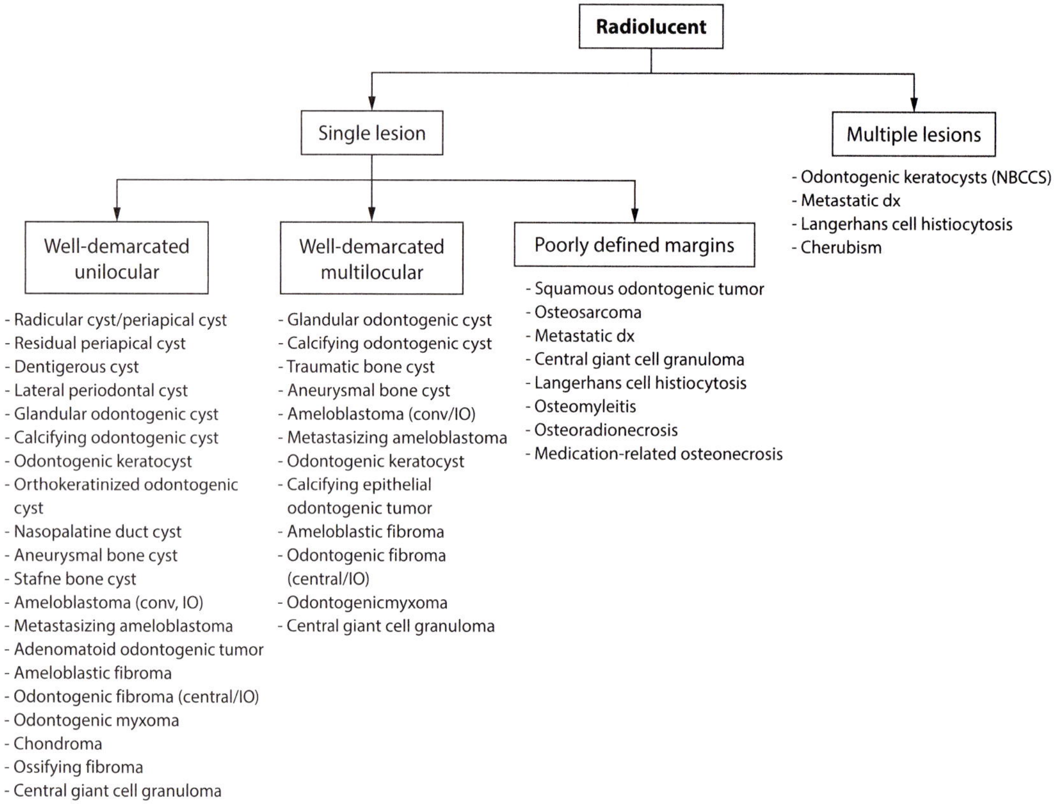

Figure 38-1 Clinical algorithm: Radiolucent lesions. (conv: conventional; IO: intraosseous; NBCCS: nevoid basal cell carcinoma syndrome)

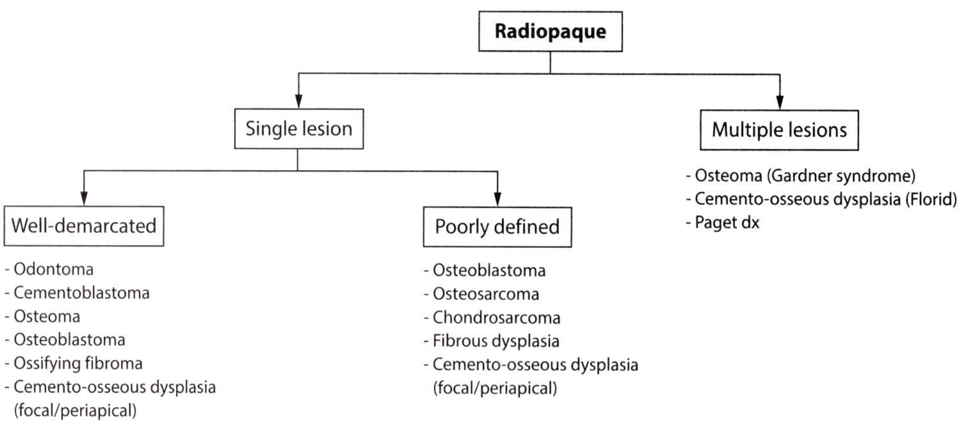

B. **Residual periapical cyst**
   1. **Clinical features**
      - Remnant of cyst left in jaw after the associated tooth has been extracted
      - Generally asymptomatic
   2. **Radiographical features**
      - Radiolucent, well-demarcated, and unilocular
   3. **Histopathological features**
      - Same as periapical cyst
   4. **Treatment**
      - Enucleation and curettage
   5. **Prognosis**
      - Excellent

C. **Inflammatory collateral cyst: mandibular buccal bifurcation cyst**
   1. **Clinical features**
      - Found on the buccal surface of erupting mandibular first molars, although some cases have involved mandibular second molars
      - Common in the developing tooth ages of 5 to 13 years
      - Localized swelling and foul-tasting discharge at the location of the erupting tooth
   2. **Radiographical features**
      - Radiolucent, single lesion, and well-demarcated
      - Associated with the erupting mandibular molars listed above
   3. **Histopathological features**
      - Nonspecific, cyst lined by nonkeratinizing stratified squamous epithelium with chronic inflammatory cell infiltrate in the connective tissue wall
   4. **Treatment**
      - Enucleation but extraction of the associated tooth is unnecessary
   5. **Prognosis**
      - Excellent

Odontogenic Cysts: Developmental

A. **Eruption Cyst (soft tissue equivalent of the dentigerous cyst)**
   1. **Clinical features**
      - Occurs during tooth eruption process in children less than 10 years of age.
      - Bluish cyst appears under the gingiva, can sometimes be painful.
   2. **Radiographical features**
      - Not typically necessary but can confirm presence of erupting tooth.
      - Diagnosis usually made clinically.
   3. **Histopathological features**
      - Surface oral epithelium with underlying inflammatory infiltrate
   4. **Treatment**
      - Usually not needed, resolves when tooth erupts through the cyst.
      - If cyst remains after tooth eruption, then simple excision.
   5. **Prognosis**
      - Excellent

B. **Dentigerous Cyst**
1. **Clinical features**
   - Second most common of all odontogenic cysts.
   - Most common between ages of 10 and 30 years.
   - Associated with the crown of any unerupted tooth, most often the mandibular third molars.
   - May grow extensively and associated with painless expansion of bone.
2. **Radiographical features**
   - Radiolucent, well-demarcated, and unilocular
   - Associated with crown of unerupted tooth
3. **Histopathological features**
   - Fibrous capsule surrounded by inflammatory infiltrate
4. **Treatment**
   - Extraction of affected tooth with enucleation and curettage.
   - If larger cyst, may consider two-stage approach with prolonged decompression with drain prior to formal treatment.
5. **Prognosis**
   - Excellent, very low recurrence rate

C. **Glandular odontogenic cyst**
1. **Clinical features**
   - Middle-aged adults, rarely less than 20 years of age.
   - Approximately 80% occur in mandible, generally anterior.
   - Small cysts can be asymptomatic, but larger ones can expand to produce pain/ paresthesia.
   - Histopathological variants resemble central mucoepidermoid carcinoma when incisional biopsy is not adequate.
2. **Radiographical features**
   - Radiolucent, single lesion, well-demarcated, unilocular or multilocular
3. **Histopathological features**
   - Lined with stratified squamous epithelium with small microcysts and clusters of mucous cells present.
   - Hobnail cells and *MAML2* gene arrangements help exclude diagnosis of mucoepidermoid carcinoma.
4. **Treatment**
   - Generally, enucleation and curettage, consideration of en bloc resection
5. **Prognosis**
   - Variable recurrence rates reported, but some greater than 30% as there is potential for locally aggressive behavior.

D. **Calcifying odontogenic cyst (Gorlin cyst)**
1. **Clinical features**
   - Variable clinical behavior, age, and location
   - Mean age of 30 years
   - Can be intraosseous or extraosseous
2. **Radiographical features**
   - Radiolucent, single lesion, well-demarcated, unilocular or multilocular.
   - Irregular calcifications can be present.
3. **Histopathological features**
   - Cystic lining with eosinophilic ghost cells, which often calcify

4. **Treatment**
    - Enucleation and curettage for intraosseous
    - Excision for extraosseous
5. **Prognosis**
    - Good

E. **Odontogenic keratocyst (OKC)**

1. **Clinical features**
    - Potentially aggressive behavior, previously known by WHO as a tumor, but *most recently* (2022) lesion is categorized as a cyst.
    - 60% of cases are diagnosed between the ages of 10 and 40 years.
    - Majority involve the posterior body and ramus of mandible.
    - If multiple, evaluate for nevoid basal cell carcinoma syndrome (NBCCS, Gorlin syndrome):
        - Autosomal dominant
            - Multiple basal cell carcinomas
            - Multiple odontogenic keratocyst
            - Skin cysts, palmar/plantar pits
            - Calcified falx cerebri
            - Increased head circumference
            - Rib/vertebral malformations
            - Hypertelorism (mild)
            - Spina bifida
2. **Radiographical features**
    - Radiolucent, single lesion, well-demarcated, unilocular or multilocular
3. **Histopathological features**
    - Parakeratinized epithelial lining, with hyperchromatic palisaded basal cell layer
    - Critical for diagnosis as otherwise very similar to periapical and dentigerous cysts
4. **Treatment**
    - Controlled decompression with intraoral drain (if large to reduce size).
    - Enucleation and curettage with extraction of involved teeth, +/− peripheral ostectomy.
    - Topical 5-fluorouacil to target proliferating cells after peripheral ostectomy has replaced Carnoy for its biocompatibility.
5. **Prognosis**
    - Locally aggressive behavior, up to 30% recurrence rate (peripheral budding).
    - Most recurrences happen within the first 5 years.

F. **Orthokeratinized Odontogenic Cyst (OOC)**

1. **Clinical features**
    - Not a subvariant of the OKC, has clinicopathological differences.
    - Predominant in young adults and most common in posterior mandible.
    - No association with a syndrome as in OKC.
2. **Radiographical features**
    - Radiolucent, single lesion, well-demarcated, unilocular or multilocular
    - Vary in size from 1 to 7 centimeters
3. **Histopathological features**
    - Orthokeratinized epithelial lining, no palisaded basal cell layer.
    - The prominent palisaded basal cell layer seen in an OKC is not present.

4. **Treatment**
    - Controlled decompression with intraoral drain (if large to reduce size)
    - Enucleation and curettage with extraction of involved teeth, +/− peripheral ostectomy
5. **Prognosis**
    - Excellent, very low risk of recurrence

G. **Gingival cyst (soft tissue equivalent of the lateral periodontal cyst)**
1. **Clinical features:**
    - Common lesions, reported in 25% to 35% of all newborns.
    - Usually less than 3 months of age.
    - Cysts are 2 to 3 mm in diameter and more common in the maxillary alveolus.
2. **Radiographical features**
    - Typically unnecessary
3. **Histopathological features**
    - Thin flattened epithelial lining with keratinaceous debris
4. **Treatment**
    - No treatment as spontaneously involute with rupture of tooth
5. **Prognosis**
    - Excellent

H. **Lateral periodontal cyst**
1. **Clinical features**
    - Asymptomatic, only found on radiograph
    - Occurs in the age of 40 to 70 years, rarely seen in those less than 30 years
    - About 80% occur with mandibular anterior teeth
2. **Radiographical features**
    - Radiolucent, single lesion, well-demarcated, and unilocular
    - Lateral to roots of *vital* teeth
    - Usually less than 1 centimeter in size.
3. **Histopathological features**
    - Thin epithelial lining with foci of glycogen-rich clear cells
4. **Treatment**
    - Enucleation with preservation of tooth
5. **Prognosis**
    - Excellent

Nonodontogenic Cysts

A. **Nasopalatine duct cyst**
1. **Clinical features**
    - Most common nonodontogenic cyst; however, only occurring in approximately 1% of the population.
    - Forms during fusion of primary and secondary palate.
    - Most common in 30 to 60 years of age, rare less than 10 years of age despite being of embryological origin, with a male predominance.
    - Common symptoms include intermittent swelling, drainage, and pain of the anterior palate.

2. **Radiographical features**
   - Heart-shaped radiolucent lesion, single lesion, well-demarcated, and unilocular
   - Above roots of central incisors
3. **Histopathological features**
   - Variable depending on proportion of respiratory (nasal) epithelium and squamous (oral) epithelium.
4. **Treatment**
   - Enucleation
5. **Prognosis**
   - Excellent

B. **Simple bone cyst (Traumatic bone cyst/Solitary bone cyst)**
1. **Clinical features:**
   - Considered a pseudocyst as it lacks a true epithelial lining.
   - Does not necessarily have traumatic history; theories include:
     - Venous obstruction
     - Local disturbance in bone growth
     - Ischemic marrow necrosis
     - Altered calcium metabolism
   - Most common between ages 10 and 20 years, and male predominance.
   - Often found on routine radiographic exam due to lack of clinical symptoms.
   - Affects mandible more than maxilla.
   - 18G-needle aspiration yields nothing or scant blood.
2. **Radiographical features**
   - Radiolucent, single lesion, well-demarcated, or multilocular
   - Can scallop roots of adjacent teeth
   - Can range from 1 to 10 centimeters in diameter
3. **Histopathological features**
   - Thin, vascular, connective tissue membrane with no epithelial lining
4. **Treatment**
   - Surgical exploration of cyst alone will often induce healing process
5. **Prognosis**
   - Excellent

C. **Aneurysmal bone cyst**
1. **Clinical features**
   - Only 2% of cases involve the jaw, often in patients less than 30 years of age, and affects mandible more than maxilla.
   - Rapid swelling of jaw can occur with pain and malocclusion.
   - 18G-needle aspiration can yield blood.
2. **Radiographical features**
   - Radiolucent, single lesion, well-demarcated, unilocular or multilocular
   - Can have "soap bubble" appearance
3. **Histopathological features**
   - Blood-filled space surrounded by connective tissue
   - No epithelial lining
4. **Treatment**
   - Generally curettage, possible sclerotherapy
   - Resection rare, only in severe cases
5. **Prognosis**
   - Excellent

Odontogenic Tumors: Benign Epithelial

A. **Ameloblastoma, Unicystic**
   1. **Clinical features**
      - Second decade and male predilection
      - Over 90% are found in the posterior body of mandible and ramus
      - Mimics a dentigerous cyst
   2. **Radiographical features**
      - Well-circumscribed radiolucency that surrounds the crown of an unerupted tooth
      - Resembles closely to the dentigerous cyst
   3. **Histopathological features**
      - Depending on the ameloblastic epithelium infiltration level can be divided into 1 of 3 subtypes:
        - Luminal
        - Intraluminal
        - Mural
   4. **Treatment**
      - Lesion is suggestive of an odontogenic cyst.
      - Debate over enucleation and curettage versus resection with clear margins.
   5. **Prognosis**
      - Recurrence rates are 10% to 20% with enucleation and curettage alone.

B. **Ameloblastoma, conventional solid or multicystic**
   1. **Clinical features**
      - Benign locally aggressive neoplasm.
      - Rare before the age of 10, with prevalence in the third to seventh decades of life.
      - About 85% occur in the mandible, most commonly in molar/ramus region.
      - Slow, painless expansion of jaw.
      - Mutation of genes in MAPK pathway observed in 90% of all lesions.
   2. **Radiographical features**
      - Multilocular radiolucent lesion with possible "soap bubble" appearance.
      - Often has buccal and lingual cortical expansion.
   3. **Histopathological features**
      - The epithelium demonstrates peripheral columnar cells exhibiting reversed polarization; *piano key* appearance
      - Multiple subtypes:
        - Follicular
        - Plexiform
        - Acanthomatous
        - Granular cell
        - Desmoplastic
        - Basal cell variant
   4. **Treatment**
      - Optimal method has been controversial.
      - Most favor resection with 1 cm past radiographic extent of tumor.
      - May consider recurrent ameloblastoma treatment with BRAF-targeted therapy with confirmed *MAPK* gene mutation in lesion.
   5. **Prognosis**
      - Good with regular clinical and radiographic surveillance

C. **Ameloblastoma, peripheral (extraosseous)**
   1. **Clinical features**
      - Middle-age adult, male predilection, and often in the mandibular premolar and maxillary molar regions
      - Sessile or pedunculated gingival mass, not ulcerated
   2. **Radiographical features**
      - Limited utility since extraosseous
   3. **Histopathological features**
      - Ameloblastic epithelium below the lamina propria
   4. **Treatment**
      - Surgical excision
   5. **Prognosis**
      - Recurrence rate 15% to 20%

D. **Metastasizing ameloblastoma**
   1. **Clinical features**
      - An ameloblastoma that metastasizes, despite benign histopathological appearance.
      - Mean age of 45 years, slightly male predominance.
      - Primary site is mandible and metastatic is lung and cervical lymph nodes.
   2. **Radiographical features**
      - Radiolucent, single lesion, well-demarcated, unilocular or multilocular
   3. **Histopathological features**
      - No cytologic changes from the conventional form other than the fact it is metastatic.
   4. **Treatment**
      - Depends on stage
   5. **Prognosis**
      - Fair/poor

E. **Adenomatoid odontogenic tumor**
   1. **Clinical features**
      - Two-thirds in teenage females
      - Two-thirds are in association with impacted canines
      - Majority occur in the anterior maxilla
   2. **Radiographical features**
      - Radiolucent, well-demarcated, and unilocular
      - Seldom exceed greater than 3 cm in diameter
      - May contain small snowflake calcifications that helps differentiate from dentigerous cyst
   3. **Histopathological features**
      - Variable duct-like structures within fibrous stroma
   4. **Treatment**
      - Enucleation
   5. **Prognosis**
      - Excellent

F. **Calcifying epithelial odontogenic tumor (Pindborg tumor)**
   1. **Clinical features**
      - Uncommon, accounts for less than 1% of all odontogenic tumors
      - Generally occur between 30 and 50 years of age
      - More common in mandible than maxilla
      - Painless, slowly progressive swelling

2. **Radiographical features**
    - Radiolucent, well-demarcated, and multilocular
3. **Histopathological features**
    - Large areas of amyloid-like extracellular material, forming concentric rings known as "Liesegang ring" calcifications (Congo red staining)
4. **Treatment**
    - Resection with small margin of normal bone
5. **Prognosis**
    - Good, a 15% recurrence rate
    - Tumors being treated by curettage alone report the highest frequency

G. **Squamous odontogenic tumor**
1. **Clinical features**
    - Variable age
    - Variable location
2. **Radiographical features**
    - Radiolucent with poorly defined margins
3. **Histopathological features**
    - Patches of squamous epithelium in fibrous stroma
4. **Treatment**
    - Conservative local excision or curettage
5. **Prognosis**
    - Excellent

Odontogenic Tumors: Mixed Epithelial and Mesenchymal

A. **Ameloblastic Fibroma**
1. **Clinical features**
    - Generally occur less than 30 years of age
    - Male predominance
    - Most common in posterior mandible
2. **Radiographical features**
    - Radiolucent, single lesion, well-demarcated, unilocular or multilocular
3. **Histopathological features**
    - Odontogenic epithelium in mesenchymal stroma
4. **Treatment**
    - Initial: enucleation and curettage
    - Recurrence: en bloc resection
5. **Prognosis**
    - Good, but close surveillance needed, up to 18% recur

B. **Odontoma**
1. **Clinical features**
    - Commonly occurs during 10 to 30 years of age
    - Asymptomatic, found on routine dental radiographical screening
2. **Radiographical features**
    - Radiopaque, single lesion, and well-demarcated
    - Two types:
        - Compound-appears as small tooth-like structures
        - Complex-enamel and dentin, no resemblance to tooth
3. **Histopathological features**
    - Irregular tooth-like structures in an enamel matrix

4. **Treatment**
   - Enucleation
5. **Prognosis**
   - Excellent

Odontogenic Tumors: Mesenchymal

A. **Odontogenic Fibroma (Intraosseous)**
   1. **Clinical features**
      - More common after age of 40 years, strong female predilection.
      - Most commonly located in posterior mandible or anterior maxilla.
      - Generally asymptomatic, may cause bony expansion or loose teeth.
   2. **Radiographical features**
      - Radiolucent, single lesion, well-demarcated, unilocular (when small), or multilocular (when large)
   3. **Histopathological features**
      - Fibroblasts in collagen matrix
   4. **Treatment**
      - Enucleation and vigorous curettage
   5. **Prognosis**
      - Good

B. **Peripheral odontogenic fibroma (extraosseous)**
   1. **Clinical features**
      - Soft tissue version of the odontogenic fibroma
      - Can occur at variable ages
      - Slow growing gingival mass with normal overlying mucosa, most are 0.5 to 1.0 centimeter in size
   2. **Radiographical features**
      - None, extraosseous
   3. **Histopathological features**
      - Same as central
   4. **Treatment**
      - Surgical excision
   5. **Prognosis**
      - Excellent

C. **Odontogenic myxoma**
   1. **Clinical features**
      - More commonly occurs in mandible, average age is 25 to 30 years, slight female predilection
      - Painless expansion of bone (when large)
   2. **Radiographical features**
      - Radiolucent, single, well-demarcated, unilocular or multilocular
      - "Soap bubble" pattern; appears similar to ameloblastoma
   3. **Histopathological features**
      - Stellate cells in loose myxoid stroma
   4. **Treatment**
      - Resection as often locally aggressive
   5. **Prognosis**
      - Good, but close follow-up needed as average recurrence rate is about 25%

D. **Cementoblastoma**
   1. **Clinical features**
      - Solitary lesion found in continuity with a tooth root
      - Majority occur in molar/premolar region of mandible, with pain and swelling present in 70% of cases
      - Most common less than 30 years of age
   2. **Radiographical features**
      - Radiopaque and well-demarcated
      - Associated with root
   3. **Histopathological features**
      - Cementoblasts
   4. **Treatment**
      - Extraction of tooth with attached mass
   5. **Prognosis**
      - Excellent

E. **Cemento-ossifying fibroma**
   1. **Clinical features**
      - The 2022 WHO update reclassified this lesion as odontogenic due to its origins from periodontal ligament progenitor cells.
      - Occurs only in tooth-bearing areas of the jaws.
      - Broad age range with peak in the third and fourth decades of life, slight female predilection.
      - Mandible far more affected than maxilla.
   2. **Radiographical features**
      - Radiolucent or radiopaque (can be mixed), and well-demarcated unilocular
   3. **Histopathological features**
      - Woven bone and cementum-like material surrounded by fibrous connective tissue
   4. **Treatment**
      - Enucleation and curettage
   5. **Prognosis**
      - Good

Nonodontogenic Tumors: Primary

A. **Osteoma**
   1. **Clinical features**
      - Young adults
      - Asymptomatic, slowly growing
      - Usually found at mandible body and condyle
      - Gardner syndrome:
         - Autosomal dominant (chromosome 5).
         - Colonic polyposis, multiple osteomas of the jaws, skin fibromas, impacted teeth.
         - Close surveillance with colonoscopy is needed as there is a high rate of malignant transformation of colonic polyps.
   2. **Radiographical features**
      - Radiopaque and well-demarcated
      - Can have multiple lesions in Gardner syndrome

3. **Histopathological features**
   - Normal appearing bone (either cancellous or compact)
4. **Treatment**
   - Observation or surgical excision (if symptomatic)
5. **Prognosis**
   - Excellent

B. **Osteoblastoma**
1. **Clinical features**
   - Commonly dull pain, tenderness, and swelling are presenting features
   - Majority occur less than 30 years of age, with a slight mandibular and female predilection
2. **Radiographical features**
   - Radiopaque, single lesion, well-demarcated or poorly defined
3. **Histopathological features**
   - Irregular bony trabecular pattern
4. **Treatment**
   - Local excision and curettage
5. **Prognosis**
   - Good, with recurrence uncommon

C. **Osteosarcoma**
1. **Clinical features**
   - Most common between ages 10 and 20 years
   - 6% of all osteosarcomas arise in the jaws, with an equal incidence in both mandible and maxilla
   - Swelling, pain, loosening of teeth
2. **Radiographical features**
   - Radiolucent, single lesion, poorly defined margins or radiopaque, single lesion, poorly defined
   - Noted sunburst appearance and widening of the periodontal ligament
3. **Histopathological features**
   - Osteoblastic, chondroblastic, or fibroblastic depending on the amount of osteoid, cartilage, or collagen produced
4. **Treatment**
   - Radical resection usually with pre- and postoperative chemotherapy
5. **Prognosis**
   - Fair

D. **Chondroma**
1. **Clinical features**
   - Most common between ages 30 and 50 years
   - Most commonly located in anterior maxilla or condyle
   - Painless, slow growing
2. **Radiographical features**
   - Radiolucent, single lesion, well-demarcated, unilocular with central area of radiopacity
3. **Histopathological features**
   - Mature hyaline cartilage
4. **Treatment**
   - Resection
5. **Prognosis**
   - Good

E. **Chondrosarcoma**
   1. **Clinical features**
      - Occurs in older adults
      - More common in maxilla than mandible
      - Painless swelling
   2. **Radiographical features**
      - Radiopaque, single lesion, poorly defined
   3. **Histopathological features**
      - Three grades exist:
         - Grade 1, similar to chondroma
         - Grade 2, increased cellularity
         - Grade 3, increased cellularity with spindle cell proliferation
   4. **Treatment**
      - Radical resection
      - Tends to be less responsive to radiation or chemotherapy
   5. **Prognosis**
      - Dependent on histologic grade

F. **Metastatic disease**
   1. **Clinical features**
      - Older adults, may be initial presentation of primary malignancy
      - Breast most common, then lung, then prostate
      - May present with pain, paresthesia, nonhealing extraction sites
   2. **Radiographical features**
      - Radiolucent, generally multiple
      - Although can have single lesion, poorly defined margins
   3. **Histopathological features**
      - Consistent with primary malignancy
   4. **Treatment**
      - Depends on primary malignancy
   5. **Prognosis**
      - Depends on primary malignancy

Nonodontogenic Tumors: Fibro-Osseous Lesions

A. **Fibrous Dysplasia**
   1. **Clinical features:**
      - Generally asymptomatic
      - May cease or "burn out" after puberty
      - Two subtypes:
         - Monostotic:
            - Most common form of the disease, 80%.
            - Equal male and female predilection with diagnosis in second decade.
            - Maxilla is more affected than mandible with growth extending into the zygoma, sphenoid, ethmoid, and frontal bones.
            - Lesions tend to stabilize after skeletal maturation.
         - Polyostotic: McCune-Albright syndrome: café au lait skin lesions, endocrinopathies such as precocious puberty, pituitary or thyroid abnormalities.

2. **Radiographical features**
   - Radiopaque, single lesion, poorly defined
   - "Ground glass" appearance
3. **Histopathological features**
   - Irregular bony trabeculations in fibrous stroma
4. **Treatment**
   - Observation or surgical excision; dependent on size, location, symptom severity
5. **Prognosis**
   - Variable, depending on location and extent of disease

B. **Cemento-osseous dysplasia**

1. **Clinical features**
   - Strong female predominance.
   - More common in African Americans, in the fourth-fifth decades of life.
   - Teeth are vital with associated lesions.
   - Three subtypes:
     i. Focal: posterior mandible
     ii. Periapical: anterior mandible, around tooth root
     iii. Florid: diffuse involvement
2. **Radiographical features**
   - Radiopaque, single lesion, well demarcated or poorly defined
   - Extent depends on subtype as florid can have multiple lesions
3. **Histopathological features**
   - Spicules of bone and cementum intermixed within connective tissue
4. **Treatment**
   - Generally, none needed
5. **Prognosis**
   - Good

C. **Central giant cell granuloma tumor**

1. **Clinical features**
   - Majority occur less than 30 years of age.
   - Majority occur in the mandible.
   - Can cross midline in anterior maxilla.
   - Similar features to Brown tumors of hyperparathyroidism.
   - Nonaggressive lesions grow slowly, are painless, and do not resorb tooth roots.
   - Aggressive lesions will be symptomatic, fast growing, and occur in younger patients.
2. **Radiographical features**
   - Radiolucent, single lesion, well-demarcated, unilocular or multilocular lesions or ill defined
3. **Histopathological features**
   - Multinucleated giant cells in loose cellular stroma
   - Has similar features to brown tumors of hyperparathyroidism
4. **Treatment**
   - Closely resembles brown tumor and hyperparathyroidism should be ruled out in all cases
   - Medical: intralesional steroids, calcitonin, or interferon
   - Surgical: aggressive curettage (usually treated surgically)
5. **Prognosis**
   - Good

Manifestations of Systemic Conditions

A. **Langerhans cell histiocytosis**
   1. **Clinical features**
      - Most common in children
      - Males more than females
      - Dull pain common
   2. **Radiographical features**
      - Radiolucent, single or multiple lesions, poorly defined
      - Teeth may have "floating in air" appearance
   3. **Histopathological features**
      - Histiocytes intermixed with plasma cells, lymphocytes, giant cells
   4. **Treatment**
      - Radiation or chemotherapy
   5. **Prognosis**
      - Poor

B. **Cherubism**
   1. **Clinical features**
      - Autosomal dominant
      - Most common during 2 to 5 years of age, can enlarge with growth and become stable by puberty
      - Painless, bilateral cheek swelling due to expansion of posterior mandible
   2. **Radiographical features**
      - Radiolucent, multiple lesions, upper and lower jaws
   3. **Histopathological features**
      - Vascular fibrous tissue containing giant cells
   4. **Treatment**
      - Observation versus surgical excision depending on symptom severity
   5. **Prognosis**
      - Variable

C. **Paget disease**
   1. **Clinical features**
      - Male predominance
      - More common in Caucasians than African Americans
      - Usually occurs older than 50 years of age
      - Chronic, slowly progressive
      - Can have cranial neuropathies if foramina are involved
   2. **Radiographical features**
      - Radiopaque, multiple lesions; "cotton-wool" appearance
   3. **Histopathological features**
      - Uncontrolled osteoblastic and osteoclastic activity
   4. **Treatment**
      - Bisphosphonates, calcitonin (slows bone turnover)
   5. **Prognosis**
      - Chronic disease, rarely causes death

D. **Osteomyelitis**
   1. **Clinical features**
      - More common in mandible than maxilla
      - Fever, leukocytosis, swelling, lymphadenopathy

2. **Radiographical features**
   - Radiolucent, single, poorly defined margins
3. **Histopathological features**
   - Necrotic bone, surrounding inflammation
4. **Treatment**
   - Surgical debridement followed by intravenous antibiotics
5. **Prognosis**
   - Variable

E. **Osteoradionecrosis**
1. **Clinical features:**
   - Complication from head and neck radiation, leaving bone hypocellular and hypoxic
   - Can be very painful
2. **Radiographical features**
   - Radiolucent, single, poorly defined margins
3. **Treatment**
   - If mild, good oral hygiene, debridement as needed
   - If severe, may require surgical resection with vascularized flap reconstruction
4. **Prognosis**
   - Variable, dependent on severity

Medication-Related Osteonecrosis of the Jaw (MRONJ)

1. **Clinical features**
   - Occurs in patients undergoing dental procedures after receiving PO/IV bisphosphonate therapy, or other antiresorptive (ie, RANK ligand inhibitor, denosumab) or antiangiogenic medications
   - No history of radiation therapy
   - Can be painful
2. **Radiographical features**
   - Radiolucent, single, poorly defined margins
3. **Treatment**
   - Variable, can range from good oral hygiene, debridement, to surgical resection and reconstruction
4. **Prognosis**
   - Variable, dependent on severity

Questions

1. Treatment that involves resection with clear margin is required for which tumor?
   A. Odontogenic fibroma
   B. Squamous odontogenic
   C. Calcifying epithelial odontogenic
   D. Ameloblastic fibroma
   E. Adenomatoid odontogenic

2. Which lesion has a unilocular radiolucent appearance?
   A. Calcifying odontogenic cyst
   B. Cemento-osseous dysplasia
   C. Ameloblastic fibroma
   D. Cementoblastoma
   E. Osteosarcoma

3. A well-defined radiolucent lesion surrounding the crown of an unerupted tooth is associated with
   A. Ameloblastoma, unicystic
   B. Calcifying odontogenic cyst
   C. Odontogenic fibroma
   D. Glandular odontogenic cyst
   E. Odontogenic myxoma

4. Which lesion has histopathological overlap with mucoepidermoid carcinoma?
   A. Adenomatoid odontogenic tumor
   B. Nasopalatine duct cyst
   C. Aneurysmal bone cyst
   D. Squamous odontogenic tumor
   E. Glandular odontogenic cyst

5. A radiolucent lesion associated with the root of a vital tooth is
   A. Dentigerous cyst
   B. Glandular odontogenic cyst
   C. Calcifying odontogenic cyst
   D. Periapical cyst
   E. Lateral periodontal cyst

Bibilography

Jing W, Xuan M, Lin Y, et al. Odontogenic tumours: a retrospective study of 1642 cases in a Chinese population. *Int J Oral Maxillofac Surg*. Jan 2007;36:20-25.

Neville BW, Damm DD, Allen CM, Chi AC. *Oral and Maxillofacial Pathology*. 5th ed. St. Louis MS: Elsevier; 2022.

Ochsenius G, Escobar E, Godoy L, Penafiel C. Odontogenic cysts: analysis of 2,944 cases in Chile. *Med Oral Patol Oral Cir Bucal*. Mar 2007;12:E85-91.

Ruggiero SL, Dodson TB, Aghaloo T, Carlson ER, Ward BB, Kademani D. American Association of Oral and Maxillofacial Surgeons' Position Paper on Medication-Related Osteonecrosis of the Jaws-2022 Update. *J Oral Maxillofac Surg*. 2022;80(5):920-943.

Soluk-Tekkesin M, Wright JM. The World Health Organization Classification of Odontogenic Lesions: A Summary of the Changes of the 2022 (5th) Edition. The World Health Organization Classification of Odontogenic Lesions: A Summary of the Changes of the 2022 (5th) Edition. *Turk Patoloji Derg*. 2022; 38(2):168-184.

Chapter 39
Carotid Body Tumors and Vascular Anomalies

Paragangliomas

Anatomy and Physiology

- Paraganglia are cells that facilitate baroreceptive and chemoreceptive reflexes of cardiovascular system.
  - Either branchiomeric (distributed along arteries and cranial nerves associated with a branchial arch) or intravagal.
  - Chief cells (type I) are derived from neural crest and are capable of secreting neurotransmitters.
  - Sustentacular cells (type II) are similar to Schwann cells surrounding autonomic ganglia.
  - In paragangliomas, cell arrangement is known as *Zellballen*, consisting of tumor nests of type I cells surrounded by type II cells in a fibrovascular stroma.
- The carotid body is a distinct oval chemoreceptor (oxygen, pH, and carbon dioxide) posterior to carotid bifurcation; afferent reflex is mediated by Hering nerve (branch of the glossopharyngeal nerve).

Epidemiology and Genetics

- Represent 1 in 10,000 of extracranial head and neck tumors; 80% are carotid body or jugulotympanic tumors, 5% are vagal tumors.
- 10% of patients with sporadic paraganglioma will have a concurrent second paraganglioma.
- Association with living at high altitude and chronic hypoxemia.
- 1% to 3% secrete catecholamines; evaluate with plasma-free metanephrines or 24-hour urine fractionated metanephrines.
- Malignant paragangliomas are rare, have propensity for regional nodal and distant spread, primarily to the lungs, liver, and bones.
  - Orbital and laryngeal most likely to be malignant (25%), followed by vagal (10%), jugulotympanic (5%), and carotid body tumors (3-6%)
  - Malignancy confirmed by presence of tumor in lymph nodes or distant metastatic sites
- Hereditary susceptibility related to mutations at several loci on chromosomes 11 and 1, named PGL1 (11q23), PGL2 (11q11.3), *PGL3* (1q21-23), and PGL4 (1p36).
- Mutations in succinate dehydrogenase (*SDH*) subunits D, C, and B are responsible for PGL1, PGL3, and PGL4, respectively; gene for PGL2 has not been identified.

- SDH is part of mitochondrial respiratory chain (Krebs cycle); has been proposed that mutations interfere with oxygen-sensing mechanism leading to an apparent hypoxic state and hypoxia-induced hyperplasia.
- Patients with PGL develop tumors at an earlier age than sporadic cases.
- Other tumor syndromes with a predisposition to paragangliomas include Neurofibromatosis type I (*NF1*), MEN type 2 (*RET*), and von Hippel-Lindau (*VHL*).
- PGL1, PGL2, and PGL3 are inherited in an autosomal dominant fashion with variable expressivity and reduced penetrance; paternally transmitted genes only lead to tumor development.
- PGL1 and PGL4 are associated with pheochromocytomas.
- PGL4 is more often malignant while PGL3 is exclusively benign.

Classification and Clinical Presentation

- Carotid body tumor
  - Present as slowly enlarging asymptomatic deep neck mass at level of carotid bifurcation most commonly in fifth and sixth decades of life.
  - Laterally mobile but fixed vertically (Fontaine sign).
  - May be pulsatile or associated with bruit.
  - Cranial neuropathies are rare, involve advanced disease extending to jugular foramen (CN X or CN XII palsy).
  - Average tumor doubling time is 5 years.
  - Shamblin classification
    - Type I—Localized tumor, easily separated from the carotid
    - Type II—Tumor adherent to carotid or partially encases external or internal carotid
    - Type III—Tumor completely encases one or more of external or internal carotid
- Jugulotympanic paraganglioma
  - Present in fifth and sixth decades of life, overwhelming female predominance.
  - Tympanic paragangliomas present with pulsatile tinnitus and conductive hearing loss; red-blue middle ear mass that blanches with pneumatic otoscopy (Brown sign).
  - Jugular paragangliomas originate within jugular bulb and have propensity for early skull base invasion and involvement of jugular foramen cranial nerves (CN IX – XII) in approximately 50% of patients.
  - Fisch classification
    - Class A—Tumors arising from tympanic plexus and confined to middle ear
    - Class B—Tumors arising from inferior tympanic canal with middle ear or mastoid invasion, intact jugular bulb, and carotid canal
    - Class C—Tumors arising in the dome of the jugular bulb and involving overlying cortical bone
    - Class D—Tumors with intracranial extension
- Vagal paraganglioma
  - Typically arise from inferior (nodose) ganglion but can arise from middle or superior ganglion associated with CN X.
  - 3:1 female predominance.
  - Inferiorly based tumors will extend into poststyloid compartment of parapharyngeal space.
  - Superiorly based tumors often present with dumbbell appearance with intracranial component in posterior cranial fossa.
  - Associated with cranial neuropathies in up to 50%.

Differential Diagnosis

- Schwannoma, neurofibroma, lipoma, salivary gland neoplasm, arteriovenous malformation

Diagnosis and Management

- Best initial imaging study is contrast-enhanced CT or MRI.
  - Mass splays internal carotid artery (ICA) and external carotid artery (ECA): consider carotid body tumor (Lyre sign).
  - Mass pushes ICA and ECA anteromedially: consider vagal paraganglioma.
  - Mass pushes ICA and ECA laterally: consider sympathetic trunk tumor.
  - If mass is above the bifurcation, unlikely to be carotid body tumor even if it splays ICA and ECA.
  - MRI appearance of carotid body tumor described as "salt and pepper" which results from combination of hyperintense hemorrhage signal and hypointense signal voids from high-flow vessels.
  - Appearance of "halo" between carotid vessels and tumor suggests a good plane of separation.
- Genetic testing should be offered to all patients with paragangliomas to guide management and identify at-risk family members.
- Surgical management
  - Typically recommended for small tumors (< 5 cm) in young, healthy patients.
  - If carotid sacrifice is a possibility (ie, Shamblin type III), consider CT angiography to evaluate collateral flow and preoperative balloon occlusion testing.
  - Preoperative embolization is controversial: no convincing evidence that it reduces intraoperative blood loss or increases operative time; decision to embolize must be weighed against risk of stroke (0-2%).
  - Keys to successful surgery include proximal and distal control of vessels, identification and preservation of cranial nerves (CN X and XII), and tumor dissection in a periadventitial plane.
  - Sacrifice of the ECA is occasionally necessary.
  - Vascular surgeon should be available for ICA repair or reconstruction if indicated.
  - Complications include cranial nerve damage (permanent in 20% of carotid body tumors, unavoidable in vagal paragangliomas), baroreflex failure (tachycardia and labile blood pressure due to loss of carotid sinus reflex, particularly in those with bilateral surgery).
- Radiation therapy
  - Preferred for unresectable cases, poor operative candidates, or patient preference
  - Cytostatic (rather than cytotoxic) effect; tumor will not shrink in size
  - Risks include carotid atherosclerosis, radiation-induced malignancy, mucositis, possible recurrent tumor growth
- Observation typically reserved for those who are poor candidates for surgery or radiation, those of advanced age, or those with metastatic tumors in which locoregional control would only be palliative.
- Patients with bilateral paragangliomas should undergo surgical resection of smaller tumor first; if there is unilateral preoperative cranial nerve weakness, radiation should be considered for the functional side.

Congenital Vascular Anomalies

Vascular Tumors: Hemangiomas and other Vascular Neoplasms

- Hemangiomas
  - Either congenital (present at birth) or infantile (not present at birth)
  - Congenital hemangiomas classified as either rapidly involuting (RICH) or noninvoluting (NICH)
  - Infantile hemangiomas are the most common vascular tumor; affect 1 in 10 white infants in North America, more common in females (3:1), and low birth weight
  - Infantile hemangiomas represent placental endothelial metastasis and are positive for glucose transporter-1 (GLUT1)
  - Diagnosis is made clinically, rarely by biopsy; ultrasound can be used to rule out vascular malformation and will appear hypoechoic, well-defined, and heterogenous in texture
  - Three phases of growth
    - Proliferation—1 month—10 months
    - Involution—12 months—5 to 6 years (50% by 5 years, 90% by 9 years)
    - Involuted—after 3 to 10 years, may see residual sequela of skin atrophy and telangiectasias
  - Three distributions
    - Focal—solitary lesion, usually red and vascular
    - Multifocal—multiple lesions; if greater than 5, should evaluate for liver/GI involvement with ultrasound
    - Segmental—usually follows trigeminal nerve distribution often involving large areas of the face; greater than 50% of patients with V3 involvement will have subglottic hemangioma
  - PHACES syndrome involves anomalies of posterior cranial fossa, hemangiomas (segmental), arteries (intracranial or cervical), cardiac (heart and aorta), eyes, and sternum.
  - Hemangiomas can be observed if no rapid growth, asymptomatic, and without involvement of eye, nose, lips, or airway.
  - Propranolol (2 mg/kg/day) is first-line oral therapy.
  - Steroids can be considered for hemangiomas refractory to propranolol or for intralesional injection in small focal lesions.
  - Lasers have limited role; pulsed dye laser can be used at end of involution to reduce appearance of residual vascular markings.
  - Indications for surgical excision include large lesions likely to leave large amounts of fibrofatty tissue after involution, ulcerative lesions that fail medical management, or symptomatic periorbital or airway hemangiomas.
- Other vascular neoplasms
  - Kaposiform hemangioendothelioma (KHE)
    - Typically seen in infants and children
    - Histological overlap between benign hemangioma and Kaposi sarcoma (negative HHV-8 stain in KHE)
    - Intermediate risk of malignant transformation
    - Commonly associated with Kasabach-Merritt phenomenon (thrombocytopenic coagulopathy)
  - Tufted angioma (TA)
    - About 50% occur in first year of life, 25% are congenital
    - Most commonly presents as a large, deep red or purple plaque on neck, shoulder, or trunk

- Typically benign, but risk of Kasabach-Merritt phenomenon
- Managed with topical corticosteroids with or without pulsed dye laser, rarely surgical excision

- Pyogenic granuloma (PG)
  - Presents as solitary, red, pedunculated, and friable lesion with rapid exophytic growth
  - Benign and sporadic, associated with pregnancy
  - Preferred treatment is complete excision or laser ablation
- Hemangiopericytoma
  - Tumors derived from pericytes surrounding blood vessels and capillaries
  - Most common in middle-aged adults, typically present with pain
  - Indolent but malignant potential similar to hemangioendothelioma
  - Preferred treatment is surgical excision; no demonstrated benefit to radiation, unclear benefit of chemotherapy

Vascular Malformations: Capillary, Venous, Lymphatic, and Arteriovenous

- In contrast to vascular tumors, lesions are present at birth and grow with child.
- Histology shows dilation of abnormal vascular channels rather than cell proliferation.
- Capillary malformations
  - Typically salmon patches (nevus simplex) or port-wine stains (nevus flammeus)
  - Located superficially within reticular dermis
  - Port-wine stain occurs in 0.3% of newborns, typically in trigeminal nerve distribution
  - Associated with Sturge-Weber syndrome (structural and vascular abnormalities of the face and leptomeninges) when in the ophthalmic distribution, should undergo screening MRI or CT to rule out intracranial pathology
  - Treatment with pulsed dye laser can help with reducing red discoloration (chromophore is hemoglobin); Nd:YAG laser can be used on thicker lesions or lesions that have darkened with age
- Venous malformations
  - Consist of localized to diffuse ectatic veins with abnormal collections of irregular venous channels
  - Incidence is 1:10,000; usually sporadic
  - May be superficial (intradermal or subcutaneous) or deep (intramuscular or intraosseous)
  - Superficial lesions present as a bluish compressible mass without audible bruit; may enlarge with dependent positioning, with Valsalva maneuver, or increased cardiac output states
  - Diagnosis made with Doppler echocardiography or MRI
  - Treatment is indicated if symptomatic (may cause pain associated with phleboliths); either surgical excision or sclerotherapy (ethanol, OK-432, sodium tetradecyl sulfate, bleomycin, or doxycycline)
  - Nd:YAG laser can be used on superficial lesions
- Lymphatic malformations
  - Usually cystic; thought to be result of maldevelopment of lymphatics with failure of connection to venous system.
  - Microcystic malformations present as clear vesicles throughout subcutaneous tissue above the level mylohyoid involving oral cavity, oropharynx, tongue, salivary glands, or pre-epiglottic space.

- Macrocystic lesions are multilocular but large translucent masses under normal or bluish skin below the level of the mylohyoid.
- Typically diagnosed by physical exam with transillumination, CT, or MRI.
- Treatment is with surgery or sclerotherapy.

- Arteriovenous malformations
  - High-flow communications between arteries and veins.
  - Becomes clinically evident in childhood or during puberty; rapid expansion may follow pregnancy or trauma.
  - Present with warmth to palpation, palpable thrill, audible bruit.
  - Diagnosis is with angiography or MRA.
  - Indications for intervention include pain, expansion, ulceration, bleeding, or cardiac side effects.
  - Treatment is with intra-arterial embolization combined with surgical excision.

Questions

1. Approximately what percentage of paragangliomas actively secrete catecholamines?
   A. 1% to 3 %
   B. 10% to 20%
   C. 50%
   D. > 80%

2. Paragangliomas are associated with all of the following familial syndromes, except
   A. Von Hippel-Lindau (VHL)
   B. Neurofibromatosis type 1 (NF1)
   C. Neurofibromatosis type 2 (NF2)
   D. Multiple endocrine neoplasia type II (RET)

3. A carotid body tumor which partially encases the external carotid artery is which type, according to the Shamblin classification?
   A. Type I
   B. Type II
   C. Type III
   D. Type IV

4. Which is *not* a treatment for infantile hemangiomas?
   A. Corticosteroids
   B. Surgery
   C. Propranolol
   D. CO_2 laser

5. Which vascular lesion is associated with Kasabach-Merritt phenomenon?
   A. Infantile hemangioma
   B. Arteriovenous malformations
   C. Kaposiform hemangioendothelioma
   D. Pyogenic granuloma

Bibliography

Boedeker CC, Hensen EF, Neumann HP, et al. Genetics of hereditary head and neck paragangliomas. *Head Neck*. 2014;36(6):907-916.

Buckmiller L, Richter G, Suen J. Diagnosis and management of hemangiomas and vascular malformations of the head and neck. *Oral diseases*. 2010;16(5):405-418.

Cass ND, Schopper MA, Lubin JA, Fishbein L, Gubbels SP. The changing paradigm of head and neck paragangliomas: what every otolaryngologist needs to know. *Ann Otol Rhinol Laryngol*. 2020;129(11):1135-1143.

Colletti G, Valassina D, Bertossi D, Melchiorre F, Vercellio G, Brusati R. Contemporary management of vascular malformations. *J Oral Maxillofac Surg*. 2014;72(3):510-528.

Cox JA, Bartlett E, Lee EI. Vascular malformations: a review. *Semin Plast Surg*. 2014 May;28(2):58-63.

Majewska A, Budny B, Ziemnicka K, Ruchała M, Wierzbicka M. Head and neck paragangliomas—a genetic overview. *Int J Mol Sci*. 2020;21(20):7669.

Moore MG, Netterville JL, Mendenhall WM, Isaacson B, Nussenbaum B. Head and neck paragangliomas: an update on evaluation and management. *Otolaryngol–Head Neck Surg*. 2016;154(4):597-605.

Netterville JL, Jackson CG, Miller FR, Wanamaker JR, Glasscock ME. Vagal paraganglioma: a review of 46 patients treated during a 20-year period. *Arc Otolaryngol–Head Neck Surg*. 1998;124(10):1133-1140.

Netterville JL, Reilly KM, Robertson D, Reiber ME, Armstrong WB, Childs P. Carotid body tumors: a review of 30 patients with 46 tumors. *Laryngoscope*. 1995;105(2):115-126.

North PE, Waner M, Mizeracki A, Mihm Jr MC. GLUT1: a newly discovered immunohistochemical marker for juvenile hemangiomas. *Hum Pathol*. 2000;31(1):11-22.

Pellitteri PK, Rinaldo A, Myssiorek D, et al. Paragangliomas of the head and neck. *Oral Oncol*. 2004;40(6):563-575.

Shamblin WR, ReMine WH, Sheps SG, Harrison Jr EG. Carotid body tumor (chemodectoma): clinicopathologic analysis of ninety cases. *Am J Surg*. 1971;122(6):732-739.

Taïeb D, Kaliski A, Boedeker CC, et al. Current approaches and recent developments in the management of head and neck paragangliomas. *Endocrine Rev*. 2014;35(5):795-819.

Van Den Berg R. Imaging and management of head and neck paragangliomas. *Eur Radiol*. 2005;15:1310-1318.

Williams MD. Paragangliomas of the head and neck: an overview from diagnosis to genetics. *Head Neck Pathol*. 2017;11:278-287.

Chapter 40
TNM Classification

Introduction

The TNM system describes a cancerous tumor's involvement at the primary site (T), as well as spread to regional lymph nodes (N) and distant metastasis (M).

Objectives of Staging System

The TNM staging system was created to describe cancer in a uniform fashion and provide physicians a common language to discuss the disease. This allows for a better understanding of prognosis and accurate patient counseling. Treatment protocols can be devised based on the treatment results of similar tumors. Finally, it is useful for stratifying cancers for clinical research and for measuring outcomes of various treatment options.

History

The American Joint Committee on Cancer (AJCC) was formed in 1959, unifying previous classification systems and providing a foundation for our current staging system. Since then, the AJCC has continued to update a stage classification system for all anatomic sites and subsites. The most recent eighth edition was published in 2017.

Definitions of TNM Categories

T describes the extent of the primary tumor. There are seven categories: TX (primary tumor cannot be assessed), T0 (no evidence of primary tumor), T*is* (tumor in situ), T1, T2, T3, and T4. Within the head and neck, the size of the tumor generally defines the T stage. Notable exceptions include vocal fold mobility in larynx cancer. Depth of invasion is now included within the AJCC eighth edition staging system for oral cavity cancer and is considered a separate entity to tumor thickness. Modifiers "a" (less severe) and "b" (more severe) can be used within some T categories to further describe the tumor.

N describes spread of the cancer to regional lymph nodes in five categories: NX (regional lymph nodes cannot be assessed), N0, N1, N2, and N3. This is basically described by size of the lymph nodes and is modified by location of the involved nodes. Evaluation of surgically excised lymph nodes by a pathologist can further affect N stage. Specifically, the eighth edition of the

Table 40-1 Lips and Oral Cavity

Stage	*Description*
T1	≤2 cm with DOI ≤5 mm
T2	≤2 cm with DOI >5 mm OR >2 cm and ≤4 cm with DOI ≤10 mm
T3	>4 cm and/or DOI >10 mm
T4a	Invades cortical bone, inferior alveolar nerve, floor of mouth/skin, mandible/maxilla, maxillary sinus, or extrinsic tongue muscles
T4b	Invades masticator space, pterygoid plates, skull base, or encases ICA

AJCC includes the additional modifier of extranodal extension (ENE) to denote spread of tumor outside of the capsule of a lymph node on histopathologic sectioning. Pathology reports will further specify ENE based on millimeters of extension beyond the capsule of the lymph node (ie, minor ≤ 2 mm and major ≥ 2 mm).

M describes the presence of distant metastasis, either as MX, M0, or M1. A patient with a metastasis beyond the regional lymph nodes has M1 disease. M0 describes no evidence of metastasis after an appropriate evaluation. MX designates that a metastatic workup has not been completed.

Prefix modifiers are also used to further describe the staging. The "c" prefix refers to staging based on clinical examination (ie, cTNM). The "p" prefix refers to staging based on pathological examination after surgical resection (ie, pTNM). In those circumstances where classification is performed during or after initial multimodality treatment, a "y" prefix is used for either cTNM or pTNM. A "r" prefix denotes a recurrence following treatment.

The current staging system, including sites and subsites, is summarized in the following tables (detailed descriptions can be found in the updated AJCC manual). These are divided into four categories:

A. Lips, oral cavity, pharynx, and larynx (Tables 40-1 to 40-7)
B. Nasal cavity and paranasal sinuses (Tables 40-8 and 40-9)
C. Major salivary glands (Table 40-10)
D. Thyroid gland (Table 40-11)

Nodal staging (Tables 40-12 to 40-15) and stage groupings (Tables 40-16 to 40-18) are shown in subsequent tables.

Table 40-2 Nasopharynx

Stage	*Description*
T1	Confined to nasopharynx or extension to oropharynx/nasal cavity
T2	Parapharyngeal extension and/or adjacent soft tissue
T3	Invades bony structures, pterygoid structures, and/or paranasal sinuses
T4	Intracranial extension, cranial nerves, hypopharynx, orbit, infratemporal fossa or masticator space

Table 40-3 Oropharynx

Stage	*Description*
T1	≤2 cm
T2	>2 cm and <4 cm
T3	>4 cm or lingual epiglottis extension
T4a	Invades larynx, extrinsic tongue muscles, medial pterygoid, hard palate, or mandible
T4b	Invades lateral pterygoid, pterygoid plates, lateral nasopharynx, skull base, or carotid

Table 40-4 Hypopharynx

Stage	*Description*
T1	≤2 cm and one subsite
T2	>2 cm <4 cm or adjacent subsite
T3	>4 cm, fixed hemilarynx, or esophageal mucosa extension
T4a	Invades cartilage, hyoid, thyroid gland, esophageal muscles, or central compartment soft tissue
T4b	Invades prevertebral fascia, carotid, or mediastinum

Table 40-5 Supraglottic Larynx

Stage	*Description*
T1	One subsite
T2	Adjacent subsite spread
T3	Cord fixation or adjacent structure invasion
T4a	Beyond larynx through thyroid cartilage
T4b	Prevertebral fascia, carotid, or mediastinum

Table 40-6 Glottic Larynx

Stage	*Description*
T1a	One vocal cord
T1b	Both vocal cords
T2	Supra/subglottis or impaired mobility
T3	Cord fixation/paraglottic space/inner thyroid cartilage
T4a	Beyond larynx
T4b	Prevertebral fascia/carotid/mediastinum

Table 40-7 Subglottic Larynx

Stage	*Description*
T1	Subglottis
T2	Extends to cords
T3	Cord fixation/paraglottic space
T4a	Beyond larynx
T4b	Prevertebral fascia/carotid/mediastinum

Table 40-8 Nasal Cavity and Ethmoid Sinuses

Stage	*Description*
T1	One subsite
T2	Two subsites/adjacent region
T3	Orbit medial wall/floor, maxillary sinus, palate, cribriform
T4a	Anterior orbit, skin, pterygoid plates, frontal/sphenoid sinus
T4b	Orbital apex, dura, brain, CN, nasopharynx, clivus

Table 40-9 Maxillary Sinus

Stage	*Description*
T1	Mucosa
T2	Hard palate and/or middle meatus
T3	Subcutaneous tissue, posterior wall, orbit floor/medial wall, pterygoid fossa, ethmoid
T4a	Anterior orbit, skin, pterygoid plates, infratemporal fossa
T4b	Orbital apex, dura, brain, CN, nasopharynx, clivus

Table 40-10 Major Salivary Glands

Stage	*Description*
T1	≤2 cm
T2	>2 and <4 cm
T3	>4 cm or extraparenchymal extension
T4a	Skin, mandible, ear canal, facial nerve
T4b	Skull base, pterygoid plates, carotid

Table 40-11 Thyroid

Stage	*Description*
T1	≤2 cm
T1a	≤1 cm
T1b	>1–2 cm
T2	>2–4 cm
T3	>4 cm or minimal ETE
T3a	>4 cm limited to thyroid
T3b	Strap muscle invasion
T4a	Subcutaneous tissue, larynx, trachea, esophagus, RLN
T4b	Prevertebral fascia, carotid/mediastinal vessels

Table 40-12 Regional Nodes (Oral cavity/Larynx etc.)

Stage	*Description*
N0	No nodes
N1	Ipsilateral ≤3 cm
N2a	Ipsilateral >3 <6 cm
N2b	Multiple ipsilateral ≤6 cm
N2c	Bilateral/contralateral ≤6 cm
N3a	>6 cm
N3b	Clinically overt ENE

Table 40-13 Staging for Regional Lymph Nodes (Non-viral Cervical Nodal Metastasis With Unknown Primary)

Clinical Staging	
N1	Ipsilateral ≤ 3 cm, no ENE
N2a	Ipsilateral > 3 cm and < 6 cm, no ENE
N2b	Ipsilateral multiple ≤ 6 cm, no ENE
N2c	Bilateral or contralateral ≤ 6 cm, no ENE
N3a	> 6 cm, no ENE
N3b	Any lymph node with clinical ENE
Pathologic Staging	
N1	Ipsilateral ≤ 3 cm, no ENE
N2a	Ipsilateral > 3 cm and < 6 cm, no ENE or Ipsilateral ≤ 3cm with ENE
N2b	Ipsilateral multiple ≤ 6 cm, no ENE
N2c	Bilateral or contralateral ≤ 6 cm, no ENE
N3a	> 6 cm, no ENE
N3b	> 3 cm with pathologic ENE or Any multiple ipsilateral/bilateral/contralateral with ENE

ENE = extranodal extension.

Table 40-14 Regional Nodes (Nasopharynx)

Stage	*Description*
N0	No nodes
N1	≤6 cm unilateral cervical or retropharyngeal
N2	≤6 cm bilateral cervical
N3	>6 cm and/or below cricoid

Table 40-15 Regional Nodes (HPV+ Oropharynx)

Stage	*Description*
cN0	No nodes
cN1	Ipsilateral ≤6 cm
cN2	Contralateral/bilateral ≤6 cm
cN3	Any node >6 cm
pN0	No nodes
pN1	1–4 nodes
pN2	≥5 nodes

Table 40-16 Stage Groupings

Stage	T	N	M
Stage I	T1	N0	M0
Stage II	T2	N0	M0
Stage III	T3	N0	M0
	T1-3	N1	M0
Stage IVa	T4a	N0, N1	M0
	Any T	N2	M0
IVb	Any T	N3	M0
	T4b	Any N	M0
IVc	Any T	Any N	M1
Oropharynx (HPV+)			
Clinical Staging			
Stage	T	N	M
Stage I	T0-2	N0, N1	M0
Stage II	T0-2	N2	M0
	T3, T4	N0, N1	M0
Stage III	T3, T4	N2	M0
Stage IV	Any T	Any N	M1
Pathologic Staging			
Stage	T	N	M
Stage I	T0-T2	N0-N1	M0
Stage II	T0-T2	N2	M0
	T3-T4	N0-N1	M0
Stage III	T3-T4	N2	M0
Stage IV	Any T	Any N	M1
Nasopharynx			
Stage	T	N	M
Stage I	T1	N0	M0
Stage II	T1	N1	M0
	T2	N0	M0
	T2	N1	M0
Stage III	T1-2	N2	M0
	T3	N0-2	M0
Stage IVa	T4	N0-2	M0
	Any T	N3	M0
Stage IVb	Any T	Any N	M1

Table 40-17 Stage Groupings (Viral and Non-Viral-Related Cervical Unknown Primary)

HPV+/p16+ Unknown Primary			
Stage	T	N	M
Stage I	T0	N1	M0
Stage II	T0	N2	M0
Stage III	T0	N3	M0
Stage IV (Clinical)	T0	N1-3	M1
Stage IV (Pathologic)	T0	N1-2	M1
EBV+ Unknown Primary			
Stage	T	N	M
Stage I	N/A	N/A	M0
Stage II	T0	N1	M0
Stage III	T0	N2	M0
Stage IVa	T0	N3	M0
Stage IVb	T0	N1-3	M1
Non-Viral Unknown Primary			
Stage	T	N	M
Stage I	N/A	N/A	N/A
Stage II	N/A	N/A	N/A
Stage III	T0	N1	M0
Stage IVa	T0	N2	M0
Stage IVb	T0	N3	M0
Stage IVc	T0	N1-3	M1

Table 40-18 Thyroid Stage Grouping

Differentiated Thyroid Cancer			
Stage	T	N	M
Under 55 y - Stage I	Any T	Any N	M0
Under 55 y - Stage II	Any T	Any N	M1
55 y and older - Stage I	T1	N0	M0
	T2	N0	M0
Stage II	T1	N1	M0
	T2	N1	M0
	T3a/T3b	Any N	M0

(Continued)

Table 40-18 Thyroid Stage Grouping (*Continued*)

Stage III	T4a	Any N	M0
Stage IVa	T4b	Any N	M0
Stage IVb	Any T	Any N	M1
Medullary Thyroid Cancer			
Stage	T	N	M
Stage I	T1	N0	M0
Stage II	T2	N0	M0
	T3	N0	M0
Stage III	T1-3	N1a	M0
Stage IVa	T4a	Any N	M0
	T1-3	N1b	M0
Stage IVb	T4b	Any N	M0
Stage IVc	Any T	Any N	M1
Anaplastic Thyroid Cancer			
Stage	Description		
Stage IV	All anaplastic thyroid cancer is Stage IV		

Bibliography

American Joint Committee on Cancer. *Cancer Staging Manual*. 8th ed. New York, NY: Springer-Verlag; 2017.

Questions

1. A 65-year-old patient with hoarseness is noted to have a 1-cm lesion on the left vocal cord, extending toward the anterior commissure. The vocal cord is mobile, and no neck masses are noted on examination or imaging. A computed tomography (CT) chest is unremarkable. Biopsy reveals squamous cell carcinoma. Which answer best describes the TNM staging?
   A. T1aN0M0
   B. T1bN0M0
   C. T2N0M0
   D. TXN0M0
   E. Unable to determine based on the information provided

2. A 70-year-old former smoker presented with hoarseness and dysphagia for 3 months. Laryngoscopy shows a tumor of the right false vocal cord extending to true vocal cord and medial wall of pyriform sinus on the same side. The vocal cord is mobile and there is no contralateral spread. CT neck reveals a right larynx mass with extension into the paraglottic space and a 1.8-cm lymph node on the right at level III. Biopsy confirms squamous cell carcinoma. Chest and brain imaging are negative. Which answer best describes the TNM staging?
   A. T1N0M0
   B. T1N1M0
   C. T2N1M0
   D. T2N2M0
   E. T3N1M0

3. A 49-year-old woman is evaluated for a left-sided thyroid mass. On ultrasound, it measures 16 mm × 14 mm, and no enlarged lymph nodes are identified. A chest X-ray (CXR) is negative, and needle aspiration confirms papillary thyroid cancer. Which answer best describes the TNM staging?
   A. T1aN0M0
   B. T1bN0M0
   C. T2N0M0
   D. T3N0M0
   E. T4N0M0

4. A 75-year-old smoker is seen for an ulcerative mass of the right oral tongue and floor of the mouth. It measures 3.5 cm in greatest diameter and invades through cortical bone of the mandible. There are multiple right-only cervical lymph nodes, the largest of which is 2 cm. A positron emission tomography (PET) scan shows no evidence of distant disease. A biopsy shows squamous cell carcinoma. Which answer best describes the TNM staging?
   A. T3N1M0
   B. T3N2aM0
   C. T3N2bM0
   D. T4aN2aM0
   E. T4aN2bM0

5. A 25-year-old man is evaluated for a right parotid mass. It measures 3 cm in greatest dimension. Imaging shows no evidence of spread to regional lymph nodes or beyond. At surgery, the tumor is noted not to extend beyond the parotid parenchyma. Final histology reveals adenoid cystic carcinoma. Which answer best describes the TNM staging?
   A. T1N0M0
   B. T1N1M0
   C. T2N0M0
   D. T2N1M0
   E. T3N0M0

Chapter 41
Cutaneous Malignancies of the Head and Neck

Nonmelanoma Skin Cancer (NMSC) Classification

- Greater than 80 histologic subtypes
  - Basal cell carcinoma (BCC) accounts for 70% to 75%
  - Cutaneous squamous cell carcinoma (cSCC) accounts for 20%
  - Merkel cell carcinoma (MCC) accounts for 5%
- Overall excellent prognosis (90% 5-year survival rate)
- Subset of aggressive NMSC
  - 10% locally recur
  - 3% to 5% develop regional metastasis
  - 2500 deaths per year
- $4.8 billion/year spent in NMSC diagnosis and treatment in the United States
- Lacking large prospective NMSC registries

NMSC Risk Factors

- Environmental
  - Sun exposure (ultraviolet radiation; UVR) remains leading cause
  - Fitzpatrick type I: fair skin, red/blonde hair, marked freckling, moles
  - Tanning booths
- Genetics
  - Xeroderma pigmentosa (XP): rare, autosomally recessive disease associated with cutaneous cancers secondary to inability to repair DNA damaged by UVR
  - Fanconi anemia: autosomal recessive aplastic anemia, lacks DNA repair mechanism
  - Basal cell carcinoma: PTCH1 (patched 1) mutation on chromosome 9q
    - Encodes sonic hedgehog receptor
    - Nevoid BCC syndrome
      - ◊ Also known as Gorlin syndrome
      - ◊ Rare, autosomal dominant disease
      - ◊ Can present with palmar pits, odontogenic keratocysts, and musculoskeletal abnormalities
  - Avoid radiation in these at-risk patient populations

- Immunosuppression (solid organ transplant [SOT], lymphoproliferative disorders, human immunodeficiency virus infection/acquired immunodeficiency syndrome, iatrogenic)
  - Work closely with transplant team to decrease level of immunosuppression
  - mTOR inhibitors may reduce skin cancer risk in SOT patients
- Merkel cell carcinoma: Polyomavirus (MCPyV)

NMSC Work-Up

- History
  - Change in lesion color, size, or shape
  - Bleeding, ulceration, or pain
  - Personal and family history of skin cancer
  - Sun exposure, occupation, sunburns, tanning booth use
  - Immunosuppression
  - Previous "moles" removed
- Physical exam
  - Full body skin exam to include draining lymphatics
  - Cranial nerve exam to assess perineural spread
- Thorough 12-point review of systems
- Biopsy
  - Shave biopsies reserved for nonpigmented superficial lesions
  - Narrow margin (1-3 mm) excisional biopsy is indicated for concerning lesions that appear more than superficial
  - Full-thickness punch or incisional biopsy indicated for lesions not amenable to excisional biopsy due to large size or location
  - Wide margin excision without diagnosis is discouraged because it may preclude further workup and treatment such as sentinel node biopsy
  - Fine-needle aspiration for concerning metastatic lymph nodes
- Radiographic imaging
  - Contrasted CT scan (or MRI with gadolinium for patients with contrast allergy) to assess cervical and parotid bed lymphadenopathy for advanced NMSC to include regional metastasis, involvement of bone, perineural invasion, or concern for deep tissue extension
  - Additional dedicated radiographic studies as warranted for positive review of systems
  - PET/CT
    - Considered for advanced metastatic disease
    - Warranted in patients with regional nodal metastasis of unknown origin
    - Used to restage patients with tumor recurrence
- Advanced NMSC should be discussed at a multidisciplinary oncology tumor board to include review of clinical trials.

Basal Cell Carcinoma (BCC)

Overview

- Most common cutaneous cancer
- Twice as common as cSCC

- 2.8 million cases diagnosed per year
- No formal American Joint Committee on Cancer Staging

Low-Risk BCC

- Nodular (most common) or superficial (second most common) subtype
- No perineural invasion
- Well-defined borders
- Primary disease
- No prior radiation
- Less than 10 mm diameter on the cheek, forehead, scalp, or neck (M-area)

High-Risk BCC

- ≥ 10 mm diameter on the cheek, forehead, scalp, or neck (M-area)
- Involvement of the H-area (central face, eyelids/brows, periorbital, nose, cutaneous lips, chin, mandible, preauricular/postauricular region, temple, or ear)
- Immunosuppression
- Perineural invasion
- Recurrent disease
- Poorly defined borders
- Aggressive subtype
  - Morpheaform
  - Basosquamous
  - Sclerosing
  - Mixed infiltrative
  - Micronodular

Treatment

- Low-risk BCC
  - Surgery is gold standard.
    - 4 mm margin for low-risk BCC (well circumscribed; < 2 cm diameter) with postoperative margin assessment
    - Mohs micrographic surgery reserved for positive margin clearance if necessary
  - Curettage and electrodesiccation (C&E)
    - Reserved for low-risk BCC
    - Fast and cost-effective but precludes histologic evaluation
    - Operator dependent
    - Not applicable in hair-bearing regions such as the scalp
  - Primary radiation for nonsurgical candidates
  - Adjuvant radiation
    - For positive, unresectable margins
    - Consideration for extensive perineural invasion or large nerve involvement
    - Recommend multidisciplinary oncology board discussion
    - Contraindicated for patients with genetic conditions predisposing to cutaneous cancers and connective tissue disorders
- High-risk BCC
  - Mohs micrographic surgery preferred for high-risk BCC
    - Allows intraoperative assessment of 100% of excised margins
    - Lower recurrence rate compared to traditional surgery but costly

- Standard excision with postoperative margin assessment
- Primary radiation for nonsurgical candidates

- Nodal metastasis
  - Rare
  - Treatment
    - Therapeutic neck dissection
    - Radiation
    - Consideration of hedgehog inhibitor (see following discussion)
    - Clinical trial
    - Recommend multi-disciplinary oncology board discussion
- Topical therapy
  - Reserved for patients deemed unfit for surgery or radiation
  - 5-Fluorouracil (5-FU)
  - Imiquimod
  - Photodynamic therapy (PDT)
  - Cryotherapy
- Intralesional interferon α-2B
  - Effective for low risk, superficial BCC
  - Rarely utilized due to expense and challenging regimen (three injections/week × 3 weeks)
  - Side effects: flu-like symptoms
- Systemic therapy
  - Hedgehog inhibitor (HHI)
    - Vismodegib
    - Sonidegib
    - FDA approved for locally advanced recurrent BCC not amenable to surgery or radiation
    - Can be considered in neoadjuvant setting as can allow for downstaging of tumors for BCCs in sensitive locations
    - Side effects
      - ◊ Muscle spasms
      - ◊ Dysgeusia
      - ◊ Alopecia
      - ◊ Nausea
      - ◊ Weight loss
      - ◊ Fatigue
      - ◊ Elevated creatine kinase
  - Immune checkpoint inhibitors (ICI)
    - Cemiplimab, PD-1 inhibitor
    - FDA approved for locally advanced patients who fail surgery, radiation, and/or HHI therapy

Follow-up and Prevention

- 30% to 50% patients develop recurrence in 5 years.
- Annual examination to include full-body exam Q6-12 months for the first 2 years and then reduce visits as deemed appropriate if no recurrence.
- Imaging as clinically indicated.
- Patient education
  - Self-exam
  - Sunscreen use

- Peak sun avoidance (10 am-2 pm)
- Concerning signs/symptoms

Cutaneous Squamous Cell Carcinoma (CSCC)

Overview

- Second most common cutaneous cancer worldwide
- Head and neck cSCC automatically deemed at least "high-risk" based on anatomical location
- 700,000 new cases per year
- 200% increase in incidence over past 30 years

Staging now based on eighth edition American Joint Commission on Cancer (AJCC) TNM staging system

- Specific to cSCC of the head and neck
  - T-stage is based on size, degree of PNI, and degree of invasion (into subcutaneous fat, bone, skull base)
  - N-stage is based on size, number, laterality, and extranodal extension (ENE) of lymph nodes
  - M-stage is based on presence of any distant metastases

Histology

- Actinic keratosis (AK) considered premalignant
- cSCC in situ: Bowen disease
- Aggressive variants at risk for recurrence:
  - Acantholytic (adenoid)
  - Adenosquamous (mucin)
  - Desmoplastic
  - Metaplastic (carcinosarcomatous)

Low-Risk cSCC

- ≤ 2 cm if on trunk or extremities
- No perineural invasion, lymphatic, or vascular invasion
- Well-defined borders
- Primary disease
- No prior radiation
- Well to moderate histologic differentiation
- Depth less than 2 mm and no invasion beyond subcutaneous fat

High-Risk cSCC

- Any head and neck location
- Size 2 to 4 cm on trunk or extremities
- Immunosuppression
- PNI less than 0.1 mm
- Recurrent disease
- Poorly defined borders
- Rapid growth
- Neurologic symptoms

- Depth 2 to 6 mm
- Aggressive subtype (see Histology section)

Very High-Risk cSCC

- Size greater than 4 cm in any location
- Depth of invasion (DOI) greater than 6 mm or invasion beyond subcutaneous fat
- Poorly differentiated histology
- Desmoplastic features
- Prognostic nutritional index (PNI) ≥ 1 mm OR tumor within nerve sheath of nerve deeper than dermis
- Any LVI

Treatment

- Diffuse AK/field cancerization and cSCC in situ
  - Cryotherapy
  - Topical 5-FU
  - Imiquimod
  - PDT
  - C&E
- Low-risk invasive cSCC
  - Surgery is gold standard
    - 4 to 6 mm margin with postoperative margin assessment
    - Mohs micrographic surgery reserved for positive margin clearance if necessary
  - C&E for nonhair-bearing area
  - Primary radiation for nonsurgical candidates
- High-risk invasive cSCC
  - Mohs micrographic surgery with complete circumferential margin assessment
  - Standard excision with postoperative margin assessment
    - Margin size is topic of a debate. Generally, 6 to 10 mm margins for high to very-high risk lesions.
  - Primary radiation with or without systemic therapy for nonsurgical candidates
  - Sentinel lymph node biopsy (see following discussion) may be considered for high-risk patients who present with clinically and radiographically node-negative disease
- Nodal metastasis
  - Treatment options
    - Therapeutic neck dissection to remove all at-risk draining echelons with preservation of critical structures unless involved with cSCC
      - ◊ Temple, high cheek, and forehead cSCCs warrant parotidectomy along with a modified radical neck dissection (I-IV) for stage III regional disease.
      - ◊ For posterior scalp and neck cSCCs, tumors behind an imaginary coronal plane through the external auditory canal warrant posterolateral neck dissection which extends to midline posteriorly and removes level V, suboccipital, and retroauricular nodes.
  - Radiation
  - Clinical trial
  - Recommend multidisciplinary oncology board discussion
- Adjuvant radiation
  - May consider for one positive node without extracapsular extension (ECE)
  - ≥ 2 positive nodes

  - 1 node greater than 3 cm
  - Any ECE
  - Incompletely excised/unresectable nodal disease
  - Unresectable positive margin
  - Consideration for extensive perineural invasion or large nerve involvement
  - Recommend multidisciplinary oncology board discussion to include discussion of clinical trials
  - Contraindicated for patients with genetic conditions predisposing to cutaneous cancers and connective tissue disorders
- Adjuvant chemoradiation
  - Consider for positive, unresectable primary margin
  - Any node with ECE
  - Incompletely excised/unresectable nodal disease
  - Recommend multidisciplinary oncology board discussion to include discussion of clinical trials
  - Cytotoxic chemotherapeutic agents
    - Cisplatin
    - Carboplatin
    - Paclitaxel
    - 5-FU
  - EGFR inhibitors
    - Cetuximab (most common)
    - Gefitinib
    - Erlotinib
    - Panitumumab
    - Lapatinib
  - Advantage of systemic therapy added to radiation in the adjuvant setting remains to be determined with prospective comparative clinical trials.
    - TROG 05.01 trial did not demonstrate survival benefit of postoperative chemoradiaton (CRT) over radiation (RT).
- Satellite lesions and in-transit metastases warrant aggressive treatment, ideally in the setting of a multidisciplinary oncology board well-versed in cutaneous cancers
- Immune checkpoint inhibitors
  - Cemiplimab.
  - Pembrolizumab.
  - First-line therapy for distant metastatic and unresectable cSCC; patients who have failed traditional surgery and/or radiation; patients in whom surgery would be functionally debilitating/morbid.
  - ICIs in immunosuppressed populations are still under investigation.
  - ICIs can be considered in the neoadjuvant setting for tumors with rapid growth, in transit mets, lymphovascular invasion, borderline resectable disease, or if surgery alone may not be curative.

    In a phase II clinical trial of stage II to IV cSCC tumors published in 2022, Gross et al demonstrated a 51% pathologic complete response to neoadjuvant cemiplimab

Follow-up and Prevention

- Annual examination to include full-body exam and at-risk nodal basins.
- Q3-12months for 2 years.
- Q6-12months for next 3 years, then annual.
- Imaging as clinically indicated.

- Patient education
  - Sunscreen use
  - Peak sun avoidance (10 am-2 pm)
  - Concerning signs/symptoms
- Nicotinamide may be effective in reducing development of new cSCC lesions.
- Retinoids (acitretin, isotretinoin) have been helpful in some high-risk patients for the prevention of future AK and cSCC.

Merkel Cell Carcinoma (MCC)

Overview

- Rare, aggressive neuroendocrine cutaneous carcinoma of the elderly
- Overall poor prognosis
  - High rates of local recurrence: 27% nodal and 7% distant metastasis
  - Overall 5-year survival 30% to 65%
- Firm, red to violaceous, nontender papule or nodule
- Rapid growth
- Most common area of metastasis: regional nodes
- Propensity for neurotropic spread and local recurrence

Histology

- Traditional hematoxylin and eosin (H&E) staining: small round blue cells; neuroendocrine granules; intercellular junctions; rigid spinous processes; paranuclear intermediate filaments
- MCC-specific immunohistochemical staining often required because 40% MCC stain negative on H&E
  - Cytokeratin (CK)-20 positive
  - Neuroendocrine markers positive: CD117; S-100; CD45; panCK
  - Thyroid transcription factor (TTF)-1 negative (differentiates from small-cell lung cancer)

Staging based on AJCC TNM staging system

- T-Stage based on tumor diameter and invasion into surrounding fascia, muscle, cartilage, and bone
- N-Stage
  - Regional metastasis (N1)
  - In-transit metastasis between primary MCC and draining echelon
    - N2 if no associated nodal disease
    - N3 if associated nodal disease
- M-stage related to location of distant metastasis

Treatment

- Surgery
  - Wide local excision (1-2 cm margin) is gold standard.
  - Therapeutic neck dissection remains standard of care for patients with Stage III regional disease.
    - All at-risk echelons should be resected with preservation of critical structures unless involved with MCC.
    - Temple, high cheek, and forehead MCC warrant parotidectomy along with a modified radical neck dissection (I-IV) for stage III regional disease.

- Posterior scalp and neck MCC warrant posterolateral neck dissection.
  - ◊ Extends to midline
  - ◊ Removes level V, suboccipital, and retroauricular nodes
- Sentinel lymph node biopsy (SLNB)
  - Considered the most sensitive staging modality for regional metastasis.
  - 33% to 40% of localized Stage I/II MCC with negative clinical and radiographic exam harbor metastatic, stage III regional disease.
  - Minimal invasive procedure to evaluate the first draining echelon nodes for occult/micrometastatic MCC.
  - Alternative to selective neck dissection for staging of localized MCC.
  - Indicated for patients with a clinically and radiographically N-zero neck.
  - Gold standard is to use preoperative radioactive colloid and intraoperative blue dye for localization.
  - SPECT-CT increased nodal yield in the head and neck region over traditional planar lymphoscintigraphy.
  - Safe in the parotid region when performed in experienced hands and with facial nerve monitoring.
  - Traditionally, patients with a positive SLNB underwent completion lymphadenectomy (CL) within 1 to 2 weeks of biopsy.
  - Negative SLNB can be observed, or MCC patients can receive adjuvant radiation for high-risk regional recurrence.
- Radiation therapy
  - Primary therapy limited to large, unresectable disease or nonsurgical candidates
  - Adjuvant therapy for high-risk patients
    - Primary site indications
      - ◊ Narrow/positive margins
      - ◊ Tumor greater than 1 cm
      - ◊ Immunosuppression
      - ◊ Perineural invasion/lymphovascular invasion
      - ◊ Head and neck subsite
  - Regional lymphatics indications
    - + SLNB
    - Multiple positive nodes
    - Extranodal spread
  - Palliative therapy
    - Unresectable or extensive disease
- Systemic therapy
  - Reserved for stage IV distant metastatic disease (M1)
  - Considered for patients failing traditional surgery and/or radiation, or patients in whom surgery would be functionally debilitating
  - Clinical trials preferred
  - Chemotherapy
    - Cisplatin or carboplatin with or without etoposide
    - Topotecan for elderly patients
    - Used if checkpoint immunotherapy contraindicated
  - Checkpoint immunotherapy
    - Cetuximab
    - Pembrolizumab
    - Avelumab
    - Can also consider in neoadjuvant setting

- Side effects
  - ◊ Hypothyroidism
  - ◊ Panhypopituitarism
  - ◊ Type 1 Diabetes
  - ◊ Crohn disease
  - ◊ Pneumonitis
  - ◊ Myasthenia Gravis

Follow-up and Prevention

- Annual examination to include full-body exam and at-risk nodal basins
- Q3-6 months for 3 years
- Q6-12 months thereafter
- Imaging as clinically indicated
- Patient education
  - Sunscreen use
  - Peak sun avoidance (10 am-2 pm)
  - Concerning signs/symptoms

Bibliography

Gross ND, Miller DM, Khushalani NI, et al. Neoadjuvant cemiplimab for Stage II to IV cutaneous squamous-cell carcinoma. *N Engl J Med*. 2022 Oct 27;387(17):1557-1568.

Lin A, Schmalbach CE. Surgery in the era of immunotherapy for advanced head and neck non-melanoma skin cancer. *Curr Oncol Rep*. 2023 Jul;25(7):735-742.

National Comprehensive Cancer Network Clinical Practice Guidelines in Oncology: Basal Cell Carcinoma. V3.2024. Available at: https://www.nccn.org/professionals/physician_gls/pdf/nmsc.pdf. Accessed 1/3/2024.

National Comprehensive Cancer Network Clinical Practice Guidelines in Oncology: Squamous Cell Carcinoma. V1.2024. Available at: https://www.nccn.org/professionals/physician_gls/pdf/squamous.pdf. Accessed 9/11/2023.

National Comprehensive Cancer Network Clinical Practice Guidelines in Oncology: Merkel Cell Carcinoma. V1.2024. Available at: https://www.nccn.org/professionals/physician_gls/pdf/mcc.pdf Accessed 22/11/2023.

Schmalbach CE, Malloy KM. Head and neck cutaneous cancer. *Otolaryngol Clin North Am*. 2021 Apr;54(2):xv-xvi.

Schmalbach CE, Ow TJ, Choi KY, et al. American Head and Neck Society position statement on the use of PD-1 inhibitors for treatment of advanced cutaneous squamous cell carcinoma. *Head Neck*. 2023 Jan;45(1):32-41.

Questions

1. The most sensitive modality for staging of Merkel cell carcinoma is
   A. Sentinel lymph node biopsy
   B. Contrasted CT
   C. Fused PET/CT
   D. MRI

2. Which of the following cutaneous cancers are associated with the polyomavirus?
   A. Squamous cell carcinoma
   B. Basal cell carcinoma
   C. Melanoma
   D. Merkel cell carcinoma

3. Which of the following basal cell carcinomas is categorized as high risk?
   A. Nodular
   B. 8 mm BCC of the cheek
   C. 3 mm auricular BCC
   D. 12 mm BCC of the forehead

4. Which systemic therapy should be considered for immunosuppressed organ transplant patients with life-threatening, rapidly growing cSCC?
   A. Checkpoint inhibitors
   B. BRAF inhibitors
   C. mTOR inhibitors
   D. Tyrosine kinase inhibitors

5. Sentinel node biopsy is considered standard of care for which of the following NMSCs?
   A. Bowen disease
   B. Advanced squamous cell carcinoma
   C. Advanced basal cell carcinoma
   D. Merkel cell carcinoma

Chapter 42
Malignant Melanoma of the Head and Neck

Essentials of Otolaryngology—Head and Neck Surgery

Incidence

- 100,640 estimated new cases of cutaneous melanoma in the United States in 2024.
- 8290 estimated deaths from cutaneous melanoma in the United States in 2024.
- 20% to 30% of melanomas are located in the head and neck region.
- Alarming increases in incidence (5% per year) and mortality (2% per year).
- Highest incidence in geographic areas with high sun exposure and populations with fair skin.

Risk Factors

- Sun exposure
  - (a) Frequent, intermittent exposure to intense sunlight appears to be the highest risk factor.
  - (b) Ultraviolet light causes a photochemical reaction in DNA, leading to the formation of pyrimidine (thymine and cytosine) dimers.
  - (c) Ultraviolet B (290-310 nm).
    - More potent cause of DNA damage
  - (d) Ultraviolet A (320-400 nm).
    - More abundant in natural sunlight than UVB
    - Can also cause oxidative DNA damage
  - (e) Visible light may also contribute to the pathogenesis.
  - (f) Sunscreen is protective.
    - Should be labeled "broad spectrum", that is, protection against both UVA and UVB light
    - Should be at least sun protection factor (SPF) 15, and preferably 30 or greater
- Tanning beds
  - (a) Produce mostly UVA radiation, but some models increase UVB fraction.
  - (b) Evidence supports an increased risk of malignant melanoma with use of tanning beds.

- Fair skin (Fitzpatrick type I), blond or red hair
- Family history of melanoma
- Freckling of the upper back
- History of three or more blistering sunburns before the age of 20 years
- History of three or more years at an outdoor job as a teenager
- Presence of actinic keratoses

Hereditary Syndromes

- Familial Melanoma/dysplastic nevus syndrome
  (a) Multiple atypical moles
  (b) Lifetime risk of melanoma approaches 100%
  (c) Genetic defect = *CDKN2A* gene at chromosome 9p21, which encodes p16(INK4a) and p14ARF
- Xeroderma pigmentosa
  (a) Autosomal recessive
  (b) 1000-fold increased risk of skin cancer, often before the age of 10
  (c) Early onset freckling (before 2 years of age)
  (d) Caused by a heterogeneous group of defects in the nucleotide excision repair pathway → cannot appropriately repair the constant DNA damage (specifically, thymine dimers) caused by UV exposure

Molecular Biology of Sporadic Melanoma

- Ras-Raf-Mek-Erk pathway
  (a) Important pathway in regulation of cell proliferation.
  (b) Activating NRAS mutations are the most common Ras family mutations.
  (c) Activating BRAF mutations are found in 50% to 70% of cutaneous melanomas.
  (d) Several **BRAF inhibitors** and **MEK inhibitors** approved by the Food and Drug Administration (FDA) to treat malignant melanomas with activating mutations in BRAF.
- c-kit
  (a) Tyrosine kinase receptor for stem cell factor.
  (b) Activating mutations and amplifications cause constitutive activation of growth and proliferation pathways.
  (c) More commonly found in melanoma unrelated to sun exposure, namely acral or mucosal melanoma.
  (d) Imatinib: A combined Abelson murine leukemia viral oncogene (ABL), c-kit, platelet-derived growth factor receptor (PDGFR) inhibitor, very successful in treating GI stromal tumors and chronic myelogenous leukemias. Imatinib or other kit inhibitors may have activity in melanomas with activating c-kit mutations (more common in acral lentiginous and mucosal melanomas).
- Mutation burden and neoantigens
  (a) Based on The Cancer Genome Atlas (TCGA) and other studies, melanoma carries a higher mutation burden compared to many other cancers.
  (b) Somatic mutations may give rise to potential tumor-specific neo-antigens, which may promote immunogenicity and response to immunotherapy.

Premalignant Lesions

Up to 80% of malignant melanomas may arise in a preexisting lesion.

- Congenital nevi
  (a) Has characteristics of benign nevus (mole), but present at birth
  (b) May or may not develop coarse surface hairs ("congenital hairy nevus")
  (c) Occurs in 1% to 2% of newborns
  (d) May be part of a rare syndrome, neurocutaneous melanosis, where patients also develop melanotic neoplasms of the central nervous system
  (e) Large or "giant" nevi (> 20 cm) have approximately 10% lifetime risk of conversion to melanoma
- Dysplastic nevus/atypical mole
  (a) Generally larger than normal moles, with irregular/indistinct borders.
  (b) Often heterogeneous coloration.
  (c) Controversy over malignant potential exists.
  (d) Dysplastic nevi should be followed closely or removed if there is a high suspicion for melanoma, or if malignant characteristics of the lesion evolve.
- Lentigo maligna (Hutchinson melanotic freckle)
  (a) Melanoma *in situ*.
  (b) Preinvasive phase (radial growth only) of *lentigo maligna melanoma* (vertical growth, as well).
  (c) Large, thin, flat, irregular pigmented lesion.
  (d) Frequently on the face and neck, areas of sun-damaged skin.
  (e) Rate of progression is generally low, but reports vary between 2% and 33%.

Melanoma Subtypes

- Lentigo maligna melanoma
  (a) Least common, 5% to 10% of all cases.
  (b) Prolonged radial growth (years to decades).
  (c) Lentigo maligna becomes lentigo maligna melanoma once it invades into the papillary dermis.
- Superficial spreading
  (a) Most common, 75% of cases.
  (b) Initial radial growth phase, with progression to vertical growth phase (often with ulceration or bleeding).
  (c) Cells are very uniform in appearance.
  (d) Smaller lesions generally have good prognosis due to lack of vertical growth.
- Nodular
  (a) 10% to 15% of all cases.
  (b) No radial growth phase: rapid vertical growth.
  (c) Commonly ulcerated.
  (d) Small lesions are often thick and have a poor prognosis.
- Acral lentiginous
  (a) Found predominantly on the soles, palms, and beneath the nail plate.
  (b) Sun exposure does not seem to be a risk factor.
  (c) Approximately 10% of cases overall, but most common among African Americans, Latin Americans, Native Americans, and Japanese.
- Desmoplastic
  (a) Rare variant of melanoma, but the most common site is head and neck.
  (b) Appearance is variable and often amelanotic.

(c) Histology: spindle-shaped tumor cells among a fibrous stroma, may show neuron-like differentiation. Categorized as pure (> 90% desmoplasia) or mixed (< 90% desmoplasia).
(d) High affinity for perineural spread, and lower rate of lymphatic metastasis compared to typical melanomas.
(e) Wide margins and adjuvant radiation are required to optimize locoregional control.

- Mucosal melanoma
  (a) Less than 1% of melanomas, but ~10% of all head and neck melanomas.
  (b) A brief review of mucosal melanoma is provided at the end of this chapter.

Differential Diagnosis

Benign Lesions

- Seborrheic keratosis
  (a) Light brown lesions, "stuck-on" appearance
- Pigmented actinic keratosis
- Benign melanocytic lesions
  (a) Mongolian spot: congenital patch of melanocytes, completely benign
  (b) Blue nevus
    - A rest of melanocytes; rare lesion, but more common in Asian patients. There are rare cases of melanoma arising from blue nevi.
    - Two variants exist:
      - Common blue nevus: common in head and neck
      - Cellular blue nevus: atypical lesions, can be difficult to differentiate from melanoma
  (c) Melanocytic nevus
    - Hamartomatous lesion composed of melanocytes
    - Spitz nevus
      - Childhood lesion composed of large or spindle-shaped melanocytes. Can have a phase of rapid growth, but it is benign. Can be difficult to differentiate from childhood melanoma.
      - Reports exist describing metastases from atypical spitz nevi, but it is debated whether these are Spitz nevi or malignant melanomas
  (d) Nevus of Ota: melanocytic hamartoma in the V2/V3 distribution
  (e) Nevus of Ito: similar to nevus of Ota, except occurring in shoulder region
- Lentigo maligna
- Atypical (dysplastic) nevus

Malignant Lesions

- Basal cell carcinoma
- Keratoacanthoma
  (a) Low-grade malignancy that resembles well-differentiated squamous cell carcinoma
- Squamous cell carcinoma
- Sebaceous carcinoma
- Merkel cell carcinoma
  (a) Neuroendocrine carcinoma of the skin

Histologic Appearance of Malignant Melanoma

- Malignant melanoma is often characterized by:
  (a) Enlarged cells with cytologic atypia.
  (b) Large, pleomorphic, hyperchromic nuclei.
  (c) Prominent nucleoli.
  (d) "Pagetoid" growth (upward, out of the basal layer) is commonly observed; this can also occur in melanocytic nevi; however, more extensive lateral spread and cytological atypia favor the diagnosis of melanoma.
  (e) Presence of melanin on hematoxylin and eosin (H&E) stain or with the aid of Fontana stain.
- However, melanomas can be "amelanotic."
- The histologic pattern and differentiation of melanoma can vary greatly.
- Melanoma has been called a "great mimicker," and belongs in the differential diagnosis of any undifferentiated tumor.
- Commonly used immunohistochemical markers:
  (a) HMB-45, S-100, Melan-A, and Vimentin.
  (b) Cytokeratin is usually negative.
- **Depth of invasion** has an important impact on prognosis.
- **Number of mitoses** has also been shown to be associated with prognosis; however, it is unclear if this is independent of depth of invasion and other adverse features. Mitotic index is no longer part of the American Joint Committee on Cancer (AJCC) staging system.

Evaluation

History and Physical Examination

- Thorough history to determine risk of melanoma (see risk factors).
- Common characteristics of malignant melanoma (ABCDE checklist):
  (a) **A**symmetry, **B**order irregularities, **C**olor variegation, **D**iameter greater than 6 mm or recent increase in size, **E**volution—changes in size, color, texture, etc.
- Dermatologist may use dermoscopy (10× magnification), a Wood lamp (UV light that enhances pigmented lesions), or reflectance confocal microscopy (RCM—allows *in vivo* visualization down to the papillary dermis) to aid diagnosis.
- A thorough physical examination of the head and neck is always warranted, but there are several important considerations specific to malignant melanoma.
  (a) **Location** has a significant impact on prognosis.
  (b) Generally, head and neck melanoma carry a worse prognosis than other sites.
  (c) Specific subsites of the head and neck are associated with a worse prognosis:
    - (worst) scalp > ear > cheek > neck (improved)
  (d) Note signs of aggressive/advanced disease:
    - Ulceration
    - Nodularity
    - Satellite lesions
  (e) Thorough examination of the draining lymph node basin is required.
    - Include parotid lymph nodes, especially for anterior scalp, temple, or cheek melanomas
    - Occipital nodes, especially for retroauricular or posterior scalp lesions

Imaging

- Stage I or II disease: **chest X-ray** (CXR) is often obtained, and is the only imaging study necessary unless suspicion for distant metastasis exists based on clinical examination or laboratory findings.
- **CT with IV contrast** of the head and neck is used to evaluate the extent of locoregional disease. Therefore, obtain it in any patient with thick lesions, evidence of local invasion, or evidence on clinical examination for regional metastasis.
- Metastatic imaging work-up includes:
  (a) CT chest, abdomen, pelvis with IV contrast.
  (b) MRI of the brain.
  (c) PET and PET-CT have been shown to be highly sensitive for the detection of systemic metastasis, and may replace whole-body CT scan.
- **Consider** metastatic screening in the following patients:
  (a) Patients with thick melanomas (> 4 mm), satellitosis, ulceration, or recurrent lesions
- Metastatic evaluation is **required** in the following patients:
  (a) Patients with regional metastases (stage III)
  (b) Patients with signs or symptoms of metastatic disease on examination or laboratory evaluation
  (c) Patients with known systemic disease (stage IV)

Other

- Baseline CBC, basic chemistry panel, total protein, albumin.
- Elevated alkaline phosphatase may signify metastatic disease to bone or liver.
- Elevated ALT/AST may signify metastatic disease to the liver.
- Elevated lactate dehydrogenase (LDH) is nonspecific, but may signify the presence of metastasis. It is also a useful marker to follow for the development of metastatic disease during follow-up. Recommended in any patient at risk for systemic disease.

Biopsy

- All lesions suspicious for malignant melanoma should undergo biopsy by a method that will give a definitive diagnosis and provide information on depth of invasion.
- Needle biopsies of the primary tumor are *not* adequate.
- Shave biopsy is discouraged and may not provide adequate information regarding depth of invasion.
- **Excisional biopsy**
  (a) Acceptable if lesion is very small
  (b) Excise with narrow (1-2 mm) margins → follow-up wide excision of margins necessary if pathologic review yields malignant melanoma
  (c) Excision of large lesions may disrupt lymphatic drainage, altering results on lymphoscintigraphy
- **Incisional** or **punch biopsies** through the thickest portion of tumor is recommended.
  (a) Allows adequate assessment of depth of invasion.
  (b) Does not disrupt border of tumor to determine appropriate margins for wide local excision.
  (c) Does not affect lymphatic drainage of the lesion if lymphoscintigraphy is necessary.

Staging

- The most important prognostic factors in malignant melanoma are depth of invasion, ulceration, satellitosis, degree of lymph node involvement, and distant metastasis.

Table 42-1 Definitions of Clark levels and Breslow thickness for malignant melanoma

Clark Levels	*Level of Invasion*
Level I	Epidermis only (*carcinoma in situ*)
Level II	Papillary dermis (not to papillary-reticular interface)
Level III	Fills/expands papillary dermis to reticular interface
Level IV	Reticular dermis
Level V	Subcutaneous tissue
Breslow Thickness	
Stage I	0.75 mm or less
Stage II	0.76-1.50 mm
Stage III	1.51-4.0 mm
Stage IV	4.1 mm or greater

- The following features should be reported upon pathologic review, according to guidelines published by the College of American Pathologists:
  - Breslow thickness
  - Clark level
  - Ulceration
  - Presence of microsatellites
  - Peripheral and deep margin status
  - Mitotic rate (number of mitosis/mm^2)
  - Presence of lymphovascular invasion
  - Neurotropism
  - Presence of tumor-infiltrating lymphocytes
  - Presence of tumor regression
  - Pathologic staging per AJCC guidelines
- A description of Clark levels and Breslow thickness (Table 42-1) is presented here as these are commonly referenced; however, the current standard of evaluation and prognostication is proposed in the staging system developed by the American Joint Committee on Cancer (AJCC, 8th edition) (Tables 42-2 and 42-3).

Table 42-2 TNM Staging Definitions for Melanoma of the Skin

Definition of Primary Tumor (T)		
T Category	*Thickness*	*Ulceration Status*
Tx, primary tumor thickness cannot be assessed (eg, diagnosis by curettage)	Not applicable	Not applicable
T0, no evidence of primary tumor (eg, unknown primary or completely regressed melanoma)	Not applicable	Not applicable

(*Continued*)

Table 42-2 **TNM Staging Definitions for Melanoma of the Skin (*Continued*)**

Tis (melanoma *in situ*)	Not applicable	Not applicable
T1	≤ 1.0 mm	Unknown or unspecified
T1a	< 0.8 mm	Without ulceration
T1b	< 0.8 mm	With ulceration
	0.8-1.0 mm	With or without ulceration
T2	>1.0-2.0 mm	Unknown or unspecified
T2a	>1.0-2.0 mm	With ulceration
T2b	>1.0-2.0mm	With or without ulceration
T3	> 2.0-4.0 mm	Unknown or unspecified
T3a	> 2.0-4.0 mm	With ulceration
T3b	> 2.0-4.0 mm	With or without ulceration
T4	> 4.0 mm	Unknown or unspecified
T4a	> 4.0 mm	With ulceration
T4b	> 4.0 mm	With or without ulceration
	Definition of Regional Lymph Node (N)	
	Extent of Regional Lymph Node and/or Lymphatic Metastasis	
N Category	*Number of Tumor-Involved Regional Lymph Node*	*Presence of In-Transit, Satellite, and/or Microsatellite Metastases*
NX	Regional nodes not assessed (eg, SLN biopsy not performed, regional nodes previously removed for another reason) **Exception:** pathological N category is not required for T1 melanomas, use cN.	No
N0	No regional metastases detected	No
N1	One tumor-involved node or in-transit, satellite, and/or microsatellite metastases with no tumor-involved nodes	
N1a	One clinically occult (ie, detected by SLN biopsy)	No
N1b	One clinically detected	No
N1c	No regional lymph node disease	Yes
N2	Two or three tumor-involved nodes in-transit, satellite, and/or microsatellite metastases with one tumor-involved node	
N2a	Two or three clinically occult (ie, detected by SLN biopsy)	No

(*Continued*)

Table 42-2 TNM Staging Definitions for Melanoma of the Skin (*Continued*)

N2b	Two or three, at least one of which was clinically detected	No
N2c	One clinically occult or clinically detected	Yes
N3	Four or more tumor-involved nodes or in-transit, satellite, and/or microsatellite metastases with two or more tumor-involved nodes, or any number of matted nodes without or with in-transit, satellite, and/or microsatellite metastases	
N3a	Four or more clinically occult (ie, detected by SLN biopsy)	No
N3b	Four or more, at least one of which was clinically detected, or presence of any number of matted nodes	No
N3c	Two or more clinically occult or clinically detected and/or presence of any number of matted nodes	Yes
	Definition of Distant Metastasis (M)	
	M Criteria	
M Category	*Anatomic Site*	*LDH Level*
M0	No evidence of distant metastasis	Not applicable
M1	Evidence of distant metastasis	See below
M1a	Distant metastasis to skin, soft tissue including muscle, and/or nonregional lymph node	Not recorded or unspecified
M1a(0)		Not elevated
M1a(1)		Elevated
M1b	Distant metastasis to lung with or without	Not recorded or unspecified
M1b(0)	M1a sites of disease	Not elevated
M1b(1)		Elevated
M1c	Distant metastasis to non-CNS visceral sites with or without M1a or M1b sites of disease	Not recorded or unspecified
M1c(0)		Not elevated
M1c(1)		Elevated
M1d	Distant metastasis to CNS with or without	Not recorded or unspecified
M1d(0)	M1a, M1b, or M1c sites of disease	Normal
M1d(1)		Elevated

SLN, sentinel lymph node biopsy.

Table 42-3 Stage Groups for Melanoma of the Skin

Clinical (cTNM)			
When T is...	*And N is...*	*And M is...*	*Then the clinical stage group is...*
Tis	N0	M0	0
T1a	N0	M0	IA
T1b	N0	M0	IB
T2a	N0	M0	IB
T2b	N0	M0	IIA
T3a	N0	M0	IIA
T3b	N0	M0	IIB
T4a	N0	M0	IIB
T4b	N0	M0	IIC
Any T, Tis	≥N1	M0	III
Any T	Any N	M1	IV
Pathological (pTNM)			
When T is...	*And N is...*	*And M is...*	*Then the clinical stage group is...*
Tis	N0	M0	0
T1a	N0	M0	IA
T1b	N0	M0	IA
T2a	N0	M0	IB
T2b	N0	M0	IIA
T3a	N0	M0	IIA
T3b	N0	M0	IIB
T4a	N0	M0	IIB
T4b	N0	M0	IIC
T0	N1b, N1c	M0	IIIB
T0	N2b, N2c, N3b, or N3c	M0	IIIC
T1a/b - T2a	N1a or N2a	M0	IIIA
T1a/b - T2a	N1b/c or N2b	M0	IIIB
T2b/T3a	N1a - N2b	M0	IIIB
T1a-T3a	N2c or N3a/b/c	M0	IIIC
T3b/T4a	Any N ≥N1	M0	IIIC
T4b	N1a - N2c	M0	IIIC
T4b	N3a/b/c	M0	IIID
Any T, Tis	Any N	M1	IV

Used with the permission of the American College of Surgeons. Amin MB, Edge SB, Greene FL, et al. (Eds.) AJCC Cancer Staging Manual, 8th Ed. Springer New York, 2017.

- Note that AJCC staging includes clinical and pathologic staging. Pathologic staging incorporates pathologic information about the regional lymph nodes after lymph node biopsy/neck dissection, subdividing stage III disease into the categories shown. Only pathologic stage is presented here, as sentinel lymph node biopsy has become routine for intermediate thickness melanomas at most centers.
- Testing for BRAF mutation status is indicated for advanced-stage melanoma.

Treatment

Surgery

Primary Lesion

- A diagnosis of malignant melanoma often requires wide local excision of the primary lesion. For patients with advanced resectable locoregional disease, neoadjuvant immunotherapy should be considered before wide local excision (NADINA phase III trial, Blank et al, NEJM 2024). Surgery may not be employed if systemic metastases are present and palliative resection is not warranted.

Margins

- General guidelines:
  (a) **1-cm** margin for tumors less than 1 mm thick
  (b) **Consider greater than 1 cm** margin for lesions with 1 to 2 mm thickness
  (c) **2-cm** margin for tumors greater than 2 mm thick, or ulcerated
- Recommendations of 1 to 2 cm are often not feasible due to functional and cosmetic considerations in the head and neck.
- Depth of resection varies based on the region of the head and neck involved. Some important considerations:
  (a) **Scalp lesions:** resected to the calvarial periosteum; the outer table of the cranium can be included if lesion is thick and encroaches upon the periosteum.
  (b) **Auricular lesions** often require partial or total auriculectomy depending on the size of the tumor and presence or absence of satellitosis.
  (c) Lesions that involve the **ear canal** may require lateral temporal bone resection.
  (d) **Facial lesions** are often resected down to the level of the facial mimetic muscles, unless lesion is thicker and requires resection of muscle or even facial bone.
  (e) **Lesions overlying the parotid gland** resected down to parotid-masseteric fascia, unless thickness requires that a superficial parotidectomy be included in resection.

Cervical Lymph Nodes

- **Therapeutic neck dissection**
  (a) There is now strong evidence to support neoadjuvant immune checkpoint therapy for patients with positive regional lymphatic disease (NADINA phase III trial, Blank et al, NEJM 2024).
  (b) Patients with evidence of lymphatic metastasis on clinical examination or imaging require a neck dissection (again, strong evidence to plan neck dissection *after* neoadjuvant immunotherapy—NADINA phase III trial, Blank et al, NEJM 2024).
  (c) Anterior scalp, temple, ear, or facial melanomas with evidence of regional disease require a **superficial parotidectomy** as well. Chin and neck melanomas do not require parotidectomy.
  (d) For posterior scalp, posterior ear, or retroauricular melanomas with evidence of regional disease, the **postauricular and suboccipital nodes** must be included in the neck dissection.

- **Sentinel lymph node biopsy**
  (a) Sentinel lymph node biopsy has been shown to improve disease-free survival for patients with intermediate thickness melanoma (Multicenter Selective Lymphadenectomy Trial-I).
  (b) Sentinel lymph node biopsy is recommended for patients with T2 or T3 tumors (depth 1-4 mm) and no evidence on clinical examination of lymph node metastasis ("N0 neck")
  (c) Also indicated for lesions extending to Clark levels IV or V, or for lesions with evidence of ulceration (eg, T1b), regardless of the thickness of the lesion.
  (d) The parotid lymph nodes and neck levels IB, II, III, and IV are at risk when primary lesions involve the anterior scalp (anterior to a vertical line drawn superiorly from the external auditory canal), temple, facial lesions, and ear.
  (e) Posterior scalp (posterior to a vertical line drawn superiorly from the external auditory canal) and retroauricular lesions drain to the posterolateral neck—levels II, III, IV, and V—along with the retroauricular and suboccipital lymph nodes.
- **Technical aspects of sentinel lymph node biopsy**
  (a) **Lymphoscintigraphy**, or lymphatic mapping, is performed 1 to 24 hours prior to sentinel node biopsy.
  (b) Dermal layer of the bed of primary lesion (or region of recent resection if excisional biopsy was performed) is injected with Technecium-99-labeled sulfur colloid or Technecium (99mTc) Tilmanocept, which binds to CD206 receptors on the surface of macrophages and dendritic cells.
  (c) Two-dimensional nuclear imaging, or three-dimensional SPECT/CT is performed to map the lymph nodes draining the site of the lesion.
  (d) **Sentinel lymph node biopsy** is then performed.
    - If lymphoscintigraphy was performed just before surgery, no additional radiotracer is injected.
    - If lymphoscintigraphy was performed the day before, additional tracer is injected 1 hour before surgery.
    - Isosulfan blue can be injected into the primary site at the time of surgery as an adjunctive method to identify sentinel nodes.
    - A hand-held gamma probe is used to identify the sentinel lymph node.
    - The sentinel node, ideally identified with the guidance of the lymphatic map, the gamma probe, and visualized with uptake of isosulfan blue, is removed.
    - If localization is to the parotid region, superficial parotidectomy may be necessary if searching for intraparotid nodes poses higher risk of facial nerve injury.
    - Additional nodes (usually ~ 3-4 lymph nodes) are removed until the reading from the gamma probe in the surgical bed is reduced to 10% of the highest reading from the resected lymph nodes.
    - Sentinel lymph nodes undergo standard sectioning with H&E staining, as well as additional sectioning with IHC evaluation using HMB-45, S-100, and Melan-A.
  (e) The role of completion neck dissection after a sentinel lymph node is found to be positive for metastatic melanoma is controversial. **Completion lymph node dissection improves regional disease control and has prognostic value, but was not associated with improved melanoma-specific survival (Multicenter Selective Lymphadenectomy Trial-II).** The impact of completion neck dissection on locoregional control and disease-specific survival for head and neck-specific melanoma is not clear. Completion neck dissection, if performed, should include parotidectomy or removal of the postauricular/suboccipital nodes if the location of primary disease places these regions at risk of metastasis.

Reconstruction

- Choose from "reconstructive ladder" (secondary intention → primary closure → skin graft → regional flap → free flap) depending on location and size of defect.
- DO NOT perform a complex reconstruction (ie, regional or free flap) until the margin status has been defined on the final pathologic report.
- If necessary, place a dressing or skin graft over large/complex wounds and return to the OR for reconstruction after margins have been deemed negative.

External Beam Radiation

- May be considered in the following settings to improve local-regional control:
  (a) Postoperative radiation following resection/neck dissection of palpable lymphatic disease
  (b) Radiation to regional lymph nodes for patients with T1b-T4, N0 disease who cannot undergo sentinel lymph node biopsy or neck dissection.
  (c) Radiation to regional recurrence in patients who have previously undergone neck dissection.
  (d) Radiation to primary site in patients at high risk of local failure (eg, T4 lesions, desmoplastic melanoma, etc.)
- Hypofractionated treatment schedule (6 Gy fractions up to a total dose of 30 Gy) is most effective.

Chemotherapy

- Systemic therapy is employed to treat melanoma in the following settings:
  (a) For patients at high risk for the development of distant metastasis (ie, Stage IIb, III, or recurrent disease)
  (b) Patients with known distant metastases (ie, Stage IV disease)
  (c) For patients with clinical Stage III disease (clinical N+), neoadjuvant ipilimumab + nivolumab has been shown to be more effective than postoperative adjuvant immunotherapy **(NADINA phase III trial, Blank et al, NEJM 2024)**
- **Available therapies:**
  (a) **Immune Checkpoint Inhibitors**: This class of agents has become the predominant therapeutic option for patients with cutaneous melanoma. Immune signaling pathways contain several natural mechanisms to repress immune responses ("checkpoints"). Tumor cells can take advantage of these mechanisms to evade destruction by immune cells. Immune checkpoint *inhibitors* have been developed to re-establish/enhance immune activation toward tumor cells. Several immune checkpoint inhibitors have been approved to treat cutaneous melanoma (listed below).
- **Ipilimumab**: a monoclonal antibody that blocks cytotoxic T lymphocyte antigen-4 (CTLA-4), approved to treat unresectable or metastatic melanoma. CTLA-4 is found on the surface of T cells, and when activated leads to downregulation of T-cell activity. Inhibition of CTLA-4 promotes the T-cell response to tumor cell antigens.
- **Pembrolizumab:** humanized monoclonal antibody designed to block the PD-1 receptor, which is expressed by immune cells. Activation of PD-1 by the ligands PD-L1 and PD-L2 (which may be upregulated on cancer cells) leads to immune suppression. Thus, inhibition of PD-1 enhances antitumor immune activity.
- **Nivolumab:** also inhibits PD-1. Nivolumab is approved for patients with stage IV or unresectable stage III, but also as adjuvant therapy for patients with stage III disease who have undergone complete resection of lymph node disease.

- The **combination of nivolumab with ipilimumab** has also been approved.
- **Relatlimab:** a monoclonal antibody that inhibits lymphocyte activation gene-3 (LAG-3). Despite its name, LAG3 transmits inhibitory signals to T cells. Relatlimlab is combined with nivolumab (combination called opdualag) to treat cutaneous melanoma.
- **MAP kinase (Ras-Raf-MEK-ERK) pathway inhibitors**
  (a) **Vemurafenib:** small molecule selective inhibitor of BRAF which is approved to treat unresectable or metastatic melanoma with activating mutations in BRAF (eg, BRAF V600E mutations).
  (b) **Dabrafenib:** BRAF inhibitor used to treat patients with tumors containing activating BRAF mutations.
  (c) **Trametinib, Cobimetinib:** MEK inhibitors, approved to treat patients with tumors containing BRAF mutations.
  (d) **Dabrafenib and Trametinib** have been approved as single agents and in combination. **Vemurafenib in combination with cobimetinib** has also been approved in combination.
- Other Chemotherapeutic agents approved to treat cutaneous melanoma
  (a) **Dacarbazine** and derivatives
    - Alkylating agent, FDA approved for the treatment of advanced melanoma → 10% to 20% response rate
  (b) **Other immunotherapy agents**
- **Interferon α-2b / Peginterferon α-2b:** cytokine normally produced by lymphocytes. FDA approved for treating malignant melanoma. Mechanism of action not well understood—modulates immune response to cancer cells.
- **Interleukin-2:** Biologic modifier similar to INFα-2b.
- **Talimogene laherparepvec "T-Vec"**: Genetically modified live oncolytic herpes virus that replicates within cancer cells and produces GM-CSF. This agent is injected directly into tumors, which causes cell lysis and release of tumor antigens. GM-CSF helps recruit immune cells, leading to an augmented immune response. T-Vec is approved for the local treatment of unresectable cutaneous, subcutaneous, and nodal lesions in patients with melanoma that has recurred after the initial surgery.

Follow-Up

- Recommendations vary, but typical follow-up schedules are every 3 to 6 months for 4 years, and annually thereafter.
- Periodic LDH and CXR recommended.
- Frequency of examination, laboratory testing, and radiologic examinations should increase for more advanced stages.

Other Considerations in Head and Neck Melanoma

Desmoplastic Melanoma

- Often nonpigmented, initially benign appearing.
- Rare, spindle-cell variant with a propensity for perineural spread.
- Occur in older patients, in heavily sun-damaged skin.
- 4% of melanomas, and tend to have a very high tumor mutation burden
- These lesions can be purely desmoplastic in nature (> 90% desmoplastic), or can have elements of both desmoplastic and conventional melanoma features (mixed desmoplastic).

- Pure desmoplastic melanomas metastasize to regional lymph nodes very infrequently, and therefore, sentinel lymph node biopsy is not recommended.
- Considerations for sentinel lymph node biopsy for mixed desmoplastic lesions are the same as for conventional cutaneous melanoma.
- Excision with wide margins (2 cm or greater if feasible).
- Adjuvant radiotherapy is recommended to optimize locoregional control.
- Recent data have supported neoadjuvant immune checkpoint inhibitor treatment.
- Desmoplastic melanoma shows high rates of response to PD-1 inhibitors.

Mucosal Melanoma

- Rare variant of melanoma, but most common site is in the head and neck.
- Most common sites: nasal > paranasal sinuses > oral cavity > nasopharynx.
- Prognosis: (best) Nasal > oral cavity > paranasal sinuses (worst).
- Disease can be indolent with vague symptoms, thus patients often present with an advanced stage of disease.
- Often amelanotic.
- Depth of invasion has not been shown to be a predictor of prognosis.
- Treatment:
  (a) Surgical resection.
  (b) Therapeutic neck dissection for clinically positive lymph nodes.
  (c) Elective neck dissection not recommended.
  (d) Radiation at high dose (> 54 Gy) and standard fractionation can improve local-regional control.
- Many patients succumb to distant metastasis.

Unknown Primary Melanoma

- Melanoma identified in cervical lymph nodes or parotid nodes with no evidence or history of a primary lesion.
- Thorough history and physical examination necessary to identify potential primary lesion, and metastatic workup indicated.
- Theorized that primary lesions can spontaneously regress.
- Treat with surgical resection/neck dissection and postoperative hypofractionated radiation (ie, treat as a Stage III melanoma).

Bibliography

American Joint Committee on Cancer (AJCC). Melanoma of the skin. In: Amin MB, Edge S, Green F, et al. (eds). *AJCC Cancer Staging Manual*. 8th ed. New York, NY: Springer; 2017.

Blank CU, Lucas MW, Scolyer RA, et al. Neoadjuvant nivolumab and ipilimumab in resectable stage III melanoma. *N Engl J Med*. 2024 Jun 2. Epub ahead of print.

Faries MB, Thompson JF, Cochran AJ, et al. Completion dissection or observation for sentinel-node metastasis in melanoma. *N Engl J Med*. 2017 Jun 8; 376(23):2211-2222.

Long GV, Stroyakovskiy D, Gogas H, et al. Combined BRAF and MEK inhibition versus BRAF inhibition alone in melanoma. *N Engl J Med*. 2014 Nov 13;371(20):1877-1888.

Morton DL, Thompson JF, Cochran AJ, et al (MSLT Group). Final trial report of sentinel-node biopsy versus nodal observation in melanoma. *N Engl J Med*. 2014;370(7):599-609.

Questions

1. Which of the following is *not* a risk factor for the development of head and neck melanoma?
   A. Fitzpatrick type I skin type
   B. Ultraviolet A exposure from tanning booths
   C. Presence of multiple nevi on the cheeks
   D. Four blistering sunburns in the teenage years

2. What is the proper margin, if feasible, for an ulcerated lesion with 1.75 mm depth of invasion?
   A. 0.5 cm
   B. 1 cm
   C. 1.5 cm
   D. 2 cm

3. You are planning to resect an ulcerated malignant melanoma that has 2.1 mm depth of invasion from the left anterior parietal scalp of a 40-year-old male patient. He has no cervical or parotid lymphadenopathy and no suspicious nodes on imaging. What is the most appropriate next step in management?
   A. Wide local excision with 2-cm margin
   B. Wide local excision with 1-cm margin, elective neck dissection
   C. Wide local excision with 2-cm margin, with sentinel lymph node biopsy
   D. Wide local excision with 2-cm margin, radiation therapy to the draining lymph node basin, including the parotid gland

4. You resect a cheek melanoma with 2.5 mm depth of invasion with 2 cm margins, and you perform a sentinel lymph node biopsy which shows 2 of 4 lymph nodes positive for melanoma cells. What is the most appropriate next step?
   A. Reconstruction of the cheek defect along with mandatory parotidectomy and neck dissection
   B. Postoperative radiation to the surrounding neck lymph nodes
   C. Medical oncology referral for consideration for adjuvant PD-1 inhibitor therapy
   D. Consideration for combination trametinib and dabrafenib

5. A patient presents with a large, left preauricular melanoma with three palpable lymph nodes in the left neck. Imaging and FNA confirm neck metastases without evidence of distant disease. Which of the following is the most appropriate treatment plan?
   A. Radical resection with sentinel lymph node biopsy
   B. Neoadjuvant ipilimumab and nivolumab, followed by wide surgical resection of the primary disease along with parotidectomy and neck dissection
   C. Palliative chemotherapy
   D. Neoadjuvant vemurafenib followed by auriculectomy and posterolateral neck dissection

Chapter 43
Tumors of the Oral Cavity

In this chapter we review the etiology, staging, and management of malignant tumors of the oral cavity. We also cover oral cavity anatomy, as well as both benign and premalignant oral lesions that should be considered in the differential diagnosis of oral cancer.

Anatomy

The oral cavity extends from the cutaneous-vermilion junction of the lips to the anterior tonsillar pillars. The posterior border of the oral cavity also includes the circumvallate papillae inferiorly and the junction of the hard and soft palate superiorly. The oral cavity is divided into seven anatomic subsites:

- Lips
- Oral tongue, anterior two-thirds
- Floor of mouth
- Buccal mucosa
- Gingiva (alveolar ridges), upper and lower
- Retromolar trigone (RMT)
- Hard palate

Salivary Glands and Ducts

- Parotid (Stenson): orifice lateral to second molars. Produce two-thirds of mouth's saliva when stimulated.
- Submandibular (Wharton): orifice in midline floor of mouth adjacent to lingual frenulum. Produce two-thirds of mouth's saliva when unstimulated.
- Sublingual (Rivinus): multiple orifices draining into floor of mouth or submandibular duct.
- Produce an average of 1500 mL saliva per day; this amount is reduced by radiotherapy and medications (primarily anticholinergics).
- Saliva is 99.5% water, with an electrolyte composition of sodium 10 mEq/L, potassium 26 mEq/L, chlorine 10 mEq/L, and bicarbonate 30 mEq/L, and organic components including glycoprotein and amylase (which is distinct from pancreatic amylase). Saliva pH varies from 6.2 to 7.4.

Teeth

- Deciduous teeth: 20
- Adult teeth: 32, numbered superiorly right to left (1-16), and inferiorly left to right (17-32)

Tongue

Surface

- Papillae: very small protrusions covering the anterior two-thirds of the tongue. There are four types: filiform (no taste function, increase tongue's surface area and texture), fungiform (diffuse, responsible for taste, touch, and temperature), and foliate (lateral tongue, taste), and circumvallate (large, form a V-shape at the junction of the anterior and posterior portions of the tongue).
- Sulcus terminalis: groove at the anterior margin of the circumvallate papillae
- Foramen cecum: pit at the apex of the sulcus terminalis from which the embryologic thyroid begins its descent
- Frenulum: anterior fold of mucous membrane that attaches the anterior inferior aspect of the tongue to the floor mouth and gingiva. Wharton salivary ducts open on either side of the frenulum. May be congenitally short (tongue-tie), decreasing tongue mobility.
- Lingual tonsil: lymphoid tissue extending over the base of the tongue (considered to be in oropharynx), posterior to the circumvallate papillae. Size varies among individuals.
- Valleculae: depressions on either side of the midline glossoepiglottic fold extending to the level of the hyoid bone. (Considered to be in oropharynx.)

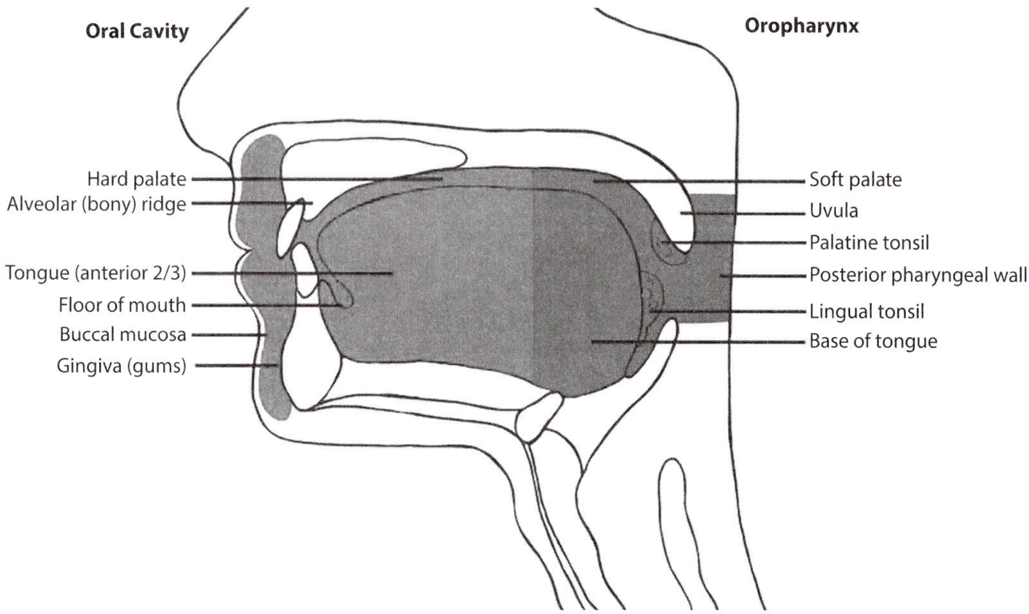

Figure 43-1 The oral cavity is separated from the oropharynx by several anatomy landmarks, including the posterior border of the hard palate, the circumvallate papillae (anterior two-thirds oral tongue and base of the tongue), and the anterior tonsillar pillars. Oral cavity is indicated by red, and oropharynx by blue. (Satgunaseelan et al., 2022, MDPI, Basel, Switzerland, open access, CC BY license)

Muscles of the Tongue

- Extrinsic: genioglossus, hyoglossus, styloglossus, and palatoglossus
- Intrinsic: superior and inferior longitudinal, vertical, and transverse; the superior longitudinal and transverse muscles originate from the fibrous lingual septum, which defines the midline
- Controlled by cranial nerve XII

Sensory Innervation

- Taste (oral tongue):

  Papillae → Afferent fibers → lingual nerve → chorda tympani (branch of facial nerve) → geniculate ganglion → intermediary nerve → nucleus solitarius

- Touch, pain, temperature (oral tongue): lingual nerve → CN V_3
- Taste (tongue base): taste receptors → CN IX → inferior petrosal ganglion → nucleus solitarius
- Touch, pain, temperature (tongue base): CN IX

Vascular Supply

- Lingual artery: third branch of the external carotid; supplies blood to the tongue, tonsils, and floor of the mouth, including the sublingual salivary glands
- Lingual vein: travels with hypoglossal nerve (veins of Ranine), making the nerve vulnerable during attempts to control bleeding

Lymphatic Drainage

- Anterior (oral) tongue: to level I (submental and submandibular), II (jugulodigastric), III, and IV (middle and lower jugular); midline drains to nodes on both sides
- Posterior (oropharyngeal) tongue: drains to both ipsilateral and contralateral deep cervical (jugulodigastric and retropharyngeal) nodes

Retromolar Trigone

- Triangulated region of gingiva overlying the ascending ramus of the mandible. The base of the triangle sits behind the last molar, and the apex is the maxillary tuberosity.
- Represents a watershed area, near the buccal mucosa, tonsillar fossa, glossopharyngeal sulcus, lateral floor of mouth, tongue base, soft palate, and, deeply, the masticator space.

Hard Palate

Consists of the palatine process of the maxilla and horizontal plates of the palatine bones. Covered with stratified squamous epithelium attached firmly to underlying bone. Contains five foramina:

- Greater palatine foramina convey the descending palatine branches of V2 and the descending palatine arteries (third division of the maxillary artery). Depressions palpable 1 cm medial to second molar.
- Accessory palatine foramina: posterior to the greater palatine foramina convey the lesser descending palatine arteries to the soft palate.
- Incisive foramen: in the midline of the anterior palate; transmits the incisural artery to the anterior septum and the nasopalatine nerve, which provides sensation to the mucosa posterior to the maxillary central incisors and the anterior hard palate.

Vascular Supply

Arterial

Maxillary artery → Descending palatine artery → Greater palatine artery: Hard palate

Maxillary artery → Descending palatine artery → Lesser palatine artery: Soft palate

Venous

Hard palate veins → Pterygoid plexus → Internal jugular

Muscles of Mastication

- Include the masseter, temporal, and lateral and medial pterygoid. Only the lateral pterygoid muscle assists in lowering the jaw
- Blood supply: branches of maxillary artery
- Nerve supply: V3 (motor branch)

Benign or Premalignant Lesions and Disorders

Oral Cavity

Lesions of the Oral Cavity

- Aphthous ulcer (canker sore): white spot with erythematous halo on the flexible, nonkeratinizing mucosa. Often triggered by local trauma; usually resolves within 7 to 10 days.
- Leukoplakia (white plaque): white hyperkeratotic lesion that may or may not be associated with dysplastic change on histologic examination. Occurs most frequently on the lip (vermilion); other locations, in descending frequency, include the buccal mucosa, mandibular gingiva, tongue, floor of the mouth, hard palate, maxillary gingiva, lip mucosa, and soft palate. Less than 10% of isolated leukoplakia will prove to be carcinoma or severe dysplasia on biopsy. Severe dysplasia (carcinoma in situ) has an approximately 20% risk of progressing to invasive carcinoma.
- Erythroplakia (red plaque): granular erythematous area, often encountered in association with leukoplakia. Half of these lesions demonstrate severe dysplasia or carcinoma *in situ* on biopsy.
- Nodular leukoplakia (mixed white and red plaques) has greater malignant potential than isolated leukoplakia, with risk similar to that of erythroplakia; may be seen in association with frank invasive cancer.
- Median rhomboid glossitis: smooth reddish area of the midline of the tongue devoid of papillae, sometimes with a corresponding lesion along the hard palate; may be associated with candida overgrowth.
- Fordyce granules: painless, pinpoint yellow nodules that occur bilaterally on the posterior buccal mucosa or at the vermillion border of the lips. Result from enlargement of ectopic sebaceous glands

- Hairy tongue involves hyperplasia of filiform papillae that may be black, blue, brown, or white depending on microflora and nicotine staining. This temporary condition is often associated with candida overgrowth and usually resolves with proper oral hygiene.
- Epulis is a nonspecific term for tumor-like masses of the gingiva. Epulis cases associated with pregnancy, which are most common, are pyogenic granulomas; others are usually giant cell reparative granulomas. The latter lesions appear on histologic examination as reticular and fibrous connective tissue with numerous giant cells, with radiographs showing cuffing or sclerotic margins of bone. Rare cases at birth resemble granular cell myoblastoma. Treatment is by excision and curettage of any underlying bony defect.
- Ranula is a mucocele of the sublingual gland that presents in the floor of the mouth. *Plunging ranula* penetrates the mylohyoid muscle and presents as a soft submandibular neck mass. Excision should include the entire sublingual gland to prevent recurrence, with care taken to protect the submandibular duct and the lingual nerve.
- Necrotizing sialometaplasia is a benign, ulcerous lesion on the posterior hard palate caused by trauma to the minor salivary glands. Closely resembles and can often be clinically misdiagnosed as malignancy. Lesions usually heal within 6 to 10 weeks. Torus palatini is a benign excessive bone growth in the midline of the palate which can continue to enlarge beyond puberty. Occasionally it must be removed to prevent denture irritation.

Developmental Conditions Affecting the Oral Cavity

- Cleft palate is due to failure of fusion of facial tissues during development and is associated with a characteristic vocal resonance and nasal regurgitation of liquids.
- Macroglossia (tongue enlargement) can result from several causes:
  (a) Benign tumors: hemangioma, lymphangioma
  (b) Storage diseases: amyloidosis, Von Gierke disease (glycogen storage disease type I), Hurler syndrome (mucopolysaccharidosis)
  (c) Other congenital conditions: Pierre Robin (relative macroglossia due to micrognathia), Down syndrome
  (d) Infection: actinomycosis or tertiary syphilis
  (e) Benign cysts

Tumors of the Mandible (Excluding Carcinoma)

- Mandibular tori: benign bony exostoses commonly seen on the lingual or buccal aspect of the anterior mandible
- Odontogenic fibroma presents as a circumscribed radiolucency with smooth borders around the crown of unerupted teeth. Radiographically, it resembles a dentigerous cyst. Treatment by excision is nearly always curative.
- Ameloblastoma: neoplasm of enamel origin that presents in the third or fourth decade, most commonly affecting the molar region. These tumors are slow growing and painless, expanding surrounding bone, but have a rare potential for malignant transformation. Treatment is complete surgical excision.
- Malignant ameloblastoma: histology is similar to ameloblastoma but demonstrates invasion, atypical mitotic figures, and pleomorphism. These tumors have a high propensity for local recurrence and may have regional or distant metastases.
- Cementomas: lesions that form cementum (bone-like connective tissue that covers the tooth root) and usually arise at the root tip in young adults. The radiographic appearance can vary from radiolucent to densely radiopaque. Treatment is simple enucleation.
- Ameloblastic odontoma: tumor composed of ameloblasts (enamel) and odontoblasts (dentin). It appears as an irregular radiopaque mass, often between tooth roots, and is associated with unerupted teeth. Simple enucleation is sufficient.

- Adenoameloblastoma: well-encapsulated follicular cyst, occurring most commonly in the anterior maxilla of adolescent girls in association with impacted teeth. A rare malignant variant exists. Treatment is excision as there is a low risk of recurrence
- Ameloblastic fibroma: slow-growing, painless lesion seen in the molar area of the mandible in adolescents and children. It contains both epithelial and mesenchymal tissue and is radiographically similar to an ameloblastoma.
- Ameloblastic sarcoma: malignant fast-growing, painful, and aggressive variant of ameloblastic fibroma that occurs most commonly in young adults. Treatment is surgical excision. Recurrence is common.
- Ewing sarcoma: rapidly growing tumor with local pain and swelling that most commonly occurs between ages 10 and 25 years. The mandible is the most common site in the head and neck. Multidisciplinary management includes surgery, chemotherapy, and radiation therapy. Survival is about 50%.
- Osteogenic sarcoma: rapidly growing, aggressive malignant tumor of bone, occurring primarily in adolescents and young adults. Survival of the mandibular variant is better than that arising in long bone. Multidisciplinary management includes surgery, chemotherapy, and radiation therapy.
- Benign salivary gland tumor: painless, slow-growing mass apparent externally in a location corresponding to a major salivary gland (eg, below the ear for the parotid). Distinguished from malignant tumors by their slow growth, mobility (nonfixation to skin), and absence of neural palsies.

Odontogenic Cysts

- Radicular cyst: most common, called a "periapical cyst" when it involves the tooth root. Presenting as a radiolucent area on X-ray, this cyst is secondary to dental infection and usually asymptomatic. Treatment is extraction or root canal therapy.
- Dentigerous (follicular) cyst: developmental abnormality caused by a defect in enamel formation. It is always associated with an unerupted tooth crown, most commonly in the mandibular third molar or maxillary cuspid. Ameloblastomas form in the cyst wall.
- Odontogenic keratocyst mimics dentigerous cysts if associated with a tooth root. Diagnosis is based on histology, and treatment is excision. Curettage and partial excision result in a high rate of recurrence.

Malignancy of the Oral Cavity

According to the World Cancer Research Fund International, in 2022, there were approximately 389,000 new cases of oral cavity cancer worldwide, with 27,570 occurring in the United States alone. Oral cavity malignancies are at least two times more common in men than in women.

- The oral cavity is the most common site of head and neck cancer (30%).
- Squamous cell carcinomas (SCCs) account for 90% of malignant neoplasms arising within the oral cavity.
- Minor salivary gland malignancies, distributed throughout the oral cavity, are the second most common. Of these, mucoepidermoid carcinoma, followed by low-grade adenocarcinoma and adenoid cystic carcinoma, are the most common.

Etiology and Epidemiology

- Tobacco and alcohol are major risk factors for oral cancer. The combined use of tobacco and alcohol has a multiplicative rather than an additive effect in enabling the development of oral cancers. The risk level is proportional to the amount and length of exposure.

- The primary carcinogenic molecules in tobacco are polycyclic hydrocarbons and nitrosamines.
- In Asian countries, betel (or areca) nut chewing is another significant risk factor.
- Other risk factors include Plummer-Vinson syndrome, wood dust exposure, and poor oral and dental hygiene.

Molecular Biology

- Molecular findings support the concept of "field cancerization," first proposed by Slaughter in 1953 to explain the development of multiple primary tumors and frequent local recurrence. In this model, a "field" of squamous mucosal cells across the entire upper aerodigestive tract is genetically altered by chronic exposure to tobacco, alcohol, or other carcinogens. These alterations lead to dysplastic epithelial changes from which cancers can arise.
- Genetic alterations are the result of inactivation of tumor suppressor genes (eg, p53, retinoblastoma, p16) or activation of proto-oncogenes to oncogenes (eg, RET, EGFR, RAS).
- The progressive accumulation of several mutations ultimately results in the progression from normal mucosa to dysplasia to carcinoma.

TNM Staging (8th Edition)

The tumor (T), lymph node (N), metastasis (M), or TNM system is a clinical staging schema based on the extent of disease as determined by physical examination and imaging prior to initial treatment. TNM staging provides a useful estimation of prognosis, aids in treatment selection, and permits the assessment of treatment outcomes. The American Joint Committee for Cancer (AJCC) coordinates and periodically updates the criteria for assessment and staging. N stage is determined either by clinical or, following surgery with lymphadenectomy, pathological criteria.

TNM Staging for Oral Cavity

Primary Tumor (T) Staging For Oral Cavity (Table 43-1)

- Tx: Primary tumor cannot be assessed
- Tis: Carcinoma in situ
- T1: Tumor ≤ 2 cm, ≤ 5 mm depth of invasion (DOI)
- T2: Tumor ≤ 2 cm with DOI > 5 and ≤ 10 mm or
- Tumor > 2 cm and ≤ 4 cm with DOI ≤ 10 mm
- T3: Tumor > 4 cm or DOI > 10 mm deep
- T4a: Moderately advanced local disease. Lip: through cortical bone, involvement of inferior alveolar nerve, floor of mouth, or skin of face. Oral cavity: invades adjacent structures only (eg, through cortical bone of the mandible/maxilla, or involves the maxillary sinus or skin of face). Superficial erosion of bone/tooth socket (alone) by a gingival primary is not sufficient to classify a tumor as T4.
- T4b: Very advanced local disease. Tumor involves the masticator space, pterygoid plates, or skull base and/or encases the carotid artery.

Clinical Regional Lymph Node (N) Staging for Oral Cavity

- Nx: regional lymph nodes cannot be assessed
- N0: no regional lymph node metastasis
- N1: metastasis in a single ipsilateral node measuring ≤ 3 cm and no extranodal extension [ENE(-)]
- N2a: metastasis in a single ipsilateral node > 3 and ≤ 6 cm and ENE(−)
- N2b: metastasis in multiple ipsilateral nodes, none > 6 cm and ENE(−)

Table 43-1 Prognostic Groups According to TNM Categories for Oral Cavity, AJCC 8th Edition Staging

	N Category			
T Category	*N0*	*N1*	*N2a-c*	*N3a,b*
T0	I	III	IVA	IVB
T1	II	III	IVA	IVB
T2	III	III	IVA	IVB
T3	IVA	IVA	IVA	IVB
T4	IVB	IVB	IVB	IVB

- N2c: metastases in bilateral or contralateral nodes, none > 6 cm and ENE(−)
- N3a: metastasis larger than 6 cm in one or more nodes and ENE(−)
- N3b: metastasis in any node and clinically overt ENE(+)

Pathologic Regional Lymph Node (pN) Staging for Oral Cavity

- Nx: Regional lymph nodes cannot be assessed.
- N0: No regional lymph node metastasis.
- N1: Metastasis in a single ipsilateral lymph node, ≤ 3 cm and ENE(−).
- N2a: Metastasis in a single ipsilateral, ≤ 3 cm and ENE(+); or a single ipsilateral lymph node > 3 cm and ≤ 6 cm without ENE.
- N2b: Metastasis in multiple ipsilateral lymph nodes, none larger than 6 cm and ENE (−).
- N2c: Metastasis in bilateral or contralateral lymph nodes, none > 6 cm and ENE (−).
- N3a: Metastasis in a lymph node larger than 6 cm and ENE (−).
- N3b: Metastasis in a single ipsilateral node larger than 3 cm and ENE(+); or metastasis in multiple ipsilateral, contralateral, or bilateral lymph nodes, any with ENE(+); or a single contralateral node of any size and ENE(+).

Distant Metastasis (M) for Oral Cavity

- Mx: distant metastasis cannot be assessed
- cM0: no distant metastasis
- cM1: distant metastasis
- pM1: distant metastasis, microscopically confirmed

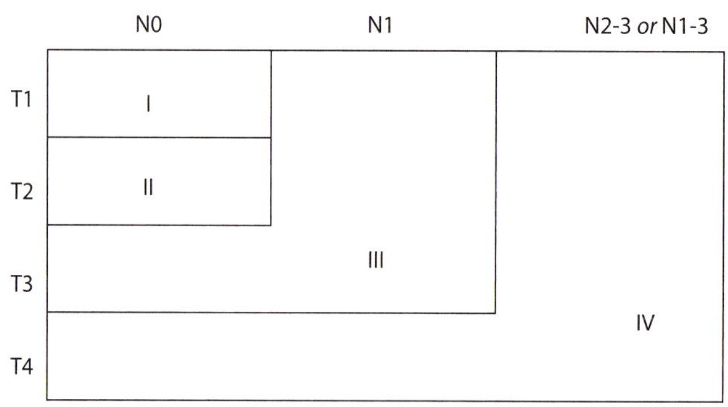

Figure 43-2 TNM staging for the oral cavity. Roman numerals indicate stage.

Evaluation and Treatment of Carcinoma of the Oral Cavity

Signs and Symptoms

- Early signs and symptoms may include a nodule, ulcerative lesion of the lip or mucosa, odynophagia, dysphagia, otalgia, and trismus.
- Cranial nerve dysfunction (eg, lower teeth numbness from invasion of the inferior alveolar nerve), severe dysphagia, unintentional weight loss, and hemoptysis are observed in more advanced disease.
- The presence of positive lymph nodes decreases the chance of cure by 50%.

Diagnostic and Imaging Studies

- Malignancy is confirmed by histologic evaluation of a tissue biopsy from the primary site and/or cytologic evaluation of a fine-needle aspirate from an enlarged lymph node.
- A computed tomography (CT) scan or contrast-enhanced magnetic resonance imaging (MRI) of the soft tissue of the neck defines the size and location of the primary tumor and involvement of surrounding anatomical structures and lymph nodes.
- Chest imaging by X-ray or CT is important for identifying distant metastases or a primary lung cancer.
- For patients who may require radiation therapy, the need for dental care should be evaluated by dental X-rays and consultation with a dentist. Any necessary dental work should be performed prior to radiation to reduce risk of osteoradionecrosis.
- For patients with stage III or IV disease, ^{18}F-fluorodeoxyglucose positron emission tomography (FDG-PET), usually combined with CT, surveys the whole body for sites of metabolically active tissue, helping to delineate regional nodal and distant metastases or identify unknown primary malignancy.
- FDG-PET may also aid in assessing response to treatment. At 3 to 4 months after the end of radiation, this imaging approach provides 97% to 100% predictive value.

Multidisciplinary Treatment Planning

Optimal care of patients with oral and pharyngeal cancer occurs within a multidisciplinary, collaborative setting, involving experts in the fields of head and neck surgery, radiation and medical oncology, radiology, and pathology. The management of aesthetic and functional outcomes requires close coordination with reconstructive surgeons, speech pathologists, dentists, oral surgeons, physical therapists, and maxillofacial prosthodontists.

General Principles of Treatment

Selecting an appropriate treatment regimen requires balancing multiple concerns: the extent and location of the tumor, clinical stage at diagnosis, and the overall medical condition of the patient.

T1-2, N0 Oral Cavity

- Surgical resection of the primary site with neck dissection (minimum levels 1-3) is the preferred treatment.
  - No positive nodes, or one positive micrometastatic node, and no pathologic adverse features (ENE, positive margins, close margins, perineural invasion [PNI], lymphovascular invasion [LVI]): consider observation with no further adjuvant treatment
  - Positive node(s) without adverse pathologic features: consider adjuvant RT
  - Positive margins or extranodal extension: consider adjuvant chemotherapy and RT

- Data showing the efficacy of sentinel lymph node biopsy for oral cavity cancer were established based on multiple European clinical trials and are being assessed with an ongoing trial in the United States (NRG HN006).
- Definitive RT can be considered in select cases in which the patient is deemed not a surgical candidate or refuses surgery.

T1-2, N1-3; T3-T4a, N0-3 Oral Cavity

- Surgical resection of the primary site with ipsilateral or bilateral (N2c or midline primary site) levels 1 to 3 neck dissection.
  - No adverse pathologic features: consider RT
  - Positive margins or extranodal extension: consider adjuvant chemotherapy and RT
- Radiation therapy can be considered for patients who are not surgical candidates or who refuse surgery.

M1 Disease

- Can consider locoregional control (surgical resection of primary site and neck dissection) followed by a combination of chemotherapy and radiation therapy
- Can consider pembrolizumab or pembrolizumab-chemotherapy for recurrent/metastatic disease (see KEYNOTE-048 below)

T4b, "unresectable" disease, or patient unfit for surgery

- Involvement of the following anatomic sites should be evaluated when considering resectability: carotid artery, prevertebral fascia, skull base, cervical vertebrae, dermal metastases, and the pterygoid muscles
- Concurrent chemotherapy and radiation therapy, or consider induction chemotherapy followed by RT

Radiotherapy and Chemoradiotherapy

- Intensity-modulated radiotherapy (IMRT) utilizes multiple beams of variable radiation intensity to deliver escalated doses to the tumor while decreasing doses to nearby organs at risk. Proton beam radiation allows for high precision targeting of tumors using pencil beam scanning.
- Oral cavity cancer is treated primarily with surgery unless the patient declines surgery, the patient is not a candidate for surgery, or the disease is deemed unresectable.
- Postoperative, combined chemoradiotherapy improves locoregional control, disease-free survival, and overall survival in patients with positive resection margins from the primary tumor or extranodal extension (ENE) of disease in one or more lymph nodes.
- The addition of chemotherapy to radiation can result in significant treatment-related toxicities that may not be well tolerated in patients with poor performance status and multiple comorbidities.

Specific Agents

- Induction chemotherapy with cisplatin and fluorouracil alone or in combination with docetaxel does not appear to enhance survival in locally advanced SCC of the head and neck compared to concomitant chemoradiation.
- For recurrent/metastatic head and neck squamous cell carcinoma, KEYNOTE-048 demonstrated that first-line pembrolizumab and pembrolizumab-chemotherapy had improved survival benefit compared to cetuximab-chemotherapy.
- Cetuximab is a monoclonal antibody against the ligand-binding site of the epidermal growth factor receptor (EGFR).

Management of the N0 Neck

In oral squamous cell carcinoma, occult cervical metastasis is common. While the rate depends on the primary tumor's site, depth of invasion, and size, many patients are at risk for regional failure. Current standards for managing N0 neck disease include:

- Expectant management (reserved for those with oral cavity cancers that are thin lesions, typically < 2 mm)
- For patients with greater than 20% risk of occult metastases, elective cervical lymphadenectomy is preferred over elective radiotherapy, as histopathologic examination of the dissected specimen allows identification of patients with no metastasis, micrometastasis, or a single node without ECS. In certain situations, these patients can potentially be spared radiation therapy.
- If a neck dissection is indicated, levels 1 to 3 should be performed at minimum. Involvement of level 4 with malignancy is approximately 10%.
- Sentinel lymph node mapping is alternate option to elective neck dissection that requires nuclear medicine support and surgical expertise. If the sentinel node is positive, then completion neck dissection is recommended.

Second Primary Malignancy in Head and Neck Squamous Cell Carcinoma

- The incidence of second primary tumors is approximately 5% to 10%, including both synchronous (found simultaneously with the initial head and neck cancer) and metachronous (develops after treatment) tumors.
- Approximately 50% of second primaries arise within the head and neck, while the lung is the next most common site (20%).
- Patient entry into formal programs for cessation of tobacco and alcohol consumption should be prioritized.

Distant Metastasis

- Distant metastasis (DM) develops in approximately 15% of patients with head and neck cancer, with about 5% to 7% present at diagnosis.
- Distant metastasis is correlated with the following factors: higher nodal stage, the number of lymphatic metastases, and advanced T stage.
- Patients with ENE, multiple positive lymph nodes, and locoregional recurrence have a significantly higher risk for developing DM.
- Screening for the presence of distant metastasis may include plain chest X-ray, chest CT scan, or PET/CT scan, depending on the presumed risk and treating center.
- For an isolated pulmonary metastasis, resection may be indicated.

Follow-up

- Most patients who die from head and neck cancer do so as a result of local or regional failure. Therefore, after definitive treatment, regular follow-up examinations are crucial. When recurrence is identified early, salvage therapy may be more effective.
- Follow-up intervals are not standardized. Recurrences usually present in the first 2 years after treatment, so a head and neck examination may be performed every 4 to 6 weeks during the first year and every 3 months during the second year. During years 3 to 5, follow-up may continue at 4- to 6-month intervals.
- Because the incidence of developing a second primary cancer remains constant at about 4% to 5% per year, routine tumor surveillance visits should be performed every 6 to 12 months for life.

- If the patient should become symptomatic at any time between visits, the surgeon should perform a thorough examination and order any ancillary tests and procedures that might be necessary.
- New pain or mass that persists is an indicator of tumor recurrence and should serve as a warning sign for the head and neck oncologist.
- Posttreatment surveillance imaging may be tailored to each patient's disease stage and risk of recurrence.

Carcinoma of the Oral Cavity

Carcinoma of the Oral Tongue

- The oral tongue is the most common site of oral cavity SCC (40%).
- Cancer of the tongue most often arises along the lateral borders.
- Risk factors include tobacco, alcohol, immunosuppression, and possibly poor oral hygiene.
- Depth of tumor invasion greater than 2 to 4 mm and perineural invasion are correlated with higher rates of regional metastasis, recurrence, and mortality.
- The incidence of SCC of the tongue in young patients has increased in the United States, from 4% in 1971 to 18% in 1993. In this young population, no clinical features or risk factors (age, substance abuse) have been clearly identified, and an increased genetic susceptibility to carcinogenesis has been postulated.
- Thorough oral cavity examinations by dentists, oral surgeons, otolaryngologists, and primary care physicians, especially in patients with risk factors, are critical for early detection.
- Erythroplakia (red, inflammatory lesion) is the most common presentation of early SCC.
- Late symptoms include tongue fixation, decreased tongue sensation, alteration in speech and swallowing, and cervical lymphadenopathy.
- Most lesions are amenable to biopsy in the office for tissue diagnosis.
- Regional metastases occur with primary nodal drainage to levels I-III (Figure 43-3).
- The incidence of nodal metastases depends on the size of the primary tumor and depth of invasion; 25% to 33% are clinically detectable, and 20% to 25% are occult.
- Tumors on the midline dorsum or ventral surface of tongue carry a greater risk of bilateral cervical lymph node metastases, and therefore bilateral neck dissection should be considered.

Oral Tongue Cancer Treatment

- For early T1-T2 lesions, partial glossectomy and reconstruction by primary closure, acellular dermal matrix, skin graft, or healing by secondary intention is preferred. For patients not suitable for surgery, external beam radiation with or without brachytherapy may be used.
- For extensive local disease, near-total or total glossectomy with free tissue transfer reconstruction may be necessary.
- Total glossectomy is associated with significant morbidity including impaired swallowing and gastrostomy dependence. Aspiration may be a chronic issue, and in some cases, total laryngectomy may be considered.
- For T4 tongue cancers, chemoradiation may be considered. However, bone involvement requires surgical resection.

Management of Mandibular Invasion in Oral Tongue Cancer

- Tumors extending superficially to the gingiva should be resected with periosteum as the deep margin.

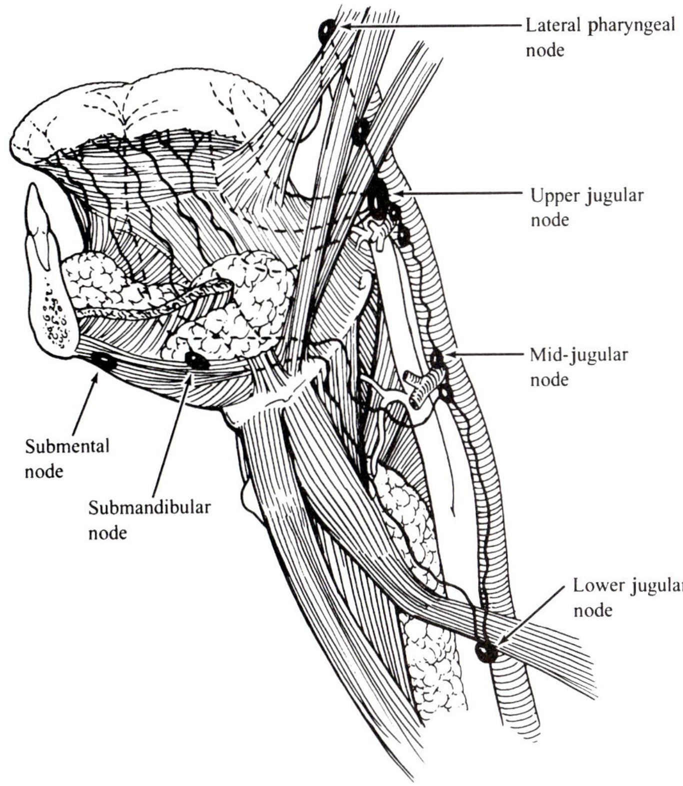

Figure 43-3 Lymphatic drainage of the oral tongue and oropharynx.

- Tumors involving periosteum require at least a marginal mandibulectomy, which may include a horizontal rim of alveolar ridge, or oblique resection of the upper and inner cortex.
- Patients with an edentulous mandible are more likely to require a segmental mandibulectomy because of decreased bone stock and increased risk for fracture with marginal mandibulectomy.
- For mandibular invasion into the medullary space of the bone, segmental mandibulectomy is indicated.

Management of the Neck in Oral Tongue Cancer

- The most frequent sites of metastasis for SCC of the oral tongue include the upper jugular nodes (73%), submandibular nodes (18%), middle jugular nodes (18%), and submental nodes (9%).
- Sentinel lymph node biopsy is accurate for staging the regional lymphatics in patients with T1-T2, N0 oral cavity cancers.
- For primary tumors with greater than 2 to 4 mm depth of invasion, elective treatment of the neck with either surgery or radiation is recommended.
- Selective neck dissection should include at least levels I-III (supraomohyoid neck dissection).

- For midline dorsum or ventral tongue cancers, bilateral neck dissections or sentinel node mapping should be performed.
- For patients with less than 2 to 4 mm depth of invasion or carcinoma in situ, observation is appropriate.

Oral Tongue Cancer Outcomes

- Five-year locoregional control rates of 91%
- Five-year survival rates
  (a) Stage I, II: 60% to 75%
  (b) Stage III, IV: 25% to 40%
  (c) Following salvage treatment for regional metastasis: 35% to 40%
- ECS reduces survival: 5-year disease-specific and overall survival rates for patients with pathologically negative necks (pN–) were 88% and 75%; for pN+/ECS– patients, 65% and 50%; and for pN+/ECS+ patients, 48% and 30%.

Carcinoma of the Lip

- The lip can be subdivided into cutaneous, vermilion (dry and wet), and mucosal subunits. The cutaneous and vermilion components are divided by the "red border."
- The mucosal lip is the second most common subsite of oral cavity SCC (16.5%).
- For the cutaneous lip, tumors occur on the lower lip in 95% of cases. BCC is more common on the upper lip than the lower lip, but SCC is still the most common cancer of the cutaneous upper lip.
- Risk factors include sunlight exposure, lack of pigmented layer, and tobacco smoking.
- Tends to be diagnosed early because of its prominent location.
- Symptoms of lip cancer:
  (a) Early: blistering, crusting, ulceration, or leukoplakia
  (b) Late: swelling, pain, and/or tenderness of the jaw, numbness or paresthesia of the lip and/or chin
- Regional metastasis occurs in approximately 10% of patients, usually later in the course of disease as compared to other oral cavity sites.
- Lymphatic drainage is primarily to submental (1A) and submandibular (1B) nodes.
- Bilateral metastasis is a concern for lesions near the midline.

Lip Cancer Treatment

- The goals of treatment, in order of importance, include: (1) complete eradication of tumor, (2) maintenance or restoration of oral competence, and (3) acceptable cosmesis.
- Small (T1, T2) lesions are treated with either surgery (preferred) or radiation only.
- Large (T3, T4) lesions usually require multimodal therapy.
- Clinically apparent lymphadenopathy or extensive disease calls for neck dissection.
- In reconstruction, proper alignment of the vermilion border is critical upon closure, which is done in four layers. The size of the defect/extent of resection determines the type of reconstruction procedure:
  (a) If less than one-fourth to one-third of the lip is involved: primary closure, facilitated by V-shaped "wedge" excision.
  (b) One-fourth to one-half: bilateral advancement or "lip-switch" flaps. The flap type should be Abbe for reconstructions close to the oral commissure and Estlander for those involving the oral commissure.
  (c) One-half to two-thirds: Karapandzic flap
  (d) Two-thirds to total: local flap reconstruction (Bernard-Burrow or Gillies fan flap) or free tissue transfer

- Postoperative radiation therapy is indicated in high-risk patients with locally advanced disease (T3-T4), perineural invasion at the primary site, positive margins, or lymph node metastases.
- Primary radiation is an option for patients unsuitable for or unwilling to undergo resection.

Lip Cancer Outcomes

- Local and regional control is greater than 90% in patients without cervical lymph node involvement.
- Five-year rates of survival (overall, 91%) based on AJCC 7th edition staging (as is all the survival control data in this chapter):
  (a) Stage I-II greater than 90% with surgery or radiation
  (b) Stage III-IV 30% to 70%
- Carcinoma of the upper lip or oral commissure is associated with 10% to 20% lower survival.
- Recurrent disease, mandibular invasion, and lymph node involvement carry a poor prognosis.

Carcinoma of the Floor of the Mouth (FOM)

- FOM is the third most common site for oral cavity tumors.
- Small lesions isolated to the FOM may be relatively asymptomatic, while more extensive lesions may invade the mandible or extend to the root of the tongue.
- Invasion of hypoglossal, lingual, or mental nerves results in decreased tongue mobility, alterations in speech and swallowing, and decreased sensation over the tongue, lip, or skin of the cheek.
- Tumor may track along the submandibular duct or obstruct its orifice, resulting in distension of the submandibular gland.
- Cervical metastasis is most frequently seen in the submandibular (64%), upper jugular (43%), and submental nodes (7%).
- Bilateral metastases may be seen for tumors approaching the midline.

FOM Cancer Treatment

- Management of the primary tumor, mandible involvement, and cervical lymphatics is similar to that described for oral tongue cancer.

FOM Cancer Outcomes

- Recurrence at the primary site (41%) is twice as common as failure in the neck (18.5%).
- Five-year survival rates for patients with cancer of the FOM:
  (a) Stage I: 64% to 80%
  (b) Stage II: 61% to 84%
  (c) Stage III: 28% to 68%
  (d) Stage IV: 6% to 36%

Carcinoma of the Retromolar Trigone

- The true incidence of RMT carcinoma is difficult to determine because tumors affecting the RMT often involve adjacent sites.
- A thin layer of mucosa and underlying soft tissue overlies the mandible, and bony involvement may develop early.
- Involvement of the inferior alveolar nerve (V3) may occur early due to close proximity to the mandibular foramen.

- At presentation, regional metastases are common: 10% to 20%.
- Lymphatic drainage is predominantly to the upper jugular lymph nodes (level II).

RMT Cancer Treatment

- For stage I or II tumors surgery is preferred to avoid the possibility of mandibular osteoradionecrosis with radiation treatment.
- Management of advanced lesions often requires a combination of surgery and radiation.
- If only the periosteum is involved or if there is minimal cortical erosion, marginal mandibulectomy may be possible.
- The majority of advanced tumors with bone invasion require composite resection. The approach may be transcervical after raising a soft-tissue flap over the bone, or translabial (lip-splitting incision) with a lateral mandibulotomy.
- Reconstruction of segmental mandibular defects typically requires free tissue transfer such as a fibula osteocutaneous free flap.
- Reconstruction using only a mandibular bar to span the bony defect is suboptimal owing to high rates of hardware infection and extrusion over time.
- Obturators may be necessary if the resection involves a significant portion of the palate.
- In patients with a significant risk of nodal disease, unilateral elective neck dissection (levels I-III) should be performed.

RMT Cancer Outcomes

- Locoregional control and disease-free survival are better with surgery and radiotherapy versus radiotherapy alone.
- Five-year locoregional control (following surgery and radiotherapy)
  (a) Stages I-III: 87%
  (b) Stage IV: 62%
  (c) Overall: 71%
- Five-year disease-specific survival (following surgery and radiotherapy)
  (a) Stages I-III: 83%
  (b) Stage IV: 61%
  (c) Overall: 69%

Carcinoma of the Alveolar Ridge Gingival Mucosa

- Gingival cancers constitute 10% of all malignancies in the oral cavity.
- Most commonly arise in edentulous areas or at the free margin of the gingiva of the lower alveolar ridge.
- Approximately 40% of patients will have invasion of the mandible or maxilla at the time of diagnosis. Superficial bone invasion does not constitute a T4 tumor stage.
- Open tooth sockets or small defects in the edentulous mandibular ridge provide ready access for tumor invasion into bone. Cancers of the upper alveolar ridge may extend through bone into the nasal cavity or maxillary sinus.
- Lymphatic drainage for alveolar ridge cancers is most often to level I (submandibular and submental) and level II (upper deep jugular nodes). Regional metastases are clinically detectable in 25% to 30% while occult metastases occur in 15%.

Gingival Cancer Treatment

- Small cancers of the alveolar ridge can be resected transorally. The defect may be closed with a local rotational flap from buccal mucosa (facial artery myomucosal flap), skin grafting, or healing by secondary intention.

- For larger tumors, especially those invading bone, partial maxillectomy (for lesions of the upper alveolar ridge) or mandibulectomy (for those of the lower ridge) is often required.
- Management of mandibular invasion requires reconstruction similar to that described for other oral cavity cancer.
- Larger defects involving the maxillary sinus can be reconstructed with an obturator or dental prosthesis, temporalis muscle flap, or free tissue transfer.
- Radiation therapy as primary modality is not recommended because of the close proximity of tumor to the underlying bone, unless the patient is an unsuitable operative candidate.

Management of the Neck in Gingival Cancer

- Therapeutic, comprehensive treatment of the neck is indicated in all patients who have clinically positive neck disease, and recommended in those with advanced T stage, radiologic or histologic evidence of mandibular invasion, and/or decreased tumor differentiation, even if the primary cancer is early stage.
- For patients with extensive nodal disease, perineural invasion, lymphovascular invasion, or inadequate margins of resection, adjuvant postoperative radiation or chemoradiation is recommended.

Gingival Cancer Outcomes

- Local and regional control is 70% to 80% with 5-year survival rates of 50% to 65%.
- The presence of mandibular cortical invasion decreases 5-year survival from 85% to 68%.
- Cervical metastases also decrease 5-year survival (86% versus 59%).

Carcinoma of the Hard Palate

- Only half of all tumors are SCCs; minor salivary gland tumors are also common.
- Can be confused with necrotizing sialometaplasia, a benign mucosal inflammatory lesion.
- Most carcinomas manifest as a granular superficial ulceration of the hard palate; the mucoperiosteum provides a barrier to tumor spread.
- In more advanced lesions, tumor may extend through the periosteum of bone into adjacent regions of the oral cavity, such as the paranasal sinuses and floor of the nose. This often occurs via the incisive foramen anteriorly and the greater and lesser palatine foramina posteriorly.
- Cervical nodal metastases are present at diagnosis in 10% to 25%.
- Lymph node basins include the retropharyngeal, upper jugular, and submandibular.
- Careful assessment of the trigeminal nerve is crucial, and perineural invasion to the Gasserian ganglion should be evaluated with MRI.

Hard Palate Cancer Treatment

- Standard initial treatment is wide local excision to obtain negative surgical margins. Radiation is generally reserved for adjuvant treatment.
- Postoperative radiotherapy is recommended in advanced disease or in cancers with adverse pathologic features mentioned previously to decrease local and regional recurrence.
- For tumors that partially erode bone, infrastructure maxillectomy may be necessary.
- For extensive involvement of the adjacent bony and soft tissue structures, a total maxillectomy, with or without orbital exenteration, or resection of cheek skin may be required.
- Elective treatment of the neck is generally not performed because of the low rate of occult metastases in early-stage disease.

Palatal Reconstruction

- For small and/or superficial defects of the hard palate, acellular dermal grafting or healing by secondary intention may be sufficient.
- Larger hard palate or infrastructure maxillectomy defects are commonly restored using an obturator with or without a skin graft, or using local flap reconstruction. The obturator is fabricated from a synthetic polymer and provides oronasal separation, which can yield normal speech and swallowing function.
- Obturators allow direct visualization of the surrounding primary site for tumor surveillance. Adjustments are needed to fit the prosthesis to avoid leakage of air or oral intake into the sinonasal cavity.
- Composite defects may require reconstruction with free tissue transfer to reconstruct bone and soft tissue defects. When bone is needed, flaps are derived from fibula, scapular, or iliac crest; in other cases, flaps are created from the radius.

Palatal Cancer Outcomes

- Local recurrence rate is 53% while regional recurrence rate is 30%.
- Five-year survival: 44% to 75%.

Carcinoma of the Buccal Mucosa

- In the United States, less than 10% of all oral cavity cancer occurs at this site. A high incidence of buccal carcinoma in India is attributed at least in part to the prevalent practice of chewing "pan," a combination of betel nut, lime, and tobacco.
- Unusual features of buccal SCC are that it more often arises from preexisting leukoplakia and more frequently presents as verrucous carcinoma, a more indolent variant, compared to other locations in the oral cavity.
- The buccinator muscle and buccal fat pad are easily invaded and provide little or no barrier to tumor spread.
- Invasion of the mandible, hard palate, maxillary sinus, cheek skin, or pterygoid muscles may occur with advanced disease.
- Advanced tumor thickness correlates with increased morbidity and mortality.
- Nodal metastases are most common in the buccinator, submental, and submandibular lymph nodes.

Buccal Carcinoma Treatment

- While early-stage cancers can be managed with radiation alone, surgical resection is preferred.
- Small, early-stage lesions can be resected transorally, while more extensive lesions may require a cheek flap approach, marginal or segmental mandibulectomy, resection of cheek skin, or partial maxillectomy.
- Reconstructive options for early-stage lesions include healing by secondary intention or closure with acellular dermal grafts, skin grafts, mucosal advancement flaps, or buccal fat pad if not involved.
- For more extensive defects, a regional flap (eg, pectoralis major, temporalis muscle) or free tissue transfer (eg, radial forearm, fibula, scapula) may be necessary.
- For advanced lesions with an N0 neck, elective supraomohyoid neck dissection is recommended.
- Adjuvant therapy (radiation or chemoradiation) is recommended for patients with advanced-stage and/or adverse pathologic features mentioned earlier.

Buccal Carcinoma Outcomes

- Locoregional recurrence ranges from 43% to 80%.
- Five-year survival
  - (a) Stage I: 78%
  - (b) Stage II: 66%
  - (c) Stage III: 62%
  - (d) Stage IV: 50%

Bibliography

Bernier J, Domenge C, Ozsahin M, et al. Postoperative irradiation with or without concomitant chemotherapy for head and neck cancer. *N Engl J Med*. 2004;350:1945-1962.

Burtness B, Harrington KJ, Greile R, et al. Pembrolizumab alone or with chemotherapy versus cetuximab with chemotherapy for recurrent or metastatic squamous cell carcinoma of the head and neck (KEYNOTE-048): a randomized, open-label phase 3 study. *The Lancet*. 2019; 394:1915-1928.

www.wcrf.org. World Cancer Research Fund International.

Lorch JH, Golou-beva O, Haddad RI, et al. TAX 324 Study Group. *Lancet Oncol*. 2011;12:153-159.

Yao M, Graham MM, Hoffman HT, et al. The role of post-radiation therapy FDG PET in prediction of necessity for post radiation therapy neck dissection in locally advanced head and neck squamous cell carcinoma. *Int J Radiat Oncol Biol Phys*. 2004;59:1001-1010.

Questions

1. Elective neck dissection for a T2N0M0 cancer of the midline floor of mouth should include which neck levels?

   A. Unilateral levels I, II, III

   B. Bilateral levels II, III, IV

   C. Bilateral level I

   D. Unilateral levels II, III, IV

   E. Bilateral levels I, II, III

2. Common risk factors for cancer of the oral tongue include tobacco and alcohol. Which additional factor is associated with it?

   A. Human papillomavirus 6 and 11

   B. Epstein-Barr virus

   C. Ingestion of smoked fish

   D. Betel nut

   E. Human papillomavirus 16 and 18

3. A patient presents with a 2 cm floor of right lateral floor of mouth lesion. PET-CT demonstrates an FDG-avid, 2 cm lymph node in right level 1B. In addition to surgical excision of the primary site, which neck dissection should be performed?
   A. Right supraomohyoid neck dissection
   B. Right levels 2 to 4 neck dissection
   C. Bilateral supraomohyoid neck dissection
   D. Bilateral levels 2 to 4 neck dissection
   E. Left supraomohyoid neck dissection

4. What is the clinical staging of a 4 cm tumor involving the oral tongue and floor of mouth with a 3 cm level 2 lymph node that is fixed and immobile?
   A. T3N1
   B. T2N2a
   C. T2N3b
   D. T2N3a
   E. T3N3b

5. The most common site of oral cavity cancer is
   A. Mucosal lip
   B. Oral tongue
   C. Retromolar trigone
   D. Buccal mucosa
   E. Gingiva

Chapter 44
Tumors of the Oropharynx

Tumors of the Oropharynx

In this chapter we review benign and malignant tumors of the oropharynx. We first cover the anatomy of the oropharynx, which will lay the framework for understanding the types of tumors or nontumor conditions that can arise in the anatomic site.

Anatomy

The oropharynx begins anteriorly at the circumvallate papillae and anterior tonsillar pillars and extends posteriorly to include the soft palate, tonsillar fossa, posterior pharyngeal wall, and the base of the tongue. It extends from the junction of the hard and soft palate superiorly to the hyoid bone and vallecula inferiorly. The oropharynx is divided into four anatomic subsites:

- Soft palate and uvula
- Palatine tonsil/tonsillar fossa
- Posterior pharyngeal wall
- Base of tongue

Soft Palate

- Muscles
  (a) Palatoglossus (anterior pillar): approximates palate to tongue and narrows oropharyngeal opening
  (b) Palatopharyngeus (posterior pillar): raises larynx and pharynx, closing oropharynx
  (c) Musculus uvulae: shortens uvula
  (d) Levator veli palatini: raises soft palate to contact posterior pharyngeal wall
  (e) Tensor veli palatini: pulls soft palate laterally giving rigidity to palate; opens Eustachian tube (originates on its cartilage)
- Motor innervation
  (a) CN V3 motor division > pharyngeal plexus > tensor veli palatini
  (b) CN X > pharyngeal plexus > remainder of palatal muscles
- Sensory innervation: CNs V2, IX, X
- Blood supply: (see Hard Palate under Oral Cavity in Chapter 43)

Palatine Tonsils

- Consist of lymphoid tissue (contiguous with that of the lingual tonsils) containing germinal centers surrounding 6 to 20 epithelium-lined crypts.
- Lies between palatoglossus muscle anteriorly and palatopharyngeus muscle posteriorly.
- From medial to lateral, the layers of the tonsillar fossa are the pharyngobasilar fascia, superior constrictor muscle, and buccopharyngeal fascia.
- Development
  - Form from the epithelial lining of the second pharyngeal pouch.
  - Lymphatic cells infiltrate during the 16th week of gestation.
- Sensory innervation: V2 (lesser palatine nerve via greater palatine canal > lesser palatine foramen), IX (tonsillar branches)
- Blood Supply
  - Arterial:
  - Venous: lingual and pharyngeal veins

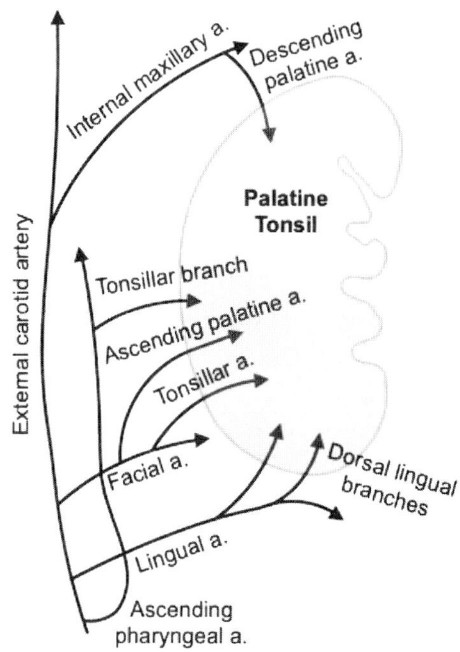

- Immunology
  - Part of the mucosal-associated lymphoid tissues (MALT). Antigens within the tonsil are presented to B cells and T-helper cells. Activated B cells proliferate and differentiate to produce antibodies (all Ig types) and memory B cells.
  - Tonsillar tissues' immunologic function remains controversial.
  - Microbes commonly present in the adult mouth and oropharynx:
    - Bacteria: Staphylococci (first oral microbe in neonate; from skin contamination), nonhemolytic streptococci, lactobacilli, *Actinomyces, Neisseria, Bacteroides,* Spirochetes (associated with gingivitis)
    - Viruses: myxovirus, adenovirus, picornavirus, coronaviruses, human papillomavirus (HPV; some strains cause oral cancer)

Posterior Oropharyngeal Wall

- Layers: mucosa > submucosa > pharyngobasilar fascia > muscle > buccopharyngeal fascia
- Pharyngeal muscles (origins and insertions):
  (a) Pharyngeal constrictors (all insert into the median pharyngeal raphe)
    i. Superior constrictor: medial pterygoid plate, mandible, and base of tongue
    ii. Middle constrictor: originates on the hyoid bone and stylohyoid ligament
    iii. Inferior constrictor: origin is on the oblique line of thyroid cartilage
  (b) Pharyngeal and laryngeal elevators (shorten pharynx)
    i. Salpingopharyngeus: temporal bone and Eustachian tube; merges with the palatopharyngeus muscle
    ii. Stylopharyngeus: styloid process; merges with palatopharyngeus muscle
    iii. Stylohyoid: styloid process to hyoid bone
- Posterior oropharyngeal wall includes: superior constrictor, superior aspect of middle constrictor
- Motor innervation
  (a) CN IX > stylopharyngeus
  (b) CN X > pharyngeal plexus > remainder of pharyngeal muscles
- Sensory innervation: CN IX
- Passavant ridge: soft tissue projection that becomes endoscopically visible upon constriction of the superior end of the superior constrictor during swallowing
- Lateral pharyngeal bands: lymphoid tissue just behind the posterior tonsillar pillars

Base of Tongue

- Anteriorly begins at circumvallate papillae. Extends laterally to glossotonsillar sulcus. Substantial lymphatic tissue.
- Muscles (see tongue under oral cavity in Chapter 43)
- Motor innervation: CN XII
- Sensory innervation:
  - Touch and gag (visceral afferent), as well as taste sensations: CN IX > nucleus solitarius
  - Taste sensation arises from the circumvallate papillae and mucosa of the epiglottis and vallecula
- Blood supply: lingual artery and vein

Noncancerous Lesions and Disorders of the Oropharynx

Lesions and Disorders of the Soft Palate

- Inflammatory conditions of the oral cavity and have overlap with the oropharynx: aphthous ulcers, leukoplakia, erythroplakia, thrush.
- Cleft palate may also affect the soft palate, leading to eustachian tube disorder (recurrent otitis media and conductive hearing loss) because of failure of the tensor veli palatini to open the eustachian tubes on swallowing.
- Congenital elongation of the uvula.
- Squamous papilloma: small, white or pink, cauliflower-like benign growth on the mucosa caused by low-risk strains of HPV (usually 6 and 11).

- Minor salivary gland tumor: more likely to be malignant than tumors of the major salivary glands. Presenting symptoms include trismus, dysphagia, and dysphonia. Benignancy distinguished by the same features as for major gland tumors.
- Uvular angioedema or angioneurotic edema (Quincke disease): severe, acute swelling of the uvula. Often in association with acute bacterial tonsillitis, it can also result from trauma (heroic snoring, burn from hot food or beverage), allergy, angiotensin-converting enzyme (ACE) inhibitors, or inherited C1 esterase deficiency. ACE inhibitor-induced angioedema is more common in those of African descent and can occur at any time following initiation of therapy. Severe swelling may be preceded by sentinel swelling. Usually treated with antihistamines and/or corticosteroids; in extreme cases, tracheotomy may be required.

Lesions and Disorders of the Palatine Tonsils

- Acute tonsillitis
- Tonsilloliths: calcifications in the tonsillar crypt; can cause halitosis, irritable cough, and a foreign body sensation
- Peritonsillar abscess
- Mononucleosis
- Tumor in the parapharyngeal space: most often extensions of benign parotid tumors or minor salivary glands (prestyloid space). May also arise from nerves (vagal schwannomas, sympathetic trunk schwannomas, and vagal paragangliomas) or lymphovasculature (vascular malformation, lymphoma) in the poststyloid space. Usually have no symptoms other than an intraoral mass. Rapid growth, extension beyond the parapharyngeal space, and/or pain suggest malignancy.

Lesions and Disorders of the Tongue Base

- Lingual tonsillar hypertrophy: often associated with sleep-disordered breathing. Can also cause difficult intubation or endoscopy, or more rarely, dysphagia or upper airway obstruction. Associated with previous adenotonsillectomy, laryngopharyngeal reflux, obesity, and medications such as phenytoin.
- Lingual tonsillitis.
- Lingual thyroid (failure of descent).
- Thyroglossal duct cyst: small, soft mass at the front midline of the neck. Formed from cells and tissues remaining after the formation of the thyroid gland during embryonic development.
- Benign vallecular cysts: accumulation of fluid in the lymphoid tissue between the base of the tongue and the epiglottis. Both types of cysts may require removal to alleviate difficulty swallowing or breathing.
- Minor salivary gland tumors (usually malignant).

Lesions and Disorders of the Oropharyngeal Walls

- Inflammation of the lateral pharyngeal bands: usually acute, associated with infection. When chronic, may be associated with laryngopharyngeal reflux.
- Cobble-stoning of posterior wall: inflammation of lymphoid tissue from persistent allergic rhinitis and postnasal drip.
- Eagle syndrome: rare type of atypical facial pain characterized by sharp pain upon swallowing, moving the jaw, or turning the neck. Results from elongation (defined at $\geq$ 3 cm) or calcification of the styloid process.

Malignancy of the Oropharynx

The global incidence of head and neck cancer (HNC) has increased over time despite a decrease in tobacco use, due to a rise in the incidence of human papillomavirus (HPV)-related tumors of the oropharynx. It is estimated that by 2030, approximately 50% of all HNCs will be HPV-related tumors of the oropharynx.

- Squamous cell carcinomas (SCCs) account for 90% of malignant neoplasms arising within the oropharynx.
- The next most common malignancy is lymphoma, primarily of the palatine tonsils and base of the tongue, due to abundant lymphoid tissue as part of Waldeyer ring.
- Minor salivary gland malignancies.
- Multiple primary tumors may be encountered.

Etiology

- Chronic tobacco and alcohol use are the major etiologic factors for HPV– oropharyngeal SCC (OPSCC).
- HPV-related oropharyngeal squamous cell carcinoma (HPV+ OPSCC) accounts for greater than 70% of oropharyngeal carcinoma in the United States.
- Oral HPV infection is associated with a higher number of any sex and oral sex partners and host immunosuppression. Tobacco increases the risk of persistent oral HPV infection.
- HPV causes malignancy by integration of genes for oncoproteins E6 and E7 into host DNA; these proteins inactivate tumor suppressors p53 and Rb, respectively.
- Worldwide, over 90% of HPV+ OPSCC are caused by high-risk HPV16.
- Protein p16 expression is upregulated in HPV+ OPSCC, and is a surrogate marker of HPV, not a direct biomarker.
- Initially, HPV+ OPSCC was most frequently seen in middle-aged, white males. However, its prevalence is increasing over time across all genders and races.
- HPV vaccines have the potential to eradicate HPV-associated malignancy, so widespread adoption has become a major public health goal.
- Genetic causes of oropharyngeal cancers include Li-Fraumeni syndrome and Fanconi anemia, both of which are rare.

Evaluation of Oropharyngeal Cancer

Presentation

- Early signs and symptoms may include odynophagia, dysphagia, foreign body sensation, oral bleeding, referred otalgia, or a neck mass.
- Cancers of the oropharynx can become quite large before the patient develops symptoms, so these tumors may present at an advanced stage. Commonly extends to adjacent sites and may be misclassified.
- Cervical lymph node metastasis, most commonly along the jugular chain (levels II-IV), is present in greater than 50% of all patients. The retropharyngeal nodes are another potential site of lymph node metastasis.
- HPV+ OPSCC often presents with cervical lymphadenopathy and either a small or inapparent primary tumor.
- A hallmark of HPV+ OPSCC is the appearance of cystic neck lymph nodes, which should not be mistaken for a branchial cleft cyst. Cystic neck lymph nodes may also represent HPV-negative head and neck cancers and papillary thyroid cancer.

Diagnostic and Imaging Studies

- Malignancy is confirmed by histologic evaluation of a tissue biopsy from the primary site and/or cytologic evaluation of a fine-needle aspirate from an enlarged lymph node.
- p16 immunohistochemistry (IHC) should be performed to determine if the tumor is associated with HPV in regions with a high attributable fraction (AF) of HPV+ OPSCC. In regions with lower AF, direct HPV testing is recommended to determine that HPV is etiologically responsible.
- For biopsy specimens from the oropharynx, p16 IHC may be sufficient for diagnosis, but additional HPV-specific testing should be done if considering clinical trials or in regions with low AF.
- For biopsy specimens from a cervical metastasis in the context of an unknown primary, both p16 IHC and HPV-specific testing are required for diagnosis of HPV+ OPSCC.
- The histopathology of HPV+ OPSCC tends to be nonkeratinizing and basaloid, while that of HPV- OPSCC is frequently keratinizing.
- A computed tomography (CT) scan or contrast-enhanced magnetic resonance imaging (MRI) of the soft tissue of the neck defines the size and location of the primary tumor and involvement of surrounding anatomical structures and lymph nodes.
- MRI may be more helpful for tumors that are endophytic/invasive.
- Chest CT is important for identifying distant metastases or a primary lung cancer.
- ^{18}F-fluorodeoxyglucose positron emission tomography (FDG-PET) is helpful to evaluate for distant metastases in locoregionally advanced cancer, to identify an unknown primary malignancy, and for patients planned for definitive radiation (RT).
- FDG-PET may also aid in assessing response to treatment. At 3 to 4 months after the end of RT, this imaging approach provides 97% to 100% predictive value.

Staging of Oropharyngeal Cancer

Staging for HPV+ and HPV− OPSCC is distinct.

Table 44-1 Primary Tumor (T) for HPV+ and HPV− Oropharyngeal Cancer, 8th Edition AJCC

T	*HPV+ OPSCC*	*HPV− OPSCC*
Tx	primary tumor cannot be assessed	
T0	no evidence of primary tumor	N/A
Tis	N/A	carcinoma in situ
T1	tumor size < 2 cm	
T2	tumor size 2-4 cm	
T3	tumor size > 4 cm or extension to lingual epiglottis	
T4a	T4a and T4b combined as T4	invasion of larynx, deep/extrinsic tongue muscles, medial pterygoid muscle, hard palate or mandible
T4b		invasion of lateral pterygoid muscle, pterygoid plates, nasopharynx or skull base; encasement of carotid artery

N/A: not applicable

Table 44-2 Regional Lymph Node (N) for HPV+ Oropharyngeal Cancer, 8th Edition AJCC

N	*Clinical (cN)*	*Pathological (pN)*
Nx	lymph nodes not assessed	
N0	no lymph node metastasis	
N1	metastasis in ≥ 1 lymph node, ipsilateral, all ≤ 6 cm	metastasis in ≤ 4 lymph nodes
N2	metastasis in contralateral or bilateral lymph nodes, all ≤ 6 cm	metastasis in > 4 lymph nodes
N3	metastasis in lymph node > 6 cm	N/A

N/A: not applicable

Table 44-3 Regional Lymph Node (N) for HPV− Oropharyngeal Cancer, 8th Edition AJCC

N	*Clinical (cN)*	*Pathological (pN)*
Nx	lymph nodes not be assessed	
N0	no lymph node metastasis	
N1	metastasis in 1 lymph node, ipsilateral, ≤ 3 cm, no extranodal extension (ENE−)	
N2a	metastasis in 1 lymph node, ipsilateral, ≥ 3 cm and ≤ 6 cm, and ENE−	cN1 with pathologically positive ENE (pENE+) or cN2a
N2b	metastasis in > 1 lymph node, ipsilateral, all ≤ 6 cm, and ENE−	
N2c	metastases in bilateral or contralateral lymph node(s), all ≤ 6 cm, and ENE−	
N3a	metastasis in lymph node > 6 cm and ENE−	
N3b	any ENE+	cN2-3 with pENE+

Table 44-4 Prognostic Groups (Stages I-IV) according to T, Clinical N, and M Categories for HPV+ Oropharyngeal Cancer, 8th Edition AJCC*

T Category	*cN Category*			
	N0	*N1*	*N2*	*N3*
T0	N/A	I	II	III
T1	I	I	II	III
T2	I	I	II	III
T3	II	II	II	III
T4	III	III	III	III

*Any M1 is stage IV.

Table 44-5 Prognostic Groups (Stages I-IV) according to T, Pathologic N, and M Categories for HPV+ Oropharyngeal Cancer, 8th Edition AJCC

T Category	*pN Category*		
	N0	*N1*	*N2*
T0	N/A	I	II
T1	I	I	II
T2	I	I	II
T3	II	II	III
T4	II	II	III

Primary Treatment of Oropharyngeal Cancer

- Early-stage OPSCC with small primary tumors (cT1-2) without nodal disease or with a single ≤ 3cm positive cervical lymph node can be treated with primary site surgery and neck dissection or definitive RT.
- Locally advanced, resectable OPSCC with large primary tumors (cT3-4) or those with multiple, contralateral, or large positive cervical lymph nodes may be treated with upfront surgery or definitive chemoradiation (CRT).
- Both surgery and RT must address the cervical nodes because the risk of occult metastasis from oropharyngeal tumors is high.
- For locally advanced, unresectable OPSCC, palliative treatment with a combination of RT and/or chemotherapy and/or immunotherapy is indicated.
- Treatment is determined in a multidisciplinary fashion, including head and neck surgeons, radiation oncology, medical oncology, and speech-language pathology.
- Patient selection to choose two rather than three treatment modalities is recommended as the morbidities are multiplicative rather than additive.

Surgery for OPSCC

- Transoral surgical procedures are preferred over open surgery, given decreased morbidity and postoperative complications. Transoral procedures include transoral robotic surgery (TORS), transoral laser microsurgery, or standard headlight oropharyngectomy.

Table 44-6 Prognostic Groups (Stages I-IV) according to TNM Categories for HPV- Oropharyngeal Cancer, 8th Edition AJCC*

T Category	*N Category*			
	N0	*N1*	*N2a-c*	*N3a,b*
T1	I	III	IVA	IVB
T2	II	III	IVA	IVB
T3	III	III	IVA	IVB
T4a	IVA	IVA	IVA	IVB
T4b	IVB	IVB	IVB	IVB

*Any M1 is stage IVC

- Open surgery with mandibulotomy or pharyngotomy is generally reserved for salvage cases.
- Elective neck dissection, for cN0, or selective neck dissection should be performed, given the high risk of occult metastasis. The external carotid artery or its branches, the ipsilateral lingual, facial, and ascending pharyngeal arteries should be ligated to decrease the risk of life-threatening postoperative hemorrhage.
- Adverse pathological features of pT3-4, greater than 1 positive cervical lymph node, positive nodal disease in levels IV or V, perineural invasion, or lymphovascular invasion are indications for adjuvant RT.
- Extranodal extension and positive margins (not amenable to re-resection) are indications for adjuvant CRT.
- Contraindications for surgery include invasion of the pterygoid process, nasopharynx, skull base, or encasement of the carotid artery. Extensive tongue base involvement that crosses midline is also a contraindication, given significant functional impairment.
- Salvage neck dissection may be performed for clinically detectable residual disease following treatment. HPV+ neck disease may take longer to resolve, even after a complete response to primary RT, so the optimal time for salvage neck dissection is controversial.
- Determination of candidacy of primary surgical therapy is based upon access (eg, tori, mouth opening, bony anatomy), footprint of tumor (lateralized, not involving the soft palate or deep into the tongue musculature), and favorable neck (no gross ENE or high number of lymph nodes which are predictive of ENE).
- *Transoral Robotic Surgery (TORS):* TORS decreases morbidity associated with surgery and has lower rates of positive margins in comparison to other surgical techniques for oropharynx tumors.
- Contraindications to TORS include poor mouth opening and a medialized carotid artery for tonsil primaries.

HPV+ OPSCC

- Survival outcomes for HPV+ OPSCC are equivalent between surgery and definitive RT or CRT for early tumors and locally advanced tumors, respectively.
- For locally advanced tumors, definitive CRT is generally the preferred treatment given morbidity associated with surgery.
- Patients with clinically obvious extranodal extension should be treated with definitive CRT to limit the morbidity associated with trimodality therapy.

HPV− OPSCC

- Overall survival is higher for both early and locally advanced HPV− OPSCC treated with surgery in comparison to definitive RT or CRT, respectively.
- Surgery, when feasible, is the preferred treatment for HPV− OPSCC.

Outcomes of Oropharyngeal Cancer

- HPV+ OPSCC has a significantly better prognosis than HPV− OPSCC.
- Patients with HPV+ OPSCC with greater than 10 pack-year history of smoking have intermediate prognoses, between those for HPV+ and HPV− OPSCC.

HPV+ OPSCC

- Five-year overall survival based on AJCC 8th edition staging:
  - Stage I: 96%
  - Stage II: 78%
  - Stage III: 67%

HPV– OPSCC

- Five-year overall survival based on AJCC 8th edition staging:
  - Stage I-II: 63%
  - Stage III: 58%
  - Stage IV: 35%

Carcinoma of the Soft Palate

- Comprises less than 2% of all mucosal head and neck cancers.
- Occurs most frequently on the oral/anterior surface of the soft palate. More readily visible and symptomatic earlier than those in other oropharyngeal subsites.
- Relatively high likelihood of additional primary tumors; rates of second primary tumors and metachronous tumors are ~13% and ~26%, respectively.
- Cancer may appear as an area of leukoplakia, erythroplakia, or raised lesion.
- Primary tumors often extend to the tonsil, tonsillar pillars, nasopharynx, or hard palate.
- Cervical metastasis is clinically present in up to 50% of patients, with bilateral metastases in 5% to 15%. The propensity for regional metastasis is high (> 40%) even for small midline lesions.
- For the soft palate, tumor thickness is correlated with regional metastasis and survival.
- Lymphatic spread most commonly affects the upper jugular nodes (level II), as well as levels III, IV, and retropharyngeal nodes.

Soft Palate Cancer Treatment

- Small primary tumors can be treated surgically by a transoral approach or by RT.
- Larger primary tumors are more commonly treated with RT or CRT to preserve tissue and prevent velopharyngeal insufficiency.
- Both sides of the neck should be surgically dissected and/or treated with RT in more advanced cases, given the increased risk for bilateral cervical lymph node metastases.
- Reconstruction of the soft palate is difficult from a functional standpoint.
- For small defects, reconstruction may not be required or may be performed using local flaps.
- Larger defects are best reconstructed by free tissue transfer with thin, pliable soft tissue such as a radial forearm flap.

Carcinoma of the Tonsil and Tonsillar Pillars

- Most common site for carcinoma of the oropharynx.
- Asymptomatic during early stages; later symptoms include dysphagia, odynophagia, otalgia, neck mass, and/or trismus.
- Invasion of adjacent structures is common; these include the soft palate, retromolar trigone, tongue base, mandible, and pterygoid muscles.
- Clinically positive lymphadenopathy ranges from 66% to 76%.
- Lymphatic drainage is primarily to ipsilateral levels II-IV and the retropharyngeal lymph nodes. Low risk of contralateral lymph node involvement (5%-10%) unless tumor extends toward midline.

Tonsillar Cancer Treatment

- Tumor exposure is the main challenge to surgical resection. Access to the tonsil and lateral oropharynx is facilitated using robotics, which has increased the use of transoral excision for early-stage cancers.

- Surgery for advanced tumors or extensive bony invasion (for those that are treatment failures, not candidates for CRT or for HPV– OPSCC) includes:
  - Anterior mandibulotomy and mandibular swing: generally require free tissue transfer for reconstruction
  - Composite resection of primary tumor and posterior mandible for large tumors involving multiple subsites with mandibular invasion.

Reconstruction Following Tonsillar Tumor Resection

- Small defects may be restored by primary closure, healing by secondary intention, or transfer of the buccal fat pad to ensure safe covering of the internal carotid artery.
- For closure of large mucosal defects involving the lateral oropharynx and tongue base, regional pedicled flaps provide excellent soft tissue bulk and adequate skin. Most commonly, these derive from the pectoralis major; other sources include latissimus dorsi and trapezius muscle.
- Larger soft tissue defects of the lateral oropharynx and tongue base are best repaired using free tissue transfer with radial forearm or anterolateral thigh flap.
- Composite defects may be reconstructed with fibula, iliac crest, or scapular osteocutaneous flaps.

Carcinoma of the Base of the Tongue

- Less common than carcinoma of the oral tongue.
- Tonsil tissue at base of tongue may give rise to lymphoma in addition to SCC.
- The most common presenting signs are referred otalgia and odynophagia.
- Subsites due to poor visualization of the tongue base and nonspecific symptoms. Palpation of the tongue base is critical for accurate diagnosis and to assess the extent of tumor.
- Tumor may invade the adjacent structures of the larynx, tonsil, soft palate, and hypopharynx. Invasion into vallecula/epiglottis may cause obstructive symptoms.
- High rate of lymphatic metastases regardless of T stage (60%-70%); most commonly to levels II-IV. Bilateral lymphadenopathy in ~20% at presentation.

Tongue Base Cancer Treatment

- In patients not candidates for CRT or treatment failures, surgical approaches for larger, deeper, or more caudally located tumors include:
  - Mandibular swing or composite resection (see section on Tonsillar Cancer)
  - Median mandibulo-glossotomy: involves division of the mandible at the symphysis and the tongue along the medial raphe. Allows access to small tumors isolated to the mid-portion of the tongue base. Lateral exposure is limited.
  - Suprahyoid pharyngotomy: approach to the tongue base through a transcervical incision. Divide suprahyoid musculature from hyoid bone and enter the pharynx immediately above the hyoid bone. Is useful for smaller neoplasms of the tongue base without extension to other sites or more inferior neoplasms unable to be accessed transorally.
- Laryngectomy may be necessary to prevent chronic aspiration in patients undergoing total glossectomy.
- Options for reconstruction of the tongue base are similar to other sites in the oropharynx noted above. For total glossectomy defects, flaps with sufficient bulk include pedicled pectoralis major or anterolateral thigh, or rectus abdominis free flap.

Bibliography

Fakhry C, Lacchetti C, Perez-Ordonez B. Human papillomavirus testing in head and neck carcinomas: ASCO Clinical Practice Guideline Endorsement Summary of the CAP Guideline. *J Oncol Pract.* 2018;14:613-617.

Fakhry C, D'Soiza G. HPV and Head and Neck Cancers Springer Nature. 2015.

Lechner M, Liu J, Masterson L, Fenton TR. HPV-associated oropharyngeal cancer: epidemiology, molecular biology and clinical management. *Nat Rev Clin Oncol.* 2022;19:306-327.

Mehanna H, Taberna M, von Buchwald C, et al. Prognostic implications of p16 and HPV discordance in oropharyngeal cancer (HNCIG-EPIC-OPC): a multicentre, multinational, individual patient data analysis. *Lancet Oncol.* 2023;24:239-251.

Patients with Oropharyngeal Squamous Cell Carcinoma: Impact of the Tumor HPV Status. Cancers (Basel). 2021;13.

Questions

1. Which of the following is NOT a risk factor for oropharyngeal malignancy?
   A. Fanconi anemia
   B. HPV 6
   C. Tobacco exposure
   D. Immunosuppression

2. A patient with a cystic neck mass undergoes fine-needle aspiration that shows malignancy, and p16 testing is positive. Which of the following could be the diagnosis?
   A. Cutaneous squamous cell carcinoma
   B. HPV-related oropharynx squamous cell carcinoma
   C. Salivary gland clear cell carcinoma
   D. All of the above

3. A patient is diagnosed with HPV+/p16+ oropharynx cancer of the palatine tonsil. On exam, the primary tumor is ~2 cm and confined to the tonsil, and there is a single ipsilateral lymph node that is < 3 cm, that is immobile and clearly fixed to underlying musculature. What is the most appropriate initial treatment modality?
   A. Surgery including transoral resection of primary tumor and ipsilateral neck dissection
   B. Definitive radiation
   C. Definitive chemoradiation
   D. None of the above

4. High-risk HPV16 is associated with what percentage of HPV+ OPSCC?
   A. 50%
   B. 75%
   C. 90%
   D. 100%

5. Elective neck dissection for a T2N0M0 tumor of the soft palate should include which levels?
   A. Ipsilateral Ib-IV
   B. Ipsilateral II-IV
   C. Ipsilateral II-IV, contralateral II-III
   D. Bilateral II-IV

Answer Key to Multiple Choice Questions:

1. B: HPV 6
2. D: All of the above
3. C: Definitive chemoradiation
4. C: 90%
5. D: Bilateral II-IV

Chapter 45
Tumors of the Larynx, Hypopharynx, and Upper Esophagus

Anatomy

Larynx Anatomy and Boundaries

- Supraglottis
  - (a) Third and fourth branchial arch derivative with no midline fusion.
  - (b) Blood supply is from superior laryngeal arteries.
  - (c) Bilateral lymphatic drainage.
  - (d) Superior surface of epiglottis to lateral margin of ventricle at junction of false vocal fold with true vocal fold.
  - (e) Quadrangular membrane is a fibroelastic membrane that extends from epiglottis to arytenoids and corniculate cartilage.
  - (f) Subsites include suprahyoid epiglottis, infrahyoid epiglottis, aryepiglottic folds, arytenoids, ventricle, false vocal folds.
- Glottis
  - (a) Sixth branchial arch derivative.
  - (b) Blood supply is from inferior laryngeal arteries.
  - (c) Extends 1 cm below apex of ventricle.
  - (d) Conus elasticus is a fibroelastic membrane that extends from cricoid cartilage to vocal ligament; limits spread of cancer laterally.
  - (e) Broyles' ligament is the insertion of vocalis tendon to thyroid cartilage; potential area for tumor spread to thyroid cartilage (absence of perichondrium in this area).
  - (f) Subsites include true vocal folds (including anterior/posterior commissure).
- Subglottis
  - (a) Sixth branchial arch derivative.
  - (b) Blood supply is from inferior laryngeal arteries.
  - (c) Extends from glottis to inferior border of cricoid cartilage.
- Pre-epiglottic space (Figure 45-1)
  - (a) Anterior to epiglottis
  - (b) Extends from hyoepiglottic ligament/vallecula to thyroid cartilage/thyroepiglottic ligament; bounded anteriorly by thyroid membrane
  - (c) Contains fibrofatty tissue
  - (d) Contiguous with paraglottic space
- Paraglottic space (Figure 45-2)
  - (a) Space outside conus elasticus and quadrangular membrane

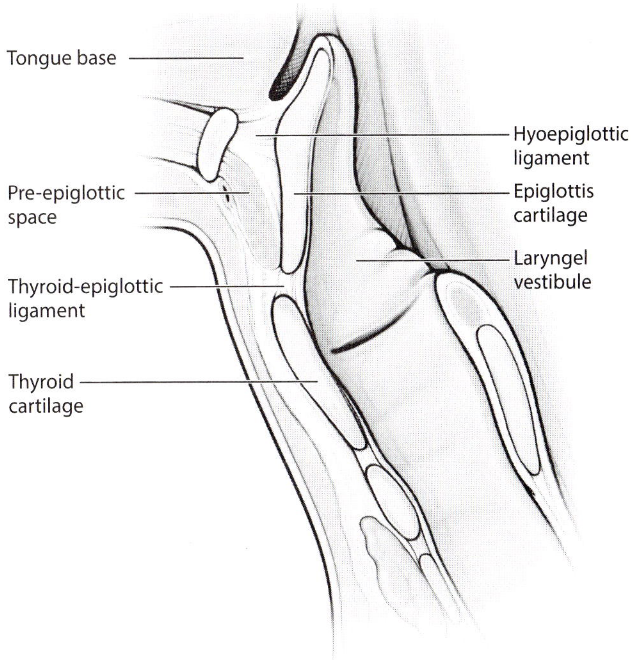

Figure 45-1 Sagittal view of larynx.

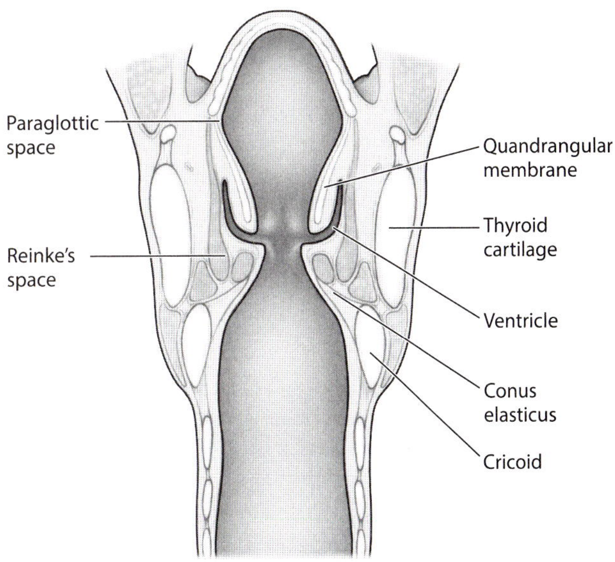

Figure 45-2 Coronal sagittal view of larynx.

(b) Contains fibrofatty tissue
(c) May allow for submucosal, transglottic spread of tumor

- Reinke space
  (a) Superficial lamina propria of true vocal fold

Hypopharynx Anatomy

The hypopharynx extends from the superior border of the hyoid to the lower border of the cricoid cartilage. It includes three subsites:

(a) Pyriform sinuses (or fossa): extend from the pharyngoepiglottic folds to the upper end of the cervical esophagus; bounded laterally by the thyroid cartilage and medially by the surface of the aryepiglottic fold and the arytenoid and cricoid cartilages
(b) Posterior hypopharyngeal wall
(c) Postcricoid space: extends from the arytenoid cartilages to the inferior aspect of the cricoid and connects the right and left pyriform sinuses, forming the anterior wall of the hypopharynx

Upper Esophagus Anatomy

The esophagus extends from the cricoid cartilage to the cardia of the stomach. In adults, this distance is 38 to 40 cm. Subsites of the esophagus include:

(a) Upper esophageal sphincter
(b) Body (subdivided into cervical, thoracic, and intra-abdominal)
(c) Lower esophageal sphincter

Muscles

- Layers: outer longitudinal, inner circular (no serous membrane)
- Composition varies longitudinally: upper 5 cm, skeletal (striated) muscle; upper-mid portion has overlapping striated and smooth muscle; lower half is smooth muscle
- Innervation: myenteric plexus of Auerbach within muscle layers (parasympathetic ganglion cells)
- Bolus transit: the upper one-third (containing striated muscle), has the most rapid peristalsis—less than 1-second transit, while movement through the lower two-thirds takes approximately 3 seconds. Gravity plays only a minor role in normal swallowing.

Upper Esophageal Sphincter (UES)

- Composed primarily of the cricopharyngeal muscle, as well as the cervical esophagus and inferior pharyngeal constrictor.
- At rest, it is tonically contracted; actively dilated by laryngeal elevation during swallowing.
- Dehiscence between the cricopharyngeus and the inferior constrictor, termed the Killian dehiscence, can weaken with age, leading to Zenker diverticulum.
- The lateral dehiscence inferior to the cricopharyngeus, termed the Killian-Jamieson space, allows branches of the inferior thyroid artery to pass through.

Lower Esophageal Sphincter (LES)

- Closure prevents reflux of gastric contents into esophagus.
- Not a true anatomic structure, but an active zone of high pressure extending 1 to 2 cm above and below the diaphragm that relaxes during passage of the peristaltic wave.
- LES function is controlled by parasympathetic tone (acetylcholine) and gastrin.
- Sphincteric function is assisted by the sling created by the diaphragmatic crura surrounding the esophageal hiatus (the opening in the diaphragm through which the esophagus passes). This effect is lost with a hiatal hernia.

Premalignant and Benign Disorders of the Larynx, Hypopharynx, and Upper Esophagus

Premalignant Laryngeal Lesions

- Spectrum from hyperplasia → atypia → dysplasia (mild/moderate/severe) → carcinoma in situ (CIS)
  (a) *Mild dysplasia*: cellular abnormalities; limited to basal one-third of epithelium
  (b) *Moderate dysplasia*: cellular abnormalities; up to two-thirds of epithelium thickness
  (c) *Severe dysplasia*: cellular atypia; greater than two-thirds of epithelium thickness
  (d) *CIS*: intraepithelial neoplasm; no basement membrane or stromal invasion
- Interval to malignant transformation variable (3-10 years)
  (a) Mild/moderate dysplasia: roughly 7% to 11% lesions undergo malignant transformation
  (b) Severe dysplasia: roughly 18% lesions undergo malignant transformation.
    - Clinically, severe dysplasia and CIS behave similarly
- Biopsy is gold standard of diagnosis
  (a) Techniques include incisional biopsy, excisional biopsy, or micro-flap excision
- Treatment for early lesions
  (a) Endoscopic excision is the preferred treatment.
  (b) Radiation
    - Effective alternative particularly for elderly, frail patients and multifocal lesions
  (c) Both surgery and radiation have excellent local control rates with early lesions.
  (d) Requires close, life-long follow-up to detect recurrent and second primary lesions.

Benign Disorders of the Hypopharynx

- Supraglottitis: presents as odynophagia and/or dysphagia, hoarse or muffled voice, and sometimes drooling. Caused by bacterial infection and treated with appropriate antibiotics, often supplemented with corticosteroids. May require intubation and/or epinephrine when breathing is affected.
- Anterior cervical osteophyte: usually asymptomatic; can cause dysphagia, hoarseness, and dyspnea. Common in the elderly. Treated with anti-inflammatory drugs, or in cases of severe effects on dietary intake, surgery.
- Medialization of the carotid artery: Usually asymptomatic but can appear as a mass in the posterior pharyngeal wall, requiring care (preferably imaging) in differential diagnosis. Presents risk of injury upon intubation. In extreme cases, can cause hoarseness or upper respiratory distress.

Benign Disorders of the Esophagus

- Barrett esophagus: characterized by metaplasia of the normal squamous mucosa of the distal esophagus to a columnar epithelium like the epithelial lining of the stomach, which may progress to dysplasia and eventually adenocarcinoma (0.5% of cases become malignant per year). Results from chronic gastroesophageal reflux, which is associated with obesity, smoking, and long-term, heavy alcohol consumption.
- Achalasia: neurogenic motility disorder in which the LES fails to relax during swallowing, causing dysphagia and regurgitation.
- Zenker diverticulum: outpouching of the esophagus. Symptoms include regurgitation of undigested food, dysphagia, aspiration, or recurrent pneumonias.
- Leiomyomas: benign tumors resulting from hyperproliferation of smooth muscle. Larger tumors can cause dysphagia, chest pain, esophageal obstruction, and regurgitation. Do not recur following resection.

Table 45-1 Prognostic Groups according to TNM Categories for Larynx and Hypopharynx/ Upper Esophagus Cancer, AJCC 8th Edition Staging

T Stage	*N Stage*			
	N0	*N1*	*N2a-c*	*N3a-b*
T1	I	III	IVa	IVb
T2	II	III	IVa	IVb
T3	III	III	IVa	IVb
T4	IVa	Iva	IVa	IVb

Malignancy of the Larynx, Hypopharynx, and Upper Esophagus

Epidemiology and Risk Factors

Laryngeal Cancer

- Second most common malignancy of upper aerodigestive tract (Table 45-1).
- 40% arise in the supraglottis, 59% in the glottis, and 1% in the subglottis.
- Squamous cell carcinoma (SCC) represents 85% to 95% of laryngeal malignancies.
- M:F ratio 4:1.
- Risk factors
  - (a) Current smokers have 10- to 20-fold increased risk.
    - Approximately 60% risk reduction after 10+ years of smoking cessation.
  - (b) Alcohol.
  - (c) Prior head and neck SCC.
  - (d) Recurrent respiratory papillomatosis: 3% to 7% undergo malignant degeneration to SCC.
    - Typically related to human papillomavirus (HPV) types 6 and 11.
  - (e) Relationship of HPV types 16 and 18 is not established.
  - (f) Environmental factors reported in literature such as exposure to wood dust, paint, asbestos, nickel, leather products, and diesel fumes.
  - (g) Gastroesophageal reflux.

Hypopharyngeal Cancer

- Over 90% of hypopharyngeal cancer is SCC.
- Risk factors for hypopharyngeal cancer include chronic tobacco and alcohol use.
- Similar to larynx cancer, the etiologic role of HPV types 16 and 18 is not established.
- In the United States, pyriform sinus carcinoma predominates (accounting for 60%-70% of cases), while in Europe, postcricoid carcinomas predominate.

Upper Esophageal Cancer

- Over 90% of esophageal cancer is SCC or adenocarcinoma.
- Risk factors for esophageal SCC include tobacco and alcohol use, achalasia, caustic injury, Plummer-Vinson syndrome, history of head and neck cancer, history of radiation therapy to the mediastinum, low socioeconomic status, and nonepidermolytic palmoplantar keratoderma (tylosis).
  - (a) Plummer-Vinson syndrome is a rare disorder that affects women between the ages of 30 and 50 years and consists of iron deficiency anemia, dysphagia, mucosal webs, weight loss, angular stomatitis, and atrophic glossitis.

- Risk factors for adenocarcinoma include Barrett esophagus, acid reflux, tobacco use, and history of radiotherapy to the mediastinum.
- More than 75% of adenocarcinomas occur in the distal esophagus, while SCC is more evenly distributed throughout.
- The most common site for primary esophageal cancer is the lower third of the esophagus followed by the middle third, and rarely the cervical esophagus.
  (a) Carcinoma involving the cervical esophagus most commonly results from extension of hypopharyngeal cancer inferiorly into the cervical esophagus (from the lower border of the cricoid cartilage to the thoracic inlet).

TNM Staging (8th Edition)

The tumor (T), lymph node (N), metastasis (M) (TNM) system is a clinical staging schema based on the extent of disease as determined by physical examination and imaging prior to initial treatment. TNM staging provides a useful estimation of prognosis, aids in treatment selection, and permits the assessment of treatment outcomes. The American Joint Committee for Cancer (AJCC) coordinates and periodically updates the criteria for assessment and staging (currently in its 8th edition). Tumors of the larynx and hypopharynx/upper esophagus are staged according to distinct T classifications but identical N classifications. N stage is determined either by clinical (cN) or, following surgery with lymphadenectomy, pathological criteria (pN).

Primary Tumor (T) Staging for Larynx

- Supraglottic SCC
  (a) T1: limited to one subsite
  (b) T2: more than one subsite of supraglottic larynx or spread outside of supraglottic larynx, without vocal fold fixation
  (c) T3: vocal fold fixation or invasion of adjacent structures (postcricoid, pre-epiglottic space, paraglottic space, inner cortex of thyroid cartilage)
  (d) T4a: (moderately advanced) invades thyroid cartilage or beyond larynx
  (e) T4b: (very advanced) invades prevertebral fascia, encases carotid artery, or invades mediastinum
  (f) Tumor spreads typically to base of tongue or pre-epiglottic space
  (g) Roughly 25% to 50% have cervical nodal metastases at time of presentation (level II-IV)
    - Incidence based on T stage: T1 (10%), T2 (29%), T3 (38%), T5 (57%)
    - Incidence of occult nodal metastasis increases based on T stage: T1 (0%), T2 (20%), T3 (25%), T4 (40%)
- Glottic SCC
  (a) T1: limited to vocal folds with normal vocal fold movement
    - T1a: one vocal fold
    - T1b: bilateral vocal folds
  (b) T2: extends to subglottis or supraglottis or impaired vocal fold mobility
  (c) T3: vocal fold fixation or invasion of adjacent structures (paraglottic space, inner cortex of thyroid cartilage)
  (d) T4a: (moderately advanced) invades thyroid cartilage or beyond larynx
  (e) T4b: (very advanced) invades prevertebral fascia, encases carotid artery, or invades mediastinum

(f) Incidence of cervical metastasis is low and correlates with T stage: T1/T2 (< 5%), T3/T4 (20%-25%)
(g) Cervical metastasis typically unilateral and in levels II-IV
(h) Transglottic lesions extend into subglottis/supraglottis and have higher rates of nodal metastasis and cartilage invasion

- Subglottic SCC
  (a) T1: limited to subglottis
  (b) T2: involves vocal folds with normal or impaired mobility
  (c) T3: involves vocal folds with fixation
  (d) T4a: (moderately advanced) invades cricoid or thyroid cartilage or beyond larynx
  (e) T4b: (very advanced) invades prevertebral fascia, encases carotid artery, or invades mediastinum
  (f) Rare, aggressive, and often poorly differentiated
  (g) Can present with airway obstruction, stridor, or dyspnea
  (h) Higher risk of spread to level VI nodes
  (i) May also present with metastasis to superior mediastinum (associated with stomal recurrence after treatment with total laryngectomy)

Primary Tumor (T) Staging for Hypopharynx/Upper Esophagus

- T1: tumor smaller than 2 cm, limited to one subsite
- T2: tumor size between 2 and 4 cm and/or involves more than one subsite
- T3: tumor size larger than 4 cm or any size tumor that fixates the larynx
- T4: tumor invades adjacent structures (eg, thyroid/cricoid cartilage, carotid artery, soft tissues of the neck, prevertebral fascia/muscles, thyroid, esophagus)

Clinical Lymph Node (N) Staging for Larynx and Hypopharynx

- Nx: regional lymph nodes cannot be assessed
- N0: no regional lymph node metastasis
- N1: metastasis in a single ipsilateral node measuring less than 3 cm
- N2a: metastasis in a single ipsilateral node measuring between 3 and 6 cm
- N2b: metastasis in multiple ipsilateral nodes, none greater than 6 cm
- N2c: metastases in bilateral or contralateral nodes, none greater than 6 cm
- N3: metastasis larger than 6 cm in one or more nodes

Pathologic Lymph Node (N) Staging for Larynx and Hypopharynx

- Nx: regional lymph nodes cannot be assessed
- N0: no regional lymph node metastasis
- N1: metastasis in a single ipsilateral lymph node, smaller than 3 cm and without extranodal extension (ENE)
- N2: metastasis in a single ipsilateral lymph node, smaller than 3 cm or less with ENE; or between 3 and 6 cm without ENE; or metastases in multiple ipsilateral lymph nodes, none larger than 6 cm without ENE; or metastasis in bilateral or contralateral lymph nodes, none larger than 6 cm in greatest dimension without ENE
- N2a: metastasis in a single ipsilateral or contralateral lymph node 3 cm or smaller and with ENE; or metastasis in a single ipsilateral lymph node between 3 and 6 cm in size without ENE
- N2b: metastasis in multiple ipsilateral lymph nodes, none larger than 6 cm without ENE
- N2c: metastasis in bilateral or contralateral lymph nodes, none larger than 6 cm without ENE

- N3: metastasis in a lymph node larger than 6 cm without ENE; or metastasis in a single ipsilateral lymph node larger than 3 cm with ENE; or metastasis in multiple ipsilateral, contralateral, or bilateral lymph nodes, with any ENE
- N3a: metastasis in a lymph node larger than 6 cm without ENE
- N3b: metastasis in a single ipsilateral node larger than 3 cm with ENE; or metastasis in multiple ipsilateral, contralateral, or bilateral lymph nodes, with any ENE

Distant Metastasis (M) for Larynx and Hypopharynx

- Mx: distant metastasis cannot be assessed
- M0: no distant metastasis
- M1: distant metastasis

Malignancy of the Larynx, Hypopharynx, and Upper Esophagus: Clinical Evaluation

Signs and Symptoms

- Glottic tumors present earlier as they are more often symptomatic at a smaller size
  (a) Hoarseness/Dysphonia (most common symptom)
  (b) Odynophagia (second most common symptom)
  (c) Referred otalgia
  (d) Dyspnea/Stridor
  (e) Dysphagia/Aspiration (Late manifestations typically in larger supraglottic tumors)
  (f) Hemoptysis
  (g) Weight loss
  (h) Globus sensation

History

- Pertinent risk factors
- Duration of symptoms
- Comorbidities
- History of prior cancers
- Dysphagia, malnutrition, dehydration, weight loss
- Dyspnea, stridor

Physical Examination

- Comprehensive head and neck examination
- Voice characteristics
- Neck examination for lymphadenopathy
- Dental evaluation
- Flexible laryngoscopy
- Videostroboscopy

Diagnostic and Imaging Studies

- Pathologic diagnosis
  (a) Endoscopy with biopsy to obtain tissue diagnosis, assess tumor extent, assess candidacy for conservation laryngeal surgery
  (b) Fine-needle aspiration (FNA) of palpable neck node

- Imaging
  (a) Computed tomography (CT) or magnetic resonance imaging (MRI) of neck
    - Extent of disease
    - Spread of tumor to pre-epiglottic, paraglottic, postcricoid areas
    - MRI more sensitive for cartilage invasion
  (b) CT chest
    - Exclude pulmonary metastases
    - Isolated pulmonary nodule more likely to be second primary than metastatic laryngeal cancer
  (c) PET-CT
    - Consider for advanced disease as it alters management in 20% to 30% of head and neck cancer patients
    - May also assist in assessing response to treatment, as at 3 to 4 months after completion of radiation, approaches 97% to 100% negative predictive value.
- Laboratory studies
  (a) Electrocardiography (ECG) for preoperative clearance
  (b) Prealbumin and albumin for nutritional status
  (c) Complete blood count (CBC), electrolyte panel, liver function tests

Treatment of Malignant Tumors of the Larynx, Hypopharynx, and Upper Esophagus

Optimal care of patients with larynx, hypopharynx, or upper esophageal cancer occurs within a multidisciplinary, collaborative setting, involving experts in the fields of head and neck surgery, radiation and medical oncology, radiology, and pathology. The management of aesthetic and functional outcomes requires close coordination with reconstructive surgeons, speech-language pathologists, dentists, oral surgeons, physical therapists, and maxillofacial prosthodontists. Selecting an appropriate treatment regimen requires balancing multiple concerns including the extent and location of the tumor, clinical stage at diagnosis, and the overall medical condition of the patient.

Treatment of Early-Stage Laryngeal Cancer (Stage I-II)

- Treated with single modality
- Treatment individualized to patient depending mainly on stage and subsite
  (a) Radiation
    - Radiation field depends on subsite
    - *Advantages*: useful in poor surgical candidates, avoids upfront tracheotomy in certain patients
    - *Disadvantages*: mucositis, laryngeal edema, dysphagia, xerostomia, risk of chondronecrosis
    - Usually involves 6-week course of treatment (total 60-70 Gy)
    - Local control rates 90% to 98% with T1 or certain T2 lesions with good voice outcomes
    - Higher failure rates of up to 30% with T2 lesions that have impaired vocal fold mobility
  (b) Surgery: transoral laser microsurgery (TLM)
    - Surgical management has shifted from open partial laryngectomy to transoral laser microsurgery (TLM).

- Transoral robotic partial laryngectomy has emerged as a viable option in select cases and with specialized surgical expertise.
- Transoral excision is optimally used as a single modality; therefore patient selection and high rate of negative margins are critical.
- *Advantages*: similar local control rates to radiation, saves radiation for possible recurrence.
- *Disadvantages*: poorer voice outcomes compared to radiation.
- *Indications*: T1 or T2 lesions with limited involvement of contralateral vocal fold, infraglottic extension, and arytenoid involvement.
- *Contraindications*: vocal fold fixation, interarytenoid involvement, poor pulmonary status, and difficult endoscopic exposure.
- 5-year disease-free survival with T1-T2 glottic cancer is 88%.

(c) Surgery: open conservation laryngeal surgery

- Supraglottic laryngectomy
  - *Indications*: T1-T2 and N0-1 with normal vocal fold mobility, tumor limited to supraglottis 2 to 5 mm from anterior commissure
  - *Contraindications*: vocal fold fixation, interarytenoid involvement, poor pulmonary status, thyroid cartilage invasion
  - *Advantages*: minimal effect on voice, possibility of avoiding radiation, permits pathologic staging
  - *Disadvantages*: applicable to select patients only, may require initial tracheotomy, requirement for postoperative swallowing therapy (almost all patients have dysphagia/aspiration)
  - Postoperative radiation associated with significantly impaired swallowing function
- Supracricoid laryngectomy can be considered in select T3 patients that are not candidates for transoral excision
  - Defect reconstructed with cricohyoidopexy (CHP) or cricohyoidoepiglottopexy (CHEP) if epiglottis is spared
  - *Indications*: good pulmonary function, limited thyroid cartilage or epiglottic involvement
  - *Contraindications*: involvement of both cricoarytenoid joints, infraglottic extension to cricoid cartilage, invasion of hyoid bone or posterior arytenoid mucosa

(d) Management of neck

- Elective treatment of neck in cN0 patients
  - Glottic: not indicated in T1-2 glottic cancer (0%-5% incidence of occult metastasis); indicated in T3-T4 glottic lesions especially those with transglottic involvement
  - Supraglottic: 30%-50% incidence of occult neck disease for supraglottic cancer with bilateral drainage patterns; patients should have bilateral level II-IV neck dissections for cN0 neck, or bilateral necks should be incorporated into radiation fields
- Clinical neck disease (cN+)
  - Comprehensive neck dissection or definitive radiation is recommended regardless of tumor site or T stage.
- Assessment of the neck after definitive chemoradiation
  - Planned neck dissection is not necessary if there is complete response to treatment on posttreatment PET-CT. Level 1 evidence indicates that PET/CT surveillance at 12 weeks after chemoradiation offers equivalent survival to planned neck dissection.

Treatment of Advanced-Stage Laryngeal Cancer (Stage III-IV)

- Advanced stage disease (T2N+, T3 and T4 disease) is typically managed with a multimodal approach.
- Current treatment emphasizes organ preservation, achieved with concurrent chemoradiation for most T3 lesions or conservation laryngeal surgery for highly select T3 lesions.
- Total laryngectomy with adjuvant therapy is indicated for advanced T4 lesions or nonfunctional larynx.
- Treatment considerations include patient's comorbidities and goals, physician's expertise, and anticipated functional outcomes.
  (a) Landmark trials
    - VA larynx study (1991)
      - Compared induction chemotherapy (cisplatin/5-FU) with definitive radiation versus total laryngectomy and postoperative radiation.
      - In the induction chemotherapy arm, patients with no response to chemotherapy underwent total laryngectomy and postoperative radiation, while patients with partial or complete response underwent radiotherapy.
      - No difference in survival was seen between the two groups (68% 2-year survival for both groups).
      - 64% laryngeal preservation in induction chemotherapy group.
      - Pattern of recurrence differed between the two groups with the nonsurgical group having more locoregional recurrence and surgical group having more distant disease.
      - Patients with T4 cancers were more likely to need salvage laryngectomy.
    - RTOG 91-11 study (2003)
      - Compared three nonsurgical treatment arms: induction chemotherapy (cisplatin/5-FU) with radiation, concurrent chemoradiation (cisplatin), and radiation alone
      - Included patients with stage III or IV disease (T2, T3, and low-volume T4 but excluded T4 with gross cartilage invasion)
      - Comparable incidence of toxic effects including mucositis, nausea/vomiting, and neutropenia with induction chemotherapy followed by radiation and concurrent chemoradiation
      - Laryngectomy-free survival and locoregional control better in concurrent chemoradiation group: 88% at 2 years
    - 10-year follow-up to RTOG 91-11
      - Concurrent group had improved locoregional control and laryngeal preservation compared with induction and radiation monotherapy groups
      - Laryngectomy-free survival improved in both induction and concurrent groups (both superior to radiotherapy alone group)
      - Notably, no difference in overall survival between the three groups at 10-year mark, potentially due to long-term toxicity in concurrent group

  (b) Definitive chemoradiation
    - Current evidence endorses nonoperative treatment of many T3 and T2N+ cancers with concurrent cisplatin and radiation.
    - Success of chemoradiation treatment depends on adherence to protocol as efficacy of radiation dramatically decreases with treatment interruptions.
    - Patients who are ineligible for cisplatin may be substituted for concurrent carboplatin or cetuximab and radiation.

(c) Total laryngectomy and neck dissection with adjuvant therapy
  - Recommended for patients with T4a disease with disease penetration through cartilage, as these patients were not eligible for organ preservation studies.
  - Retrospective evidence indicates that total laryngectomy provides improved locoregional control over (chemo)radiation treatment.
  - Additionally, patients with severe airway compromise requiring tracheostomy at diagnosis are poor candidates for organ preservation.

(d) Subglottic laryngeal cancer, special considerations
  - Usually presents at advanced stage
  - Neck dissection should include level VI (pretracheal and unilateral or bilateral paratracheal) and hemithyroidectomy or total thyroidectomy due to risk of local spread and peristomal recurrence

(e) Postoperative concurrent chemoradiation
  - RTOG 9501 and EORTC 22931 studies in 2004
  - High-risk patients with all sites of head and neck SCC
    - Meta-analysis of both studies showed improved overall survival with adjuvant chemoradiation for patients with positive margins or ENE

(f) Voice rehabilitation after total laryngectomy
  - Tracheosophageal prosthesis (TEP) considered to have best voice outcomes
  - Esophageal speech
    - Difficult to learn
    - Requires trapping, swallowing, and expulsion of air to create voice via vibration of pharyngoesophageal mucosa
  - Electrolarynx
    - Considered too mechanical by many patients

Treatment of Hypopharyngeal Cancer

- The rich lymphatic network in the submucosal tissue surrounding the hypopharynx allows early spread to regional lymph nodes (60%-75% at presentation) and direct extension into adjacent soft tissues.
  (a) Carcinoma of the medial aspect of the hypopharynx often extends into the larynx and has a greater propensity for contralateral metastasis than lesions of the lateral wall.
  (b) Posterior cricoid cancers may invade into the cricoarytenoid muscles and cartilage of the larynx.
  (c) Lateral hypopharyngeal cancers may extend superiorly to the oropharynx and nasopharynx, inferiorly to involve the esophagus, or deep into the prevertebral fascia.
- A characteristic feature of hypopharyngeal cancer is its tendency for submucosal spread, which must be taken into consideration during resection to obtain a negative margin.
- Management of hypopharyngeal carcinoma remains challenging and controversial; treatment selection depends on stage, subsite, patient performance status, and institutional preference.
- For T1-T2N0 lesions, radiation is the primary treatment, as surgery requires laryngectomy; radiation may also be used to treat bilateral cervical nodal basins as well as retropharyngeal nodes with improved morbidity.
- For selected small, superficial tumors, emerging surgical technologies allow transoral resection, including CO_2 laser microsurgery and robotics (for those in the pyriform sinus).

These procedures are combined with elective or therapeutic neck dissection and followed by adjuvant radiation.
- T2-3 and T1N+ lesions are treated by a variety of strategies; the National Comprehensive Cancer Network (NCCN) guidelines recommend:
  (a) Induction chemotherapy with subsequent treatment dependent on response
  (b) Chemoradiation
  (c) Surgery including total laryngopharyngectomy and neck dissection with adjuvant therapy as indicated
- Treatment of T4 tumors may involve:
  (a) Induction chemotherapy with subsequent treatment dependent on response
  (b) Chemoradiation
  (c) Surgery including total laryngopharyngectomy and neck dissection with adjuvant therapy as indicated
- Postcricoid tumors usually present at an advanced stage and therefore require total laryngopharyngectomy, or if involving the cervical esophagus, laryngopharyngoesophagectomy.
- In advanced cases, postoperative (chemo)radiation improves local and regional control and enhances survival.
- Indications for postoperative radiation include cervical lymphadenopathy and advanced tumor stage, while those for postoperative chemoradiation include positive surgical margins and ENE.

Treatment of Esophageal Cancer

- Cancer involving the cervical esophagus may extend to involve the larynx and trachea
  (a) Tracheoesophageal fistula may result from invasion of cancer through the posterior wall of the trachea.
  (b) Distal esophageal cancer may extend inferiorly to involve the esophagogastric junction.
- At diagnosis, more than 50% of patients have metastases or an unresectable primary tumor.
- Early-stage disease is treated surgically with a transthoracic or transhiatal approach for partial or total esophagectomy
- Transcervical approach is utilized for upper cervical esophagus or inferior extension from hypopharynx.
- Laryngectomy with or without partial tracheal resection may be necessary for upper cervical esophageal cancer.
- Endoscopically placed stents may be deployed for palliative treatment of dysphagia in advanced-stage disease.
- Primary radiation may be used as an alternative treatment in patients who are poor surgical candidates.
- No improvement in survival has been demonstrated with preoperative radiation
  (a) Adjuvant radiation improves local disease control.
- Preoperative chemotherapy may result in a reduction in primary tumor size and regional and distant metastases, but no survival benefit has been demonstrated.
  (a) Postoperative chemotherapy may also treat regional and distant metastases but results in increased toxicity, morbidity, and no improvement in survival.
- Concurrent chemoradiation is useful as primary treatment modality in patients with unresectable disease

Reconstruction After Surgical Treatment

- Partial laryngopharyngectomy or total laryngectomy with partial pharyngectomy for primary, untreated patients may be reconstructed by primary pharyngeal closure.
  (a) For partial laryngopharyngectomy defects with insufficient remaining pharyngeal mucosa (or circumferential defects), free tissue reconstruction with fasciocutaneous flaps (eg, radial forearm, anterolateral thigh) is indicated as a pharyngeal patch
- Total laryngopharyngectomy or total laryngopharyngectomy with esophagectomy may be reconstructed with a free jejunal autograft or gastric pull-up.

Major Complications of Treatment

- Surgery
  (a) Pharyngocutaneous fistula (PCF)
    - Increased incidence in previously radiated patients
      - Regional or free-flap reconstruction reduces PCF incidence in these patients
    - Treatment: optimize nutrition, thyroid hormone supplementation, local wound care, debridement, possible flap closure

  (b) Stomal stenosis
    - May be secondary to stomal recurrence
    - May require patient to wear appliance such as laryngectomy tube

  (c) Dysphagia secondary to pharyngeal stenosis
- Chemoradiation
  (a) Esophageal stenosis secondary to scarring or radiation
  (b) Dysfunctional larynx
    - Can result from severe local side effects after chemoradiation
    - May require tracheotomy, g-tube, or total laryngectomy

Follow-up After Definitive Treatment

- Local or regional disease progression is most common cause of death in patients with head and neck cancer.
  (a) Regular follow-up examinations are crucial after definitive treatment as early detection of recurrence permits effective salvage therapy.
- Follow-up intervals are not standardized.
  (a) As recurrences usually present in the first 2 years after treatment, head and neck examinations are performed every 4 to 6 weeks during the first year, every 3 months during the second year, and every 4 to 6 months during years 3 to 5.
  (b) As the incidence of developing a second primary cancer remains constant at about 4% to 5% per year, routine surveillance visits should be performed every 6 to 12 months for life.
- If the patient should become symptomatic at any time between visits, the surgeon should perform a thorough examination and order any ancillary tests and procedures as necessary.
  (a) Pain is a sensitive indicator for tumor recurrence and should serve as a warning sign for the head and neck oncologist.
- Posttreatment imaging is controversial; in the absence of symptoms or abnormal physical examination findings, the NCCN recommends against routine imaging studies.

Bibliography

Bernier J, Domenge C, Ozsahin M, et al. Postoperative irradiation with or without concomitant chemotherapy for head and neck cancer. *N Engl J Med*. 2004;350:1945-1962.

Department of Veterans Affairs Laryngeal Cancer Study Group, et al. Induction chemotherapy plus radiation compared with surgery plus radiation in patients with advanced laryngeal cancer. *N Engl J Med*. 1991;324(24):1685-1690.

Forastiere AA, Ismaila N, Wolf GT. Use of larynx-preservation strategies in the treatment of laryngeal cancer: American Society of Clinical Oncology clinical practice guideline update summary. *J Clin Oncol*. 2018;36(11):1143-1169.

Olson C, Alexander R, Stinnett S. Dysplastic lesions of the larynx. *Otolaryngol Clin North Am*. 2023;56(2):233-246.

Pfister DG, Spencer S, Adelstein D, et al. Head and neck cancer, version 2.2020, NCCN clinical practice guidelines in oncology. *J Natl Compr Cancer Netw*. 2020;18(7):224-234.

Questions

1. Based on results of the landmark RTOG 9501 and EORTC 22931 trials, indications for adjuvant chemoradiation after surgical resection of head and neck cancers include
   A. Extranodal extension
   B. Angiolymphatic invasion
   C. Positive margins
   D. Perineural invasion
   E. A, C

2. Established risk factors for hypopharyngeal squamous cell carcinoma include
   A. Alcohol
   B. Tobacco
   C. Plummer-Vinson syndrome
   D. Gastroesophageal reflux disease
   E. A, B, D

3. A 45-year-old man presents with a 6-month history of worsening odynophagia and otalgia. He is noted on physical examination to have an ulcerated mass over the lingual epiglottis extending to the false vocal fold on the left. He is also noted to have some decreased mobility of his right vocal fold. On imaging, he is noted to invasion of the paraglottic space and bilateral enlarged lymph nodes with largest being 3.5 cm in size. What is the clinical stage for this patient?
   A. T3N2c
   B. T3N1
   C. T2N1
   D. T3N2b
   E. T2N2c

4. The RTOG 91-11 study specifically excluded what type of patient with laryngeal cancer?
   A. Patients with N3 disease
   B. Patients with T4a primary tumors with gross thyroid cartilage invasion
   C. Patients with any T4a primary tumors
   D. Patients with bilateral/contralateral neck nodes
   E. A, D

5. A 27-year-old man presents with a history of dysphonia and a whitish lesion of the true vocal fold that was biopsied and noted to be severe dysplasia. What is the approximate rate of malignant transformation?
   A. 10%
   B. 20%
   C. 40%
   D. 50%
   E. 60%

Chapter 46
Chemotherapy and Immunotherapy for Head and Neck Cancer

Overview of Systemic Therapies in Head and Neck Squamous Cell Carcinoma

- The head and neck primary sites in which head and neck squamous cell carcinoma (HNSCC) may arise include the oral cavity (OC), oropharynx (OPC), larynx, hypopharynx, sinonasal cavity, and paranasal sinuses.
- The role of cytotoxic chemotherapy was first established in HNSCC in the 1970s when agents such as cisplatin, 5-fluorouracil (5-FU), methotrexate, and bleomycin showed activity in HNSCC.
- The role of systemic therapy in definitive treatment of HNSCC is first determined by whether treatment is in the postoperative (adjuvant) setting or given definitively (ie, as the primary treatment) with concurrent radiotherapy (RT) in patients who do not have surgery.
- In the 1990s, it became clear that combining chemotherapy with RT improves disease control and survival compared to RT alone. Moreover, the benefits of adding chemotherapy appeared limited to concurrent treatment with RT—concurrent chemoradiotherapy (CRT)—but not neoadjuvant or adjuvant chemotherapy alone.[1]
- The modern approach to CRT most often combines daily RT with weekly low-dose chemotherapy. The historical approach combined RT with bolus cisplatin (100 mg/m^2 every 3 weeks). Weekly cisplatin (40 mg/m^2) was compared with bolus cisplatin in two trials (JCOG1008 in the adjuvant setting, ConCERT trial in the definitive setting) and found weekly cisplatin to be noninferior in terms of efficacy and associated with less toxicity, and has since been adopted as the preferred modality of treatment. When patients are cisplatin-ineligible due to pre-existing medical conditions (severe baseline hearing loss, CrCl < 40 mL/minute, or baseline peripheral neuropathy) or cisplatin-intolerant due to cisplatin-related toxicity, alternative chemotherapy regimens can be used with a preference for carboplatin-based treatment.
- While there is no current role for neoadjuvant chemotherapy in patients with locally advanced HNSCC for whom an upfront operative approach is planned, there is an emerging role for anti-PD-1 immune checkpoint inhibitor (ICI) treatment that recently showed improved event-free survival (EFS) in patients with stage III or IVA HNSCC (phase 3 KEYNOTE-689 study [NCT03765918]).
- For unresectable recurrent and/or metastatic (R/M) HNSCC, anti-PD-1 ICI treatment with or without chemotherapy (based on whether the PD-L1 combined positive score

Table 46-1 The Most Common Systemic Therapies Used in Standard of Care (SOC) Treatment of Head and Neck Cancer and Their Mechanisms of Action

Drug Group	*Agent*	*Target(s)*	*MOA*
Platinum	Cisplatin Carboplatin	DNA alkylator	Causes double-strand DNA breaks
Taxane	Paclitaxel Docetaxel	Microtubule inhibitor	Impairs mitosis
DNA antimetabolite	5-Fluorouracil	Pyrimidine antimetabolite	Incorporation into DNA during synthesis phase causes synthesis arrest
	Gemcitabine	Purine antimetabolite	
EGFR (HER1) inhibitor	Cetuximab Panitumumab	Monoclonal antibody-targeting EGFR	Decreases downstream growth signaling. Cetuximab also elicits antibody-dependent cell-mediated cytotoxicity
	Afatinib	Tyrosine kinase inhibitor targeting EGFR	
Immune checkpoint blockade	Pembrolizumab Nivolumab Toripalimab	PD-1 inhibitor	Reinvigorates exhausted T cells

[CPS] is low versus high) is the mainstay first line of treatment. Anti-PD-1 ICI treatment combined with cetuximab, a monoclonal antibody directed at epidermal growth factor receptor (EGFR), is an alternative first-line option for ICI-eligible patients who are ineligible for or expected to have difficulty tolerating chemotherapy. Cetuximab with chemotherapy is an alternative first-line option for patients who are ineligible for ICI.

- While the biologic underpinnings and treatment outcomes of HNSCC driven by human papillomavirus (HPV) are known to be distinct from HNSCC not associated with HPV, at present the use of systemic therapies, namely cytotoxic chemotherapy and anti-PD-1 ICI treatment, is similar regardless of HPV status.
- Clinical trials should be considered whenever they are available.

Definitive Treatment of HNSCC

- Definitive concurrent CRT is indicated in locoregionally advanced disease without distant metastasis, that is, Stage III, IVA, or IVB as determined by the American Joint Committee on Cancer (AJCC) 8th edition Staging System.
- The preferred concurrent CRT is weekly cisplatin throughout the course of radiation. But in patients who are cisplatin ineligible, the most frequently used alternative regimens are weekly carboplatin with or without weekly paclitaxel or cetuximab.
- In the definitive treatment setting, 8-year overall survival (48%) and progression-free survival (42%) are improved when concurrent chemotherapy is administered along with radiation in the appropriate patient population (Stage III-IVB tumors).[2] Survival is progressively better with more chemotherapy delivery during concurrent CRT but is also associated with greater toxicity.[3]

Adjuvant Treatment of HNSCC

- Adjuvant CRT is considered for patients whose final pathology identifies positive margins and/or extranodal extension (ENE). Based on a pooled analysis of EORTC 22931 and RTOG 9501, two large, randomized trials that compared adjuvant RT alone to concurrent CRT, both of these pathological high-risk features were found to identify patients who might benefit from the addition of concurrent chemotherapy to postoperative RT (PORT). EORTC 22931 defined margins as positive if tumor involved the tissue edge and margins as close if tumor cells were ≤ 5 mm from the tissue edge. RTOG 9501 defined margins as positive if tumor cells were present less than 0.1 mm from the tissue edge. A common practice is to consider tumor present ≤ 1 mm from the tumor edge as a positive margin. ENE is considered present if tumor cells are visualized penetrating through or residing beyond the lymph node capsule.[4-6]
- Based on eligibility criteria for EORTC 22931 and RTOG 9501, pathological features beyond margins and ENE may indicate a role for adjuvant CRT, including but not limited to greater than two lymph nodes involved, involvement of level 4 or 5 lymph nodes (OC and OPC only), extensive perineural invasion (PNI), and extensive lymphovascular invasion (LVI). In post-hoc analyses, the utility of these additional pathological features as individual predictors of survival was not reported, and thus, conclusions about their individual utility to determine the potential benefit of CRT cannot be assessed. Although the post-hoc analysis of EORTC 22931 and RTOG 9501 is compelling, these results must be interpreted with caution to ensure that the presence of positive margins or ENE is not the only two high-risk pathological features that warrant consideration for adjuvant CRT over RT. Rather, consideration of each patient's tumor, which includes all pathological features assessed, is necessary to individualize treatment to each patient.
- The same chemotherapeutics that can be used as radiosensitizing chemotherapy in definitive treatment may also be used in the adjuvant setting with a preference given for cisplatin whenever possible.

Special Considerations for HPV-Associated HNSCC

Definitive Treatment of HPV-Associated OPC

- HPV-associated OPC has had a distinct AJCC staging system from HPV-independent OPC since the 8th edition was published in 2019. This change was made to reflect the overall better prognosis in HPV-associated OPC than HPV-independent HNSCC.
- It is important to remember that the good cancer-related outcomes in HPV-associated OPC that were established in earlier trials (eg, RTOG 0129) enrolled patients staged according to AJCC 7th edition when HPV-associated OPC was staged the same as HPV-independent OPC. Therefore, even though the AJCC 8th edition has been in use since 2017, patient selection for treatment—that is, definitive RT versus definitive CRT—requires determining both the AJCC 8th edition stage to provide a patient with a more accurate estimate of prognosis, and AJCC 7th edition stage to optimally select patients for CRT versus RT.

- Concurrent cisplatin-based CRT causes significant acute- and long-term treatment-related toxicity. Therefore, after it became clear that HPV-associated OPC was associated with much higher cure rates than their HPV-independent counterparts, a major effort was undertaken to de-escalate treatment intensity in these good-prognosis patients. Several de-escalation clinical trials have been conducted with the goal of finding a lower intensity regimen for treatment while not compromising the high cure rates of HPV-associated OPC. To date, the two largest de-escalation trials (RTOG 1016 and De-ESCALaTE) randomized patients with locally advanced HPV-associated OPC to standard RT with either cisplatin or cetuximab. These de-escalation trials have overall yielded disappointing results, showing in that, both in assessing recurrence rates (De-ESCALaTE, 2-year recurrence rate 16.1% vs 6.0%; RTOG 1016, 5-recurrence rate 17.3% vs 9.9%;) and overall survival (De-ESCALaTE, 2-year OS (overall survival) 89.4% vs 97.5%; RTOG 1016, 5-year OS 77.9% vs 84.6%), cetuximab is an inferior radiosensitizer compared to chemotherapy in HPV-associated tumors. There was also little difference in acute (77.4% vs 81.7%) or long-term (16.5% vs 20.4%) toxicity between the two arms.[7,8]

Adjuvant Treatment of HPV-Associated OPC

- Adjuvant treatment of HPV-associated OPC has a slightly different approach from its HPV-independent counterpart because HPV-associated OPC is associated with a better overall prognosis. De-escalation approaches to de-intensify treatment have also been prospectively evaluated. EA3311 was a pivotal trial evaluating adjuvant treatment of HPV-associated OPC. This was a large, randomized phase 2 study that comprised 360 patients eligible for analysis. After resection for HPV-associated OPC, patients were stratified into *low-* (T1-T2 resected with negative [> 3 mm] margins, N0-N1 and no ENE), *intermediate-* (T1-T2 resected to negative or close [< 3 mm] margins, N1-N2 with ≤ 1 mm ENE, or up to four positive nodes), and *high-risk* (positive margins, > 1 mm of ENE, and/or ≥ 5 metastatic lymph nodes) groups based on pathology. Low-risk patients (N = 38, Arm A) were observed, high-risk patients (N = 113, Arm D) received standard adjuvant CRT (66 Gy + weekly cisplatin 40 mg/m^2), and intermediate-risk patients (N = 208; n = 100 to 50 Gy [Arm B] and n = 109 to 60 Gy [Arm C]) were randomized to receive 50 Gy (reduced dose) versus 60 Gy (standard adjuvant dose) of radiation alone. Three-year PFS (progression free survival) estimates indicate that survival was comparable among all four groups (Arm A: 96.9%, Arm B: 94.9%, Arm C: 93.5%, Arm D: 90.7%) with a trend toward worse survival in high-risk patients. This trial indicates that when patients with HPV-associated tumors have been surgically staged, treatment de-escalation can be considered in the form of omitting chemotherapy or using lower doses of RT in approximately 60% of patients.[9,10]

Other Special Considerations

Organ Preservation

- A fundamental tenet of treating patients with any cancer is the balance of disease control with treatment toxicity. Patients with head and neck cancer are an exceptionally susceptible group to both acute and long-term treatment-related toxicity due primarily to the unique anatomical regions involved, namely, delicate organs that are essential for breathing, eating, and drinking. To this end, patient selection for surgical versus nonsurgical curative intent approaches with similar rates of long-term disease control is essential and requires robust multidisciplinary care.

- Larynx cancer is a common disease site in which organ preservation is preferred if there is sufficient preoperative laryngeal function. An essential component of organ-preserving treatment is the prompt implementation of salvage surgery in the event of tumor recurrence. This approach showed equal efficacy in the VA larynx study, which randomized 332 patients with advanced larynx SCC to sequential induction chemotherapy then radiation (IC → RT) versus surgery then radiation (surgery → RT) and found similar 2-year OS 68% vs 68%.[11] RTOG 91-11 randomized 520 patients with advanced larynx SCC to concurrent CRT (n = 174), sequential induction chemotherapy then RT (n = 174, IC → RT), and RT alone (n = 172). All 5- and 10-year cancer-related outcomes supported the use of concurrent CRT (5-year OS 55.1%), with numerically similar survival in sequentially treated patients (5-year OS 58.1%) and RT-treated patients (5-year OS 53.8%) but significantly worse rates of local control (LC), locoregional control (LRC), and distant control (DC) in patients who received RT alone (LC 71.1% vs 53.6%, LRC 67.7% vs 51.2%, and DC 86.4% vs 78.0%, respectively).[12]
- Oropharyngeal cancer is another anatomical site in which organ preservation is often preferred for advanced cancers. In the United States, most oropharyngeal cancers are HPV-associated, and based on the ORATOR-1 trial survival outcomes are similar between surgically treated patients and those treated with definitive CRT (3-year OS 88.2% vs 87.2%, 3-year PFS 85.3% vs 87.3%) without significant differences in quality of life (QoL) at 3 years according to results of preplanned analysis of prospectively collected MD Anderson Dysphagia Inventory (MDADI).[13]
- Organ preservation for hypopharyngeal lesions has not been prospectively assessed, but resection of advanced hypopharyngeal lesions often results in severe functional impairment that may lead to serious long-term effects of treatment, including chronic aspiration and permanent feeding tube dependence. Therefore, definitive CRT is often strongly considered for these patients.
- Oral cavity tumors are an important exception to the general rule that organ-preserving approaches provide patients with comparable cancer-related outcomes with surgical management. Various retrospective studies have demonstrated inferior survival outcomes in patients with oral cavity tumors who receive definitive CRT compared to those who undergo surgical resection followed by pathology-informed adjuvant therapy. [14]

Induction Chemotherapy

- Induction chemotherapy (IC) with high-dose multiagent chemotherapy is administered before proceeding to CRT and most often consists of doceTaxel, cisPlatin, 5-FU (TPF).[15,16]
- In large randomized trials, TPF was associated with improved cancer-related outcomes compared to PF (cisPlatin, 5-FU)[15,16] but studies that randomized patients to CRT versus IC followed by CRT did not indicate an overall survival benefit with IC, and therefore it is not a standard approach to treating HNSCC with the exception of nasopharyngeal cancer (NPC) as is described below.[17,18]

- Anecdotally, IC is used in selected cases of non-NPC HNSCC, such as when a tumor is growing rapidly and encroaching upon vital structures, which is a clinical scenario often seen in aggressive sinonasal carcinoma.

Systemic Therapy for Recurrent and/or Metastatic Head and Neck Cancer

- Stage IVC represents distant metastatic disease and is generally considered incurable. In addition, unresectable locoregionally recurrent disease is typically incurable. Thus, the goal of systemic therapy when not paired with RT is palliative.
- The preferred first-line therapy for R/M HNSCC is based on data from KEYNOTE-048, which showed that pembrolizumab (anti-PD-1 ICI treatment) improves OS compared to the EXTREME regimen (cisplatin, 5-FU, cetuximab). In the KEYNOTE-048 regimen participants received combination cisplatin, 5-FU, and pembrolizumab every 3 weeks for 6 cycles then pembrolizumab maintenance therapy every 3 weeks to complete 2 years of treatment; participants could also receive pembrolizumab every 3 weeks without chemotherapy at the investigator's discretion if their PD-L1 was high; participants in KEYNOTE-048 receiving the EXTREME regimen received chemotherapy plus cetuximab received the combination until intolerability or progression; however, in the landmark EXTREME regimen trial (cisplatin/5-FU versus cisplatin/5-FU/cetuximab) participants received a maximum of 6 cycles of combination chemotherapy plus cetuximab before moving on to cetuximab maintenance therapy.[19,20] This trial showed that immunotherapy-based regimens are more effective than cetuximab-based regimens for first-line treatment of R/M HNSCC, and that higher PD-L1 CPS is associated with better survival in patients who receive immunotherapy. However, cisplatin and 5-FU can cause significant AEs that make treatment difficult to tolerate, and therefore, carboplatin plus paclitaxel is often selected as the chemotherapy pair for pembrolizumab based on KEYNOTE-B10, which showed similar rates of efficacy compared with cisplatin plus 5-FU (median OS 13.1 vs 13.0 months) but better tolerability. [19,21]
- Patients who are not fit for chemotherapy can be considered for anti-PD-1 treatment plus cetuximab based on phase 2 clinical trial data showing ORR 45%, median OS 18.4 months, and median PFS 6.5 months for pembrolizumab plus cetuximab (N = 33) in IO- and cetuximab-naïve patients, and ORR 22.2%, median OS 9.7 months, and median PFS 3.4 months for nivolumab plus cetuximab (N = 45) in the subsequent line setting. A phase 3 trial to confirm clinical benefit of this regimen is not yet underway.[22,23]
- Patients who progress on immunotherapy or are ineligible for immunotherapy can be offered cetuximab with chemotherapy based on the EXTREME (platinum, 5-FU, cetuximab) and TPExtreme (platinum, docetaxel, cetuximab) trials.[20,24] In the TPExtreme trial, 541 participants were randomized to the EXTREME or TPEx regimen. Participants in the EXTREME regimen arm (N = 270) received up to 6 cycles of chemotherapy plus cetuximab then cetuximab maintenance, and in the TPEx arm (N = 269) received up to four cycles of chemotherapy plus cetuximab then cetuximab maintenance. Median OS and PFS were comparable (13.4 months in EXTREME arm vs 14.5 months in TPEx arm, 6.2 months vs 6.0 months, respectively), and G3 and G4 events were less frequent in the TPEx arm (73% and 33% vs 87% and 46%). These data support the use of either

TPEx or EXTREME. The efficacy of these regimens in the post-ICI setting is not clearly defined but limited data indicate similar rates of response to cetuximab-containing regimens in the post-ICI setting compared to the pre-ICI era.
- Because survival remains poor for most patients, even with first-line immunotherapy, clinical trials should always be considered when available.

Nasopharynx Cancer

- Nasopharyngeal cancer is a unique entity among head and neck cancers because most cases are associated with Epstein-Barr virus infection, although some cases may be HPV-associated or virus-negative as in the case of nasopharyngeal radiation-related tumors, which may be seen in patients previously treated with RT for a separate HNSCC primary tumor.
- Given the location of nasopharyngeal tumors, resection is often not an option for treat ment but can occasionally be pursued after thorough multidisciplinary tumor board discussion.
- Unlike in non-NPC tumors, induction chemotherapy with gemcitabine and cisplatin followed by concurrent CRT is associated with improved overall survival compared to CRT alone. A phase 3 trial (N = 480 patients) randomized N = 238 patient to receive concurrent CRT and N = 242 to receive IC followed by concurrent CRT, and showed statistically significant improvement in 3-year OS (90.3% vs 94.6%) and 3-year recurrence-free survival (85.3% vs 76.5%).[25] Recent data from the randomized CONTINUUM trial (N = 425 patients) indicate that anti-PD-1 ICI plus IC (N = 210) compared to IC alone (N = 215) improves 3-year event-free survival (86% vs 76%) but these data are too premature to assess the impact of this regimen on OS thus the current SOC remains induction therapy with gemcitabine and cisplatin without ICI.[26]
- R/M NPC is treated in the first line with combination ICI plus chemotherapy (toripalimab, gemcitabine, and cisplatin) based on the randomized JUPITER-02 trial (N = 289) that showed an overall survival benefit when anti-PD-1 ICI was added to chemotherapy (median OS NR [not reached] vs 33.7 months).[27]

Areas of Clinical Investigation

- CRT plus immunotherapy: The rationale for this combination is that RT may enhance immunotherapy activity by numerous theorized mechanisms, including the abscopal effect. Unfortunately, this combination was shown to be ineffective in JAVELIN-100, NRG-HN004, and KEYNOTE-412, but NRG-HN005 and EA3161 are expected to report data in the coming years.
- Neoadjuvant immunotherapy in resectable HNSCC: There is strong biological rationale for neoadjuvant immunotherapy in solid tumors, partially focused on the opportunity to reinvigorate the full complement of exhausted T cells within the tumor immune microenvironment. When a tumor has been resected the exhausted but potentially tumor-specific intratumoral T cells are also removed with it, which could theoretically limit the efficacy of immunotherapy postoperatively. A recent study (KEYNOTE-689) of neoadjuvant/adjuvant immunotherapy with pembrolizumab in

advanced, resectable HNSCC was reported to have met its primary endpoint. These data have not been released but may be practice-changing for patients with advanced HNSCC planned for surgical resection.

- De-escalation with an assay to detect measurable residual disease (MRD): An attractive approach to improving early detection of recurrent tumors is the use of an MRD assay following completion of curative-intent treatment. This assay could either be a circulating tumor HPV DNA (ctHPVDNA) assay in HPV-associated tumors, or a mutation- or methylation-based assay that could be either tumor informed or tumor uninformed. Tumor-informed assays leverage the unique mutational and/or methylation profile of each individual patient's tumor to improve detectability of MRD in circulation. The assay would be serially monitored after completing curative-intent treatment. This concept is being actively studied and has accurately stratified patients who will versus will not experience recurrence, but it remains unknown if the application of this approach will lead to improved clinical outcomes.
- Induction chemotherapy plus ICI: This approach has not yet been studied in randomized prospective trials. A recent single-arm phase 2 trial of anti-PD-1 (camrelizumab) plus TPF induction for locally advanced hypopharyngeal SCC (cT3-4aN0-2M0) showed promising results with ORR 82.4% and 2-year OS, PFS, and larynx preservation rates of 83.0%, 77.1%, and 70.0%, respectively. These data warrant further prospective study of induction chemotherapy plus ICI.[28]
- Novel systemic therapies for R/M HNSCC: Exploration of bispecific antibody therapies and antibody-drug conjugate (ADC) therapies is active and promising. Bispecific antibodies under investigation include those targeting EGFR/TGFβ, EGFR/LGR5. ADCs under investigation include those targeting Trop2, Nectin-4, and tissue factor.[29]

References

1. Lacas B, Carmel A, Landais C, et al. Meta-analysis of chemotherapy in head and neck cancer (MACH-NC): An update on 107 randomized trials and 19,805 patients, on behalf of MACH-NC Group. *Radiother Oncol.* 2021;156:281-293.
2. Nguyen-Tan PF, Zhang Q, Ang KK, et al. Randomized phase III trial to test accelerated versus standard fractionation in combination with concurrent cisplatin for head and neck carcinomas in the radiation therapy oncology group 0129 trial: long-term report of efficacy and toxicity. *J Clin Oncol.* 2014;32:3858–3867.
3. Ang K, Zhang Q, Wheeler RH, et al. A phase III trial (RTOG 0129) of two radiation-cisplatin regimens for head and neck carcinomas (HNC): impact of radiation and cisplatin intensity on outcome. *J Clin Oncol* [Internet]. 2024;28:5507.
4. Bernier J, Domenge C, Ozsahin M, et al. Postoperative irradiation with or without concomitant chemotherapy for locally advanced head and neck cancer [Internet]. *N Engl J Med.* 2004;350: 1945-1952.
5. Bernier J, Cooper JS, Pajak TF, et al. Defining risk levels in locally advanced head and neck cancers: a comparative analysis of concurrent postoperative radiation plus chemotherapy trials of the EORTC (#22931) and RTOG (#9501). *Head Neck.* 2005;27:843-850.
6. Cooper JS, Zhang Q, Pajak TF, et al. Long-term follow-up of the RTOG 9501/intergroup phase III trial: postoperative concurrent radiation therapy and chemotherapy in high-risk squamous cell carcinoma of the head and neck. *Int J Radiat Oncol Biol Phys.* 2012;84:1198-1205.
7. Mehanna H, Robinson M, Hartley A, et al. Radiotherapy plus cisplatin or cetuximab in low-risk human papillomavirus-positive oropharyngeal cancer (De-ESCALaTE HPV): an open-label randomised controlled phase 3 trial. *Lancet.* 2019;393:51-60.

8. Gillison ML, Trotti AM, Harris J, et al. Radiotherapy plus cetuximab or cisplatin in human papillomavirus-positive oropharyngeal cancer (NRG Oncology RTOG 1016): a randomised, multicentre, non-inferiority trial. *Lancet.* 2019;393:40-50.
9. Ferris RL, Flamand Y, Weinstein GS, et al. Phase II randomized trial of transoral surgery and low-dose intensity modulated radiation therapy in resectable p161 locally advanced oropharynx cancer: An ECOG-ACRIN Cancer Research Group Trial (E3311). *J Clin Oncol* [Internet]. 2021;40:138-149.
10. Burtness B, Flamand Y, Quon H, et al. Long-term follow up of E3311, a phase II trial of transoral surgery (TOS) followed by pathology-based adjuvant treatment in HPV-associated (HPV+) oropharynx cancer (OPC): A trial of the ECOG-ACRIN Cancer Research Group. 2024;43(23):2559-2565.
11. Department of Veterans Affairs Laryngeal Cancer Study Group, Wolf GT, Fisher SG, Hong WK, et al. Induction chemotherapy plus radiation compared with surgery plus radiation in patients with advanced laryngeal cancer. *N Engl J Med.* 1991;324:1685-1690.
12. Forastiere AA, Zhang Q, Weber RS, et al. Long-term results of RTOG 91-11: a comparison of three nonsurgical treatment strategies to preserve the larynx in patients with locally advanced larynx cancer. *J Clin Oncol.* 2013;31:845-852.
13. Nichols AC, Theurer J, Prisman E, et al. Randomized trial of radiotherapy versus transoral robotic surgery for oropharyngeal squamous cell carcinoma: long-term results of the ORATOR trial. *J Clin Oncol* [Internet]. 2022;40:866-875.
14. Spiotto MT, Jefferson G, Wenig B, Markiewicz M, Weichselbaum RR, Koshy M. Differences in survival with surgery and postoperative radiotherapy compared with definitive chemoradiotherapy for oral cavity cancer: A National Cancer Database analysis. *JAMA Otolaryngol Head Neck Surg.* 2017;143:691-699.
15. Lorch JH, Goloubeva O, Haddad RI, et al. Induction chemotherapy with cisplatin and fluorouracil alone or in combination with docetaxel in locally advanced squamous-cell cancer of the head and neck: long-term results of the TAX 324 randomised phase 3 trial. *Lancet Oncol.* 2011;12:153-159.
16. Szturz P, Vinches M, Remenár É, et al. Prognostic factor analysis and long-term results of the TAX 323 (EORTC 24971) study in unresectable head and neck cancer patients. *Eur J Cancer.* 2021;156:109-118.
17. Haddad R, O'Neill A, Rabinowits G, et al. Induction chemotherapy followed by concurrent chemoradiotherapy (sequential chemoradiotherapy) versus concurrent chemoradiotherapy alone in locally advanced head and neck cancer (PARADIGM): a randomised phase 3 trial. *Lancet Oncol.* 2013;14:257-264.
18. Cohen EEW, Karrison TG, Kocherginsky M, et al. Phase III randomized trial of induction chemotherapy in patients with N2 or N3 locally advanced head and neck cancer. *J Clin Oncol.* 2014;32:2735-2743.
19. Burtness B, Harrington KJ, Greil R, et al. Pembrolizumab alone or with chemotherapy versus cetuximab with chemotherapy for recurrent or metastatic squamous cell carcinoma of the head and neck (KEYNOTE-048): a randomised, open-label, phase 3 study. *Lancet.* 2019;394:1915-1928.
20. Vermorken JB, Mesia R, Rivera F, et al. Platinum-based chemotherapy plus cetuximab in head and neck cancer [Internet]. *N Engl J Med.* 2008.
21. Dzienis M, Cundom J, Fuentes CS, et al. Pembrolizumab plus carboplatin and paclitaxel as first-line therapy for recurrent/metastatic head and neck squamous cell carcinoma (KEYNOTE-B10): a single-arm Phase IV Trial. *J Clin Oncol.* 2024;42:2989-2999.
22. Chung CH, Bonomi M, Steuer CE, et al. Concurrent cetuximab and nivolumab as a second-line or beyond treatment of patients with recurrent and/or metastatic head and neck squamous cell carcinoma: Results of phase i/ii study. *Cancers* (Basel). 2021;13:1-16.
23. Sacco AG, Chen R, Worden FP, et al. Pembrolizumab plus cetuximab in patients with recurrent or metastatic head and neck squamous cell carcinoma: an open-label, multi-arm, non-randomised, multicentre, phase 2 trial. *Lancet Oncol.* 2021;22:883-892.

24. Guigay J, Aupérin A, Fayette J, et al. Cetuximab, docetaxel, and cisplatin versus platinum, fluorouracil, and cetuximab as first-line treatment in patients with recurrent or metastatic head and neck squamous-cell carcinoma (GORTEC 2014-01 TPExtreme): a multicentre, open-label, randomised, phase 2 trial. *Lancet Oncol*. 2021;22:463-475.
25. Zhang Y, Chen L, Hu G-Q, et al. Gemcitabine and cisplatin induction chemotherapy in nasopharyngeal carcinoma. *N Engl J Med*. 2019;381:1124-1135.
26. Liu X, Zhang Y, Yang KY, et al. Induction-concurrent chemoradiotherapy with or without sintilimab in patients with locoregionally advanced nasopharyngeal carcinoma in China (CONTINUUM): a multicentre, open-label, parallel-group, randomised, controlled, phase 3 trial. *Lancet*. 2024;403:2720-2731.
27. Mai HQ, Chen QY, Chen D, et al. Toripalimab plus chemotherapy for recurrent or metastatic nasopharyngeal carcinoma: The JUPITER-02 Randomized Clinical Trial. *JAMA*. 2023;330:1961-1970.
28. Gong H, Tian S, Ding H, et al. Camrelizumab-based induction chemoimmunotherapy in locally advanced stage hypopharyngeal carcinoma: phase II clinical trial. *Nat Commun*. 2024;15.
29. Park JC, Shin D. Current landscape of antibody-drug conjugate development in head and neck cancer. *JCO Precis Oncol*. 2024;8:e2400179.

Questions

1. A patient with oral cavity SCC undergoes surgery and reconstruction revealing a pT3N1 tumor. Adjuvant chemoradiotherapy can be considered in all of the following situations EXCEPT
   A. Positive margins
   B. Residual gross tumor
   C. Extranodal extension present
   D. One focus of lymphovascular invasion
   E. None of the above

2. A patient with HPV-associated oropharyngeal cancer is AJCC 8th edition Stage I (cT2N1), AJCC 7th edition Stage IVA (cT2N2a). Definitive chemoradiotherapy should be considered as the nonsurgical treatment approach.
   A. True
   B. False

3. A patient is being offered definitive chemoradiotherapy for Stage IVA p16-negative oropharyngeal cancer. The patient has severe hearing loss at baseline and uses hearing aids to communicate, and also has severe peripheral neuropathy from prior chemotherapy received to treat breast cancer. Which of the following is not a reasonable radiosensitizing chemotherapy option?
   A. Cisplatin
   B. Carboplatin
   C. Carboplatin plus paclitaxel
   D. Paclitaxel
   E. Docetaxel
   F. None of the above

4. A patient with advanced oral cavity squamous cell carcinoma undergoes composite resection and reconstruction. Final pathology reveals PNI but no positive margins or ENE. He received adjuvant radiotherapy. Two years later he presents with new oral pain. Exam revealed a locally recurrent tumor. Cross-sectional imaging reveals numerous new lung nodules, and transthoracic percutaneous biopsy proves metastatic carcinoma. Patient is restaged ACJJ Stage IVC oral cavity carcinoma. PD-L1 CPS is assessed and found to be high (75%). He has no history of autoimmune disease. Which of the following are reasonable first-line treatment options?
   A. Carboplatin plus 5-FU plus pembrolizumab
   B. Carboplatin plus paclitaxel plus pembrolizumab
   C. Pembrolizumab
   D. Cetuximab plus carboplatin plus 5-FU
   E. None of the above

5. A patient presents with 6 months of nasal congestion and is found to have a tumor within the right Fossa of Rosenmuller. Biopsy is positive for nasopharyngeal carcinoma, EBV positive. Cross-sectional imaging reveals pathologically enlarged cervical lymphadenopathy but no distant metastases. Which of the following is the appropriate first step in management?
   A. Induction chemotherapy
   B. Concurrent chemoradiotherapy
   C. Induction chemoimmunotherapy
   D. Radiotherapy
   E. Surgical resection
   F. None of the above

Chapter 47
Radiation Therapy for Head and Neck Cancer

Background

- Radiation induces double-strand breaks within DNA, killing tumor cells.
- Normal tissues have a greater ability to repair radiation-induced damage as compared to tumor cells.
  - This difference is exploited by fractionating radiation therapy.
- For head and neck (H&N) cancer, radiation is usually delivered 5 days a week over 6 to 7 weeks.
- Each daily radiation treatment for a patient is the same as the day prior. Treatment breaks are highly discouraged due to tumor repopulation during breaks.
- Active smoking during radiation diminishes treatment effectiveness.

Radiation Dose

- The unit of radiation is Gray (Gy), and 1 Gy is equal to 1 joule (J) of energy absorbed per kilogram of matter.
- Daily doses of radiation are usually in the range of 1.8 to 2.0 Gy/day.
- Total radiation doses depend on tumor type and histology, but in general:
  - 50 to 56 Gy is used to sterilize microscopic disease such as in the clinically negative neck at risk for lymphatic nodal spread.
  - 60 to 63 Gy is used either in the postoperative setting to control microscopic residual disease within the postoperative bed or in definitive settings to cover regions at high risk of microscopic disease extension. This dose is also used for intermediate-risk areas in the neck such as lymph node levels with involved nodal disease.
  - 66 Gy is typically used for postoperative positive margins or regions where extranodal extension was present.
  - 70 Gy is used to control gross tumor with curative intent.
- Typically, a treatment plan will simultaneously dose different anatomic regions within each daily fraction.
  - For example, when treating an oropharyngeal cancer, one can give gross tumor 2 Gy per fraction, while giving high-risk nodal areas 1.8 Gy per fraction, while giving the uninvolved low neck 1.6 Gy per day in 35 daily fractions.
  - This provides a total dose of 70 Gy to the primary tumor and gross lymph nodes, 63 Gy to high-risk areas, and 56 Gy to low-risk areas.

Radiation Therapy Techniques

Three-Dimensional Conformal Radiation Therapy (3D-CRT)

- A form of photon (X-ray) radiation that refers to the use of CT-based radiation planning.
- The tumor and avoidance structures are contoured on axial CT images.
- Radiation therapy is planned, usually with two to six beams, with the goals of treating the tumor and avoiding critical structures.
- In the modern era, this is used primarily in palliative H&N RT or treatment of early-stage larynx cancer.

Intensity Modulated Radiation Therapy (IMRT)

- IMRT is a form of photon radiation that generally provides a significant advantage over 3D-CRT, and is now standard of care in H&N radiation therapy.
- IMRT uses many beams or arcs (known as VMAT or volumetric arc therapy) to deliver thousands of tiny beams of radiation from many angles to conform radiation dose around critical normal structures such as the major salivary glands, pharyngeal constrictor muscles, or the spinal cord to deliver a high dose to targets.

Proton Therapy

- Proton therapy employs the use of a particle accelerator to deliver RT with hydrogen ions. The dose absorption in tissue can have favorable physical properties; however, it is not uniformly favored over IMRT for technical reasons.
- The strongest indications for proton therapy include use for pediatric, chordoma, ocular, and re-irradiation cases.

Image-Guided Radiation Therapy (IGRT)

- IGRT refers to the incorporation of three-dimensional imaging prior to radiation delivery.
- Prior to each treatment, a CT imaging study (aka "Simulation" or "mapping") is performed in the treatment position to confirm alignment of the target volumes.

Role of Radiation in Head and Neck Cancers

- Radiation therapy (RT) plays a critical role in the management of head and neck cancer.
- RT can be used as curative intent treatment alone or with combined chemotherapy which sensitizes both cancer cells and normal cells to the effects of radiation.
- RT is frequently used postoperatively for patients with an elevated risk of recurrence based on stage and pathologic findings. Postoperative RT is most effective if started within 6 weeks of surgery but rarely starts prior to 4 weeks post-op due to concerns with delayed healing.
- Preoperative radiation is not routinely used in head and neck cancer.

Toxicity

- Toxicity is highly correlated with the site treated, RT dose, fractionation schedule, and prioritization of normal tissue during RT planning.
- RT-induced skin toxicity
  - Skin toxicity is common, especially when neck radiation is included in the treatment plan.
  - RT targeting subdermal structures such as primary tumor or lymph nodes may damage basal dermal progenitor cells.
  - Desquamation may begin within 4 weeks as damaged basal skin cells are not replaced.

  - Following RT, skin toxicity may worsen for several days.
  - Mild/moderate dermatitis and desquamation will generally self-resolve within 2 to 3 weeks unless superimposed infection is present.

Acute Complications

- Mucositis/Pain
  - May occur by third week of RT.
  - Usually resolves within 2 to 4 weeks after RT completion.
  - Prevalence varies by anatomic site, RT dose, and use of systemic therapy.
  - Most oral or oropharynx RT cases will get grade 2 or higher mucositis.
  - Odynophagia is a significant cause of weight loss and gastrostomy tube placement.
  - Mucositis appears as white ulcerated patches of the oral cavity, may be confused with thrush.
  - Management:
    - Meticulous oral hygiene
    - Aggressive pain management
      - ◊ Mucosal lidocaine HCL 2% (cheaper and similarly effective to compounded "magic mouthwash")
      - ◊ NSAIDs
      - ◊ Nonopioid analgesics such as gabapentin and pregabalin
      - ◊ Short and/or long-acting oral or transdermal narcotic
- Fungal infection (candidiasis)
  - Due to disruption of mucosal barriers, typically at least 2 weeks after starting RT
  - Symptoms include
    - White plaque that can often be wiped off revealing bleeding/irritated mucosa
    - Pain/burning out of proportion to mucositis
    - Altered taste (also very common from RT)
  - Management
    - Fluconazole 200 mg PO on day 1 and then 100 mg daily for a total of 7 to 14-day course.
    - Nystatin or clotrimazole lozenges can be effective but treatment failure is higher.
- Dysgeusia
  - Occurs at low RT dose to base of tongue, often early in treatment
  - Results in bland or noxious taste
  - Most patients experience taste recovery within 3 months of RT; permanent lack of taste is rare
- Dysphagia
  - Results from tumor destruction of pharyngeal or laryngeal structures in combination with (acute) inflammation or (chronic) fibrosis from radiation
  - Management
    - Referral to specialist for swallow evaluation
    - Gastrostomy tube indicated for short-term feeding in many patients
- Xerostomia
  - May manifest early in treatment if salivary glands are proximate to treatment targets
  - Worst in the months after treatment, may continue to improve for 2 years
  - Management
    - Oral rinse with a solution of one-fourth teaspoon baking soda and one-eighth teaspoon salt mixed in one cup of warm water; biotene mouthwash.
    - Xylimelt lozenges, OTC.
    - Humidified air at bedtime.

    - Pilocarpine or cevimeline is indicated in refractory severe xerostomia but has mixed results.
    - Thickened secretions benefit from guaifenesin extended release 600 mg to 1.2 g po every 12 hours as needed.
    - Glycopyrrolate/scopolamine is avoided in most non-end-of-life situations as they can make secretions harder to expectorate.

Late Complications

- Dental problems arise as a consequence of xerostomia.
  - Predisposes to dental caries as saliva has bactericidal properties.
  - Prevention/Management
    - Meticulous dental care
    - Treat xerostomia
    - Prescription fluoride toothpaste or dental trays
    - Restoration/root canal/gum grafting as needed—no significant increased risk for poor outcome posttreatment
    - Extractions or dental implants (eg, bone manipulation) are associated with increased risk of osteonecrosis if the area received greater than 4000 cGy of radiation; consult a radiation oncologist if these procedures are under consideration
- Osteoradionecrosis (ORN) of jaw
  - Rare toxicity occurring from RT in addition to mechanical insult or RT alone
  - May occur as early as 3 months post-RT
  - Management includes possible combination of
    - Meticulous oral hygiene
    - Surgical debridement
    - Culture of wound and long-term antibiotics
    - Pentoxifylline 400 mg PO BID (contraindicated if active cancer present) until ORN improves
    - Vitamin E 1000 IU daily
    - Hyperbaric oxygen in refractory cases
- Trismus
  - Results from fibrosis of pterygoid muscles, temporomandibular joint (TMJ), or oral soft tissues from surgery or RT
  - Management
    - Trismus exercises managed by speech therapist, physical therapist, head and neck surgeon, or others
    - Possible adjunctive stretching device use (Therabite or Orastretch)
- Lymphedema of the neck
  - Results from surgery and/or RT to the neck
  - Typically peaks in the months following treatment and is present in the submental region
  - Management
    - Decongestive physical therapy by a trained lymphedema specialist
- Hearing change
  - Often caused by cisplatin
  - Can also result from high-dose RT to cochlea for nasopharynx or skull base cancers
  - Inflammation in the eustachian orifice secondary to radiation can cause middle ear effusion

  - Management
    - Referral for formal otology and possible hearing aids
    - Middle ear effusion often self-resolves; otherwise, myringotomy may be performed
- Hypothyroidism
  - Occurs in up to one-third of patients with bilateral neck RT, lower risk in unilateral neck treatment
  - Annual thyroid function testing in asymptomatic patients beginning at 1 year post RT
  - Management
    - Levothyroxine

Role of Radiation Therapy in Specific Disease Sites

Larynx Cancer

- RT alone is often used for early-stage larynx carcinoma, T1-2N0.
- In these settings narrow field irradiation, consisting of a field extending from the hyoid bone down to the cricoid is often used; 3D RT or IMRT may be used, local control is greater than 90%
- Larynx preservation with chemoradiation is typically an option for patients with locally advanced laryngeal tumors, with T3 and select T4a and/or positive lymph nodes, provided that the airway is stable, pretreatment swallow function is largely intact, and there is no deep thyroid cartilage invasion.
- Concurrent chemoradiation has shown the best rates of larynx preservation, with an 88% rate of larynx preservation at 2 years in RTOG 91-11.[1]
- Survival is equivalent for patients receiving laryngectomy or larynx preservation so long as early surgical salvage is considered for patients with residual or recurrent disease.
- Indications for postoperative radiation include T4 primary (not T3 like other HN subsites), pN1 disease, PNI, LVI, and close margin. Indications for adjuvant chemoradiation include positive margin or extranodal extension.

Hypopharynx Cancer

- Concurrent chemoradiation is the preferred approach when attempting larynx preservation in patients with hypopharyngeal cancer.
- Given the rich lymphatic network of the hypopharynx, nodal and distant metastases occur at higher rate than larynx cancer.

Nasopharynx Cancer

- Nasopharynx is always managed nonoperatively.
- Patients have a high rate of level II, V, and retropharyngeal nodal involvement.
- Disease frequently spreads from nasopharynx into skull, and thus, a detailed cranial nerve exam is important in all patients.
- PET/CT and MRI studies are useful parts of the staging process.
- Epstein-Barr virus is responsible for endemic cases; viral DNA titers should be drawn pretreatment and in surveillance.
- For T1-2N0 tumors, radiation alone can be considered.
- For T3+ or node-positive disease, cisplatin-based chemoradiation is favored.
- Three cycles of induction chemotherapy are typically given prior to chemoRT for advanced EBV+ disease.[2] Induction or adjuvant chemotherapy is often considered for advanced EBV-negative disease.

Oral Cavity Tumors

- Oral cavity cancers are generally managed surgically, with consideration of radiation as an adjuvant therapy based on the final pathologic results.
- Indications for postoperative radiation include T3/T4 primary, pN1 disease, PNI, LVI, close margin. Indications for adjuvant chemoradiation include positive margin or extranodal extension.
- Depth of invasion alone, without other risk factors present (see above), does not typically represent an independent indication for adjuvant radiation in T1-T2N0 oral cavity cancer.[3]
- For small early-stage (T1-2N0) well-lateralized tumors of the buccal mucosa, retromolar trigone, and gingiva, radiation therapy to the primary site and ipsilateral neck can be considered.
- For cancers of midline structure, the bilateral necks should be managed with neck dissection +/– bilateral neck radiation if risk factors are present.

Oropharynx Cancer

- The incidence of oropharyngeal carcinoma is increasing due to an increase in HPV-associated tumors, with estimates that currently around 90% of all newly diagnosed tumors are associated with HPV.
- Data demonstrates that HPV-associated tumors carry a favorable prognosis.
- In the HN005 study which evaluated T1-2N1M0 or T3N0-N1M0 (AJCC 8th edition) oropharyngeal squamous cell carcinoma and ≤ 10 pack-year smoking history, 2-year PFS was 98.1%.
- It should be noted that HPV-associated tumors in smokers with a greater than 10 pack-year history of smoking have a worse prognosis than nonsmokers.[4]
- Current trials are aimed and potentially de-escalating therapy for HPV-associated tumors; however, recent data from NRG HN005 failed to demonstrate equivalence of de-escalated radiation or systemic therapy approaches in an unselected cohort of HPV+ oropharynx cases.[5]
- As of early 2025, it is recommended to only offer de-escalated definitive treatment in the setting of a clinical trial.
- Patients with T1-2N0 disease can be treated with radiation alone. Controversy exists about the requirement for concurrent chemotherapy in the setting of a single involved LN less than 3 cm in size. Multiple nodes or T3 disease are indications for definitive chemoradiation.
- Patients with small, well-lateralized tumors with no or minimal nodal disease can be considered for ipsilateral only irradiation.

Salivary Gland Tumors

- Salivary gland tumors are primarily managed surgically when feasible, with adjuvant therapy based on the results of final pathology.
- Radiation is generally recommended in patients with T3+ disease, high-grade tumors, node-positive tumors, positive margins, perineural invasion, and in patients with recurrent tumors.
- For adenoid cystic carcinomas, adjuvant irradiation should always be considered.
    - Given the high propensity for perineural spread of this disease, it is generally advised to radiate the pathway of at-risk nerves to their location at the base of skull.

- For example, in an adenoid cystic carcinoma of the parotid, irradiation would be given to the path of the V2 and 7th cranial nerves to the base of skull, to decrease the rate of relapse due to growth of tumor cells along the nerve.

Postoperative Radiation Therapy

- Radiation therapy is often offered to patients postoperatively, depending on the final pathologic results.
- Potential indications for irradiation include:
  - Close (< 3-5mm) or positive margins
  - Extracapsular extension of lymph nodes
  - Multiple nodes positive
  - T3-T4 primary tumors
  - Perineural invasion
  - Lymphovascular invasion
- In the case of positive margins or extracapsular extension of lymph nodes, chemotherapy (preferably with cisplatin) concurrently with irradiation should be considered.[6]
- The timing of radiation in the postoperative setting matters, and data have shown improved outcomes when radiation is completed by 12 weeks.[7]
- This implies that radiation, which is usually 6 to 6 ½ weeks in length, should optimally start 5 to 6 weeks postsurgery.

Palliative Radiation

- Palliative radiation can be used for de novo or previously radiated H&N cancers causing symptoms or at high risk of causing symptoms.
  - Common symptoms that may benefit include pain, bleeding, or obstruction
- Numerous radiation fractionation schedules with varying equivalent intensities of radiation exist.
  - Palliative RT may be as few as three fractions delivered weekly or 20 fractions delivered daily; some paradigms include twice daily treatment as well.
  - In general palliative RT remains an option for most patients who have received a single prior course of radiation, though patient performance status, expected survival, and other available therapies should be considered prior to its use.

Re-irradiation

- Failures arising in an irradiated field are difficult to manage.
- The ideal treatment in this situation is surgical resection.
- Often, however, if surgery is not possible, and a repeat course of irradiation therapy is the only potentially curative option.
- Re-irradiation is potentially curative for a minority of patients. In highly selected patient populations, it is associated with a 2-year locoregional control of approximately 50%.[8]
- Re-irradiation therapy has a potentially high likelihood of toxicity, and patient selection is paramount.
- The time interval between the initial course of irradiation and the consideration of re-irradiation is of critical importance, and retreatment within less than 6 months is not considered.
- Recurrences that occur in the field less than 1 year after the initial course of irradiation are likely somewhat radiation resistant and represent persistent disease; these are not optimal candidates for re-irradiation.

- The ideal patient has a small recurrence or new primary cancer with very limited or no nodal disease in an area that was previously irradiated several years ago.
- Effort must be made to limit overlap, and in the case of re-irradiation we have typically only treated gross tumor alone with no elective irradiation.
- We have also typically re-irradiated in conjunction with radiosensitizing chemotherapy.
- Consideration should be given to hyperfractionated irradiation when performing re-irradiation—that is, breaking the daily dose of irradiation into two fractions given 6 hours apart.
    - This has been shown to lead to less late toxic effects in patients receiving reirradiation for nasopharyngeal cancer.[9]
    - The downside of this approach is the logistical issues of requiring a patient to come to the radiation center twice daily.
- One can also consider re-irradiation in the adjuvant setting, generally advised only for positive (< 1 mm margin) or extranodal extension. Adjuvant reirradiation was tested in a randomized trial and shown to lead to an improvement in locoregional control and disease-free survival, although no overall survival benefit was noted. Toxicity was significant with nearly 40% of patients having Grade 3-4 late toxicity at 2 years.[10]

Neck Dissection Following Definitive Chemoradiation

- The practice of elective neck dissection for patients undergoing chemoradiation has generally fallen out of favor due to high rates of neck dissection which showed no residual tumor.
- Prospective study has supported our current approach of performing a 12-week post-therapy PET/CT scan and observing patients with PET-negative disease.[11]

Questions

1. Patients found to have extracapsular extension following surgical resection should be treated with adjuvant
   A. Concurrent chemoradiation
   B. Conventionally fractionated radiation alone
   C. Accelerated radiation alone
   D. Observation

2. The dose of radiation traditionally used for gross disease is
   A. 50 Gy
   B. 60 Gy
   C. 70 Gy
   D. 80 Gy

3. Radiation therapy is usually given in daily doses of
   A. 1 Gy/day
   B. 1.5 Gy/day
   C. 2 Gy/day
   D. 2.5 Gy/day

4. Which is true in general about larynx preservation?
   A. Rates of larynx preservation are generally less than 50%.
   B. Larynx preservation allows a substantial percentage of patients to preserve their larynx; however, this comes at the cost of inferior survival.
   C. Induction chemotherapy followed by radiation offers the best chance of larynx preservation.
   D. The rate of larynx preservation in patients with gross penetration through the thyroid cartilage is less than 50%.

5. Studies have demonstrated that surgery and postoperative radiation should be completed in what time period for optimal results?
   A. 9 weeks
   B. 12 weeks
   C. 15 weeks
   D. 17 weeks

References

1. Forastiere AA, Goepfert H, Maor M, et al. Concurrent chemotherapy and radiotherapy for organ preservation in advanced laryngeal cancer. *N Engl J Med*. 2003;349(22):2091-2098.
2. Zhang Y, Chen L, Hu GQ, et al. Gemcitabine and cisplatin induction chemotherapy in nasopharyngeal carcinoma. *N Engl J Med*. 2019;381(12):1124-1135. doi:10.1056/NEJMoa1905287.
3. Ebrahimi A, Gil Z, Amit, M, et al. Depth of invasion alone as an indication for postoperative radiotherapy in small oral squamous cell carcinomas: An International Collaborative Study. *Head Neck*. 2019;41(6):1935-1942.
4. Ang KK, Harris J, Wheeler R, et al. Human papillomavirus and survival of patients with oropharyngeal cancer. *N Engl J Med*. 2010;363(1):24-35.
5. Yom SS, Harris J, Caudell JJ, et al. Interim futility results of NRG-HN005, a randomized, phase II/III non-inferiority trial for non-smoking p16-positive oropharyngeal cancer patients. *Int J Radiat Oncol Biol Phys*. 2024;120(2):S2-S3.
6. Bernier J, Cooper JS, Pajak TF, et al. Defining risk levels in locally advanced head and neck cancers: a comparative analysis of concurrent postoperative radiation plus chemotherapy trials of the EORTC (#22931) and RTOG (# 9501). *Head Neck*. 2005;27(10):843-850.
7. Rosenthal DI, Mohamed ASR, Garden AS, et al. Final report of a prospective randomized trial to evaluate the dose-response relationship for postoperative radiation therapy and pathologic risk groups in patients with head and neck cancer. *Int J Radiat Oncol Biol Phys*. 2017;98(5):1002-1011.
8. Romesser PB, Cahlon O, Scher ED, et al. Proton beam reirradiation for recurrent head and neck cancer: multi-institutional report on feasibility and early outcomes. *Int J Radiat Oncol Biol Phys*. 2016;95(1):386-395.
9. You R, Liu YP, Xie YL, et al. Hyperfractionation compared with standard fractionation in intensity-modulated radiotherapy for patients with locally advanced recurrent nasopharyngeal carcinoma: a multicentre, randomised, open-label, phase 3 trial. *Lancet*. 2023;401(10380):917-927.
10. Janot F, de Raucourt D, Benhamou E, et al. Randomized trial of postoperative reirradiation combined with chemotherapy after salvage surgery compared with salvage surgery alone in head and neck carcinoma. *J Clin Oncol*. 2008;26(34):5518-5523.
11. Mehanna H, Wong W-L, McConkey CC, et al. PET-CT Surveillance versus Neck Dissection in Advanced Head and Neck Cancer. *N Engl J Med*. 2016;374(15):1444-1454.

Chapter 48
Tumor Biology of Head and Neck Cancer

Advanced sequencing modalities combined with increased computing power and artificial intelligence are making an impact for characterization of head and neck cancers, and this information will be critical for estimating prognosis and determining appropriate therapy. The Cancer Genome Atlas (TCGA), supported by the National Cancer Institute (NCI), has provided detailed information about common gene defects and expression patterns, as well as protein expression profiles found in head and neck squamous cell carcinoma (HNSCC). Although similar data are emerging for some salivary cancer types and molecular analyses of thyroid cancers are rapidly evolving, we will limit discussion here to HNSCC.

Human papillomavirus (HPV)-associated (HPV+) HNSCC should be considered a different disease from tobacco-associated or sporadic HNSCC that arises in nonsmokers. Compared to HPV-negative disease, HPV+ HNSCC have improved survival, occur in a younger cohort with different risk factors, and have a distinct set of molecular defects driving the tumor. Because of these differences, HPV− and HPV+ HNSCC will be presented separately. Within HPV+ HNSCC there are two subtypes, one with good prognosis and one with poor prognosis.

HPV-Negative HNSCC

Although betel (areca) nut is a major driver of oral SCC in Southeast Asia, tobacco use is the major etiologic factor in the United States and western countries. Tobacco carcinogens drive genetic alterations (eg, mutations, deletions, amplifications) that cause progressive epithelial changes ultimately resulting in cancer. Common or distinct genetic events observed in HPV-negative HNSCC and involved pathways are categorized below. **Percentages listed are among HPV-negative HNSCC.**

A. *Tumor suppressors* (inactivating mutations, deletions, or epigenetic silencing)
  i. P53: proliferation, apoptosis, genome maintenance
    a. Mutation: 79%
    b. Deletions: 1%
  ii. CDKN2A (p16INK4a): proliferation
    a. Mutation: 25%
    b. Deletion: 33%
    c. Methylation: 32%

- iii. FAT1: migration, proliferation
  - a. Mutation: 25%
  - b. Deletions: 8%
- iv. NOTCH1: differentiation
  - a. Mutation: 19%
  - b. Deletions: 2%
- v. CASP8: apoptosis
  - a. Mutation 12% (linked with HRAS activation)
  - b. Deletions: 1%
- vi. Let-7c miRNA: differentiation
  - a. Copy number loss: 35%
  - b. Deletions: 1%
- vii. NSD1: chromatin modifier
  - a. Mutations: 12%
  - b. Deletions: 1%

B. *Oncogenes* (activating mutations, amplification, overexpression)
- i. PIK3CA: proliferation, survival
  - a. Mutation: 16%
  - b. Amplification: 20% (large amplicon 3q26-ter, not clear if PIK3CA is the target)
- ii. 11q13: amplification of multiple genes—32%
  - a. CCND1(cyclin D1): proliferation
  - b. EMS1 (cortactin): migration, invasion, proliferation
  - c. FADD: apoptosis (role as oncogene questionable)
- iii. EGFR: proliferation, survival
  - a. Amplification: 12%
  - b. Overexpression: 75%
- iv. FGFR1: proliferation, survival
  - a. Amplification: 12%
- v. HRAS: proliferation, migration, survival
  - a. Mutation: 6% (linked with CASP8 mutations)
- vi. MYC: proliferation, survival
  - a. Amplifications: 13%

The most commonly amplified and deleted chromosomal regions and involved genes are

A. *Commonly amplified regions*
- i. 11q13: 32%
  - a. Genes in amplicon: cyclin D1, EMS1 (cortactin), FADD
- ii. 3q26-ter: 20%
  - a. Genes in amplicon: PIK3CA, p63, h-TERC, SOX2, others
- iii. 8q24: 14%
  - a. Genes in amplicon: POU5F1B (functional isoform OCT4), MYC
- iv. 7p11: 12%
  - a. Genes in amplicon: EGFR
- v. 8p11: 12%
  - a. Genes in amplicon: FGFR1

B. *Commonly deleted regions*
- i. 9p21: 33%
  - a. Genes in deleted region: CDKN2A (encoding p16INK4a and ARF)

Major Biological Pathways Altered in HPV-negative HNSCC and Genetic Alterations Driving These Pathways

Common names of genes are given m=mutation, a=amplification, d=deletion

For amplification/deletions, chromosomal region is listed (eg, d:9p21 = deletion of chromosomal region 9p21)

A. Proliferation/cell cycle: p53 (m), CDKN2A ($p16^{INK4a}$, m, d:9p21), CCND1 (cyclin D1, a:11q13), EMS1 (cortactin, a:11q13), EGFR (a:7p21), FGFR (a:8p11), FAT1 (m), PIK3CA (m, a:3q26-ter), HRAS (m), MYC (a:8q24)
B. Survival/apoptosis: p53 (m), PIK3CA (m, a:3q26-ter), HRAS (m), EGFR (a:7p11), FGFR1 (a:8p11), CASP8 (m)
C. Differentiation: NOTCH (m), p63 (a:3q26-ter),
D. Migration: EMS1 (a:11q13), HRAS (m), FAT1 (m)

HPV+ HNSCC

HPV-associated HNSCC are epidemiologically, biologically, and clinically different compared to HPV-negative head and neck cancers. In addition to retention of HPV genes, molecular differences distinguishing HPV+ from HPV-negative HNSCC include distinct gene expression, as well as mutational, structural (amplification and deletion), and methylation profiles. Since major HPV oncoproteins E6 and E7 inactivate p53 and Rb, respectively, HPV+ HNSCCs almost always harbor wild-type p53 and express high levels of CDKN2A, which encodes $p16^{INK4a,}$ the Rb upstream regulator. Irrespective of HPV status, head and neck squamous cancers demonstrate losses of 3p and 8p and gains of 3q and 8q chromosomal regions, suggesting commonalities of molecular pathogenesis with HPV-negative HNSCC. Recent analysis suggests that there are two subtypes of HPV+ HNSCC that are driven by distinct HPV carcinogenesis programs and most reliably identified by activity of the NF-kB transcription factor. Tumors with high NF-kB activity are more sensitive to radiation therapy and have improved survival, while tumors lacking mutations have poor survival equivalent to HPV-negative HNSCC.

Genetic events found in HPV+ HNSCC are listed below. **Percentages listed are amongst HPV+ HNSCC.**

A. *Tumor suppressors* (inactivating events)
   i. NOTCH1: differentiation
      a. Mutation: 6%
   ii. TRAF3: NF-kB inhibition and activation of immunity
      a. Mutations: 5%
      b. Deletions: 11%
   iii. CYLD: NF-kB inhibition and activation of immunity
      a. Mutations: 12%
      b. Deletions: 3%
   iv. let-7c miRNA: differentiation
      a. Copy number loss: 17%
B. *Oncogenes* (activating events)
   i. PIK3CA: proliferation, treatment resistance, cell survival
      a. Mutation: 28%
      b. Amplification: 26% (large amplicon at 3q, not clear if PIK3CA is the target)
   ii. E2F1: proliferation, cell survival
      a. Focal amplifications: 14%
   iii. FGFR3: angiogenesis, cell migration

a. Activating FGFR3-TACC3 fusion: 6%
b. Mutations: 11%
iv. MYC: proliferation, cell survival
a. Hotspot for HPV integration/amplification: 4%
v. TP63: epithelial stemness, epithelial differentiation
a. Hotspot for HPV integration/amplification: 4%

The most commonly amplified and deleted chromosomal regions and involved genes are

A. *Commonly amplified regions*
i. 3q: 27%; genes in amplicon (possible targets): PIK3CA, p63, h-TERC, SOX2, others
ii. 8q: 17%; Genes in amplicon: POU5F1B (functional isoform OCT4), MYC
B. *Commonly deleted regions*
i. 3p: 11%

Major Biological Pathways Altered in HPV+ HNSCC and Genetic Alterations Driving These Pathways

Names of genes are given; m=mutation, a=amplification, d=deletion, f=fusion

A. Proliferation/cell cycle: p53(inactivated by HPV E6), Rb (inactivated by HPV E7), PIK3CA (m, a:3q26-ter), E2F1 (focal a), MYC (focal a)
B. Survival/apoptosis: PIK3CA (m, a:3q26-ter), FGFR3 (FGFR3-TACC3 f)
C. Immunity and NF-kB pathway activation: TRAF3 and CYLD (focal d and m)
D. Differentiation: NOTCH1 (m), p63 (a:3q26-ter)

Differences Between HPV+ and HPV− HNSCC Protein Expression and Activation; RPPA

Using reverse phase protein array (RPPA), our group evaluated expression of 137 total and phosphorylated proteins in 29 HPV+ and 12 HPV− prospectively collected HNSCCs. 33 proteins and 8 phosphoproteins were expressed in tumors in HPV-dependent manner. Four major pathways that distinguish HPV+ from HPV− HNSCCs include: (1) DNA repair, (2) cell cycle, (3) apoptosis, and (4) PI3K/AKT/mTOR.

A. DNA repair is the largest functional category of differentially expressed proteins (12 of 41 differentially expressed proteins [29%], including PARP1, BRCA2, PCNA, and XRCC1) with total protein levels significantly upregulated in HPV+ as compared to HPV− tumors.
B. Cell cycle: Due to HPV E7-dependent downregulation of Rb, which in turn unleashes transcriptional activity of E2F1, HPV+ tumors express lower levels of Rb and higher levels of S and G2/M cyclins E1 and B1. In contrast, HPV− HNSCC expresses higher levels of cyclin D1 and corresponding higher levels of phospho-Rb.
C. Increased markers of **apoptosis,** including cleavage of caspases 3 and 7, were found in HPV+ tumors.
D. PI3K/AKT/mTOR: Mutant PIK3CA in HPV+ tumors preferentially activates the mTOR, but not AKT pathway. Direct Akt targets, including phospho-Raf, phospho-GSK3β, and phospho-TSC2, were expressed at relatively lower levels in HPV+ tumors.

Brief Mechanistic Description for Major Players in HPV+ and HPV– HNSCC

- **P53** is one of the two major tumor suppressors in human cancer, and p53 tumor-suppressing activity must be altered by some means in all or nearly all cancers. P53 functions in response to abnormal proliferative signals, DNA damage, viral infection, and other cellular stresses resulting in cell cycle arrest or death. HPV– HNSCC inactivate p53 through mutation in the vast majority of cases, while tumors driven by HPV express the E6 viral oncoprotein to degrade and inactivate p53. P53 inhibits **survival** and **proliferation** of cancer cells and is an effector of **DNA damage response**.
- **Retinoblastoma (Rb)** is the other major tumor suppressor in human cancer, and like p53 its function is universally, or nearly universally, inhibited in tumors. Unlike p53, there are few mutations in Rb in HNSCC; however, Rb is inhibited in nearly all HPV– HNSCC by loss of CDKN2A (p16) or amplification of CCND1 (cyclin D1). HPV+ tumors inactivate Rb through expression of the viral oncoprotein, E7. Rb is a major regulator of **cell cycle and proliferation**.
- **CDKN2A ($p16^{INK4a}$)** binds and inhibits cyclin-dependent kinase 4 and 6 (CDK4/CDK6) preventing their ability to phosphorylate and inhibit Rb. Loss of $p16^{INK4a}$ allows CDK4 or CDK6 (see below) to inactivate Rb, which promotes **proliferation**. Of interest and clinical utility, p16 is highly expressed in HPV+ HNSCC due to Rb inactivation by HPV E7, **and expression of p16 is used as a surrogate marker for HPV positivity of HNSCC.**
- **CCND1 (cyclin D1)** binds to CDK4 or CDK6 activating them to phosphorylate and inactivate Rb. Cyclin D1 family member, cyclin D2, is also amplified in a small percentage of HNSCC (3%). Overexpression of cyclin D1 inhibits Rb, which promotes **proliferation**.
- **E2F1** is a transcription factor that regulates the expression of many genes to **promote proliferation**. E2F1 is inhibited by Rb by binding and preventing its transactivation activity. E2F1 is amplified in 14% of HPV+ tumors.
- **HPV16 E6 oncoprotein** in combination with a cellular protein, E6-associated protein (E6AP), ubiquitinates p53, resulting in its degradation, therefore **inhibiting apoptosis and supporting genome instability and inappropriate proliferation.**
- **HPV16 E7 oncoprotein** inactivates Rb via direct binding, ubiquitination, and proteasome-dependent degradation, resulting in release and activation of transcriptional factor E2F family members driving expression of S-phase genes, **deregulating cell cycle, and promoting proliferation**
- **FAT1** is a protocadherin that inhibits WNT (wingless-related integration site) signaling by inhibiting β-catenin. Mutations in FAT1 allow β-catenin signaling which promotes **proliferation and migration** and has a role in stem cell maintenance.
- **NOTCH1** is a transmembrane receptor that signals after binding of ligands: Delta-like-1 and Jagged-1. For signaling, NOTCH is cleaved by γ-secretase releasing a portion of the Notch intracellular domain that translocates to the nucleus. NOTCH1 can function as an oncogene or tumor suppressor depending on cell context. In HNSCC, mutations are inactivating, suggesting that NOTCH1 acts as a tumor suppressor. Notch signaling plays a role in cellular **differentiation.**
- **EGFR** (epidermal growth factor receptor) is a receptor tyrosine kinase activated by binding to epidermal growth factor (EGF) or other ligands. EGFR family members include HER2 which is amplified in a small percentage of HNSCC (3%). Signaling through EGFR promotes **survival and proliferation**.

- **FGFR1** (fibroblast growth factor receptor 1) is a receptor tyrosine kinase activated by binding to its ligands, fibroblast growth factors. Signaling through FGFR1 promotes **survival and proliferation**.
- **FGFR3** (fibroblast growth factor receptor 3) is a receptor tyrosine kinase that plays an important role in the regulation of **cell proliferation and apoptosis**.
- **PIK3CA** is the catalytic subunit of the phosphoinositide 3-kinase that converts phosphatidylinositol 4,5-biphosphate (PIP2) to phosphatidylinositol 3,4,5-triphosphate (PIP3). PTEN is a tumor suppressor that catalyzes the opposite conversion of PIP3 to PIP2 and is lost in a low percentage of HNSCC. Activation of PIK3CA results in PI3K signaling through AKT, mTOR, and other targets to promote **proliferation and survival**.
- **HRAS** is an oncogene activated by binding to GTP stimulated by upstream signaling from receptor tyrosine kinases and other receptors. Ras is inactivated by hydrolysis of GTP to GDP, and mutations in HRAS prevent its ability to hydrolyze GTP leaving it continuously in an active state. HRAS signals through PI3K, RAF, and MAPK, and RALGDS to promote **proliferation and survival**.
- **MYC** is an oncogenic transcriptional factor that regulates numerous important cellular processes, including transcription, **replication, cell cycle, and apoptosis.**
- **TRAF3 and CYLD: TRAF3** is a member of the TNF receptor-associated factor (TRAF) protein family and **CYLD** is the gene whose inactivation is responsible for cylindromatosis. These proteins have important similarities and important roles in activating type I interferon response against DNA viruses. They also inhibit the NF-kB pathway. Inactivation of TRAF3 or CYLD occurs exclusively in HPV+ HNSCC, most likely representing a mechanism for escape of **both innate and acquired anti-viral responses**.
- **Let-7c microRNA (miRNA)** is a candidate tumor suppressor that controls cell **proliferation and differentiation.**

Questions

1. Which one of the following is not a tumor suppressor gene?
   A. p53
   B. FAT1
   C. NOTCH1
   D. EGFR

2. Which type of HNSCC is associated with better survival?
   A. HPV+ NF-kB low activity
   B. HPV+ NF-kB high activity
   C. HPV-negative with smoking history 15 pack-years
   D. HPV-negative non-smoker

3. Which gene is not commonly altered in HPV-negative HNSCC?
   A. EGFR
   B. CYLD
   C. CDKN2A
   D. PIK3CA

4. Which one of the following is not an oncogene?
   A. FGFR1
   B. HRAS
   C. TRAF3
   D. PIK3CA
5. Activation of which pathway best distinguishes the two subtypes of HPV+ HNSCC
   A. EGFR
   B. MAPK
   C. NF-kB
   D. p53

Chapter 49
Skull Base Surgery

Introduction

Advances in surgical technique as well as strategies to deliver both neoadjuvant chemotherapy and adjuvant radiation therapy have drastically improved outcomes in patients with malignant tumors invading the skull base in the last few decades. In addition, more complete knowledge of pathology and radiology has better delineated those who would benefit from surgical intervention near the skull base. Head and neck surgeons, neurosurgeons, and in some instances, ophthalmologic oncologists, work together to address tumors of the head and neck that abut or extend into the intracranial space.

Approaches

Surgical approaches to the skull base are broadly named after the cranial fossa at which they are directed, namely, anterior, middle, and posterior. Lesions of the midline such as the region of the sella turcica and clivus require a central approach. Far lateral approaches are utilized for access to the region of the brain stem and medulla (Figure 49-1). Expanded endonasal approaches to sinonasal malignancies involving the skull base have also been described for anterior skull base malignancies.

Anatomy

Anterior Skull Base

The anterior skull base is defined as the bony partition between the frontal lobes in the anterior cranial fossa and the midline and paramedian facial structures including nasal cavity and eyes.

The gyri of the frontal lobes overlie most of the anterior cranial fossa; the ocular gyri and gyrus rectus lie lateral to the midline. The floor of the anterior cranial fossa is composed of ethmoid, sphenoid, and frontal bones. Anteriorly, it forms the crista galli and cribriform plate of the ethmoid bone and covers the upper nasal cavity. The crista galli defines the midline of the anterior skull base. Posteriorly, it forms the planum sphenoidale. Laterally, the frontal bone and lesser wing of the sphenoid form the roof of the orbit and the optic canal, blending medially into the anterior clinoid process. The cribriform plate is the thinnest portion of the ethmoid bone and transmits the first cranial nerve to the olfactory fossa through multiple foramina.

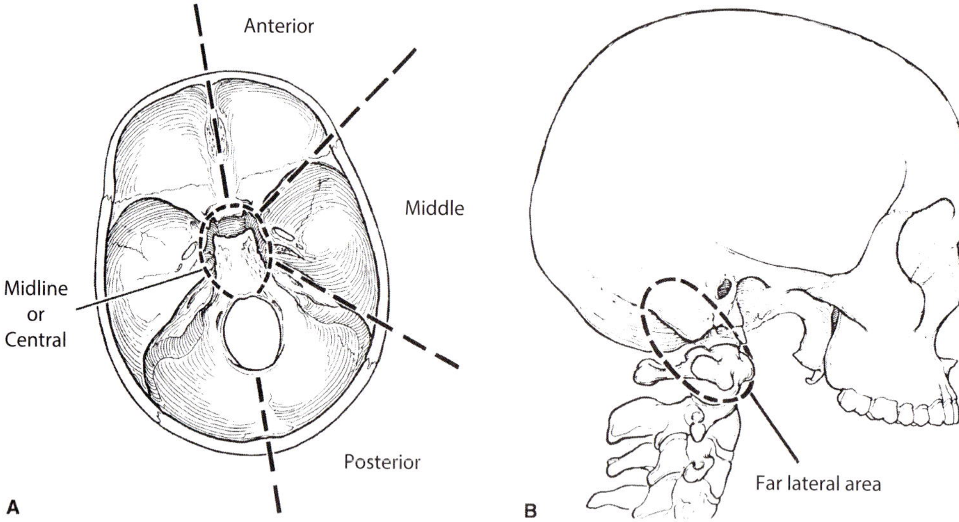

Figure 49-1 **A.** Diagram outlining the various regions of cranial base surgery. *(Reproduced with permission from Donald PJ. Presentation and preparation of patients with skull base lesions. In: Donald PJ, ed. Surgery of the Skull Base. Philadelphia, PA: Lippincott-Raven; 1998:74.)* **B.** The far lateral approach.

Infratemporal Fossa

The infratemporal fossa is located inferiorly to the temporal fossa. The boundaries of the infratemporal fossa include the maxillary sinus anteriorly, the parotid gland posteriorly, the ascending ramus of the mandible and the temporalis muscle laterally, the zygomatic arch and the greater wing of the sphenoid superiorly as well as the pterygoid fascia medially. The roof of the infratemporal fossa is the floor of the middle cranial fossa. It also includes the parapharyngeal space, which contains the internal carotid artery (ICA), internal jugular vein, CN IX to XII, and the masticator space that contains the maxillary and mandibular branches of the trigeminal nerve, the internal maxillary artery, the pterygoid venous plexus, and the pterygoid muscles. The infratemporal fossa is connected to the middle cranial fossa via multiple foramina: carotid canal, jugular foramen, foramen spinosum, foramen ovale, and foramen lacerum.

Middle Cranial Fossa

The middle cranial fossa contains the temporal lobe of the brain. The anterior wall of this fossa is penetrated medially by the superior orbital fissure and the optic canal. The floor of the middle cranial fossa is composed of temporal bone and, to a small extent, the lesser wing of the sphenoid. Both petrous pyramids of the temporal bone meet in the middle where they articulate with the sphenoid bone that is aerated by the sphenoid sinus and indented superiorly by the sella turcica.

The Gasserian ganglion situated in Meckel cave and the mandibular branch (V3) of the trigeminal nerve exiting through the foramen ovale are the key anatomical structure of the middle fossa. Meckel cave and the trigeminal ganglion are located medially near the apex of the petrous bone. Along the anterior border of the petrous bone are also the Glasscock and Kawase triangles.

The boundaries of Glascock triangle form a line from the foramen spinosum to the arcuate eminence/facial nerve hiatus laterally, the greater superficial petrosal medially, and V3 anteriorly. Kawase triangle is made by the greater superficial petrosal nerve laterally, the petrous ridge

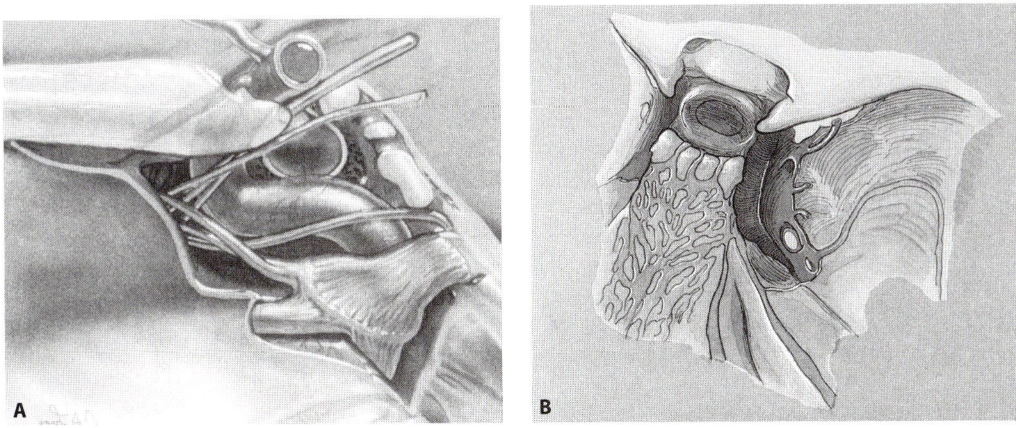

Figure 49-2 **A.** The cavernous sinus showing the cranial nerves and the ICA. **B.** The venous connections to the cavernous sinus.

medially, and the arcuate eminence at the base. The petrous carotid artery is found beneath the greater superficial petrosal nerve. V3 travels inferiorly to the infratemporal fossa. The foramen rotundum is also medially located and carries V2 to the pterygopalatine fossa. Foramen spinosum houses the middle meningeal artery. The internal carotid artery runs under the Gasserian ganglion and is separated from it by a thin plate of bone.

The cavernous sinus receives the internal carotid artery as it ascends the foramen lacerum. It is located laterally to the sphenoid sinus and contains the third, fourth, and sixth cranial nerves, the former two in a double fold of dura in its lateral wall and the latter in a sparse adventitia of the lateral wall of the ICA (Figure 49-2). In addition, numerous extracranial veins and dural venous sinuses connect in the cavernous sinus including the superior and inferior petrosal sinuses posteriorly and the sphenoparietal sinus anteriorly. The cavernous sinus connects to the contralateral sinus via the circular sinus around the pituitary and the basilar plexus across the clivus.

Temporal Bone/Petrous Apex

The temporal bone has four parts: mastoid, squamosa, tympanic, and petrous. The petrous apex is shaped like a pyramid and is located between the middle and posterior fossae. The petrous apex forms three surfaces, anterior (temporal), posterior (posterior fossa), inferior (occipital).

Anterior Surface The anterior superior surface forms the middle fossa floor. The arcuate eminence is the bulge along the superior surface overlying the superior semicircular canal. The facial hiatus transmits the greater superficial petrosal nerve and exits anterolaterally to the arcuate eminence.

Posterior Surface The posterior surface of the petrous apex is the anterolateral wall of the posterior cranial fossa. It extends medially from the posterior semicircular canal and the endolymphatic sac to the petroclinoid ligament and the canal for the abducens nerve (Dorello canal). It is bounded superiorly and inferiorly by the superior and inferior petrosal sinuses. The internal auditory (IAC) canal lies midway across its surface. The lateral portion of the IAC is divided into a superior and an inferior portion by a horizontal ridge called the transverse or falciform crest. The facial nerve and superior vestibular nerve are superior to this crest, while the cochlear nerve and inferior vestibular nerve are inferior to this crest. The facial nerve is located anterior to the superior vestibular nerve and is separated by a vertical ridge of bone called Bill bar.

The endolymphatic duct lies on the posteroinferior face of the temporal bone. The vestibular aqueduct enters the temporal bone lateral to the operculum and travels to the inferior surface of the vestibule.

Inferior Surface The inferior surface is bounded by the jugular bulb and the inferior petrosal sinus. It contains the carotid canal situated anterior to the jugular foramen and medial to the styloid process. It proceeds superiorly to the petrous apex and turns 90 degrees anteromedially. The digastric ridge runs in the sagittal plane, medial to the mastoid tip, and intersects with the stylomastoid foramen. The styloid process is anterior to the stylomastoid foramen. The jugular foramen is medial to the styloid process. The jugular bulb lies in the lateral compartment. The mastoid compartment contains cranial nerves nine, ten, and eleven. The cochlear aqueduct enters medially between the jugular fossa and the carotid canal. The spine of the sphenoid is anterior to the vertical segment of the carotid canal. The cartilaginous portion of the Eustachian tube begins medial to the spine of the sphenoid. The hypoglossal canal is medial and inferior to the jugular foramen.

Clinical Investigation

History and Physical Exam

A thorough history should be obtained, with particular attention to timing, progression, and quality of symptoms, as well as aggravating or alleviating factors. The most common symptoms associated with base of skull neoplasms are anosmia, blindness, or diplopia when the orbit or cavernous sinus is invaded, facial numbness when the trigeminal nerve is involved, and dysphagia or hoarseness with involvement of the jugular foramen. Facial pain usually indicates a locally advanced malignancy with perineural spread. Trismus is an important symptom as it is common in sinus malignancies with posterior extension or pharyngeal carcinomas with involvement of the pterygoid region. Rare presenting symptoms seen mostly in locally advanced disease include headache and clear rhinorrhea (CSF leak).

For patients who have had previous treatment, past operative and pathology reports, laboratory tests, and records of previous examinations should be reviewed.

Physical exam should be performed in a systematic fashion as outlined below.

- Face/scalp skin: examined for any premalignant or malignant lesions. Any scars of previous skin excisions should be noted and discussed with the patient.
- Eyes: The symmetry of the orbits should be compared, and any proptosis or differences in scleral show should be noted. Ectropion can be found in cases of facial nerve paralysis. The conjunctiva should be evaluated for erythema or irritation. Pupil size and reactivity as well as visual field testing are important. Extraocular mobility should be evaluated in eight directions (up, down, right, left, and diagonally right up, right down, left up, left down). Spontaneous nystagmus should be evaluated by having the patient wear Frenzel lenses, while gaze nystagmus is elicited by having the patient follow the examiner's finger performing a "cross" type movement. Positional nystagmus is provoked by the Dix-Hallpike maneuver.
- Ears: The skin of the pinna and the external auditory canal should be evaluated as well as the postauricular skin. The tympanic membrane should be evaluated with pneumatic otoscopy and microscopic otoscopy when evaluation with handheld otoscope is suspicious. Tuning fork evaluation is an essential part of the otologic exam.
- Nasal cavity/nasopharynx: Anterior rhinoscopy with or without decongestion will reveal abnormalities of the septum, turbinates, and nasal mucosa. When pathology is

noted, rigid endoscopy provides a better visualization of the paranasal sinus meatus to evaluate extent of disease. The nasopharynx should be evaluated endoscopically with focus on the Eustachian tubes, Fossa of Rosenmuller, posterior and lateral pharyngeal wall, and palate mucosa and mobility.

- Oral cavity/oropharynx: Carefully evaluate oral mucosa, teeth, and tongue. Tongue should be evaluated for movement, atrophy, or fasciculations. In the case of hypoglossal nerve dysfunction, the tongue will deviate toward the lesion. The drainage from the parotid and submandibular ducts should be evaluated while massaging the corresponding salivary glands. The oropharynx begins at the boundary of the hard and soft palate superiorly and the circumvallate papillae inferiorly. The mucosa of the palatine tonsils, the lingual tonsils, the soft palate, and the lateral and posterior pharyngeal walls should be evaluated carefully with direct visualization, mirror exam, and or fiberoptic endoscopy. The movement of the palate as well as the presence of a gag reflex should be noted. The base of tongue and tonsils should be palpated and any asymmetry noted.
- Larynx: Evaluation of vocal cord mobility and laryngeal sensation is important in evaluation of skull base lesions. Videostroboscopy can provide detailed information related to anatomy and function when needed.
- Neck: Careful palpation should be performed. Mobility, location, and size should be noted. Vertically fixed masses raise suspicion for carotid body tumor.
- Cranial nerves: A full cranial nerve exam is imperative in all skull base cases.

Radiography

CT/MRI scan: Complementary and essential in every case, images should be obtained in axial, coronal, and sagittal planes. Fine-cut CT scan has the advantage of detecting bone erosion. MRI with Gadolinium-based intravenous contrast with fat-suppression software is employed to differentiate fat from tumor tissue. More recently, diffusion-weighted imaging (DWI) has been utilized to further distinguish benign from malignant skull base lesions. MRI can narrow down the differential diagnosis for lesions of the cerebellopontine angle and the petrous apex as seen below:

Tumor	T_1	T_1-*Gad*	T_2
Vestibular schwannoma	Iso or mildly hypointense	Marked enhancement	Moderately hyperintense
Meningioma	Iso or mildly hypointense	Marked enhancement	Hypo to hyperintense
Cholesteatoma (epidermoid)	Hypointense (variable)	No enhancement	Hyperintense
Arachnoid cyst	Hypointense	No enhancement	Hyperintense
Lipoma	Hyperintense	No enhancement	Intermediate
Cholesterol granuloma	Hyperintense	No enhancement	Hyperintense

- Angiogram: Useful for hypervascular lesions such as glomus tumors, carotid body tumors, or juvenile angiofibromas. Also useful in cases of suspected carotid artery invasion. Balloon test occlusion should be considered for assessing cerebral perfusion through the noninvolved internal carotid artery. Patients who will require sacrifice of the internal carotid artery should be tested to determine the need for bypass during surgery.
- PET CT: Positron emission tomography is useful in detecting local, regional, and distant metastatic disease. Utilization of CT with PET scan enables accurate cross-sectional localization of SUV (standard uptake value) avidity.

Preparation

While some tumors of this region (ie, angiofibromas, vestibular schwannomas, meningiomas, and paragangliomas) can sometimes be diagnosed by radiographic imaging, others will require a pathological diagnosis. In the case of deep tumors where fine-needle aspiration may not be feasible, diagnosis can often be obtained with a interventional radiology CT-guided biopsy. When this is not feasible, an endoscopic skull base biopsy should be considered for lesions of the paranasal sinuses, anterior skull base, or pterygopalatine fossa. Due to the complexity of anatomy and surgical planning in this area, tissue diagnosis before embarking on a definitive resection is paramount as negative margin surgery often involves sacrifice of critical structures. Unresectability criteria for skull base tumors include invasion of the brain stem, involvement of both internal carotid arteries, involvement of both cavernous sinuses, extensive invasion of brain parenchyma, and invasion of the spinal cord. Invasion of the optic chiasm would lead to bilateral blindness and is a relative contraindication. Patient factors such as distant metastasis, multiple comorbidities, and lack of consent should also be considered. Of critical importance is consideration of pathology for which neoadjuvant therapy or definitive nonsurgical therapy is effective.

Extensive surgery of the skull base can call for placement of a tracheostomy, lumbar drain, temporary tarsorrhaphy or gold weight in eyelids, anesthetic vascular monitoring, and or installation of scalp electrodes to monitor brain activity if carotid artery clamping is anticipated.

Anterior Skull Base Tumors and Surgical Approaches

Differential Diagnosis of Anterior Skull Base Masses[1]

Benign masses of the anterior skull base:

I. Benign mass-occupying lesions
   a. Hamartomas
II. Sinonasal papillomas
   a. Exophytic papilloma
   b. Oncocytic papilloma
   c. Inverted papilloma
III. Benign vascular lesions
   a. Juvenile nasopharyngeal angiofibroma
   b. Hemangioma
   c. Arteriovenous malformation
   d. Venous malformation
   e. Paraganglioma
IV. Congenital midline masses
   a. IgG4-related ophthalmic disease
   b. Tolosa-Hunt syndrome
V. Other rare benign neoplasms and lesions
   a. Rosai-Dorfman disease
   b. Lipoma
   c. Pleomorphic adenoma
   d. Phosphaturic mesenchymal tumor
   e. Solitary fibrous tumor
   f. Glomangiopericytoma
   g. Eosinophilic angiocentric fibrosis

Malignant masses of the anterior skull base:

VI. Sinonasal squamous cell carcinoma (SCC)
   a. De novo SCC
   b. Inverted papilloma-transformed SCC
VII. Minor salivary gland tumors of the sinonasal tract
   a. Adenocarcinoma (intestinal vs nonintestinal, renal-cell like)
   b. Adenoid cystic carcinoma
   c. Mucoepidermoid carcinoma
   d. Acinic cell carcinoma
VIII. Sinonasal sarcoma
   a. Rhabdomyosarcoma
   b. Osteosarcoma
   c. Fibrosarcoma
   d. Biphenotypic sinonasal sarcoma
   e. Leiomyosarcoma
   f. Angiosarcoma
   g. Ewing sarcoma
   h. Synovial Sarcoma
   i. Malignant peripheral nerve sheath tumor
   j. Hemangiopericytoma
   k. Kaposi Sarcoma
IX. Sinonasal neuroectodermal and neuroendocrine carcinomas
   a. Olfactory neuroblastoma
   b. Sinonasal undifferentiated carcinoma
      i. Sinonasal undifferentiated carcinoma
      ii. NUT carcinoma
      iii. SWI/SNF complex-deficient sinonasal carcinomas
   c. Neuroendocrine carcinoma
   d. Mucosal melanoma
X. Nasopharyngeal carcinoma
XI. Sinonasal lymphoma
   a. B-cell lymphoma
   b. T-cell lymphoma
   c. Extramedullary plasmacytoma
XII. Metastatic tumors
   a. Germ cell tumors
   b. Carcinosarcoma
   c. Teratocarcinosarcoma

Surgical Approaches to the Anterior Skull Base

Craniofacial Resection (Figure 49-3):

1. Lateral rhinotomy incision or midface degloving.
2. Medial maxillary ostectomy with registering of fixation plates first.
3. Can extend to total maxillectomy if tumor is extensive.
4. Ethmoidectomy and medial maxillectomy.

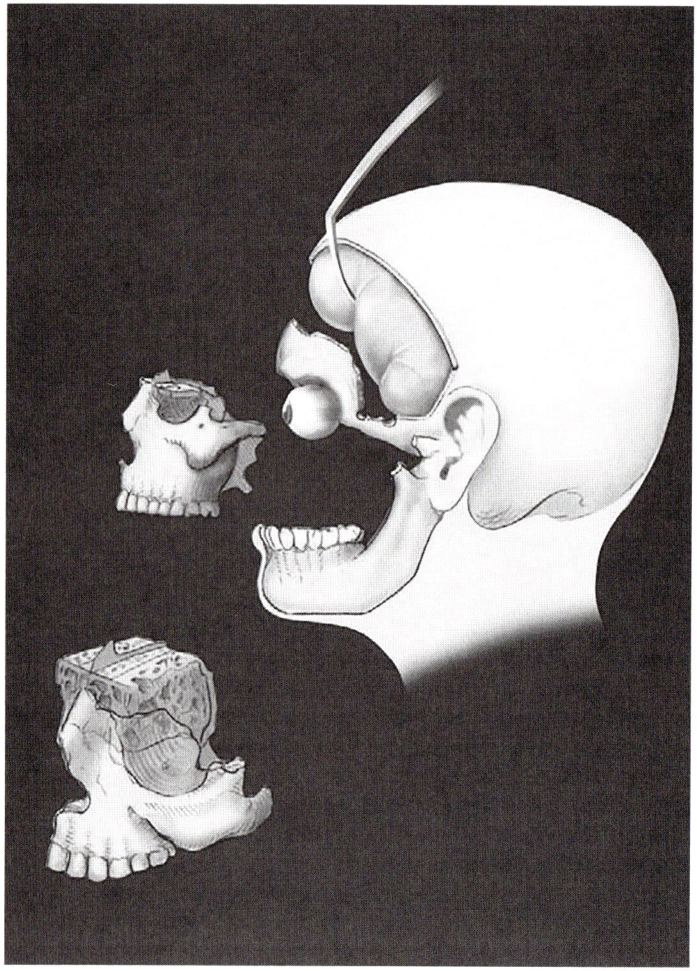

Figure 49-3 Anterior craniofacial resection with sparing of the orbit.

5. If tumor invades the posterior maxillary wall, remove.
6. If pterygomaxillary space invaded, drill pterygoid plates and remove soft tissue with adequate margin.
7. Drill out anterior wall and floor of sphenoid sinus.
8. Small portions of the lateral sphenoid wall and the medial cavernous sinus can be removed with care not to disrupt the ICA.
9. Palatal muscles can be removed if involved.
10. The Eustachian tubes are removed if the lateral wall of the nasopharynx is involved.
11. At the completion of the extracranial portion, margins are checked. Only the anterior cranial floor should have residual tumor.
12. Bicoronal flap raised with preservation of the pericranium.
13. Posterior scalp is raised to give appropriate length to pericranial flap.

14. Two parallel incisions are made in the calvarial periosteum on either side of the frontal skull to the origin of the temporalis muscle. Incisions are connected across the vertex posterior to the scalp incision. The flap is elevated down to the supraorbital rims.
15. The pericranial flap is pedicled on the supraorbital and supratrochlear vessels.
16. Neurosurgeon performs a small craniotomy to extirpate intracranial extent of tumor.
17. Tumor invading dura or brain should be cleared by a margin of 5 mm.
18. The neurosurgeon delineates the circumference of tumor penetrating the anterior fossa floor and clears areas involved with a margin of 5 to 10 mm.
19. Multiple frozen sections are obtained to ensure clear margins.
20. The dura is repaired with dural graft matrix, temporalis fascia, fascia lata, lyophilized dura, or bovine pericardium grafts.
21. The pericranial flap is placed under the dural reconstruction and wedged between the healthy dura and beyond the posterior extremity of the defect and the residual anterior fossa floor at this site.
22. A dacryocystorhinostomy can be considered with placement of sialastic stent through the lacrimal pucta if the duct has been severed.
23. Free microvascular flaps are used in many skull base surgery cases, including those requiring a total maxillectomy, facial skin, orbit, extensive resection of the infratemporal fossa, as well as those cases with anticipated need for radiation therapy.
24. Orbital exenteration is usually indicated with gross invasion of the extraocular muscles, optic nerve, with consideration of exenteration with periorbital fat invasion depending on the feasibility of obtaining negative margins.
25. Orbital exenteration: periorbita is incised over the superior and lateral orbital rims. Dissection continues along the roof of the orbit and lateral walls until the superior orbital fissure (SOF) and the optic foramen are exposed. Lidocaine is injected around these structures to prevent autonomic-induced cardiac arrhythmias. The neurovascular structures of the SOF are carefully ligated and divided. The optic nerve and ophthalmic artery are also ligated and divided. The extraocular muscles are transected at the orbital apex. In patients with sinonasal carcinoma, en bloc resection is associated with improved recurrence-free survival; however, there has been gradual acceptance of close margin surgery with trimodality therapy.[1]

Expanded Endonasal Endoscopic Approach to Anterior Skull Base

- Benefits include the avoidance of large transfacial and scalp incisions, better visualization through magnification and angled scopes as well as avoidance of brain retraction.
- Can be combined with craniotomy approach (cranioendoscopic resection).
- Recent case series have quoted a 5-year survival of up to 60% in endoscopic management of sinonasal malignancies, which is comparable to that achieved with the traditional craniofacial approach.[2] Outcomes are most dependent on pathology of the malignancy.
- Endoscopic and open approaches have comparable outcomes in negative margin resection and cancer outcomes. Benefits of the endoscopic approach compared to open include decreased perioperative mortality, decreased postoperative complications, and shorter hospital stays.[3] Drawbacks include limited exposure for larger, complex tumors near the orbit and with invasion of the brain. In addition, in large sinonasal tumors with skull base extension, endoscopic approaches can lead to a much more challenging reconstruction.[4,5]

- For more lateral exposure, endoscopic approaches via the pterygopalatine fossa and infratemporal fossa may be employed.
- Contraindications include:
  1. Orbital involvement
  2. Involvement of far lateral maxillary sinus
  3. Dural involvement lateral to the orbit
  4. Extensive brain invasion
  5. Cavernous sinus or carotid involvement
  6. Lesion lateral to the cavernous carotid or superolateral to the optic nerve
- In sinonasal malignancies the site of origin of the tumor should be removed en bloc with adequate margins.
- Watertight closure of the skull base defect is paramount.
- The reconstructive ladder should be considered when planning skull base reconstruction, including free mucosal flaps, pedicled flaps, and even free flaps if necessary. The Hadad-Bassagasteguy flap (pedicled nasoseptal mucosal flap) has been shown to reduce incidence of CSF leak. There are also other pedicled mucosal flaps available within the sinonasal cavity, which may be chosen based on tumor location or prior surgery that may compromise preferred pedicled flaps. While the workhorse pedicled flap is the nasoseptal flap, other pedicled intranasal flaps include the middle turbinate flap and the posterior pedicled inferior turbinate flap. As mentioned above, a pericranial flap may be employed for a large anteriorly based skull base defect. Temporoparietal fascia and or muscle flaps may also be used for the anterior skull base, but require tunneling through the infratemporal fossa, or rarely, for especially large defects with supraorbital extension, transposition via a supraorbital epidural corridor.[6]
- Procedure[7]
  1. Nasoseptal flap harvested and tucked into nasopharynx.
  2. Tumor is debulked endonasally to visualize margins, origin, and site of skull base involvement.
  3. Maxillary sinus antrostomies, ethmoidectomy, and sphenoidotomy performed for identification of landmarks of the nasal cavity and visualization of the optic and carotid canals.
  4. May resect posterior wall of frontal sinus, medial wall of orbits, roof of sphenoid, and septum if needed for adequate margins.
  5. A Draf III procedure is performed to remove the floor of the frontal sinus.
  6. The nasal septum is transected below the tumor to the sphenoid rostrum.
  7. The anterior and posterior ethmoid arteries are ligated and divided at skull base.
  8. The anterior skull base is drilled thin and elevated; it is removed from the crista galli to the planum sphenoidale and from the medial orbital wall to the contralateral medial orbital wall.
  9. The dura is cauterized and opened around tumor with adequate margin.
  10. Cortical blood vessels are elevated, and olfactory roots are transected.
  11. Margins are confirmed through multiple frozen sections.
  12. Closure of dural defect done in multilayered fashion. Can use dural graft matrix in the subdural space followed by fascia graft followed by nasoseptal flap. This is later secured in place using fibrin glue followed by gelfoam or fat.
  13. Reconstruction is buttressed with nasal packing; the use of nasal trumpets can reduce the risk of pneumocephalus while preserving nasal airway. In certain cases tracheotomy can also be used to divert the flow of air and prevent pneumocephalus.

Surgery of the Infratemporal Fossa

Three approaches described by Fisch et al.

Type A: access to the temporal bone

Indications

(a) Glomus tumors
(b) Salivary gland cancers
(c) Squamous cell carcinoma
(d) Cholesteatoma
(e) Neurinoma
(f) Meningioma
(g) Rhabdomyosarcoma, teratoma, myxoma

Type B: access to the clivus

Indications

(h) Chordoma
(i) Chondroma
(j) Squamous cell carcinoma
(k) Dermoid/epidermoid cysts
(l) Meningioma, craniopharyngioma, plasmacytoma, arachnoid cyst, and craniopharyngeal fistulae

Type C: access to the parasellar region and nasopharynx

Indications

(m) Salvage surgery for squamous cell carcinoma
(n) Adenoid cystic carcinoma around Eustachian tube
(o) Advanced juvenile nasopharyngeal angiofibroma

Open Approach to the Infratemporal Fossa

1. C-shaped incision from the temporal region extending 4 cm postauricularly, then down into the neck.
2. A periosteal flap pedicled on the EAC anteriorly is created.
3. EAC is transected at the bony cartilaginous junction deep to the periosteal flap.
4. The lateral EAC is everted and closed.
5. The periosteal flap is rotated anteriorly and sutured to the closed EAC.
6. The neck dissection is performed, and cranial nerves IX, X, XI, XII, internal carotid artery and internal jugular vein are exposed.
7. The facial nerve is identified at the stylomastoid foramen.
8. A mastoidectomy removing the mastoid tip, entire bony auditory canal, medial canal skin, tympanic membrane, and middle ear contents is performed.
9. The facial nerve is translocated anteriorly at the stylomastoid foramen.
10. The mandibular condyle is mobilized, and the glenoid fossa is exposed.
11. The internal carotid artery is dissected from the neck to the skull base to its position below the cochlea.
12. The posterior and middle fossa dura can be opened to expose the cranial cavity when intracranial extension is present.
13. Can sacrifice the labyrinth and/or cochlea to access the internal carotid artery, the petrous apex, the clivus, or the anterior brain stem.
14. Several techniques can be applied for reconstruction including recontouring with allogenic tissue matrix, temporalis muscle-fascia flap or microvascular free flap.
15. A layered closure is performed and a pressure dressing applied for 24 hours.

Middle Fossa Tumors and Surgical Approaches

Differential Diagnosis of Middle Fossa Masses

I. **Tumors of the middle cranial fossa**
1. Chordoma
2. Chondrosarcoma
3. Meningioma
4. Trigeminal schwannoma
5. Osteosarcoma
6. Cholesteatoma
7. Cholesterol granuloma
8. Squamous cell carcinoma
9. Lymphoma

Surgical Approaches to Middle Cranial Fossa

Combined approach, involving infratemporal fossa approach with a small, low, middle fossa craniotomy:

- Incision begins near the midline of the calvarium, 2 cm behind the hairline. It is carried inferiorly in front of the ear for parotid, sinus, and neck lesions or behind the ear for lesions of the temporal bone or clivus.
- The flap is elevated forward to the level of the lateral orbital rim and angle of the mandible.
- The external auditory canal (EAC) is severed across the bony cartilaginous junction.
- The temporal branch of the facial nerve is protected by elevating a patch of temporal fascia deep to the branch during the skin elevation.
- The ICA and internal jugular vein are identified in the neck to obtain proximal vascular control.
- The temporalis muscle is elevated through an incision made in the pericranium about 2 cm outside the periphery of its origin. The muscle is elevated to its insertion in the coronoid process of the mandible.
- The arch of the zygoma and the condyle of the mandible are removed (Figure 49-4).
- Under magnification, the tympanomeatal flap is raised and the middle ear is entered anteriorly, exposing the opening of the Eustachian tube.
- Using a small cutting burr, cuts are made within the tympanic annulus at 2 o'clock and 7 o'clock. The superior cut is directed superiorly into the middle ear, across the tensor tympani canal anterior to the cochleariform process into the superior part of the protympanum. The inferior cut is made across the hypotympanum into the mouth of the Eustachian tube.
- The external canal is then drilled down to the level of the dura into the squamosal part of the temporal bone superiorly and inferiorly through the thickness of the external canal into the glenoid fossa.
- The cut through the glenoid fossa is only about 2 mm deep and is directed toward the foramen spinosum where the middle meningeal artery is ligated.
- Neurosurgery performs small craniotomy through greater wing of the sphenoid and squamous temporal bone connecting the cut in the external auditory canal posteriorly to the pterygoid plates anteriorly.
- When bone flap is removed, a greenstick fracture occurs so that the protympanum is fractured across and the internal carotid artery is exposed as it enters the posterior wall of the bony Eustachian tube.

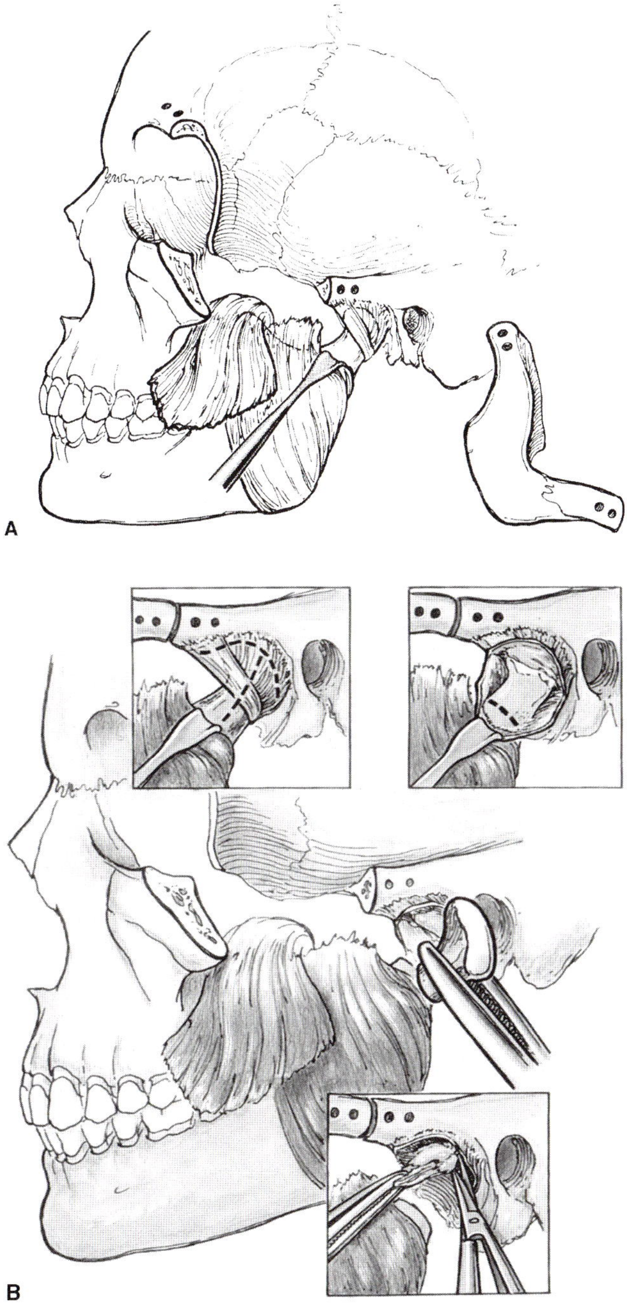

A

B

Figure 49-4 **A.** Bony excision complete. *(Reproduced with permission from Donald PJ. Infratemporal fossa-middle cranial fossa approach. In: Donald PJ, ed. Surgery of the Skull Base. Philadelphia, PA: Lippincott-Raven; 1998:324).* **B.** Condylectomy: Lateral aspect of the temporomandibular joint capsule is opened and connected to the mandibular neck. The condylar neck is transected and the condyle removed. The meniscus and attached soft tissue are removed. *(Reproduced with permission from Donald PJ. Infratemporal fossa-middle cranial fossa approach. In: Donald PJ, ed. Surgery of the Skull Base. Philadelphia, PA: Lippincott-Raven; 1998:325).*

- The internal carotid artery can be dissected from the fibrous ring at the opening of the carotid canal through the vertical and horizontal portions all the way to the cavernous sinus if involved with tumor.
- The tumor is removed en bloc and frozen sections are checked to ensure margins are negative.
- The carotid artery may be grafted if sacrifice necessary to clear margins versus leaving microscopic disease on the carotid adventitia.
- The Eustachian tube is removed subcranially to expose the nasopharynx. In involved the entire Eustachian tube and the clivus can be excised.
- Dura is closed with fascia grafts, and nasopharynx is separated from cranial cavity with either a pedicled temporalis muscle flap or a rectus abdominis free flap.
- Finally, the craniotomy bone flap and zygomatic arch are plated into position.

The Far Lateral Approach to the Middle Cranial Fossa

Indication: This approach is appropriate for tumors originating from clivus, upper posterior neck, or extending posteroinferiorly from the temporal bone.

1. Incision is a question mark beginning high in the occiput and coursing around the postauricular area descending to the upper neck.
2. Trapezius, splenius capitis, semispinalis capitis, and longissimus capitis are separated from the basio-occiput exposing the cervical spine.
3. The bone of the spinous processes of the cervical spine is carefully drilled with care not to injure the vertebral artery.
4. Usually the vertebral artery can be taken safely if invaded by tumor.
5. If vertebral artery sacrifice is anticipated, a preoperative balloon occlusion test should be performed to establish the safety of sacrificing the artery.
6. If not sacrificed the artery is mobilized to the foramen magnum and the atlanto-occipital joint is exposed.
7. The lateral mass of the atlas is drilled away with care not to injure the occipital emissary vein and the hypoglossal canal.
8. Occipital craniotomy is performed.
9. Can extend resection up to the temporal bone with a mastoidectomy to expose the jugular bulb.
10. Neurosurgeon can perform an occipital-spinal fusion if concern for spinal instability.
11. A fascial graft can be used for dural closure if necessary.
12. The occipital bone graft is replaced and the muscles are reapproximated before closure.

Masses of the Temporal Bone

- Glomus tumors are the most common lesions in this area.
  - Glomus tumors are paragangliomas that arise from paraganglionic tissue derived from the migration of neural crest cells during embryonic development.
  - May present with hearing loss, pulsatile tinnitus, vertigo, cranial nerve neuropathies (V, VI, VII, IX, X, XI, and XII), aural pain, or neck mass.
  - Physical examination includes a full neurologic exam and otomicroscopic evaluation.
  - 1% of paragangliomas display physiologically significant catecholamine secretion. Presence of tachycardia, arrhythmias, flushing, or labile hypertension should prompt analysis of 24-hour urine specimen for vanillylmandelic acid, metanephrine, and normetanephrine levels.

- Audiogram is required part of initial evaluation.
- CT scan, arteriography, MRI with gadolinium and MRA are useful to evaluate bone invasion, vascularity, and soft tissue extension, respectively.
- Two major classifications:
  - Fisch classification:[8]
    - ◊ Class A: limited to mesotympanum
    - ◊ Class B: limited to hypotympanum, mesotympanum and mastoid
    - ◊ Class C: involvement of infralabyrinthine components and extending to petrous apex
      - * Type C1: limited involvement of the vertical portion of the carotid canal
      - * Type C2: invading the vertical portion of the carotid canal
      - * Type C3: invasion of the horizontal portion of the carotid canal
    - ◊ Class D: intracranial extension
      - * Type D1: intracranial extension less than 2 cm in diameter
      - * Type D2: intracranial extension greater than 2 cm in diameter
- Glasscock-Jackson classification
  - Glomus tympanicum:
    - I. Small mass limited to the promontory filling the middle ear
    - II. Tumor completely filling middle ear space
    - III. Tumor filling middle ear extending into mastoid
    - IV. Tumor filling middle ear and extending into mastoid or through tympanic membrane to fill external auditory canal
  - Glomus jugulare:
    - I. Involving jugular bulb, middle ear and mastoid
    - II. Extending under internal auditory canal
    - III. Extending into petrous apex, may have intracranial extension
    - IV. Extending beyond petrous apex into clivus or infratemporal fossa, may have intracranial extension
- Other tumors of the temporal bone:
  - EAC
    - Benign
      - ◊ Pleomorphic adenoma
      - ◊ Ceruminous adenoma
        - * Malignant
          1. Squamous cell carcinoma
          2. Basal cell carcinoma
          3. Sarcoma
          4. Melanoma
          5. Lymphoma
          6. Adenocarcinoma
          7. Adenoid cystic carcinoma
          8. Ceruminous adenocarcinoma
  - Middle ear and mastoid
    - Benign
      1. Paraganglioma
      2. Myxoma
      3. Lipoma
      4. Hemangioma
      5. Schwannoma

      6. Neurofibroma
      7. Ostema
      8. Chondroblastoma
      9. Giant cell tumor
      10. Meningioma
      11. Teratoma
    - Malignant
      1. Squamous cell carcinoma
      2. Basal cell carcinoma
      3. Adenocarcinoma
      4. Carcinoid tumor
      5. Rhabdomyosarcoma
      6. Malignant paraganglioma
      7. Malignant schwannoma
      8. Hemangiopericytoma
      9. Osteosarcoma
      10. Chondrosarcoma
      11. Malignant germ cell tumor

- Staging of SCC of the temporal bone determines surgical approach
  - T1: limited to EAC, no bone erosion—sleeve resection or lateral temporal bone resection
  - T2: limited bony EAC erosion—lateral temporal bone resection
  - T3: full-thickness EAC erosion with limited less than 5 mm soft tissue involvement or middle ear involvement or facial paresis—subtemporal temporal bone resection
  - T4: erosion of cochlea, petrous apex, medial wall of middle ear, carotid canal, jugular foramen dura, and greater than 5 mm soft tissue involvement—total temporal bone resection
- Lateral temporal bone resection:
  1. C-shaped postauricular incision curved into a cervical neck crease.
  2. In ear canal incision is made in the cartilaginous EAC encompassing the lesion.
  3. Auriculectomy or partial auriculectomy may be required.
  4. Stepped incision is made through the fascia, muscle, and periosteum.
  5. Flap elevated anteriorly to the root of the zygoma.
  6. Elevation of the soft tissues over the mastoid done in a subperiosteal plane.
  7. Ear canal is sectioned at the bony cartilaginous junction and closed in multiple layers.
  8. The temporalis muscle and the temporoparietal fascia can be preserved and reflected forward to be used later in reconstruction.
  9. Mastoidectomy with skeletonization of the facial nerve, tegmen, sigmoid sinus, and bony ear canal is performed.
  10. Extended facial recess approach is performed and dissection continues into glenoid fossa anteriorly. The incudostapedial joint is sectioned and the incus is removed.
  11. The tensor tympani is sectioned.
  12. The stylomastoid foramen is decompressed and the digastric muscle is exposed.
  13. A chisel is used to lightly cantilever the mobilized specimen.
  14. Parotidectomy and supraomohyoid neck dissection is performed for staging in a majority of patients.
  15. A rotational flap or rectus free flap may be required for closure if auriculectomy performed.

- Subtotal temporal bone resection removes the temporal bone lateral to the petrous apex including the otic capsule and includes mobilization of the petrous carotid artery and an infratemporal fossa dissection.
- Total temporal bone resection includes resection of the petrous apex with or without resection of the petrous carotid artery. It involves an extensive infratemporal fossa dissection with mobilization or resection of the petrous carotid artery and middle and posterior fossa craniotomy.

Tumors of the Internal Auditory Canal and the Cerebellopontine Angle

- 90% of tumors at the cerebellopontine angle are vestibular schwannomas.
- 10% are either meningiomas, arachnoid cysts, cholesteatomas, facial neuromas, or metastatic lesions.
- Vestibular schwannomas are benign tumors of the superior and inferior vestibular nerves that originate at the junction of the Schwann cells and astrocytes, typically in the internal auditory canal. Their growth rate is 1 to 4 mm per year on average.
- 95% occur in a sporadic fashion, while 5% are associated with neurofibromatosis type 2 or familial vestibular schwannoma.
- Up to one-third of vestibular schwannomas remain stable in size when monitored over time.
- Hearing loss with gradual progression is the most common presenting symptom but 20% of patients can present with sudden-onset sensorineural hearing loss (SNHL).
- Tinnitus is present in up to 70% of patients presenting with an acoustic tumor.
- Facial nerve deficits are observed in 10% of patients.

Approaches to the Internal Auditory Canal and Cerebellopontine Angle

- **Three approaches have been described:**

1. Translabyrinthine approach
   a. Advantages
      i. Minimized cerebellar retraction and potential subsequent atrophy
      ii. Less postoperative headaches
      iii. Visualize facial nerve prior to tumor dissection
   b. Disadvantages
      i. Up to 21% incidence of CSF fistula
      ii. Loss of residual hearing
      iii. Longer exposure time
2. Retrosigmoid approach
   a. Advantages
      i. Quicker approach
      ii. 50% hearing preservation in tumors less than 2 cm
   b. Disadvantages
      i. Twenty-three percent incidence of postoperative headache.
      ii. Requires cerebellar retraction with possible subsequent atrophy.
      iii. 7% to 21% incidence of CSF fistula.
      iv. In larger tumors, dissection precedes identification of the facial nerve.

3. Middle cranial fossa approach
    a. Advantages
        i. 50% to 75% chance of hearing preservation
        ii. Minimal risk of CSF fistula
    b. Disadvantages
        i. Slight increased risk to facial nerve if tumor originates on inferior vestibular nerve
        ii. Requires some temporal lobe retraction which could pose additional risks in the elderly

Translabyrinthine Approach

This approach was first introduced in 1904 by Panse, but did not become a standard approach until its reintroduction by William House.

Technique

1. A curved postauricular incision is made 3 cm behind the postauricular crease.
2. A complete mastoidectomy is performed.
3. The sigmoid sinus is skeletonized, and only a very thin wafer of bone is left covering the sinus (Bill island).
4. Dura is exposed anterior and 2 cm posterior to the sinus allowing compression of the sinus for improved exposure.
5. A complete labyrinthectomy is performed.
6. The internal auditory canal is skeletonized 180 degrees.
7. All bone covering the dura from the sigmoid sinus to the porus acousticus is removed as well as the bone covering the middle fossa dura.
8. The jugular bulb is skeletonized.
9. The intralabyrinthine segment of the facial nerve is identified together with the vertical crest (Bill bar) which separates the facial nerve from the superior vestibular nerve in the lateral-most aspect of the IAC.
10. The dura over the IAC and posterior fossa is incised.
11. The superior vestibular nerve together with the tumor is reflected off the facial nerve.
12. Tumor debulking proceeds with bipolar cautery, CO_2 laser, or Cavitron ultrasonic surgical aspirator (CUSA) together with microdissection.
13. The epitympanum is filled with temporalis fascia and open air cell tracts are occluded with bone wax.
14. Mastoid cavity is packed with abdominal fat.
15. Three-layer closure of incision.

Transotic Approach

The transotic approach as described by Fisch is a modification of the translabyrinthine approach. It adds additional exposure anterior to the IAC and decreases the risk of a post-operative CSF fistula. In addition to the steps of a translabyrinthine approach, the following components are added:

Technique

1. A 4-cm-by-4 cm craniotomy is performed immediately posterior to the sigmoid sinus.
2. A dural flap is created and retracted.
3. Arachnoid is incised and CSF is drained from the cisterna magna.
4. The cerebellum is covered with a cottonoid and retracted posteriorly with a flat blade retractor.

5. The CPA is now visualized.
6. At this point, tumor can be excised, vestibular nerve sectioned, or the trigeminal, facial, or vestibular nerve can be decompressed.
7. Tumor is debulked with bipolar cautery, Cavitron ultrasonic aspirator, or CO_2 laser.
8. Once adequate exposure of the posterior face of the petrous bone and operculum is exposed, the dura overlying the IAC is incised and elevated.
9. The IAC is skeletonized from posterosuperiorly.
10. The operculum is an important landmark which identified the entry point of the endolymphatic duct.
11. Remaining anteromedial to the endolymphatic duct while approaching the IAC decreases the risk of entry into the labyrinth with resultant deafness.
12. In general, up to 7 mm of bone can be removed safely from the medial aspect of the IAC.
13. Once the facial nerve is identified, the remainder of the tumor is peeled off of the nerve and excised.
14. All exposed air cells are occluded with bone wax.
15. Fascia is placed over the IAC.
16. The dural flap over the CPA is closed.
17. The craniotomy defect is filled with bone chips, or a cranioplasty is performed, with hydroxyapatite cement and the wound closed.

Retrolabyrinthine Approach

Originally described by Hitselberger and Pulec in 1972 for section of the fifth nerve, use of this approach has been expanded. Presently, its use is limited to vestibular nerve sections and management of hemifacial spasm by microvascular decompression. There are minimal advantages to this approach and a significant disadvantage of limited visualization.

Technique

1. A postauricular incision is made and a layered flap created.
2. A cortical mastoidectomy is performed.
3. The dura is skeletonized along posterior fossa and superiorly along the middle fossa dura.
4. The facial nerve, labyrinth, and incus are identified.
5. The sigmoid sinus is decorticated and retrosigmoid air cells are removed to expose the retrosigmoid dura.
6. A dural flap is made parallel to the sigmoid sinus (behind the endolymphatic sac) up to the level of the superior petrosal sinus.
7. The cerebellum is retracted and the arachnoid incised, exposing the seventh to eighth nerve complex.
8. The vestibular nerve is sectioned or a nerve decompression performed.
9. The tumor is removed or the nerve sectioned.
10. The wound is closed with silk sutures on the dura; abdominal fat may be used to obliterate the surgical defect prior to layered closure.

Approaches to the Petrous Apex

Evaluation of the patient with pathology at the petrous apex must include consideration of lesions involving the clivus, pituitary, nasopharynx, sphenoid, temporal bone, and meninges.

Lesions of the Petrous Apex

- Cholesteatoma
  - Arise from the foramen lacerum from the epithelial elements congenitally included in Sessel pocket of the cephalic flexure of the embryo.
  - Ninety-four percent of cases present with hearing loss.
- Mucocele
- Metastatic tumor
- Mesenchymal tumor (chondroma)
- Osteomyelitis, including malignant external otitis and mastoiditis
- Clival tumor (chordoma)
- Glomus tumor
- Nasopharyngeal tumors
- Meningioma
- Neurinoma (trigeminal or acoustic)
- Aneurysm of the ICA
- Cholesterol granuloma
- Histiocytosis X

Symptoms

- Cranial neuropathy
  - Nerves III, IV, V, VI, VII, and VIII
  - Jugular foramen syndrome of nerves IX, X, and XI
  - Hypoglossal foramen XII
- Headache (often retro-orbital or vertex)
- Tinnitus, hearing loss
- Eustachian tube dysfunction; serous effusion
- Meningitis
- Gradenigo syndrome (otorrhea, lateral rectus palsy, trigeminal pain)

Goals of Surgical Management

1. Provide exposure or permit easy access for exteriorization.
2. Preserve residual hearing.
3. Preserve facial function.
4. Preserve the ICA.
5. Protect the brain stem.
6. Prevent CSF leakage.

Approaches

A. Infracochlear
B. Supralabyrinthine
C. Retrolabyrinthine
D. Middle cranial fossa
E. Trans-sphenoid
F. Partial labyrinthectomy
G. Transcochlear
H. Infratemporal fossa

The Transcochlear Approach

This approach provides access to the skull base medial to the porus acusticus and anterior to the petrous apex and brain stem.

Technique

1. An extended postauricular incision is made.
2. A cortical mastoidectomy is performed.
3. The facial nerve is skeletonized from the stylomastoid foramen to the geniculate ganglion.
4. Bone covering the posterior fossa dura, sigmoid sinus, and middle fossa dura is removed.
5. A labyrinthectomy is performed.
6. The chordae tympani and greater superficial petrosal nerves are divided and the facial nerve is mobilized posteriorly.
7. The stapes and incus are removed and the cochlea is drilled out.
8. The dissection is bounded by the carotid artery anteriorly, the superior petrosal sinus above, the jugular bulb below, and the sigmoid sinus posteriorly; the medial extent is the petrous apex just below Meckel cave.
9. Following tumor removal, the wound may be filled with harvested fat and closed in layers.

Surgery for Vertigo

Only in persistent incapacitating vertigo which has failed medical management surgical intervention considered.

1. Ménière disease
   a. Symptoms, signs, medical treatment
      i. Fluctuating hearing loss.
      ii. Episodic vertigo.
      iii. Tinnitus.
      iv. Aural pressure.
      v. Fifteen percent to 30% bilateral.
      vi. Medical management includes low-salt diet (< 2000 mg/d), diuretics, stress reduction, vestibular rehabilitation therapy.
      vii. Other possible medical therapies include corticosteroids (both systemic and intratympanic) and Meniett therapy (micropressure therapy).
      viii. Differential diagnosis includes autoimmune inner ear disease, tertiary syphilis, vestibular schwannoma, perilymphatic fistula, basilar migraine.
   b. Surgical options
      i. Endolymphatic shunt or sac decompression 60% to 75% success rate drops to 50% at 5 years; 1% to 3% hearing loss.
      ii. Intratympanic gentamycin (three-fourths cc gentamycin 40 mg/mL mixed with one-fourth cc of bicarbonate 0.6M); 85% to 90% success rate. Limit use to unilateral disease. Two to six treatments up to 20% incidence of SNHL.
      iii. Labyrinthectomy used in patients with unilateral disease with nonserviceable hearing in the affected ear; 85% success rate.
      iv. Vestibular neurectomy used in patients with unilateral disease and serviceable hearing bilaterally; 90% success rate; 10% incidence of SNHL.
2. Benign paroxysmal positional vertigo
   a. Signs, symptoms, medical treatment
      i. Vertigo induced by head motion and lasts for less than 1 minute. Resolves over weeks to months. Frequently recurrent.

- ii. Hallpike demonstrating rotatory nystagmus with 5 to 10 seconds latency and 10 to 30 seconds duration is pathognomonic.
- iii. Vertigo is secondary to posterior semicircular canal debris.
- iv. Canalith repositioning maneuver is effective 74% to 91% of the time.

b. Surgical options
   - i. *Singular neurectomy:* 90% success rate with 25% risk of complete or partial hearing loss
   - ii. *Posterior semicircular canal occlusion:* 90% success rate with 20% risk of hearing loss

3. Perilymphatic fistula
   a. Signs, symptoms, medical treatment
      - i. SNHL
      - ii. Vertigo
      - iii. Symptoms exacerbated with Valsalva or loud noises
      - iv. Site of leak around stapes footplate and round window
      - v. Treat initially with bed rest and stool softeners

   b. Surgical options
      - i. Exploratory tympanotomy and closure of fistula by denuding surrounding mucosa and sealing small pieces of fascia.
4. Unilateral labyrinthine injury (trauma, vascular, viral, tumor)
   a. Signs, symptoms, medical treatment
      - i. Manage with vestibular rehabilitation therapy

   b. Surgical options
      - i. Labyrinthectomy
      - ii. Vestibular neurectomy via retrosigmoid, middle cranial fossa, or translabyrinthine approaches, 85% success rate
5. Superior canal dehiscence syndrome
   a. Signs, symptoms, medical treatment
      - i. Vertigo and oscillopsia in response to Valsalva or loud noises
      - ii. Chronic disequilibrium or positional vertigo
      - iii. Autophone
      - iv. Possible mild conductive hearing loss

   b. Surgical options
      - i. Plug superior semicircular canal via middle cranial fossa approach

   c. Resurface superior semicircular canal via the middle cranial fossa approach

Complications and Outcomes

Most series quote a complication rate of approximately 50% in complicated skull base surgical resections. One of the most common complications is cerebrospinal fluid leak that can lead to tension pneumocephalus and meningitis. CSF leaks commonly resolve spontaneously but should be repaired if not resolved in 7 to 10 days. Although the efficacy of prophylactic antibiotics for CSF leak is still in question the practice of continuing perioperative antibiotics until resolution is commonplace. The likelihood of this complication is diminished with the use of vascularized free-flap reconstruction of the skull base. Wound complications including wound dehiscence, infection, craniotomy bone flap loss, and free-flap failure are also common.

Functional and cosmetic results can be enhanced by the use of therapeutic devices and prosthetics. Orthognathic retraining and the use of an active rehabilitation mandibular exercise program, for example, can often address trismus.

Mortality after resection of tumors of the skull base has been reported mostly in the context of vascular sacrifice of the carotid artery. This complication has been known to occur despite preoperative balloon occlusion tests. Fortunately, a majority of lesions can be resected utilizing the aforementioned approaches without requiring vascular sacrifice, decreasing the risk of vascular complications. Myocardial infarction, pulmonary embolism, and cerebral edema make up the remainder of the commonest causes of perioperative death and occur mostly in the elderly with multiple medical comorbidities.

Current data support the use of surgical resection of skull base lesions, followed by radiation therapy for high-risk pathology, dural invasion, or positive margins on final pathology.[1] When employing these techniques multiple institutions report an average of approximately 50% overall survival at 5 years. Again, the most critical factor in long-term outcome is the pathology of the tumor. Emphasizing that although there have been significant improvements in the field, new modalities of therapy for high-risk tumors should continue to be pursued to improve on these results.

References

1. Kuan EC, Wang EW, Adappa ND, et al. International consensus statement on allergy and rhinology: sinonasal tumors. *Int Forum Allergy Rhinol.* 2024;14:149-608.
2. Shah JP, Levyn H, Valero C, et al. Skull base surgery for malignant tumors: the 2nd international collaborative study (1995-2015). Head Neck. 2024;46(11):2762-2775.
3. Graffeo CS, Dietrich AR, Grobelny B, et al. A panoramic view of the skull base: systematic review of open and endoscopic endonasal approaches to four tumors. *Pituitary.* 2014;17:349-356.
4. Shah JP, Levyn H, Valero C, et al. Skull base surgery for malignant tumors: The 2nd international collaborative study (1995–2015). *Head Neck.* 2024;46:2762-2775.
5. Hannan CJ, Kelleher E, Javadpour M. Methods of skull base repair following endoscopic endonasal tumor resection: a review. *Front Oncol.* 2020;10.
6. Har-El G. Anterior craniofacial resection without facial skin incisions-a review. *Otolaryngol–Head Neck Surg.* 2004;130:780-787.
7. Oldring D, Fisch U. Glomus tumors of the temporal region: surgical therapy. *Am J Otol.* 1979; 1(1):7-18.

Questions

1. Which of the following is a contraindication to an extended endoscopic approach to anterior skull base tumors?
   A. Extension through lateral maxillary sinus wall
   B. Involvement of the cavernous sinus
   C. Orbital involvement
   D. Tumor extension superolateral to orbital nerve
   E. Dural involvement
   F. A, B, C, and D are correct

2. Which of these cerebellopontine angle lesions has the characteristic MRI finding of high signal intensity on both T1 and T2-weighted images?
   A. Lipoma
   B. Cholesterol granuloma
   C. Arachnoid cyst
   D. Vestibular schwannoma
   E. Meningioma

3. Which one of the following is considered a "relative," rather than "absolute" contraindication to surgery of the skull base?
   A. Invasion of both cavernous sinuses
   B. Invasion of the optic chiasm
   C. Invasion of bilateral carotid arteries
   D. Invasion of the spinal cord
   E. Invasion of the brain stem

4. Which of these approaches is ideal for small intracanalicular tumors where hearing preservation is a priority?
   A. Middle fossa approach
   B. Retrosigmoid approach
   C. Translabyrinthine approach
   D. Retrolabyrinthine approach

5. Which is the most important predictor of 5-year survival in the resection of skull base malignancies?
   A. A watertight dural seal
   B. Tumor-free margins at the end of resection
   C. The use of postoperative radiation therapy
   D. The use of free-flap reconstruction
   E. The use of laser for resection of the tumor

Part 5
Laryngology

Chapter 50
Anatomy and Physiology of the Larynx

Anatomy

The larynx is an anatomical structure bridging the upper aerodigestive tract and the lower airways. Within the larynx, the vocal folds act as the principal valve dynamically controlling the aperture.

Laryngeal Cartilages and Surrounding Structures

A. *Hyoid bone* is the cranial-most component.
   i. Significance:
      a. U-shaped bone with a central body and superiorly projecting greater and lesser cornua
      b. Suspended from the mandible by muscular attachments and from base of the skull by stylohyoid ligaments
   ii. Action/Function:
      a. Provides stability to the larynx and pharynx
      b. Acts as site of attachment for cervical strap, digastric, extrinsic tongue, middle pharyngeal constrictor, and hyolaryngeal elevator muscles
   iii. Embryological origin: derived from mesenchyme of the second and third pharyngeal arches

a. The body and lesser horns (cornua) are derived from the second pharyngeal arch.
b. The greater horns (cornua) are derived from the third pharyngeal arch.
iv. Insertion: N/A. The only "free-floating" bone in the human body

B. *Thyroid cartilage* is the largest component of the laryngeal skeleton.
   i. Significance:
      a. Shield-shaped, formed from two alae (laminae) fused anteriorly with a posterior opening
      b. Forms the Adam's apple, a prominent feature that is more pronounced in males
      c. For gender reaffirming surgery, patients who are transitioning from man to woman undergo "chondrolaryngoplasty" to reduce the size of the Adam's apple
   ii. Action/Function:
      a. Provides anterior support and protection for the larynx.
      b. Posteriorly, each ala has superior and inferior cornua.
         1. Thyrohyoid ligament connects the superior cornua to the hyoid bone.
         2. Inferior cornua articulate with the cricoid cartilage.
   iii. Embryological origin: derived from mesenchyme of the fourth pharyngeal arch

C. *Cricoid cartilage* is the strongest of the laryngeal cartilages.
   i. Significance:
      a. The only complete and rigid ring in the airway
      b. Shaped like a signet ring with a lower height anteriorly than posteriorly
      c. Key landmark for emergency procedures like cricothyroidotomy
   ii. Action/Function: provides robust support and forms the base of the larynx
   iii. Embryological origin: derived from mesenchyme of the sixth pharyngeal arch

D. *Epiglottic cartilage*:
   i. Significance: leaf shaped; maintains the structural integrity of the epiglottis
   ii. Action/Function:
      a. Attaches to the inside of the thyroid cartilage anteriorly and projects superiorly and posteriorly above the glottic aperture.
      b. The petiole is the point of attachment to the thyroid cartilage.
      c. The inferior aspect of the epiglottis has fenestra that allows blood vessels to cross through the cartilage.
   iii. Embryological origin: derived from mesenchyme of the fourth pharyngeal arch

E. *Arytenoid cartilages* are the primary moving parts of the larynx.
   i. Significance
      a. Pyramidal shaped, with broad bases that articulate with the posterior superior surface of the cricoid cartilage via shallow ball and socket joints
      b. Vocal process:
         1. Anterior projection of each arytenoid
         2. Site of attachment for thyroarytenoid muscle
      c. Muscular process
   ii. Action/Function: muscles that open and close the glottis act by moving the arytenoids
   iii. Embryological origin: derived from mesenchyme of the sixth pharyngeal arch

Laryngeal Joints

A. *Cricoarytenoid joint:*
   i. Significance: synovial joint; abduction of the vocal cords and tension adjustment

   ii. Action/Function: Motion is primarily rotational about a variable vertical axis, with minor gliding/sliding motion secondarily.
      a. Arytenoid rotates externally to move vocal process upward and outward.
      b. Arytenoid rotates internally to move the vocal process medially and inferiorly.
   iii. Embryological origin: Derived from mesenchyme of the 6th pharyngeal arch
B. *Cricothyroid joints:*
   i. Significance: synovial joint, adjusts the length and tension of the vocal cords
   ii. Action/Function: primary motion is rotational, akin to a bucket (cricoid) on a handle (inferior cornua), with minimal sliding
   iii. Embryological origin: derived from mesenchyme of fourth and sixth pharyngeal arches

Extrinsic Ligaments

A. *Thyrohyoid membrane*:
   i. Significance:
      a. Connects thyroid cartilage and hyoid bone
      b. Pierced on lateral surface by superior laryngeal vessels and internal branch of superior laryngeal nerve
   ii. Action/Function:
      a. Connects thyroid cartilage and hyoid bone, maintaining the position of the larynx relative to the hyoid during swallowing and speech
      b. Provides a passageway for the superior laryngeal vessels and the internal branch of the superior laryngeal nerve
   iii. Embryological origin: derived from mesenchyme of third and fourth pharyngeal arches
   iv. Origin/Insertion: spans between the upper border of the thyroid cartilage and the lower border of the hyoid bone
B. *Cricothyroid membrane*:
   i. Significance:
      a. Relatively avascular and easily accessible, may be pierced in emergency cricothyrotomy for airway access
      b. Forms part of the conus elasticus
   ii. Action/Function:
      a. Connects the anterior surfaces of cricoid and thyroid
      b. Provides a passageway for the human communicating nerve (external SLN to the TA-LCA muscle complex)
   iii. Embryological origin: derived from mesenchyme of fourth and sixth pharyngeal arches
   iv. Origin/Insertion: extends between the cricoid and thyroid cartilages

Intrinsic Ligaments and Membranes

A. *Quadrangular membrane*:
   i. Significance: forms the upper part of the elastic membrane, the fibrous internal framework of the supraglottic larynx
   ii. Action/Function: provides internal structure to the supraglottic airway
   iii. Embryological origin: derived from mesenchyme of fourth and sixth pharyngeal arches

iv. Origin/Insertion:
   a. Extends from epiglottis postero-laterally to the arytenoids and corniculate cartilages
   b. Extends inferiorly to the false vocal fold

B. *Conus elasticus*:
   i. Significance: forms lower portion of elastic membrane (below the ventricle)
   ii. Action/Function: provides internal structure to the subglottic airway
   iii. Embryological origin: derived from mesenchyme of fourth and sixth pharyngeal arches
   iv. Origin/Insertion:
      a. Inferior attachment: superior border of the cricoid cartilage
      b. Superior anterior attachment: internal surface of apex of the thyroid cartilage
      c. Superior posterior attachment: vocal process of the arytenoid cartilage

C. *Vocal ligament*: the free upper edge of the conus elasticus
   i. Significance: anterior and posterior macula flavae are condensations at each end of vocal ligament
   ii. Action/Function:
      a. Allows vocal fold vibration and regulates tension to control pitch
      b. Provides structural support to the vocal folds
      c. Flavae are believed to produce essential extracellular matrix components of lamina propria
   iii. Embryological origin: derived from mesenchyme of fourth and sixth pharyngeal arches
   iv. Origin/Insertion:
      a. Inserts onto the anterior thyroid cartilage as Broyle ligament
      b. Extends from the vocal process of the arytenoid cartilage to the thyroid cartilage

Extrinsic Laryngeal Muscles (Table 50-1)

Table 50-1 Key Aspects of Extrinsic Laryngeal Muscles

A. Depressor muscles	
Significance:	Paired muscles depressing pharynx and larynx during swallowing/speech
Action/Function:	*Sternohyoid:* Depresses hyoid bone, indirectly lowering the larynx *Omohyoid:* Depresses and stabilizes hyoid bone, lowering the larynx *Thyrohyoid:* Depresses hyoid bone and elevates the larynx
Origin (embryo):	*Sternohyoid and Omohyoid:* Derived from the third pharyngeal arch *Thyrohyoid:* Derived from mesenchyme of the fourth pharyngeal arch
Origin/Insertion:	*Sternohyoid:* Origin: Manubrium of the sternum and the first costal cartilage Insertion: Oblique line of the thyroid cartilage *Omohyoid:* Origin: Superior border of the scapula near the suprascapular notch Insertion: Inferior border of the hyoid bone *Thyrohyoid:* Origin: Oblique line of the thyroid cartilage Insertion: Lower border of the body and greater horn of the hyoid bone.

(*Continued*)

Table 50-1 Key Aspects of Extrinsic Laryngeal Muscles (*Continued*)

Innervation:	*Sternohyoid and Omohyoid:* Ansa cervicalis (C2, C3) *Thyrohyoid:* C1 via hypoglossal nerve
B. Elevator muscles:	
Significance:	Paired muscles elevating pharynx and larynx during swallowing, speech
Action/Function:	*Geniohyoid:* Elevates hyoid bone and pulls it forward, raising the larynx *Digastric:* Elevates the hyoid bone and the larynx *Anterior Belly:* Depresses the mandible when the hyoid bone is fixed; raises the hyoid bone when the mandible is fixed *Posterior belly:* Elevates and stabilizes hyoid during swallowing, speech *Mylohyoid:* Elevates hyoid bone and floor of the mouth, raising the larynx *Stylohyoid:* Elevates and retracts hyoid bone, elongating mouth floor
Origin (embryo):	*Geniohyoid:* Derived from the paraxial mesoderm (occipital myotomes) *Mylohyoid, Digastric anterior belly:* Mesenchyme of first pharyngeal arch *Stylohyoid, Digastric posterior belly:* Mesenchyme second pharyngeal arch
Origin/Insertion:	*Geniohyoid:* Origin: Inferior mental spine on the inner surface of the mandible Insertion: Body of the hyoid bone *Digastric:* *Anterior belly:* Arises from digastric fossa of the mandible *Posterior belly:* Arises from mastoid notch of the temporal bone Insertion: Intermediate tendon connected to the hyoid bone *Mylohyoid:* Origin: Mylohyoid line on the inner surface of the mandible Insertion: Body of the hyoid bone and median raphe
Innervation:	*Geniohyoid:* C1 *Mylohyoid, digastric (anterior belly):* V3 *Stylohyoid, digastric (posterior belly):* VII
C. Pharyngeal constrictor muscles:	
Significance:	*Superior constrictor:* Does not attach to the larynx
Action/Function	Three paired muscles that contract sequentially during swallowing
Origin (embryo):	Primarily derived from the sixth pharyngeal arches
Origin/Insertion:	*Superior constrictor:* Pterygoid hamulus, pterygomandibular raphe, mylohyoid line of mandible *Middle constrictor:* Arises from the hyoid bone and stylohyoid ligament *Inferior constrictor:* Arises from the oblique line on the thyroid cartilage
Innervation:	Pharyngeal plexus, primarily via the vagus nerve
D. Cricopharyngeus muscle:	
Significance:	Continuous circular muscle surrounding the esophageal inlet Inferior fibers of the inferior constrictor muscle
Action/Function:	Forms the pharyngoesophageal segment (upper esophageal sphincter)
Origin (embryo):	Derived from mesenchyme of the fourth and sixth pharyngeal arches
Origin/Insertion:	Arises from the lateral aspects of the cricoid cartilage of the larynx Attaches to the posterolateral external surface of the cricoid cartilage
Innervation:	Recurrent laryngeal nerve and fibers from the pharyngeal plexus

Intrinsic Laryngeal Muscles (Table 50-2)

Table 50-2 Key Aspects of Intrinsic Laryngeal Muscles

A. Thyroarytenoid muscle:	
Significance:	Dual functionality in both tension and relaxation of vocal fold
Action/Function:	*Medial* (vocalis muscle) controls the length, tension, and stiffness *External* adducts the vocal folds
Origin (embryo):	Derived from mesenchyme of the sixth pharyngeal arch
Origin/Insertion:	Origin: Anterior interior surface of the thyroid cartilage Insertion: Vocal process and anterior surface of the arytenoid cartilage
Innervation:	Recurrent laryngeal nerve
B. Lateral cricoarytenoid muscle:*	
Significance:	The primary muscle involved in vocal fold adduction
Action/Function:	Pulls the muscular process, rotating the arytenoid cartilage inward This moves the vocal process inward and inferiorly
Origin (embryo):	Derived from mesenchyme of the sixth pharyngeal arch
Origin/Insertion:	Origin: Lateral aspect of the cricoid arch Insertion: Muscular process of the arytenoid cartilage
Innervation:	Recurrent laryngeal nerve
C. Interarytenoid muscle:	
Significance:	The only unpaired laryngeal muscle
Action/Function:	Connects the arytenoid cartilages, facilitating vocal fold adduction Oblique fibers constrict the laryngeal inlet; Transverse fibers close the posterior glottis
Origin (embryo):	Derived from mesenchyme of the sixth pharyngeal arch
Origin/Insertion:	Spans between the arytenoid cartilages, connecting them directly
Innervation:	Receives ipsilateral and contralateral innervation from recurrent and superior laryngeal nerves
D. *Aryepiglottic muscle:*	
Significance:	Small muscle in the free edge of the aryepiglottic fold
Action/Function:	Narrows laryngeal inlet by pulling epiglottis toward arytenoid cartilages
Origin (embryo):	Derived from mesenchyme of the sixth pharyngeal arch
Origin/Insertion:	Origin: Apex of the arytenoid cartilage Insertion: Lateral margin of the epiglottis and the aryepiglottic fold
Innervation:	Recurrent laryngeal nerve and superior laryngeal nerve
E. Posterior cricoarytenoid muscle:	
Significance:	Two bellies, horizontal and vertical, with distinct roles
Action/Function:	Horizontal belly: Abducts and stabilizes the vocal cords Vertical belly: Lengthens the vocal fold and stabilizes the arytenoid

(*Continued*)

Table 50-2 **Key Aspects of Intrinsic Laryngeal Muscles (*Continued*)**

Origin (embryo):	Derived from the mesoderm of the sixth pharyngeal arch
Origin/Insertion:	Origin: Posterior cricoid lamina Insertion: Muscular process of the arytenoid cartilage
Innervation	Recurrent laryngeal nerve
F. *Cricothyroid muscle:*	
Significance:	Only muscle not innervated by the recurrent laryngeal nerve
Action/Function:	Closes the cricothyroid space and Increases distance between anterior commissure and posterior cricoid Increases length and tension in the vocal fold to raise vocal pitch Minor vocal fold adduction activity
Origin (embryo):	Derived from mesenchyme of the fourth pharyngeal arch
Origin/Insertion:	Origin: Anterior arch of the cricoid cartilage Insertion: Thyroid cartilage
Innervation:	External branch of the superior laryngeal nerve—ONLY

Compartments of Laryngeal Lumen

A. *Vestibule*: from the inlet of the larynx to the edges of the false vocal folds
   i. Anterior boundary: laryngeal surface of the epiglottis
   ii. Posterior boundary: interarytenoid area
   iii. Lateral boundary: false vocal folds
B. *Ventricle (ventricle of Morgagni)*: a deep recess between the false and true vocal folds
   i. Saccule is a conical pouch that ascends from the anterior part of the ventricle.
   ii. Numerous minor salivary glands open into the ventricle.
C. *Glottis (rima glottidis)*: the space between the free margins of the true vocal folds
   i. Radial sector (teardrop shaped) when the vocal folds are abducted widely
   ii. Narrows to a slit during phonation
      a. Closes completely during swallow, Valsalva, and cough
D. *Pyriform sinus*: a pharyngeal recess within the thyroid lamina but lateral to paraglottic space

Divisions of the Larynx

A. *Supraglottis:* from the tip of the epiglottis to the beginning of squamous epithelium at the junction between the lateral wall and the floor of the ventricle
B. *Glottis:* the true vocal folds and the posterior commissure
   i. Membranous vocal fold: from anterior commissure to vocal process of arytenoid
      a. Composed of laminar soft tissue: muscle, vocal ligament, lamina propria, and epithelium
      b. From anterior commissure to the vocal process of the arytenoid cartilage
      c. Vibration of epithelium and lamina propria over vocal ligament and muscle produces the voice
   ii. Cartilaginous vocal fold: arytenoid cartilages
   iii. Posterior commissure: mucosa and the underlying interarytenoid muscle

C. *Infraglottis:* from the undersurface of the true vocal fold to the superior cricoid edge
D. *Subglottis:* from the undersurface of the true vocal folds to the inferior cricoid edge

Spaces in the Larynx

A. *Paraglottic space*: between thyroid ala, conus elasticus, and quadrangular membrane
B. *Preepiglottic space*: bounded by the vallecula, thyroid cartilage, thyrohyoid membrane, and epiglottis

Laryngeal Mucosa

A. Stratified squamous epithelium over superior and medial surface of vocal folds.
B. Ciliated pseudostratified columnar epithelium elsewhere.
C. The tissue between the vocal fold epithelium and muscle is a specialized extracellular matrix known as lamina propria.
   i. The vocal fold lamina propria has three layers that allow the vocal fold mucosa (epithelium and superficial layer of the lamina propria) to vibrate freely over the underlying vocal ligament. (Figure 50-1)
      a. *Superficial:* very loose fibrous tissue and rich in hyaluronic acid and water
      b. *Middle layer:* denser, with more elastic fibers
      c. *Deep*: cross-linked collagen, progressively denser toward the TA-LCA muscle

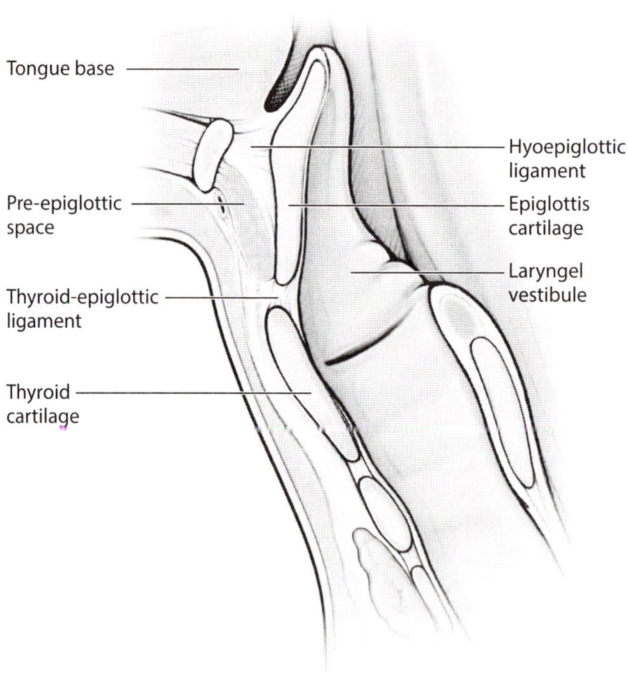

Figure 50-1

D. Hirano's Body Cover Theory of the vocal folds:
   i. Epithelium and superficial layer of the lamina propria form the vibratory "Cover"
   ii. Intermediate and deep layers of the lamina propria compose the "Transition," providing elasticity and support
   iii. Vocalis muscle forms the "Body," ensuring stability and tension control

Nerve Supply

Two branches of the vagus nerve

A. *Superior laryngeal nerve* (SLN)
   i. Exits vagus at nodose ganglion and divides into two branches
      a. Internal (sensory) branch pierces thyrohyoid membrane and carries afferent sensation from the supraglottic and glottic larynx.
      b. The external (motor) branch supplies cricothyroid muscle and contributes to the human communicating nerve.
B. *Recurrent laryngeal nerve* (RLN)
   i. Motor nucleus is the nucleus ambiguous.
   ii. Majority of motor innervation to all ipsilateral intrinsic laryngeal muscles except cricothyroid.
   iii. Interarytenoid muscle receives bilateral innervation.
   iv. Sensory fibers from the subglottis and trachea to nucleus solitarius.
   v. Longer course on left side: Fibers descend into chest with vagus nerve, and then loop around the ligamentum arteriosum to ascend in tracheoesophageal groove.
   vi. Right RLN fibers leave vagus and loop upward around the subclavian artery to ascend in tracheoesophageal groove.
   vii. On both sides, RLN enters larynx near cricothyroid joint.
   viii. Extralaryngeal branching may be encountered.
   ix. Embryonic branchial arch system causes the circuitous routes of the RLNs.
      a. RLN is the nerve of the sixth segmental arch.
      b. Left artery of sixth arch is the ductus arteriosus (ligamentum arteriosum).
      c. Right artery of the sixth arch disappears, so that right RLN loops around the fourth arch, which becomes the subclavian artery.
      d. Nonrecurrent RLN is associated with anomalous retroesophageal subclavian.
C. *Intralaryngeal nerves:*
   i. *Galen nerve*: Connects the SLN and RLN (motor and sensory)
   ii. Human communicating nerve: Arises from external branch of the SLN and pierces the cricothyroid membrane to innervate the larynx (motor and sensory)
   iii. Interarytenoid nerve (superficial and deep): nerves from bilateral RLN that traverse the interarytenoid muscle (motor and sensory)
   iv. Intralaryngeal branches of the RLN: three branches of the RLN are routinely seen: branch to the interarytenoid muscle, PCA, and the TA-LCA muscle complex

Blood Supply and Lymphatic Drainage

A. Superior laryngeal artery: arises from the superior thyroid artery, a branch of external carotid
B. Inferior thyroid artery: arises from the thyrocervical trunk
C. Superior thyroid vein drains into internal jugular vein

D. Inferior thyroid vein drains into the innominate vein
E. Glottic lymphatic drainage: very sparse, and only ipsilateral
   i. The limited lymphatic drainage reduces the likelihood of tumor spread to lymph nodes, such as for squamous cell carcinoma, often resulting in more localized disease
F. Supraglottic lymphatics drain: to upper jugular lymph nodes, some contralateral crossover
G. Infraglottic lymphatics drain: to pretracheal or lower jugular nodes with some contralateral crossover

Embryology

A. Fourth week of embryologic development: Respiratory diverticulum appears as a thickening on the ventral wall of the foregut, just caudal to the fourth branchial arch.
B. Diverticulum elongates to form the larynx, trachea, and lungs.
C. The laryngeal cartilages arise from the fourth and sixth branchial arches.
D. The cricothyroid muscle is derived from the fourth arch and is supplied by the superior laryngeal nerve.
E. All other intrinsic laryngeal muscles are from the sixth arch, supplied by the recurrent laryngeal nerve.
   i. The laryngeal lumen becomes obliterated by mesenchyme during the sixth week, but begins to recanalize during the 10th week.

Development

A. At birth, the larynx is at the level of the second or third vertebra, and epiglottis is in contact with the soft palate.
   i. This creates two separate channels in the aerodigestive tract: one for food and the other for swallowing.
   ii. This arrangement is characteristic of mammals, allowing for respiration via obligate nasal breathing during feeding.
B. After birth, the larynx gradually descends in the neck.
C. By 4 to 6 months, the epiglottis is no longer in contact with the soft palate.
   i. One common cavity in the pharynx
   ii. Increased risk of aspiration during swallow
D. By the age of 6 to 8 years, the larynx descends to the level of the fifth cervical vertebrae.
   i. The pharyngeal space is a good resonating chamber for phonation and versatile organ for resonant phonation.
E. During adolescence in males, the larynx doubles in anterior-posterior diameter and undergoes a second descent, resulting in a deeper voice than that of females.
F. By age 7, a tri-laminar lamina propria has developed.
G. Ossification:
   i. *Hyoid bone*: Begins shortly after birth in six centers, complete by 2 years of age
   ii. Thyroid cartilage: Begins at puberty, at inferior margin, progressing cranially

   iii. Cricoid cartilage begins in young adulthood in the posterior superior area and progresses caudally
   iv. Arytenoid cartilages calcify in the third decade
H. The larynx descends with age due to weakening muscles and connective tissues, especially in men.
   i. In elderly men, it can significantly drop (2-3 cm) compared to its position in youth.
   ii. This necessitates careful consideration during tracheostomy placement.

Protection of the Lower Airway: Primary and Phylogenetically Oldest Function

A. Prevention of aspiration during the swallow
   i. The supraglottis (aryepiglottic folds and ventricular vocal folds), along with glottis (true vocal folds) constrict the laryngeal inlet during swallowing.
   ii. True vocal fold closure is the last barrier to aspiration, and material passing the true vocal folds into the trachea defines aspiration
B. Cough: to clear foreign matter from the lower airway, the larynx
   i. Vocal fold close during compressive phase
   ii. Subglottic pressure builds up due to expiration against closed vocal folds
   iii. Burst of air opens glottis and removes any secretions or other materials in the glottis and supraglottic area (expulsive phase)
C. Variation of glottic resistance according to respiratory demand
   i. Vocal folds open during inspiration, wider with deep breathing or panting
   ii. Varying degree of vocal fold adduction seen during exhalation
      a. Degree of closure determines the rate of passive exhalation. This provides the lower airways with back pressure allowing an "auto-PEEP" function.
D. Valsalva maneuver: Larynx closes tightly with inflated lungs
   i. Stabilizes thorax for muscular actions (eg, heavy lifting)
   ii. Increases intra-abdominal pressure for defecation, vomiting, and childbirth

Reflexes

A. Reflex closure in response to tactile or chemical stimulus.
B. Laryngospasm with strong stimulus or reduced threshold (anesthesia, hypoxia/hypercarbia).
C. Arrhythmia, bradycardia, and occasionally cardiac arrest may result from stimulating the larynx, as with intubation.
   i. This could be an exaggeration of responses that alter heart rate in response to respiratory cycle. These responses can be blocked with atropine.
D. Episodic prolonged apnea and subsequent sudden infant death may be due to hyperactive laryngeal reflex.

Phonation

A. Mechanism:
   i. The vocal folds are adducted by the laryngeal muscles, creating a seal that blocks the airway, allowing subglottic pressure to build during exhalation.
   ii. Once subglottic pressure exceeds the resistance of the closed vocal folds, they are pushed apart from the bottom up, forming a small opening (glottis) through which air can escape.

   iii. As air flows through the narrow glottis, the resulting negative pressure (Bernoulli effect) starts drawing the vocal folds back toward each other.
   iv. The Bernoulli effect and natural elastic tension in the vocal folds (myoelastic forces) complete their closure from the bottom up, progressively sealing the glottis.
   v. With the glottis closed, subglottic pressure builds again, and the cycle repeats rapidly, typically hundreds of times per second.
   vi. Stroboscopy leverages Talbot law to capture and display vocal fold vibrations as a slow-motion sequence, enabling detailed visual analysis of vocal fold function. (see "Clinical Evaluation" section G)
B. Requirements for normal phonation:
   i. Appropriate vocal fold approximation
   ii. Too loose → breathiness
   iii. Too tight → strained voice
   iv. Adequate expiratory force
   v. Control of length and tension
   vi. Some degree of vocal fold mucosal pliability is needed for sustained sound production
   vii. Adequate vocal fold bulk—(TA-LCA muscle complex may become atrophic with aging or neuropathy)
   viii. Resonance of vocal tract
C. *Acoustics*: The voice is a complex waveform (not sinusoidal). It has a variety of formats and subharmonics.
   i. Increase in aperiodic components of the wave results in dysphonia.
D. *Resonance*: The cavities of the supraglottis, hypopharynx, oropharynx, oral cavity, and nasopharynx modulate the sound signal by acting as resonance chambers that filter sound and selectively amplify certain frequencies.
E. *Articulation*: The palate, tongue, teeth, pharynx, and lips shape vocal sound into vowels and create consonants.

Clinical Evaluation of Hoarseness—History and Physical

A. Define what the patient means
   i. "Hoarseness" is a generic term used by patients to report their symptoms, while "Dysphonia" is a clinical diagnosis[1]
      a. Change in sound of the voice
      b. Increased effort in speaking
      c. Vocal fatigue
      d. Change in volume of the voice
B. Establish time course
   i. Onset: gradual or sudden
   ii. Duration: acute or chronic
   iii. Stable, declining, improving, or fluctuating
C. Medical history to assess causes, contributing factors:[1]
   i. Traumatic: Trauma to the neck or larynx, intubation injury
   ii. Surgery: Prior surgery of the head, neck, or chest
   iii. Inflammatory: Acute or chronic laryngitis, allergy, rhinitis
   iv. Autoimmune: Granulomatosis with polyangiitis, sarcoidosis, rheumatoid arthritis

v. Infections: Viral, bacterial, fungal infections
vi. Endocrinologic: Hypothyroidism, diabetes, puberty, menopause, andropause
vii. Gastrointestinal: Gastro-esophageal reflux disease, laryngopharyngeal reflux
viii. Neurologic and psychologic: Neurodegenerative diseases, stress, anxiety, depression
ix. Neoplastic: Cancer, metastatic cancer, and other neoplasms
x. Congenital: Laryngeal web, vocal fold cyst, laryngeal cleft
xi. Musculoskeletal: Cervicalgia, muscle tension
xii. Behavioral: Vocal fold nodules, cyst, or polyp, vocal misuse or overuse
xiii. Medication: Antihistamines, anticoagulants, ACEi, antipsychotics, diuretics, steroids
xiv. Substance use and environmental irritants: Tobacco smoke, alcohol and drug abuse, chemical pollutants, dust

D. Voice history
  i. Previous voice problems
    a. Past voice issues, diagnoses, treatments, and outcomes
  ii. Professional or occupational demands on voice
    a. Vocal demands based on profession
    b. Professional voice user identification (eg, teacher, singer)
    c. Upcoming vocal commitments that may affect treatment
  iii. Vocal training
    a. History of vocal training, duration, types of exercises
    b. Multiple teachers or inconsistent training involvement
  iv. Vocal abuse: shouting, speaking over noise, screaming
    a. Behaviors like shouting, speaking over noise, screaming
    b. Specific events or habits contributing to vocal strain
  v. Validated patient-reported outcome measurement tools (PROMS)
    a. Such as: Voice Handicap Index and Reflux Symptom Index (see section H below)

E. Physical—Perceptual analysis:
  i. Quantify hoarseness:
    a. GRBAS Rating Scale: each parameter rated on a scale of 0 (normal) to 3 (severe):[2]
      1. Grade (severity)
      2. Roughness
      3. Breathiness
      4. Asthenia (weakness)
      5. Strain
    b. CAPE-V: visual analog scale (0-100 mm), with lower scores indicating better voice quality:[3]
      1. Overall severity
      2. Roughness
      3. Breathiness
      4. Strain
      5. Pitch
      6. Loudness
    c. CAPE-V Sentences (eg, "The blue spot is on the key again", "How hard did he hit him?" and "We were away a year ago")

F. Examine the larynx endoscopically—indirect mirror examination generally inadequate.
   i. Clinicians should perform laryngoscopy when:
      a. hoarseness does not resolve after 4 weeks,
      or,
      b. serious underlying cause is suspected:[1]
         1. Tobacco or alcohol use
         2. Concomitant neck mass
         3. Trauma
         4. Hemoptysis
         5. Dysphagia
         6. Odynophagia
         7. Otalgia
         8. Airway compromise
         9. Accompanying neurologic symptoms
         10. Unexplained weight loss
         11. Worsening hoarseness
         12. Immunocompromise
         13. Possible aspiration of foreign body
         14. Neonatal hoarseness,
         15. After intubation or neck surgery
G. Video and audio recording provide a comprehensive documentation, facilitating playback for detailed assessment:
   i. Flexible transnasal laryngoscopy:
      a. Generally well tolerated
      b. Allows assessment during connected speech and other tasks
      c. Distal chip images are clearer than fiberoptic examinations
   ii. Rigid endoscopy:
      a. Transoral: 90- or 70-degree Hopkins rod telescope
      b. Allows brighter image and higher degree of magnification
      c. Cannot view during connected speech
      d. Tolerance may be limited by gag reflex
   iii. Stroboscopy:
      a. Strobe light frequency is timed slightly off the vocal frequency, capturing sequential phases of vibration to create a composite image approximating the full glottic cycle (Talbot law)
      b. This imaging allows the clinician to:
         1. Assess the pliability of vocal fold for potential stiffness or reduced flexibility
         2. Detect adynamic segments, submucosal lesions, or other structural abnormalities
         3. Analyze the symmetry, periodicity, and completeness of glottic closure during vibration
      c. It may be less reliable in cases of severely aperiodic or chaotic vocal fold vibrations.
   iv. High-speed video:
      a. Provides true slow-motion visualization of vocal fold vibration, mostly used for research
   v. Audio recording: Passage reading for connected speech:
      a. Provides a phonetically diverse sample for consistent voice analysis

b. Useful for detecting subtle changes in vocal quality over time
c. The Rainbow Passage: The most commonly used

H. Objective measures of voice:
  i. Phonetogram: Determines frequency and loudness range
  ii. Acoustic analysis:[4]
    a. Fundamental frequency: Indicates the number of vocal fold vibrations/cycles per second (determinant of basic pitch). Normal values: males: 85 to 180 Hz; females: 165 to 255 Hz
    b. Jitter: Measures frequency instability (pitch variation). Normal values: less than 1% for both males and females
    c. Shimmer: Measures amplitude instability (loudness variation). Normal values: less than 3% to 5% for both males and females
    d. Noise-to-Harmonics Ratio (NHR): Assesses the ratio of noise to harmonic sound. Normal values: Less than 0.2% for both males and females
  iii. Spectral analysis:
    a. Energy distribution: Assesses harmonic structure and noise presence. Normal Values: not fixed; varies by individual voice characteristics
  iv. Cepstral analysis:
    a. Cepstral peak prominence (CPP): measures clarity and strength of harmonic structure. Normal values: males: 10 to 12 dB, females: 9 to 11 dB
  v. Electroglottography: monitors electrical impedance across the glottis to document changes in glottal closure during phonation
  vi. Aerodynamic measures: Measures airflow and subglottic pressure during phonation
    a. Subglottic pressure: Measures the pressure beneath the vocal folds during phonation. Normal values: varies depending on the individual's voice and intensity of speech. Mostly used in research
    b. Airflow rate: Assesses the amount of air passing through the vocal folds during phonation. Normal values: range between 100 to 200 mL/s for normal speech. Mostly used in research
    c. Maximum phonation time (MPT): measures the longest duration a patient can sustain a vowel sound on one breath. Normal values: males: 25-35 seconds, females: 15 to 25 seconds. Clinically useful measurement

I. Quality of life measures (patient-reported outcome measures)
  i. Aims to quantify the patient's experience with their laryngeal disorder(s).
  ii. Patient reports their experience with common complaints/situations that laryngeal disordered patients have previously reported.
  iii. Laryngology patient-reported outcome measures now exist to quantify the patient experience with the following functions:
    a. Voice: voice handicap index-10 (VHI-10), voice handicap index (VHI), voice-related quality of life (V-RQOL)[5]
    b. Singing: singing voice handicap index-10 (SVHI-10), singing voice handicap (SVHI)
    c. Swallowing: eating assessment tool 10 (EAT-10), MD Anderson dysphagia inventory (MDADI)
    d. Breathing: dyspnea index (DI)
    e. Cough: Cough severity index (CSI), Leicester cough questionnaire
    f. Symptoms associated with reflux: reflux symptom index (RSI)

References

1. Stachler RJ, Francis DO, Schwartz SR, et al. Clinical practice guideline: hoarseness (Dysphonia) (Update). *Otolaryngology–Head and Neck Surgery*. 2018 Mar;158(1 Suppl).
2. Hirano M. Phonosurgical anatomy of the larynx. In: Ford CN, Bless DM, editors. *Phonosurgery: Assessment and Surgical Management of Voice Disorders*. New York, NY: Raven Press;1991:25-42.
3. Kempster GB, Gerratt BR, Verdolini Abbott K, Barkmeier-Kraemer J, Hillman RE. Consensus auditory-perceptual evaluation of voice: development of a standardized clinical protocol. *Am J Speech-Language Pathol*. 2009 May;18(2):124-32.
4. Kent RD, Ball MJ, editors. *Voice Quality Measurement*. San Diego, CA: Singular Publishing Group; 2000.
5. Rosen CA, Lee AS, Osborne J, Zullo T, Murry T. Development and validation of the Voice Handicap Index-10. *Laryngoscope*. 2004 Sep;114(9):1549-1556.

Questions

1. Injury to the external branch of the superior laryngeal nerve during thyroid surgery typically results in which of the following?
   A. Unilateral vocal cord paralysis and inability to phonate
   B. Loss of abduction and adduction of the vocal cords
   C. Impaired tension of the vocal cords, leading to difficulty reaching higher pitches "pitch ceiling" and vocal fatigue
   D. Bilateral vocal cord paralysis, leading to airway compromise
   E. None of the above

2. According to the AAO-HNS Clinical Practice Guidelines on Hoarseness (dysphonia), which of the following is most appropriate when evaluating a patient with persistent hoarseness for more than 4 weeks without an obvious cause?
   A. Immediate initiation of proton pump inhibitors (PPIs) for suspected laryngopharyngeal reflux
   B. Routine prescription of oral corticosteroids to reduce vocal fold inflammation
   C. Referral for laryngoscopy to rule out structural or functional abnormalities of the vocal folds
   D. Ordering a CT scan of the head and neck for patients with hoarseness lasting more than 2 weeks
   E. Empiric use of antibiotics to manage potential bacterial infection contributing to hoarseness

3. Which of the following are all extrinsic muscles of the larynx?
   A. Sternohyoid, cricothyroid, omohyoid, thyrohyoid
   B. Digastric, mylohyoid, stylohyoid, thyroarytenoid
   C. Superior constrictor, middle constrictor, inferior constrictor, interarytenoid
   D. Thyrohyoid, omohyoid, mylohyoid, stylohyoid
   E. None of the above

4. Which of the following statements about voice measures is correct?
   A. Jitter measures cycle-to-cycle frequency fluctuations, with a normal value of ≤ 1%
   B. Shimmer measures cycle-to-cycle frequency fluctuations, with a normal value of ≤ 0.4%
   C. Maximum phonation time (MPT) measures the amplitude instability in vocal fold vibrations
   D. Fundamental frequency measures the perturbation in the peak-to-peak timing of each glottal pulse

5. What are the five layers of the vocal fold?
   A. Epithelium, superficial lamina propria, intermediate lamina propria, deep lamina propria, vocalis muscle
   B. Epithelium, intermediate lamina propria, thyroid cartilage, deep lamina propria, cricothyroid muscle
   C. Epithelium, arytenoid cartilage, cricoid cartilage, superficial lamina propria, vocalis muscle
   D. Epithelium, hyoid bone, thyroid cartilage, intermediate lamina propria, vocalis muscle

Chapter 51
Disorders of the Larynx

Various pathologies can affect the voice, swallowing, and breathing. This chapter highlights some of the most common laryngeal conditions.

Common Causes of Hoarseness and Dyspnea

1. Vocal Fold Inflammation

Acute Laryngitis

Common Causes

A. Infectious: laryngeal inflammation directly from infection or as a result of coughing related to an upper or lower airway infection
   i. Bacterial: *Moraxella catarrhalis, Haemophilus influenza, Streptococcus pneumonia, Staphylococcus aureus*
   ii. Viral: parainfluenza, influenza, herpes simplex virus
   iii. Fungal: *Candida albicans*

B. Postviral: ulcerative laryngitis

C. Noxious chemical exposure

D. Angioedema

E. Phonotrauma: shouting and loud talking and/or protracted voice use, excessive coughing

F. Allergy

G. Irritants: environmental chemicals in the air or inhaled substances such as unfiltered cigarettes or vapor creating devices, smoke from fires

H. Inhaler use, for example, Advair

I. Radiation treatment

Diagnosis

A. History of sudden onset of hoarseness

B. History of inciting factor (voice abuse, upper respiratory infection [URI] resulting in excessive coughing, reflux symptoms)

C. Laryngopharyngeal reflux (LPR) may not manifest symptoms of gastroesophageal reflux disease (GERD), such as classic heartburn or indigestion

D. No dyspnea (this suggests another diagnosis)

E. Reflux should be suspected if hoarseness occurs after a patient has gone to bed soon after a large meal, or after drinking alcohol. A foul taste in the mouth on awakening is another sign of nocturnal reflux like nocturnal laryngospasm and/or morning hoarseness with antecedent voice abuse

Physical Examination

A. *Routine head and neck examination*: seeks signs of URI, sinusitis, and tonsillitis
B. Voice may be rough, weak, or breathy and increased effort is required to speak
C. Laryngeal examination: rule out other causes of hoarseness:
   i. Assure normal vocal fold motion
   ii. Rule out lesions on vocal fold
   iii. Look for infraglottic edema, which may be suggestive of chronic laryngopharyngeal reflux disease
   iv. Unilateral or bilateral mid-membranous vocal fold ulcers are suggestive of ulcerative laryngitis

Natural History

A. Generally resolves spontaneously over 1 to 2 weeks (ulcerative laryngitis may take longer to heal)
B. May evolve into chronic condition depending on the etiology. For example, ulcers on the vocal folds may develop into scar if not healed well
C. Laryngitis precipitated by one factor may be prolonged by other factors, such as pre-existing laryngopharyngeal reflux or poor vocal habits

Treatment: Symptomatic and Supportive

A. Vocal hygiene—total voice rest is rarely needed but reduced voice use for a limited time period is thought to be of benefit
B. Hydration
C. Decongestant for nasal obstruction
D. Cough suppression
E. Mucolytic
F. Avoid drying antihistamines
G. H_2 blockers or proton pump inhibitors (PPIs) if acid reflux suspected with GERD/LPRD behavior modification
H. Steroids only for urgent need to use voice (performance, etc.)

Laryngopharyngeal Reflux Disease

A. *Symptoms*: globus, dysphonia, dysphagia, chronic cough, throat clearing, and mucous; only 25% to 35% have heartburn
B. *Pathophysiology*: intermittent patency of pharyngoesophageal segment and/or reflexive symptoms due to acid exposure of the lower esophageal sphincter, worse with physical exertion and increased intra-abdominal pressure
C. *Diagnosis*:
   i. Clinical symptoms with resolution with empiric trial (full-dose medication management and behavioral modification implementation)
   ii. Endoscopy
      a. Vocal folds edema, thick mucous, infraglottic edema, interarytenoid swelling, diffuse edema, and erythema
   iii. 24-hour pH probe
      a. Improved results with impedance measuring (detects acid and nonacid reflux along the entire length of esophagus, gold standard)

b. Similar information can be obtained from intraesophageal pH monitoring (Bravo); however, a procedure (EGD) is required for implementation, and only distal esophageal pH results are provided, but it does often provide a longer period of pH data than 24 hours

D. *Treatment*
   i. Empiric LPR trial
      a. BID proton pump inhibitor taken 30 minutes prior to breakfast and dinner
      b. Can add H_2 blocker at nighttime
      c. Can add alginate therapy after meals and QHS (provides a barrier between the upper aerodigestive tract and the stomach)
      d. Minimum of 2 to 3 months duration
      e. Patient compliance with medication timing and diet/lifestyle changes should be assessed
   ii. Diet modification
   iii. Behavioral modification
   iv. Esophagoscopy to rule out Barrett esophagitis
   v. Surgical management
      a. Fundoplication

2. Vocal Fold Lesions

Vocal Nodules

A. Cause: typically a result of phonotraumatic vocal behavior such as the following:
   i. Phonating too loudly, too much, or with improper vocal technique
   ii. Severe/protracted coughing
B. Epidemiology:
   i. Frequently occur in young children or adult females, not common in adult males.
   ii. Vocal fold lesions like nodules can be an occupational hazard for singers and grade school teachers.
   iii. Singers may have small lesions of the vocal folds that do not disrupt the vocal fold vibration nor voice quality and thus need no treatment.
C. Diagnosis:
   i. History
      a. Voice is chronically dysphonic, often characterized by increased effort, raspy voice quality, and changes in the singing voice.
      b. Singers may report reduced vocal range, instability in their passaggio (transition from chest register to head register), or require longer warm-up before singing.
   ii. Physical
      a. Laryngoscopy and video stroboscopy reveal bilateral, usually symmetric subepithelial lesions in the middle portion of the membranous vocal folds. Upon stroboscopic evaluation the mucosal wave (vibration of the vocal fold mucosa) is typically preserved, and glottal closure is an hourglass shape.
      b. These lesions are always subepithelial and will have normal overlying epithelium, and thus, a malignancy concern should be minimal.
      c. By definition, vocal nodules resolve or significantly get smaller with voice therapy and reduction of voice demands. If the patient has had high-quality voice therapy AND was compliant with voice therapy and the vocal fold lesions do not change, the diagnosis is NOT vocal nodules.

D. Treatment
   i. The cornerstone of treatment is voice therapy. Vocal nodules will resolve if vocal habits are corrected and this process may require weeks or months.
   ii. In-office steroid vocal fold injections can be considered as an adjunct treatment to help reduce the edema and inflammation surrounding the vocal fold nodules.
   iii. Surgery for symptomatic lesions persisting after adequate voice therapy in a compliant patient.
      a. Vocal fold lesions that still cause symptoms after voice therapy in a compliant patient may require surgery; by definition, these are not vocal nodules.
   iv. Treatment decisions should be based on vocal function, not appearance.

Vocal Fold Polyp

A. Fibrovascular mid-membranous subepithelial lesion of the vocal fold that results from phonotraumatic vocal behavior
B. *Primary symptom*: dysphonia
   i. Bleeding into polyp can cause sudden enlargement
C. Diagnosis:
   i. *History*: chronic dysphonia, increased effort with speaking
   ii. *Laryngoscopy*: subepithelial mass that can be broad-based or pedunculated, normal overlying epithelium, can be translucent or hemorrhagic. Stroboscopy reveals preserved mucosal wave and hourglass closure on phonation. Polyp can be unilateral or bilateral.
D. Treatment:
   i. *Surgery:* phonomicrosurgical excision via direct microlaryngoscopy.
   ii. *Laser:* angiolytic lasers that can be delivered through a flexible fiber system such as the KTP laser and blue light laser performed in-office or via microlaryngoscopy.
   iii. *Voice therapy*: vocal fold polyps usually do not regress with therapy, but voice may improve. Voice therapy prior deciding if surgery is necessary is important. Postoperative voice therapy is recommended for voice rehabilitation and to minimize the chance of recurrent lesions.

Vocal Fold Cysts

A. *Etiology*: possibly congenital, or acquired by vocal trauma
B. *Pathophysiology*: vocal impairment due to the lesion
   i. *Cysts*: fluid or mucoid-filled lesions that can occur in either the subepithelial space or on the vocal ligament
C. *Presentation*: chronic dysphonia; voice quality may vary depending on changes in fluid levels within the cyst
D. Diagnosis:
   i. Stroboscopy is very helpful to characterize the location and functional impact of the cyst on vocal fold vibration. Ligamentous vocal fold cysts tend to cause severe impairment of the mucosal wave and are difficult to diagnose in the office due to their deeper anatomic location, and thus, the definitive diagnosis is often made during microlaryngoscopy.
E. Treatment:
   i. *Voice therapy*: helps with patient symptoms but does not help with lesion regression. Voice therapy prior deciding if surgery is necessary is important. Postoperative voice therapy will help with voice rehabilitation.
   ii. *Surgery:* excision via microlaryngoscopy and microflap technique. Ligamentous vocal fold cysts require more extensive dissection which results in a higher risk of scarring and delayed recovery postoperatively compared to other lesions.

Contact Ulcer and Vocal Fold Granuloma

A. Laryngeal ulcers and granulomas typically appear on the vocal process of the arytenoid cartilage, but may occasionally be seen on the free edge of the vocal fold.
B. *Causes*: vocal abuse, throat clearing, intubation, glottal incompetence (vocal fold atrophy with secondary hyperfunction in voicing), and laryngopharyngeal reflux.
C. Diagnosis:
   i. *History*:
      a. Pain with phonation that can often radiate to the ipsilateral ear
      b. Foreign body sensation
      c. Hoarseness
      d. Frequent throat clearing
      e. History of intubation
      f. Acid reflux symptoms
   ii. Physical examination
      a. Vocal fold granuloma associated with vocal process of the vocal fold
      b. Stroboscopy can be helpful to identify evidence of glottal incompetence
D. Treatment:
   i. Control of acid reflux:
      a. Please refer to the section on laryngopharyngeal reflux disease.
      b. Worthwhile to try even in patients without symptoms of GERD.
   ii. Vocal hygiene
   iii. Voice therapy if vocal abuse/misuse detected
   iv. *Surgical removal*: Only for symptomatic lesions which do not respond to medical therapy, or when a tumor or other pathology is suspected
      a. Recurrence rate is high if the underlying cause of vocal process granuloma has not been addressed, for example, chronic cough, reflux, and voice misuse.
   v. Botulinum toxin injection of the thyroarytenoid-lateral cricoarytenoid muscle complex can be considered in refractory cases or as adjunct to surgical removal. Significant dysphonia results from the injection, and this patient should be prepared for this outcome.

Sulcus Deformity of the Vocal Fold

A. *Etiology:* congenital or acquired presumably due to vocal misuse.
B. *Pathophysiology:* loss of lamina propria resulting in the vocal fold epithelium along the free edge of the vocal fold tethering toward or in direct contact with the vocal ligament. Can occur unilaterally or bilaterally, for the entire vocal fold length or a segment, and can have an associated vocal fold lesion (cyst, polyp, fibrous mass).
C. *Presentation*: chronic dysphonia, higher vocal pitch, increased vocal effort.
D. *Diagnosis:* can be seen on office endoscopy but may require microlaryngoscopy with direct palpation for confirmation. On stroboscopy, evidence of glottal insufficiency is often seen and impairment of mucosal wave is common.
E. *Treatment*
   - Augmentation can be helpful to increase vocal volume and reduce effort of phonation. For patients with severe dysphonia, surgery will provide symptom improvement but not result in a normal voice.
   - Improving the mucosal wave impairment is a major challenge in laryngology. Approaches include excision, collagen or steroid injection, Gray mini-thyrotomy, or mucosal elevation with submucosal grafting.

Epithelial Dysplasia

A. Keratosis and leukoplakia are epithelial lesions of laryngeal epithelium that can be associated with malignancy.
B. *Etiology*: Smoking is the only strongly suspected etiology. Other suggested causes included LPRD, voice misuse/abuse, glottal insufficiency.
C. *Presentation*: dysphonia.
D. *Physical examination*: Thickened epithelium, white or reddish patches
  i. *Stroboscopy*: Lesions can impair glottal closure and/or mucosal wave.
  ii. Can consider narrow band imaging to further delineate the lesion.
E. *Diagnosis*: requires biopsy for histology. However, a trial of conservative measures may be indicated if malignancy is not strongly suspected.
F. Treatment:
  i. *Conservative*: cessation of smoking, antireflux therapy, and voice therapy
  ii. Direct microlaryngoscopy with biopsy or microflap excision of lesion
  iii. Periodic follow-up to detect recurrence, or possible new lesions
G. *Complications*: Excision can cause scarring with chronic dysphonia.

Recurrent Respiratory Papillomatosis: Benign Epithelial Growths Caused by Human Papilloma Virus

A. RRP are benign epithelial growths of the larynx caused by human papilloma virus (HPV), most common subtypes 6 and 11. The lesions most commonly arise from epithelium transition zones where stratified squamous epithelium transitions to respiratory epithelium, but papilloma may involve trachea or even distal bronchi.
B. Epidemiology:
  i. Juvenile onset
    a. Maternal transmission from mothers with genital warts. (Cesarean section does not reduce the incidence of transmission.)
    b. Risk factors are thought to be first-born child, young mother, and vaginal delivery.
  ii. Adult onset
    a. Sexual transmission has been implicated.
C. *Presentation*:
  i. Children: usually present with stridor and dyspnea
  ii. Adults: present with dysphonia
D. Diagnosis:
  i. Can usually be strongly suspected with office examination
  ii. Definitive diagnosis requires microlaryngoscopy and biopsy
E. Treatment:
  i. Suspension microlaryngoscopy and excision are usually required. Microdebrider, angiolytic lasers such as KTP laser or blue light laser, or CO_2 laser are most commonly used, but microsurgical instruments are also used, particularly for small, isolated lesions. Surgery is not curative, but can improve function (voice and breathing).
  ii. Office-based laser procedures under local anesthesia can be used in many adults.
  iii. Adjunctive approaches should be considered for moderate or severe cases including oral indole-3-carbinol, intralesional injection of cidofovir, or intralesional injection or intravenous bevacizumab or biosimilar. Intravenous bevacizumab is not curative but has a high rate of disease control while patient receives regular treatments (every 6-12 weeks).

- iv. Recurrence is common. Repeated surgery can lead to permanent scarring and webbing.
- v. Malignant transformation may occur, particularly with subtypes 16 and 18.
- vi. Tracheotomy should be avoided if possible, as there are concerns for distal spread of lesions due to epithelial change of the airway at the trach site.
- vii. Routine screening (low-dose CT) chest imaging is wise to monitor for pulmonary disease.

3. Neurologic Disorders

Vocal Fold Paralysis

A. Presentation
- i. Symptoms vary greatly depending on unilateral versus bilateral and the position of the vocal fold(s)
- ii. Unilateral paralysis
  - a. Dysphonia (breathy and weak), vocal fatigue, decreased projection, decreased range, shortness of breath with speaking, high-pitched (compensatory falsetto)
  - b. Coughing and choking during swallowing, particularly with liquids
  - c. *Occasionally asymptomatic* if the immobile vocal fold is situated in a median position, allowing for complete glottic closure on phonation
- iii. Bilateral vocal fold paralysis
  - a. Depends on position of vocal folds:
    - Medialized: normal voice with stridor and dyspnea
    - Lateralized: weak voice, may also have dysphagia

B. Etiology
- i. *Cancer*: lung, thyroid, esophagus, and other
- ii. *Surgery*: thyroidectomy, cervical spine, intrathoracic
  - a. Thyroidectomy is most common cause of bilateral vocal fold paralysis
- iii. *Cardiovascular*: aortic aneurysm, patent ductus surgery, cardiac valve surgery, enlarged atrium (Ortner syndrome)
- iv. *Inflammatory*: collagen vascular disorders, sarcoidosis, Lyme disease, and syphilis
- v. *Central lesions*: Arnold-Chiari malformation, multiple sclerosis, cerebellar stroke (Wallenberg), etc
  - a. Isolated vocal fold paralysis due to other central lesions (such as stroke) is rare, as other cranial nerves are usually affected
  - b. *Idiopathic*: in about 20% of cases

C. Pathophysiology
- i. Position of paralyzed vocal fold may be lateral, paramedian, midline. The vocal fold may medialize over time (~6 months).
  - a. Nerve injuries regenerate to varying degrees, and partial injuries are common.
  - b. Regenerated or repaired nerve does not restore motion, but can restore muscular tone.
  - c. Regenerating neurons often show synkinesis and thus the vocal fold is not technically "paralyzed," but the vocal fold does not move due to incomplete recovery or misdirected recovery.
- ii. If source of the vocal fold paralysis is a central or high vagal lesion, the presumption is that the vocal fold tends to be more lateral and have less tone

D. Diagnosis
- i. Differentiate vocal fold paralysis from mechanical fixation
  - a. Mechanical fixation can occur from posterior glottis stenosis, crico-arytenoid joint fixation (arthritis or injury), or dislocation.

   b. Laryngeal electromyography (LEMG) can help to determine nerve injury and identify the stage of reinnervation if present.
      1. Absence of EMG activity or presence of synkinetic activity predicts poor recovery.
   c. Laryngoscopy (direct or flexible) with palpation of the vocal process to assess for mobility

E. Treatment
   i. For unilateral paralysis, goal is to improve glottal closure to reduce glottic insufficiency.
   a. Voice therapy if there is minimal or no glottic insufficiency
   b. Vocal fold injection augmentation:
      1. Can be done awake or asleep through the mouth, or through the neck
      2. The ideal long-term substance would be well tolerated and permanent. Currently, no injectable substance is perfect for the treatment of vocal fold paralysis.
         - Teflon injection was the most widespread treatment through the 1970s, but is no longer used as granulomas eventually developed in many patients and the removal of these "Teflon granulomas" are very destructive to the larynx.
         - Hyaluronic acid (HA) comes in a variety of formulations and some can last up to 6 to 9 months, requires no preparation but is not FDA approved for the larynx.
         - Carboxymethylcellulose lasts 1 to 2 months, requires no preparation and is FDA approved.
         - Calcium hydroxylapatite, lasts approximately 12 to 18 months, requires no preparation and is FDA approved.
         - Autologous fat, harvested by liposuction or open harvest. Unpredictable survival—sometimes dissipates within a short time, but may survive for years and represents an autologous long-term solution. Procedure is done under general anesthesia.
         - Silk protein-HA, the newest injectable material on the market, lasts at least 12 months. However, there is a concern about inflammation upon injection and has not been studied with long-term follow-up.
   c. Medialization laryngoplasty (Type I thyroplasty)
      1. Vocal fold medialized by a permanent implant using either Gore-Tex strips or silastic block placed in paraglottic space, via a window in thyroid cartilage.
         - Usually performed under local anesthesia with light IV sedation, so that voice results can be monitored during the procedure
         - Complications:
            - Postoperative airway obstruction due to edema (rare).
            - Late extrusion of implant (rare).
            - Failure to achieve adequate voice, usually because implant is too high or too anterior. Also, implant may seem adequate intraoperatively, but prove to be too small after resolution of vocal fold edema or subsequent muscle atrophy.
            - Medialization laryngoplasty is not effective for patients with a lateralized arytenoid resulting in a "open" posterior glottis. This condition requires reposition of the arytenoid cartilage to optimize laryngeal function (voice, airway protection, and swallowing).

d. *Arytenoid adduction:* Mimics the action of the lateral cricoarytenoid muscle
   1. *Indications*: large glottal gap due to a lateralized vocal process.
   2. Often performed in combination with medialization laryngoplasty.
   3. Muscular process of the arytenoid cartilage is exposed by transecting the attachments of the inferior constrictor muscles to the thyroid ala, and reflecting the pyriform fossa mucosa.
   4. Suture through muscular process is passed through anterior thyroplasty window, and traction is applied to rotate arytenoid internally.

e. *Laryngeal reinnervation:* Most commonly, a branch of the ansa cervicalis is anastomosed to the distal recurrent laryngeal nerve. An alternate approach is to use a neuromuscular pedicle. Reinnervation by either technique is reported to restore bulk and tone to the reinnervated muscles, but not vocal fold motion. This technique has not been shown to be more effective than static medialization.

ii. Treatment for bilateral vocal fold paralysis
   a. Improves airway while trying to minimize the negative impact on voice
      1. Tracheotomy is the gold standard. Speech is still possible with digital occlusion of the tracheotomy tube or use of a Passy-Muir valve.
      2. Arytenoidectomy:
         - External or endoscopic (total) rarely needed or performed
         - Medial removes medial portion of arytenoid cartilage while attempting to preserve membranous vocal fold for phonation
      3. Transverse cordotomy involves a destructive incision across the width of the vocal fold at the vocal process to enlarge the airway. This incision can be enlarged posteriorly in the arytenoid and/or anteriorly into the membranous vocal fold depending on the airway needs of the patient.
      4. Suture lateralization can be performed to enlarge the airway if there is no abnormality of the joint and if vocal fold motion recovery is expected.
      5. Reinnervation can restore abductor function in expert hands with an extensive reinnervation procedure.
      6. Laryngeal "pacing" with an implantable stimulator is still experimental but promising.

Vocal Fold Paresis

A. *Symptoms*: dysphonia, vocal fatigue, decreased projection, decreased range, shortness of breath with prolonged speaking

B. *Pathophysiology*: partial denervation leading to weakening of vocal fold movement

C. *Diagnosis*:
   i. Laryngoscopy: unilateral or bilateral vocal fold motion impairment: range of motion (adduction and/or abduction) and/or speed of motion. The vocal fold(s) may also have an appearance of decreased "bulk" or "tone"; this can be seen as a "bowed" appearance of the vocal fold(s). Sometimes supraglottic findings may be seen suggestive of subtle vocal fold paresis: ipsilateral "ventricular show" on the paretic side coupled with contralateral false vocal fold compensatory hyperadduction.
   ii. Laryngeal EMG can assist in diagnosis of subtle vocal fold paresis.

D. *Treatment*:
   i. Observation
   ii. Voice therapy
   iii. Augmentation with either injection or medialization laryngoplasty

Laryngeal Dystonia (Formerly Spasmodic Dysphonia): Focal Dystonia of the Larynx

A. *Pathophysiology*: intermittent involuntary spasms of intrinsic laryngeal muscles during speech
B. *Etiology*: unknown. Problem is thought to occur in the basal ganglia
C. Presentation:
   i. Adductor form:
      a. Most common
      b. Strained and strangled voice with frequent voice breaks
      c. Breaks commonly occur at onset of words beginning with vowels (eg, "—eggs")
   ii. Abductor form:
      a. About 1 in 10 patients with laryngeal dystonia (LD)
      b. Whispering or breathy voice
      c. Voice breaks between plosive consonants and vowels (eg, "pu—pp—y")
D. *Diagnosis*: based on the perceptual assessment, sentence reading, and laryngeal examination to rule out anatomic pathology
   i. One or more of these vocal tasks are normal: laugh, cry, shout, whisper, sing, or yawn. Dysphonia is task specific.
   ii. Laryngeal examination shows normal laryngeal anatomy and normal function for non-speech tasks.
E. Treatment modalities:
   i. Speech therapy alone has very limited efficacy.
   ii. EMG-guided botulinum toxin A injection of the thyroarytenoid-lateral cricoarytenoid muscle complex is currently the most widely used treatment for adductor LD.
      a. Very small amounts of toxin are injected on one or both sides of the larynx to weaken, but not paralyze the muscle.
      b. Injection can be percutaneous, usually with EMG guidance, or through a working channel of a flexible laryngoscope.
      c. The effective dose varies amongst patients and can be established by trial and error and titration.
      d. Botulinum toxin A is effective for abductor SD, and requires injection into the posterior cricoarytenoid muscle. This injection can be performed either by rotating the larynx or through the posterior lamina of the cricoid cartilage across the glottis.
   iii. Surgical treatment:
      a. Selective laryngeal adductor denervation-reinnervation, transects adductor branches of the RLNs and reinnervates them with branches of the ansa cervicalis.
      b. Lateralization thyroplasty (Isshiki type 2) has been reported to be effective for adductor SD.

Essential Tremor of the Vocal Tract

A. *Pathophysiology*: involuntary, rhythmic oscillations (~4 Hz) of the laryngeal muscles.
B. *Etiology*: Problem is thought to occur in the ventral thalamus.
C. Presentation: Shaky voice quality, reduced speech intelligibility, increased vocal effort, can be accompanied by head and hand tremors. Thought to be age-related.
D. *Diagnosis*: Laryngeal exam can demonstrate diffuse vocal tract tremor on sustained vowel phonation; oscillation of the larynx can be noted on phonation with neck palpation. Head and hand tremor may be noted as well.

E. Treatment modalities:
   i. Speech therapy for mild cases
   ii. Botulinum toxin A injection of the thyroarytenoid-lateral cricoarytenoid muscle complex is currently the most widely used treatment. Similar to laryngeal dystonia, the effective dose can be determined by trial and error. Other injection locations can be tried: false vocal fold, strap muscles and/or inter-arytenoid muscle.
   iii. Vocal fold injection laryngoplasty may be considered for those with concurrent vocal fold atrophy to reduce vocal effort.

4. Laryngeal Infections

Candidiasis

A. *Risk factors*: powdered inhaled steroids for asthma or chronic obstructive pulmonary disease (COPD), immune compromise, and antibiotic therapy
B. Diagnosis:
   i. History of progressive voice change, pain with swallowing
   ii. Examination of larynx shows white patches on bright red mucosa
   iii. May appear to be leukoplakia of the vocal folds
C. Treatment:
   i. Systemic antifungal treatment. Nystatin swish and swallow is ineffective as it does not reach the larynx.
   ii. Withhold steroid or switch to a nonsteroidal inhaler.
   iii. Biopsy necessary for persistent lesions to rule out dysplastic lesions.

Epiglottitis: Infectious Inflammation and Edema of the Supraglottis

A. *Pathophysiology*: The swollen epiglottis obstructs the airway, with rapidly progressive dyspnea. If untreated, death can occur within a few hours.
B. *Etiology*: Usually *Haemophilus influenzae*, although it may be caused by other bacteria or viruses. The occurrence of epiglottitis has decreased steadily in the United States since the *H. influenzae* type B vaccine became a routine childhood immunization in the late 1980s.
C. *Presentation*: sore throat, dysphagia and drooling, fever, stridor, dyspnea (relieved somewhat by leaning forward), "hot potato" voice
D. Diagnosis:
   i. Primarily based on history.
   ii. Point tenderness at the hyoid level in midline is a characteristic sign.
   iii. Examination should be careful and gentle to avoid stimulating a gag, which can precipitate sudden upper airway obstruction. Do not use a tongue blade. Flexible endoscopy can usually be used in adults.
   iv. Imaging should not delay treatment when diagnosis is strongly suspected.
      a. In doubtful cases, with mild dyspnea, a lateral soft tissue neck X-ray demonstrates the swollen epiglottis ("thumb print" sign)
      b. A CT scan may demonstrate the rare occurrence of an abscess of the epiglottis. However, when the diagnosis is strongly suspected, treatment should not be delayed to obtain imaging.
      c. Any patient who is sent for imaging for suspected epiglottitis should be continuously attended by a physician capable of emergency airway management.
   v. Blood cultures are more likely than mucosal cultures to document the pathogen.
E. Treatment:
   i. Establish airway in the operating room, under controlled conditions, with tracheotomy or orotracheal intubation.

   ii. Selected adults who present more than 8 hours after onset without severe stridor may be managed without intubation or tracheotomy, but with close monitoring.
   iii. Intravenous antibiotics and steroids.

Croup (Acute Laryngotracheobronchitis)

A. Croup primarily occurs in children between the ages of 1 and 3 years.
B. *Cause*: Virus, parainfluenza types 1 to 4, *H influenzae*, streptococci, staphylococci, or pneumococci are often cultured.
C. Symptoms:
   i. Congestion and barking cough, with hoarseness, progressing to stridor.
   ii. With increasing obstruction, suprasternal retractions and accessory muscle use can be seen.
   iii. Agitation and tachycardia are signs of hypercarbia.
   iv. Circumoral pallor and cyanosis are late signs.
D. Diagnosis:
   i. *History*
   ii. *Imaging*: "steeple" sign on soft tissue anteroposterior (AP) image (subglottic narrowing due to edema)
E. *Treatment*: Depends on severity
   i. Cool mist inhalation may result in quick resolution
   ii. Steroids
   iii. Hospitalization for persistent and significant distress
   iv. Humidified oxygen, intermittent racemic epinephrine
   v. Antibiotics if indicated by fever and/or culture
   vi. Airway intervention if obstruction is severe (severe croup may actually be bacterial tracheitis)
   vii. Recurrent croup is an indication for operative endoscopy, due to possible anomaly such as subglottic stenosis, cyst, laryngeal cleft, or hemangioma

Laryngeal Tuberculosis (TB)

A. *Etiology*: an infection by *Mycobacterium tuberculosis*. Can be spread from pulmonary TB or an isolated, primary infection of the larynx
B. *Presentation*: dysphonia, dysphagia, pain with swallowing. Often laryngoscopy exam can be mistaken for a laryngeal mass. Unilateral vocal fold immobility may be observed
C. Diagnosis:
   i. High index of suspicion if the patient has a history of pulmonary TB, recent travel history, being born in a country with high incidence of TB, or immunosuppression.
   ii. Laryngeal culture and biopsy: laryngeal tissue can be sent for acid-fast bacilli (AFB) staining. However, a negative AFB stain does not definitive rule out laryngeal TB. Must wait for mycobactcrium culture to confirm, which can take 6 weeks. Laryngeal biopsy helps to rule out malignancy. In cases of laryngeal TB, necrotizing granulomas can be seen.
D. Treatment:
   i. Refer to Pulmonary Medicine and Infectious Disease for systemic TB treatment to rule out pulmonary TB.
   ii. See patient for follow-up after completion of TB treatment. Some may require voice rehabilitation due to vocal fold scarring or vocal fold paralysis from the infection.

Staphylococcus Laryngitis

A. *Etiology*: Thought to be a chronic bacterial colonization of the larynx by *Staphylococcus aureus*. It's most likely sinonasal in origin.
B. *Presentation*: primarily dysphonia. These patients often report a longstanding history of sinonasal issues. Laryngoscopy exam shows yellow exudate coating the larynx. Sometimes, thick, yellow mucus can be seen in the nasal cavity as well.
C. Diagnosis:
   i. Primarily based on clinical history laryngoscopy exam.
   ii. Can consider doing a laryngeal culture, but risk of contamination from oropharyngeal flora is high.
   iii. If sinonasal source is suspected, doing a CT sinus would be helpful to assess for chronic rhinosinusitis (CRS).
D. Treatment:
   i. Oral antibiotic treatment long-term (1-2 months). Antibiotic choice should cover MRSA, for example, trimethoprim and sulfamethoxazole.
   ii. Topical sinonasal treatment, for example, saline sinus rinse and topical nasal corticosteroids. In patients with CRS refractory to medical treatment, sinus surgery may be required to clear the laryngeal bacterial colonization.

5. **Systemic Diseases Affecting the Larynx**

Sarcoidosis

A. This is a systemic granulomatous disease that usually affects the lungs. Laryngeal involvement is not common. Granulomatous masses can cause hoarseness, while mediastinal adenopathy or neural involvement can cause vocal fold paralysis or paresis. Sometimes the sarcoidosis is limited to the larynx only.
B. *Presentation*: hoarseness, globus sensation, occasionally dyspnea. Laryngoscopy exam can show significant *supraglottic* swelling. Discrete masses are rarely seen.
C. *Diagnosis*:
   i. Diagnosis requires laryngeal biopsy, showing non-necrotizing granulomas.
   ii. Fungal infections and other granulomatous diseases must be excluded.
   iii. Serum angiotensin-converting enzyme (ACE) and calcium levels may be elevated in systemic sarcoidosis, but they are usually negative in isolated laryngeal sarcoidosis.
D. *Treatment*:
   i. Systemic steroids for acute airway edema
   ii. Intralesional steroid injection on a serial basis for isolate laryngeal sarcoidosis
   iii. Large lesions may require excision, debulking, or even tracheotomy
   iv. Consider rheumatology or pulmonology referral for consideration of other systemic treatment such as methotrexate and azathioprine

Rheumatoid Arthritis

A. Rheumatoid arthritis can cause inflammatory fixation of the cricoarytenoid (CA) joint and/or inflammatory vocal fold lesion (Bamboo nodules) on the vocal folds.
B. *Presentation*: hoarseness, pain, and referred otalgia. Bilateral CA joint fixation can cause stridor and dyspnea.
C. *Diagnosis*:
   i. Patient may have a clinical history of rheumatoid arthritis.
   ii. Physical examination shows unilateral or bilateral vocal fold immobility.
   iii. Bamboo nodules have the unique appearance of having multiple lesions within the vocal fold in a horizontal fashion, shaped like bamboo.

iv. Serology: elevated erythrocyte sedimentation rate and rheumatoid factor.
v. High-resolution CT scan can show erosion of joint and soft tissue swelling.
vi. Palpation of the CA joints may show stiffness of the joints. CA joint involvement occurs in very severe, late-stage RA patients.

D. *Treatment*:
i. Serial steroid injections can be performed into the CA joints to reduce stiffness, potentially restoring some form of motion.
ii. In cases of bilateral CA joint fixation not responding to serial steroid injections, glottal balloon dilation, or even a posterior cordotomy can be offered to the patient to enlarge the glottal airway. Tracheotomy would be a last resort.
iii. Bamboo nodules can be managed with serial steroid injections. Voice therapy can be considered. In general, surgery should be avoided.
iv. These patients should be referred to rheumatology for consideration of systemic treatment for their rheumatoid arthritis.

Granulomatosis with Polyangiitis (GPA)

A. This is an autoimmune vasculitis that primarily affects the lungs and kidneys. In up to 20% of cases, the larynx is affected, with exophytic granulation tissue that often progresses to subglottic stenosis.
B. *Presentation*: cough, hoarseness, stridor. Many have a prior diagnosis of GPA.
C. *Diagnosis*:
i. Biopsy shows necrotizing granulomas and capillary thrombosis.
ii. Antinuclear antibody (ANA) may be positive, but antineutrophil cytoplasmic antibody (C-ANCA) is more sensitive.
D. *Treatment*:
i. *Medical*: Systemic steroids for acute airway symptoms. Will need to be followed by rheumatology for other systemic treatment options
ii. *Surgical*: Stenosis is treated with radial excision, balloon dilation, and steroid injection. Recurrence can be quite rapid if the underlying GPA is not well controlled. Airway patency can be maintained with serial subglottic steroid injections in the office.

Amyloidosis

A. Abnormal deposition of amyloid, a type of protein, within tissues. This can be isolated to the larynx or systemic secondary to other conditions such as renal failure and multiple myeloma. Needs to rule out extramedullary plasmacytoma.
B. *Presentation*: most commonly chronic hoarseness, shortness of breath and stridor in extreme cases.
C. *Diagnosis*: Laryngeal examination shows deposits of amyloids in the larynx, which can involve the false folds, ventricles, true vocal folds, and subglottis.
D. *Biopsy*: Specimens should be processed with Congo red stain and viewed under polarized light to show apple green birefringence.
E. *Treatment*:
i. Endoscopic CO_2 laser debulking of the amyloid deposits that negatively impact function should be considered.
ii. Total removal is impossible but recurrence is very slow.

6. Laryngeal Trauma

A. *Pathophysiology*:
i. Laryngeal fractures are not common, since the larynx is protected posteriorly by the spine, and anteriorly by the chin and sternum.

ii. Laryngeal fractures usually result from a direct anterior blow. Other cause of laryngeal fracture includes a crushing injury, for example, from strangulation.
iii. Such trauma can also injure the cervical spine and cervical esophagus.

B. *Presentation*:
   i. Dysphonia or aphonia
   ii. Dyspnea, increased work of breathing, and stridor
   iii. Cough and hemoptysis
   iv. Dysphagia and odynophagia
   v. Neck pain

C. *Physical signs*:
   i. Loss of neck contour due to flattening of thyroid cartilage
   ii. Neck hematoma
   iii. Subcutaneous emphysema
   iv. Loss of normal laryngeal crepitus

D. *Management*: determined by stability of the airway
   i. Acute airway distress
      a. Proceed directly to operating room for awake tracheotomy with local anesthesia, followed by direct laryngoscopy under general anesthesia to assess the extent of endolaryngeal injury.
      b. Orotracheal intubation is not recommended, as laryngeal distortion makes this difficult, and the tube may create a false passage and intubation can worsen the laryngo-tracheal injury.
   ii. Stable airway:
      a. Flexible laryngoscopy to assess airway patency, vocal fold motion, and look for lacerations and exposed cartilage.
      b. If flexible laryngoscopy examination is normal, manage conservatively with observation, humidification, and steroids.
      c. If flexible laryngoscopy examination shows hematoma, swelling, decreased vocal fold motion, or other distortion, perform CT scan only if airway is patent. If CT shows displaced fracture, proceed to surgical repair. Otherwise, conservative management with steroids, humidified air, and observation.
      d. If examination shows lacerations or exposed cartilage, proceed to operating room for detailed evaluation, and endoscopic and/or open repair of injuries. Key principles are airway management and restoration of external laryngeal framework. Acute surgical repair is superior to delayed/chronic repair.
   iii. *Surgical repair*:
      a. If mucosal laceration is present, endoscopic suture of the laceration should be considered. Local flaps or free mucosal grafts may be used to close defects. Steroids can be injected to help reduce edema and scarring.
      b. If an arytenoid cartilage is completely avulsed and displaced, it is better to remove it than attempt to reposition it.
      c. Laryngeal cartilage fractures should be reduced and fixed with mini-plates (similar size to mid-face repair).
      d. Laryngeal stents may be used to add stability, but can stimulate granulation tissue. Should be considered in severely comminuted fracture to provide stability.

7. **Laryngeal and Tracheal Stenosis**
   A. *Etiology*: traumatic, for example, prolonged intubation, autoimmune disease such as GPA, or idiopathic. Symptoms and treatment vary depending on location, severity, and etiology of the stenosis. Supraglottic stenosis is much less common than glottis/subglottic/trachea

B. *Presentation*: Exertional dyspnea, stridor, +/– dysphonia
C. Diagnosis:
   i. Prior history of intubation, neck trauma, or autoimmune disease
   ii. Office endoscopy to evaluate supraglottic, glottic airway, and vocal fold motion. Subglottis can be visualized by asking the patient to tuck his/her chin toward chest
   iii. Awake bronchoscopy under local anesthesia in the office to evaluate the upper airway
   iv. CT scan to evaluate subglottic and tracheal airway, and cricoarytenoid joints
   v. Direct laryngoscopy and bronchoscopy to determine extent of lesion, palpate CA joints, and evaluate the posterior commissure
D. *Treatment*:
   i. Supraglottic stenosis
      a. Endoscopic excision of scar
      b. Serial in-office steroid injections to maintain the airway patency
   ii. Glottic stenosis
      a. Posterior glottic stenosis typically presents as dyspnea and stridor. Anterior glottic web typically causes dysphonia.
      b. Posterior glottic stenosis can be managed with glottal enlargement procedure such as posterior cordotomy. Anterior glottic web can be treated with endoscopic excision and keel stenting.
   iii. Subglottic stenosis
      a. Endoscopic surgery typically entails laser incision or excision of scar, balloon dilation, and steroid injection.
      b. Open surgery entails cricotracheal resection.
      c. Serial in-office steroid injections can be performed to maintain airway patency.
   iv. Tracheal stenosis
      a. Similar to subglottic stenosis, can be managed with endoscopic dilation or open resection

Common Causes of Upper Cervical Esophageal Dysphagia

1. Upper Cervical Esophageal Abnormalities

Zenker diverticulum

A. Symptoms: Usually solid dysphagia, postprandial regurgitation, halitosis, neck swelling, aspiration, gurgling after eating
B. Pathophysiology: pseudodiverticulum at Killian triangle between inferior constrictor and cricopharyngeus
   i. Discoordination between UES and pharyngeal contraction causing increased intraesophageal pressure
   ii. More frequently in men, seventh to eighth decade, and left side
C. Diagnosis: Barium swallow demonstrates diverticulum above the CP muscle; gastroscopy is optional.
D. Treatment
   i. Open diverticulectomy with cricopharyngeal myotomy
      a. Risks include mediastinitis, RLN injury, hematoma, infection
      b. Decreased recurrence with CP myotomy compared to endoscopic procedures
      c. Requires nasogastric tube for 2 to 5 days post op

- ii. Endoscopic
  - a. Requires exposure to perform the procedure with a bivalve laryngoscope, which is difficult to place in patients with prominent teeth, cervical kyphosis, and retrognathia
  - b. 5% conversion rate to open
  - c. Can use electrocautery, CO_2 laser, stapler
  - d. 5% recurrence rate
  - e. Can consider feeding postoperative day 0/1
  - f. Z-POEM (peroral endoscopic myotomy) is another minimally invasive technique to divide the septum separating the diverticulum and esophagus

Cricopharyngeal Muscle Dysfunction (CPMD)

- A. Symptoms: dysphagia to solids > liquids, globus sensation, food sticking
  - i. Pathophysiology: hypertrophy of cricopharyngeus muscle/inability of CP muscle to relax during swallowing
  - ii. Diagnosis:
    - a. Barium swallow will show cricopharyngeus bar
    - b. Manometry: tonic contraction of cricopharyngeus without relaxation
  - iii. Treatment
    - a. Dietary modification to a soft diet
    - b. Balloon or rigid dilation
    - c. Botulinum toxin injection
      - Can be injected in office or in operating room
      - Risk of intralaryngeal muscle diffusion and vocal fold paralysis
      - Doses of 50 to 100 Units split into 3 to 4 injection sites
    - d. Endoscopic myotomy
      - Performed with bivalve endoscope
      - Similar to management of Zenker diverticulum, exposure is most important part of surgery
      - Most commonly use CO_2 laser
      - Incise through mucosa and cricopharyngeus
      - Leaves buccopharyngeal fascia and areolar tissue intact, which prevents pharyngeal leak
    - e. Open myotomy
      - Similar approach to Zenker's
      - Can place bougie prior to surgery to provide cutting surface
      - Remove portion of muscle to prevent rehealing

Bibliography

Hirano M. Phonosurgical anatomy of the larynx. In: Ford CN and Bless DM editors. *Phonosurgery*. New York, NY: Raven Press; 1991.

Mallur PS, Shapiro J. Evaluation and examination of the patient with dysphagia. In: Fried MP, Tan M eds. *Clinical Laryngology: The Essentials 1st Edition*. New York, NY: Thieme Medical. 2014.

Rosen CA, Gartner-Schmidt J, Hathaway B, et al. A nomenclature paradigm for benign mid-membranous vocal fold lesions. *Laryngoscope*. 2012;122(6):1335-1341.

Siu J, Tam S, Fung K. A comparison of outcomes in interventions for unilateral vocal fold paralysis: a systematic review. *Laryngoscope*. 2016;126(7):1616-1624.

Woodson GE. Spontaneous laryngeal reinnervation after recurrent laryngeal or vagus nerve injury. *Ann Otol, Rhinol Laryngol*. 2007;116(1):57-65.

Questions

1. What are the most common subtypes of HPV involved in RRP?
   A. 6, 16
   B. 11, 18
   C. 6, 11
   D. 16, 30

2. What type of vocal cord lesions are associated with rheumatoid arthritis?
   A. Singer nodules
   B. Bamboo nodules
   C. Reinke edema
   D. Teacher nodes

3. A patient with adductor laryngeal dystonia will have the most difficulty with which of the following words?
   A. Mama
   B. Puppy
   C. Elephant
   D. Rainbow
   E. Candle

4. The arytenoid adduction procedure mimics the action of which muscle?
   A. Cricothyroid
   B. Interarytenoid
   C. Thyroarytenoid
   D. Lateral cricoarytenoid
   E. Posterior cricoarytenoid

5. Laryngeal stroboscopy is most useful in the diagnosis of
   A. Laryngeal dystonia
   B. Laryngeal paralysis
   C. Epiglottitis
   D. Vocal fold sulcus
   E. Laryngopharyngeal reflux

Part 6
Pediatrics

Chapter 52
Embryology of Clefts and Pouches

Correlation Between Age and Size of Embryo

Weeks	*Millimeters*
2.5	1.5
3.5	2.5
4	5
5	8
6	12
7	17
8	23
10	40
12	56
16	112
5-10 mo	160-350

Development of the Branchial Arches

The first 8 weeks constitute the period of greatest embryonic development of the head and neck. There are five arches that are named either pharyngeal or branchial. Between these arches are the grooves or clefts externally and the pouches internally. Each pouch has a ventral or dorsal wing. The derivatives of the arches are usually of mesoderm origin. The groove is lined by ectoderm, and the pouch is lined by endoderm (Figure 52-1).

Each arch has an artery, nerve, and cartilage bar. These nerves are anterior to their respective arteries, except in the fifth arch where the nerve is posterior to the artery. (Embryologically, the arch after the fourth is called the fifth or sixth arch depending on the theory one follows. For simplicity in this synopsis, it is referred to as the fifth arch.) Caudal to all the arches lies the 12th nerve. The sternocleidomastoid muscles are derived from the cervical somites posterior and inferior to the above arches.

There are two ventral and two dorsal aortas in early embryonic life. The two ventral aortas fuse completely, whereas the two dorsal ones only fuse caudally (Figure 52-2A). During the course of embryonic development, the first and second arch arteries degenerate. The second arch artery has an upper branch that passes through a mass of mesoderm, which

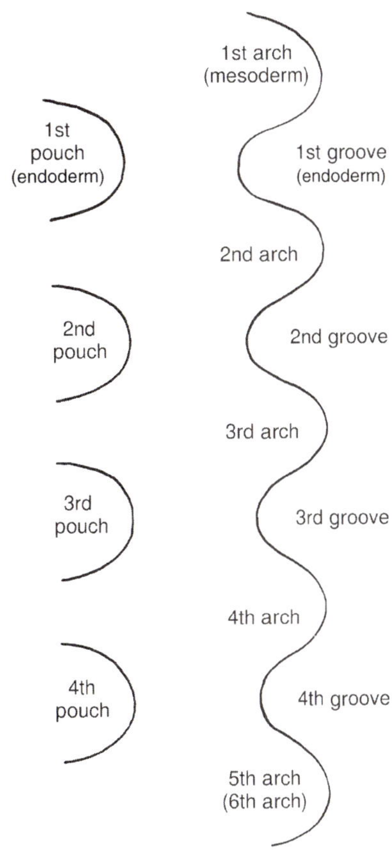

Figure 52-1 Pouches and grooves.

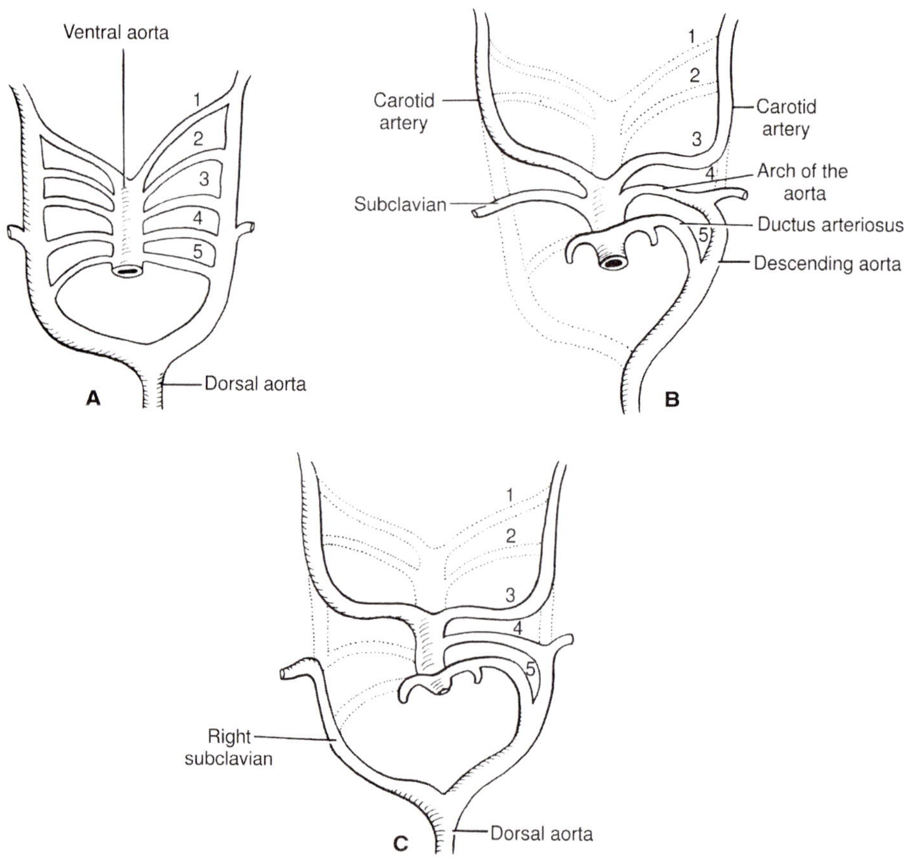

Figure 52-2 Development of the embryonic arteries.

later chondrifies and ossifies as the stapes. This stapedial artery usually degenerates during late fetal life but occasionally persists in the adult. The third arch artery is the precursor of the carotid artery on both left and right sides. The left fourth arch artery becomes the arch of the aorta. The right fourth arch artery becomes the proximal subclavian. The rest of the right subclavian and the left subclavian are derivatives of the seventh segmental arteries. The left fifth arch artery becomes the pulmonary artery and ductus arteriosus. The right fifth arch artery becomes the pulmonary artery with degeneration of the rest of this arch vessel (Figure 52-2B).

Should the right fourth arch artery degenerate and the right subclavian arise from the dorsal aorta instead, as shown in Figure 52-2C, the right subclavian becomes posterior to the esophagus, thus causing a constriction of the esophagus without any effect on the trachea (dysphagia lusoria). The innominate artery arises ventrally. Hence when it arises too far from the left, an anterior compression of the trachea results (anomalous innominate).

The fifth arch nerve is posterior and caudal to the artery. As the connection on the right side between the fifth arch artery (pulmonary) and the dorsal aorta degenerates, the nerve (recurrent laryngeal nerve) loops around the fourth arch artery, which subsequently becomes the subclavian. On the left side, the nerve loops around the ductus arteriosus and the aorta. Table 52-1 lists the branchial arches and their derivatives.

Arch → Nerve
Arch → Artery
Arch → Cartilage bar

(Nerve anterior to artery except in fifth arch)

Arch: mesoderm differentiates → Muscles, bones, vessels, cartilage

Four primitive aortas → Two ventral → Fused ventrally
Four primitive aortas → Two dorsal → Fused dorsally

Table 52-1 Branchial Arches and Their Derivatives

Arch	*Ganglion or Nerve*	*Derivatives*
First (mandibular)	Semilunar ganglion V3	Mandible Head, neck, manubrium of malleus Body and short process of incus Anterior malleal ligament Sphenomandibular ligament Tensor tympani Mastication muscles, mylohyoid Anterior belly of digastric muscle Tensor palati muscle
Second (hyoid)	Geniculate ganglion VII	Manubrium of malleus Long process of incus All of stapes superstructure except footplate and annular ligament (vestibular portion) Stapedial artery Styloid process Stylohyoid ligament Lesser cornu of hyoid Part of body of hyoid Stapedius muscle Facial muscles Buccinator, posterior belly of digastric muscle Styloid muscle Part of pyramidal eminence Lower part of facial canal
Third	IX	Greater cornu of hyoid and rest of hyoid Stylopharyngeus muscle, superior and middle constrictors; common and internal carotid arteries
Fourth	Superior laryngeal nerve	Thyroid cartilage, cuneiform, inferior pharyngeal constrictor, cricopharyngeus, cricothyroid muscles, aorta on the left, proximal subclavian on the right
Fifth[a]	Recurrent laryngeal nerve	Cricoid, arytenoids, corniculate, trachea, intrinsic laryngeal muscles, inferior constrictor muscle, ductus arteriosus

[a]Often called the *sixth arch* from the standpoint of evolution and comparative anatomy.

Derivatives of the Pouches

A. Each pouch has a ventral and a dorsal wing. The fourth pouch has an additional accessory wing. The endodermal lining of the pouches proliferates into glandular organs.

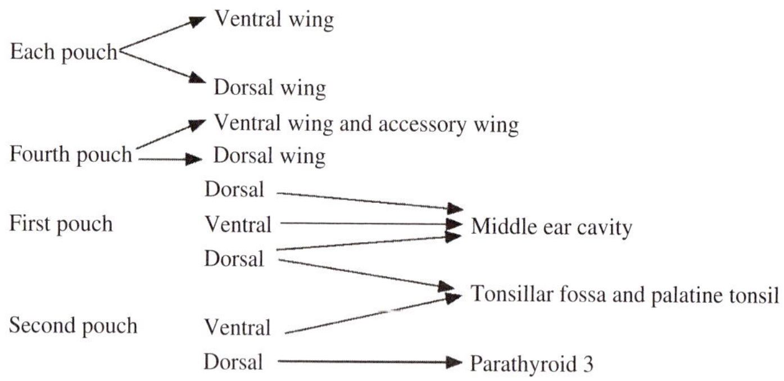

B. During embryonic development the thymus descends caudally, pulling with it parathyroid 3. Consequently, parathyroid 3 is inferior to parathyroid 4 in the adult.
C. The ultimobranchial body becomes infiltrated by cells of neural crest origin, giving rise to the interfollicular cells of the thyroid gland. These cells secrete thyrocalcitonin.
D. As these "out-pocketing" pouches develop into glandular elements, their connections with the pharyngeal lumen, referred to as pharyngobranchial ducts, become obliterated. Should obliteration fail to occur, a branchial sinus (cyst) is said to have resulted.
E. The second pharyngobranchial duct (between the second and third arches) is believed to open into the tonsillar fossa, the third pharyngobranchial duct opens into the pyriform sinus, and the fourth opens into the lower part of the pyriform sinus or larynx. An alternative school of thought believes that branchial sinuses and cysts are not remnants of patent pharyngobranchial ducts but, rather, are remnants of the cervical sinus of His.
F. The cutaneous openings of branchial sinuses, if present, are always anterior to the anterior border of the sternocleidomastoid muscle. The tract always lies deep to the platysma muscle, which is derived from the second arch (Figure 52-3).
   i. Course of a second arch branchial cyst
      a. Deep to second arch derivatives and superficial to third arch derivatives
      b. Superficial to the 12th nerve and anterior to the sternocleidomastoid
      c. In close relation with the carotid sheath but superficial to it
      d. Superficial to the ninth nerve, pierces middle constrictor, deep to stylohyoid ligament, and opens into tonsillar fossa
   ii. Course of a third arch branchial cyst
      a. Again, subplatysmal and opens externally, anterior to the sternocleidomastoid muscle
      b. Superficial to the 12th nerve, deep to the internal carotid artery and the ninth nerve
      c. Pierces the thyrohyoid membrane above the internal branch of the superior laryngeal nerve and opens into the pyriform fossa

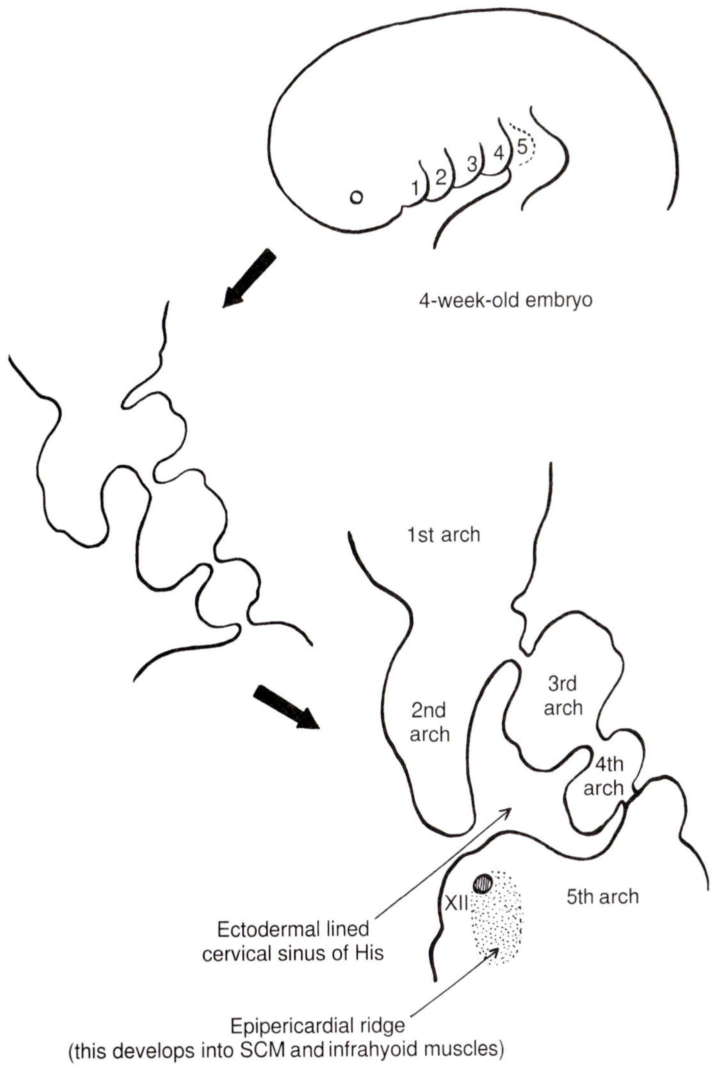

Figure 52-3 Pharyngobranchial ducts.

iii. Course of a fourth arch branchial cyst

a. Right

1. The tract lies low in the neck beneath the platysma and anterior to the sternocleidomastoid muscle.
2. It loops around the subclavian and deep to it, deep to the carotid, lateral to the 12th nerve, inferior to the superior laryngeal nerve; opens into the lower part of the pyriform sinus or into the larynx.

b. Left

1. Because the fourth arch vessel is the adult aorta, the cyst may be intrathoracic, medial to the ligamentum arteriosus and the arch of the aorta.

2. It is lateral to the 12th nerve, inferior to the superior laryngeal nerve.
3. It opens into the lower pyriform sinus or into the larynx.

Arches

First Arch (Mandibular Arch), Meckel Cartilage

Meckel cartilage →	Upper part →	Malleus head and neck; incus body, short process
	Intermediate →	Anterior malleal ligament
		Sphenomandibular ligament
	Lower →	Mandible
Mesoderm →	Tensor tympani, masticator muscles, anterior belly of digastric muscle, tensor palati muscle	
Nerve →	(V) Semilunar ganglion	
Artery →	"Degenerates"	

Second Arch (Hyoid Arch)

Reichert cartilage →	Manubrium of malleus
	Long process of incus
	Lenticular process
	Stapes superstructure (except vestibular part of footplate)
	Pyramidal eminence
	Styloid process, stylohyoid ligament
	Lesser cornu of the hyoid
	Part of the body of the hyoid
	Lower half of facial canal
Mesoderm →	Platysma, stapedius muscle and tendon, facial muscles, auricular muscle, posterior belly, stylohyoid muscle
Nerve →	Facial nerve (VII) geniculate ganglion
Artery →	Ventral, second aortic arch "degenerates" (persistent stapedial artery)

Third Arch

Cartilage bar →	Greater cornu of the hyoid, part of body of the hyoid
Mesoderm →	Stylopharyngeus muscle nerve
Nerve →	(IX) Superior and inferior ganglia
Artery →	Common and internal carotid arteries

Fourth Arch

Cartilage bar	→	Thyroid cartilage, cuneiform cartilage
Mesoderm	→	Inferior pharyngeus constrictor muscle, cricothyroid muscle, cricopharyngeus muscle
Nerve	→	Superior laryngeal nerve (jugular and nodose ganglion)
Artery: Left	→	Aorta
Right	→	Proximal subclavian (the rest derived from seventh segmental artery)

Fifth Arch

Cartilage bar	→	Cricoid, arytenoid, corniculate
Mesoderm	→	Intrinsic muscles of larynx (except cricothyroid); trachea
Artery: Left	→	Pulmonary → Ductus arteriosus
Right	→	Pulmonary
Nerve	→	Recurrent laryngeal nerve

Embryology of the Thyroid Gland

In a 4-week-old embryo, a ventral (thyroid) diverticulum of endodermal origin can be identified between the first and second arches on the floor of the pharynx. It is also situated between the tuberculum impar and the copula. (The tuberculum impar together with the lingual swellings becomes the anterior two-thirds of the tongue, and the copula is the precursor of the posterior one-third of the tongue.) The ventral diverticulum develops into the thyroid gland. During development, it descends caudally within the mesodermal tissues. At 4.5 weeks the connection between the thyroid diverticulum and the floor of the pharynx begins to disappear. By the sixth week it should be obliterated and atrophied. Should it persist through the time of birth or thereafter, a thyroglossal duct cyst is present. This tract travels either superficial to, through, or just deep to the hyoid and reaches the foramen cecum (Figure 52-4).

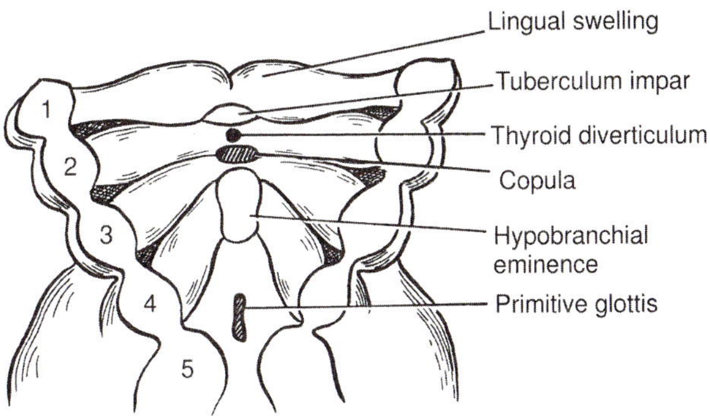

Figure 52-4 4-week-old embryo.

Table 52-2 Embryonic Development of the Tongue

Age (Weeks)	*Structure*
4	Tuberculum impar, lingual swellings, copula
7	Voluntary muscles, nerve XII, papillae, tonsillar tissues
8-20	Circumvallate papillae
11	Filiform and fungiform papillae

Embryology of the Tongue

The tongue is derived from ectodermal origin (anterior two-thirds) and entodermal origin (posteriorly). At the fourth week, two lingual swellings are noted at the first arch, and a swelling, the tuberculum impar, appears between the first and second arches. These three prominences develop into the anterior two-thirds of the tongue. Meanwhile, another swelling is noted between the second and third arches, called the copula. It develops into the posterior one-third of the tongue. At the seventh week, the somites from the high cervical areas differentiate into voluntary muscle of the tongue. The circumvallate papillae develop between the 8th and 20th weeks and the filiform and fungiform papillae develop at the 11th week (Table 52-2).

Embryology of Tonsils and Adenoids

A. Palatine tonsil (8 weeks) develops from the second pouch (ventral or dorsal).
B. Lingual tonsil (6.5 weeks) develops between the second and third arch ventrally.
C. Adenoids (16 weeks) develop as a subepithelial infiltration of lymphocytes.

Embryology of Salivary Glands

A. Parotid gland (5.5 weeks) is of ectodermal origin, derived from the first pouch.
B. Submaxillary gland (6 weeks) is of ectodermal origin, derived from the first pouch.
C. Sublingual gland (8 weeks) is of ectodermal origin, derived from the first pouch.

Embryology of the Nose

The nasal placode is of ectodermal origin and appears between the middle of the third and fourth weeks of gestation (Figure 52-5A). It is of interest to note that at this stage the eyes are laterally placed, the auricular precursors lie below the mandibular process, and the primitive mouth is wide. Hence, abnormal embryonic development at this stage may result in these characteristics in postnatal life.

At the fifth week, the placodes become depressed below the surface and appear as invaginated pits. The nasal pit extends backward into the oral cavity but is separated from it by the bucconasal membrane (Figure 52-5B). This membrane ruptures at the seventh to eighth week of gestation to form the posterior nares. Failure in this step of development results in choanal atresia. The nasal pit extends backward as well as upward toward the forebrain area. Epithelium around the forebrain thickens to become specialized olfactory sensory cells.

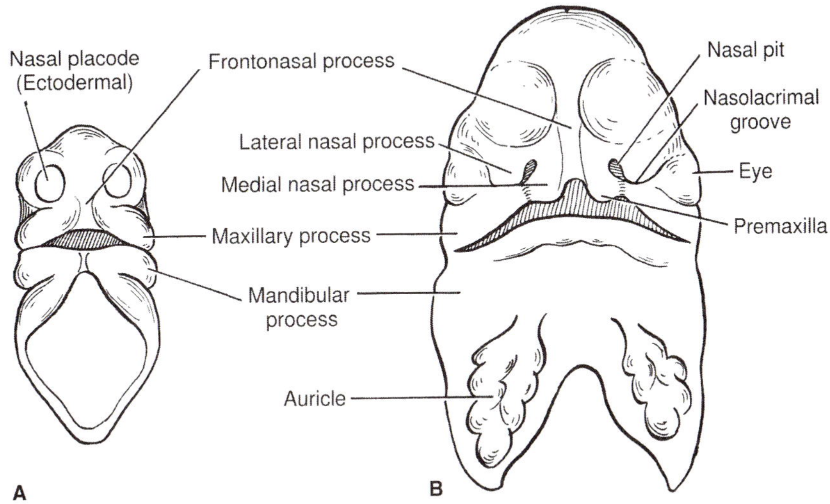

Figure 52-5 Development of the nasal placode. **(A)** 4-week-old embryo; **(B)** 5-week-old embryo.

Anteriorly, the maxillary process fuses with the lateral and medial nasal processes to form the anterior nares. The fusion between the maxillary process and the lateral nasal process also creates a groove called the nasolacrimal groove. The epithelium over the groove is subsequently buried, and, when the epithelium is resorbed, the nasolacrimal duct is formed, opening into the anterior aspect of the inferior meatus. The duct is fully developed at birth.

The frontonasal process (mesoderm) is the precursor of the nasal septum (Figure 52-6). The primitive palate (premaxilla) located anteriorly is also a derivative of the frontonasal process (mesoderm). Posteriorly (Figure 52-7), the septum lies directly over the oral cavity until the ninth week, at which time the palatal shelves of the maxilla grow medially to fuse with each other and with the septum to form the secondary palate. The hard palate is formed by the eighth to ninth week (Figure 52-8), and the soft palate and the uvula are completed by the 11th to 12th week.

From the 8th week to the 24th week of embryonic life, the nostrils are occupied by an epithelial plug. Failure to resorb this epithelium results in atresia or stenosis of the anterior nares.

Along the lateral wall of the nasal precursor, the maxilloturbinal is the first to appear, followed by the development of five ethmoturbinals and one nasoturbinal. Table 52-3 gives the derivatives of each embryonic anlage, and Table 52-4 gives a timetable of their development.

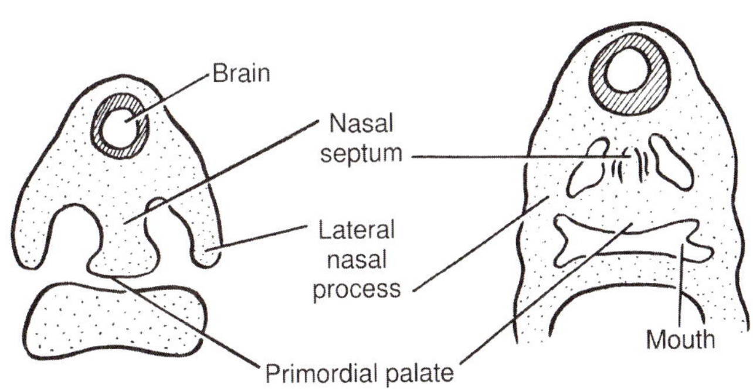

Figure 52-6 Development of the nasal septum (see text).

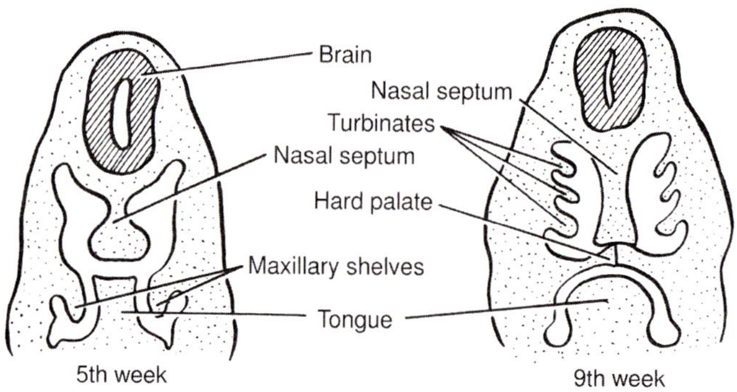

Figure 52-7 Further development of the nasal septum (see text).

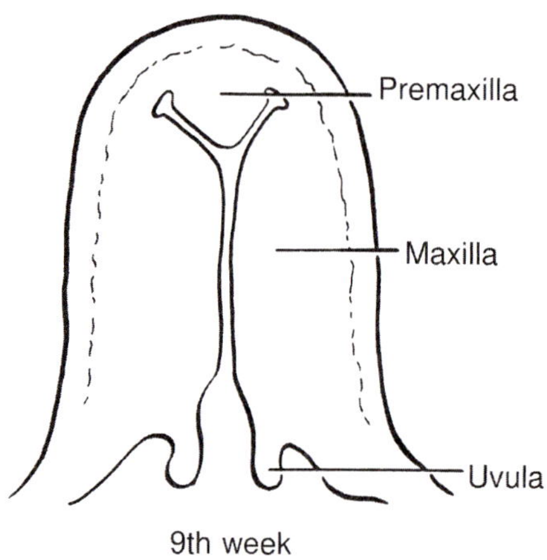

Figure 52-8 Parts of the palate.

Table 52-3 Embryonic Anlagen and Their Derivatives

Anlagen	*Derivatives*
Maxilloturbinal	Inferior concha
First ethmoturbinal	Middle concha
Second and third ethmoturbinals	Superior concha
Fourth and fifth ethmoturbinals	Supreme concha
Nasoturbinal	Agger nasi area

Table 52-4 Timetable of Nasal Development

Structures	*Time of Development (Week)*
Inferior concha formed	7
Middle concha formed	7
Uncinate process formed	7
Superior concha formed	8
Cartilage laid down	10
Vomer formed and calcified	12
Ethmoid bone calcified	20
Cribriform plate calcified	28
Perpendicular plate, crista galli calcified	After birth

Embryology of the Larynx

Figure 52-9 depicts the embryonic development of the larynx between the 8th and 28th weeks of fetal life.

The entire respiratory system is an outgrowth of the primitive pharynx. At 3.5 weeks, a groove called the laryngotracheal groove develops in the embryo at the ventral aspect of the foregut. This groove is just posterior to the hypobranchial eminence and is located closer to the fourth arch than to the third arch. During embryonic development, when a single tubal structure is to later become two tubal structures, the original tube is first obliterated by a proliferation of lining epithelium, then, as resorption of the epithelium takes place, the second tube is formed and the first tube is recannulized. Hence, any malformation involves both tubes. This process of growth accounts for the fact that more than 90% of tracheoesophageal fistulas are associated with esophageal atresia. During development the mesenchyme of the foregut grows medially from the sides, "pinching off" this groove to create a separate opening. With further maturation, two separate tubes, the esophagus and the laryngotracheal apparatus, are formed.

This laryngotracheal opening is the primitive laryngeal aditus and lies between the fourth and fifth arches. The sagittal slit opening is altered to become a T-shaped opening by the growth of three tissue masses. The first is the hypobranchial eminence, which appears during the third week. This mesodermal structure gives rise to the furcula, which later develops into the epiglottis. The second and third growths are two arytenoid masses, which appear during the fifth week. Later, each arytenoid swelling shows two additional swellings that eventually mature into the cuneiform and corniculate cartilages.

As these masses grow between the fifth and seventh weeks, the laryngeal lumen is obliterated. At the ninth week, the oval-shaped lumen is reestablished. Failure to recannulize may result in atresia or stenosis of the larynx. The true and false cords are formed between the 8th and 10th weeks. The ventricles are formed at the 12th week.

The two arytenoid masses are separated by an "interarytenoid notch," which later becomes obliterated. Failure of this obliteration to occur results in a posterior cleft up to the cricoid cartilage and opening into the esophagus. This is a culprit of severe aspiration in the newborn.

Table 52-5 outlines the muscular and cartilaginous development of the larynx.

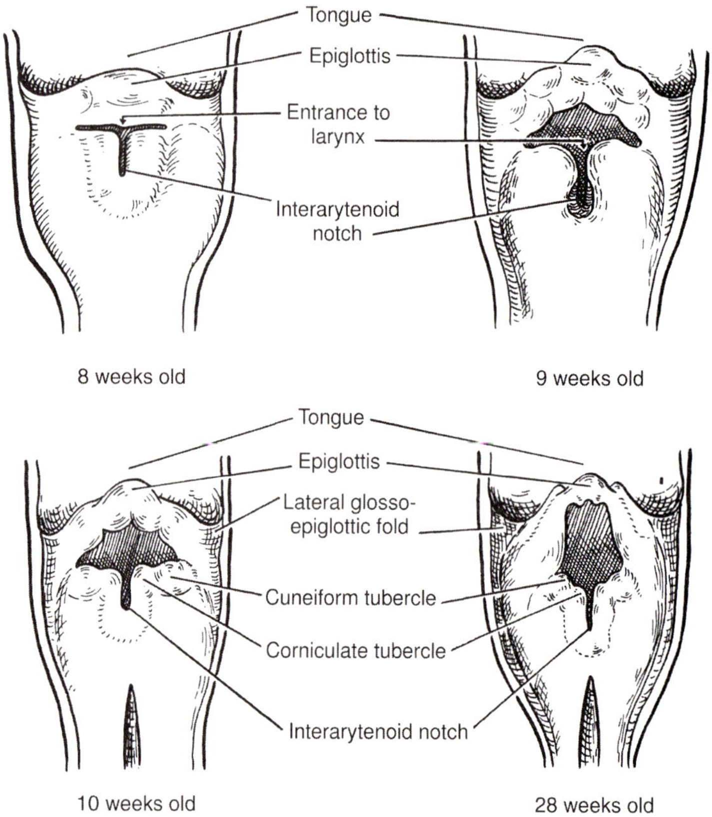

Figure 52-9 Development of the fetal larynx.

Table 52-5 Laryngeal Muscular and Cartilaginous Development With Embryonic Age

Development	*Age (weeks)*
Muscular	
Inferior pharyngeal constrictor and cricothyroid muscles formed	4
Interarytenoid and postcricoarytenoid muscles formed	5.5
Lateral cricoarytenoid muscle formed	6
Cartilaginous	
Development of epiglottis (hypobranchial eminence)	3
Thyroid cartilage (fourth arch) and cricoid cartilage (fifth arch) appear	5
Chondrification of these two cartilages begins	7
Development and chondrification of arytenoid (fifth arch) and corniculate (fifth arch) (vocal process is the last to develop)	12
Chondrification of the epiglottis	20
Development of the cuneiform cartilage (fourth arch)	28

Table 52-6 Development of Paranasal Sinuses

Sinus	*Characteristics*	*Age*
Maxillary	Arises as a prolongation of the ethmoid infundibulum	12 wk
	Pneumatizes	At birth
	Reaches stable size	18 y
Frontal	Arises from the upper anterior area of the middle meatus	Starts at late fetal life or even after birth
	Pneumatizes	After 1 y
	Full size	20 y
Sphenoid	Arises from the epithelial outgrowth of the upper posterior region of the nasal cavity in close relation with the sphenoid bone	Starts at third fetal month
	Pneumatizes	During childhood
	Full size	15 y
Ethmoid	Arises from the evagination of the nasal mucosa into the lateral ethmoid mass	Sixth fetal month
	Pneumatization completed	7 y
	Full size	12 y

The laryngeal muscles are derivatives from the mesoderm of the fourth and fifth arches and hence are innervated by the 10th nerve. The infant larynx is situated at a level between the second and third cervical vertebrae. In the adult, it lies opposite the body of the fifth cervical vertebra.

Table 52-6 outlines the development of the paranasal sinuses.

Ossification of Laryngeal Skeleton

Hyoid → Ossification from six centers → Starts at birth; completed by 2 years

Thyroid → Starts at 20 to 23 years; starts at inferior margin
- Extends posteriorly at each ala
- Superior margin never ossified

Cricoid → Starts at 25 to 30 years
- Incomplete
- Starts at inferior margin

Arytenoids → Starts at 25 to 30 years

Middle Ear Cleft

Embryology of the ear and congenital deformities (Tables 52-7A and B)

Table 52-7A Embryology of the Ear

Week	*External Ear*	*Middle Ear*	*Inner Ear*	*Facial Nerve*
3-5	Ectoderm—first branchial groove Endoderm—first branchial pouch	Second branchial pouch—middle ear space, second mesenchymal arch—stapes arch	Neuroectoderm + ectoderm—otic placode evolves to otic pit, vesicle, and endolymphatic duct and sac; ventral—vestibule; dorsal—cochlea, acoustic ganglion; superior—vestibular; inferior—cochlear, otic capsule from mesenchyme tissue	Primordial facial–acoustic—sensory fibers: chordae tympani nerve, nervus intermedius, geniculate ganglion, greater superficial petrosal nerve
6-9	First to second arch form hillocks of His First arch 1 tragus 2 helical crus 3 helix Second arch 4 antihelix 5 antitragus 6 lobule	Malleus and incus—single mesenchymal mass, mesenchymal stapes footplate; Meckel's cartilage—head and neck of malleus, body and short process of incus; Reichert cartilage—manubrium of malleus, long process of incus, stapes arch	Semicircular canals, macula divides: upper—utricle, lower—saccule; cochlea—2.5 turns wk 6-8.5	VII and VIII separate, extends to facial muscles, fallopian canal evolves as sulcus 9th wk, and fuses with Reichert cartilage
10-14	Hillocks fuse—auricle	Stapes arch formed, four mucosal pouches formed: anterior—anterior pouch of von Trolch; medius—petrous and epitympanium; superior—posterior pouch of von Trolch, mastoid; posterior—oval and round window niche, sinus tympani	Vestibular end organs formed, otolithic membrane, macula, cochlea tectorial membrane, scala tympani, fissula ante fenestram, fossula post fenestram	Extensive facial branching, location anterior in relation to external ear
15-20	Auricle recognizable, tympanic ring formed	Ossicles adult size, ossification begins	Membranous labyrinth complete without end organs, ossification begins at 14 sites	Located anterior and superficial, migration posterior

(*Continued*)

Table 52-7A Embryology of the Ear (*Continued*)

Week	*External Ear*	*Middle Ear*	*Inner Ear*	*Facial Nerve*
21-28	(External auditory canal) EAC epithelial core reabsorbs, complete 28th wk	Drum formed 28th wk; ectoderm—squamous; mesoderm—fibrous; entoderm—mucosal	Ossification complete 23rd wk; last to ossify fissula ante fenestrum, fossula post fenestrum; cochlea structures formed	Fallopian canal closes and ossifies
30-Birth	Auricle and ear canal continued to grow to age 9 y	Middle ear air space formed; tympanic ring ossifies by age 3; eustachian tube grows 17-36 mm	Membranous and bony labyrinth adult size; endolymphatic sac grows until adulthood	Facial nerve lateral until mastoid tip formed at age 3; 25% fallopian canals dehiscent
Grade	*Microtia*	*Atresia*		
I	Slight deformity of pinna	EAC normal—atretic, ossicles—deformed or fixed, abnormal course of facial nerve		
II	Deformed cartilage framework of pinna	Atresia, absent tympanic bone, small middle ear space, deformed ossicles, facial nerve anterior and lateral		
III	Soft tissue remnant of pinna	Middle and inner ear deformities		
IV	Anotia	Severe inner ear deformities: Scheibe—collapse of cochlear duct, deformed organ of corti; Michel aplasia—absent inner ear		

Congenital deformities incidence: microtia 0.13-6 per 1000 live births; atresia 1.2-5.5 per 1000 births; ossicular abnormalities 2% of patients having stapes surgery; bilateral deformities 10%; congenital hearing loss: sensorineural 85%; conductive 15% with external deformities in 50%.
Common syndromes associated with conductive hearing loss: mandibulofacial dysostosis (Treacher Collins); hemifacial microsomia; oculoauricular vertebral dysplasia (Goldenhar); craniofacial dysostosis (Crouzon disease).
Data from Sataloff RT. *Embryology and Anomalies of the Facial Nerve and Their Surgical Implications.* New York, NY: Raven Press; 1991.

Table 52-7B Microtia–Atresia

External ear deformities
- Preauricular pits and sinuses:
- Etiology: failure of complete closure first and second branchial arch hillock
- Incidence: white 0.18%, black 1.49%
- Pathology: epithelial-lined tract, may be associated with chronic inflammation, may extend to tragus or scaphoid fossa
- Management: observation unless infected; excision of complete fistula tract

Auricular deformities:
- Microtia grade I-IV often associated with atresia grade I-IV; protruding ear–cupped ear–deep conchal bowl; helical and antihelical rim deformities
- Management: dependent on severity of deformity; otoplasty—reconstruction

(*Continued*)

Table 52-7B Microtia–Atresia (*Continued*)

Evaluation congenital hearing loss and deformities: Audiology: birth—otoacoustic emissions (OAE); brain stem-evoked response audiometry (BERA); play audiometry at the age of 18 mo Expected hearing loss: Atresia: 60-70 dB conductive loss Stapes fixation: 50-65 dB conductive loss; presence of a carhart notch may suggest abnormal course of facial nerve Ossicular abnormalities: 25-50 dB conductive loss Facial nerve impinging on stapes: 20-35 dB conductive loss Radiology: conductive hearing loss—computed tomography (CT), thin 0.6 mm sections, axial and coronal views prior to surgery Sensorineural hearing loss—early childhood CT 0.6 mm, MR I < 1 mm of the cochlea and labyrinth, axial and coronal
Management Amplification: 6 mo of age hearing aids, sound stimulation Cochlear implant: age 1-2 y with profound sensorineural hearing loss Bone anchored hearing device considered for nonsurgical patients—age 6 y Surgical reconstruction: external and middle ear Reconstruction of pinna prior to EAC and middle ear; age 5-8 y, depending on size of opposite ear. Four stages: 1. Bury carved rib cartilage skeleton of pinna. 2. Construct lobule. 3. Elevate helical rim and graft postauricular sulcus. 4. Construct conchal bowl and tragus, may be combined with atresia surgery. Atresia, middle ear reconstruction: indications—conductive hearing loss > 30 dB, bone conduction < 20 dB, aerated and accessible middle ear space. reconstruction 70% tympanoplasty—ear canal, drum, and ossicular chain, stapes and oval window 17%, 60% have additional ossicular abnormalities, facial nerve covers the oval window 13% requiring fenestration of the horizontal canal. Alternative treatment: bone-anchored auricular prosthesis and hearing aid; no treatment with normal or aidable opposite ear.

Bibliography

Anson BJ, Donaldson JA. *The Ear: Developmental Anatomy and Surgical Anatomy of the Temporal Bone*. 3rd ed. Philadelphia, PA: WB Sanders Company; 1981:23-57.

Isaacson G, ed. Congenital anomalies of the head and neck. *Otolaryngol Clin North Am*. 2007;40:1-8.

Jahrsdoerfer R. Congenital malformations of the ear. *Ann Otolaryngol*. 1980;89:348-353.

Lambert PR. Congenital aural atresia. In: Bailey, ed. *Head & Neck Surgery–Otolaryngology*. Philadelphia, PA: Lippincott–Raven; 1998:1997-2010.

Sataloff RT. *Embryology and Anomalies of the Facial Nerve and Their Surgical Implications*. New York, NY: Raven Press; 1990.

Questions

1. The ultimobranchial body is responsible for cells that produce
   A. Insulin
   B. Parathyroid hormone
   C. Thyrocalcitonin
   D. Amylase
   E. Thyroxine

2. What is the precursor to the nasal septum?
   A. Medial nasal process
   B. Lateral nasal process
   C. Frontonasal process
   D. Maxillary process
   E. Ethmoturbinal

3. The anterior two-thirds of the tongue are derived from
   A. Endoderm
   B. Ectoderm
   C. Mesoderm
   D. Neural crest cells
   E. Thyroid cells

4. Which nerve is associated with the fourth branchial arch?
   A. Hypoglossal nerve
   B. Facial nerve
   C. Glossopharyngeal nerve
   D. Superior laryngeal nerve
   E. Trigeminal nerve

5. Cutaneous openings of branchial arch sinus tracts are always anterior to
   A. Hyoid bone
   B. Submandibular gland
   C. Sternocleidomastoid muscle
   D. Angle of the mandible
   E. Recurrent laryngeal nerve

Chapter 53
Cleft Lip and Palate

Overview

- Cleft lip and/or cleft palate is the most common congenital malformation of the head and neck, occurring in 1:700 live births.
- Annual multidisciplinary team evaluation is gold standard of care and includes experienced medical, surgical, dental, and allied health professionals for care coordination.
- Each patient should be evaluated for additional congenital anomalies or comorbidities, neurodevelopmental disorders, and psychosocial concerns.

Anatomy

- Lip (Figure 53-1)
  (a) Muscle: orbicularis oris
    - Innervated by CN VII
    - Creates complete sphincter around mouth
  (b) Primary blood supply: superior labial artery
  (c) Landmarks:
    - Vermilion: mucosal lip of external dry mucosa and internal wet mucosa of oral cavity
    - Vermilion-cutaneous (v-c) junction: muco-epithelial junction between cutaneous and mucosal lip; small discrepancy during cleft lip repair can be easily visible
    - Lip roll (also "white roll"): 2 mm convexity outlining vermilion-cutaneous junction due to bulging of orbicularis oris
    - "Cupid's bow": comprised of two vermilion high points (bilateral peaks at insertion of philtral ridges to v-c junction) and central low point, critical during cleft lip repair
    - Philtrum: central depression of upper lip
      - Philtral ridges: paramedian vertical columns formed at fusion plane between maxillary and frontonasal prominences
      - Philtral dimple: midline dimple above central portion of cupid's bow formed by decussation of the muscles to contralateral philtral column and attachment of orbicularis oris to dermis
- Palate
  (a) Muscles:
    - Innervated by CN X except tensor veli palatini (innervated by V3)
    - Soft palate includes levator veli palatini, tensor veli palatini, musculus uvulae

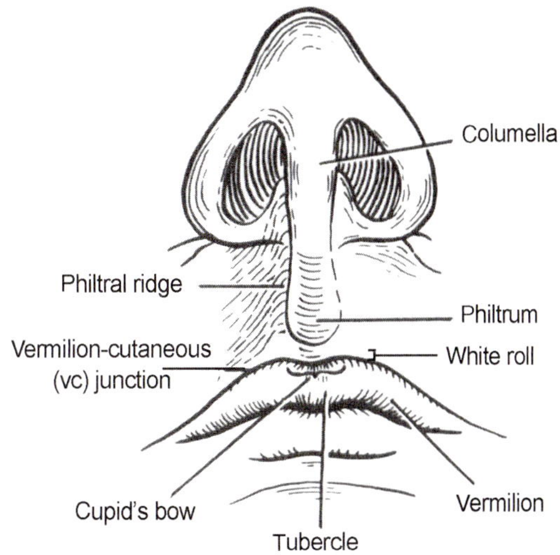

Figure 53-1 Anatomy of the lip. *(Reproduced with permission from Lee KJ, ed. Essential Otolaryngology. 7th ed. Stamford, CN: Appleton & Lange; 1999.)*

- Contiguous with adjacent palatoglossus and palatopharyngeus (anterior and posterior tonsillar pillars, respectively)

(b) Primary blood supply:
- Hard palate: greater palatine artery
- Soft palate: descending palatine branch of facial artery, palatine branch of ascending pharyngeal artery, lesser palatine artery

(c) Landmarks
- Hard palate: bony palate including premaxilla centrally and vertical segments of palate bone posteriorly
- Soft palate: muscular palate as above
- Incisive foramen: divides primary palate (anterior to incisive foramen, includes alveolus) and secondary palate (includes hard palate posterior to incisive foramen and soft palate)
- Greater palatine foramen: for greater palatine vessels and nerve, located at posterolateral aspect of hard palate bilaterally
- Lesser palatine foramen: for lesser palatine nerve
- "Space of Ernst": potential space posterior to greater palatine neurovascular bundle to assist in mobilization of palatal tissue

Embryology (Figure 53-2)

- Lip
  (a) Gestational week 4: paired maxillary prominences arise from first pharyngeal arches and frontonasal prominence (only unpaired prominence) from mesenchyme ventral to forebrain
  (b) Gestational week 5: nasal placodes invaginate to form medial and lateral nasal prominences

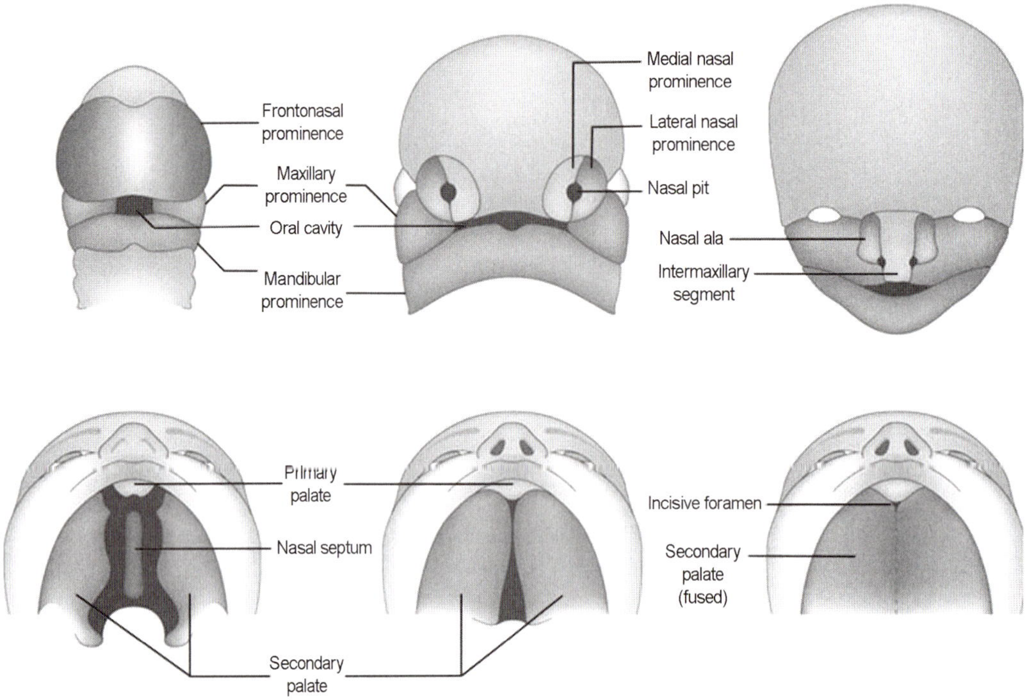

Figure 53-2 Embryologic development of the midface. The upper row is a frontal view of lip development during gestation and the lower row is an axial view of palatal development during gestation. *(Reproduced with permission from Dixon MJ, Marazita ML, Beaty TH, Murray JC. Cleft lip and palate: understanding genetic and environmental influences. Nat Rev Genet. Mar 2011;12(3):167-178.)*

(c) Gestational weeks 6 to 7: medial growth of paired maxillary prominences meet paired medial nasal prominences and frontonasal prominence to form upper lip
  - Disruption → clefting of lip and/or nose
- Palate
  (a) Gestational weeks 5 to 12: fusion of paired medial nasal prominences forms premaxilla (includes four incisor tooth buds), fuse to maxillary prominences
    - Disruption → clefting of primary palate
  (b) Gestational weeks 5 to 6: soft palate musculature migrates toward midline from both sides of developing oropharynx
  (c) Gestational weeks 6 to 7: palatal shelves extend medially from maxillary prominences
  (d) Gestational weeks 9 to 10: soft palate muscles oriented horizontally
  (e) Gestational weeks 8 to 12: palatal shelves fuse to form secondary palate from anterior (incisive foramen) to posterior (uvula)
    - Disruption → clefting of secondary palate

Epidemiology/Incidence

- Incidence varies widely depending on geographic origin, race, ethnicity, gender, environmental exposures, and socioeconomic status.
  (a) Increased risk by ethnic descent: Native American > Asian > United States > European > African

(b) Cleft lip more common in males, isolated cleft palate more common in females

- Etiology often "multifactorial," though increased risk with family history in first-degree relatives
- Majority of clefts are unilateral, majority of unilateral cleft lips are left-sided
- Increased incidence of associated syndrome with isolated cleft palate

Etiology

- Nonsyndromic
  (a) 70% of cleft lip with or without cleft palate
  (b) 50% of isolated cleft palate
- Syndromic
  (a) van der Woude syndrome
    - Autosomal dominant (*IRF6* gene on chromosome 1)
    - Most common syndromic cause of cleft lip +/− palate
    - Lower lip pits (90% penetrance) and cleft lip and/or cleft palate
  (b) Pierre Robin Sequence (PRS)
    - May be syndromic (with other associated abnormalities) or nonsyndromic
    - Classic triad: micrognathia → glossoptosis → cleft palate (U-shaped)
    - Stickler syndrome
      - Autosomal dominant (mutations in genes involved in collagen production)
      - Flattened facial appearance, eye abnormalities (severe myopia, glaucoma, cataracts, retinal detachments), cleft palate (and PRS), hearing loss, joint abnormalities (hypermobile; kyphosis/scoliosis/platyspondyly)
      - Need ophthalmology evaluation
  (c) 22q11.2 deletion syndrome (Velocardiofacial syndrome, DiGeorge syndrome)
    - Cleft palate (overt or submucous), velopharyngeal dysfunction without cleft palate
    - Also cardiac anomalies, unique facial characteristics, learning disabilities, medial displacement of carotid arteries, immunodeficiency (thymus), hypocalcemia
  (d) Others: mandibulofacial dysostosis (Treacher-Collins), Trisomy 21, CHARGE, craniofacial microsomia, Crouzon, Apert, Nager
- Environmental risks
  (a) Teratogens: retinoids, tobacco, alcohol abuse, illicit drugs, nitrate compounds, organic solvents, lead, anticonvulsants
  (b) Nutrition: inadequate folic acid (vitamin B9), vitamins B6 and B12
  (c) Amniotic band sequence
  (d) Increasing birth order has higher risk of clefting

Classification

- Multiple classification schemes exist
  (a) Tessier classification widely used for complex craniofacial clefts
  (b) Veau classification for cleft palate
    - I: soft palate only
    - II: soft palate and hard palate to incisive foramen (secondary palate)
    - III: soft palate, hard palate, and alveolus (secondary and primary palate) unilaterally, typically involving unilateral lip as well
    - IV: soft palate, hard palate, and alveolus bilaterally, typically involving bilateral lip as well

- May describe lip and/or palate and include
  - (a) Anatomical involvement
    - Isolated lip
    - Lip and alveolus
    - Lip and palate (includes alveolus)
    - Isolated palate
  - (b) Laterality: unilateral (left or right) versus bilateral
    - Unilateral cleft palate: nasal septum contiguous with noncleft side palatal shelf
    - Bilateral cleft palate: nasal septum/vomer isolated from bilateral palatal shelves but contiguous with premaxilla
  - (c) Completeness:
    - Complete cleft lip: extends into nasal sill
    - Incomplete cleft lip: involves muscle, skin, and mucosa but intact nasal sill/floor
    - Simonart band: soft tissue (may be skin only) bridge at nasal sill
    - Alveolar involvement may be complete or incomplete (ie, notch)
  - (d) Severity
    - Width description
    - Microform/minorform cleft lip: subtle or "occult" cleft, typically has philtral ridge or depression due to dehiscence or misinsertion of orbicularis oris without overt skin involvement, asymmetric high point of Cupid bow, irregular v-c junction, and/or vermilion notch
    - Submucous cleft palate
    - Palatal mucosa intact with dehiscence and aberrant insertion of levator veli palatini
    - Features: bifid uvula, hard palate notch, zona pellucida (translucent or "bluish" region in central soft palate due to thin layers of mucosa only)
  - (e) Additional atypical features

Management

- Multidisciplinary care
  - (a) Gold standard of care
  - (b) Team requires coordinator, surgeon, orthodontist, speech-language pathologist
    - Required to have access to psychology, social work, audiology, genetics, pediatric dentistry, otolaryngology, and pediatrics
  - (c) Visits typically annual for entire team
    - Initial visit prenatally, as newborn or within first year depending on team structure
- Early
  - (a) Prenatal diagnosis can be made at anatomy evaluation (16-20 weeks)
    - Typically for fetal cleft lip (possible palate)
    - Can discuss surgery timeline, expectations, associated anomalies, delivery plan with parent(s) proactively
    - Isolated cleft palate not typically diagnosed prenatally
    - Micrognathia with potential airway complications also diagnosed prenatally
  - (b) After birth
    - Airway
      - Typically intervention only needed for Robin sequence (micrognathia) or sequelae of craniofacial syndromes

    - May involve positioning changes, nasopharyngeal airway, surgery (tracheotomy, mandibular distraction osteogenesis, tongue-lip adhesion)
- Feeding
  - Isolated cleft lip or with alveolus may be able to breastfeed or use standard bottle
  - Palatal involvement limits ability to create suction → modified bottle incorporates passive flow, rate of flow controlled by valve
  - Speech language pathology, lactation referrals
  - Monitor weight gain
- Referrals
  - Presurgical orthopedics
    - Typically begin within first 2 weeks of life
    - Include nasoalveolar molding (NAM), lip taping, lip adhesion
    - Can be time-intensive
  - Genetics
  - Confirm results of newborn hearing screen, refer to audiology if indicated
- Management from childhood to adhulthood
  (a) Surgical timeline in Figure 53-3
    - Goals of repair: to restore function and anatomic features including cosmesis of involved structures (lip, palate, and/or alveolus)
  (b) Ongoing assessments with speech language pathology
    - Increased need for speech/language/articulation therapy
    - At risk for velopharyngeal dysfunction and potential secondary speech surgery
  (c) Ongoing assessments with dentistry, orthodontics
    - Increased need for orthodontic intervention in preparation for or after alveolar bone grafting
    - At risk for poor midface growth, class III malocclusion → may require orthognathic surgery at skeletal maturity
  (d) Ongoing assessments with audiology
    - Ongoing Eustachian tube dysfunction in children with cleft palate
    - Craniofacial syndromes commonly have associated hearing loss
  (e) Ongoing assessments with psychology
  (f) Social media impact increasing

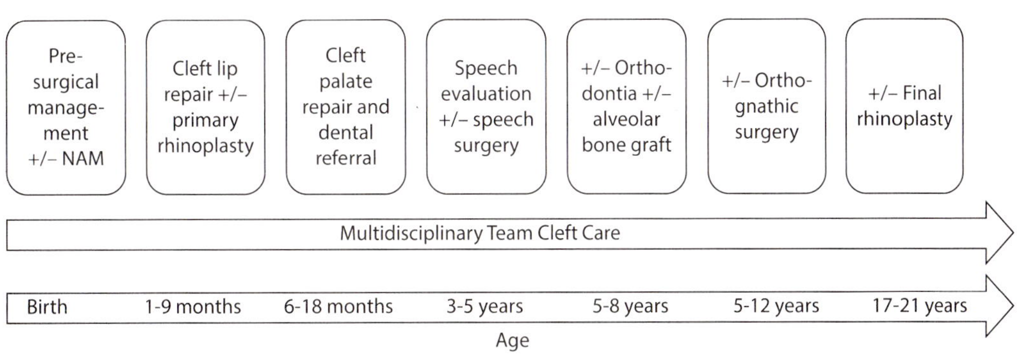

Figure 53-3 Timeline for the management of patients with cleft lip/palate. The multidisciplinary cleft team facilitates management throughout the years.

Surgical Repair

- Cleft Lip
  - (a) Timing
    - Rule of 10s: > 10 weeks, > 10 lb, > 10 hemoglobin
    - Usually performed at age 3-4 months: delay early anesthesia exposure, improves accuracy of repair, and parental acceptance of malformation
  - (b) Goals
    - Restore function of orbicularis oris (competence, complete sphincter)
    - Alignment and recreation of lip and nose landmarks
    - Also columellar length in bilateral cleft lip
  - (c) Unilateral cleft lip
    - Relevant anatomy
      - Orbicularis oris
        - ◊ Dehiscent
        - ◊ Abnormal attachments to base of nasal sill on cleft side and columellar base on noncleft side
      - Lower lateral cartilage
        - ◊ Equal lengths on cleft and noncleft sides
        - ◊ Lateral steal: lateral crus longer and medial crus shorter on cleft side
        - ◊ Alar base displaced inferiorly, laterally, and posteriorly on cleft side
      - Nasal tip
        - ◊ Displaced
        - ◊ Cleft side dome lower → flattening or hooding of nostril
      - Septum
        - ◊ Caudal nasal septum and columella are deviated to noncleft side
      - Maxilla hypoplastic on cleft side
      - Absent/dehiscent nasal floor on cleft side in complete cleft
    - Surgical techniques
      - Multiple techniques and adaptations described (Figure 53-4)
        - ◊ Straight line
        - ◊ Triangular or geometric flap
        - ◊ Advancement-rotation (Millard, Mohler, Noordhoff)
          - * Rotate noncleft side (medial lip, philtrum)
          - * Advance cleft side (lateral lip)
        - ◊ Anatomic subunit (Fisher)
      - Often includes primary rhinoplasty
        - ◊ Early intervention of nasal deformity → decreases nasal asymmetries and allows symmetric growth
        - ◊ Technique
          - * Release lower lateral cartilages from skin and soft tissue envelope via lateral and medial approaches
          - * May use alar base suture to set width and position
          - * Reposition dome and lower lateral cartilages with sutures to create alar symmetry and tip projection
      - May include gingivoperiosteoplasty
      - Outcomes
        - ◊ Millard technique or its adaptations most commonly used in United States with increasing use of Fisher technique

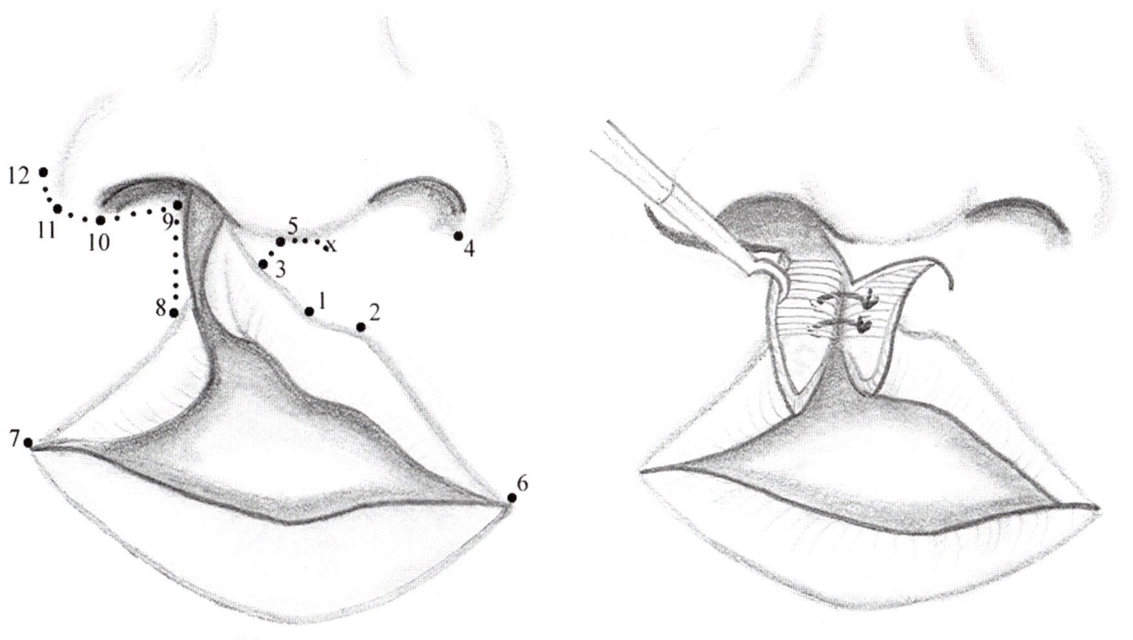

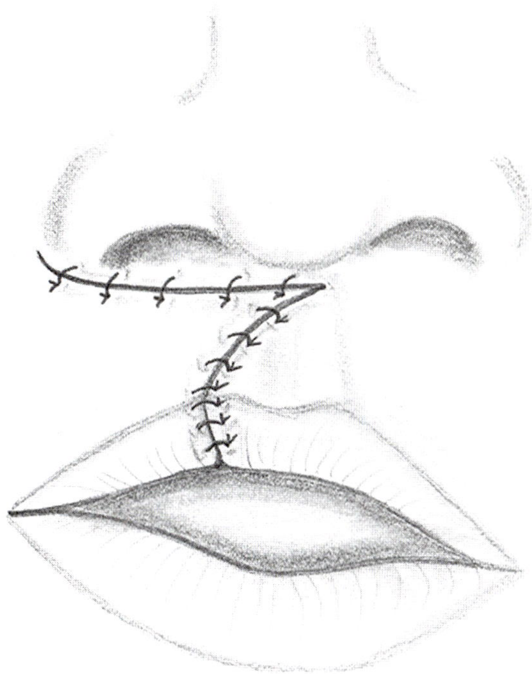

Figure 53-4 Markings for a unilateral cleft lip repair using the rotation-advancement technique. The orbicularis oris muscle fibers are approximated and the lip is closed. *(Reproduced with permission from Tibesar RJ, Black A, Sidman JD: Surgical repair of cleft lip and palate. Otolaryngol Head Neck Surg. 2009 Dec;20(4):245-255.)*

(d) Bilateral cleft lip
- Relevant anatomy
  - Premaxilla isolated and frequently protrudes anteriorly and superiorly (can increase tension on or even preclude lip repair)
  - Orbicularis dehiscent and only in lateral lip segments
    - ◊ Prolabium (central soft tissue of lip, with premaxilla) does not contain orbicularis or white roll
  - Short or absent columella
    - ◊ Decreases projection of nasal tip
  - Absent nasal floors in complete clefts
  - Wide nasal tip, wide alar bases
- Surgical techniques (Figure 53-5)

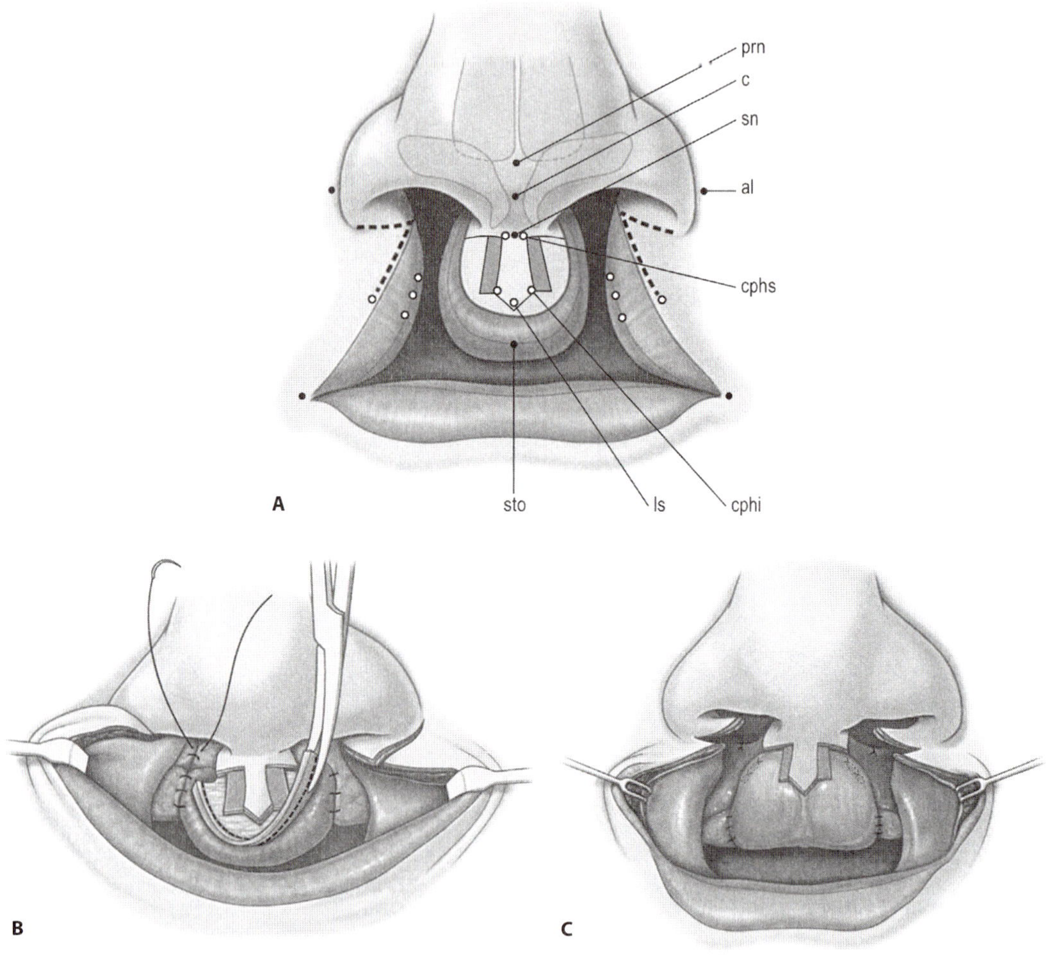

Figure 53-5 The markings for a bilateral cleft lip repair. The orbicularis oris muscle fibers are approximated and the flaps are closed to reconstruct the lip. *(Reproduced with permission from Neligan PC, Rodriguez ED, Losee JE, editors: Plastic Surgery. Philadelphia: Saunders-Elsevier; 2012.)*

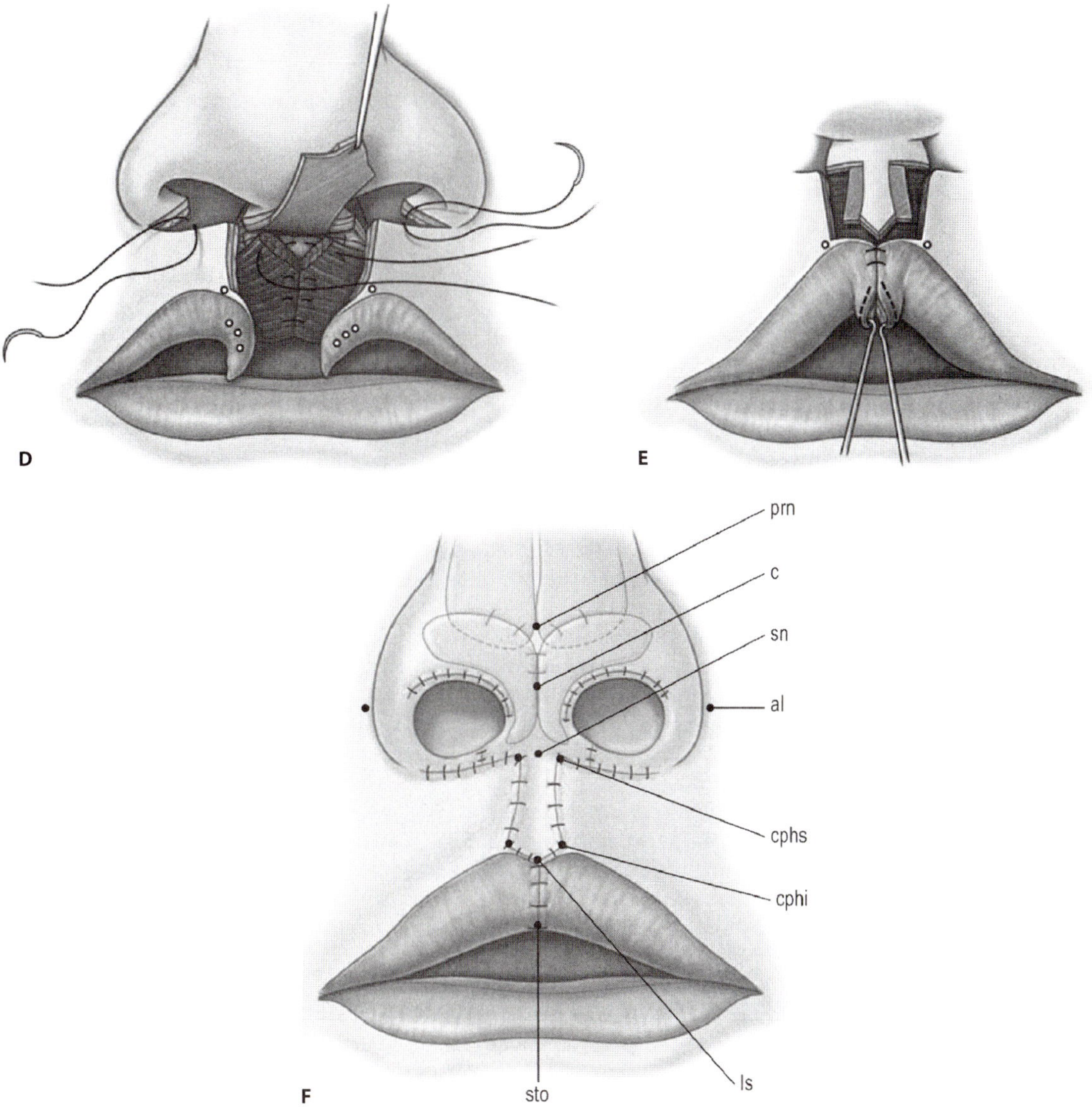

Figure 53-5 (*Continued*)

- Multiple techniques described (primarily Millard and Mulliken)
- Critical to reapproximate orbicularis oris across central premaxilla
- Need to reduce width of prolabium
- Presurgical orthopedics (especially NAM) can yield increased columellar length, improved premaxillary and lateral arches alignment
  - ◊ Lip adhesion may be needed prior to definitive lip repair for symmetry, to stabilize premaxilla/prevent further protrusion.
  - ◊ Secondary columellar lengthening is an option.

  - Often includes primary rhinoplasty (technique similar to unilateral)
  - May include gingivoperiosteoplasty

(e) Postoperative
- Goals: prevent infection or tension, provide wound care, control pain, and promote adequate nutrition
  - May use arm restraints to protect sutures/closure.
  - Nasal conformer/stent may be used to maintain shape.
  - Feeding guidelines vary by surgeon.
- Complications: uncommon
  - Often associated with increased tension of closure, infection, or underlying poor nutrition
  - Include lip dehiscence, poor cosmesis ("whistle deformity" or vermilion notch, misalignment of white roll or v-c junction), orbicularis oris muscle discontinuity, nasal asymmetry

Cleft palate

- Timing

(a) Overt cleft palate
- Best speech outcomes achieved when palate repair is performed less than 12 months of age, when possible (most repairs performed between 6 and 16 months of age in United States)
  - Two-stage repair with early soft palate closure + delayed hard palate closure to minimize potential negative impact on maxillary growth also considered, not as common practice in United States
- Airway implications may drive timing decision-making but important to balance increased risk of compensatory articulation errors in setting of delayed palate repair
  - Common concern in setting of PRS
  - Early airway management in PRS (ie, mandibular distraction) may improve timing of palate repair

(b) Submucous cleft palate
- Recommendation to repair with evidence of velopharyngeal dysfunction
  - May have normal velopharyngeal function, thus not all patients with SMCP require intervention
- Typically after age 3 to 4 years, given need for adequate language development, may require articulation therapy for adequate evaluation

- Goals

(a) Restore functional anatomy of palate, primarily feeding and speech
- Prevent nasal regurgitation
- Create suction for feeding
- Establish velopharyngeal closure during speech

(b) Re-establish separate oral and nasal cavities

(c) Restore functional anatomy of tensor veli palatini, primarily Eustachian tube function

- Relevant anatomy (Figure 53-6)

(a) Cleft involving hard palate
- Nasal mucosa of vomer contiguous with oral hard palate mucosa along cleft margin in unilateral

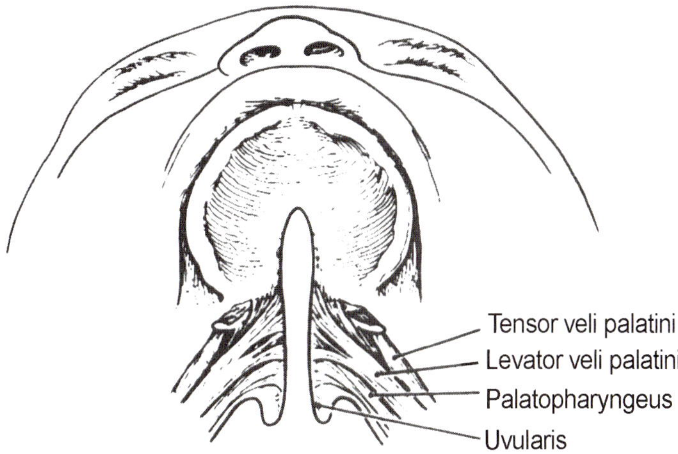

Figure 53-6 Schematic diagram of clefting of the secondary palate. Note the abnormal attachment of the levator veli palatini to the posterior edge of the hard palate instead of meeting in the midline. *(Reproduced with permission from Meyers AD. Biological Basis of Facial Plastic Surgery. New York, NY: Thieme Medical Publishers; 1993.)*

- Vomer isolated in bilateral, need to re-establish nasal floor bilaterally and often includes bilateral vomer flaps

(b) Cleft involving soft palate
- Levator veli palatini muscle dehiscent, reoriented anteriorly at medial aspect and attached to posterior hard palate
  - Cannot create velopharyngeal closure due to inability to move intact levator "sling" for palatal elevation
- Tensor veli palatini aponeurosis disrupted in midline, often thinner with aberrant insertion on anterior levator muscle
  - Cannot dilate Eustachian tube

(c) Submucous cleft palate
- Three classic features
  - Bifid uvula
  - Hard palate notch
  - "Zona pellucida": blue/gray region in midline soft palate representing nasal and oral mucosa only due to absent levator muscle
- Palatal mucosa intact, though underlying muscular anatomy similar to cleft involving soft palate

- Surgical techniques

(a) Multiple techniques and adaptations described
- Surgeon may adapt technique based on cleft width

(b) Hard palate closure
- May involve vomer flaps
- Elevation of mucoperiosteal flaps via Bardach (two-flap), V-Y pushback, von Langenbeck, etc.

- All typically incorporate "straight line closure" of soft palate as well
- Axial pedicled flaps based on greater palatine artery in subperiosteal plane
- Often results in exposure of hard palate bone laterally to heal by remucosalization alone
- Reapproximated in midline

○ Bilateral buccal flaps can be incorporated in primary repair to decrease hard palate elevation (popularized by Mann)

(c) Soft palate closure

○ Intravelar veloplasty (Figure 53-7)
- Involves dissection of levator muscle to recreate separate closure layer (advanced dissection described in Sommerlad procedure)
- Results in "straight-line closure"

○ Double-opposing Z-plasty or "Furlow palatoplasty" (Figure 53-8)
- Indications
◊ Commonly used for isolated cleft palate of soft palate only or SMCP
◊ Added to above hard palate closure techniques for "6-flap palatoplasty"

○ Four flaps
◊ Two posteriorly based myomucosal flaps (one nasal, one oral) + two anteriorly based mucosa-only flaps (one nasal, one oral)
◊ Flaps transposed in nasal layer and oral layer, no separate muscle closure
◊ Reorients levator muscle posteriorly, potential secondary consequence of lengthening palate as well given nature of Z-plasty

- Postoperative

(a) Goals

○ Minimize tension on closure
- Feeding guidelines vary by surgeon, but common; may modify feeding regimen with open cup, liquid diet, etc.
- Often use arm restraints to protect sutures/closure
- Avoidance of pacifiers, specific bottles, utensils, etc., by surgeon preference

○ Adequate pain control and hydration/nutrition

○ Infection is rare

(b) Complications

○ Airway, especially in setting of Robin sequence

○ Oronasal fistula (uncommon)

○ Velopharyngeal dysfunction

Additional Associated Diagnoses

- Hearing and otologic disease

(a) 95% of patients with cleft palate will have Eustachian tube dysfunction, typically chronic otitis media with effusion (COME)

○ Typically due to anatomical change of tensor veli palatini muscle

○ Frequently treated with tympanostomy tubes
- May coordinate with palatoplasty
- Early tube placement prior to palatoplasty may be indicated pending NBHS results/need for diagnostic ABR testing, other hearing concerns

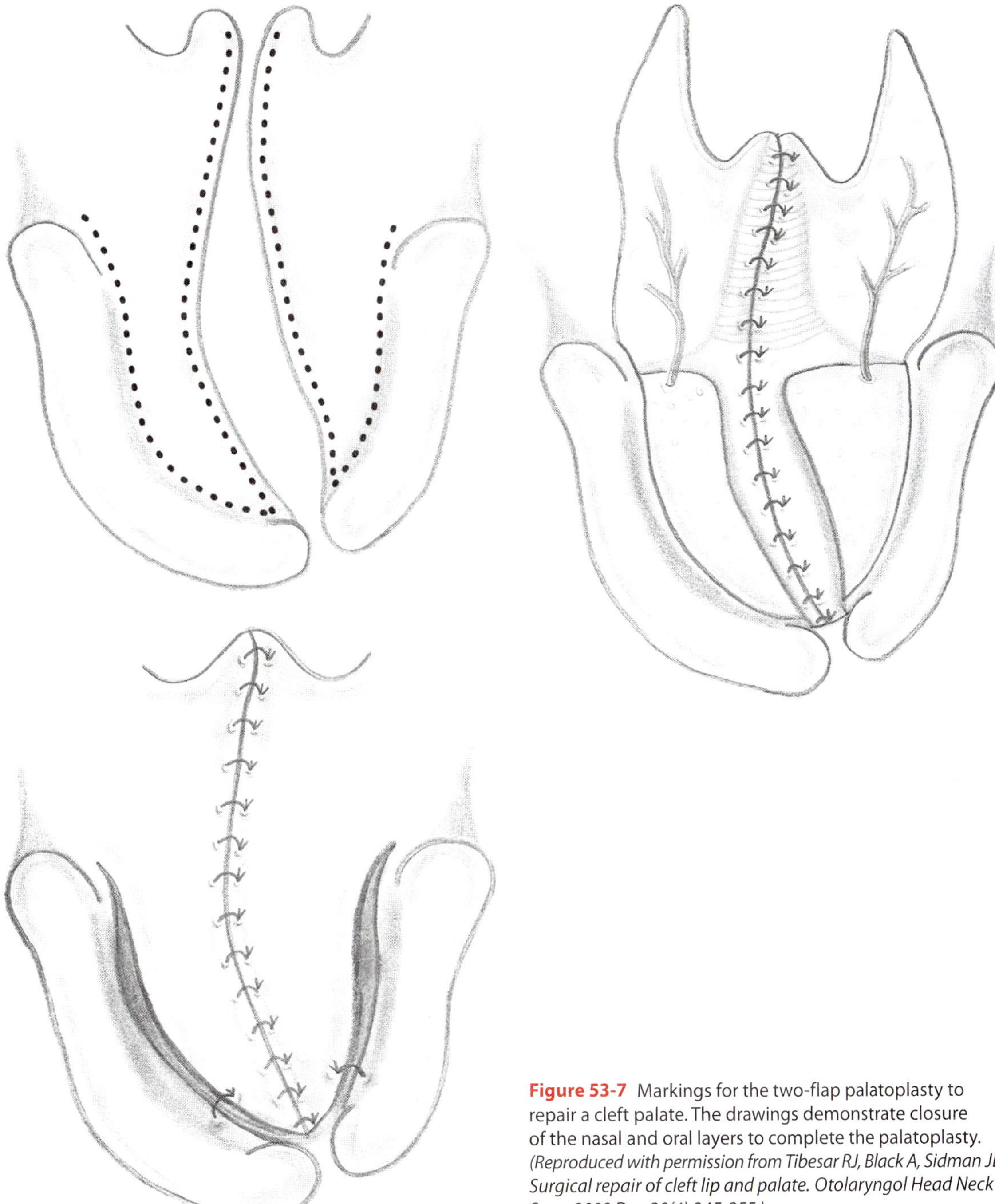

Figure 53-7 Markings for the two-flap palatoplasty to repair a cleft palate. The drawings demonstrate closure of the nasal and oral layers to complete the palatoplasty. *(Reproduced with permission from Tibesar RJ, Black A, Sidman JD: Surgical repair of cleft lip and palate. Otolaryngol Head Neck Surg. 2009 Dec;20(4):245-255.)*

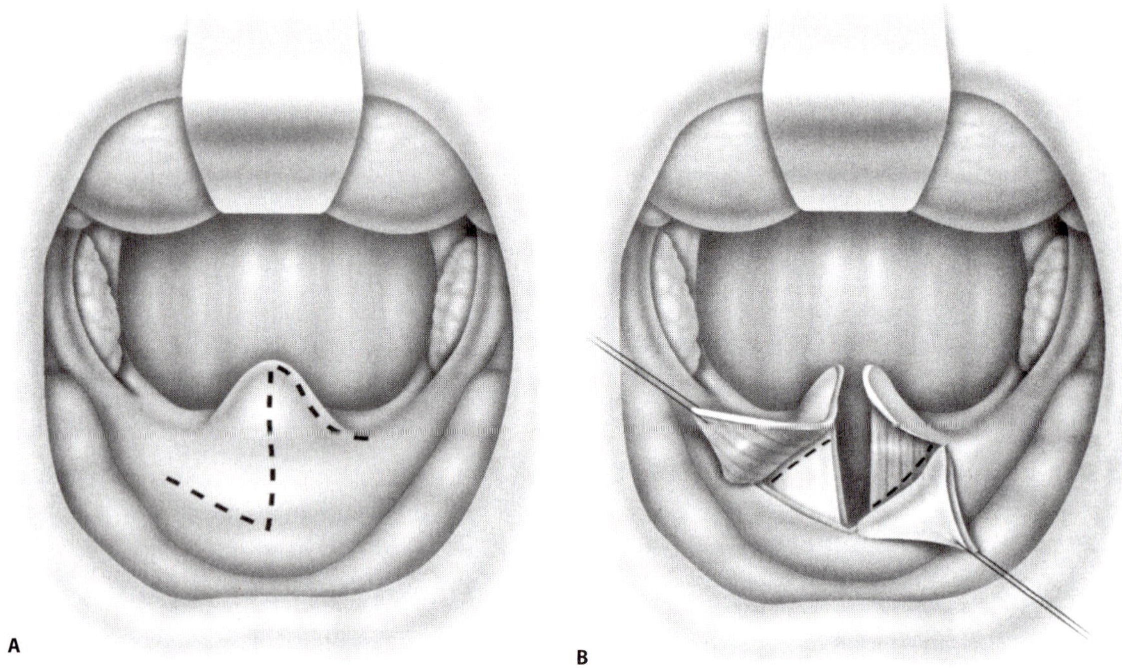

Figure 53-8 The steps involved in completing the Furlow double-opposing Z-plasty. *(Reproduced with permission from Muntz HM. Current techniques for treatment of velopharyngeal insufficiency. Otolaryngol Head Neck Surg. 2001 Dec;12(4): 204-209.)*

  - Early tube placement prior to palatoplasty may result in chronic tube otorrhea (often referred to as "milk otorrhea")
  - Common to require more than 1 set of tubes
- Palatoplasty anticipated to improve Eustachian tube function with time
  - Some evidence suggests that technique (specifically Furlow) may improve outcome
- Need for monitoring long term given potential risk for cholesteatoma, TM retraction, and associated hearing loss

(b) Ongoing audiologic evaluation important given increased risk for articulation, language disorders
- Increased need, especially in patients with syndromic craniofacial diagnoses (ie, Stickler syndrome in PRS)

- Obstructive sleep apnea (OSA)
  (a) Increased risk of OSA in patients with cleft and craniofacial diagnoses
  (b) Warrants frequent screening for patients, though may underestimate prevalence
  (c) Recommendation for polysomnography prior to surgical intervention
  (d) May result from surgical intervention, especially pharyngeal surgery (ie, pharyngeal flap)

- Speech
  (a) Annual screening and/or intervention for language, articulation, and resonance disorders
    - SLP is required member of ACPA-approved cleft team.
  (b) Velopharyngeal dysfunction (VPD)
    - Incomplete closure of palate and pharyngeal wall
      - Normal in /m/, /n/, and /ng/
      - Abnormal for all other productions
      - Results in hypernasal resonance, nasal air emission, and/or nasal turbulence
      - May demonstrate nasal regurgitation as well
    - Includes velopharyngeal insufficiency (anatomic), incompetence (motor impairment), and/or mislearning (neuromotor/planning)
    - Most common associated diagnosis is cleft palate
      - Occurs in 10% to 40% of patients with repaired cleft palate
      - May have decreased risk with prior double-opposing Z-plasty technique
      - Noncleft VPD associated with 22q11.2 deletion syndrome, additional neurological diagnoses, Trisomy 21; may occur postadenoidectomy
    - Evaluation
      - Perceptual speech evaluation by SLP
      - Objective speech measurements including nasometry, pressure flow
      - MRI of velum
      - Functional evaluation including nasopharyngoscopy and/or video fluoroscopy in multidisciplinary team approach
        - ◊ Useful tool(s) to guide surgical planning based on closure pattern
        - ◊ Can identify medialized carotids, asymmetry, residual adenoid/tonsil hypertrophy
    - Management
      - Speech therapy for compensatory articulation errors, may be needed pre- and postsurgery
      - Nasopharyngeal bulb or palatal lift appliances may be nonsurgical options
      - Surgery
        - ◊ Palatal revision and/or lengthening
          - ∗ Double-opposing Z-plasty
          - ∗ Buccal flaps
        - ◊ Posterior pharyngeal augmentation (injection pharyngoplasty)
          - ∗ Variable results (can migrate, extrude, resorb)
          - ∗ Injectable material, fat, or implant options
          - ∗ May be helpful after prior pharyngeal surgery for localized gaps
        - ◊ Sphincter pharyngoplasty (Figure 53-9)
          - ∗ Bilateral superiorly based myomucosal flaps (palatopharyngeus vs superior constrictor) transposed medially to augment posterior pharyngeal wall at site of expected VP closure
          - ∗ Not a functional sphincter
        - ◊ Pharyngeal flap (Figure 53-10)
          - ∗ Central superiorly based myomucosal flap inset into soft palate
          - ∗ Obstructs central pharynx, can restrict palatal movement
          - ∗ Higher incidence of postoperative OSA than other interventions

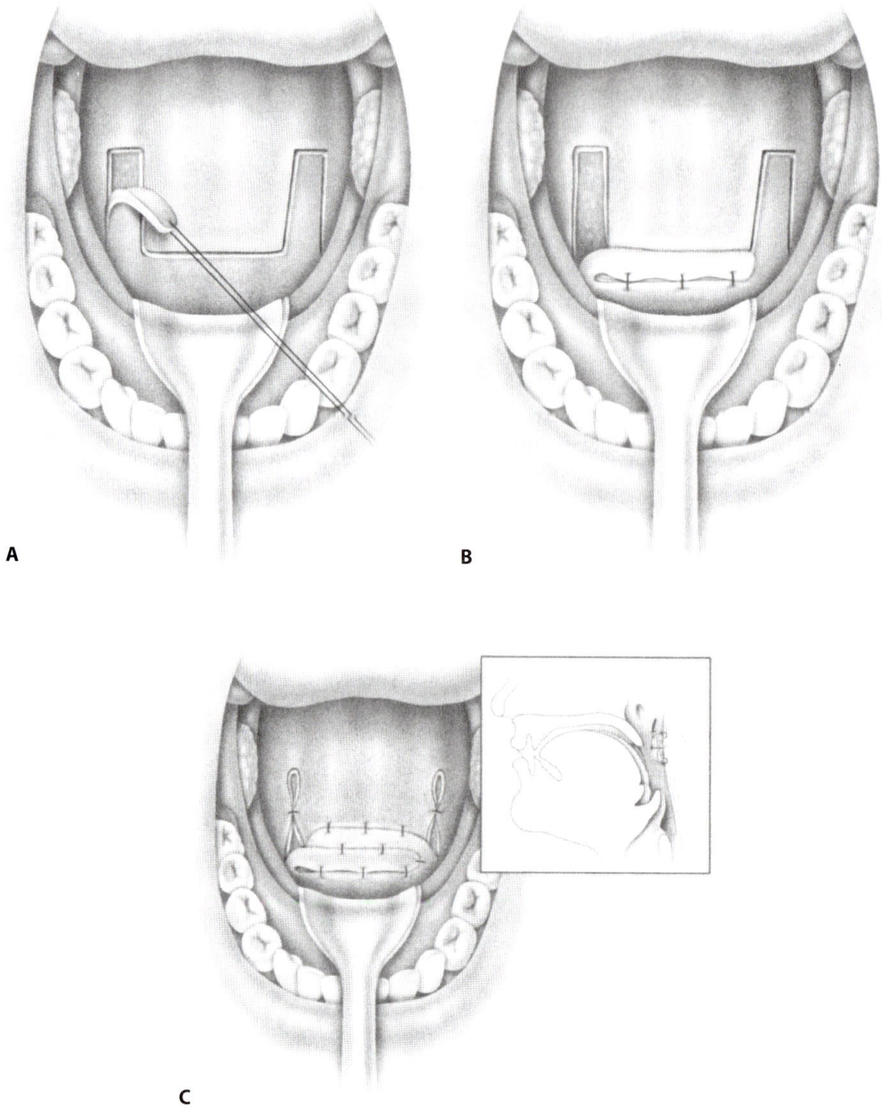

Figure 53-9 The steps involved in completing a sphincter pharyngoplasty. *(Reproduced with permission from Muntz HM. Current techniques for treatment of velopharyngeal insufficiency. Otolaryngol Head Neck Surg. 2001 Dec;12(4):204-209.)*

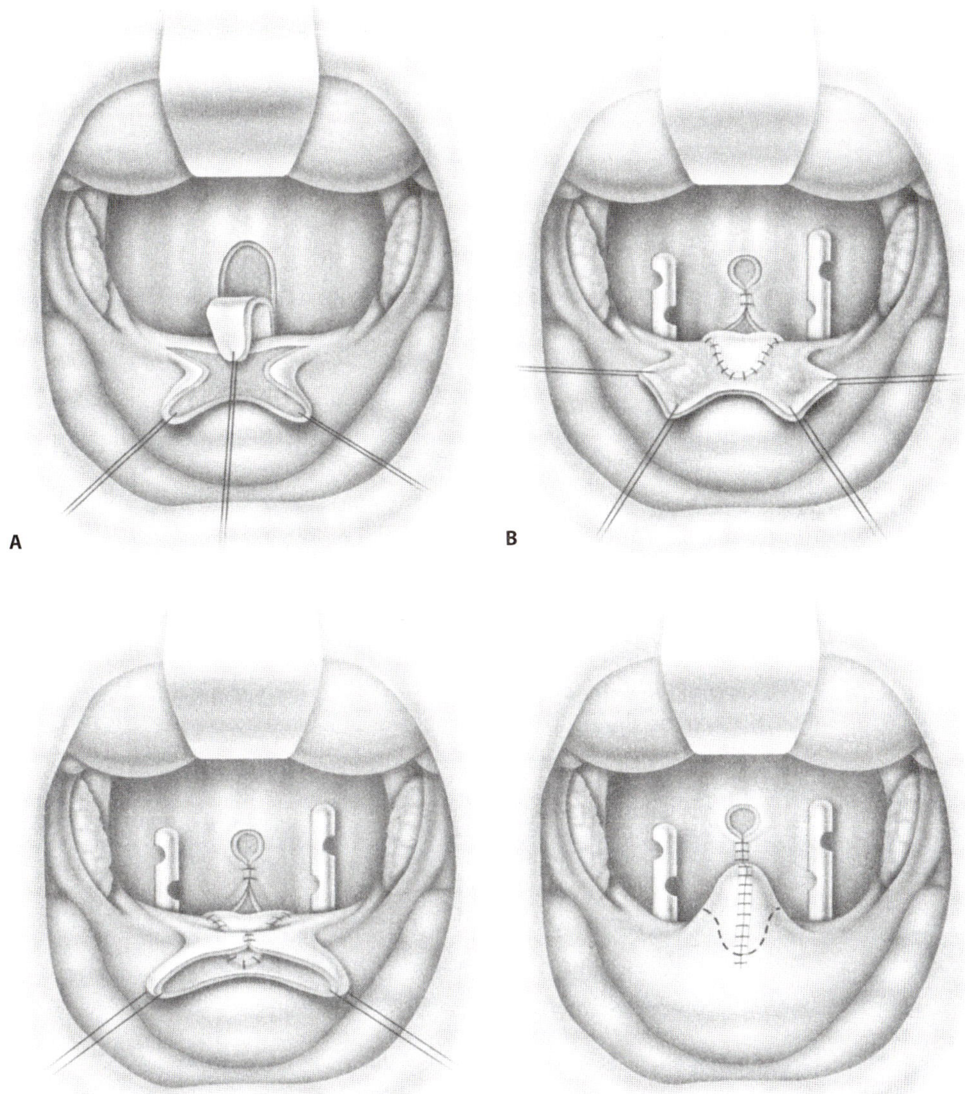

Figure 53-10 The steps involved in completing a superiorly based pharyngeal flap. *(Reproduced with permission from Muntz HM. Current techniques for treatment of velopharyngeal insufficiency. Otolaryngol Head Neck Surg. 2001 Dec;12(4): 204-209.)*

Acknowledgment

I would like to acknowledge Ryan Belcher, MD and Steven Goudy, MD for their work on the 12th edition chapter on Cleft Lip and Palate.

Bibliography

Belcher RH, Goudy SL. Cleft lip and palate. In: Chan Y, Goddard JC, eds. *K. J. Lee's Essential Otolaryngology*. 12th ed. McGraw Hill Education; 2019.

Dixon MJ, Marazita ML, Beaty TH, Murray JC. Cleft lip and palate: understanding genetic and environmental influences. *Nat Rev Genet*. 2011;12(3):167-178.

Losee JE, Kirschner RE. *Comprehensive Cleft Care*. 2nd ed. Thieme; 2016.

Muntz HM. Current techniques for treatment of velopharyngeal insufficiency. *Operative Tech Otolaryngol*. 2001;12:204-209.

Sykes JM, Senders CW. Pathologic anatomy of cleft lip, palate and nasal deformities. In: Meyers AD, ed. *Biol Basis Facial Plast Surg*. 1993;5:57-71.

Questions

1. In a patient with a unilateral cleft lip and cleft nasal deformity, the caudal septum
   A. Is unaffected with respect to its anatomic position
   B. Deviates to the cleft side
   C. Deviates to the noncleft side
   D. Deviates ipsilateral to the cartilaginous and bony septum

2. The posterior boundary of the primary palate is the
   A. Anterior border of the soft palate
   B. Incisive foramen
   C. Base of the uvula
   D. Alveolar ridge

3. An associated syndrome is most commonly seen in patients with
   A. Cleft of the secondary palate only
   B. Cleft lip only
   C. Cleft lip and palate
   D. Cleft lip with or without cleft palate

4. A child with normal palatal anatomy would be expected to have
   A. Nasal air emission during /m/ ('m' sound) production
   B. Hard palate notch
   C. Ankyloglossia
   D. Glossoptosis

5. Chronic otitis media is observed in _____ of children with cleft palate.
   A. 95%
   B. 80%
   C. 60%
   D. 20%

6. In a family with a child with a unilateral cleft lip and a parent with lip pits, you would expect to confirm a diagnosis of ___ which is inherited in an ____ pattern.
   A. 22q11 deletion syndrome; autosomal dominant
   B. 22q11 deletion syndrome; autosomal recessive
   C. Stickler syndrome; autosomal dominant
   D. Stickler syndrome; autosomal recessive
   E. van der Woude syndrome; autosomal dominant
   F. van der Woude syndrome; autosomal recessive

Chapter 54
Pediatric Otolaryngology

General Information

This chapter focuses on otolaryngologic issues in children. The chapter is divided into (1) ears and hearing; (2) nose, nasopharynx, and paranasal sinuses; (3) mouth and upper digestive tract; (4) airway; and (5) head and neck.

Ears and Hearing

Outer Ear (Pinna, External Auditory Canal [EAC], Tympanic Membrane [TM])

Developmental Anatomy

A. Prenatal development
   i. 5 weeks' gestation
      a. Auricle develops from first (mandibular) and second (hyoid) arches that give rise to six Hillocks of His.
      b. Controversial, but first Hillock gives rise to tragus, second to helical crus, third to remainder of helix, fourth to antihelix, fifth to antitragus, sixth to lobule. Lobule is last to form and some feel it is not derived from Hillocks.
   ii. 8 weeks' gestation
      a. Cartilaginous (outer third) of EAC derived from invagination of concha cavum (first branchial groove)
      b. Bony EAC (inner two-thirds) derived from invagination of meatal plug (solid epithelial core) from primary meatus to primitive tympanic cavity to form meatal plate
   iii. 21 weeks' gestation
      a. Epithelial cells resorb to canalize bony EAC. Incomplete resorption results in atresia or stenosis.
      b. Tympanic membrane has three layers:
         1. Outer epithelial layer from ectoderm of first branchial groove.
         2. Middle fibrous layer.
         3. Inner mucosal layer from endoderm of first pharyngeal pouch.
         4. Pars tensa composed of three layers. Pars flaccida composed of two (outer and inner) layers. Perforations in pars tensa that heal and look thin are composed of outer and inner layers (missing middle layer) and should be called dimeric membrane (rather than monomeric membrane which is a misnomer).

B. Postnatal development
   i. Medial EAC ossifies by 2 years of age and reaches adult size by 9 years of age.
   ii. TM almost adult size at birth but horizontally oriented. Becomes more vertical as EAC lengthens.
   iii. Pinna is 80% of adult size by age 5, adult size by age 9. Lobule may continue to grow thereafter.

Signs and Symptoms

Visible lesion, drainage, infection, abnormally shaped pinna

Clinical Assessment

Close inspection of pinna and remainder of head and neck for associated features as described below.

Pathologies

Congenital

A. Preauricular tag
   i. Most common ear anomaly
   ii. Due to supernumerary hillock formation
   iii. May be associated with branchio-oto-renal (BOR) syndrome involving hearing loss, branchial cleft cyst, and renal anomalies or other craniofacial syndromes
   iv. May be removed electively
B. Preauricular pit
   i. Likely due to failure of fusion of hillocks
   ii. Most commonly at helical root. Pit below tragus more likely to be first branchial cleft anomaly
   iii. May be associated with BOR
   iv. Acute infection warrants antibiotics and drainage if necessary
   v. Definitive excision after resolution of inflammation. Removal of entire tract plus cartilage at base of tract is necessary to prevent postoperative infection and recurrence
C. Protruding ears
   i. Larger than average distance from helical rim to mastoid.
   ii. Usually bilateral.
   iii. Due to under development of antihelix and deep conchal bowl.
   iv. Elective otoplasty at 5 or 6 years of age. Leave both ears undraped and address more severely deformed ear first. Mustarde suture recreates antihelical fold. Furnas suture sets back conchal bowl. Cartilage scoring, retropositioning of the helical tail, and suture techniques without incisions have also been described.
D. Microtia
   i. Clinical features
      a. Prevalence 1:600 to 12,000
      b. More often male, unilateral, right side
      c. More common in Hispanic, Aboriginal, Asian, and Andean descent
      d. Associations:
         1. Syndromic (60%): Oculo-auriculo-vertebral spectrum (OAVS) (ie, Goldenhar/hemifacial microsomia-holoprosencephaly, facial asymmetry, macrostomia, oral cleft, microphthalmia, vertebral anomaly, limb reduction, polydactyly, renal and cardiac anomaly; Treacher Collins (bilateral condition); BOR; Townes-Brocks; Miller; Meier-Gorlin
         2. Other: Aural atresia, hearing loss (90%), facial nerve palsy
      e. Absence of lobule is unusual and more likely associated with retinoic embryopathy and CHARGE syndrome

ii. Assessment
   a. Clinical examination to rule out concomitant atresia or syndrome.
   b. Weerda classification selected by *AM J Med Genetics* for reporting:
      1. First degree: All components present. Length more than 2 standard deviations (SD) below normal. Reconstruction only occasionally requires additional skin or cartilage.
      2. Second degree: Some components present. Length more than 2 standard deviations (SD) below normal (ie, rudimentary helix). Partial reconstruction requires some additional skin and cartilage.
      3. Third degree: Structures present but not recognizable (ie, peanut ear). Also includes anotia. Total reconstruction requires skin and large amounts of cartilage
   c. Bone conduction auditory brain stem response (ABR) prior to 4 months of age to avoid anesthetic and capitalize on open sutures to achieve ear-specific thresholds

iii. Management
   a. Counselling involving parents and child.
   b. Nonsurgical
      1. Masking with longer hair
      2. Adhesive retained prosthesis
   c. Surgical
      1. Bone-anchored auricular prosthesis (BAAP)
         - Advantages: Good for burns, auricular avulsion, failed microtia repair
         - Disadvantages: Requires removal of auricular remnant precluding future microtia repair, daily make-up application, replacement due to degradation
      2. Microtia repair
         - Reconstruction at 5 or 6 years of age or older, so rib is large enough to match other side. Reconstructed ear should grow with child
         - Performed 3 to 4 months prior to atresia repair when using a rib graft, or afterward when using synthetic implants
         - Three types of implant material:
           (a) Autogenous rib graft
               - Three-staged approach (Brent method)
                 - *Stage 1: harvest rib cartilage, place framework*
                 - *Stage 2: transpose lobule*
                 - *Stage 3: elevate auricle for projection using skin graft*
               - Two-staged approach (Nagata method)
                 - *Stage 1: harvest rib cartilage, place framework, transpose lobule*
                 - *Stage 2: elevate auricle for projection using skin graft*
               - Advantages: Maintenance free after healed
               - Disadvantages: Bleeding, infection, skin or cartilage loss, poor cosmetic result, pneumothorax
           (b) Synthetic implant
               - Medpore/Su-Por
                 - Advantages: can perform as early as age 3, fewer stages, no ribdonor, site morbidity, less variability in carving
                 - Disadvantages: foreign body, varied success, limited long-term data, extrusion
           (c) Irradiated rib
               - Largely abandoned due to high rate of resorption

E. Aural atresia
   i. Clinical features
      a. Incidence 1:20,000 live births
      b. More often nonsyndromic, male, unilateral, right side
      c. Associations
         1. Goldenhar (hemifacial microsomia), Apert, Crouzon, Pfeiffer, Treacher Collins, Duane, Turner, trisomies 13,14,15,18, 21,22
         2. Renal dysgenesis
   ii. Assessment
      a. Bone conduction auditory brain stem response (ABR) prior to 4 months of age to avoid anesthetic and capitalize on open sutures to achieve ear-specific thresholds
      b. CT imaging (high resolution, low-dose, nonenhanced) of temporal bone if canal stenosis to rule out canal cholesteatoma or if there is drainage from canal or pit near canal. Otherwise, defer imaging until prior to surgical repair due to risk of sedation
   iii. Management
      a. Monitor hearing carefully. Early amplification where appropriate
      b. Treat occult ear infections
      c. Unilateral atresia:
         1. Early repair only if canal cholesteatoma
         2. Early air conduction hearing aid in side with patent EAC. Bone conduction hearing aid (adhesive or headband) on atretic side
      d. Bilateral atresia:
         1. Early bone conduction hearing aid (adhesive or headband)
      e. Surgical management:
         1. Percutaneous abutment retained bone conduction aid (ie, BAHA, Ponto)
            - Bone conduction threshold must be 40 to 45 dB in at least one ear to be effective
            - Usually one stage but may be two stages in young children with thin calvaria (delayed placement of abutment on screw until osseointegration complete)
            - Advantages: superior and more consistent hearing compared to atresia repair, no risk to facial nerve, not dependent on patent auditory canal, no risk of restenosis or drainage, no water precautions necessary
            - Disadvantages: failure to osseointegrate, soft tissue infection, cosmesis
         2. Transcutaneous magnet retained bone conduction aid (ie, Osia, Sentio, Bonebridge)
            - Advantages: as per percutaneous abutment retained device but with improved cosmesis
            - Disadvantages: skin breakdown, discomfort at magnet site, poorer gain than percutaneous options, dislodgement during physical activities
         3. Atresia repair:
            - Usually delayed until over 5 years of age
            - Performed after microtia repair with a rib graft to minimize injury to skin flap, or before using synthetic implants to prevent implant exposure and infections
            - Likelihood of significant improvement in hearing following surgery associated with anatomical findings on CT imaging (Jahrsdoerfer criteria). Score of 8 or better out of 10 predicts better outcomes:
               (a) Stapes present (2 points)
               (b) Oval window patent (1 point)

(c) Round window patent (1 point)
(d) Incus-stapes connection (1 point)
(e) Malleus-incus complex (1 point)
(f) Facial nerve position (1 point)
(g) Middle ear space aerated (1 point)
(h) Mastoid pneumatized (1 point)
(i) External ear appearance (1 point)

- Advantages: Creates EAC to house hearing aid which is often required
- Disadvantages: Canal restenosis (most common complication up to 25%), persistent otorrhea, sensorineural hearing loss (SNHL), facial nerve palsy, high revision rate (15%-20%), degradation of audiological results over time due to TM lateralization and/or ossicular chain fixation, tympanic membrane perforation external canal cholesteatoma, need for frequent ear cleaning

F. First branchial cleft cyst, Work type I (see Head and Neck section)

Infectious

A. Otitis externa
  i. Acute
    a. Change from acidic to alkaline environment predisposes to bacterial infection
    b. Most commonly *Pseudomonas aeruginosa, Staphylococcus aureus*, mixed flora
    c. Symptoms include moderate to severe otalgia (tender tragus), itching, aural fullness, hearing loss, otorrhea
    d. Diagnosis based on symptoms of rapid-onset ear canal inflammation (otalgia, itching, fullness) and signs (tender, diffuse canal edema or erythema)
    e. Beware malignant otitis externa (osteomyelitis) in diabetic and immunocompromised patients. Requires addition of parenteral antibiotics
    f. Treatment includes debridement, analgesia, acidifying agents (acetic acid) and/or topical antibiotic/steroid drops +/– otowick if significant canal edema
  ii. Chronic
    a. Same bacteria as acute otitis externa
    b. Symptoms include itching, mild discomfort, drainage
    c. Treatment same as acute otitis externa. Prolonged treatment with topical antibiotics can lead to otomycosis (*Aspergillus* and *Candida*) which may require topical clotrimazole
    d. Cream containing betamethasone and clotrimazole

Traumatic

A. Auricular hematoma
  i. Associated with wrestling. Left untreated, may result in "cauliflower ear"
  ii. Requires incision and drainage and sandwiching of pinna between two dental rolls for 7 to 14 days to prevent re-accumulation of blood under perichondrium
  iii. Antibiotic prophylaxis
  iv. Suspect abuse if identified in nonambulatory infant
B. Auricular laceration and avulsion
  i. Laceration
    a. Copious irrigation, debridement, primary closure, antibiotics, rabies, or tetanus prophylaxis if indicated, bolster if perichondrium raised off cartilage

- ii. Avulsion
    - a. Less than 1.5 cm: reattach missing segment or primary closure
    - b. Greater than 1.5 cm: composite graft from opposite ear or local flap
    - c. Complete: options include microvascular reimplantation, banking of de-epithelialized cartilage under temporalis fascia for later reconstruction, reconstruction using costal cartilage, or auricular prosthesis

C. Exostoses
- i. Overgrowth of immature lamellar bone likely due to cold water exposure
- ii. Bilateral, multiple, broadly based lesions in medial half of external auditory canal
- iii. Surgical removal only if symptomatic (ie, conductive hearing loss, infection)

D. Osteoma
- i. Overgrowth of cancellous bone
- ii. Unilateral, pedunculated lesions in outer half of external auditory canal
- iii. Surgical removal only if symptomatic (ie, conductive hearing loss, infection)

E. Keratosis obturans
- i. Desquamation of hyperplastic epithelium leading to EAC obstruction
- ii. Symptoms include inflammation, otalgia, and hearing loss
- iii. Treatment includes acetic acid irrigations or surgical removal

Neoplastic

A. Benign
- i. Dermoid
    - a. Two cell layers (mesoderm and ectoderm)
    - b. May cause hearing loss and recurrent otitis externa
    - c. Surgical removal if symptomatic
- ii. Pilomatricoma (formerly pilomatrixoma, calcifying epithelioma of Malherbe)
    - a. Benign neoplasm from hair cortex cells
    - b. More common in Caucasian females
    - c. Painless, superficial, firm, bluish discoloration over skin
    - d. Diagnosis may require ultrasound to demonstrate calcification
    - e. Treatment options include observation versus surgical excision
- iii. Fibrous dysplasia
    - a. Monostotic (70%), polyostotic (24%) or Albright syndrome (6%)
    - b. Symptoms include temporal bone mass, otorrhea, conductive hearing loss
    - c. CT demonstrates lesion with ground-glass appearance
    - d. Surgery only if symptomatic
- iv. Langerhans cell histiocytosis
    - a. Clonal proliferation of Langerhans cells
    - b. Symptoms include postauricular swelling, temporal bone mass, otorrhea, conductive hearing loss, aural polyp
    - c. CT demonstrates punched-out lytic lesions
    - d. Bone scan recommended to assess the number of sites affected
    - e. Pathology demonstrates Birbeck granules
        1. Treatment options
            - Monostotic disease: surgery with possible addition of steroids
            - Polyostotic disease: chemotherapy or radiation

B. Malignant
- i. Rhabdomyosarcoma
    - a. Aggressive tumor of striated muscle (15% have distant metastases at diagnosis)
    - b. 3% occur in temporal bone

c. Three types:
   1. Embryonal (most common type in head and neck)
   2. Alveolar (more common in adolescents)
   3. Pleomorphic
   4. Sclerosing (rare, poor prognosis)

d. Symptoms include mass in ear canal, polyp, discharge, bleeding, pain, hearing loss, facial nerve palsy
e. CT or MRI demonstrate enhancement and destruction
f. Diagnosis based on biopsy. Pathology shows small round blue cells with hyperchromatic nuclei, large polygonal tumor cells with abundant eosinophilic cytoplasm with cross-striations. Molccular genetics of embryonal rhabdomyosarcoma shows deletion of short arm of chromosome 11 (11p15)
g. Treatment includes chemotherapy and radiation (see Head and Neck section)

ii. Ewing sarcoma
   a. Aggressive tumor of bone
   b. Less than 6% of Ewing sarcoma involves temporal bone
   c. Diagnosis based on biopsy. Pathology demonstrates sheets of small round blue cells with scant cytoplasm and inconspicuous nucleoli. Molecular genetic translocation t(11:22)(q24;q12) pathognomonic
   d. Treatment includes chemotherapy, radiation +/– surgical decompression if compressive symptoms (see Head and Neck section)

iii. Leukemia and lymphoma
   a. 20% of leukemia patients have temporal bone involvement
   b. Infiltration of tympanic membrane, middle ear, mastoid, petrous apex
   c. Diagnosis based on biopsy. Pathology demonstrates small round blue cells
   d. Improves with treatment of underlying disease. Treat secondary infections

iv. Other
   a. Chondrosarcoma
   b. Liposarcoma
   c. Hemangiosarcoma

Middle Ear (Ossicles, Eustachian Tube [ET])

Developmental Anatomy

A. Prenatal development
   i. 3 weeks' gestation
      a. First pharyngeal pouch forms tubotympanic recess. At 7 weeks' gestation, tubotympanic recess becomes constricted by second branchial arch to form Eustachian tube and tympanic cavity
   ii. 4 to 6 weeks' gestation
      a. Ossicles begin to develop. At 8 weeks' gestation, malleoincudal and incudostapedial joints form. Ossicles are adult size and shape at birth
         1. First arch (mandibular arch) gives rise to head of malleus, short process, and body of incus, tensor tympani tendon
         2. Second arch (hyoid arch) gives rise to manubrium of malleus, long process of incus, stapes superstructure, stapedius tendon. Stapes footplate derives from otic capsule
   iii. 21 weeks' gestation
      a. Mastoid antrum appears

B. Postnatal development
   i. Eustachian tube doubles in length from birth to adulthood
   ii. Mastoid tip poorly developed at birth. Facial nerve is therefore more superficial and prone to surgical injury. Pull of sternocleidomastoid lengthens mastoid tip over time
   iii. Mastoid air cells grow in first 2 to 3 years of life

Signs and Symptoms

A. Otorrhea
B. Conductive hearing loss
C. Otalgia
D. Disequilibrium

Clinical Assessment

A. Otoscopic examination including pneumatic otoscopy
B. Audiological testing including tympanometry
C. CT and/or MRI

Pathologies

Congenital

A. Ossicular anomalies
   i. Suspect when conductive hearing loss and normal otoscopic examination
   ii. Syndromic
      a. Apert/Crouzon (see below)
         1. Ankylosis of malleus and incus to lateral wall, deformed stapes
      b. Beckwith-Wiedemann
         1. Overgrowth disorder (macroglossia or hemihypertrophy) with a predisposition to tumor development (Wilms tumor, hepatoblastoma)
         2. May also have hypoglycemia, abdominal wall defects, visceromegaly, adrenocortical cytomegaly, and renal anomalies
         3. Due to mutation or deletion on chromosome 11p15
         4. CT demonstrates anterior bony fixation of malleus and stapes fixation. Also have ear lobule crease
      c. Branchio-otorenal (BOR) syndrome (see below)
         1. Fused malleoincudal complex
      d. CHARGE syndrome (see below)
         1. Abnormally shaped incus and stapes, ossicular chain fixation, absent stapedius tendon, absent stapes footplate.
      e. Congenital stapes footplate fixation (aka x-linked stapes gusher, Phelp syndrome) (see below)
         1. Stapes fixed to oval window. Therefore, manipulation may lead to dead ear
      f. DiGeorge
         1. **C**ardiac anomalies, **A**bnormal facies, **T** cell deficit due to thymic hypoplasia, **C**left palate, **H**ypocalcemia due to hypoparathyroidism (acronymCATCH22)
         2. Due to mutations in *TBX1* gene on chromosome 22q11
         3. CT demonstrates ossicular malformations and Mondini malformation
      g. Goldenhar (aka oculo-auriculo-vertebral dysplasia)
         1. Prevalence 1/45,000
         2. May be caused by mutation in 14q32 leading to first and second branchial arch anomalies

3. Clinical features (unilateral):
    - Epibulbar dermoids: benign white tumors over sclera
    - Conductive hearing loss, facial nerve deviation
    - Vertebral anomalies (hemi or fused)
    - Parotid agenesis
    - Cleft lip/palate and hypoplastic mandible
4. Ossicles may be fused as one block which is commonly fused to wall of hypoplastic middle ear cavity. May also have absent ossicles
5. Treatment:
    - Ophthalmology consultation
    - Conventional or bone anchored hearing aids
    - Correction of cleft lip/palate and mandible

h. Hurler
1. Inherited mucopolysaccharidosis, whereby lack of lysosomal enzymes leads to inability to degrade glycosaminoglycans or mucopolysaccharides which in turn accumulate in tissue
2. Due to mutation on chromosome 4p16 encoding alpha-L-iduronidase
3. Thick mucosa in middle ear due to lysosomes filled with glycosaminoglycans (Hurler cells). Hurler cells have also been found in middle ear ossicles, spiral ganglion neurons, the organ of Corti, and the vestibulocochlear nerve

i. Klippel-Feil (see below)
1. Deformed head of the malleus, rudimentary head of the incus, short or absent long process of the incus or absent incus, missing parts of stapes or complete absence, fixed stapes footplate (risk of gusher at surgery)

iii. Nonsyndromic
a. Congenital stapes ankylosis (accounts for 50%-70% of stapes fixation)
1. Management initially with hearing aids
2. Stapedectomy when older

b. Juvenile otosclerosis (15% develop symptoms as children)
1. Progressive hearing loss from 10 years of age
2. Usually bilateral (90%)
3. Family history in one-half of patients

B. Cholesteatoma
i. Keratinized squamous epithelium in middle ear or mastoid space
ii. Pressure and degradative enzymes erode soft tissue and bone
iii. Clinical features
a. Congenital
1. Well-circumscribed pearly white mass behind intact tympanic membrane in absence of otorrhea, perforation, or prior otologic surgery
2. Likely results from persistent epithelial rests at the time of neural groove closure between third and fifth weeks' embryogenesis
3. Usually undiagnosed until 2.5 to 5 years of age
4. More often male (3:1), unilateral (97%)
5. Present as hearing loss or facial nerve paralysis

b. Acquired
1. Primary acquired
    - Negative middle ear pressure creates retraction pocket leading to buildup of keratinous debris (usually in pars flaccida)
2. Secondary acquired
    - Due to migration of keratin through TM perforation into the middle ear space, implantation of keratin from prior surgery or trauma.

3. Present as foul-smelling ear with persistent discharge through perforated tympanic membrane and keratin in middle ear space. Hearing loss, vertigo, or facial nerve paralysis possible if left untreated

iv. Diagnosis
a. Fine-cut (0.625-mm thickness) CT temporal bone without contrast.
b. MRI shows lesion to be isointense on T1 (cholesterol granuloma is intense on T1) without enhancement from contrast and hyperintense on T2. Diffusion-weighted imaging is sensitive/specific for recurrent/persistent postsurgical disease.

v. Management
a. Surgical removal with goal of obtaining dry, safe ear. Hearing preservation is secondary.
b. Small lesions removed through transcanal approach. Larger lesions may require tympanomastoidectomy. Canal wall may be left up, taken down to reach diseased areas, or reconstructed to obliterate the mastoid space.

C. Vascular anomalies
i. Aberrant or dehiscent internal carotid artery
a. Anteroinferior quadrant of tympanic membrane
b. Symptoms of pulsatile tinnitus
ii. High-riding jugular bulb
a. Posteroinferior quadrant of tympanic membrane
b. Venous pulsatile tinnitus (up to 28% of secondary pulsatile tinnitus)
c. Do not perform myringotomy if there is any suspicion of this finding
iii. Persistent stapedial artery

Infectious

A. Acute otitis media (AOM) (AAP Clinical Practice Guideline, 2013)
i. Most common bacterial infection of childhood
ii. Diagnosis based on any one of the following:
a. Rapid onset of inflammation in middle ear
b. Moderate to severe bulging of TM
c. Mild bulging of TM and recent ear pain (< 48 hours) or intense erythema
d. New onset otorrhea not due to otitis externa
iii. Most common organisms
a. *Streptococcus pneumoniae* (35%)
b. *Hemophilus influenzae* (nontypeable: ie, not type B, etc.) (25%)
c. *Moraxella catarrhalis* (10%)
d. *d. Staphylococcus aureus* and *Streptococcus pyogenes*
e. Anaerobes (newborns)
f. Gram-negative enteric organisms (infants)
g. Viral
iv. Incidence of beta-lactamase-producing organisms is 20% to 30%
v. Predisposing factors
a. Male
b. First nations/Inuit
c. Craniofacial abnormality
d. Immunodeficiency
e. Bottle propping
f. Day care
g. Smoke exposure
h. Sibling with history of recurrent AOM
i. Infection in child less than 6 months of age

vi. Complications
  a. Intratemporal (within temporal bone)
    1. Conductive hearing loss
    2. TM perforation
    3. Mastoiditis
    4. Facial nerve palsy
    5. Labyrinthitis
    6. Petrositis
    7. SNHL
    8. Bezold abscess (abscess in sternocleidomastoid muscle)
  b. Intracranial (within cranium)
    1. Meningitis: Recurrent meningitis due to AOM warrants evaluation using imaging for cochlear or temporal bone malformation
    2. Sigmoid sinus thrombosis
    3. Otitic hydrocephalus
    4. Epidural abscess
    5. Subdural abscess
    6. Intracranial abscess

vii. Management:
  a. Exclusive breastfeeding for first 6 months of life
  b. Avoid tobacco smoke
  c. Influenza vaccine after 6 months of age (up to 55% reduction in AOM)
  d. Pneumococcal conjugate vaccine (29% reduction in AOM if given before 24 months of age)
  e. Assess and treat pain
  f. Antibiotic therapy
    1. May closely observe without antibiotics if
      - Parents are reliable
      - Age 6 months to 2 years and unilateral nonsevere AOM. (Severe = moderate otalgia, otalgia lasting 48 hours, fever 39°C)
      - Age more than 2 years and nonsevere bilateral AOM
      - No head/neck anomalies, immunodeficiency, chronic cardiac, or pulmonary disease
      - Give antibiotics if worsens or fails to improve after 48 to 72 hours
    2. Treatment with antibiotics if fails to fulfill above criteria
      - First-line treatment if no previous antibiotics: high-dose amoxicillin (azithromycin, cefdinir, cefuroxime, or ceftriaxone if penicillin allergic)
      - If failure of initial antibiotic treatment: amoxicillin-clavulanate (ceftriaxone or clindamycin if penicillin allergy)
      - Do not prescribe prophylactic antibiotics
    3. Myringotomy and tubes for recurrent AOM
      - 3 episodes in 6 months
      - 4 episodes in 1 year with one episode in preceding 6 months

B. Otitis media with effusion (OME) (AAO-HNSF Clinical Practice Guideline 2016 (Update))
  i. Diagnosis
    a. Middle ear fluid without signs of infection or inflammation
    b. Conductive hearing loss
    c. Otoscopy shows retraction, amber fluid, air bubbles, meniscus
    d. Pneumatic otoscopy to assess mobility of TM
    e. Flat tympanogram (type B)

- ii. Predisposing factors
  - a. Acute otitis media
  - b. Poor Eustachian tube function (ie, cleft palate)
- iii. Management
  - a. Observation with serial audiograms (90% resolve within 3 months)
  - b. Tympanostomy tube indications:
    1. Chronic bilateral OME (> 3 months) with hearing loss
    2. Chronic unilateral or bilateral OME with vestibular or behavioral problems, ear discomfort, poor school performance
    3. Children at risk (sensory, physical, cognitive, behavioral deficits) with OME of any duration that is unlikely to resolve (flat tympanograms)

Traumatic

- A. Perforation due to foreign body
  - i. Most heal spontaneously
  - ii. Vertigo or SNHL warrants audiological assessment. Consider middle ear exploration
- B. Temporal bone fracture
  - i. Less common in children.
  - ii. Most likely to be longitudinal or mixed fractures. According to newer more clinically relevant Little classification more commonly sparing the otic capsule
  - iii. Less likely to be associated with facial nerve palsy or SNHL

Neoplastic

- A. Benign
  - i. Choristoma
    - a. Aggregates of normal tissue (such as salivary or neural) in an abnormal location
  - ii. Paraganglioma (glomus jugulare and glomus tympanicum)
    - a. Derived from chemoreceptive cells of neural crest origin along parasympathetic nerves
    - b. Usually benign. Rarely can be malignant
    - c. Slow growing, expansile, locally destructive
    - d. CT angiography shows lesion, blood supply, extent of bone destruction. MRI shows avidly enhancing salt-pepper appearance
    - e. Pathology shows clusters of chief cells called *zellballen*
    - f. Complete surgical resection optimal with adjuvant chemo/radiation for nonresectable or malignant disease. Test for catecholamine secretion preoperatively
  - iii. Fibrous dysplasia
  - iv. Langerhans cell histiocytosis (see below)
- B. Malignant
  - i. Rhabdomyosarcoma
  - ii. Ewing sarcoma
  - iii. Leukemia and lymphoma
  - iv. Chondrosarcoma
  - v. Liposarcoma
  - vi. Hemangiosarcoma
  - vii. Adenocarcinoma
  - viii. Fibrosarcoma

Inner Ear (Cochlea, Vestibule, Internal Auditory Canal [IAC])

Developmental Anatomy

A. Prenatal development
  i. 3 weeks' gestation
    a. Otic placode appears. Later invaginates to become otocyst/otic vesicle which develops into membranous labyrinth
  ii. 5 weeks' gestation
    a. Endolymphatic duct (first to develop), cochlear duct, and vestibular precursor form on otocyst
    b. Otocyst has two parts:
      1. Pars superior: becomes ampulla and semicircular canals. Semicircular canals develop in following order (superior, posterior, lateral)
      2. Pars inferior: becomes saccule and cochlea
  iii. 6 weeks' gestation
    a. Cochlear duct grows from saccule. At 10 weeks reaches full 2.5 turns. At 20 weeks reaches full adult size. At 21 weeks organ of Corti becomes functional

B. Postnatal development
  i. Endolymphatic sac and duct grow until age 3 to 4 years

Signs and Symptoms

A. Speech delay
B. Behavioral problems
C. Disequilibrium

Clinical Assessment

A. History
  i. Risk factors for childhood permanent hearing loss [Joint Committee on Infant Hearing (JCIH), 2019]. Neonates who pass the infant hearing screen but possess these risk factors should undergo audiologic monitoring usually 6 months until 3 years of age.
    a. Family history of permanent childhood hearing loss
    b. In-utero infections such as CMV and TORCH, mother with Zika
    c. Stigmata of syndrome known to include hearing loss or Eustachian tube dysfunction
    d. Craniofacial anomalies
    e. Syndromes associated with progressive hearing loss (ie, Alport, Jervell, and Lange-Nielsen, neurofibromatosis, osteopetrosis, Pendred, Usher, Waardenburg)
    f. Neurodegenerative disorders (ie, Charcot-Marie Tooth, Friedrich ataxia, Hunter)
    g. Postnatal infections associated with hearing loss such as bacterial and viral (herpes, varicella) meningitis or encephalitis
    h. Admission of more than 5 days to a NICU
    i. Hyperbilirubinemia requiring serum exchange transfusion
    j. Asphyxia or hypoxic ischemic encephalopathy, ECMO
    k. Ototoxic medications (including chemotherapy), loop diuretics, aminoglycosides for more than 5 days.
    l. Head trauma
    m. Recurrent or persistent OME for at least 3 months
    n. Caregiver concern regarding hearing, speech, language, or developmental delay

B. Auditory function tests
   i. Physiological tests
      a. Otoacoustic emissions (OAE): Low-intensity sounds produced by outer hair cells of the cochlea as they expand and contract. Used as infant hearing screen and to test for functional hearing loss. Drawback is that OAEs can estimate hearing sensitivity only within a limited range of frequencies.
      b. Auditory brain stem response (ABR): Auditory evoked potential generated by brief click or tone pip transmitted via insert earphone. Waveform peaks denote functionality of different parts of auditory pathway.
      c. Tympanometry: Test of middle ear function. Not as useful in infants (< 6 months old) due to increased compliance of EAC
   ii. Behavioral tests
      a. Visual reinforcement audiometry (VRA): Responses in soundfield (not ear specific) are rewarded visually (ie, clapping clown). Used for children 8 months to 3 years of age
      b. Conditioned play audiometry: Ear-specific responses. Used for children 3 to 5 years of age
      c. Conventional audiometry: Ear-specific air conduction (AC) and bone conduction (BC) thresholds. Used for children greater than 5 years of age
C. Vestibular testing (see Chapter 14)
D. Imaging the temporal bone
   i. Low-dose fine cut (0.625 mm) temporal bone CT scan is the standard.
   ii. MRI may be helpful for internal auditory canal (IAC) (ie, number of nerves on sagittal section), endolymphatic sac, patency of cochlear duct, mass lesions.

Pathology/Treatment/Complications

Congenital Hearing Loss

A. Genetic: nonsyndromic
   i. Autosomal recessive
      a. Connexins (GJB2 and GJB6 encoding connexins 26 and 30, respectively)
         1. Most common genetic nonsyndromic SNHL
         2. 35delG mutation accounts for 80% of connexin 26 mutations
         3. Dysfunctional gap junctions impair potassium ion recycling in stria vascularis
      b. Enlarged vestibular aqueduct (EVA)
         1. May also have sensorineural hearing loss (mild to profound, audiogram flat or downsloping high-frequency loss), conductive hearing loss (low frequency), may be isolated or associated with Mondini malformation
         2. May have sudden hearing loss with head trauma
         3. Do not have SLC26A4 mutation or thyroid problems
      c. Mitochondrial A1555G mutation
         1. Maternally inherited mutation in mitochondrial 12S RNA
         2. 15% of patients in United States with SNHL due to aminoglycosides have this mutation. Much more common in Mongolia
      d. Otoferlin mutation/auditory dyssynchrony
         1. Mutation in *OTOF* gene causes vesicle membrane fusion problem
         2. Causes auditory dyssynchromy: present OAE, absent ABR, variable auditory thresholds
   ii. Autosomal dominant
      a. Wolfram
         1. Most common cause of dominantly inherited low-frequency SNHL
         2. Progressive hearing loss

B. Genetic: syndromic (over 400 types in total)
  i. Autosomal recessive
    a. Pendred
      1. 2% of profound congenital SNHL
      2. Mutations in SLC26A4 or PDS lead to defect in iodine-chloride transporter
      3. SNHL (unilateral or bilateral, progressive), Mondini malformation
      4. Associated with thyroid goiter (euthyroid), thyroid malignancy
      5. Test for SLC26A4, TSH, T3, T4. Do not remove thyroid unless malignancy present
    b. Usher
      1. 3% of deaf population, 50% of deaf/blind population
      2. Mutations in MYO7A, USH2A, and others lead to defective tip links and Usherin protein
      3. SNHL, vestibular dysfunction, retinitis pigmentosa
      4. Three types:
        - USH1 (MYO7A mutation) (40% of cases): profound congenital bilateral SNHL, absent vestibular function, early retinitis pigmentosa by 10 years of age
        - USH2 (USH2A mutation) (60% of cases): moderate SNHL, normal vestibular function, later onset retinitis pigmentosa
        - USH3 (3% of cases, mostly Norwegian): progressive SNHL, variable vestibular function
    c. Jervell and Lange-Nielsen
      1. 1/1000 of profoundly deaf population
      2. Mutation in KVLQT1 leads to dysregulation of potassium channel
      3. Severe/profound SNHL, prolonged QT, and large T waves on ECG
      4. Presents as 20 to 30-year-old healthy person with sudden onset of syncope and sudden death
      5. Treat with beta blocker
      6. Test first-degree relatives for Ward-Romano syndrome due to similar cardiac problem without hearing loss
    d. Biotinidase deficiency
      1. 1/60,000
      2. Lack enzyme to recycle biotin
      3. Leads to hair loss, hearing loss, seizures, hypotonia, coma, and death
      4. Tested as part of infant screening program because it is preventable with dietary replacement
  ii. Autosomal dominant
    a. Waardenburg
      1. Most common inherited congenital deafness (2%)
      2. Mutation in neural crest cells leads to defective intermediate layer of stria vascularis
      3. Clinical features
        - White forelock (25% of cases, varying age of first appearance)
        - Hearing loss (unilateral or bilateral, EVA in 50%)
        - Synophores (eyebrows grow together)
        - Dystopia canthorum (lateral displacement of inner canthi)
        - Blue eyes or heterochromia iridis (different colors)
        - Pinched nose
        - Hirschsprung disease (absent ganglia in distal colon)
        - Limb defects

4. Four types:
   - WS1 (most common): PAX3 mutation, dystopia canthorum, hearing loss (20%)
   - WS2A (Tietz syndrome): MITF mutation, no dystopia canthorum, hearing loss (50%)
   - WS3 (Klein-Waardenburg): Unilateral ptosis, eyelid and limb anomalies
   - WS4 (Shah-Waardenburg): SOX10 mutation, Hirschsprung

b. Apert/Crouzon
1. Craniosynostosis of coronal suture leads to prominent forehead and flat occiput. Large fontanelles close at later age
2. Due to mutation in *FGFR2* gene on chromosome 26
3. 70% normal intelligence, 30% delayed
4. Fused vertebrae (40%)
5. Conductive hearing loss, ankylosis of malleus and incus to lateral wall, and deformed fixed stapes footplate, wide cochlear aqueduct, absent internal auditory canal (prohibits cochlear implantation)
6. Downslanting palpebral fissures
7. Proptosis and exposure keratitis
8. Apert involves syndactyly (fingers and toes 2,3,4 fused in mid-digital mass), whereas Crouzon does not
9. Treatment includes eye care for keratitis, craniofacial surgery, and Tessier procedure for separating fused digits

c. Branchio-otorenal (aka Melnick-Fraser)
1. 2% of deaf children, 1/40,000
2. Autosomal dominant. Many mutations are de novo and are specific to individual families. High penetrance, variable expressivity, successive anticipation (worse with every generation)
3. Due to mutation in *EYA1* gene on chromosome 8q13
4. Clinical diagnosis based on three major, two major/two minor, or one major and first-degree relative with diagnosis:
   - Major criteria
     (a) Hearing loss (conductive, SNHL, or mixed). Often mild and goes undiagnosed, therefore audiogram recommended in all patients with a family history of branchial anomalies
     (b) Preauricular pits
     (c) Branchial cleft cyst or fistula
     (d) Renal dysplasia/malformed calyces, aplasia, polycystic kidneys
   - Minor criteria
     (a) External ear
     (b) Middle ear
     (c) Inner ear
     (d) Tags, facial asymmetry, palatal abnormalities
5. Temporal bone features pathognomonic (1) fused malleoincudal complex; (2) facial nerve on medial side of cochlea; (3) hypoplastic apical turn of cochlea; (4) funnel-shaped internal auditory canal; and (4) patulous Eustachian tube; and (5) medially displaced carotid arteries
6. Confirmatory diagnosis by genetic testing for EYA1 mutation (only 40% have mutation in *EYA1* gene)
7. Treatment includes hearing screen, hearing aid if loss is diagnosed, genetics in family members

d. CHARGE
   1. Stands for **C**oloboma of the eye, **H**eart defects, **A**tresia choanae, **R**etardation of growth/development, **G**enitourinary abnormalities, **E**ar anomalies, and deafness
   2. Due to sporadic microdeletions in *CHD7* gene on chromosome 8 (only 50% of patients have this mutation)
   3. Clinical diagnosis based on major and minor criteria:
      - Major criteria
        (a) Coloboma of the eye (cleft of iris, retina, macula, or disc, not eyelid), microphthalmos, anophthalmos
        (b) Ear anomalies: outer (wide ear with little or no lobe, antihelix discontinuous with tragus)
        (c) Ear anomalies: middle (abnormally shaped incus and stapes, ossicular chain fixation, absent stapedius tendon and stapes footplate, and conductive loss)
        (d) Ear anomalies: inner (absent oval window, Mondini malformation, hypoplastic or absent semicircular canals)
        (e) Choanal atresia
        (f) Cranial nerve anomalies (missing olfactory nerve, abnormal facial nerve course, and facial palsy, swallowing difficulties, aspiration)
      - Minor criteria
        (a) CHARGE behavior (perseverance, obsessive, compulsive)
        (b) Growth hormone deficiency
        (c) CHARGE facies, prominent forehead, arched eyebrows, thick nostrils, facial asymmetry
        (d) Cleft lip and palate
        (e) Tracheoesophageal fistula
        (f) Heart defects such as tetralogy of Fallot
        (g) Renal anomalies (absent, small, misplaced)
        (h) Genitourinary (small penis, undescended testes, small labia, small or missing uterus)

e. Neurofibromatosis type 2 (NF2)
   1. Autosomal dominant
   2. Mutation in tumor-suppressor gene schwannomin on chromosome 22 leads to abnormal production of protein merlin
   3. Hearing loss around age 20 years, tinnitus, imbalance, vertigo
   4. Diagnostic criteria:
      - Bilateral vestibular schwannomas
      - First degree relative with NF2 PLUS patient has unilateral vestibular schwannoma OR two other tumors (neurofibroma, meningioma, glioma, schwannoma)
      - Unilateral vestibular schwannoma AND two other tumors (mentioned above)
      - Multiple meningiomas PLUS unilateral vestibular schwannoma OR any two of schwannoma, glioma, neurofibroma, cataract

f. Otosclerosis (aka otospongiosus)
   1. Endochondral bony sclerosis of stapes footplate to oval window
   2. Autosomal dominant, incomplete penetrance (25%)
   3. 1% of Caucasian adults
   4. More common in females
   5. Conductive and sensorineural hearing loss

g. Stickler
    1. Myopia, cataracts, retinal detachment
    2. Progressive mixed hearing loss (80%)
    3. Midface hypoplasia
    4. Robin sequence
    5. Hypermobile joints and arthritis
h. Treacher-Collins (aka mandibulofacial dysostosis)
    1. Mutation in chromosome 5q leads to abnormal treacle protein
    2. May be due to maternal sensitivity to vitamin A
    3. Bilateral features
    4. Diagnostic criteria:
        - Microtia (also has aural atresia, conductive hearing loss, sensorineural hearing loss, and vestibular dysfunction)
        - Midface hypoplasia (underdevelopment of zygomatic arch)
        - Downsloping palpebral fissures
        - Coloboma of outer third of lower eyelid with absence of lashes
        - Micrognathia (may have cleft palate, velopharyngeal insufficiency)
i. Klippel-Feil
    1. Failure of segmentation of cervical vertebrae leading to fused appearance
    2. Due to mutations in *GDF6* gene on chromosome 8q22, *MEOX1* gene on chromosome 17q21, and *GDF3* gene on chromosome 12p13
    3. CT demonstrates narrow downsloping external auditory canals, deformed head of the malleus, rudimentary head of the incus, short or absent long process of the incus or absent incus, missing parts of stapes or complete absence, fixed stapes footplate (risk of gusher at surgery), dehiscence of facial nerve, absence of one or all semicircular canals, cochlear malformation or absence

C. X-linked
    i. Nonsyndromic
        a. Congenital fixation of stapes footplate with perilymphatic gusher
            1. Most common x-linked deafness
            2. Due to mutation of *POU3F4* gene on Xq21 locus
            3. Affected males have stable hearing at birth, then progressive mixed hearing loss or sensorineural loss which is often bilateral (75%)
            4. Carrier females have mild hearing loss and less severe middle ear anomalies
            5. Family history of hearing loss
            6. Large internal auditory canal, absent lamina cribrosa
            7. Entry into cochleovestibular apparatus leads to gush of perilymphatic fluid which can lead to a dead ear
    ii. Syndromic
        a. Alport
            1. Mostly due to x-linked mutation in COL4A5. 15% autosomal recessive due to mutations in COL4A3 or COL4A4
            2. Progressive high-frequency sensorineural hearing loss
            3. Retinal flecks, anterior lenticonus (protrusion of the lens), spherophakia (spherical lens), congenital cataracts
            4. Glomerulonephritis, hematuria, and progressive renal failure
        b. Deafness dystonia (rare)
            1. Hearing loss, blindness, dystonia, mental deterioration

c. Norrie (rare)
   1. Hearing loss, blindness, mental deterioration

d. Otopalatodigital (rare)
   1. Conductive hearing loss due to ossicular malformations
   2. Cleft palate
   3. Broad fingers, large spaces between toes

e. Wildervanck
   1. Familial
   2. Affects females only
   3. Mixed hearing loss
   4. CN6 palsy
   5. Fused cervical vertebrae

D. Chromosomal
   i. Down syndrome
      a. Most common chromosomal anomaly
      b. 90% are trisomy 21. 5% are due to translocations
      c. Superior helix folded over, stenotic external auditory canal, middle ear and mastoid disease, sensorineural hearing loss, hypoplastic lateral semicircular canal bony island, superior semicircular canal dehiscence, narrow internal auditory canal, cochlear nerve stenosis, large vestibular aqueduct
   ii. Turner syndrome
      a. Absence of one X chromosome
      b. Short stature
      c. Conductive and sensorineural hearing loss
      d. Webbed neck
      e. Shield chest
      f. Gonadal dysgenesis

E. Environmental
   i. Fetal alcohol
      a. Microcephaly, mental retardation, seizures
      b. Narrow forehead, eyelid ptosis, midface hypoplasia, short nose
      c. Conductive and sensorineural hearing loss

Infectious Hearing Loss

A. Congenital TORCH infections
   i. Clinical features
      a. **T**oxoplasmosis
      b. **O**ther: syphilis, varicella, parvovirus B19 ("Fifth disease," "slapcheek")
      c. **R**ubella: Developmental delay, meningoencephalitis, SNHL, cataracts, retinopathy, glaucoma, patent ductus arteriosus, pulmonary artery stenosis
      d. **C**ytomegalovirus: Most common infectious cause of congenital SNHL. Severe symptoms in 5%. Intrauterine growth retardation (IUGR), microcephaly, large cerebral ventricles, intracerebral calcification, SNHL, retinitis, hepatosplenomegaly, thrombocytopenia, jaundice. "A neonatal dried blood spot can be tested for CMV DNA using PCR in children older than three weeks."
      e. **H**erpes

B. Meningitis: Streptococcus is the most common, but any organism may cause hearing loss

C. Mumps

Traumatic

A. Ototoxic medications
  i. Clinical features
    a. Chemotherapeutics (cisplatin, carboplatin)
    b. Loop diuretics (furosemide). May be reversible
    c. Aminoglycoside antibiotics. Predisposition to hearing loss if A1555G mutation in maternally inherited mitochondrial DNA
B. Noise
C. Temporal bone fracture

Management

A. Early identification is crucial (universal newborn hearing screening)
B. Amplification
C. Cochlear implantation
D. Sign language

Neoplastic

A. Acoustic neuroma (see Neurofibromatosis).

Nose, Nasopharynx, and Paranasal Sinuses

Developmental Anatomy

A. Prenatal development
  i. 3 weeks' gestation
    a. Anterior neuropore at skull base persists medial to optic recess
    b. Fonticulus nasofrontalis
      1. Space between inferior part of frontal bone and nasal bones
      2. Entrapped tissue becomes extranasal encephalocele (meninges with or without brain tissue)
    c. Prenasal space
      1. Potential space posterior to nasal bones
      2. 3 to 8 weeks' gestation: dura projects through foramen cecum (hole in skull base) and down through prenasal space. As foramen cecum closes, the diverticulum retracts into the cranium. Entrapped tissue becomes intranasal glioma (no meningeal connection) or intranasal encephalocele (retains meningeal connection)
  ii. 4 weeks' gestation
    a. External nasal development
    b. Neural crest proliferation creates nasal placode. Adjacent cells give rise to medial and lateral nasal processes
      1. Medial nasal process: joins maxillary process to form columella and philtrum. Overgrowth leads to pyriform aperture stenosis
      2. Frontal prominence: joins medial nasal/maxillary processes to form frontonasal process which develops into frontal/nasal bones, ethmoids, cartilaginous nose.
    c. Nasal pits invaginate and nasobuccal membrane ruptures (5-6 weeks') forming nasal cavities. Failure to rupture leads to choanal atresia

d. Nasal septum development
e. Grows downward from nasofrontal process
f. Fuses to palatine process anteriorly (at 9 weeks') then posteriorly (at 12 weeks'). Septomaxillary ligament joining septum to anterior nasal spine, pulls on maxilla

iii. 10 to 16 weeks' gestation
a. Paranasal sinus development
b. Maxillary sinus (10 weeks)
1. First to develop
2. Pneumatization from middle meatus into ethmoid cartilage. Extension into maxilla at 5 months
3. Radiologically visible at birth

c. Ethmoid sinus (4 months')
1. Pneumatization from middle and superior meatus into ethmoid capsule. Secondary pneumatization between birth and 2 years of age
2. Basal lamella of middle turbinate separates anterior and posterior ethmoid cells

d. Sphenoid sinus (4 months')
1. Sphenoethmoid recess becomes constricted
2. Secondary pneumatization between 6 and 7 years of age
3. Sphenoid and frontal sinuses commonly absent in Down syndrome

e. Frontal sinus (4 months')
1. Begins with mucosal invaginations
2. Secondary pneumatization at 6 months to 2 years, but not radiologically visible until 6 years of age

B. Postnatal development
i. Vomer and perforated portions of cribriform plate ossify by 3 years of age.
ii. Adenoids peak in size from 3 to 5 years of age and regress by 8 years of age.
iii. Maxillary sinus floor is superior to nasal floor at birth, same level as nasal floor at 8 years of age, and 5 mm below nasal floor by adulthood.
iv. Ethmoid, sphenoid, and frontal sinuses continue to grow as above.
v. External nasal dimensions mature by 13 years of age in females and 15 years of age in males.

Signs and Symptoms

A. Infants are obligate nasal breathers for several weeks, so nasal obstruction leads to respiratory distress.
B. After they begin to breathe orally, obstruction manifests as sleep apnea and feeding difficulties.
C. Purulent rhinorrhea.
D. Mass effect.

Clinical Assessment

A. Complete head and neck examination noting dysmorphic features
B. Examine from anteriorly to posteriorly and then superiorly to inferiorly
C. Anterior rhinoscopy for septum, vestibule, and anterior nasal cavity
D. Flexible nasopharyngoscopy for nasal passage, nasopharynx, oropharynx, and larynx
E. Physical examination may be limited for sinus pathology
F. X-ray, CT, or MRI depending on suspected pathologies

Pathology/Treatment/Complications

Congenital

A. Pyriform aperture stenosis
   i. Clinical features
      a. Due to overgrowth of nasal process of maxilla
      b. Presentation similar to choanal atresia
      c. May be associated with single central incisor, holoprosencephaly, or pituitary deficiency
   ii. Diagnosis
      a. Based on physical examination and CT scan
      b. MRI brain for pituitary abnormalities
   iii. Management
      a. Close observation and conservative measures such as suction, nasal saline (one side at a time), decongestants, steroids
      b. Airway compromise warrants balloon dilation or sublabial incision and drillout of pyriformapertures
B. Nasolacrimal duct obstruction/cyst
   i. Clinical features
      a. Due to failed canalization of caudal nasolacrimal duct
      b. 90% unilateral
      c. Symptoms appear at 1 to 3 weeks of age. These include epiphora, medial canthal discharge, and noninjected conjunctiva
   ii. Diagnosis
      a. Cystic lesion in inferior meatus
   iii. Management
      a. Usually resolves spontaneously by 9 months as cyst ruptures into nasal passage
      b. Marsupialization
      c. Associated duct stenosis may require dilatation
C. Choanal atresia/stenosis
   i. Clinical features
      a. Failure of resorption of bucconasal membrane of Hochstetter at 5 weeks'
      b. 1:5000 live births
      c. Twice as common in females than males
      d. Twice as likely to be unilateral than bilateral
      e. Majority are mixed bony and membranous
      f. 50% of patients have other congenital anomalies
      g. Associated with CHARGE and Treacher-Collins (see above)
      h. Bilateral atresia presents in newborn as "cyclical cyanosis" with airway obstruction and cyanosis at rest that resolves with crying and agitation (due to open-mouth posture)
      i. Unilateral atresia presents later in life as unilateral nasal obstruction and thick, stringy, unilateral nasal discharge
   ii. Diagnosis
      a. Classic consultation is for "inability to pass suction catheter through nose." However, flexible nasopharyngoscopy with direct visualization is required.
      b. CT scan of choanae confirms diagnosis and extent of atresia. The nose should be suctioned and decongested with oxymetazoline prior to imaging.
   iii. Management
      a. Oral airway or McGovern nipple (feeding nipple with end cut off) while infant is obligate nasal breather.

b. Bilateral choanal atresia almost always requires early surgical repair.
c. Unilateral atresia can be repaired when problematic, usually prior to starting school.
d. Endoscopic (preferred) or transpalatal repair with or without placement of stents.
e. Syndromic choanal atresia or patients with multiple-level obstruction may have poorer outcomes and require tracheotomy.

D. Nasal encephalocele/glioma/dermoid
  i. Encephaloceles and gliomas develop due to failure of closure of foramen cecum at 3 weeks' gestation.
    a. Encephalocele (no communication with skin)
      1. At root of nose, maintain communication with subarachnoid space
      2. 1:35,000 live births
      3. 35% have other abnormalities
      4. Four types
        - Nasal
          (a) Nasofrontal: between nose and forehead
          (b) Nasoethmoid: between nose and ethmoid
          (c) Nasoorbital: between nose and orbit
        - Frontal
        - Atretic/parietal
        - Occipital
    b. Glioma (no communication with skin)
      1. No communication with subarachnoid space.
      2. 15% have fibrous stalk continuous with dura.
  ii. Dermoid (communication with skin/pit in nasal dorsum)
    a. Midline mass or pit (most common congenital mass)
    b. Ectodermal and mesodermal elements
    c. May pass through foramen cecum to cranial fossa
  iii. Diagnosis
    a. Encephalocele is soft and compressible, transilluminates, and has positive Furstenberg test (expands with crying, Valsalva maneuver, or compression of jugular veins)
    b. Gliomas are firm, noncompressible, do not transilluminate, and have negative Furstenberg test
    c. Imaging important to assess communication with intracranial space. CT for bony skull base defect. MRI for CSF communication
  iv. Management
    a. Antibiotics for infection
    b. Surgical excision for definitive management
    c. Involve neurosurgery if intracranial connection

E. Tornwald cyst
  i. Clinical features
    a. Persistence of pharyngeal bursa (first described by Mayer, then Luschka)
    b. Present as midline nasopharyngeal cyst or chronic crusting
  ii. Diagnosis
    a. Clinical or using MRI or CT
  iii. Management
    a. Surgical excision or marsupialization

F. Primary ciliary dyskinesia
  i. Clinical features
    a. Defective dynein arms lead to poor mucociliary clearance, otitis media, sinusitis, and bronchiectasis.
    b. May be due to autosomal recessive mutations in DNAI1 and DNAH5 (38%).
    c. Can be associated with Kartagener syndrome (50%)
      1. Sinusitis, bronchiectasis
      2. Situs inversus
      3. Infertility
  ii. Diagnosis requires ciliary biopsy from noninflamed nasal or tracheal mucosa
  iii. Management is symptomatic (washing and suctioning nasal cavity and sinuses)

G. Cystic fibrosis
  i. Clinical features
    a. Most common fatal autosomal recessive disorder (1/2000 live births)
    b. Mutations in *CFTR* gene (delta F508 most common) cause defect in cell membrane chloride ion transport
    c. Increased mucus viscosity impairs clearance leading to infection
    d. Suspect in children under 10 years of age with nasal polyps
    e. Nasal obstruction and chronic sinusitis (30%)
      1. Most common bacteria cultured are *S aureus* (47%) and *P aeruginosa* (26%) (*P aeruginosa* more common in patients older than 8 years of age). Both of these bacteria found in same sinus in only 7% of patients, suggesting separate specimens should be obtained from several sinuses.
      2. Sinus bacteria highly predictive of pulmonary bacteria in children over 8 years of age.
    f. Persistent productive cough, bronchitis, bronchiectasis
    g. Pancreatic insufficiency, fat malabsorption, coagulopathy (due to vitamin K deficiency), meconium ileus
    h. Cirrhosis and hepatomegaly
    i. Nephrolithiasis
    j. Infertility
    k. Reduced bone density
    l. Venous thrombosis
  ii. Diagnosis
    a. Clinical symptoms of CF in one organ system
    b. Evidence of dysfunctional cystic fibrosis transmembrane conductance regulator protein evidenced by any of the following:
      1. Elevated sweat chloride level (first line, diagnostic if greater or equal to 60 mmol/L)
      2. Genetic testing (used if sweat chloride intermediate, less than 60 mmol/L)
      3. Abnormal nasal potential difference (false negative if inflammation)
      4. Immunoreactive trypsin test (IRT) during neonatal screening (identifies 50% of cases)
    c. CT shows bilateral pansinusitis
  iii. Treatment
    a. Medical management
      1. Nasal steroid sprays
      2. Nasal irrigation with saline and mucolytics (dornase alfa)
      3. Topical, nebulized (tobramycin), oral (macrolide) antibiotics
      4. CFTR modulator therapy

b. Surgical management (endoscopic sinus surgery)
    1. For alleviation of nasal obstruction after failure of maximal medical therapy.
    2. Unclear if sinonasal surgery improves pulmonary function.
    3. Check coagulation preoperatively.

Trauma

A. Septal deviation
    i. Neonatal septal deviation
        a. Relatively common
        b. Most improve spontaneously
        c. Severe deviations with airway compromise should be corrected early
    ii. Acquired septal deviation
        a. Impact of early surgery on facial growth controversial. Conservative therapy with minimal removal of cartilage advocated
B. Septal hematoma
    i. Nasal obstruction
    ii. Diagnosed on examination
    iii. Management
        a. Drainage and nasal packing to minimize risk of abscess, perforation, and saddle nose deformity
C. Septal abscess
    i. Nasal obstruction, pain, and fever
    ii. Leads to cartilage loss and saddle nose deformity
    iii. Management
        a. Drainage, packing, and antibiotics (to cover *S pneumoniae* and group A beta-hemolytic *streptococci*)
        b. Suspect child abuse in children under 2 years of age
D. Nasal fractures
    i. Most common facial fracture of childhood
    ii. Greenstick fractures common
    iii. Rule out septal hematoma/abscess or CSF leak
    iv. Diagnosis
        a. Based on clinical examination
        b. Radiographs not helpful
    v. Management
        a. Closed reduction if obvious cosmetic deformity
        b. Reduce immediately before swelling occurs or 5 to 7 days after trauma when swelling subsides
E. Nasoethmoid fractures
    i. Uncommon in children
    ii. Rule out intracranial and cervical spine injuries
    iii. May require reconstructive surgery
F. Orbital floor fractures
    i. Clinical features
        a. Hypoesthesia of infraorbital nerve
        b. Inferior rectus muscle entrapment
        c. Enophthalmos
        d. Globe injuries
    ii. Management
        a. May require reconstructive surgery

G. Nasal foreign body
  i. Associated with malodorous rhinorrhea, often unilateral
  ii. Button/disk batteries must be removed immediately due to risk of necrosis and septal perforation

Infectious/Inflammatory

A. Rhinitis of infancy
  i. May cause airway obstruction and feeding difficulties in infants
  ii. Onset at birth or within first month of life
  iii. Seasonal variation, more common in fall and winter
  iv. May be due to RSV, chlamydia, GERD, meconium aspiration
  v. Management
    a. Bulb suction for nose. Ear suction used in nose is more slender and less traumatic
    b. Topical vasoconstrictor for 3 days and saline drops. If no improvement in 5 days add steroid drops or spray
    c. Culture may be helpful
    d. CT reserved for nonresponders

B. Allergic rhinitis
  i. Itchy nose with discharge and obstruction. Bruising under eyes "allergic shiners" and "supratip crease" (from rubbing nose upward) common
  ii. IgE-mediated response (type 1)
  iii. Types:
    a. Seasonal (grass, trees, pollen, ragweed)
    b. Perennial (allergens within home)
    c. Sporadic (intermittent to specific allergen)
    d. Occupational
  iv. Family history of atopy in 50% to 75% of children
  v. Examination shows pale, boggy edematous mucosa, inferior turbinate hypertrophy, thin clear rhinorrhea, +/− polyps
  vi. Diagnosis:
    a. Based on clinical history alone
    b. May confirm with skin prick test, intradermal tests, radioallergosorbent assay testing (RAST) or enzyme-linked immunosorbent assay (ELISA)
  vii. Management
    a. Avoidance
    b. Pharmacotherapy (nasal saline, decongestants, steroid sprays, antihistamines, leukotriene inhibitors, mast cell stabilizers, anticholinergics)
    c. Allergen-specific immunotherapy

C. Viral rhinitis
  i. Common in childhood
  ii. Pathogens include rhinovirus, coronavirus, adenovirus, and respiratory syncytial virus

D. Bacterial rhinitis
  i. Diphtheria: pseudomembrane formation on nasal septum
  ii. Pertussis: associated with prolonged cough
  iii. Chlamydia: red nasal mucosa in neonate with rhinorrhea. Vertical transmission from mother to child during delivery
  iv. Syphilis—congenital infection

a. First stage—presents in first 3 months of life with watery rhinorrhea which progresses to mucopurulent drainage
b. Second stage—presents later in childhood with "snuffles" and gumma formation in nasal cavity

E. Adenoid hypertrophy
i. Clinical features
a. Nasal obstruction
b. Hyponasal speech
c. "Adenoid facies": open mouth, flat midface, long lower face, high-arched palate. Open mouth posture leads to unopposed compressive action of masseter muscles on maxilla and overgrowth of molars due to lack of contact
d. Rhinorrhea
e. Sleep apnea
f. Eustachian tube dysfunction
g. Recurrent acute otitis media

ii. Diagnosis
a. Flexible nasopharyngoscopy (benefits: faster, no radiation, and allows evaluation of effect of palate location on size of choanal aperture)
b. X-ray (benefit: no scope for uncooperative children; risks: radiation, crying children elevate soft palate which makes nasal aperture look smaller, thus overestimating adenoid size)

iii. Management
a. Topical steroids and nasal saline
b. Add montelukast for mild cases
c. Surgery for moderate/severe cases
d. Recurrent obstruction following surgery responds better to nasal steroids than prior to surgery. Failure to improve warrants revision of adenoidectomy
e. Biopsy recurrent adenoid regrowth to rule out lymphoma
f. Complications of surgery include velopharyngeal insufficiency, bleeding, infection, torticollis (Grisel syndrome), nasopharyngeal stenosis, Eustachian tube injury, and atlantoaxial subluxation (ie, Down syndrome: avoid neck extension even if they have "normal" flexion/extension cervical spine X-rays)

F. Rhinosinusitis
i. Acute
a. Clinical features
1. Purulent rhinorrhea more than 10 days with fever
2. Uncomplicated infections due to:
   - *S pneumoniae* (30%)
   - *H influenzae* (20%)
   - *M catarrhalis* (20%)
   - *S pyogenes* (5%)
3. Complicated infections due to
   - Polymicrobial
   - *Streptococcus anginosus*
   - Anaerobes
   - Methicillin-resistant *S aureus* (MRSA)
4. Communicating location of infection (Chandler classification). These are not progressive and are only descriptive
   - Preseptal cellulitis
   - Orbital cellulitis (associated with chemosis)

- Subperiosteal abscess
- Orbital abscess
- Venous/cavernous sinus thrombosis

5. Risks of spread
   - Frontal bone (Pott puffy tumor)
   - Meningitis
   - Abscess (subdural, epidural, brain)

b. Diagnosis
1. Uncomplicated sinusitis based on clinical symptoms. Radiographic sinus opacification is nonspecific in young children
2. Complications require urgent CT scan

c. Treatment
1. Uncomplicated: Oral amoxicillin 10 to 14 days. Beta-lactamase inhibitor if severe symptoms or if no improvement after 72 hours
2. Complications: Intravenous antibiotics that have good soft tissue and CNS penetration. Consult ophthalmology and/or neurosurgery as required. May require urgent surgical drainage

ii. Recurrent acute

a. Clinical features
1. Free of symptoms for 2 weeks between episodes

b. Diagnosis
1. Rule out immunodeficiency, cystic fibrosis (CF), primary ciliary dyskinesia (PCD), and gastroesophageal reflux disease (GERD)
2. Assess adenoid size

c. Treatment
1. Adenoidectomy if adenoids obstructive

iii. Chronic

a. Clinical features
1. Congestion, rhinorrhea, headache, postnasal drip, cough, halitosis
2. Low-grade symptoms lasting more than 12 weeks
3. Infections due to:
   - *Staphylococcus aureus*
   - Anaerobes
   - Fungi

b. Diagnosis
1. Cultures from middle meatus/ethmoid/maxillary sinus helpful if
   - Immunocompromised
   - Systemic illness
   - Progression despite appropriate therapy
   - Suppurative complications

c. Treatment
1. Antibiotic therapy 4 to 6 weeks
2. Adenoidectomy may be helpful in younger children
3. Endoscopic sinus surgery for failed medical management. Limited to involved sinuses (usually maxillary and anterior ethmoids)

G. Nasal polyps

i. Antrochoanal polyp

a. Clinical features
1. Extends from maxillary sinus into nasal cavity
2. Most unilateral

b. Diagnosis
   1. Flexible nasopharyngoscopy
   2. CT or MRI
c. Management
   1. Endoscopic removal. Send to pathology to rule out inverting papilloma

ii. Multiple polyps
   a. Related to allergy, chronic sinusitis or cystic fibrosis (see above)

Neoplasms

Most sinonasal tumors in children are benign

A. Benign
   i. Juvenile nasopharyngeal angiofibroma (JNA)
      a. Clinical features
         1. Most common benign nasopharyngeal tumor
         2. Incidence 1:5,000 to 1:60,000
         3. Mostly males
         4. Commonly 14 to 18 years of age
         5. Originates in sphenopalatine recess. Extend laterally to pterygomaxillary space and superiorly to cavernous sinus and middle cranial fossa
         6. Nasal mass, obstruction, epistaxis, facial deformity, and proptosis
      b. Diagnosis
         1. History and examination. Biopsy contraindicated due to risk of bleeding
         2. CT, MRI, and magnetic resonance angiography (MRA) for extent
      c. Treatment
         1. Preoperative embolization 48 hours prior to minimize blood loss
         2. Surgical approach depends on extent of lesion. Approaches include
            - Endoscopic (most common)
            - LeFort I osteotomy and midface degloving
            - Lateral rhinotomy
            - Transpalatal
            - Lateral infratemporal fossa
         3. Tumors with intracranial extension require neurosurgical consultation
         4. Radiation for unresectable lesions. Risk of malignant transformation
         5. Use of hormonal therapy unclear
   ii. Fibrous dysplasia
      a. Clinical features
         1. Normal bone replaced by fibrous tissue
         2. Types:
            - Monostotic (70%)
            - Polyostotic (24%)
            - McCune-Albright syndrome (6%): multiple café au lait spots, precocious puberty.
         3. Nasal mass, obstruction, sinusitis.
         4. Often incidental finding on CT or MRI performed for other reason
      b. Diagnosis
         1. CT shows ground-glass appearance
      c. Management
         1. Surgery only if symptomatic
         2. Contouring of bone for cosmetic appearance where resection not possible

iii. Teratoma (rare)
  a. Clinical features
    1. Usually present at birth
    2. Tissue from all three germ layers present: ectoderm, mesoderm, endoderm
    3. Rare malignant potential
    4. Nasal obstruction
  b. Diagnosis
    1. CT or MRI
  c. Treatment
    1. Surgical excision

B. Malignant
  i. Rhabdomyosarcoma (see above)
  ii. Lymphoma (see above)

Idiopathic

A. Granulomatosis with polyangiitis (GPA, formerly known as Wegener granulomatosis)
  i. Clinical features
    a. Autoimmune disease
    b. Rare, less than 1:100,000
    c. Teen females more common than males
  ii. Diagnostic criteria in children require 3 of 6 features (EULAR 2010)
    a. Sinonasal (recurrent epistaxis or septal perforation) or oral inflammation
    b. Abnormal pulmonary chest x-ray or CT
    c. Abnormal urinalysis or necrotizing pauci-immune glomerulonephritis
    d. Granuloma within or around an artery on pathology
    e. Laryngotracheobronchial involvement with stenosis
    f. Positive PR3/cANCA or MPO/pANCA
  iii. Management
    a. Trimethoprim/sulfamethoxazole prevents flareups in upper respiratory tract
    b. Cyclophosphamide + prednisone for acute life-threatening exacerbations
    c. Methotrexate + prednisone for maintenance therapy

Oral cavity/Oropharynx

Developmental Anatomy

A. Prenatal development
  i. 4 week's gestation
    a. Tongue forms from mesenchymal proliferations on floor of oral cavity
    b. Anterior two-thirds develops from lateral lingual swellings (first arch) and median tuberculum impar
    c. Posterior one-third develops from copula (second arch) and hypobranchial eminence (third and fourth arches)
    d. Tongue musculature develops from occipital somites
  ii. 6 weeks' gestation
    a. Upper lateral lip forms as maxillary prominences meet nasal prominences. Upper medial lip forms as both nasal prominences meet
    b. Palatal shelves grow medially from maxillary prominences
  iii. 7 weeks' gestation
    a. Bilateral Meckel cartilages begin intramembranous ossification on lateral aspect of mandibular symphysis. This spreads anteriorly and posteriorly. Fusion at symphysis does not occur until after birth

iv. 12 weeks' gestation
   a. Medial nasal prominences fuse forming intermaxillary segment with four incisor tooth buds
   b. Secondary palate fuses from incisive foramen to uvula

B. Postnatal development
   i. All structures of the oral cavity grow postnatally
   ii. Tonsils peak in size by age 5 to 8 years

Signs and Symptoms

A. Stertor
B. Airway obstruction
C. Visible lesion
D. Feeding difficulties
E. Sialorrhea
F. Altered speech

Clinical Assessment

Direct examination of oral cavity from anteriorly and using nasopharyngoscope from posterosuperiorly

Pathology/Treatment/Complications

Congenital

A. Ankyloglossia (limited tongue mobility caused by restrictive lingual frenulum, "tongue-tie")
   i. Clinical features
      a. Anterior (lingual frenulum extends to the tip of the tongue) or posterior
      b. Congenital anomaly
      c. May interfere with breastfeeding (maternal pain, poor latch) or social/mechanical issues in older children
   ii. Diagnosis
      a. Inability of tongue to extend past red-white junction of lower lip may be predictive of success following division
   iii. Treatment
      a. Frenulectomy (division) or frenuloplasty (division plus suture closure of defect) for breastfeeding difficulties (evaluation for other sources of breastfeeding problems, lactation history prior to surgery) or social/mechanical issues

B. Ranula
   i. Clinical features
      a. Cystic lesion in anterolateral floor of mouth
      b. Due to obstruction of sublingual duct or injury of sublingual gland
      c. Plunging ranula: extends below mylohyoid muscle
   ii. Diagnosis
      a. Unilateral cystic lesion in floor of mouth
      b. Filled with thick, clear fluid
      c. Differentiate from macrocystic lymphatic malformation
      d. May require MRI or CT to confirm diagnosis
   iii. Treatment
      a. Excision of sublingual gland eradicates disease
      b. Careful preservation of submandibular duct orifice to prevent sialadenitis and lingual nerve to prevent numbness
      c. Marsupialization of cyst not recommended due to high rate of recurrence

C. Floor of mouth dermoid
  i. Well-circumscribed cyst filled with keratin
  ii. Surgical excision
D. Midline rhomboid glossitis
  i. Soft tissue mass in posterior midline tongue
  ii. Due to defect in posterior tongue development (tuberculum impar)
  iii. No treatment necessary
E. Lingual thyroid gland
  i. Clinical features
    a. Due to abnormal descent of thyroid from foramen cecum to lower neck
    b. Increases in size with age, infection, and other thyroid disorders
    c. May cause airway obstruction, speech, and feeding difficulties
    d. May be the patient's only functioning thyroid tissue
  ii. Diagnosis
    a. Thyroid scan to detect other functioning thyroid tissue lower in neck
    b. Thyroid function studies
  iii. Treatment
    a. Observation if minimal or no symptoms
    b. Thyroid suppression
    c. Surgery if fails medical management or suspicion of malignancy
F. Lingual thyroglossal duct cyst
  i. Clinical features
    a. Due to abnormal descent of thyroid from foramen cecum to lower neck
    b. Cystic swelling in base of tongue (intrinsic to musculature)
  ii. Diagnosis
    a. MRI (T2 sagittal) for location and to ensure there is normal thyroid gland in neck to decrease chances of removing only functioning thyroid
  iii. Treatment
    a. Suspension microlaryngoscopy and surgical removal using bipolar cautery (to minimize swelling), microdebrider, or laser
    b. Consider overnight intubation until swelling subsides
    c. Consider thyroid function tests postoperatively
G. Vallecular cyst
  i. Clinical features
    a. Retention cyst from obstructed minor salivary gland
    b. Cystic swelling in vallecula between tongue base and epiglottis (extrinsic to tongue musculature)
  ii. Diagnosis
    a. MRI (T2 sagittal) for location
  iii. Treatment
    a. Suspension microlaryngoscopy and surgical removal using cautery, microdebrider, or laser
    b. Consider overnight intubation until swelling subsides
H. Macroglossia
  i. Large anterior tongue
    a. Beckwith-Wiedemann
      1. Clinical features
        - Due to mutation on chromosome 11 in imprinting control region (ICR) leading to abnormal gene methylation or paternal uniparental disomy (UPD) where both paternally expressed genes are active

- Macrosomia (birthweight over 10 lb)
- Hypoglycemia
- Auricular pits
- Omphalocele
- Hepatosplenomegaly
- Tumors develop in 10% (Wilms, rhabdomyosarcoma, hepatoblastoma)

2. Treatment
   - Wedge resection of anterior tongue to allow child to close mouth

b. Glycosaminoglycan (GAG) storage diseases

1. Hurler syndrome (mucopolysaccharidosis I)
   - Autosomal recessive
   - Deficient lysosomal alpha-L-iduronidase leads to GAG storage.
   - Deafness, coarse facial features, low nasal bridge, cardiac anomalies, stunted growth.
   - Treatment includes ECG, genetic testing, urine tests for mucopolysaccharides, spine x-ray, enzyme therapy with intravenous iduronidase
2. Hunter syndrome (mucopolysaccharidosis II)
   - X-linked recessive
   - Deficient enzyme iduronate-2-sulfatase leads to storage of heparan sulfate and dermatan sulfate
   - Large head, prominent forehead, flattened nasal bridge, large tongue
   - Treatment includes testing for *I2S* gene and wedge resection of tongue where necessary

c. Congenital hypothyroidism

1. Due to myxedema of tongue
2. Diagnosed as part of neonatal screening
3. Treatment includes early thyroid replacement to reverse symptoms

ii. Large tongue base

a. Trisomy 21 (Down syndrome)

b. Treatment includes lingual tonsillectomy, midline posterior glossectomy +/− genioglossus advancement for severe obstructive sleep apnea

I. Glossoptosis

i. With retrognathia

a. Clinical features

1. Pierre-Robin sequence
   - Retrognathia leads to severe glossoptosis. Tongue prevents fusion of palate in midline causing U-shaped cleft of secondary palate
   - Mandible requires 4 to 6 months to grow and alleviate obstruction
2. Stickler syndrome
   - Most autosomal dominant mutation in collagen genes (COL)
   - Myopia before 10 years of age, retinal detachment
   - Hearing loss (mixed conductive and sensorineural)
   - Joint problems
3. Nager syndrome (acrofacial dysostosis)
   - Auricular anomalies including atresia
   - Malar hypoplasia
   - Downslanting palpebral fissures
   - Eyelid coloboma
   - Cleft palate
   - Thumb hypoplasia

4. Treacher Collins syndrome (Mandibulofacial dysostosis)
    - Most autosomal dominant mutation in *TCOF1* gene
    - Malar hypoplasia with deficient zygomatic arch
    - Eyelid coloboma
    - Hearing loss, bilateral microtia, and atresia
    - Choanal atresia

b. Treatment depends on degree of obstruction
    - Positioning on side or prone
    - McGovern nipple (nipple with tip cut off, better tolerated than oral airway)
    - Nasal trumpet
    - Tongue-lip adhesion (benefits controversial)
    - Subperiosteal release of floor of mouth (SRFM; 84% effective)
    - Mandibular advancement
    - Tracheotomy

ii. Without retrognathia
  a. Clinical features
    1. Tongue prolapses posteriorly despite mandible being in proper position.
  b. Treatment depends on degree of airway obstruction
    - Positioning on side or prone
    - McGovern nipple
    - Nasal trumpet
    - Tongue-lip adhesion (benefits controversial)
    - Subperiosteal release of floor of mouth (SRFM; 84% effective)
    - Tongue suspension or genioglossus advancement
    - Tracheotomy

J. Velopharyngeal insufficiency
  i. Clinical features
    a. Nasal air escape on consonant sounds, hypernasality on vowel sounds
    b. Compensatory misarticulations (m, n, ng, w do not require closure)
    c. May have nasal regurgitation of food
    d. 25% to 40% after cleft palate repair
  ii. Diagnosis
    a. Perceptual speech evaluation
    b. Nasometry
    c. Nasendoscopy to look for velopharyngeal closure patterns
    d. Fiberoptic endoscopic evaluation of swallowing (FEES)
  iii. Management
    a. Speech therapy: for sound-specific VPI and compensatory misarticulations
    b. Furlow palatoplasty to lengthen palate
    c. Sphincter pharyngoplasty: superomedial rotation of bilateral muscle flaps from posterior pharyngeal wall to recreate Passavant ridge
    d. Pharyngeal flap: superior rotation of midline muscle flap from posterior pharyngeal wall with attachment to soft palate
    e. Palatal lift or obturator (last resort)

Neoplastic

A. Benign
  i. Epulis (granular cell tumor)
    a. Most commonly from maxillary gingiva
    b. Mostly female (4:1)
    c. Treat with surgical excision

ii. Epignathus
    a. Teratoma from palate or pharynx in basisphenoid region (Rathke pouch)
    b. Diagnosed on prenatal ultrasound, confirmed on fetal MRI
    c. Associated with polyhydramnios, midline facial defects, airway obstruction
    d. May require EXIT procedure to secure airway
iii. Hamartoma
    a. Normal tissue in normal location growing in disorganized fashion
    b. Treat with surgical excision if problematic
iv. Choristoma
    a. Normal tissue in abnormal location
    b. Treat with surgical excision if problematic

B. Malignant
  i. Rhabdomyosarcoma: see Head and Neck section
  ii. Lymphoma: see Head and Heck section
  iii. Squamous cell carcinoma
    a. Rare in children
    b. Tongue most commonly involved, but lip, palate, or gingiva may be as well
    c. Rapid growth
    d. Early regional metastases
    e. Treatment similar to that recommended for adults

Infectious/Inflammatory

A. Tonsillitis
  i. Viral (majority of tonsillitis)
    a. Adenovirus, rhinovirus, echovirus, coxsackie, RSV, influenza, parainfluenza
    b. Epstein-Barr virus (human herpes virus 4, infectious mononucleosis)
      1. Clinical features
        - High fever and malaise
        - Grayish-white coating on tonsils
        - Petechiae at hard-soft palate junction
        - Hepatosplenomegaly
        - Develop rash with amoxicillin
      2. Diagnosis
        - CBC shows 50% lymphocytes, 10% atypical
        - ESR more likely to be elevated in EBV than bacterial infection.
        - Monospot positive (85% sensitive—less in first 2 weeks, 100% specific) If initial test negative, repeat once per week for 6 weeks
        - EBV serology: use if monospot negative after 6 weeks
  ii. Bacterial
    a. Clinical features
      1. Group A beta-hemolytic *S pyogenes* (most common)
      2. May be associated with rheumatic fever or glomerulonephritis
      3. May be cause of periodic fever, aphthous ulcers, pharyngitis, cervical adenitis (PFAFA)
        - Each episode lasts 3 days
        - At least 3 episodes
        - Reccur every 3 weeks
        - Symptom-free intervals
        - Rule out cyclical neutropenia

b. Diagnosis
   1. Sore throat plus one of exudate, adenopathy, positive RADT or GABHS culture, temperature greater than 38.3°C
   2. Rapid antigen detection test (RADT). If negative, perform throat culture. Antistreptolysin-O (ASO) titers not recommended as they only indicate prior infection
c. Treatment
   1. Antibiotics to avoid complications
   2. Tonsillectomy if 7 episodes in 1 year, 5 episodes per year for each of 2 years, or 3 episodes per year for each of 3 years

B. Peritonsillar abscess
   i. Purulent infection of Weber glands in potential space between tonsil and pharyngeal constrictor.
   ii. Due to mixture of anaerobic and aerobic bacteria.
   iii. Clinical features
      a. Trismus (best indicator)
      b. Antecedent pharyngitis
      c. Fever
      d. Odynophagia
      e. Airway obstruction
      f. Unilateral palatal enlargement and deviation of uvula to contralateral side
   iv. Diagnosis
      a. Clinical examination
      b. May attempt drainage with needle if unsure whether cellulitis or abscess
      c. CT scan of neck with contrast not routinely indicated but may help if clinical picture unclear or suspicion of spread
   v. Treatment
      a. Intravenous antibiotics +/− steroids
      b. Drainage is mainstay of therapy
      c. Recurrence rate 17%. Tonsillectomy recommended after second abscess

C. Retropharyngeal abscess
   i. Infection of lymph nodes (of Rouviere) in retropharyngeal space between visceral and alar fasciae. Usually disappear by age 5 years
   ii. Infection may extend inferiorly to mediastinum
   iii. Most common organisms
      a. Beta-hemolytic *Streptococcus*
      b. Anaerobic streptococci
      c. *Staphylococcus aureus*
   iv. Clinical features
      a. Torticollis (best indicator)
      b. Antecedent pharyngitis
      c. Fever
      d. Odynophagia
      e. Airway obstruction
      f. Sialorrhea
      g. Bulge in posterior pharyngeal wall (best appreciated with nasopharyngoscopy)
   v. Diagnosis
      a. Lateral neck x-ray shows thickening of prevertebral tissue and loss of lordosis due to spasm of prevertebral muscles. Neck must be extended to prevent false appearance of thickened tissue. Thickening greater than one-half the width of the vertebral body at the same level is pathological.

b. CT scan of neck with contrast distinguishes phlegmon (nondrainable) from abscess (drainable) and helps define the level and angle of entry for drainage.

vi. Treatment

a. Intravenous antibiotics

b. Incision and drainage of abscess (fluid filled with rim enhancement)

D. Tonsillar hypertrophy

i. Clinical features

a. May cause obstructive sleep apnea

1. Inspiratory effort in the absence of air flow
2. Signs and symptoms in children (different from adults):
   - Heroic snoring
   - Pauses
   - Gasping
   - Neck hyperextension
   - Nocturnal diaphoresis
   - Nocturnal enuresis
   - Parasomnias (tooth grinding, sleepwalking)
   - Morning headache
   - Excessive daytime sleepiness
   - Attention deficit or hyperactivity
   - Poor school performance

b. May cause dysphagia

ii. Diagnosis

a. Parental observation (use clock and count number of episodes per hour)

b. Sleep study (not oxygen saturation study) is gold standard

1. Differentiates obstructive from central apnea and degree of obstruction
2. Obstructive sleep apnea defined as apnea-hypopnea index (AHI) greater than 1 (two apneas or hypopneas in two consecutive breaths per hour) or drop in oxygen saturation to less than 92%. Many consider surgery when AHI greater than 5 per hour

iii. Indications for treatment

a. Obstructive sleep apnea with tonsil hypertrophy (grade 3 or 4)

1. Tonsillectomy and adenoidectomy (many reserve surgery for AHI greater than 5 per hour)
2. Single intraoperative dose of dexamethasone for postoperative nausea
3. No role for routine postoperative antibiotics
4. Advocate for pain control (avoid codeine)

b. Asymmetric tonsils in children with immunosuppression and solid organ transplant to rule out posttransplant lymphoproliferative disorder (PTLD)

iv. Complications of tonsillectomy and adenoidectomy

a. General anesthetic

b. Loose/chipped teeth

c. Primary bleeding (< 24 hour, 0.2%-2.2%); secondary bleeding (> 24 hour, 0.1%-3.0%)

d. Velopharyngeal insufficiency

e. Aspiration pneumonia

f. Torticollis

g. Respiratory distress/airway obstruction

h. Death

Traumatic

A. Penetrating trauma of the oral cavity
   i. Clinical features
      a. Impalement of oropharynx and palate usually from running while holding sharp object.
      b. Risk of carotid injury (higher risk if injury lateral to anterior tonsillar pillar)
   ii. Management
      a. Most injuries do not require surgical repair
      b. CT neck with contrast if concerned about carotid injury
      c. Injuries in infants who are not yet walking should alert to abuse

Larynx/Subglottis

Developmental Anatomy

A. Prenatal development
   i. 4 weeks' gestation
      a. Ventral wall of foregut (laryngotracheal groove) develops thickening
      b. Laryngotracheal groove divides into ventral (trachea) and dorsal (esophagus) components. Divided by tracheoesophageal septum
   ii. 6 weeks' gestation
      a. Laryngeal lumen obliterated by mesenchyme
   iii. 8 weeks' gestation
      a. Larynx, trachea, and esophagus are formed
   iv. 10 weeks' gestation
      a. Recanalization of larynx and trachea. Failure to do so results in laryngeal/ tracheal atresia
   v. 12 weeks' gestation
      a. Vocal cord movement detectable
   vi. Branchial arches contribute to each of the following structures
      a. Second arch: hyoid upper body and lesser horn
      b. Third arch: hyoid lower body and greater horn
      c. Fourth arch: thyroid cartilage, cricothyroid muscle (superior laryngeal nerve)
      d. Fifth arch: cricoid, cuneiform, corniculate, arytenoid cartilages. Intrinsic muscles except cricothyroid (recurrent laryngeal nerve)
B. Postnatal development
   i. Neonatal glottis measures 7 mm anteroposteriorly and 4 mm laterally
   ii. Subglottis is narrowest part measuring 4 to 5 mm in diameter
   iii. Larynx descends in neck with growth
      a. At level of C4 at birth, C5 at 2 years, C6 at 5 years, and C6-C7 at 15 years

Signs and Symptoms

A. Voice change
B. Drooling
C. Stridor (inspiratory, expiratory, biphasic)
D. Tachypnea
E. Tachycardia
F. Tracheal tug, chest wall retractions, abdominal breathing
G. Desaturation first, followed by bradycardia
H. Feeding difficulties and weight loss (burn calories by breathing and preferentially breathe rather than eat)

Clinical Assessment

A. Inspect nose for flaring, lips for cyanosis, neck for tracheal tug, chest for indrawing
B. Auscultation over trachea for stridor
C. Flexible nasopharyngoscopy for vocal cord movement and pathology
D. Direct laryngoscopy and bronchoscopy under anesthesia may be required

Pathology/Treatment/Complications

Laryngomalacia

A. Clinical features
   i. Most common cause of stridor in infants
   ii. Inspiratory stridor within first 6 weeks of life
   iii. Worse lying supine and when agitated
   iv. Improves sitting up and prone
   v. Ninety percent spontaneously resolve by 12 months
   vi. Neurologically impaired children may have progressive laryngomalacia
   vii. May be associated with airway compromise (stridor, retractions, desaturation, cyanosis), feeding difficulties, and failure to thrive
B. Diagnosis
   i. Flexible nasopharyngoscopy
      a. Short aryepiglottic folds
      b. Omega-shaped epiglottis
      c. Prolapse of epiglottis into laryngeal inlet
      d. Redundant tissue over arytenoid cartilages due to inspiration against closed glottis leading to acid reflux
   ii. 10% to 20% incidence of secondary synchronous airway lesion. More severe or atypical symptoms warrant laryngoscopy and bronchoscopy
C. Management
   i. Monitor growth on growth curve
   ii. Most do not require intervention due to high rate of spontaneous improvement
   iii. Treating gastroesophageal reflux may break the cycle and improve respiratory symptoms
   iv. Infants with severe laryngomalacia (cyanotic episodes, failure to thrive) may benefit from supraglottoplasty
   v. Beware of syndromes such as CHARGE whereby supraglottoplasty leads to epiglottic collapse and worsens respiratory distress

Vocal Cord Dysfunction

A. Clinical features
   i. Second most common laryngeal anomaly of infancy
   ii. Mostly idiopathic in infants, iatrogenic in older children
   iii. Left vocal cord more commonly affected due to longer, more circuitous route
B. Etiology
   i. Congenital
      a. Complex congenital heart disease
      b. CNS anomalies
         1. Hydrocephalus
         2. Spinal cord anomalies
         3. Nucleus ambiguus dysgenesis (usually familial and bilateral)
         4. Kernicterus

c. Other associations
1. Moebius syndrome: associated with bilateral facial nerve palsy
2. Trisomy 21 (Down syndrome)
3. Mediastinal anomalies
4. Trauma: usually improves in 4 to 6 months
5. Diaphragmatic hernia
6. Erb palsy

ii. Acquired
a. Arnold-Chiari malformation
1. Unilateral or bilateral paresis
2. May also have central sleep apnea

b. Infectious
1. Poliomyelitis
2. Guillain-Barré
3. Botulism
4. Diphtheria
5. Syphilis

c. Iatrogenic
1. Cardiac surgery
2. Thyroidectomy
3. Intubation injury

C. Diagnosis
i. MRI brain, neck, chest (entire length of recurrent laryngeal nerves)
ii. Palpation of arytenoid cartilages to rule out posterior glottic stenosis or dislocation

D. Management
i. Dependent on degree of airway compromise
ii. Spontaneous recovery may occur up to several years later
iii. Observation of no desaturations, cyanosis, or respiratory distress
iv. Chiari malformation may require decompression
v. Unilateral palsy requires feeding assessment to rule out aspiration
vi. Bilateral palsy may require tracheotomy
vii. Reserve destructive procedures such as vocal cord lateralization, anterior and posterior cricoid splits, arytenoidectomy, and posterior costal cartilage graft laryngotracheoplasty for longstanding bilateral vocal cord paralysis with respiratory distress or poor quality of life
viii. Reserve procedure such as injection laryngoplasty or reinnervation procedure unliteral paralysis who failed observation

Laryngeal Cleft

A. Clinical features
i. Incomplete fusion of posterior cricoid lamina and tracheoesophageal septum
ii. Incidence 1/10,000 to 1/20,000 live births
iii. More common in males
iv. Present with coughing with feeds (worse with thin liquids) and recurrent pneumonia
v. Associated with CHARGE, VACTERL/VATER, Opitz, Pallister Hall syndromes

B. Diagnosis
i. Video swallow study shows aspiration
ii. Rigid laryngoscopy with distraction of arytenoids is essential. Flexible nasopharyngoscopy not adequate for ruling out laryngeal cleft

iii. Benjamin and Inglis classification based on inferior extent of cleft
   a. Type I: Interarytenoid cleft down to but not below true vocal folds
   b. Type II: Extension into cricoid cartilage but not through it
   c. Type III: Extension through entire cricoid +/– into cervical trachea
   d. Type IV: Extension into thoracic trachea
   e. Deep interarytenoid notch
      1. A deep interarytenoid notch that does not extend to the vocal folds may still cause aspiration requiring treatment
   f. Type IV may be subdivided to better reflect need for different approach
      1. IVA: Extension into proximal thoracic trachea not more than 5 mm below innominate artery
      2. IVB: Extension into distal thoracic trachea more than 5 mm below innominate artery

C. Treatment
   i. Types I and II: may be injected temporarily with filler to determine the effect of treatment and temporize until endoscopic suture repair can be performed.
   ii. Types I, II, and shallow type III may be amenable to endoscopic suture repair.
   iii. Long type III and shallow type IV not extending past the innominate artery require open surgical repair. This is best performed using a transtracheal approach with placement of posterior costal cartilage graft and interposing fascia.
   iv. Long type IV requires open surgical repair. This is best performed using cricotracheal separation to obviate the need for bypass with placement of interposing fascia.

Subglottic Stenosis

A. Clinical features
   i. Congenital
      a. Due to cricoid malformation (ie, elliptical cricoid)
      b. Types of presentation
         1. No issues at birth, followed by recurrent croup
         2. Stridor at birth
         3. Failure to extubate
      c. Types
         1. Membranous
         2. Cartilaginous
   ii. Acquired
      a. Due to trauma such as prolonged intubation
      b. Exacerbated by GERD, eosinophilic esophagitis, and infection
      c. Congenital stenosis may predispose to acquired stenosis

B. Diagnosis
   i. Rigid laryngoscopy and bronchoscopy
   ii. Sizing of airway to assess degree of stenosis (Cotton-Myer grading system)
      a. Grade 1: 0% to 50% stenosis
      b. Grade 2: 51% to 70% stenosis
      c. Grade 3: 71% to 99% stenosis
      d. Grade 4: 100% stenosis
   iii. Rule out concomitant GERD, EE, and MRSA that portend poorer outcomes.

C. Management
   i. Treat GERD, EE, MRSA where present

ii. Staging of procedures
   a. Single stage: Patient does not have tracheotomy at end of procedure.
   b. Double stage: Patient has tracheotomy removed at later date.
iii. Endoscopic (scar division, balloon dilatation, steroid injection)
iv. Open laryngotracheal reconstruction (LTR)
   a. Anterior cricoid split with thyroid ala or costal cartilage graft
   b. Posterior cricoid split with costal cartilage graft
   c. Anterior and posterior cricoid splits with costal cartilage grafts
   d. Cricotracheal reconstruction (CTR)
   e. Cervical slide tracheoplasty

Subglottic Cyst

A. Acquired from intubation injury
B. Due to blocked mucous gland
C. Treatment
   i. Suspension microlaryngoscopy with excision/marsupialization of cyst
   ii. Inhaled steroid and antibiotic to facilitate healing of denuded cartilage

Subglottic Hemangioma

A. Most common neoplasm of pediatric airway
B. Arise from hematopoietic progenitor cells from placenta or stem cells followed by genetic alterations and cytokine expression (ie, MMP-9, VEGF, b-FGF, TGF-β)
C. Twice as common in females
D. Clinical features
   i. Biphasic stridor at 6 weeks of age (85% present by 6 months of age)
   ii. Progressive symptoms as lesion grows in proliferative phase
   iii. Plateau at 1 year of age
   iv. Spontaneous involution by 18 months to 2 years of age
   v. 60% of hemangiomata in "beard" distribution also have subglottic lesion
E. Diagnosis
   i. High kV AP neck x-ray shows unilateral subglottic mass (usually left side)
   ii. Rigid bronchoscopy
      a. Do not intubate prior to visualizing or lesion may become compressed and go unnoticed
      b. Vascular blush on vocal cord
      c. Rounded vascular lesion in subglottis (usually left side)
      d. Biopsy not required if in typical location in typical age group
      e. Beware rare ALK-positive histiocytic lesion which can be a mimicker
   iii. Rule out PHACES syndrome: **P**osterior fossa malformations, **H**emangioma typically involving the face, **A**rterial lesions of the head and neck, **C**ardiac abnormalities (coarctation of the aorta), **Eye** abnormalities, and **S**ternal cleft or **S**upraumbilical hernia
F. Management
   i. Minimal manipulation and awaken patient
   ii. Secure airway via intubation only if essential
   iii. Propranolol or nadolol
   iv. Intravenous or injectable steroids may be required
   v. Historically, CO_2 laser, open surgical excision, and alpha interferon were options but these are reserved for patients who fail medical management

Granular Cell Tumor

A. Benign tumor resembling hemangioma
B. Rare in children
C. Up to 10% found in larynx
D. Clinical features
   i. Hoarseness, cough, stridor, hemoptysis, dysphagia, pain
E. Diagnosis
   i. High kV AP neck x-ray.
   ii. Rigid bronchoscopy reveals yellow to gray-pink, firm, nonulcerated lesion.
   iii. Histology demonstrates large fusiform or polygonal cells with abundant pale cytoplasm and marked cell membrane. Eosinophilic granules in cytoplasm may induce pseudoepitheliomatous hyperplasia which can be confused with squamous cell carcinoma.
F. Management
   i. Surgical excision with ample margins to prevent recurrence

Neurofibroma

A. Benign tumor of Schwann cell with low malignant potential
B. Located on arytenoid cartilages or aryepiglottic folds
C. May be associated with neurofibromatosis (see above).
D. Management involves suspension microlaryngoscopy with surgical excision

Malignant Laryngeal Tumors

A. Rare in children
B. Clinical features
   i. Differential diagnosis
      a. Embryonal variant of rhabdomyosarcoma (most common)
      b. Squamous cell carcinoma
      c. Choriocarcinoma
      d. Primitive neuroectodermal tumor (PNET)
      e. NUT midline carcinoma
   ii. Progressive airway obstruction, dysphonia, dysphagia
C. Management
   i. Flexible nasopharyngoscopy
   ii. Rigid laryngoscopy and bronchoscopy with biopsy
   iii. Consider tracheotomy based on current and predicted airway obstruction
   iv. CT and MRI with metastatic workup
   v. Chemotherapy, radiation, surgery dependent on nature of malignancy

Infectious/Inflammatory

A. Laryngotracheobronchitis (croup)
   i. Clinical features
      a. Viral infection, most commonly parainfluenza
      b. Bacterial superinfection (*H. influenzae* or *S. aureus*) may follow
      c. More common in children under 2 years of age
      d. Present with barky cough and biphasic stridor
      e. Variable degree of airway compromise
      f. Recurrent croup (three or more episodes) is unusual, suspect underlying subglottic stenosis
   ii. Diagnosis
      a. High kV neck x-ray
         1. AP rather than PA, as it is easier to restrain child in this orientation and the patient is closer to the film so there is less magnification

            2. Ensure arms are down at side (unlike chest x-ray)
            3. "Steeple sign" in subglottis or loss of shouldering whereby subglottis opens laterally immediately below vocal cords to resemble how the outline of a person's neck turns into their shoulders. Easier to diagnose when patient is phonating
            4. Lateral x-ray may show narrowing
        b. Flexible nasopharyngoscopy may help rule out other etiologies
        c. No indication for routine rigid laryngoscopy or bronchoscopy
    iii. Treatment
        a. Humidification, hydration, oxygen
        b. Nebulized epinephrine
        c. Consider nebulized steroids
        d. Oral or intravenous steroids
        e. Consider heliox
        f. Recurrent croup warrants repeat high kV neck x-ray when infection resolves (minimum 6 weeks following infection) to rule out underlying subglottic pathology. Consider rigid laryngoscopy and bronchoscopy if x-ray does not resolve this question
B. Epiglottitis
    i. Clinical features
        a. Usually caused by *H. influenzae* type B (Hib)
        b. Incidence has fallen dramatically after introduction of Hib vaccine
        c. Must consider immunization status, other bacteria, leukemia, caustic injury
        d. Rapid onset sore throat, fever, inspiratory stridor, respiratory distress, drooling, "tripod position" (hands on knees) due to inability to swallow secretions.
        e. After diagnosis confirmed, avoid irritating child
    ii. Diagnosis
        a. High kV lateral neck x-ray shows "thumb sign" (widened epiglottis). Child should be accompanied in radiology suite by physician skilled at intubating
    iii. Management
        a. Intubation in the operating room with tracheotomy tray prepared
        b. Administer inhalational anesthetic
        c. Blood and airway cultures can be obtained following intubation.
C. Recurrent respiratory papillomatosis (RRP)
    i. Clinical features
        a. Most common benign neoplasm of the larynx in children
        b. Second most common cause of hoarseness in children (nodules are first)
        c. Incidence 4/100,000 in United States, 0.24/100,000 in Canada
        d. Usually diagnosed between 2 and 5 years of age
        e. May involve any transition from squamous to columnar epithelium such as mucosal abrasion, tracheotomy site, etc.
            1. Larynx (most common)
            2. Oral cavity
            3. Trachea
            4. Bronchi
    ii. Classification
        a. Juvenile (< 12 years of age)
            1. More aggressive
            2. Due to vertical transmission or sexual abuse

3. Human papillomavirus (HPV) 6 and 11 most common (same as genital condylomata), 16 and 18 less common but higher risk malignant transformation (2%-3%)
b. Adult (20-40 years of age)
1. Less aggressive
2. Sexually acquired
3. Extralaryngeal involvement in 16% of patients
iii. Diagnosis
a. Flexible nasopharyngoscopy shows exophytic protruberances on vocal fold with multiple pinpoint dimples
b. Rigid laryngoscopy with biopsy confirms diagnosis
c. Histopathology shows pedunculated, finger-like projections with fibrovascular core, covered by stratified squamous epithelium
d. PCR confirms viral subtype
e. Chest CT if pulmonary involvement
iv. Management
a. Goals of treatment:
1. Maintain patent airway
2. Preserve lamina propria to preserve voice
3. Prevent injury to trachea to decrease risk of extralaryngeal spread.
b. Multiple treatments required per year, decreases in frequency as child ages.
c. Microdebrider or laser (CO_2 and KTP) most commonly used.
d. Indications for adjuvant therapy:
1. More than six procedures per year
2. Distal spread
3. Rapid recurrence
e. Adjuvant therapies
1. Intralesional cidofovir
2. Interferon-alpha
3. Photodynamic therapy
4. Indole-3-carbinol
f. Annual biopsies to rule out malignant transformation.
g. Quadrivalent and 9-valent vaccines for prevention of HPV have decreased the incidence of RRP. Vaccine therapy for those already affected with HPV is under study.
h. IV bevacizumab (Avastin) has been shown to be effective in recent studies.

Iatrogenic

A. Intubation injury
i. Acute
a. Edema, granulation tissue, ulceration, soft scar, arytenoid dislocation
ii. Chronic
a. Granulation tissue, ulceration, fibrotic scar, arytenoid fixation

Idiopathic

A. Paradoxical vocal fold movement
i. Clinical features
a. Vocal cord adduction on inspiration, abduction on expiration
b. More common in females with social stressors (ie, athletes)

c. Inspiratory stridor and strained voice
d. Associated with laryngopharyngeal reflux
e. Often misdiagnosed as asthma

ii. Diagnosis
a. Flexible nasopharyngoscopy reveals abnormal vocal cord movement while awake and normal movement while asleep.
b. May need to perform nasopharyngoscopy while patient on treadmill to notice episode.

iii. Management
a. Reassurance.
b. Panting exercises (leads to vocal cord relaxation).
c. Topical lidocaine may have minor benefit.
d. Proton pump inhibitor.
e. Voice therapy, massage, and biofeedback.
f. Counselling by professional with experience treating conversion disorders.
g. Severe respiratory distress may warrant helium-oxygen therapy (heliox) to reduce airway turbulence, botox, or anticholinergic agents such as inhaled ipratropium.
h. Counsel family that the patient may pass out, but this will allow them to breathe again.

Tracheobronchial Tree

Developmental Anatomy

A. Prenatal development
i. Lung bud grows at distal end of laryngotracheal tube
ii. Divides into two bronchial buds which form primitive primary bronchi, lower airway, and lung parenchyma
iii. 5 weeks' gestation
a. Esophagotracheal septum regresses leading to separation of laryngotracheal tube and esophagus
b. Incomplete separation results in tracheoesophageal fistula
iv. 8 weeks' gestation
a. Tracheal cilia appear
v. 20 weeks' gestation
a. All major microscopic features of trachea are visible
vi. 24 weeks' gestation
a. Surfactant secretion begins. Sufficient quantity to prevent lung collapse by 28 to 32 weeks'

B. Postnatal development
i. Trachea lengthens and descends deeper into mediastinum
ii. Trachea grows from 4 cm at birth to 12 cm in adult
iii. Trachea becomes more firm
iv. Division of bronchioles and alveoli continues for at least 8 years

Signs and Symptoms

A. Dyspnea
B. Cough
C. Aspiration, recurrent pneumonia
D. Failure to thrive

Clinical Assessment

A. Auscultation
B. Chest x-ray (AP and lateral)
C. Fluoroscopy
D. CT
E. Rigid laryngoscopy and bronchoscopy (gold standard)
F. Some advocate flexible bronchoscopy in the awake patient in clinic but this is still under investigation

Pathology/Treatment/Complications

Congenital

A. Tracheomalacia (intrinsic tracheal narrowing)
   i. Clinical features
      a. Trachealis muscle moves anteriorly to narrow tracheal lumen
      b. Barking or honking stridor on forceful expiration
      c. Not usually associated with respiratory distress
   ii. Diagnosis
      a. Rigid bronchoscopy with spontaneous ventilation without positive pressure
      b. Rule out extrinsic pulsatile vascular compression (vascular ring or sling)
      c. May be detected on sagittal fluoroscopy
   iii. Management
      a. Reassurance and observation usually sufficient
      b. Continuous positive pressure ventilation
      c. Aortopexy to pull trachea anteriorly to decrease degree of trachealis obstruction being investigated
      d. Suturing of trachealis muscle to prevertebral fascia
      e. Tracheotomy as last resort, as pressure makes trachealis muscle weaker
B. External compression of trachea (extrinsic tracheal narrowing)
   i. Clinical features
      a. Compression of trachea (mostly anterior) narrows lumen
      b. Stridor, respiratory distress, cyanosis, recurrent or chronic lung infections
   ii. Diagnosis
      a. Rigid bronchoscopy with spontaneous ventilation without positive pressure
      b. Pulsatile vascular compression of trachea
      c. Tracheal cross-section shaped like sideways "teardrop" usually with narrow point on patient's left side
      d. CT chest with contrast and three-dimensional reconstruction of trachea and vasculature to confirm responsible vessel
   iii. Management
      a. Continuous positive pressure ventilation with slow wean
      b. Aortopexy or division of vascular ring as required
      c. Shortening of trachea (using slide tracheoplasty or resection) to alter relationship of trachea and offending vessel
      d. Tracheotomy last resort due to risk of tracheotomy tip eroding into vessel
      e. Metallic stents only in palliative cases due to high risk of erosion into vessel
C. Tracheoesophageal fistula (TEF or TOF)
   i. Clinical features
      a. Communication between trachea and esophagus
      b. Incidence 1/2500 live births

c. More common in males
d. Due to incomplete separation of foregut at 4 to 5 weeks' gestation
e. Defective signaling in Sonic Hedgehog pathway in mice
f. Associated with polyhydramnios in utero
g. Associated with VACTERL syndrome: **V**ertebral, **A**nal atresia, **C**ardiac, **T**racheoesophageal fistula, **E**sophageal atresia, **R**adial or renal atresia, **L**imb anomalies
h. Coughing with feeds, cyanotic episodes, dysphagia, regurgitation, recurrent pneumonia

ii. Diagnosis
a. Majority are proximal esophageal atresia with distal TEF
1. X-ray shows anterior bowing of trachea from distended esophageal pouch
2. Feeding tube passed through nose down esophageal atresia with injection of air into pouch. If esophageal atresia is present along with air in stomach, then a fistula exists

b. "Pullback" esophagram for H-type fistula or recurrent TEF
1. Nasogastric tube inserted into esophagus and pulled backward up esophagus as contrast is injected under force during fluoroscopy.
2. Air bronchogram (white outline of tracheobronchial tree) indicates presence of fistula.

c. Rigid bronchoscopy
1. Primary fistulae easily detected. Rule out secondary fistula
2. Secondary fistulae more difficult to detect
- May require insertion of nasogastric tube into distal esophagus with forceful injection of large volume of air while looking for bubbles in trachea
- Fogarty catheter inserted to distal esophagus, followed by inflation of balloon and slow withdrawal while investigating posterior tracheal wall is an alternative

d. Four main types of TEF
1. Proximal esophageal atresia with distal TEF (90%)
2. H-type fistula (2%-4% of primary TEF, 100% of secondary TEF)
3. Proximal TEF with distal esophageal atresia (1%)
4. Proximal esophageal atresia with TEF and distal esophageal atresia with second TEF (1%)

iii. Management
a. Thoracoscopic or open surgery
1. TEF closed at same time as esophageal atresia repair.
2. Recurrence rate 20%. Minimized by
- Less extensive mobilization of esophagus
- Absorbable sutures
- Complete division of tract rather than ligation
- Noncontiguous tracheal and esophageal suture lines
- Minimal tension on anastomosis
- Interposing tissue between layers
- Minimal postoperative trauma
- Resection of TEF tract and direct tracheopexy of trachealis to prevertebral fascia obliterates residual tracheal pouch and risk of accidentally intubating it (primary Jennings procedure).

3. Anterior intrusion of posterior trachealis muscle following TEF ligation can lead to respiratory distress but can be corrected by suturing trachealis directly to prevertebral fascia (secondary Jennings procedure).
4. Rate of vocal cord paralysis following TEF repair (usually left side) is 11%, increasing to 50% with H-type TEF repair because they occur higher in neck where nerves are closer to tracheoesophageal groove. Most patients have clinical recovery of aspiration and voice within 8 months because injured cord medializes, but only 37% recover nerve function.

b. Endoscopic
1. Reserved for recurrent fistulae following open approach (20%)
2. De-epithelialization of tract using electrical or chemical cautery with or without addition of fibrin glue
3. Success rates vary from 60% to 90% with average of two attempts required
4. Clip placed in esophagus may facilitate closure of recalcitrant TEF

c. Slide tracheoplasty or tracheal resection
1. For recalcitrant TEF unable to be closed by any other method
2. Obliteration of TEF by shortening trachea to separate tracheal and esophageal suture lines

D. Complete tracheal rings

i. Clinical features
a. Approximately 1 in 64,500 live births
b. Associated with congenital heart disease, left pulmonary artery sling, lung agenesis, duodenal atresia, and Down syndrome
c. Associated with left pulmonary artery sling (48%), intracardiac anomalies (47%), tracheal bronchus (13%), lung agenesis (9%), Down syndrome (8%), anorectal/duodenal malformation (7%), VACTERL (6%)

ii. Diagnosis
a. Flexible or rigid bronchoscopy
1. Location: helpful to place scope at proximal end of stenosis, turn off room lights, and visualize whether light is superior or inferior to clavicles. This determines whether it needs to be repaired via cervical or thoracic approach
2. Length
3. Degree of narrowing

b. CT with contrast and 3D reconstruction of trachea and vasculature helps to delineate extent of stenosis and associated cardiac anomalies, such as LPA sling (48%), VSD (15%), tetralogy of Fallot (10%), ASD (7%), etc.
c. Cardiac echocardiogram for concurrent cardiac anomalies

iii. Management
a. Depends on degree of airway compromise
b. Observation as patient outgrows stenosis (increase in diameter 0.38 mm per year). More likely to outgrow if shorter segment stenosis. Often require medical management for symptomatic episodes
c. Medical
1. Often required for symptomatic episodes during observation period
2. Steroids
3. Inhaled epinephrine
4. Heliox
5. Bag/mask ventilation
6. Laryngeal mask airway. Works well for elective surgery

7. Intubation as last resort. Should be performed by most experienced person with placement of endotracheal tube just below vocal cords. Forcing tube distally leads to edema and loss of airway

d. Extracorporeal membrane oxygenation (ECMO)
   1. May be required for acute airway obstruction as bridge to surgery

e. Slide tracheoplasty
   1. Reserved for severely symptomatic patients in first few months of life or patients with poor exercise tolerance around age 5 years
   2. Performed simultaneously with cardiac repair if required
   3. Patient usually placed on cardiac bypass or ECMO
   4. Multiple flexible bronchoscopies for bronchopulmonary lavage required following surgery
   5. Often requires several balloon dilatations until trachea relaxes

E. Sleeve trachea
   i. Clinical features
      a. Continuous smooth span of cartilage without tracheal rings or intercartilaginous ligaments
      b. Associated with Pfeiffer syndrome: autosomal dominant craniosynostosis, midface hypoplasia, proptosis, syndactyly caused by mutations in chromosome 8 or *FGFR2* gene

Infectious/Inflammatory

A. Allergic bronchopulmonary aspergillosis
   i. Clinical features
      a. Wheezing, mucous production, pulmonary infiltrates, elevated IgE
      b. Associated with reactive airway disease or cystic fibrosis
      c. May be unilateral, therefore confused with foreign body aspiration
   ii. Diagnosis
      a. Based on retrieval of cast from bronchial tree
   iii. Treatment
      a. Removal of airway casts
      b. Systemic treatment of atopy

B. Tuberculosis (TB)
   i. Granulomas may be seen in tracheobronchial tree
   ii. Diagnosis based on biopsy of lesion
   iii. Treatment as per systemic tuberculosis

Foreign Body Aspiration

A. Clinical features
   i. 1000 deaths per year in the United States
   ii. Most common cause of accidental death in children less than 1 year of age
   iii. 25% of airway foreign bodies have been present for over 2 weeks
   iv. Ingestion may be observed or unobserved. Any suspected foreign body aspiration must be thoroughly investigated
   v. Initial episode usually involves coughing, gagging, or sputtering that usually resolves as foreign body moves past vocal cords
   vi. Chronic cough, lung infection, or bronchiectasis if present for long time.
   vii. Symptoms related to level and degree of obstruction
      a. Larynx: change in voice, cough, odynophagia, airway obstruction
      b. Trachea: palpable thud, expiratory wheeze
      c. Bronchus: cough, unilateral wheeze

viii. Location in decreasing order:
  a. Right main bronchus (60%)
  b. Left main bronchus (30%)
  c. Hypopharynx (2%-5%)
  d. Trachea (3%-12%)
  e. Larynx (1%-7%)

B. Diagnosis
  i. History alone may prompt bronchoscopy even if no foreign body on x-ray
  ii. Physical findings as above
  iii. X-ray:
    a. AP and lateral
      1. Radiopaque lesion seen less than 25% of time
      2. Mediastinal shift away from foreign body
      3. Elevated contralateral hemidiaphragm
      4. Post-obstructive collapse if present for long time
      5. Pneumomediastinum
      6. Pneumothorax
    b. Inspiratory and expiratory films in lateral decubitus
      1. Dependent lung should collapse but looks hyperinflated if foreign body blocking bronchus
      2. Only in 50% of patients with foreign body (specific but not sensitive)
  iv. CT scan
    a. Some advocate CT for visualizing airway foreign bodies
    b. More sensitive than x-ray, less sensitive than bronchoscopy
    c. Risk of sending patient with airway foreign body to CT scanner
    d. May require anesthetic for CT and another for bronchoscopy
    e. Suggest using only following negative bronchoscopy where symptoms persist, to look for object in subsegmental bronchi and help plan next bronchoscopy
  v. Bronchoscopy
    a. Gold standard for diagnosis

C. Management
  i. Rigid laryngoscopy and bronchoscopy with spontaneous ventilation
  ii. Sharp edges are retrieved into bronchoscope to minimize trauma
  iii. Rarely, tracheotomy is required for removal of large foreign bodies

Esophagus

Developmental Anatomy

A. Prenatal development (see laryngeal development)
  i. Upper esophagus and upper esophageal sphincter
    a. Fourth, fifth, and sixth branchial arches give rise to striated muscle
    b. Innervated by vagal nerve and recurrent laryngeal nerve
  ii. Middle esophagus
    a. Somites and endoderm give rise to smooth and skeletal muscle
  iii. Lower esophagus and lower esophageal sphincter
    a. Mesenchyme of somites surrounding foregut
  iv. 6 weeks' gestation
    a. Circular muscle and ganglion cells of myenteric plexus form
  v. 7 weeks' gestation
    a. Blood vessels enter submucosa.

vi. 9 to 13 weeks' gestation
   a. Myenteric plexus has cholinesterase activity and ganglion cells differentiate
   b. Peristalsis begins in first trimester
vii. 16 weeks' gestation
   a. Ciliated epithelium replaced by stratified squamous epithelium
   b. Residual islands of ciliated epithelium give rise to esophageal glands

B. Postnatal development
   i. Peristalsis matures and regurgitation decreases
   ii. Pressure at lower esophageal sphincter reaches maturity at 3 to 6 weeks of age

Signs and Symptoms

A. Feeding difficulties
B. Aspiration
C. Regurgitation
D. Foreign bodies in the esophagus may present as stridor and respiratory distress

Clinical Assessment

A. X-ray to look for air in esophagus and bowel
B. Passage of nasogastric tube can demonstrate patency
C. Gastrograffin or barium swallow
   i. Stricture
   ii. Filling defect denotes foreign body
   iii. Tracheoesophageal stricture

Pathology/Treatment/Complications

Congenital

A. Tracheoesophageal fistula (see above)
B. Esophageal stenosis
   i. Usually in distal one-third.
   ii. Can occur anywhere along length of esophagus
C. Achalasia: rare in children
   i. Clinical features
      a. Decreased ganglion cells in enteric nervous system within smooth muscle
      b. Chronic aspiration and chronic pulmonary diseaseFailure to thrive
   ii. Diagnosis
      a. Chest x-ray: widened mediastinum
      b. Barium swallow
         1. "Bird-beak" deformity: dilated proximal esophagus and tapering of distal esophagus
      c. Manometry
         1. Increased tone in lower esophageal sphincter (LES)
         2. Failure of LES to relax on swallow
         3. Absence of peristalsis
   iii. Treatment
      a. Medical management to improve peristalsis and decrease LES tone
      b. Dilatation
      c. Myotomy for nonresponders

Neoplastic

Neoplastic lesions are rare in children.

Infectious/Inflammatory

A. Eosinophilic esophagitis (EE)
  i. Clinical features
    a. Chronic inflammation of esophagus due to infiltration of eosinophils
    b. Due to food or environmental allergies. May be postinfectious
    c. Other risk factors
      1. Male
      2. Allergies (food or seasonal), asthma
      3. Family history of EE
      4. Living in cold, dry climate
    d. Symptoms include
      1. Gastroesophageal reflux disease unresponsive to proton pump inhibitors
      2. Vomiting (61%)
      3. Dysphagia (39%). More common if endoscopic findings or eosinophils in blood
      4. Abdominal pain (34%)
      5. Feeding disorders (14%)
      6. Heartburn (14%)
      7. Food impaction (7%)
      8. Vague chest pain (5%)
      9. Diarrhea (5%)
      10. Failure to thrive
  ii. Diagnosis
    a. Esophagoscopy may or may not raise suspicion; therefore biopsy required
      1. Majority of children have no findings on esophagoscopy
      2. White exudate
      3. Esophageal rings ("trachealization" or corrugation)
      4. Linear furrows
      5. Pallor
      6. Congestion
      7. Loss of vascularization
    b. Biopsy
      1. Multiple biopsies required from proximal, mid, and distal esophagus
      2. Persistent esophageal eosinophilia greater than 15 eosinophils per high-power field after 2 months of proton pump inhibitor therapy or with normal pH study
      3. Degranulated eosinophils
      4. Eosinophilic microabscesses (clusters of four or more eosinophils)
      5. Eosinophils in superficial layers of squamous mucosa
      6. Patchy or diffuse distribution of eosinophils through entire length of esophageal squamous mucosa
      7. Lamina propria fibrosis
  iii. Management
    a. Referral to gastroenterologist and allergist
    b. Elimination and elemental diets to decrease allergen exposure. Must be supervised by dietician due to risk of nutritional deprivation
    c. Proton pump inhibitor +/− promotility agents for acid reflux
      1. One-third have good response to proton pump inhibitor alone

d. Swallowed topical glucocorticoid
   1. Decreases esophageal inflammation
   2. Fluticasone via metered dose inhaler without spacer is sprayed into mouth and swallowed
   3. Patients should not inhale or eat or drink for 30 minutes after
   4. Dose in children ranges from 88 to 440 μg/day in divided doses
   5. Responders do so within 1 week. Treatment continued for 8 weeks
   6. Relapse rates 14% to 91% when stopped
   7. Nonresponders should try oral viscous budesonide

e. Dupilumab

f. Careful esophageal dilatation for strictures not responsive to medical management as may lead to perforation

B. Juvenile dermatomyositis
   i. Clinical features
      a. Systemic autoimmune inflammatory muscle disorder and vasculopathy
      b. Expanded diagnostic criteria (2006 international consensus survey)
         1. Heliotrope rash over eyelids, Gottron papules over metacarpophalangeal joints, and proximal interphalangeal joints
         2. Calcinosis cutis (firm lump in skin)
         3. Symmetrical proximal muscle weakness
         4. Elevated muscle enzymes
         5. Myopathic changes on electromyopathy
         6. Abnormal muscle biopsy findings
         7. Muscle MRI and US abnormalities
         8. Nailfold capillaroscopy abnormalities
            - Dysphonia
      c. Vasculopathy may affect gastrointestinal tract

C. Stevens-Johnson syndrome
   i. Life-threatening skin condition whereby cell death leads to separation of epidermis from dermis
   ii. Hypersensitivity complex reaction due to medications, infections, and cancer

Traumatic

A. Foreign body ingestion
   i. Clinical features
      a. Dysphagia
      b. Drooling
      c. History of choking episode
      d. May cause compression of trachea and airway obstruction
      e. Diagnosis may be delayed
   ii. Diagnosis
      a. X-ray
         1. AP and lateral x-rays from mouth to anus
         2. Must rule out button battery
            - Halo sign (visible double density ring on AP film)
            - Step sign (visible step on lateral film)
            - Batteries must be removed as soon as possible
         3. Must rule out two or more magnets
            - One magnet will not cause problems but two will
            - Stick to each other through bowel wall leading to perforation

b. Contrast esophagram
   1. May help rule out radiolucent foreign body
   2. Coating marshmallow in barium may detect nonobstructive object like fishbone that may be missed with liquid contrast

iii. Treatment
   a. Rigid esophagoscopy and removal using optical forceps
   b. Esophageal button batteries require emergent removal due to risk of liquefaction necrosis, perforation and stricture. Batteries that have passed into the stomach can be followed radiographically until they pass the rectum
   c. Nasogastric tube to prevent stricture if severe circumferential injury
   d. Sucralfate may be beneficial for severe circumferential injury. Binds to exposed proteins for protection, inhibits pepsin, and binds bile salts
   e. Two or more magnets require emergent removal. May leave one magnet behind as long as there are no other magnets to be attracted to
   f. Coins most commonly lodge at thoracic inlet

B. Caustic ingestion
   i. Clinical features
      a. Accidental ingestion most common in first 3 years of life
      b. Degree of injury related to type of corrosive, amount, concentration, duration of contact
      c. Types of corrosives
         1. Alkali (NaOH, KOH, NH_4OH)
            - Found in drain cleaners and button batteries
            - Causes liquefaction necrosis that diffuses into deep tissue layers
         2. Acids (HCl, H2SO4, HNO3)
            - Cause coagulation necrosis where degree of injury is more superficial
         3. Phenol (ie, Lysol)
         4. Hypochlorous acid (HClO)
            - Found in bleach
            - Forms hydrochloric acid when oxygen is released
   ii. Assessment
      a. Determine substance ingested
      b. Intraoral signs do not correlate with esophageal exposure
      c. Assess entire patient to rule out airway involvement and perforated viscus
   iii. Management
      a. Observation if few symptoms and benign physical examination
      b. Clear liquid diet during observation with intravenous hydration if necessary
      c. Steroids
         1. May minimize injury in first 8 hours
         2. Do not give steroids if severe esophageal injury noted at time of endoscopy due to risk of perforation
      d. Antibiotics may hasten re-epithelialization
      e. Esophagoscopy
         1. If indicated, should be performed 24 to 72 hours after incident to delineate areas of injury. Earlier endoscopy may underestimate degree of injury
         2. Endoscope should not be advanced beyond area of significant injury to minimize risk of esophageal rupture
      f. Nasogastric tube passed under direct vision if severe esophageal injury
      g. Gastrostomy tube may be required
      h. Esophageal stricture may require dilatation or resection

Idiopathic

A. Gastroesophageal reflux disease (GERD)
  i. Clinical features
    a. Regurgitation of stomach contents into esophagus
    b. Very common in infants
    c. Symptoms and signs
      1. Arching of back and discomfort
      2. Cough
      3. Hoarseness
      4. Laryngospasm
      5. Bronchospasm
      6. Apneic episodes
  ii. Diagnosis
    a. Flexible nasopharyngoscopy
      1. Redundant, erythematous tissue over arytenoid cartilages
      2. Pooling of frothy clear secretions at esophageal inlet
      3. Vocal cord nodules or granulomata
      4. "Cobblestoning" of posterior pharyngeal wall (lymphatic hypertrophy)
    b. Barium swallow
      1. May show reflux of contrast or hiatus hernia
    c. Impedance probe
      1. Detects frequency and level of acid and nonacid reflux up the esophagus
    d. pH probe
      1. Detects frequency of acid reflux up the esophagus
    e. Upper GI endoscopy
      1. Allows inspection of mucosa, lower esophageal sphincter, and biopsies
  iii. Treatment
    a. Physical measures
      1. Elevate head of bed by placing wedge under mattress or book under bed frame. Extra pillows merely kink the neck and do not improve reflux
      2. Allow ample time for digestion prior to going to bed
      3. Eliminate acidic foods and caffeine (ie, spices, tomatoes, chocolate, caffeinated drinks)
      4. Thicken feeds
      5. Small frequent feeds
    b. Pharmacological
      1. Acid suppression
        - Antacids
        - H_2 blockers
        - Proton pump inhibitors: must be given on empty stomach 1 hour before meal or else do not work. Supplement with vitamin D drops to prevent decreased calcium absorption from long-term PPI use
      2. Prokinetic agents
        - Domperidone
        - Metoclopramide
        - Cisapride: for patients with unusual, debilitating problems for whom there is no alternative therapy in the United States due to risk of cardiac arrhythmia.

c. Surgical
   1. Nissen fundoplication: complete or partial wrap
   2. Feeding gastrojejunostomy (GJ) tube: poorer quality of life for patient and caregiver due to need for continuous feeds and frequent loose stools.

Head and Neck

Developmental Anatomy

A. Prenatal development
   i. Embryology in first 8 weeks' determines pathway an anomaly will follow.
   ii. Six branchial arches. External clefts lined with ectoderm, internal pouches lined with endoderm. The fifth branchial arch degenerates.
   iii. Each arch has a nerve, artery, cartilaginous bar, muscle.
      a. First arch: trigeminal nerve; malleus head/neck, anterior malleolar ligament, incus body/short process, mandible, sphenomandibular ligament; tensory tympani, tensor veli palatini, muscles of mastication, digastric anterior belly, mylohyoid
      b. Second arch: facial nerve; external carotid artery; malleus manubrium, incus long process, stapes (not vestibular side of footplate), pyramidal eminence, styloid process, hyoid lesser cornu and upper half body; stapedius tendon, muscles of facial expression, digastric posterior belly, stylohyoid
      c. Third arch: glossopharyngeal nerve; internal and common carotid arteries; hyoid greater cornu and lower half body; stylopharyngeus
      d. Fourth arch: superior laryngeal nerve; right subclavian artery, aortic arch; thyroid cartilage, cuneiform cartilage; cricothyroid membrane, inferior pharyngeal constrictors
      e. Sixth arch: recurrent laryngeal nerve; right pulmonary artery, ductus arteriosus; cricoid, arytenoid, corniculate; intrinsic laryngeal muscles (except cricothyroid)
   iv. Cysts, sinuses, and fistulae course deep to derivatives of their own branchial arch and superficial to derivatives of the next branchial arch. The origin of third and fourth branchial anomalies is controversial.
   v. Types of anomalies:
      a. Cyst (lined by mucosa or epithelium, no external opening, arises from embryonic rests trapped inside developing tissue)
      b. Sinus (from incomplete closure of pouches and clefts, communicates with single body surface that may be either the skin or the pharynx).
      c. Fistula (from incomplete closure of pouches and clefts, communicates with two body surfaces)
B. Postnatal development
   i. Majority of these structures continue to grow postnatally, with the exception of arytenoid cartilages which attain adult size at birth

Signs and Symptoms

A. Neck mass
B. Compressive symptoms
C. Fever, chills, night sweats, weight loss

Clinical Assessment

A. Complete head and neck examination including cranial nerves
B. Flexible nasopharyngoscopy
C. Imaging usually necessary for determining type and extent of lesion

Pathology/Treatment/Complications

Congenital

A. Vascular anomalies (ISSVA classification, 2018). Even though not all are congenital, the entire classification is delineated here for simplicity.
  i. Vascular tumors
    a. Benign
      1. Infantile hemangioma (IH)/hemangioma of infancy
        - Clinical features
          (a) Most common tumor of childhood (10% of Caucasians)
          (b) More common in preterm infants
          (c) Three times more common in females
          (d) Present at birth as flat discoloration with no mass
          (e) Pattern: focal, multifocal, segmental or indeterminate
          (f) Types: superficial, deep, mixed, reticular/ abortive/minimal growth or others
          (g) Three phases of growth:
            - Proliferative phase begins around 4 weeks, rapid growth until 4 months, plateau around 1 year
            - Quiescent phase between proliferation and involution
            - Involution phase can last up to 10 years
            - May be associated with Kasabach-Merritt syndrome, consumptive coagulopathy and systemic hemangiomata
            - May be associated with syndromes like: PHACE and LUMBAR
        - Diagnosis
          (a) Based on history and physical
          (b) MRI with gadolinium confirms diagnosis
          (c) Biopsy only if clinical picture unclear
          (d) Glut-1 positive on histopathology
          (e) Hemangioma in beard distribution more likely to also have subglottic hemangioma. Therefore, stridor warrants rigid bronchoscopy
        - Treatment
          (a) Observation for small lesions not at risk of causing functional or long-term cosmetic deformity
          (b) Beta-blocker (propranolol or nadolol) if loss of function such as impaired vision, ulceration, or bleeding
          (c) Short-term steroids may control growth
          (d) Pulsed dye laser for ulcerated lesions
          (e) Surgical excision for persistence following medical management. Try to resect after lesion has entered involution phase
      2. Congenital hemangioma (CH)
        - Clinical features
          (a) Fully formed at birth. Three subtypes:
            - RICH: rapidly involuting congenital hemangioma
            - NICH: noninvoluting congenital hemangioma
            - PICH: partially involuting congenital hemangioma

- Diagnosis
  (a) Glut-1 negative on histopathology
- Treatment
  (a) RICH disappear within weeks to months, but may take longer. NICH should be observed to ensure they are not RICH and then may require surgical excision in absence of involution

3. Tufted angioma
4. Spindle-cell hemangioma
5. Epithelioid hemangioma
6. Pyogenic granuloma (aka lobular capillary hemangioma)

b. Locally aggressive or borderline vascular tumors (not congenital but included here to maintain structure of ISSVA classification for completeness)
   1. Kaposiform hemangioendothelioma
   2. Retiform hemangioendothelioma
   3. Papillary intralymphatic angioendothelioma (PILA; Dabska tumor)
   4. Composite hemangioendothelioma
   5. Pseudomyogenic hemangioendothelioma
   6. Polymorphous hemangioendothelioma
   7. Hemangioendothelioma not otherwise specified
   8. Kaposi sarcoma

c. Malignant vascular tumors (for completeness)
   1. Angiosarcoma
   2. Epithelioid hemangioendothelioma

ii. Vascular malformations
   a. Simple
      1. Capillary malformations (CM)
         - Cutaneous or mucosal (aka "port-wine" stain)
         - Telangiectasia (ie, hereditary hemorrhagic telangiectasia)
         - Cutis marmorata telangiectatica (CMTC)
         - Nevus simplex/salmon patch/"angel kiss," "stork bite"
         - Reticulate CM
         - CM of CM-AVM
      2. Lymphatic malformations (LM)
         - Common (cystic) LM
         - Dysmorphogenesis of vascular channels lined by lymphatic endothelial cells.
         - Caused by mutation in *PIK3CA* gene (Osborn-Dickie mutation)
           (a) Clinical features
              - Present at birth and grow in proportion to child
              - May enlarge with viral or bacterial infection
           (b) Classification:
              - Microcystic LM: usually above myelohyoid muscle
              - Macrocystic LM: usually below myelohyoid muscle
              - Mixed cystic LM
           (c) Diagnosis
              - T2-MRI shows lesion as well as bright anomaly, no radiation
              - US or CT with contrast may also be used
           (d) Treatment
              - Antibiotics for acute infection

- Microcystic LM: surgical resection (often difficult due to infiltration into normal structures) or sclerotherapy
- Macrocystic LM: surgical resection or sclerotherapy
- Bleomycin causes less swelling but is less effective, thus requiring more injections. Useful in aerodigestive tract. Doxycycline is more effective but causes more swelling. Useful for neck and limbs
- Rapamycin useful for residual lesions following sclerotherapy. Avoid tape on skin as it can cause permanent mark on skin

- Generalized lymphatic anomaly (GLA)
- LM in Gorham-Stout disease
- Channel type LM
- Primary lymphedema

3. Venous malformations (VM)
   - Common VM
   - Familial VM cutaneo-mucosal (VMCM)
   - Blue rubber bleb nevus (Bean) syndrome VM
   - Glomuvenous malformation (GVM)
   - Cerebral cavernous malformation (CCM)
   - Familial intraosseous vascular malformation (VMOS)
   - Verrucous venous malformation (formerly verrucous hemangioma)
4. Arteriovenous malformations (AVM)
   - Clinical features
     (a) Associated with palpable thrill, bruit, hypertrichosis, hyperthermia, hyperhydrosis
     (b) Subtypes:
       - Sporadic
       - In HHT
       - In CM-AVM
     (c) Treatment
       - Embolization followed by surgical resection
5. Arteriovenous fistula
   - Sporadic
   - In HHT
   - In CM-AVM

b. Combined
c. Of major named vessels
d. Associated with other anomalies

B. Branchial cleft anomalies
   i. Clinical features
      a. Cysts are lined by mucosa or epithelium with no external opening. Present as mass that may become enlarged or infected (erythematous, warm, painful) with respiratory illness.
      b. Sinuses communicate with a single body surface. Present as skin pit that discharges sticky exudate. May become infected.
      c. Fistulae communicate with two body surfaces. Present as neck mass or recurrent thyroiditis (third branchial anomalies).
      d. First branchial anomalies (5%-25%): Work divided these postoperatively based on histology and location; however, some use this classification preoperatively (with caution) to plan surgery

1. Work I (less common)
   - Ectoderm-derived duplication of external auditory canal lined by squamous epithelium
   - Usually anteromedial to EAC but may be posterior to pinna
   - Course lateral to facial nerve. May course under annulus into middle ear and attach to umbo of malleus
2. Work II (more common)
   - Ectoderm and mesoderm derived, lined by squamous epithelium and contain adnexae and cartilage
   - Open into external auditory canal or concha as fistula or cyst and also as fistula on face at angle of mandible
   - Pass superficial (57%), deep (30%), or between (13%) branches of facial nerve. Deep to facial nerve more common in females, young children, fistulae rather than sinuses, and tracts not opening into external auditory canal

e. Second branchial anomalies (40%-95%)
   1. Present as neck mass along anterior border of sternocleidomastoid muscle
   2. Unilateral fistula (more common on right side) may be seen along anterior border of sternocleidomastoid muscle, midway between mandible and clavicle

f. Pyriform fossa abnormalities (formerly known as third and fourth branchial anomalies) (2%-8%)
   1. Present as recurrent thyroiditis, thyroid abscess, or fistula if previous incision and drainage. Most on left side of neck

ii. Diagnosis
   a. Work I anomalies: CT with contrast for relation to bony structures
   b. Work II anomalies: MRI with gadolinium to visualize parotid gland
   c. Second branchial cleft sinuses: no imaging required
   d. Second branchial cleft cysts: CT with contrast or MRI
   e. Pyriform fossa/third branchial anomalies: CT with contrast or MRI. Gas bubbles along tract are diagnostic. Confirmation of pyriform fossa fistula on laryngoscopy essential prior to surgery

iii. Treatment
   a. Antibiotics for acute infection. May require incision and drainage
   b. Surgical excision
      1. Work I anomalies: use nerve monitor. Begin with small preauricular incision and be prepared for full parotidectomy approach
      2. Work II anomalies: use nerve monitor and begin with parotidectomy approach. Mastoid tip less developed in children, thus facial nerve is superficial
      3. Second branchial cleft sinuses: place lacrimal probe in sinus, elliptical incision around sinus, and dissection of tract
      4. Second branchial cleft cysts: excise cyst and tract
      5. Pyriform fossa/third branchial anomalies: Place probe into pyriform fossa on direct laryngoscopy, open neck, identify probe, and resect tract, usually with hemithyroidectomy. Some advocate electrocautery of pyriform sinus tract alone; however, potential risk of injury to recurrent laryngeal nerve exists

C. Thyroglossal duct cyst
  i. Clinical features
    a. Midline lesion anywhere from foramen cecum at base of tongue to pyramidal lobe of thyroid gland. Extensive branching of ductal system, especially above hyoid bone
    b. Usually presents as neck mass due to upper respiratory tract infection
    c. Elevates with tongue protrusion
    d. Most contain small rim of thyroid tissue
    e. Rarely may contain the only functioning thyroid tissue or may develop into thyroid malignancy (< 1% risk)
  ii. Diagnosis
    a. Ultrasound
      1. Ensures thyroid gland is in normal location (decreases chances that cyst is only functioning thyroid tissue)
      2. May distinguish thyroglossal duct cyst from dermoid cyst. Helps consent patient and plan extent and duration of surgery. Presence of septae, irregular wall, and solid components is more indicative of thyroglossal duct cyst than dermoid cyst (SIST score)
    b. Nuclear imaging
      1. May be used when orthotopic thyroid is not evident to ensure thyroglossal duct cyst is not the only functioning thyroid tissue
  iii. Treatment
    a. Antibiotics +/− incision and drainage for acute infection
    b. Surgical excision (Sistrunk)
      1. After resolution of infection
      2. Recommend delineation of cyst, puncture with small needle to determine thyroglossal (mucus-filled) versus dermoid (keratin-filled) cyst. Thyroglossal warrants excision of all contents between strap muscles (not just following tract) down to and including pyramidal lobe of thyroid, plus resection of middle third of hyoid bone (Sistrunk procedure) with a cuff of tongue muscle to minimize chances of recurrence

D. Dermoid cyst
  i. Clinical features
    a. Usually asymptomatic lesion in midline of the neck
    b. May become acutely infected
    c. Does not elevate with tongue protrusion
  ii. Diagnosis
    a. See thyroglossal duct cyst
  iii. Treatment
    a. Antibiotics for acute infection
    b. Surgical excision (simple cystectomy)
      1. After resolution of infection
      2. Delineation of cyst, puncture with needle. Dermoid cyst warrants simple cystectomy

Neoplastic

A. Salivary gland tumors
  i. Clinical features
    a. Most common presentation is asymptomatic mass
    b. Parotid neoplasms

1. Benign (75%): pleomorphic adenoma, hemangioma
2. Malignant (25%): mucoepidermoid carcinoma, acinic cell carcinoma

c. Submandibular neoplasms
1. Majority are benign (opposite to what is seen in adults)

ii. Diagnosis
a. US to delineate infection versus neoplasm
b. MRI for diagnosis and surgical planning

iii. Management
a. Superficial versus deep lobe parotidectomy with negative margins
b. Serial surveillance MRI postoperatively to look for recurrence of malignant lesions

B. Rhabdomyosarcoma
i. Clinical features
a. Most common soft tissue malignancy of childhood
b. Arises from mesenchymal tissue, may originate in nonstriated muscle
c. 40% present by 5 years of age, 70% by 12 years of age
d. Most common sites of origin (decreasing frequency):
1. Orbit: best prognosis, rapid onset proptosis in children younger than 10 years
2. Nasopharynx: unilateral Eustachian tube dysfunction, nasal obstruction, rhinorrhea. Usually late diagnosis
3. Middle ear/mastoid: Unilateral otorrhea with aural polyp
4. Sinonasal: obstruction. Usually late diagnosis

ii. Diagnosis
a. Prompt surgical biopsy
b. Intraoperative frozen section shows small round blue cell tumor
c. Pathological subtyping requires immunohistochemistry
1. Embryonal (includes botryoid and spindle)
   - Young children
   - Due to mutations in chromosome 11
2. Pleomorphic
   - Older children and adults
3. Alveolar and undifferentiated
   - Mostly outside head and neck
   - Poor prognosis
4. Sclerosing
   - Very rare
   - Very poor prognosis

d. Staging
1. MRI or CT of primary site
   - Whichever is best for primary is usually good enough for imaging lymphadenopathy. If MRI is used for the primary and the lymph nodes are not visualized well enough, CT may be added.
2. CT chest
3. Bone scan
4. Bone marrow biopsy

iii. Treatment
a. Surgical excision if feasible with little to no mutilation
b. Chemotherapy (lasting approximately 1 year)

c. Radiation (beginning at approximately week 12)
d. Outcome
    1. Depends on site, clinical stage, and pathological subtype
    2. 5-year failure-free survival rate 81% for patients 1 to 9 years of age
    3. Lower if outside this age range

C. Lymphoma
  i. Hodgkin lymphoma
    a. Clinical features
      1. Malignancy of lymphoreticular system associated with Epstein-Barr virus
      2. Adolescents and young adults, rarely children less than 5 years of age
      3. More common in males
      4. Presents as cervical and supraclavicular neck mass
      5. Spleen is most common extranodal site (denotes disease progression)
    b. Diagnosis
      1. Lymph node excisional biopsy
        - Specimen must be sent fresh without formalin
        - Send separate specimen for flow cytometry
        - Avoid preoperative steroids because they degrade the specimen
      2. Pathology
        - Diagnosis based on presence of Reed-Sternberg cells (multinucleated giant cells)
        - Two subtypes (WHO classification)
          (a) Classical Hodgkin lymphoma (CHL)
          (b) Nodular lymphocyte-predominant Hodgkin lymphoma (NLPHL)
    c. Staging
      1. CT chest, abdomen, pelvis
      2. Whole body PET scan (detects metastases including bone lesions and gages response to therapy)
      3. Bone marrow and lumbar puncture only in select patients
    d. Treatment
      1. Dependent on stage of disease at presentation
      2. Surgery
        - For diagnosis and staging, not resection or cure
      3. Chemotherapy
        - For all stages
        - Stage determines number of courses of chemotherapy
      4. Radiation
        - Need depends on initial stage plus initial response to chemotherapy (as determined by repeat CT PET)
    e. Outcome
      1. 90% have good initial response regardless of stage
      2. Event-free survival 85% to 90%. Overall survival 95%
      3. Potential for significant late effects (cardiac, secondary malignancies, infertility)
  ii. Non-Hodgkin lymphoma (NHL)
    a. Clinical features
      1. Comprises multiple pathological entities
        - B cell such as Burkitt, Burkitt-like, and Burkitt leukemia
        - Diffuse large B cell, lymphoblastic, anaplastic large cell

2. Children age 2 to 12 years
3. Males more common
4. Immunosuppressed children more common
5. Presents as asymptomatic adenopathy
6. May involve Waldeyer ring
7. Children more commonly present with advanced disease

b. Diagnosis
1. Pathological diagnosis required
2. Each entity has own pathological appearance
3. Staged according to St. Jude/Murphy system
   - CT chest, abdomen, pelvis
   - Bone marrow aspirate and biopsy
   - Lumbar puncture

c. Treatment
1. Most entities treated with aggressive chemotherapy (CAR T-cell therapy in refractory and relapsing cases)
2. Limited role for radiation

d. Outcome
1. Prognosis depends on stage at presentation
2. Patients with CNS or bone marrow involvement have worse outcomes
3. 70% to 95% survival depending on entity

iii. Burkitt lymphoma (type of NHL)

a. Clinical features
1. A type of non-Hodgkin lymphoma
2. Associated with Epstein-Barr virus (EBV) infection
3. Almost exclusively seen in children
4. Males more commonly affected
5. Most rapidly proliferating human cancer
6. Endemic disease (associated with high malaria zones and EBV)
   - Affects maxilla, may affect mandible
   - Present with loose dentition, facial distortion, proptosis, and trismus
7. North American disease
   - Most common presentation is abdominal mass
   - 25% have head and neck involvement (asymptomatic adenopathy)
   - Nasopharyngeal and tonsillar involvement have been reported

b. Diagnosis
1. Pathology
   - Diffuse proliferation of uniform, undifferentiated cells with small nuclei. Classically described as a "starry sky pattern" because of interspersed large macrophages
2. Staging—similar to NHL

c. Treatment
1. Chemotherapy
2. Surgical debulking for bowel obstruction

d. Outcome
1. 90% have complete response to therapy initially.
2. Overall 2-year survival is 90% to 95%.
3. Children with CNS and marrow involvement do worse.

D. Histiocytosis
  i. Clinical features
    a. Three major classes:
      1. Langerhans cell histiocytosis (Histiocytosis X)
      2. Malignant histiocytosis syndrome (T-cell lymphoma)
      3. Non-Langerhans cell histiocytosis (hematophagocytic syndrome)
    b. Langerhans cell histiocytosis (Histiocytosis X)
      1. Three overlapping states of clonal proliferation of Langerhans cells
        - Eosinophilic granuloma
          (a) Localized, benign, monostotic. Excellent prognosis
        - Hand-Schuller-Christian disease
          (a) Skull lesions, exophthalmos, diabetes insipidus. Chronic course
        - Letterer-Siwe disease
          (a) Disseminated form, multiple organ involvement, presents by 3 years of age, rapidly progressive course
      2. Incidence 1/200,000
      3. May be genetic, oncologic, or autoimmune
      4. Mainly 5 to 10 years of age
      5. Males more common
  ii. Diagnosis
    a. Pathology
      1. Non-neoplastic proliferation of Langerhans cells
      2. Birbeck granules (organelles within nuclear cytoplasm)
        - Skeletal survey or bone scan
        - Serum electrolytes
        - Urine specific gravity for diabetes insipidus
      3. BRAF mutation
  iii. Treatment
    a. Debridement and curettage of focal lesions
    b. Adjuvant therapy for systemic involvement
    c. Radiation for nonresectable lesions
    d. BRAF inhibitors (promising results)

Infectious/Inflammatory

A. Atypical mycobacteria
  i. Clinical
    a. Prolonged erythema over skin that eventually turns violaceous in color
    b. May drain spontaneously
    c. Not responsive to antibiotics that cover skin flora
    d. Most commonly *Mycobacterium avium intracellulare* or *Mycobacterium scrofulaceum*
  ii. Diagnosis
    a. Culture and sensitivity, and polymerase chain reaction (PCR) may be diagnostic
    b. Avoid incision and drainage due to the risk of persistent fistulous tract
  iii. Treatment
    a. Treat empirically with clarithromycin or combined antibiotic therapy
    b. Surgery
      1. If fails to respond to antibiotics.
      2. Place incision 1 to 2 cm away from site of infection, elevate small skin flap, and curette lesion and undersurface of skin. Continue clarithromycin or combined antibiotic therapy postoperatively.

B. Cat scratch
  i. Clinical
    a. History of exposure to cats, usually kittens
    b. Caused by *Bartonella henselae* (gram-negative bacillus)
    c. Rarely have systemic involvement
  ii. Diagnosis
    a. Blood test for bacteria
  iii. Treatment
    a. Treat empirically with clarithromycin

C. Kawasaki disease (aka mucocutaneous lymph node syndrome)
  i. Clinical features
    a. Multisystem vasculitis of unknown etiology
    b. Children less than 5 years of age. Peak incidence between 1 and 2 years
    c. Most common cause of acquired heart disease in children (coronary artery aneurysm)
  ii. Diagnosis (American Heart Association) using FEBRILE acronym:
    a. Fever longer than 5 days plus 4 of the following
    b. Exanthem: generalized polymorphous nonvesicular rash
    c. Bulbar conjunctivitis: bilateral, nonexudative, painless
    d. Redness: lip erythema, fissuring and crusting, strawberry tongue, diffuse erythema of oral cavity
    e. Internal organ involvement (not part of the criteria)
    f. Lymphadenopathy: acute, nonpurulent, diameter more than 1.5 cm, unilateral
    g. Extremity changes: red or edematous palms and soles, followed by desquamation or transverse grooves across finger and toe nails (Beau lines)
  iii. Treatment (to prevent coronary complications)
    a. Aspirin and antiplatelet medications
    b. Intravenous immunoglobulin therapy (IVIG)
    c. Echocardiogram at time of diagnosis, 2 weeks later and 2 months later
    d. Corticosteroids
    e. Methotrexate
    f. Infliximab
    g. Anticoagulants if unresponsive to treatment or complications

D. Kikuchi disease (aka histiocytic necrotizing lymphadenitis)
  i. Clinical features
    a. Cervical lymphadenopathy with or without systemic signs
    b. Generally self-limited; however, may rarely be fatal
  ii. Diagnosis
    a. Biopsy may be mistaken for lymphoma or systemic lupus erythematosus
  iii. Treatment
    a. Self-limiting

Traumatic

A. Fibromatosis colli/pseudotumor of infancy/congenital torticollis
  i. Clinical features
    a. Lateral neck mass within sternocleidomastoid muscle
    b. Presents in first 6 weeks of life
    c. Associated with breech position in utero and congenital hip dysplasia

ii. Diagnosis
  a. Based on physical examination
  b. Confirmed with ultrasonography
  c. No need for CT or MRI
iii. Treatment
  a. Urgent referral to physiotherapy plus home programme (> 90% success)
  b. Botox injections to weaken affected muscle (rarely required).
  c. Surgical excision of mass with reapproximation of muscle (rarely required)

B. Facial nerve palsy
  i. Clinical presentation
    a. Risk factors
      1. Primiparous mother
      2. Large birth weight
      3. Prolonged labor
      4. Assisted (forceps or vacuum) vaginal delivery
    b. Signs of trauma, ecchymosis, fractures, laceration
  ii. Diagnosis
    a. Physical examination
  iii. Treatment
    a. 90% recover spontaneously

Acknowledgments

The authors acknowledge Dr. Robin T. Cotton and Dr. Evan J. Propst for a 12th version of this text and Dr. Kathleen Sie, from Seattle Children's Hospital, for authoring the 11th version, Dr. Paul Nathan and Dr. Sumit Gupta, Division of Hematology/Oncology, Hospital for Sick Children, for their experience regarding management of head and neck malignancies; Dr. Susan Blaser, Division of Neuroradiology, Hospital for Sick Children, for her expertise regarding temporal bone anomalies in various syndromic conditions and Dr. Sharon Cushing, Hospital for Sick Children for her updates to the section on Ears and Hearing.

Bibliography

ISSVA Classification of Vascular Anomalies ©2018 International Society for the Study of Vascular Anomalies. issva.org/classification. Accessed 21 September 2024.

Mitchell RB, Archer SM, Ishman SL, et al. Clinical Practice Guideline: Tonsillectomy in children (Update)-executive summary. *Otolaryngol Head Neck Surg*. 2019 Feb;160(2):187-205.

Rosenfeld RM, Tunkel DE, Schwartz SR, et al. Executive summary of clinical practice guideline on tympanostomy tubes in children (update). *Otolaryngol Head Neck Surg*. 2022 Feb;166(2): 189-206.

Ryan MA, Leu GR, Upchurch PA, Tunkel DE, Walsh JM, Boss EF. Systemic bevacizumab (Avastin) for juvenile-onset recurrent respiratory papillomatosis: a systematic review. *Laryngoscope*. 2021 May;131(5):1138-1146.

Year 2019 Position Statement: Principles and guidelines for early hearing detection and intervention programs. *J Early Hear Detect Interv*. 4(2);1-44.

Questions

1. Which of the following is NOT a typical clinical feature of a lingual thyroid gland?
   A. Airway obstruction
   B. Feeding difficulties
   C. Increased size with infection
   D. Hyperthyroidism
   E. Speech difficulties

2. Which of the following is NOT considered a risk factor for early childhood hearing loss according to the Joint Committee on Infant Hearing (JCIH)?
   A. Hypoxic ischemic encephalopathy
   B. Craniofacial anomalies
   C. In-utero exposure to Zika virus
   D. Vitamin D deficiency
   E. ECMO

3. Which of the following is the most common complication following atresia repair surgery?
   A. Tympanic membrane perforation
   B. Facial nerve palsy
   C. Canal restenosis
   D. Sensorineural hearing loss
   E. Cholesteatoma

4. A 7-year-old patient with eosinophilic esophagitis (EE) has persistent symptoms despite undergoing conventional therapies including proton pump inhibitors and dietary modifications. Given the lack of response, the team is considering the next step in management. Which of the following treatments should be considered next for this patient?
   A. Increase the dosage of proton pump inhibitors.
   B. Begin an elemental diet
   C. Initiate dupilumab therapy.
   D. Schedule an esophageal dilation procedure.
   E. Prescribe systemic glucocorticoids.

5. In an infant presenting with a segmental infantile hemangioma involving the beard area, which of the following is the most important consideration in the management due to associated risks?
   A. Immediate use of systemic steroids to prevent growth
   B. Assessment for potential airway obstruction and initiation of proactive airway management
   C. Surgical excision of the hemangioma to prevent further complications
   D. Application of topical timolol to reduce the size of the lesion
   E. Laser therapy to prevent permanent disfigurement

Part 7
Facial Plastic and Reconstructive Surgery

Chapter 55
Facial Plastic Surgery

Facial Analysis

Facial Landmarks (Figure 55-1)

A. Trichion – midline point of hairline
B. Glabella – most prominent portion of forehead in midsagittal plane, superior to root of the nose
C. Nasion – deepest point in the nasofrontal angle; location of nasofrontal suture
D. Radix – root of nose; contains the nasion
E. Rhinion – junction of bony and cartilaginous nasal dorsum; thinnest skin of the nose
F. Tip defining point – most anterior projection of nasal tip, corresponds to the apex of the lobular arch of the lower lateral cartilage
G. Subnasale – meeting of the columella and the upper lip
H. Stomion – midpoint of the oral fissure determined with the lips closed
I. Pogonion – anterior-most border of chin
J. Menton – inferior-most border of chin
K. Cervical point – posterior-most area of the intersection between the submental region and neck

General Facial Assessment

A. Vertical fifths (width) – facial width can be divided into five equally spaced segments
   a. Demarcated by lateral auricle, lateral canthus, medial canthus, medial canthus, lateral canthus, and lateral auricle

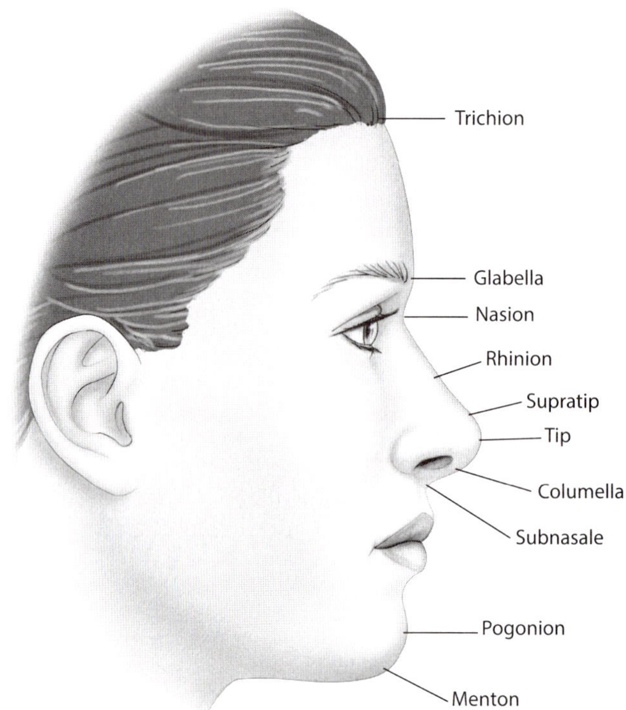

Figure 55-1 Facial anatomic landmarks. *(Adapted with permission from Taub PJ and Baker SB:* Rhinoplasty. *New York, NY: McGraw-Hill Education; 2011.)*

b. Each fifth approximates the width of one eye, which equals the intercanthal distance

B. Horizontal thirds (height) – facial height can be divided into 3 equally spaced segments demarcated by trichion, glabella, subnasale, and menton

C. Lower facial thirds – lower third of face can be further divided into thirds
   a. Subnasale to stomion = one third of lower facial height
   b. Stomion to menton = two thirds of lower facial height

D. Ideal width to length ratio of face: 3:4

Facial Angles (Figure 55-2)

A. Nasofacial angle – intercept of glabella to pogonion line (facial plane) with nasion to tip line (nasal dorsal line); ideally 30 to 40°

B. Nasolabial angle – intercept of line from the subnasale to the most anterior point on columella (columellar point) with line from the subnasale to the vermillion border of upper lip; ideally 90 to 105° in men, 95 to 120° in women

C. Nasofrontal angle – intercept of glabella to nasion line with nasion to tip line (nasal dorsal line); ideally 115 to 130°

D. Nasomental angle – intersection of nasal dorsal line with tip to pogonion line (nasomental line); ideally 120 to 132°

E. Mentocervical angle – intercept of glabella to pogonion line with menton to cervical point line; ideally 80 to 95°

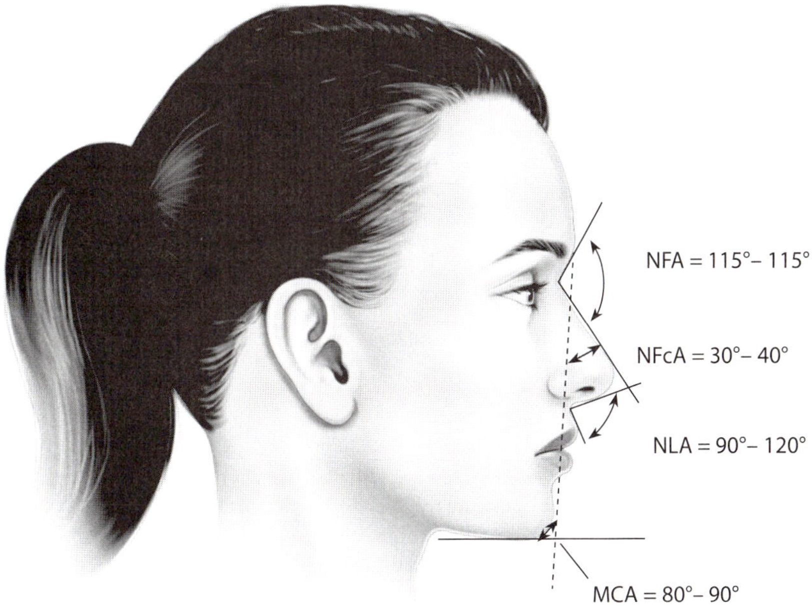

Figure 55-2 Facial Angles.

Aesthetic Facial Surgery

Chin and Midfacial Surgery

Preoperative Assessment

A. Angle's Classification of Malocclusion
   a. Class I (normal occlusion) – mesiobuccal cusp of the first maxillary molar fits in the mesiobuccal groove of the first mandibular molar
   b. Class II (retrognathia) – mesiobuccal cusp of the first maxillary molar is anterior to the mesiobuccal groove of the first mandibular molar
   c. Class III (prognathia) – mesiobuccal cusp of the first maxillary molar is posterior to the mesiobuccal groove of the first mandibular molar
B. Chin projection
   a. Anterior projection of chin assessed in relation to a line dropped from the lower lip vermilion border
      i. Women – chin ideally 1 to 2 mm posterior to this line
      ii. Men – chin ideally at or slightly anterior to this line
   b. Appropriate chin position can also be described in relation to a vertical line dropped from the nasion perpendicular to the Frankfort horizontal plane

i. Frankfort horizontal line – line drawn from superior portion of external auditory canal through the infraorbital rim
    1. Should be parallel to the floor in photos used for analysis

ii. Women – chin ideally just posterior to this line

iii. Men – chin ideally at this line

C. Differentiate microgenia from retrognathia
    a. Microgenia
        i. Small chin with normal occlusion
        ii. Can be treated with chin augmentation or sliding genioplasty
    b. Retrognathia
        i. Retrodisplaced mandible with class II occlusion
        ii. Correction of malocclusion requires sagittal split osteotomies, vertical osteotomies with bone grafting, or distraction osteogenesis

Sliding Genioplasty

A. Technique
    a. A transoral approach is used via a gingivobuccal incision extending from canine to canine. Subperiosteal dissection is performed below the level of the mental foramina. A horizontal osteotomy of the mandibular symphysis (usually below cuspid apices and mental foramina) is performed. The mobilized inferior segments are advanced, then plated or wired in the new position

B. Indications
    a. Significantly deficient lower third vertical height
    b. Severe cases of retrognathia or retrognathia with significant asymmetry

C. Advantages
    a. Ability to increase vertical height of the lower third

D. Disadvantages
    a. Longer surgical and recovery time than chin implant
    b. Higher risk of injury to dentition and mental nerve than chin implant
    c. Risk of lower lip incompetence from disruption of mentalis muscle

E. Risks and Complications
    a. Mental nerve injury
    b. Malposition
    c. Poor bony union
    d. Damage to tooth roots during osteotomy
    e. Lower lip incompetence (due to failure to re-suspend the mentalis muscle)

Chin Implants

A. Implant materials
    a. Silastic (most commonly used), expanded polytetrafluoroethylene (e-PTFE), porous polyethylene, acrylics

B. Techniques
    a. Transoral approach – the implant is placed through a midline gingival incision in the inferior vestibule
    b. Submental approach
        i. Incision placed in the submental crease. Lateral subperiosteal pockets are created to secure the implant. The implant can be suture stabilized to periosteum

ii. Advantages compared to the transoral approach: decreased contamination by oral flora, no sutures inside the mouth, improved visibility due to more direct approach
iii. Disadvantages compared to the transoral approach: external scar

C. Some bony resorption and soft tissue settling occurs postoperatively; the final augmentation is ultimately 70% of implant width

D. Risks and complications
   a. Implant migration
   b. Infection, possibly requiring explantation
   c. Bony resorption
   d. Improper size
   e. Mental nerve injury
   f. Hypertrophic scar
   g. Lower lip incompetence
   h. Implant extrusion

Lip Lift

A. Preoperative Assessment
   a. History
      i. History of injectables, fat grafting / transposition, or implants in the lips
         1. Recommended to dissolve filler – if possible – prior to lip lift
   b. Physical exam
      i. Distance between the nasal sill and the upper vermilion border
         1. Average upper lip length is 11 to 13 mm for a female and 13 to 15 mm for a male
         2. This length increases with aging
      ii. Tooth show with animation
         1. Ideal tooth show with the mouth gently opened is 3 mm
      iii. Asymmetries
      iv. Migration of any filler that has been previously placed
      v. Ideal upper lip:lower lip ratio is 1:1.6

B. Indications
   a. Increased distance between the nasal sill and vermillion border
   b. Decreased tooth show with animation
   c. Decreased red lip show

C. Technique
   a. "Bullhorn" lip lift / indirect lip lift
      i. Many variations have existed on the placement of the incisions, and whether orbicularis oris muscle is excised as well
      ii. Skin excision with the incision in the subnasal area
         1. The superior incision is placed in or 1 mm inferior to the alar-facial crease bilaterally and extends medially below the columella
            a. The incision should not extend laterally past the alar crease
            b. The highest point of the superior incision should be at the superior edge of the philtrum, just lateral to the columella
         2. The inferior incision is drawn after measuring the amount of skin to be excised, with the widest portion of skin excision medially below the columella
            a. 4 to 7 mm of skin excision on average
            b. Should leave at least 10 mm of white lip after excision
      iii. Dissection is in the sub-superficial muscular aponeurotic system (SMAS) layer

- b. Direct lip lift
  - i. Skin excision around the vermilion border with advancement of the mucosa superiorly
- D. Complications
  - a. Scarring, especially of the nasal base
  - b. Damage to the orbicularis oris, causing a change in smile
  - c. Theoretical risk of skin necrosis if lip lift is performed at the same time as rhinoplasty
    - i. This has largely been disproved

Midfacial Augmentation

- A. Indications
  - a. Accentuation of malar prominence
  - b. Adjunct to facelift for prominent nasolabial folds
  - c. Asymmetry of malar prominence from congenital deformity, surgical resection or incomplete reduction of malar fracture
- B. Evaluation
  - a. Overall aesthetic impression prioritized in evaluation
  - b. Malar region should appear full, and not fall more than 5 mm posterior to nasolabial folds on true lateral projection
- C. Technique
  - a. Intraoral approach most commonly used (canine fossa incision); a subciliary approach can also be used. The periosteum is elevated over the malar eminence and zygoma. The implant is inserted subperiosteally and secured by the confines of the pocket, or with sutures and bolster.
- D. Complications
  - a. Migration of implant
  - b. Infection, possibly requiring explantation
  - c. Intaroral exposure of implant
  - d. V2 distribution numbness (injury to the infraorbital nerve)

Aging Face Surgery

Aging Changes of the Face

- A. Thinning of papillary dermis (approximately 1% per year in adults)
- B. Decreased collagen production; shorter, more coarse collage bundles
- C. Decreased elastin production; increased fragmentation of elastin chains resulting in disordered collection of fibers
- D. Increased skin laxity and wrinkling (rhytidosis)
- E. Photodamage
- F. Dermal atrophy
- G. Soft tissue ptosis
- H. Loss of soft tissue volume including decreased subcutaneous fat
- I. Bone resorption of facial skeleton – particularly involving maxilla (medial and pyriform region), orbital rim (superomedial, inferolateral), and mandible (pre-jowl)
- J. Aging Concerns in the Upper Third
  - a. Forehead rhytids and glabellar furrows
  - b. Brow descent
- K. Aging Concerns in the Middle Third
  - a. Upper eyelid dermatochalasis (skin laxity)
  - b. Periorbital rhytids

c. Pseudoherniation of fat in lower eyelids, lower eyelid laxity
d. Nasolabial folds

L. Aging Concerns in the Lower Third
a. Nasolabial folds
b. Jowling (sagging soft tissue along mandible)

M. Aging concerns in the Neck
a. Submental skin laxity and fat deposition
b. Platysmal banding
c. Submandibular gland ptosis
d. Prominence of the anterior bellies of the digastric muscles

Forehead Lift

A. The primary goal of "forehead" or "brow" lifting is to restore the normal position of the ptotic brow in order to produce an attractive and youthful appearance. Secondary goals of forehead lifting may include improvement of the glabellar and forehead rhytids.

B. Ideal brow position
a. Medial: The eyebrow should start on a plane extended vertically from the medial canthus
b. Lateral: The eyebrow should end at a point on a line that is extended from the nasal ala through the lateral canthus of the eye. The lateral end of the brow should be on the same horizontal plane as the medial end, or slightly above
c. Superior: In men, the brow should sit at the level of the superior orbital rim and have a horizontal shape. In women, the brow should sit above the superior orbital rim with an apex located between the lateral limbus and lateral canthus

C. Techniques
a. Coronal forehead lift – a coronal incision is made 4 to 6 cm behind the anterior hairline with the incision beveled parallel to the hair follicles. The forehead tissues are elevated in a subgaleal, supraperiosteal plane to the level of the superior orbital rims. Medially, careful dissection is performed in the regions of the supraorbital and supratrochlear neurovascular bundles in order to avoid postoperative hypoesthesia. Laterally, the plane of dissection is immediately overlying the deep temporal fascia in order to avoid trauma to the frontal branch of the facial nerve which lies in the temporoparietal fascia. The corrugator and procerus muscles can be partially resected in order to reduce glabellar rhytids and the frontalis muscle can be scored to reduce forehead rhytids as appropriate. The soft tissue is then redraped and a 1 to 2 cm strip of skin and soft tissue is usually excised along the length of the incision prior to closure.
   i. Advantages
      1. Scar is well hidden within the hairline (avoid in males with alopecia)
      2. Predictable, long-lasting results
      3. Excellent exposure
      4. Ability to precisely address different muscle groups
   ii. Disadvantages
      1. More extensive dissection
      2. Elevates hairline
      3. Scalp hypoesthesia posterior to incision line
b. Pretrichial forehead lift – performed similarly to the coronal forehead lift, but the incision is placed just within the first few rows of hairs of the anterior hairline, tapering into the hairline laterally. The incision is made perpendicular to the axis of the hair follicles in order to allow the hair shafts to grow through the scar
   i. Advantages
      1. Excellent exposure

2. Shortens the height of a tall forehead by bringing the hairline down
   a. Good option for individuals with a pre-existing high hairline where elevation of the vertical height of the forehead would not be appropriate

ii. Disadvantages
   1. Potentially visible scar
   2. Alopecia from damage to hair follicles
   3. Scalp hypoesthesia posterior to incision line
   4. Contraindicated in men due to location of scar in receding hairline

c. Endoscopic forehead lift – 4 or 5 small incisions are made in the scalp posterior to the hairline. Periosteal elevators are inserted through these incisions to elevate the brow soft tissue in a subperiosteal plane. Dissection is performed down to the supraorbital rims, and laterally over the temporalis fascia. Optionally, an endoscope is introduced through an adjacent incision to allow visualization of the neurovascular bundles to avoid trauma to these structures. Curved grasping forceps and cautery may be used to resect procerus and corrugator musculature. The mobilized forehead is suspended in an elevated position using sutures with bone-tunnels or bioabsorbable screws or fixation devices.
   i. Advantages
      1. Absence of visible scars
      2. With an endoscope, can provide great visualization of the neurovascular bundle
   ii. Disadvantages
      1. Occasional problems with fixation devices (infection, palpability, tissue reaction)
      2. May be unable to achieve same degree of lift as other approaches, particularly for patients with more marked ptosis and a heavier brow
      3. More difficult visualization

d. Temporal forehead lift – modification to the endoscopic forehead lift in which just the lateral incisions are made. Dissection is performed on the deep temporal fascia.
   i. Used to lift just the lateral tail of the brow

e. Indirect forehead lift – incision is made in a horizontal rhytid on the forehead

f. Direct forehead lift – incision is made directly above the brow
   i. Advantages
      1. Most control for lifting the brow

B. Forehead lift complications
   a. Hematoma
   b. Infection
   c. Asymmetry
   d. Nerve injury (frontal branch of the facial nerve, supraorbital nerve, supratrochlear nerve)
   e. Alopecia

Upper Blepharoplasty

A. Indications
   a. Dermatochalasis — excess upper eyelid skin laxity
   b. Pseudoherniation of the central and medial fat compartments

B. Surgical anatomy
   a. Anterior lamella of the lid: skin, orbicularis oculi
   b. Middle lamella of the lid: septum
   c. Posterior lamella of the lid: eyelid retractor muscles, tarsus, conjunctiva
   d. The distance from the lash line to the upper eyelid crease is ideally 8 to 10 mm in Caucasian women and 6 to 9 mm in men

e. The upper lid may cover 3 to 4 mm of the iris but should be situated above the pupil
f. The lid crease should be at the level of the nasion
g. 2 upper fat pads (medial and central); upper lateral compartment is occupied by the lacrimal gland
    i. Medial and central fat pads are separated by superior oblique
h. Whitnall's ligament: extends from the fascia of the lacrimal gland laterally to the trochlea medially
    i. Suspends the levator palpebrae superioris muscle

C. Preoperative Assessment
  a. History
    i. Visual acuity, visual field defects, history of dry eye symptoms, ophthalmic history, glaucoma, cataracts, history of previous upper lid surgery (higher risk of lagophthalmos)
    ii. Comorbidities: Graves' disease, Sjogren's syndrome, hypertension, use of anticoagulants
    iii. Blepharochalasis – uncommon condition involving recurrent episodes of eyelid edema and inflammation. Typically occurs in younger patients.
  b. Physical Exam
    i. Assess degree of skin laxity (snap test)
    ii. Assess for ptosis
    iii. Assess for brow ptosis. Excess upper eyelid skin may be secondary to brow ptosis, which would require forehead lift.
    iv. Assess for pseudoherniation of medial and central fat compartments
    v. Visual acuity, visual field tests
    vi. Schirmer tear test – paper strip used to measure tear production (15 mm of moisture produced on strip in 5 minutes is normal), or Tear Film Break Up Time

D. Technique
  a. The patient is marked in the sitting position. The lower marking is placed in the pre-existing palpebral crease which is most commonly located 8-10 mm above the lash line. Excess skin is assessed using Green forceps. The skin excision is planned such that the lash line slightly everts without causing lagophthalmos. Generally, more skin is removed laterally than medially. In women, the lateral extent of the incision may be carried lateral to the lateral canthus. Extension beyond the orbital rim should be avoided. For patients with lateral hooding, the incision should be extended superiorly rather than violating the thicker periorbital skin. After injection of local anesthetic containing epinephrine, the skin ellipse is excised revealing the underlying orbicularis oculi muscle. A small strip of muscle may be excised to deepen the eyelid crease. If necessary, conservative resection of excess fat of the central and/or medial compartment may be performed. The incision is then closed with nonabsorbable sutures.

E. Complications
  a. Orbital hematoma – a rare but potentially catastrophic complication, as pressure from the hematoma on the optic nerve can result in permanent blindness. Permanent blindness can result if hematoma is not addressed within 60-90 minutes. Prompt recognition and decompression by opening the incision, and urgent ophthalmologic consultation are indicated. Lateral canthotomy and cantholysis should be considered if necessary for alleviation of pressure, as well as administration of mannitol, acetazolamide, and steroids.
  b. Scarring
  c. Milia – inclusion cysts along the incision line. Treated by unroofing with a needle.

d. Blepharoptosis – undiagnosed preoperative unilateral ptosis may be unmasked by the correction of upper lid laxity. Minimal ptosis (<2mm) can be treated with transconjunctival Muller muscle resection. Larger degree of ptosis is addressed best with levator resection or levator aponeurosis dehiscence repair. Ptosis can also be caused by intraoperative injury to the levator muscle, aponeurosis, or tarsal plate
e. Lagophthalmos – results from overzealous skin excision. Always leave a minimum of 20 mm of distance from lash-line to the inferior aspect of the brow. Usually resolves with time but, if persistent, may require full thickness skin grafting for correction.

Lower Blepharoplasty

A. Indications
  a. Dermatochalasis – excess lower eyelid skin laxity
  b. Pseudoherniation of the lateral, central and medial fat compartments
B. Surgical anatomy
  a. The lower lid should sit at the inferior aspect of the iris
  b. 3 lower fat pads (medial, central and lateral)
    i. Medial and central fat pads are separated by inferior oblique
    ii. Central and lateral fat pads are separated by the arcuate expansion of the inferior oblique
  c. Lockwood's ligament – extends from the lateral canthus to the medial canthus
    i. Encloses the inferior rectus and inferior oblique muscles
C. Preoperative Assessment
  a. History
    i. Visual acuity, history of dry eye symptoms, ophthalmic history, glaucoma, cataracts, history of previous upper lid surgery (higher risk of lagophthalmos)
    ii. Comorbidities: Graves' disease, Sjogren's syndrome, hypertension, use of anticoagulants
    iii. Blepharochalasis
  b. Physical Exam
    i. Assess degree of skin laxity (snap test)
    ii. Negative vector profile – globe projects anterior to the infraorbital rim. Do not remove fat in these patients
    iii. Festoons – redundant folds of lax skin or orbicularis muscle that hang from canthus to canthus
    iv. Malar bags – a reas of soft tissue fullness and edema on the lateral edge of the infraorbital ridge and zygomatic prominence. Difficult to treat with lower blepharoplasty
    v. Lid retraction test – lower lid is pulled inferiorly with finger. If medial canthus moves 3 mm or more, patient is at risk of ectropion or scleral show, and lid tightening should be considered
D. Techniques
  a. Skin flap
    i. Indicated in patients with excess skin laxity only
    ii. Surgical technique: performed through subciliary incision 2 to 3 mm below lash line. Skin flap is raised to a level just below infraorbital rim. The flap is redraped, and excess skin is trimmed leaving 1mm of redundancy to avoid postoperative ectropion. The incision is then closed with absorbable or nonabsorbable sutures
  b. Skin-muscle flap
    i. Indicated for orbicularis oculi hypertrophy, fat pseudoherniation, and excessive skin

ii. Surgical technique: performed through subciliary approach. Extends from 1 mm lateral to inferior punctum to 8 to 10 mm lateral to lateral canthus. Retention suture placed in the tarsus for superior retraction. Skin-muscle flap raised to level of orbital rim, and fat is removed if necessary just level with the infraorbital rim. Skin-muscle flap is redraped superotemporally. Redundancy excised with blade beveled caudally to excise 1 to 2 mm more muscle than skin to avoid a bulging ridge of muscle at incision line. Canthoplasty or lid shortening procedure should be performed if there is any indication of lower lid laxity to avoid postoperative ectropion

c. Transconjunctival approach
   i. Indicated when fat pseudoherniation is the dominant issue and minimal or no skin excess is present
   ii. Surgical technique: transverse incision is made through the conjunctiva. The incision can be placed 2 mm below the tarsal plate to create a pre-septal plane, or 4 mm below the tarsal plate to create a post-septal plane whereby the fat compartment is directly entered. Excess fat is resected, level with the infraorbital margin. Excess eyelid skin can be resected through a "skin pinch" where excess skin is gathered and excised below the lash line transcutaneously

E. Complications
   a. Orbital hematoma – more common in lower blepharoplasty than upper blepharoplasty
   b. Ectropion due to excess skin excision or scar retraction or lateral laxity. Risk can be decreased with simultaneous lid tightening procedure
   c. Milia
   d. Dry eye
   e. Lateral scleral show – may be present in first 1 to 2 weeks secondary to edema, improved by taping or upward massage
   f. Epiphora due to eversion or injury of lacrimal punctum
   g. Inferior oblique injury – muscle located between medial and central fat compartments. Higher risk during post-septal approach

Rhytidectomy

A. Preoperative Assessment
   a. History
      i. History of injectables, autoimmune conditions of the skin, prior radiation, prior surgery of the face and neck
      ii. Smoking history (increased risk of flap necrosis in active smokers)
   b. Physical Exam
      i. Favorable factors for surgery: good skin quality, minimal photoaging, strong facial bony structures, prominent chin and cheekbones, adequate midfacial volume, sharp cervicomental sulcus
      ii. Unfavorable factors: low-positioned hyoid (limits amount of improvement that can be made to cervicomental angle), microgenia or retrognathia, deep nasolabial folds, active smoker
      iii. Dedo classification system for the neck
         1. Class I: minimal skin laxity
         2. Class II: skin laxity alone
         3. Class III: submental jowling and submental adiposity which might benefit from submental liposuction

4. Class IV: anterior platysmal banding which might benefit from adjunctive platysmaplasty
5. Class V: congenital or acquired micrognathia which might benefit from adjunctive chin augmentation
6. Class VI: low-lying hyoid bone

B. Techniques
  a. Skin only excision: rarely used
  b. Superficial musculoaponeurotic system (SMAS) plication
    i. Elevation of anterior (temporal and preauricular) and posterior (postauricular and cervical) skin flaps. The incision courses from the temporal region (either within or just along the temporal tuft of hair), along the margin of the root of the helix, posterior to the tragus, around the lobule, and onto the postauricular surface of ear. It is commonly extended into or along the posterior hairline. The skin is elevated just deep to the hair follicles in the hair-bearing portion of the flap, and just deep to the subdermal plexus in non-hair-bearing skin. The elevation is carried medially far enough to accommodate plication sutures within the SMAS. In the neck, the elevation can be connected in the midline if desired. The SMAS is then plicated under tension with heavy sutures to provide a deep suspension. The skin flaps are then redraped and tailored prior to closure to avoid tension on the skin
      1. For men, the tragal aspect of the incision may be placed anterior to the tragus so as not to bring the hair-bearing facial skin onto the tragus
  c. SMAS imbrication
    i. After exposure of the superficial surface of the SMAS as described in the SMAS plication technique above, the SMAS itself is elevated off the parotidomasseteric fascia. The sub-SMAS plane is usually carried 1 to 2 cm beyond the anterior parotid. The SMAS is then repositioned superolaterally under tension and the overlapping SMAS is either redraped or resected (imbrication). The skin flaps are then redraped and tailored for tensionless skin closure
    ii. The SMAS imbrication technique allows for greater improvement in the jowls as compared to plication, but midface correction is limited as compared to the deep plane facelift technique
  d. Deep plane facelift
    i. The sub-SMAS plane is carried further medially than the imbrication technique, with release of the mandibular, parotid-masseteric, and zygomatic ligaments. This plane must be transitioned to a supra-SMAS plane in the superior-medial cheek directly on the anterior surface of the zygomaticus major and minor muscles. Because these muscles are innervated on their deep surfaces, the risk of facial nerve injury is limited. In the neck, a pre-platysmal and sub-platysmal plane is elevated centrally, and sub-platysmal plane elevated laterally
    ii. The deep plane facelift allows repositioning of the malar fat pad, and thus has a more dramatic effect on the nasolabial fold. The risk of facial nerve injury can be higher than the previously mentioned techniques
  e. Deep plane neck lift
    i. Deep plane facelift may be extended inferiorly to suspend the platysma superolaterally and enhance the jawline
    ii. A deep neck lift can be performed independently in a younger patient without facial rhytids with a heavier neck, for which submental liposuction alone will not result in significant benefit

iii. If performed independently, can be performed from either a submental incision alone or from a submental incision in combination with preauricular / postauricular incisions, depending on patient anatomy
iv. Dissection is in a sub-platysmal plane
v. Can incorporate any of the adjunctive techniques listed below, depending on the patient's anatomy

f. Adjunctive techniques for the neck
   i. Submental liposuction
      1. Performed through a submental incision (and sometimes through incisions at the angle of the mandible)
      2. Used for adiposity superficial to the platysma muscle
      3. Risks
         a. Irregularities that can be seen through the skin
            i. This risk can be minimized by ensuring the cannula is not facing the skin, and by leaving a small amount of subcutaneous tissue on the skin flap
   ii. Direct excision of subplatysmal fat
      1. Performed through a submental incision
   iii. Platysmaplasty – midline plication or imbrication with or without myotomy
      1. Performed through a submental incision
      2. Suturing techniques to improve the cervicomental angle by anchoring the platysma muscle down to the soft tissue overlying the hyoid
   iv. Subcapsular excision of submandibular glands for ptosis of the submandibular glands
      1. Performed through a submental incision
      2. Risks
         a. Injury to the marginal mandibular nerve
   v. Partial excision of the anterior bellies of the digastric muscles
      1. Performed through a submental incision
      2. Will improve the contouring of the jawline depending on patient anatomy

C. Complications
   a. Hematoma – occurs in 3% to 15% of cases. Manifests with unilateral pain or swelling. If untreated, necrosis of overlying skin flaps may occur causing permanent scarring and / or cutaneous irregularity. Timely evacuation is imperative
      i. Obesity (BMI >30) is a risk factor for hematoma development
   b. Skin necrosis – results from excessive skin tension, as a result of untreated hematoma, or poor local or systemic vascularity (especially with smokers). Most commonly occurs in the postauricular area. Skin loss manifests with dark eschar. Usually resolves with wound care but can result in worse scarring
   c. Alopecia – may occur in hair-bearing areas if hair follicles are traumatized during incision and / or flap elevation. Avoided by ensuring incisions are parallel to the hair follicles, minimizing cautery in hair-bearing regions and making sure the flap is not elevated too superficially
   d. Nerve injury
      i. The most commonly injured sensory nerve injury is the great auricular nerve (7% incidence), which may be encountered during flap elevation over the sternocleidomastoid
      ii. The most commonly injured motor nerve is the buccal branch of the facial nerve. Incidence of neuropraxia is 1%, and permanent nerve injury occurs in 0.1% of cases
   e. Other complications: infection, prolonged edema / ecchymosis, hypertrophic or widened scarring, pixie ear deformity, cobra neck deformity (overaggressive subplatysmal lipectomy with inadequate midline platysmaplasty)

Aesthetic Nasal Surgery

Surgical Anatomy of the Nose

A. Tip supporting mechanisms
  a. Major (3)
    i. Shape and strength of lower lateral cartilages
    ii. Attachment of medial crural footplates to caudal septum
    iii. Scroll region – attachment of upper lateral cartilage (caudal border) to lower lateral cartilage (cephalic border)
  b. Minor (6)
    i. Interdomal ligament
    ii. Cartilaginous septal dorsum
    iii. Sesamoid complex extending the support of the lateral crura to piriform aperture
    iv. Attachment of alar cartilages to overlying skin and musculature
    v. Anterior nasal spine
    vi. Membranous septum

B. Nasal valves
  a. External nasal valve – nasal sill, lower lateral cartilage, columella
  b. Internal nasal valve – septum, caudal end of the upper lateral cartilage, inferior turbinate

Nasal Analysis

A. Nasal skin
  a. Skin thickness – significantly influences final rhinoplasty results
    i. Moderate skin thickness is ideal
    ii. Thick sebaceous skin results in increased postoperative edema and limits improvement in tip definition despite contouring of underlying structures
    iii. Thin skin – easier to improve definition, but more likely to reveal minor irregularities
  b. Nasal skin is generally thick at the nasion, thinnest over the rhinion, and thick over supratip and tip

B. Frontal view
  a. Nasal thirds – assess for deviation and width
    i. Upper third: nasal bones
    ii. Middle third: upper lateral cartilages
    iii. Lower third: lower lateral cartilages
  b. Assess brow-tip aesthetic line, should be a smooth line from medial brow to ipsilateral nasal tip defining point
    i. The brow has its medial origin along a line directly vertical to the medial canthus and the nasal-alar junction
  c. Assess tip definition and width
  d. Alar-columellar margin forms a "gull in flight" outline

C. Lateral / profile view
  a. Nasal height – nasion to subnasale should be equivalent to middle 1/3 of facial length
  b. Radix
    i. Nasion should be located between the upper lid lash line and supratarsal crease
    ii. Depth should be 9-14 mm from the anterior corneal plane
    iii. Nasofrontal angle should be 115 to 130°

c. Nasal dorsum – should be parallel to and lie at or 1 to 2 mm posterior to a line drawn from the nasion to location of desired tip projection
    i. Assess for presence of hump and nature of hump (bony, cartilaginous, both)
d. Supratip break
    i. Desirable feature in the female nose
    ii. Separates dorsum from lobule
    iii. Ideally 1 to 3 mm above tip-defining point
e. Tip projection – distance from nasion to tip-defining point
    i. Goode method – distance from tip to alar margin = 0.55-0.6 the distance from the nasion to the nasal tip
    ii. Goode triangle – 3:4:5 proportion of sides of right triangle formed by columella, nasal height, and nasal dorsum
    iii. Simons method – length of subnasale to tip-defining point should equal length of subnasale to the upper lip vermilion border
f. Tip rotation – degree of inclination of nasolabial angle
    i. Nasolabial angle: intersection between subnasale to columellar point (most anterior point of columella) line and subnasale to vermilion border of upper line
    ii. Ideal values: men 95 to 105°, women 95 to 120°
    iii. More rotation is acceptable in shorter individuals
g. Columellar show – ideally 2 to 4 mm
h. Chin – assess position in relation to a line dropped from the lower vermilion border or a line dropped from the nasion perpendicular to the Frankfort horizontal plane

D. Base view
    a. Should reveal an equilateral triangle
    b. Assess for caudal septal deviation
    c. Assess size, shape, orientation and symmetry of nostril, width and length of columella, height of lobule
    d. Columella to lobule ratio should be 2:1
    e. Nasal base width should equal the intercanthal distance

E. Intranasal exam
    a. Adequacy of nasal airway, position of septum, internal and external nasal valve competence, condition of mucosa and inferior turbinates, assess for septal perforation

Rhinoplasty

A. Incisions
    a. Marginal: follows the caudal edge of lower lateral cartilage
    b. Intercartilaginous: incision between lower and upper lateral cartilage
    c. Transcartilaginous / intracartilaginous: incision through lower lateral cartilage
    d. Transcolumellar: used for open rhinoplasty, inverted-v or stairstep
    e. Hemitransfixion: unilateral incision between caudal portion of septum and medial crura
    f. Transfixion: through-and-through incision between caudal portion of septum and medial crura

B. Techniques
    a. Closed (endonasal)
        i. Non-delivery: intercartilaginous incisions

1. Advantages: no major tip support mechanisms disrupted, no external scar, preserved intact caudal rim
2. Disadvantages: limited visualization, minimal exposure of lower lateral cartilage, limited tip modification possible, potential vestibular valve scar

ii. Delivery: marginal and intercartilaginous or transcartilaginous incisions, to deliver the lower lateral cartilage as a bilaterally pedicled chondrocutaneous flap
1. Advantages: improved visualization of entire lower lateral cartilage, good access to nasal tip and dome, no external incision
2. Disadvantages: compromise one major tip support mechanism (scroll region), limited tip modification possible, higher revision rates than open

b. Open
i. Combines transcolumellar and bilateral marginal incisions to allow elevation of entire skin and soft tissue envelope (SSTE)
ii. Optimal when maximum amount of exposure is desired (eg, revision rhinoplasty, cleft rhinoplasty, teaching purposes)
iii. Necessary for significant tip work, caudal septal repositioning or replacement
iv. Advantages: improved visualization, complete exposure of nasal tip structures and cartilaginous and bony nasal dorsum, good for teaching purposes, allows for precise graft and suture placement, lower revision rates than endonasal approach
v. Disadvantages: external scar, disruption of the SSTE (one of the minor tip supporting mechanisms), increased postoperative edema and numbness

c. Dorsal preservation
i. Principles
1. Avoiding upper lateral crural resection
a. The internal nasal valve and middle vault are not disturbed in dorsal preservation rhinoplasty
2. Subperichondrial dissection
3. En bloc lowering of the dorsum
a. Because the nasal bones overlap with the septal cartilage, taking out septal cartilage at this area allows for the hump to be reduced
i. This overlap is, on average, 4 to 11 mm
ii. The dorsal hump usually sits over this area of overlap

ii. Techniques
1. Push-down
a. Lateral and transverse (radix) osteotomies and septal resection in order to lower the dorsum as a single unit to reduce a dorsal hump
i. Sidewalls displaced into the nasal cavity
2. Let-down
a. Osteotomies with a wedge resection of bone at the sidewalls, allowing the lateral aspects of the bony vault to sit on the maxilla

iii. Limitations:
1. Dorsal hump that is mostly osseous
2. Wide or inherently deformed nasal bones

iv. Dorsal preservation can be combined with either open or closed rhinoplasty approaches

C. Indications and maneuvers
a. Nasal dorsal hump
i. Dorsal hump can be bony, cartilaginous, or both
ii. Reduction of bony hump can be performed with Ruben osteotome or sequential rasping, or with dorsal preservation techniques

   iii. Reduction of a large hump without deprojecting the tip will create the illusion of a longer nose
   iv. Reducing a large hump results in an open roof deformity, which creates the illusion of a widened dorsum. Need to correct with spreader grafts and osteotomies
b. Crooked nose
   i. Goal is to create a smooth brow-nose aesthetic line
   ii. Crooked upper third is typically corrected with osteotomies
   iii. Crooked middle third may require combination of septoplasty / septal scoring, asymmetric spreader grafts, onlay grafts
   iv. Crooked lower third may require septoplasty / caudal septal repositioning, modification of lower lateral cartilages, camouflage grafts
c. Osteotomies
   i. Indications: close an open roof defect, straighten crooked nasal bones, narrow a broad upper third
   ii. Medial osteotomy
      1. Completed before lateral osteotomy
      2. Osteotome inserted between upper lateral cartilage and nasal septum and used to free the nasal bones from the perpendicular plate of ethmoid
   iii. Lateral osteotomy
      1. Low to high cut along nasomaxillary groove
      2. Started above the level of inferior turbinate to prevent internal nasal valve collapse
   iv. Intermediate osteotomies
      1. Indicated for excessively convex nasal bones
d. Tip modification
   i. Goal is to improve tip definition and shape while maintaining or improving tip support. Hence, avoid cartilage excision whenever possible
   ii. Techniques for bulbous tip
      1. Cephalic trim – removal of a strip of cartilage from the cephalic edge of the lower lateral cartilage, leaving caudal aspect intact (should leave 8-10 mm of cartilage width for support and to prevent alar collapse)
      2. Suture tip contouring – can improve tip definition without cartilage excision
      3. Lateral crural strut grafts – cartilage grafts sewn to undersurface of lateral crura to flatten contour. (Can also be used to strengthen lateral crura to alleviate external nasal valve collapse)
      4. Vertical Lobule (Dome) Division – excision of a portion of intermediate crura and reapproximation of lateral and medial crura
   iii. Changes to tip rotation and projection are best understood in the context of the Tripod or M-Arch Models
      1. Tripod Model considers conjoined medial crura and lateral crura on each side
         a. If the lateral crura are shortened or the medial crura are elongated, this will increase rotation
         b. If the lateral crura are elongated or the medial crura are shortened, this will decrease rotation
      2. M-Arch Model incorporates the intermediate crural curvature
   iv. Methods to increase tip projection
      1. Transdomal sutures, interdomal sutures
      2. Lateral crural steal
      3. Shield graft, cap graft
      4. Columellar strut or caudal septal extension graft
      5. Septocolumellar suture

v. Methods to decrease tip projection
    1. Complete transfixion incision
    2. Retrodisplacement and reposition of medial crura
    3. Medial crural overlay – incise and overlap medial crura
    4. Lateral crural overlay – incise and overlap lateral crura
    5. Vertical lobule (Dome) division

vi. Methods to increase tip rotation
    1. Reduce caudal septum anteriorly (anterior septal angle)
    2. Tongue-in-groove – anterior placement of medial crura along septum
    3. Augment premaxilla
    4. Lateral crural overlay
    5. Removal of dorsal hump (gives the illusion of tip rotation)

vii. Methods to decrease tip rotation
    1. Shorten medial crural footplate / medial crural overlay
    2. Caudal septum excision near spine (posterior septal angle)
    3. Tongue-in-groove medial crura to caudal septal extension graft
    4. Dorsal augmentation (gives the illusion of decreased tip rotation)

D. Revision rhinoplasty
  a. 5-10% of open rhinoplasties and 10% to 15% of closed rhinoplasties require revision
  b. Recommend waiting 1 year after primary rhinoplasty before doing a revision
  c. Often necessitates cartilage harvest from ear, autologous rib or cadaveric rib (as there is usually no septal cartilage remaining for grafting)

E. Complications
  a. Pollybeak deformity – abnormal fullness of the supratip region as compared to the tip
    i. Causes
      1. Inadequate cartilaginous hump removal
      2. Supratip dead space from excessive cartilaginous hump removal resulting in excessive scar formation ("paradoxical pollybeak deformity")
      3. Loss of tip support / projection
    ii. Management
      1. Soft tissue scar: steroid injection or direct excision
      2. Persistent dorsal cartilaginous hump: supratip cartilage resection
      3. Loss of tip support – reestablish tip support with cartilage grafting (columellar strut, caudal septal extension graft)
  b. Saddle nose deformity – collapse of the middle third with loss of nasal height
    i. Causes
      1. Excessive reduction of nasal dorsum
      2. Necrosis of septal cartilage
        a. Can be due to intranasal drug use, septal hematoma / abscess, or autoimmune conditions (ie, granulomatosis with polyangiitis)
    ii. Management
      1. Extended height spreader grafts
      2. Dorsal onlay graft for augmentation
  c. Open roof deformity – gap between the dorsal septum and lateral nasal wall
    i. Causes
      1. Hump reduction with inadequate lateral osteotomies
    ii. Management
      1. Lateral osteotomies
      2. Spreader grafts
      3. Dorsal onlay graft

d. Inverted-V deformity – inferomedial displacement of the upper lateral cartilages
   i. Causes
      1. Weakening of attachment of upper lateral cartilages to nasal bones
      2. Collapse of upper lateral cartilages due to over-resection of dorsum
   ii. Management
      1. Placement of spreader grafts
      2. Ensuring upper lateral cartilages adequately secured to dorsal septum
e. Alar notching or retraction
   i. Causes
      1. Over-resection of lower lateral cartilage
      2. Excessive removal of vestibular skin
      3. Poor closure of marginal incisions
   ii. Management
      1. Caudal repositioning of the lower lateral cartilages with a lateral crural strut graft
      2. Alar rim graft
      3. Composite graft
f. Rocker deformity – step-off between the nasal and frontal bones
   i. Causes
      1. Continuation of osteotomies too far superiorly into the frontal bone without back fracture
   ii. Management
      1. Transverse percutaneous osteotomies
g. Tip defects
   i. Bossae: bulbous deformity of the domes caused by irregular scarring or inadequate support, usually due to over-resection
   ii. Pinched tip: excess narrowing of nasal tip usually due to over-resection
   iii. Tip ptosis: disruption of major tip support mechanisms, poor healing, inadequate tip support
h. Persistent Nasal Obstruction
   i. Causes
      1. Persistent septal deformity
      2. Nasal valve collapse
      3. Intranasal scarring / synechiae
   ii. Management (depending on the cause)
      1. Septoplasty (persistent septal deformity)
      2. Spreader grafts (internal nasal valve collapse)
      3. Lateral crural strut grafts (external nasal valve collapse)
      4. Alar batten grafts (external nasal valve collapse)
      5. Scar lysis (intranasal scarring / synechiae)

Otoplasty

Anatomy

A. Auricle is comprised of a complex structure of fibroelastic cartilage
   a. Covered with skin that is closely adherent anteriorly, more loosely attached posteriorly

B. Important landmarks
   a. Helix
   b. Superior crus of anihelix
   c. Inferior crus of antihelix
   d. Antihelix
   e. Cymba concha and cavum concha
   f. Triaangular fossa
   g. Tragus
   h. Antitragus
   i. Lobule

Preoperative Evaluation

A. Auricular size and location
B. Auricular components and convolutions (helix, antihelix, scaphoid fossa, triangular fossa, lobule)
C. Compare to contralateral ear
D. Ideal measurements
   a. Vertical height – 6 cm
   b. Width – 55% of length
   c. Ideal auriculocephalic angle: 25 to 35°
   d. Upper third distance from helix to mastoid: 10 to 12 mm
   e. Middle third distance from helix to mastoid: 16 to 18 mm
   f. Lower third distance from helix to mastoid: 20 to 22 mm
   g. Preoperative photograph – anterior full face, posterior full head, close-up photographs of both ears
E. Most common aesthetic auricular defect: protruding ear (prominauris)
   a. Auriculocephalic angle >35°
   b. Underdeveloped antihelical fold
   c. Overdeveloped conchal cartilage
   d. Superior helix >20mm from scalp
F. Auricular molding can be done in a newborn due to high levels of maternal estrogen allowing for the cartilage to be softer
G. Timing of otoplasty
   a. Best before child starts school, age 5 to 6 years
      i. Ear is 85% to 90% of adult size, cartilage has adequate strength
      ii. Reduce teasing, anxiety

Otoplasty

A. Overdeveloped conchal bowl
   a. Furnas suture technique (conchomastoid sutures)
      i. Permanent sutures approximating conchal cartilage to mastoid periosteum
      ii. Placement of conchomastoid suture as far posteriorly to avoid narrowing of external auditory canal
      iii. When done, may reduce / eliminate need for Mustarde sutures
   b. Cartilage Sculpting Techniques (Converse, Farrior, Pitanguy)
      i. Involves variable reshaping, splitting or removal of auricular cartilage
      ii. Farrior technique includes a combination of suture and cartilage sculpting technique
      iii. Disadvantages: cartilage irregularities, asymmetries

B. Underdeveloped antihelical fold
  a. Mustarde suture technique
    i. Postauricular incision, followed by undermining in a supraperichondrial plane. 2 to 3 horizontal mattress sutures placed along the scapha to create an antihelical fold. All sutures placed prior to final tightening
    ii. Disadvantages: resilience of cartilage, suture exposure

C. Complications
  a. Inadequate correction (most common)
  b. Suture extrusion
  c. Chondritis
  d. Hematoma
  e. Telephone ear deformity: upper and lower poles of the auricle protrude relative to the middle pole due to overcorrection of the concha or undercorrection of the helix
  f. Reverse telephone ear deformity: middle pole protrudes relative to the upper and lower poles of the auricle; due to overcorrection of the helix or undercorrection of the concha
  g. Cartilage irregularities

Facial Skin Rejuvenation/Resurfacing

Principles

A. Removal of the epidermis with creation of a controlled injury to the papillary dermis or upper reticular dermis

B. Healing process stimulates production of new collagen and a resurfaced epidermis from deeper, less sun-damaged cells

Skin Anatomy

A. Epidermal layers
  a. Stratum corneum (most superficial layer)
  b. Stratum granulosum
  c. Stratum lucidum
  d. Stratum spinosum
  e. Stratum basale (deepest layer)

B. Dermal layers
  a. Papillary dermis – thin, loose collagen surrounding adnexal structures; abundant elastic fibers
  b. Reticular dermis – thick, compact collagen. Damage to this layer results in permanent scar

C. Subcutaneous layer

Skin Analysis

A. Fitzpatrick Classification of Skin Types
  a. Class I: very white, always burns, never tans
  b. Class II: white, usually burns, tans minimally
  c. Class III: white to olive, sometimes burns, often tans
  d. Class IV: brown, rarely burns, nearly always tans

- e. Class V: dark brown, very rarely burns, nearly always tans
- f. Class VI: black, never burns, always tans
- g. Fitzpatrick III through VI are at higher risk for pigmentary dyschromia

B. Glogau Classification of Photoaging
- a. Class I: minimal wrinkles only when the face is in motion
- b. Class II: wrinkles in motion
- c. Class III: wrinkles while at rest
- d. Class IV: wrinkled in all areas

Dermabrasion

A. Principles
- a. Mechanical method of removing the epidermis to create a papillary dermal wound
- b. Induces new collagen and resurfaced epidermis from deeper, less damaged cells
  - i. Re-epithelialization is complete within 7 days

B. Indications
- a. Acne scarring
- b. Facial rhytids
- c. Premalignant solar keratosis
- d. Rhinophyma
- e. Adjunct for scar revision
  - i. Should wait 6-8 weeks after surgery before performing dermabrasion on scars

C. Contraindications
- a. Active herpetic lesions

D. Advantages
- a. Inexpensive
- b. Portable
- c. Widely available
- d. Precise control of depth

E. Complications
- a. Milia
- b. Acne flares
- c. Persistent post-procedure erythema
- d. Herpes simplex infection
  - i. Pretreat any patients with history of herpes simplex virus infection
- e. Hyperpigmentation / hypopigmentation
  - i. Post-inflammatory hyperpigmentation is more common in higher Fitzpatrick skin types
    1. Treat with lightening agents (such as hydroquinone) before and after dermabrasion
    2. Can also be treated with oral steroids
  - ii. Hypopigmentation is much harder to treat

Chemical Peeling

A. Principles
- a. Chemical method of removing layers of the epidermis and dermis
- b. Removes superficial lesions and improves skin texture

B. Indications
- a. Acne scarring
- b. Facial rhytids

c. Actinic keratosis
d. Seborrheic keratosis
e. Photodamaged skin
f. Pigment irregularities
g. Adjunct for scar revision

C. Contraindications
  a. Active herpetic lesions
  b. Collagen vascular disease
  c. Pustular acne
  d. Prior radiation

D. Advantages
  a. Inexpensive
  b. Portable
  c. Widely available

E. Common peels
  a. Superficial peels – penetrate only within the epidermal layers
    i. Exfoliation of stratum corneum to stratum basale
    ii. Useful for mild sun damage, irregular pigmentation, light cross-hatch wrinkling, acne, benign keratoses
    iii. Period of recovery: 1-5 days
    iv. May require multiple sessions to obtain maximum results
    v. Will not have any frosting of the skin during treatment
    vi. Examples: glycolic acid 40% to 70%, 10% to 25% Trichloroacetic acid (TCA), Jessner's solution
      1. Jessner's solution: 14g resorcinol, 14g salicyclic acid, 14mL lactic acid in 100mL ethanol
  b. Medium depth peels – penetrate into the papillary dermis
    i. Useful for destruction of epidermal lesions, moderate sun damage, pigmentary changes, acne scarring
    ii. Period of recovery: 7 to 10 days
    iii. Will have superficial frosting with a background of erythema during treatment
    iv. Examples: Monheit peel (Jessner's solution followed by 35% TCA peel)
  c. Deep peels – penetrate into the reticular dermis
    i. Useful for severely sun-damaged skin
    ii. Period of recovery: 10 to 14 days
    iii. Will have more solid frosting without erythema during treatment
    iv. Examples: 50% TCA, Gordon Baker phenol peel
      1. Gordon Baker phenol peel: 3 mL phenol USP 88%, 2 mL tap water, 3 drops croton oil, 8 drops septicol (liquid soap)
        a. Depth is controlled by the concentration of croton oil
        b. Phenol peels cause liquefactive necrosis in the deep dermis
        c. Toxicity: cardiac arrythmias, renal and hepatic toxicity
          i. Avoid toxicity with IV hydration, application to only 1 facial subunit at a time, cardiac monitoring, and screening of patients (avoid in patients with cardiac comorbidities)

F. Complications
  a. Hyperpigmentation/hypopigmentation
  b. Cutaneous infections (bacterial, fungal, herpes simplex activation)
  c. Cardiac arrythmias (phenol peel)

d. Renal toxicity (phenol peel)
e. Melasma
f. Ectropion
g. Prolonged erythema – may indicate a potential for scarring, so should be treated with topical or oral steroids, or subcutaneous steroid injection

Laser Skin Resurfacing

A. Principles
   a. Lasers utilize the concept of selective thermolysis, which is determined by absorbance of skin constituents (chromophore, oxyhemoglobin, melanin), the power and the spot size
   b. Lasers can be divided into ablative and non-ablative
B. Ablative lasers
   a. Target and remove the epidermis and portions of the superficial dermis
   b. Induce collagen remodeling and new collagen production
   c. Advantages
      i. Produce results in a precise and controlled fashion at the appropriate depth
   d. CO_2 (carbon dioxide) laser
      i. Target chromophore: water
      ii. Wavelength: 10,600 nm
      iii. Depth of penetration: 20 to 60 um on first pass (increased depth with additional passes)
      iv. Advantages
         1. Best outcome for removing severe sun damage and correction of elastosis and deeper wrinkling
      v. Disadvantages
         1. Significant postoperative downtime
            a. 10-14 days is required for re-epithelialization, followed by erythema that may last 1-3 months
         2. Increased risk of pigmentary changes, scarring, and infection
   e. Er:YAG (Erbium:YAG) laser
      i. Target chromophore: water
      ii. Wavelength: 2940 nm
      iii. Depth of penetration: 3 to 5 um
      iv. Produces a more superficial ablation than CO_2 laser
      v. Advantages
         1. Faster healing time (5 days) with less postoperative erythema (3-4 weeks)
         2. Useful for treating more superficial rhytids
      vi. Disadvantages
         1. Less collagen remodeling and tightening
         2. Unable to manage deeper wrinkles and more severe photodamage
   f. Fractionated laser
      i. Microzones of injury surrounded by normal intervening skin; allows for rapid healing of injured tissue
         1. MTZ (microthermal injury zone) is created over approximately 12% to 20% of entire treatment area
         2. 100 um diameter area of injury is surrounded by 250 um of normal tissue
      ii. Wavelength: 1550 nm
      iii. Depth of penetration: 30 um

- iv. Advantages
  1. Decreased downtime (reservoir of undamaged skin adjacent to sites of laser injury allows for rapid re-epithelialization after treatment through migration of viable cells into wounded area)
- v. Typically, a series of multiple treatments are performed at 7-30-day intervals

g. Indications
- i. Rhytids
- ii. Dyschromia
- iii. Superficial / shallow acne scars
- iv. Elevated scars
- v. Skin lesions (lentigines, seborrheic keratoses, actinic keratoses, early superficial basal cell carcinomas)

h. Contraindications
- i. Active or recent use of isotretinoin
  1. Skin resurfacing should be delayed 6 to 12 months from last isotretinoin use to prevent scarring
- ii. Active infection
- iii. History of radiation therapy, collagen vascular disease (eg, scleroderma), history of hypertrophic scarring or keloid formation

i. Complications
- i. Milia
- ii. Infection (herpes simplex virus, bacterial, fungal)
- iii. Hyperpigmentation / hypopigmentation
- iv. Scarring
- v. Ectropion
- vi. Persistent erythema

j. Treatment protocol
- i. Skin may be prepared for up to 6 weeks prior to laser resurfacing using a combination of retinoid acid, alpha-hydroxy acid and hydroquinone
- ii. Prophylactic oral antiviral and antibiotic medications should be prescribed
- iii. Local, regional or general anesthesia is administered. Depth of tissue vaporization can be controlled by varying laser parameters and number of passes. Depth of penetration is determined to be superficial, deep or upper reticular dermis

C. Non-ablative lasers

a. Do not cause disruption or injury to the epidermis

b. Advantages
- i. Decreased downtime

c. Infrared laser
- i. Targets dermal water to induce collagen production and remodeling to improve fine lines and skin texture
- ii. ND:YAG (neodymium:YAG) laser wavelength: 1064 nm
- iii. Diode laser wavelength: 1450 nm

d. Pigment-specific laser
- i. Lightens lentigines and ephelides
- ii. QS Nd:YAG (Q-switched Nd:YAG) laser wavelength: 1064 nm and 532 nm
- iii. QS alexandrite wavelength: 755 nm
- iv. QS ruby laser wavelength: 694 nm

e. Vascular-specific lasers
- i. Target erythema, flushing and telangiectasias

f. Intense pulsed light
    i. Broad wavelength that can target both vascular and pigmentary alterations
g. Advantages
    i. Improve mild to moderate rhytids and acne scars with no external wounding
h. Disadvantages
    i. Less dramatic results as compared to ablative lasers

Aesthetic Injectables

Botulinum Toxin

A. Produced by *Clostridium botulinum* bacteria
B. Eight serotypes, with Botulinum toxin A being the most potent and most commonly used in clinical practice
    a. Type B has a quicker onset of action but shorter duration of action than type A
C. Botox (Allergen, Irvine, California) was initially approved by the Food and Drug Administration for the treatment of strabismus, blepharospasm, cervical dystonia
D. Mechanism of action
    a. Blockade of presynaptic acetylcholine release at the neuromuscular junction through cleavage of SNARE proteins
        i. Muscle fibers become functionally denervated, resulting in muscle fiber atrophy and flaccid paralysis
E. Preparation and pharmacology
    a. Botox (Allergan) is typically available in 100 or 200U vials
    b. Each vial is a lyophilized complex consisting of 100U of toxin, 0.5 mg of human albumin and 0.9 mg of sodium chloride
F. Clinical efficacy
    a. Onset of action: 6-36 hours after exposure
    b. Maximum effect: 7-14 days from exposure
    c. Duration of effect: 3-4 months
        i. New neuromuscular junctions and axonal sprouts eventually replace nonfunctional junctions and restore muscle function
G. Indications
    a. Common aesthetic regions
        i. Glabellar complex (procerus and corrugators)
            1. Procerus: horizontal forehead rhytids
            2. Corrugators: vertical forehead rhytids ("11 lines")
        ii. Frontalis muscle (horizontal forehead rhytids)
        iii. Lateral orbicularis oculi muscle ("crow's feet")
        iv. Transverse nasalis ("bunny lines")
        v. Platysma: banding in the neck
        vi. Depressor anguli oris (downturned corners of the mouth)
        vii. Mentalis muscle (chin dimpling)
        viii. Orbicularis oris ("lip flip")
    b. Other indications
        i. Synkinesis of the facial nerve
        ii. Sialocele
        iii. Migraines
        iv. Hyperhidrosis
        v. Gustatory sweating (Frey's syndrome)

H. Complications
  a. Local reaction: pain, edema, erythema, ecchymosis, headache
  b. Eyelid ptosis: from diffusion of botulinum toxin into the levator palpabrae superioris
    i. Treatment: alpha 2 agonist eyedrops to stimulate Muller's muscle
  c. Brow ptosis
  d. Immunologic reaction: acute Gell and Coombs type 1 reaction
  e. Systemic reaction: nausea, fatigue, malaise, flu-like symptoms, distant rash
  f. Therapeutic failure from circulating neutralizing antibodies

I. Contraindications
  a. Hypersensitivity to ingredients (ie, albumin)
  b. Neuromuscular disease (ie, myasthenia gravis, Lambert-Eaton syndrome)
  c. Patients treated with aminoglycosides, penicillamine, quinine, calcium channel blockers
  d. Pregnancy / lactation
  e. Relative contraindication: patients on anticoagulation therapy

Injectable Fillers

A. Indications
  a. Soft tissue augmentation to decrease the prominence of facial grooves and creases and to provide volume to atrophied tissue

B. Technique
  a. Varies for the particular facial region being addressed
  b. Intradermal injection for cutaneous rhytids
  c. Subcutaneous injection to smooth deep nasolabial folds, glabellar creases, marionette lines
  d. Supra-periosteal injection for the temple, zygomatic eminence, cheek, chin and pre-jowl

C. Materials
  a. Collagen
    i. Major structural component of skin
    ii. Bovine collagen was the first FDA-approved dermal filler
      1. Taken off of the market in 2010
      2. Required pre-treatment allergy testing
  b. Hyaluronic acid (HA)
    i. Most prominent glycosaminoglycan in the skin
    ii. Most commonly used filler material world-wide
    iii. Binds to water when injected into skin; volumizes, softens and hydrates the skin
    iv. Since 2010, all FDA-approved HA products contain lidocaine
    v. Lasts about 6 to 12 months depending on location with increased longevity in less mobile areas of the face
    vi. Advantages
      1. Predictable and lasting soft tissue augmentation
      2. Hyaluronidase available for intravascular injection, overcorrection or undesirable migration (off-label use)
  c. Synthetic fillers
    i. Poly-L-lactic acid (PLLA; Sculptra)
      1. Deep dermal or supraperiosteal injection
      2. Induces a fibroblast response resulting in collagen formation

3. Requires multiple treatments with effects lasting years
4. FDA approved for the treatment of lipodystrophy secondary to anti-retroviral therapy for HIV

ii. Calcium hydroxyapatite (CAHA)
1. Identical to mineral portion of bone
2. Subdermal or supraperiosteal injection
3. Induces collagen formation
4. FDA approved for the treatment of lipodystrophy secondary to anti-retroviral therapy for HIV

d. Autologous fat
i. Involves harvest of fat (usually from inner thighs, periumbilical area or flanks) and transfer with cannula injection
ii. Indications
1. Facial rhytids, grooves and volume loss
iii. Advantages
1. Autologous
2. Completely biocompatible
3. Available in sufficient quantities
4. Naturally integrated into host tissue
5. Potentially permanent
6. Inexpensive and simple to obtain
iv. Disadvantages
1. Results can be unpredictable
2. Viability of transferred fat varies depending on surgical technique and patient factors
v. Surgical technique
1. Harvesting of fat via liposuction
a. Infiltrate donor site with tumescent solution
b. 3 mm puncture incision, harvesting cannula with a blunt tip is attached to a 10mL Luer-lock syringe
c. Cannula is pushed through the harvest site as the surgeon uses digital manipulation to pull back on the plunger of the syringe and create gentle negative pressure
d. Once syringe is filled, it is disconnected from the cannula and replaced with a plug that seals the Luer-Lock end of the syringe
2. Refinement and transfer
a. Centrifugation can be used to separate the components of the harvested fat based on density
i. Upper portion (least dense): oil
ii. Middle portion: fatty tissue
iii. Lower portion (most dense): blood, water and aqueous element (tumescence)
iv. Recommended centrifuge speed: 3000 rotations per minute for 3 minutes
b. Decant oil layer and wick off any remaining oil using an absorbent material
c. Remove Luer-Lock plug to release densest liquid layer, leaving the fatty layer behind for transplantation
3. Transplantation and placement
a. Cannula technique preferred
b. Accuracy of volume, location and level of placement is critical to success

e. Other filler materials
   i. Autologous cell therapy
   ii. Micronized AlloDerm
   iii. Autologous fibroblasts
   iv. Silicone
   v. Polymethylmethacrylate (PMMA; ArteFill)
      1. Permanent filler
      2. Requires skin test for bovine collagen allergy prior to use
f. Complications
   i. Allergic reaction
   ii. Vascular occlusive event
      1. Can result in skin necrosis
      2. Can result in central retinal artery occlusion (intravascular injection with retrograde embolization)
         a. Presents with sudden vision loss, retinal whitening and a cherry-red spot in the central macula
         b. Results in blindness if perfusion is not restored within 90 minutes
      3. Treatment: hyaluronidase, aspirin, topical nitropaste, warm compresses, massages
   iii. Tyndall effect
      1. Bluish appearance of hyaluronic acid injected too superficially beneath the skin
         a. Treatment: express product through a needle hole or dissolve with hyaluronidase

Scar Revision

A. Principles
   a. Relaxed skin tension lines (RSTL) – created by the intrinsic tension of the skin at rest. These lines generally fall perpendicular to the underlying musculature and parallel to facial rhytids, except around the eye where RSTLs are parallel to the orbicularis oculi
   b. Lines of maximal extensibility (LME) – usually perpendicular to the RSTLs and represent the direction in which closure can be performed with the least tension. Typically, parallel to the muscle fibers
B. Approaches to scar revision
   a. Excision – excision of the scar along RSTLs, normal facial creases, and the junctions between distinct facial aesthetic units, with meticulous everted closure. Serial excision of larger scars may be performed in stages according to these principles. Usually best for scars 0 to 30 degrees from the RSTLs. Excision is often done in an ellipitical fashion with a 3:1 length to width ratio
   b. Irregularization
      i. Z-plasty – reorient a scar that does not lie in the RSTLs. This both lengthens and reorients the scar. Created by the addition of two limbs that are similar to the length of the scar, one at either end of the existing scar. These limbs are incised at angles of 30, 45, or 60° relative to the scar. This will lengthen the scar by 25, 50, and 75%, respectively. This will also reorient the scar by 45, 60 or 90°, respectively, relative to the original scar. Multiple Z-plasties can be employed along a single scar to lengthen the line. Z-plasty is usually best for scars that are oriented 30 to 60 degrees from the RSTLs

ii. W-plasty – created by a series of interdigitating triangles on either side of the scar. It distributes tension and breaks up a linear scar. Usually best for scars 60-90 degrees from the RSTLs
iii. Geometric broken line closure – involves outlining of one side of the scar to be excised with an irregular composite of rectangular, triangular, and semicircular shapes. The complimentary template for interdigitation is then outlined on the opposite side of the scar. The new scar carries an irregularly irregular pattern that is less conspicuous. Usually best for very long scars 60-90 degrees from the RSTLs

c. Resurfacing – mechanical dermabrasion or laser resurfacing can serve as a primary scar treatment modality or as an adjunct to surgical scar revision (6 weeks after scar revision)

Hair Restoration

A. Preoperative evaluation
 a. Background
  i. Male pattern baldness (androgenic alopecia) is the most common hair loss disorder (80% of men, 40% of women)
   1. Androgenic alopecia is mediated by 5-alpha reductase activity, which converts testosterone into dihydrotestosterone (DHT)
  ii. Educate patient on progressive nature of male pattern baldness
  iii. May require more than one session of hair transplantation for best results depending on amount and pattern of loss
  iv. Hair phases – anagen (growth), catagen (hair follicle detaches from blood supply), telogen (resting phase), and exogen (shedding)
 b. History
  i. Progression and timeframe of hair loss
  ii. Location of hair loss
  iii. Familial patterns of baldness to determine future hair loss patterns
  iv. Rule out other potential causes of hair loss (ie, autoimmune causes, medication-related, hormonally-related, psychologic conditions)
  v. Hair transplantation can also be performed for eyebrow and facial hair
 c. Physical exam
  i. Norwood classification of male pattern baldness:
   1. Type I – minimal to no recession of the hairline
   2. Type II – areas of recession at the frontotemporal hairline
   3. Type III – deep, symmetric recession at the temples, which are bare or only sparsely covered
   4. Type IV – hair loss is primarily from the vertex; limited recession of the frontotemporal hairline
   5. Type V – vertex hair loss region is separated from the frontotemporal region but is less distinct; the band of hair across the crown is narrow
   6. Type VI – frontotemporal and vertex regions are joined together
   7. Type VII – a narrow band of hair remains in a horseshoe shape
B. Nonsurgical treatment
 a. Minoxidil (Rogaine) – topical medication that vasodilates peripheral vessels; used frequently as an adjunct to hair transplantation
  i. Increases the diameter of existing hairs and increases the percentage of follicles in the anagen phase

b. Finasteride (Propecia) – inhibits 5-alpha reductase, thereby preventing conversion of testosterone to DHT. Improvement noted in about 2/3 of men. Must continue taking the medication for continued results
c. Platelet-rich plasma (PRP) injection
   i. Patient's own blood is centrifuged to obtain serum rich in platelets, growth factors, chemokines, and cytokines
   ii. Serum is then micro-injected into scalp areas of hair loss
   iii. Current evidence shows improvement in hair density and thickness
   iv. Requires multiple sessions
   v. Can be used to treat hair loss on its own or as an adjunct after hair transplantation to increase graft survival

C. Basic principles of hair transplantation
   a. Donor hairs taken from occipital scalp, which is less androgen-sensitive and usually preserved in male pattern baldness
   b. Follicular unit – natural bundling of 1-4 hairs; most follicular units contain 2-3 hairs
   c. Follicular unit grafting – use of microscopic dissection to isolate individual follicular units for transplantation with a minimum amount of non-hair-bearing surrounding skin
      i. Microscopic dissection minimizes amount of scalp skin around each graft, allowing for greater hair density, faster healing, and less trauma to existing hairs
      ii. Minimizes accidental transection of hair follicles, increasing hair yield by an estimated 20%
      iii. Allows for precise placement of 1-hair grafts in anterior hairline and more dense follicles posteriorly for natural appearance

D. Surgical technique
   a. Performed under local anesthesia with or without oral sedation
   b. Hairline designed in an irregularly irregular fashion with patient feedback
   c. Graft harvest techniques:
      i. Strip technique (follicular unit transplant; FUT) – single donor strip 1 cm in height excised from occipital scalp in subcutaneous plane deep to hair follicles. Length of strip determined by number of grafts needed. The donor site closed primarily with running nonabsorbable suture
         1. There are approximately 80 follicular units per cm^2 of scalp, therefore a 20 cm^2 donor strip will yield approximately 1600 grafts
      ii. Follicular unit extraction (FUE) – grafts harvested one at a time with 0.8 – 1.0 mm punches, therefore no linear donor site incision. Best for males who wear hair very short in which a scalp scar may be visible
   d. After extraction via FUT or FUE, grafts are dissected under microscopic visualization. They are stored in chilled saline and sorted by number of hairs per unit.
   e. Grafts are placed through stab incisions angled to lie naturally. Follicular units with 1 hair are placed anteriorly along the hairline
   f. More dense units are placed further posteriorly for natural feathering effect

E. Postoperative Care
   a. Transplanted hairs fall out after several weeks and re-grow 8-10 weeks later
      i. Regrowth accelerated by minoxidil
   b. Telogen effluvium – normal phenomenon; rapid hair loss of a portion of all head hair after a hair transplant
      i. Regrowth occurs after 3-4 months

F. Complications
  a. Folliculitis
  b. Graft failure
  c. Poor scarring
  d. Scalp anesthesia / dysesthesia
  e. Unnatural aesthetic result

Questions

1. What represents the junction of the bony and cartilaginous nasal dorsum?
   A. Nasion
   B. Radix
   C. Rhinion
   D. Subnasale
2. What is the ideal width to length ratio of the face?
   A. 2:3
   B. 4:5
   C. 1:2
   D. 3:4
3. Which of the following describes Fitzpatrick Class IV skin?
   A. brown, rarely burns, nearly always tans
   B. white to olive, sometimes burns, often tans
   C. white, usually burns, tans minimally
   D. dark brown, very rarely burns, nearly always tans
4. The following are all methods to increase tip rotation, except:
   A. Augment premaxilla
   B. Medial crural overlay
   C. Lateral crural overlay
   D. Reduce caudal septum anteriorly (anterior septal angle)
5. All of the following are major tip support mechanisms, except:
   A. Size, shape and resilience of medial and lower lateral crura
   B. Attachment of upper lateral cartilage to lower lateral cartilage
   C. Cartilaginous septal dorsum
   D. Medial crural footplate attachment to caudal border of quadrangular cartilage

Answers

1. C
2. D
3. A
4. B
5. C

Chapter 56
Reconstructive Head and Neck Surgery

Introduction

Reconstruction of the head and neck presents unique challenges, as it involves not only restoring physical appearance but also preserving vital functions such as speech, swallowing, and facial expressions. The complexity of this region means that successful reconstruction must address both aesthetic and functional aspects to ensure patients can reintegrate into their social and professional lives. Advances in surgical knowledge and techniques have now made it possible to replace nearly every type of tissue loss, from skin and bone to muscle and nerves. These developments have significantly improved the functional and aesthetic outcomes for patients who have undergone ablative surgery, experienced major facial trauma, or suffered from infections or inflammatory disorders.

The goal of this chapter is to provide essential insights into the principles and practices of head and neck reconstruction. We will explore the key considerations for effective tissue replacement, including the need for a comprehensive defect analysis and the selection of appropriate reconstructive techniques. From traditional methods to innovative approaches, we aim to equip surgeons with the knowledge to achieve optimal results, ensuring that both the form and function of the head and neck are meticulously restored. This chapter will serve as a guide to understanding the nuanced and multifaceted nature of head and neck reconstruction, from initial assessment to the execution of complex surgical interventions.

Reconstructive Considerations

a. Structural
   i. Bone stock for skeletal framework and/or osseointegration
   ii. Volume restoration
   iii. Soft tissue coverage of vital structures (eg, carotid artery, intracranial contents)
b. Functional
   i. Muscle continuity
   ii. Potential for a sensate tissue surface
   iii. Volume restoration (bulk of tongue to improve speech/swallow)
c. Recipient bed
   i. Previously irradiated
   ii. Presence of infectious/inflammatory material

d. Locational
   i. Ocular: corneal protection
   ii. Auricular: patency of ear canal, preservation of helical rim for glasses use
   iii. Nasal: patency of nasal airway
   iv. Lips: oral competence
   v. Mandibular: establish facial height and mastication
   vi. Lingual: aid in deglutition and speech
   vii. Laryngeal: patency of airway, prevention of pharyngocutaneous or pharyngotracheal fistula

The Reconstructive Ladder

a. Utilizes a hierarchical system tiered by complexity.
b. Surgeon chooses the technique that is most expedient for addressing the reconstructive problem with contingency plans in case of flap/graft failure or recurrence.
c. It should be noted that sometimes the simplest plan has limitations in terms of aesthetics, long-term durability, and functionality.
d. The reconstructive ladder must also be applied in the context of the patient's overall health status, wishes, and desires. All these factors will determine the final reconstructive choice.
   - Healing by secondary intention
   - Primary closure
   - Skin, cartilage, bone, nerve, and composite grafting
   - Local flaps
   - Regional flaps
   - Prosthetic reconstruction
   - Microneurovascular free tissue transfer

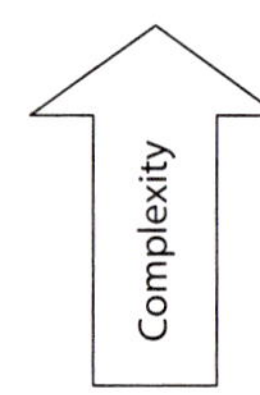

Healing by Secondary Intention

a. Development of granulation tissue in the wound
b. Myofibroblasts cause wound contraction
c. Final phase is epithelialization
d. Debris and scabbing of the wound (from desiccation) delay ultimate epithelialization
e. Poor reconstructive option for sites of the face with free edges—nasal ala, upper/lower eyelid, lips—with resulting distortion

Concave surfaces that heal well by secondary intention
Lateral forehead (temple)
Glabella
Medial canthal area
Concave areas of ear
Perinasal melolabial fold

Primary Closure

a. Key considerations include location and quantity of tissue loss, and wound tension.
    i. Certain locations are less amenable to primary closure.
        1. Floor of mouth: poor tensile strength of mucosa, may cause tongue tethering
        2. Near eye or mouth: risk of losing sphincter functionality resulting in lack of eye closure or oral competence
        3. Palate: can result in velopharyngeal insufficiency
    ii. Excessive tension is associated with greater degree of necrosis.
b. Wound tension dictated by collagen I and II, and elastin.
    i. Collagens serve as structural framework
    ii. Elastin affects the compliance of skin
c. Mechanical creep refers to the increased skin length that occurs when force is applied to approximate skin edges, which is a result of reorientation of collagen and elastin fibers.
d. Biologic creep or stress relaxation is the decrease in tension of expanded or lengthened skin that occurs when chronic stretching force is applied, which is a result in alteration of the physiology of skin.
e. Phases of wound healing:
    i. Inflammatory: starts immediately after injury and lasts between 4 and 10 days. Characterized by neutrophils which secrete acute phase cytokines, platelets which activate the extrinsic coagulation cascade causing fibrin formation, and macrophages which play a role in phagocytosis and recruitment of keratinocytes, fibroblasts, and angiogenesis.
    ii. Proliferative: starts on the third day and lasts 2 weeks. Keratinocytes migrate to the wound margin and begin proliferation to aid in reepithelialization. Granulation tissue replaces fibrin clot and serves as a scaffolding for cell migration. Fibroblasts produce type I and III collagen along with other extracellular matrix proteins. Growth factors are produced to aid in angiogenesis.
    iii. Remodeling: begins around the third week lasts up to 1 to 2 years. Type III collagen gradually becomes replaced by type I. Lymphocytes predominate cell type.
f. Wound tensile strength:
    i. 1 week: 3%
    ii. 3 weeks: 20%
    iii. 12 months: 80%

Grafts

a. Rely on recipient bed for survival which may include fat, muscle, perichondrium/periosteum, and fascia.
b. To best facilitate graft take one should:
    i. Effectively immobilize the graft relative to the recipient by use of bolsters, quilting stitches, or negative pressure wound vacs.
    ii. Avoid hematoma and other fluid accumulations that could serve as a barrier between the recipient bed and the graft.
        1. Accomplished most often through slits in the graft ("pie holes") to allow egress of fluid from the wound bed
    iii. Avoid infection.
c. Split-thickness skin graft (STSG)
    i. Harvested from large surface areas using dermatome. Includes entire thickness of epidermis and variable levels of dermis, resulting in thin, medium, and thick grafts

ii. Usual thickness varies from 0.012 to 0.016 in. Thinner grafts have less metabolic demand and exhibit more reliable neovascularization, but experience more contracture than thicker grafts.
iii. Wound care at the donor site should promote re-epithelization which occurs most quickly when the wound is kept moist. This can be accomplished with an occlusive semipermeable dressing that keeps the exudate in contact with the wound.
iv. Typical healing of skin graft:
  1. Plasma imbibition: 24 to 48 hours. Characterized by diffusion of nutrients from recipient bed
  2. Inosculation: 48 hours. Capillaries from recipient bed establish connection with capillaries from skin graft.
  3. Neovascularization: 3 to 7 days. New vessel growth into skin graft
v. Disadvantages include color and texture match and graft contracture.

d. Full-thickness skin graft (FTSG)
  i. Donor sites include postauricular and preauricular skin, upper eyelid, supraclavicular neck, and nasolabial region.
  ii. Graft is defatted, and donor site is closed primarily.
  iii. Appropriate for small (1-5 cm), visible facial defects (nasal dorsum, nasal tip).
  iv. Donor site morbidity is lower than STSG.
e. Cartilage grafts
  i. Reconstruction of the ear and nose frequently requires grafting with cartilage to restore structural support.
  ii. Can augment nasal dorsum, modify the nasal tip, address internal and external valve collapse, and much more.
f. Septal cartilage grafts
  i. Care must be taken to leave 1 to 1.5 cm caudal and dorsal struts when harvesting septal cartilage to maintain support of the nasal dorsum and tip.
g. Auricular cartilage grafts
  i. Typically harvested from the conchal bowl with no cosmetic deficit.
  ii. Composite grafts include cartilage and skin which can be used for complex defects of the nose that require structure and lining or external skin replacement
  iii. Composite grafts up to 1.5 cm may be used, but grafts 1 cm or less in diameter are more apt to survive.
h. Costal cartilage grafts
  i. Straight segments of the sixth to the eighth ribs are used for nasal dorsal reconstruction defects (eg, saddle nose deformity).
  ii. Curved and straight segments of the sixth through the eighth ribs (use of lower ribs is also described) are used for auricular reconstruction (significant tissue replacement as in microtia reconstruction).
  iii. Precise and balanced carving is central to preventing warping of cartilage over time.
i. Bone grafts
  i. Free bone grafts can be sculpted to fill donor defects. However, all free bone grafts are scaffolds that are replaced by mesenchymal cells that differentiate into osteoblasts. This limits the size and thickness of free bone grafts due to need for vascular invasion. Resorption is a common problem, and cortical bone grafts must be rigidly immobilized to reduce the incidence of this complication
j. Cortical free bone grafts
  i. Common harvest sites
    1. Split calvarium
    2. Split rib
    3. Iliac crest

ii. Applications
1. Nasal dorsal augmentation
2. Posttraumatic reconstruction of facial buttresses
3. Grafting gaps in the maxilla from large advancements (as in LeFort I advancement)
4. Orbital reconstruction (posttraumatic or after ablative surgery)
5. Mandibular reconstruction (nonirradiated field where complete mucosal coverage is possible)

k. Cancellous bone grafts
i. More quickly vascularized than cortical bone due to high concentration of osteocytes
ii. Have no structural integrity, so cannot be used for load-bearing
iii. Harvest sites
1. Iliac crest
2. Tibia
iv. Applications
1. Repair of segmental mandibular defects up to 5 cm with a bone cage or packed around a titanium fracture plate with tight mucosal closure
2. Alveolar bone grafting in cleft lip and palate
3. Frontal sinus obliteration

l. Nerve grafts
i. Nerve interposition grafts in head and neck reconstruction are primarily used for facial reanimation.
ii. Common donor sites include
1. Greater auricular nerve, which is often in the operative field and therefore easy to harvest
iii. Medial antebrachial cutaneous nerve
iv. Sural nerve (the longest graft available yielding up to 25-30 cm of length)
v. Nerve to vastus lateralis is often available during harvest of anterolateral thigh flap

Local Skin Flaps

a. Also termed random pattern flaps because they are based upon the subdermal plexus and do not have a dominant vascular supply.
b. Superior color match and texture to skin grafts.
c. Flap design considerations:
i. Mechanical properties of skin.
ii. Skin is anisotropic, meaning that its mechanical properties vary with direction.
iii. Relaxed skin tension lines (RSTLs) are lines of minimal tension, whereas lines of maximal tension are perpendicular to the RSTLs. Flaps should be designed to move in ways that minimize tension by placing flap incisions parallel to RSTLs. A traditional length-to-width ratio of 3:1 or less is used to ensure adequate flap perfusion.
iv. Aging skin is less elastic than younger skin with less ability to recoil when stretched. Elastosis that characterizes aging skin accounts for ptosis with age.
d. Commonly used designs include advancement, rotation, bilobed, island transposition, and rhomboid transposition flaps (Figure 56-1).
e. Excess tension and smoking (which causes vessel narrowing, endothelial injury, and poor oxygen-carrying capacity of red blood cells) have a negative impact on the success of flaps.

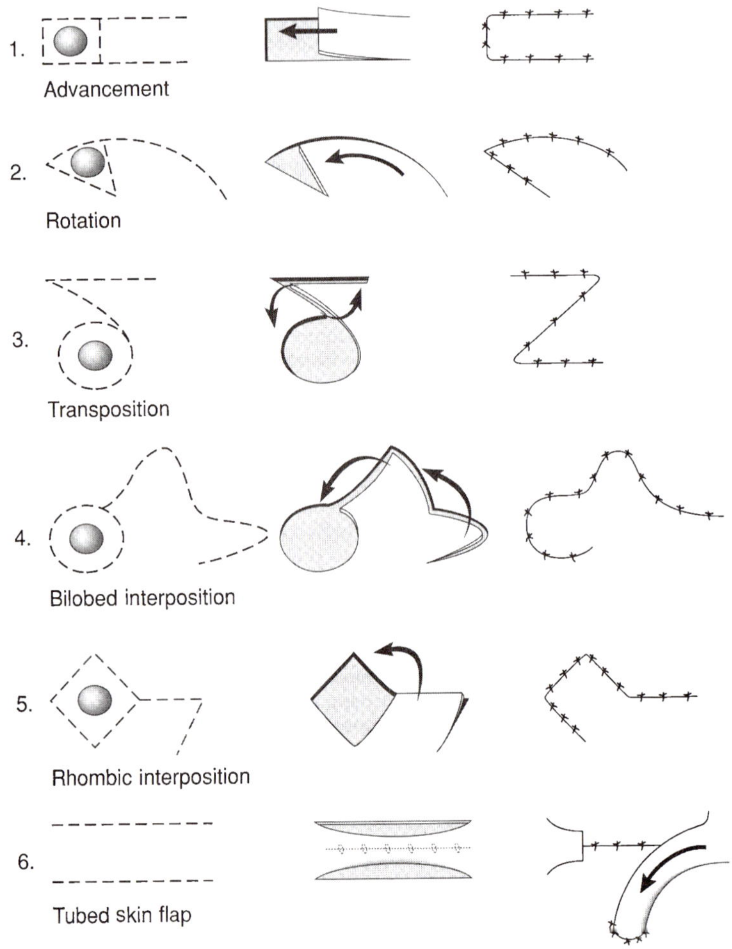

Figure 56-1 Six common local skin flaps.

Regional Flaps

a. These flaps are generally axial-pattern flaps, fasciocutaneous, or myocutaneous.
b. Paramedian forehead flap
   i. Based on the supratrochlear artery
   ii. Used in the reconstruction of nasal defects, including those that extend to the upper lip and medial cheek
c. Temporoparietal fascia flap
   i. Based on branches of the superficial temporal artery
   ii. Used as vascularized tissue bed for STSGs used in auricular, forehead, and periorbital reconstruction
   iii. May also be used for skull base reconstruction

d. Palatal island flap (buccal myomucosal flap)
   i. Based on greater palatine artery
   ii. Use for defects of the central palate, or defects of the central palate including the maxillary alveolus posterior to but not including the canine teeth
e. Temporalis flap
   i. Muscle flap based on the deep temporal artery
   ii. Used for facial reanimation, primarily in the lower face
f. Pectoralis major flap
   i. Based on the pectoral branch of the thoracoacromial artery.
   ii. Ease of dissection and versatility make this a workhorse flap with many applications.
   iii. This flap can reach as superiorly as the hard palate and superior helix. It is suitable for reconstruction of facial, oral, and pharyngeal defects below this level. It may be transferred into the neck to provide coverage of the ipsilateral carotid artery.
   iv. To transfer a thinner flap without overlying skin and subcutaneous tissue, the muscle with its overlying fascia may be transferred and then skin grafted.
   v. The flap may be tubed on itself for pharyngoesophageal reconstruction.
g. Trapezius system of flaps
   i. *Lateral island* flap
      1. Dependent on identification of a transverse cervical artery and vein that are coursing under the anterior border of the trapezius muscle and not intertwined in the branches of the brachial plexus
      2. Used to reconstruct defects of the lateral scalp, neck, and cheek
   ii. *Lower island* flap
      1. Two major pedicles include the transverse cervical artery and the dorsal scapular artery.
      2. Used for delivery of skin to the lateral scalp, neck, and cheek.
      3. It has the widest arc of rotation of the trapezius flaps.
   iii. *Superior trapezius* flap
      1. Based on paraspinous perforating branches of the intercostal vessels
      2. Used for reconstruction of the lateral neck and lower cheek
h. Latissimus dorsi flap
   i. Based on the thoracodorsal artery
   ii. Broad, thin muscle that may be transposed into the head and neck either subcutaneously or via a transaxillary approach
   iii. Used to reconstruct the lateral neck and scalp
i. Supraclavicular flap
   i. Based on supraclavicular artery branching of the transverse cervical artery
   ii. Used in reconstruction of the cutaneous neck, pharynx, trachea, parotid, and more
j. Deltopectoral flap
   i. Based on the superior most internal mammary perforators
   ii. Used in reconstruction of the cutaneous neck, pharynx, trachea, and more
k. Internal mammary artery perforator (IMAP) flap
   i. Evolution of the deltopectoral flap that is harvested based upon a single perforator from the internal mammary artery.
   ii. Indications are similar, and donor site morbidity is improved.

Free Microvascular Tissue Transfer Overview

a. Microvascular free tissue transfer is the reconstructive method that most closely replaces missing tissue.
b. The "free flap" is also to some extent free of the geometric limitations imposed by pedicles.

c. The use of microvascular free tissue transfer in the past three decades has decreased the incidence of partial flap loss and dehiscence seen in other pedicled flaps.
d. Offers significant functional and cosmetic improvement over previously available techniques in reconstruction of composite defects.
e. Possible tissue combinations include fascia, skin, fat, muscle, nerve, and/or bone.
f. Points of technique
    i. Previous treatment may affect the availability of recipient vessels, and these patients should be considered for preoperative head and neck vessel imaging.
    ii. Patients who do not have recipient vessels within the reach of the defect should be consented for vein grafts.
    iii. The external jugular vein should be preserved when possible as a potential recipient vein or vein graft.
    iv. Major arteries and veins that are to be sacrificed should be handled with care and transected some distance from their takeoffs to leave a stump for anastomosis.
    v. Enteric, muscle, and bone-containing free flaps are the most sensitive to ischemia time.
    vi. Complete dissection of the flap in situ, as well as preparation of the recipient vessels should be performed prior to pedicle transection to decrease ischemia time.
    vii. Attention to detail in flap design and insetting (pedicle geometry, tension, and kinking) should minimize the risk of vascular compromise.
g. Avoiding complications
    i. Most failures occur within 72 hours of revascularization, hence the need for vigilant monitoring.
    ii. Vessel wall dissection, disruption, and suture puncture result in endothelial discontinuity and exposure of thrombogenic subendothelial collagen.
    iii. This forms the basis for use of postoperative aspirin or heparin after revascularization to prevent thrombus formation at the anastomotic site.
    iv. Perfusion is maintained through maintenance of normal blood pressures and euvolemia.
    v. Maintenance of normothermia will minimize peripheral vasoconstriction and sympathetic outflow which are deleterious to microvascular blood flow.

Fascial and Fasciocutaneous Free Flaps

a. Temporoparietal fascia free flap
    i. Based on the superficial temporal vessels.
    ii. The temporoparietal fascia, with or without overlying skin, may be transferred as a free flap.
    iii. Split calvarial bone may be harvested with this flap to create a composite flap.
    iv. Disadvantages:
        1. Small caliber donor vessels.
        2. Superficial vessels (vein more than artery), making them vulnerable during flap harvest.
        3. Risk of injury to the frontal branch of the facial nerve.
        4. Risk of alopecia.
b. Parascapular/Scapular free flap
    i. Based on the transverse or descending cutaneous branches of the circumflex scapular artery
        1. Parascapular flap is based with the long axis of the flap vertically utilizing the descending cutaneous branch.
        2. Scapular flap is based with the long axis of the flap horizontally utilizing the transverse cutaneous branch.

ii. Provides a large cutaneous donor site that closes primarily
iii. The transverse and descending branches can each supply separate skin paddles allowing for a chimeric fasciocutaneous flap
iv. May be harvested in addition to other components of the subscapular system as part of a "Mega Flap"
v. Disadvantages:
1. Relatively short vascular pedicle, difficult to dissect full extent of subscapular length
2. Patient position can be challenging and must allow for exposure of adequate surface of the back

c. Lateral arm free flap
i. Based on the posterior branches of the radial collateral vessels.
ii. Perforators are transferred to the skin through the lateral intermuscular (brachialis-brachioradialis-triceps) septum.
iii. Sensate capabilities are provided by the posterior cutaneous nerve of the forearm and the posterior cutaneous nerve of the arm.
iv. Transfer of a portion of the humerus has been described with this flap.
v. Donor site may be closed primarily.
vi. Skin and subcutaneous tissues of the arm in this area are thicker and less pliable than the forearm.
vii. Skin in this area is the best color match for facial skin of all the free flaps.
viii. Disadvantages:
1. Pedicle dissection is more difficult than that of the forearm flap.
2. Pedicle is shorter and of smaller caliber than that of the forearm flap.
3. Lateral arm numbness.

d. Radial forearm free flap
i. Based on radial artery and its associated venae comitans or cephalic vein.
ii. Fascial or fasciocutaneous design based on the long, large-caliber radial vessels.
iii. Fasciocutaneous vessels are transmitted to the skin paddle via the lateral intermuscular septum.
iv. Sensate capabilities are provided by the lateral and medial antebrachial cutaneous nerves.
v. Versatility, pliability, and dependability make this a workhorse flap with multiple applications.
vi. Absence of a complete palmar arch precludes use of this flap, so a preoperative Allen's test must be performed to ascertain palmar arch integrity.
vii. This flap may include a monocortical segment of the radius by incorporating a cuff of the flexor pollicis longus muscle.
1. Immediate plating (load sharing) of the radial defect is required to allow faster return to function and decrease risk of pathologic fracture.
2. The segment of bone that may be harvested with this flap is inadequate for osseointegrated implants.
viii. Disadvantage:
1. Cosmetic deformity at donor site with fasciocutaneous flap harvest (forearm tendons are grafted with a STSG).
2. Potential numbness along distribution of superficial radial nerve
3. Can impact grip strength

e. Ulnar forearm free flap
i. Based on ulnar artery and its associated venae comitans or cephalic vein
ii. Indications and uses are similar to the radial forearm free flap; however, advantages of the ulnar include virtually hairless flap, and less obvious donor site as it lies on the proximal ulnar aspect of the forearm.

  - iii. Disadvantages
    1. Cosmetic deformity at donor site with fasciocutaneous flap harvest (forearm tendons are grafted with a STSG).
    2. Potential numbness along distribution of branches of ulnar nerve
    3. Can impact grip strength
- f. Thoracodorsal artery perforator (TDAP) flap
  - i. Based on a musculocutaneous perforator from the thoracodorsal artery
  - ii. Provides fasciocutaneous or musculocutaneous tissue depending on whether the latissimus muscle is included in the flap or if the overlying skin is separated from the muscle, and the perforator is dissected through the latissimus muscle
  - iii. Provides a thin, malleable flap for reconstruction
  - iv. Donor site closed primarily
  - v. Disadvantages
    1. Limited pedicle length as dissection of proximal thoracodorsal to subscapular artery is difficult
- g. Anterolateral thigh free flap
  - i. Based on the branches of the lateral circumflex femoral artery, most often the descending branch
  - ii. May be harvested as a fasciocutaneous, or musculofasciocutaneous flap including the vastus lateralis
  - iii. Sensate capability provided by lateral femoral cutaneous nerve.
  - iv. Versatility allows for multiple skin and/or muscle paddles to be harvested for complex defects.
  - v. Subcutaneous tissues may be trimmed to make the skin paddle(s) more pliable.
  - vi. Relatively inconspicuous donor site.
  - vii. Disadvantage:
    1. Variable pedicle anatomy.
    2. Bulk of flap, therefore, patient selection is a key component of the decision-making process
- h. Medial thigh free flap
  - i. Based on the septocutaneous perforators of the profunda femoris vessels.
  - ii. Sensate capability provided by lateral femoral cutaneous nerve
  - iii. Flap is less pliable than forearm flap due to thicker subcutaneous tissue but may be tubed.
  - iv. Disadvantages:
    1. Difficult pedicle dissection
    2. Variable pedicle anatomy
    3. Thickness of flap correlates with patient's body habitus
    4. Risk to nutrient artery of the femur, which is a branch of the second perforator of the profunda femoris
- i. Medial sural artery perforator (MSAP) flap
  - i. Based on perforator vessels from the either the medial or lateral branch of the medial sural artery
  - ii. Thin, pliable tissue
  - iii. Long vascular pedicle
  - iv. Potential for minimally hair-bearing skin
  - v. Pedicle requires dissection through the gastrocnemius, but preserves the majority of the muscle
  - vi. Defects of 6 cm or less can be closed primarily

1. Disadvantages
   a. Variable perforator anatomy
   b. Too much disruption of gastrocnemius can affect gait
   c. Not ideal for large defects as width should not exceed 6 cm

Muscular and Myocutaneous Flaps

a. Anterolateral thigh flap
   i. See above description
b. Latissimus dorsi free flap
   i. Based on the branches of the thoracodorsal artery to latissimus muscle.
   ii. May be harvested as a muscle only or myocutaneous flap based on the thoracodorsal artery.
   iii. The muscle component of this flap is broad and thin, making it a pliable flap that is easy to contour to defects.
   iv. The thoracodorsal artery is a branch of the subscapular artery, so the latissimus dorsi may be harvested as part of a "Mega Flap" based on the subscapular artery and incorporating the scapular tip, lateral border, parascapular skin island, and/or scapular skin island free flaps.
   v. Portion of the serratus muscle can also be incorporated if branches to the serratus muscle are preserved.
c. Rectus abdominus free flap
   i. Based on the inferior epigastric vascular pedicle.
   ii. May be harvested as a muscle only or myocutaneous flap.
   iii. Perforator flap designs allow harvesting of skin and subcutaneous flap, sparing the muscle (and avoiding abdominal wall weakness).
   iv. May be designed with several different orientations of the skin paddle
   v. Flap is less pliable than forearm flap due to thicker subcutaneous tissue, but may be tubed.
   vi. Disadvantages:
      1. Abdominal wall weakness resulting from muscle harvest is possible.
      2. Thickness of flap correlates with the patient's body habitus.
d. Gracilis free flap
   i. Muscle flap based on the terminal branch of the adductor artery, a branch of the profunda femoris.
   ii. Motor capability provided by the anterior branch of the obturator nerve.
   iii. Relatively inconspicuous donor site is closed primarily with minimal functional deficit.
   iv. A skin paddle can be transferred with this muscle, but the musculocutaneous perforators are variable and sometimes absent.
   v. Applications:
      1. Primary application is facial reanimation due to capacity for motor innervation.
      2. Disadvantage is bulk of the flap.

Osseous and Osteocutaneous Free Flaps

a. Osteocutaneous radial forearm free flap
   i. See above description
b. Fibular free flap
   i. Based on the peroneal artery and associated venae comitans.
   ii. May be transferred as a bone-only or osteocutaneous flap.

iii. Skin component perfused by septocutaneous and musculocutaneous vessels transmitted via the posterior crural septum.
iv. Sensate capability provided by lateral sural cutaneous nerve.
v. Absence of anterior tibial vessels (peroneal arteria magna) or involvement of the anterior tibial vessels with severe atherosclerotic disease precludes the use of this flap, so preoperative vessel imaging (CT angiogram or MRA) is necessary.
vi. Disadvantages:
 1. The anatomy of the skin perforators is variable.
 2. A STSG is occasionally needed to resurface the donor site in larger reconstructions.
 3. Transient ankle stiffness frequently occurs after flap harvest.

c. Iliac crest free flap
 i. Composite flap consisting of skin, subcutaneous tissue, internal oblique muscle, and iliac crest is based on the deep circumflex iliac artery.
 ii. Simultaneous harvest without patient repositioning allows for two-team approach.
 iii. Relatively inconspicuous donor site.
 iv. Disadvantages:
  1. Volume of tissue and lack of rotation of soft tissue component with respect to osseous component can make inset of this flap difficult.
  2. Significant donor site morbidities can include chronic pain and gait disturbance.
  3. Risk of hernia.

d. Osseous scapular free flaps
 i. Based on the angular branch of the thoracodorsal (scapular tip) or the peroneal branch of the circumflex scapular artery (lateral border), which are the two branches of the subscapular artery.
 ii. Soft tissue components discussed previously (see above).
 iii. Separation of the soft tissue and bone flaps is possible, allowing the most freedom of rotation for three-dimensional insetting of any composite free flap.
 iv. Relatively inconspicuous donor site with improved donor site morbidity compared to other osseous flaps.
 v. Disadvantages:
  1. Bone stock is thin and not adequate for osseointegrated implants
  2. Variable vascular anatomy
  3. Division of the teres major is necessary for pedicle dissection, and this may weaken the shoulder girdle
  4. Potential for brachial plexus injury

Visceral Free Flaps

a. Jejunal free flap
 i. Based on mesenteric arcade vessels.
 ii. May be transferred as a tubed interposition graft for segmental pharyngoesophageal reconstruction, or an open "patch graft."
 iii. Transfers a secretary mucosal surface, which is useful in cases of previous irradiation.
 iv. Flap must be inset isoperistaltically.
 v. A "sentinel loop" of "test intestine" may be developed and brought out through the neck incision for monitoring.
 vi. Disadvantages:
  1. Need for laparotomy and enteric anastomosis.
  2. Two enteric anastomoses are needed in the neck.

3. The risk of anastomotic stricture is high.
4. Risk of intrathoracic anastomotic leak.
5. A feeding jejunostomy is required.
6. The mesenteric vessels are known for their friability and tendency toward intimal separation.
7. Postoperative dysphagia caused by peristalsis that is not coordinated with native pharyngeal swallowing mechanism.
8. Poor vocal result with tracheoesophageal puncture.
9. Significant possible donor site morbidity (prolonged ileus, abdominal adhesions).

Facial Reanimation Principles

a. Patients with facial paralysis may experience diminished eye protection, nasal obstruction, difficulty with mastication, articulation, and loss of facial expression and functional losses which can lead to social and psychological isolation.
b. Reconstructive goals include the restoration of facial symmetry, amelioration of functional deficits and the return of volitional and spontaneous, emotion driven facial movements.
c. Several factors determine the type and timing of procedures to restore facial function:
    i. The etiology of the paralysis
    ii. The site of lesion
    iii. The duration of paralysis
    iv. The severity of the paralysis (complete vs incomplete)
    v. Integrity of the nerve
d. When the facial nerve is intact (Bell's palsy, Ramsay-Hunt syndrome, after vestibular schwannoma resection) the patient is observed and monitored for recovery.
    i. If uncertainty as to the integrity of the nerve exists, as in the case of temporal bone trauma, exploration is necessary.
e. Traumatic and iatrogenic transections of the facial nerve should be repaired by neurorrhaphy with or without interposition grafting, at the time of injury to optimize the chances of recovery.
f. Interposition grafting is indicated when the distance between healthy cut ends of the nerve is 1 cm or more because excessive mobilization of the nerve leads to devascularization.
    i. Common donor nerves include the greater auricular nerve, the median antebrachial cutaneous nerve, and the sural nerve which provides up to 25 cm of length.
g. When planned resection of the nerve is necessary as part of oncologic surgery, strategies for reanimation should be anticipated and implemented at the time of resection, if possible (with priority on procedures to protect the eye).
h. In general, peripheral nerve injuries distal (medial) to the pupillary line are not repaired due to sufficient neural anastomoses in the midface.
i. One year of observation is the often-cited cut-off, after which time irreversible muscle atrophy may occur, eliminating nerve re-innervation as an option for reanimation.
    i. Long-standing cases of facial paralysis (more than 1 year) are characterized by fibrosis of nerve tubules, which hampers axon regeneration.
    ii. Muscle atrophy also occurs due to denervation and is irreversible after 2 to 3 years.
    iii. In patients with an intact facial nerve and complete paralysis, a balance must be struck between allowing adequate time for potential recovery and a prolonged surveillance period where irreversible muscle atrophy occurs.
    iv. The right balance avoids premature or unneeded procedures and avoids the development of irreversible muscle changes that can only be salvaged with muscle transfers.

Nerve Transposition

a. Donor nerves are used to power the distal facial nerve when recovery in an intact nerve has not occurred or when the proximal stump of the nerve is not available for neurorrhaphy.
b. Options include input from the contralateral intact facial nerve or an ipsilateral cranial nerve.
c. The donor nerve can be sutured to the distal facial nerve main trunk or to select distal branches (buccal branches and zygomatic branches prioritized to restore smile and eye closure).
d. Cross facial nerve grafting (CFNG)
    i. Indications:
        1. Sufficient proximal motor input is lacking.
        2. Muscle atrophy has not yet occurred.
        3. One or more peripheral branches of the facial nerve is accessible on the affected side.
    ii. Considered the "gold standard" nerve input option—successful reconstruction allows the patient spontaneous, coordinated facial movements with expression of emotion.
    iii. Buccal branches of contralateral facial nerve are cut and coapted to a sural nerve graft which is tunneled across the upper lip. The distal end of the sural nerve graft is tagged.
    iv. 8 to 9 months are needed for axonal growth across the nerve graft. Axonal growth across the graft is determined by a progressing Tinel sign. The second stage is then performed coapting the nerve graft to a corresponding buccal branch on the paralyzed side.
    v. Disadvantages:
        1. Less powerful movements because of the limited number of axons available for reinnervation and two coaptation sites.
        2. Multiple stages and a prolonged time course before results are seen.
        3. Donor site morbidity can result in paresis of the "intact" side of the face.
        4. Muscle denervation continues during the time required for axonal growth across the face which could result in irreversible atrophy.
        5. Options to keep nerve stimulation to the recipient muscle must often be performed during the period between stages one and two. The term "babysitter" procedure describes the use of other ipsilateral nerve transfers to maintain nerve stimulation to facial muscles on the side of paralysis during this interval.
e. Nerve substitutions
    i. Indications are the same as those for cross-facial nerve grafting. Nerve substitutions can be used as the definitive nerve input to the distal facial nerve or serve as a "way station" along a multistaged reconstructive approach.
    ii. Facial movements result from activation of the donor cranial nerve. Mass movements may occur depending on site of repair (main trunk vs distal nerves).
    iii. Emotional expression is usually not a characteristic of this type of reanimation.
    iv. With cross-facial nerve grafting considered the "gold standard" (coordinated, emotional movements) ipsilateral nerve substitutions can serve as an intermediate procedure to prevent muscle atrophy during the 8 to 9 months when axonal regeneration occurs across the nerve grafts.
    v. The nerve substitution (12-7 or 5-7) can be performed at the same setting as the cross-facial nerve grafts.
        1. The hypoglossal-facial nerve transposition has been commonly used since initial descriptions in the late 1970s.
        2. In original descriptions the hypoglossal nerve is transected just before entering the tongue, transposed under the digastric, and sutured to the facial nerve main trunk.

3. The technique evolved to avoid hemitongue denervation and atrophy. The hypoglossal nerve can be partially transected, and an interposition graft (jump graft) connects the transected portion of the hypoglossal nerve to the facial nerve.
4. The masseteric nerve transfer is being utilized increasingly, based on several advantages the technique offers compared to the XII-VII transfer.
5. The masseteric nerve is a distal branch of the motor branch of CNV found along a line that bisects the angle between the zygomatic arch superiorly, the condyle posteriorly. The nerve has 2 to 3 branches.
6. Proximity to the ipsilateral facial nerve branches allows for nerve transposition that often does not require an interposition graft. This and the lack of two suture lines allow faster recovery of movement compared to 12-7 transposition.
7. Morbidity considered more acceptable than the hypoglossal-facial substitution.
8. Results:
   a. Movement seen after 6 to 12 months (longer recovery in 12-7 patients than 5-7 patients)
   b. Synkinesis can occur in many patients.
   c. Spontaneous, reflexive facial movements rarely achieved.
9. Other historic nerve substitutions:
   a. Spinal accessory-facial substitution
   b. Ansa hypoglossi-facial substitution

vi. At the second stage, the nerve grafts can be inset replacing the ipsilateral nerve substitution, or can be coapted to distal nerve branches, leaving the ipsilateral nerve substitution in place for "double innervation." This combination would allow spontaneous expression with no interruption in any facial tone and movements endowed by the nerve substitution.

Neuromuscular Pedicle Transfer

a. Indicated in cases of irreversible facial nerve paralysis (muscle atrophy), unsuccessful cross facial grafting, or if extratemporal facial nerve is not intact.
b. Can be powered by a CFGN which would be done as a first stage, followed by harvesting and inset of the muscle flap with coaptation of the nerve grafts to the nerve of the flap as a second stage.
c. After clinical evidence of arrival of nerve fibers to contralateral side, the microsurgical transfer of a muscle with its motor nerve is performed.
d. Can also be powered by ipsilateral cranial nerve with the masseteric nerve being an excellent option. This allows the muscle graft to be performed in one stage with microvascular and microneural anastomoses at one setting.
e. The muscle is inset from the zygomatic arch to the oral commissure on the affected side to reanimate the lower face.
f. The gold standard is the Gracilis muscle with anterior branch of the obturator nerve.
g. Other muscles described in muscle transfer:
   i. Serratus or latissimus dorsi muscle with the subscapular, long thoracic nerve
   ii. Pectoralis major muscle with the medial and lateral pectoral nerves
   iii. Abductor hallucis with a branch of the medial plantar nerve
   iv. Internal oblique with intercostal and infracostal neurovascular pedicles
   v. Trapezius muscle with its branch of the spinal accessory nerve
h. Disadvantages:
   i. Need for multiple stages
   ii. Ancillary procedures are needed for upper facial reanimation.

Muscle Transposition

a. Indications are the same as those for neuromuscular pedicle transfer.
b. Also indicated in patients who cannot or choose not to undergo neuromuscular pedicle transfer.
c. Traditional muscle transfer transposes the central third of the temporalis muscle 180 degrees over the zygomatic arch, insetting it into the oral commissure.
   i. By biting and activating the muscle, the patient accomplishes excursion of the commissure
   ii. Disadvantages
      1. Long scalp incision required
      2. Muscle bulge over the zygomatic arch
d. Results in elevation of the oral commissure occur in most patients at rest.

Static Procedures

a. Static procedures are useful adjuncts in the management of facial paralysis
b. Static slings
   i. Indications are the same as those for muscle transposition
   ii. Provide elevation of the oral commissure without volitional movement
   iii. Common materials used:
      1. Fascia lata
      2. Acellular dermal allograft
      3. Expanded Polytetrafluoroethylene (ePTFE)
c. Periorbital procedures
   i. Eye lubrication is critical-artificial tears frequently during the day; ocular lubricant and eyelid taping at night.
   ii. Browlift may be indicated to treat brow ptosis resulting in obstruction of lateral visual fields.
   iii. Upper eyelid loading-Gold or platinum *implants* are placed in the upper eyelid to correct lagophthalmos. Inability to close the eye can result in corneal drying, ulceration, and vision disturbances.
   iv. Canthoplasty procedures elevate lax lower eyelids and aid in efficiency of tear collection along with improved eye closure.
   v. Tarsorrhaphy may be indicated in severe cases of lagophthalmos when more conservative approaches are inadequate in preventing drying of the cornea.
d. Rhinoplasty
   i. Nasal obstruction may result from external valvular collapse from paralysis of the dilator naris muscle.
   ii. Rhinoplasty techniques such as alar battens or nasal valve suspension can improve airway patency.

Synkinesis

a. A late finding in patients with recovery after facial paralysis. Defined as mass movements of the face from aberrant re-innervation after facial paresis/paralysis.
b. A common finding is ocular-oral synkinesis (movement of the oral commissure during eye closure). Patients may also have platysmal involvement causing neck pain.
c. Hyperkinesis can also result in hypertonicity of certain muscle groups.
   i. Hyperkinesis of the orbicularis oris results in partial eye closure and narrowed palpebral fissure width.
d. Hyperkinesis of the midfacial muscles results in deepening of the nasolabial fold.
e. Patients may have regions of hypertonicity and regions of flaccidity.

f. Mainstays of treatment are botulinum toxin injection of hypertonic muscle groups, including orbicularis oris, mentalis, platysma on the affected side and DAO and frontalis on the contralateral side for improved facial symmetry.
g. Physical therapy exercises and massage.

Prosthetic Reconstruction

Prosthetic reconstruction complements surgical techniques in cases of major orofacial defects. Osseointegrated implants typically form the anchor for facial prostheses. Because these implants require good bone stock for stability, the importance of providing a platform for osseointegrated implants is paramount. In the case of palatal reconstruction, residual dentition can form the basis for anchoring of a prosthetic piece. Other requirements include healthy soft tissue around the implant posts, and therefore an implant site with soft tissue that is thin enough that the posts do not become buried, but robust enough to prevent exposure of the abutments. This may require thinning of subcutaneous tissues over the abutments. Patient compliance with care of the implants is necessary to prevent infection. In addition to auricular prostheses, craniofacial implants are used to improve cosmesis in patients with orbital and nasal defects, often using eyeglasses as a camouflage.

Future Trends

Composite facial allotransplantation is currently in the experimental phase and offers an opportunity for restoration of appearance and function for patients with severe disfigurement when other reconstructive options have failed or are limited. Cosmetic results are immediate, but there is a paucity of data on functional outcomes. Early acute rejection has been reported in several cases of facial transplantation, infections, and lymphoproliferative disorders resulting from immunosuppression and malignancies have been reported following facial allotransplantation with some fatalities. Reluctance to consent to donation by patient families has limited the availability of facial allotransplants. Other issues surrounding this method of facial reconstruction include the need for lifelong immunosuppression, patient selection, donor and recipient confidentiality, and cost to society. Functional outcome studies on facial allotransplantation will inform the risk-to-benefit ratio of these procedures.

Ongoing advances in tissue engineering of osseous, adipose, cartilaginous, and neural tissues hold promise for the development of customized tissues that can be transferred with little to no donor site morbidity. The ability to use software programs to model osseous defects from CT scan imaging allows for the construction of custom implants, rigid plating, and guides for contouring osseous free flaps which enhance precision and decrease operative time. These technologies coupled with intraoperative navigation can enhance the accuracy of complex craniofacial trauma reconstruction and reduce the need for revision surgery.

Bibliography

Blackwell KE. Unsurpassed reliability of free flaps for head and neck reconstruction. *Arch Otolaryngol Head Neck Surg*. 1999;125:295-299.

Butts SC, Harris S. Physiology of skin grafts and local flaps. In: *Sataloff's Comprehensive Textbook of Otolaryngology Head and Neck Surgery, Facial Plastic and Reconstructive Surgery*. Volume 3. Jaypee Brothers Medical Publishers; New Delhi, 2016:37-46.

Cummings CW. *Cummings Otolaryngology—Head and Neck Surgery*. 7th ed. (Flint PW, ed.). Elsevier/Saunders; 2021:Chapters 77-78, 1085-1118.

Ein L, Hadlock TA. Facial reanimation. In: *BJ. Bailey, Head & Neck Surgery—Otolaryngology*. 6th ed. Lippincott Williams & Wilkins; Philadelphia, 2022.

Questions

1. At 1 week following primary closure of an incision, what is the expected wound tensile strength?
   A. 3%
   B. 20%
   C. 50%
   D. 80%

2. A patient who developed Ramsay-Hunt syndrome and has had a HB VI facial nerve paralysis now for 18 months (since symptom onset). EMG shows electrical silence. The patient wants to restore movement and symmetry of the lower face—what reconstructive option would be best for this patient?
   A. 12-7 jump graft to the facial nerve trunk
   B. Static sling to elevate the commissure using fascia lata
   C. Cross facial nerve grafting
   D. Gracillis free flap powered by CN V (masseteric nerve)**

3. Which of the following statements about skin grafts is incorrect?
   A. They heal well over the fat, muscle, perichondrium, and fascia.
   B. The three phases of skin graft healing are plasma imbibition, inosculation, and neovascularization.
   C. They require immobilization and avoidance of shear to take.
   D. The thinner the graft, the greater the likelihood of take but the greater the risk of contracture.
   E. They depend on formation of a hematoma for survival.**

4. Which of the following correctly indicates the vascular supply of the scapular tip from proximal to distal?
   A. Subscapular artery > axillary artery > thoracodorsal artery > angular artery
   B. Axillary artery > subscapular artery > thoracodorsal artery > angular artery**
   C. Axillary artery > circumflex scapular artery > thoracodorsal artery > periosteal branches
   D. Subscapular artery > thoracodorsal artery > circumflex scapular artery > angular artery

5. Which of the following flaps can be harvested with an associated sensory nerve, thus potentially providing sensate properties?
   A. Radial forearm free flap**
   B. Latissimus free flap
   C. MSAP flap
   D. Parascapular flap
   E. Pectoralis flap

Chapter 57
Facial and Orbital Trauma

Facial Trauma May Consist of

- Soft tissue injuries, such as lacerations
- Visceral injuries, such as injuries to the eyes, brain, salivary glands and ducts, nerves, and blood vessels
- Bony injuries to the facial skeleton—such as injuries to the craniomaxillofacial skeleton are the focus of this chapter

Goals of Bony Facial Trauma Management:

- Restore function
- Restore form—repair cosmetic defects with a thoughtful approach that minimizes scar from the intervention

Principles

- Face is designed in such a way that trauma is less likely to impact critical structures such as the eye and brain.
  - The nose, an anterior projection of the face, often takes the brunt of the impact.
  - Sinuses act as "crumple zones" to protect the brain from force.
  - Thinner bones of the orbit's floor and medial wall absorb forces, protecting against globe rupture.
- Understanding suture lines and bony structures is important for understanding both the distribution of force that leads to fractures and how to successfully repair them.
- The face is often divided into thirds. The information in this chapter is presented in order of upper to lower thirds.
  - Upper third:
    - Frontal bone
  - Middle third:
    - Orbits, zygomas, maxillae
    - Nose, naso-ethmoid complex—may also be called the central face
  - Lower third:
    - Mandible

- **Buttresses**
  - Three paired vertical and horizontal buttresses.
  - Vertical buttresses: thicker, provide facial height, support forces of mastication.
    - Basomaxillary or medial, zygomaticomaxillary or lateral, and pterygomaxillary or posterior
  - Horizontal buttresses: thinner and weaker, provide facial projection, connect vertical buttresses.
    - frontal bone and supraorbital rims, nasal bones and inferior orbital rims, and the hard palate

Diagnosis of Facial Trauma

- Assessment of facial trauma should include a thorough physical exam.
  - Always begin with the ABCs: airway, breathing, circulation
  - Consider cervical spine injury
  - Assess neurologic status
  - Assess for other injuries
- History
  - Mechanism of injury
  - Past medical and surgical history, including:
    - Bleeding disorders, diabetes, immunosuppression, prior facial trauma, tetanus vaccination (if patient can participate)
- Physical examination
  - Eyes:
    - Pupillary response
    - Extraocular movements (look for entrapment)—may require forced duction testing
    - Enophthalmos or proptosis
    - Periorbital swelling or bruising:
      - ◊ Bilateral "raccoon eyes" develop within 1 to 3 days of trauma, predictive of anterior skull base fracture

      Subconjunctival hemorrhage
    - Chemosis
    - Intercanthal distance
    - Ophthalmology consultation to evaluate for globe injury and assess intraocular pressure
      - ◊ Required prior to any operative orbital fracture repair
  - Nose:
    - Evaluate for septal hematoma—visualize and palpate
    - Epistaxis
    - Dorsal deviation, tenderness, or palpable step-offs
    - Nasal obstruction or change in nasal appearance (by questioning of patient if able to participate in exam)
    - Clear rhinorrhea—concerning for possible CSF leak
  - Ears:
    - Hemotympanum
    - Otorrhea
    - Tuning forks—Weber and Rinne
    - Battle sign—bruising over the mastoid process can indicate skull base fracture

- Face:
  - Palpable bony step-offs or tenderness
  - Soft tissue swelling
  - Lacerations, possible foreign bodies
  - Flattening of the malar eminences
  - Mobile bony fragments or midface mobility
- Mouth:
  - Loose or missing teeth
    - ◊ Must be weary of potential aspiration
  - Dental occlusion—by exam (and questioning of patient if able to participate in exam)
    - ◊ Class I occlusion: mesio-buccal cusp of the first maxillary molar sits in the buccal groove of the first mandibular molar
      - * Ideal
    - ◊ Class II occlusion: mesio-buccal cusp of the first maxillary molar sits anterior to the buccal groove of the first mandibular molar
      - * Overbite or retrognathism
    - ◊ Class III occlusion: mesio-buccal cusp of the first maxillary molar sits posterior to the buccal groove of the first mandibular molar
      - * Underbite or prognathism
  - Intraoral lacerations
  - Fracture segment mobility
- Cranial nerves:
  - Assess optic nerve (CN 2), extraocular movements as above (CN 3, 4, 6), sensation to light touch in V1, V2, and V3 distributions (CN 5), facial movement (CN 7), and hearing (CN 8).

• **Imaging**
- Computed tomography (CT) scan is the gold standard for most facial trauma.
- Axial, coronal, and sagittal views should all be evaluated in tandem, with specific attention to the structures/potential fracture patterns below:
  - Axial—
    - ◊ Vertical orbital walls and optic canal
    - ◊ Maxillary bones
    - ◊ NOE fractures
    - ◊ Nasal bone fractures
    - ◊ Zygomatic arches
  - Coronal—
    - ◊ Orbital floor fractures
    - ◊ Medial orbital wall
    - ◊ Comminuted nasal bone fracture
    - ◊ Septal fractures
    - ◊ Zygomaticomaxillary complex fractures
    - ◊ Walls of frontal sinus
    - ◊ Pterygoid plates
  - Sagittal—
    - ◊ Orbital floor
    - ◊ Optic canal
    - ◊ Walls of frontal sinus
    - ◊ Frontal sinus outflow tract

- Orthopantomograms (also known by the brand name "Panorex") may be used for the evaluation of mandibular fractures.
  - Two-dimensional panoramic tomograms
  - Inexpensive and accessible
- CT imaging generally not required for isolated nasal bone fracture.
- Three-dimensional reconstructions may in many cases assist with surgical planning.

- **General management**
  - Consider prophylactic and postsurgical antibiotics with oral flora coverage—penicillins, cephalosporins, or clindamycin.
  - If operative repair is warranted, timing of surgical intervention is dependent on patient's trauma burden, nature of injury, patient age, and surgeon preferences.
    - In adults, repair should generally be performed within 14 days of injury, though exact timing of intervention is dependent on patient's comorbidities/trauma burden and degree of swelling.
    - Repair should be sooner than 14 days (ie, 24-72 hours) for mandibular fractures, NOE fractures and all operative pediatric facial fractures.
    - Surgical emergencies (ie, orbital floor fracture with entrapment) should be managed as such.
  - If operative repair is performed, consider use of intraoperative CT imaging to confirm adequate reduction/plate placement.
- **Upper third**
  - **Frontal fracture**
    - Classified based on:
      - ◊ Location: anterior table, posterior table, and/or nasofrontal recess
      - ◊ Nondisplaced, displaced, or comminuted
  - Potential complications of frontal sinus fracture:
    - Sinusitis
    - Meningitis
    - CSF leak
    - bone erosion
    - Mucoceles or mucopyoceles
    - Brain abscess
  - In recent years, there has been a shift to more conservative approaches to management of frontal sinus fractures.
  - **Anterior table fractures**
    - Not all anterior table fractures require surgical repair; repair is based on degree of deformity.
    - Severity determined by direct examination and palpation for contour irregularity (may need to wait 7-10 days for swelling to subside), as well as review of imaging.
    - Minimally displaced fractures without significant contour irregularity and without involvement of the frontal sinus outflow tract may be observed or later treated with injectable fillers or overlay graft if needed (camouflage).
      - ◊ Camouflage typically performed via endoscopic approach.
    - More significantly displaced and/or comminuted fractures typically require open reduction and internal fixation (ORIF).
      - ◊ Open approaches:
        - * Coronal, pretrichial, upper blepharoplasty, suprabrow, subbrow approaches (with or without trephination to assess the patency of the frontal sinus outflow tract) may be considered.

      - More extensive fractures may require a coronal or pretrichial approach.
      - Existing laceration may also be used for access.
    - ◊ Endoscopic approaches:
      - Increasing use of endoscopic technique in recent years with use of percutaneous screw, Draf IIb, or Draf III.
- **Posterior table fractures**
  - Posterior table fractures may be associated with CSF leak, dural tear, or intracranial injury (neurosurgery consultation is required), and are often associated with anterior table fractures along with comorbid severe injuries.
  - Some authors recommend exploration of all posterior table fractures while others recommend observation for displaced posterior table fractures in the absence of CSF leak.
  - This author feels operative intervention should be determined by two factors: severity of fracture (displacement/comminution) and presence of CSF leak, in consultation with neurosurgery colleagues.
  - Minimally displaced, noncomminuted fractures
    - ◊ Can often be observed
    - ◊ Repeat CT scan at 1 month and 1 year to evaluate for mucocele formation
  - Minimally displaced fractures with CSF leak
    - ◊ Can often be observed initially
    - ◊ If CSF leak persists, operative intervention is required
      - Operative intervention may include:
        - Sinusotomy
        - Dural repair
        - Sinus obliteration
  - Significantly displaced/comminuted fractures with or without CSF leak
    - ◊ Operative intervention often required and may include:
      - Dural repair
      - Sinus obliteration
        - During approach via coronal incision, it is important to maintain a pericranial flap that can be used for dural repair if needed.
        - Obliteration entails meticulous removal of all sinus and frontal sinus outflow tract mucosa.
        - The sinus and frontal sinus outflow tract are then filled autologous bone, fat, muscle, or pericranium.
          - Avoidance of use of alloplastic materials is recommended due to infection/extrusion risk.
      - Sinusotomy, that is, endoscopic Draf III
        - There is some evidence that performing a Draf III to ensure frontal sinus drainage may obviate need for sinus obliteration and decrease risk of future mucocele formation if any sinus mucosa remains.
      - Sinus cranialization
        - Consider cranialization for large posterior table fractures, especially if intracranial injury present and need for craniotomy.
        - Pericranial flap should be carefully maintained for later use.
        - Cranialization involves removal of the entire posterior table—this enables full examination and possible repair of the dura.
        - Frontal sinus outflow tract must be obliterated, and anterior table then replaced (secured with titanium plates).

- **Frontal sinus outflow tract**
  - Associated with injury to the frontal sinus floor.
  - If no posterior table displacement and sinus is draining, can consider observation with close follow-up/repeat CT imaging.
    - ◊ Low threshold for surgery if patient develops sinusitis
  - If associated posterior table injury, repair with obliteration versus endoscopic Draf III.
- **Supraorbital rim fractures**
  - These fractures may result in palpable step off and/or V1 compression, requiring reduction of the fracture and decompression of the nerve.

- **Middle third**
  - **Nasal bone and septal fractures**
    - Clinical diagnosis
      - ◊ Consider nasal reduction if dorsal irregularity or nasal obstruction; this should be driven by patient's symptoms and cosmetic concerns.
      - ◊ Reduction may be closed or open (ie, septorhinoplasty)
      - ◊ Closed reduction should ideally take place within 2 weeks of the nasal fracture.
        - * Before bone heals and osteotomies are required
        - * Before swelling has started or after it has subsided (usually 5-10 days postinjury)
        - * May require use of Asch forceps for reduction of the septum
      - ◊ Delayed, open septorhinoplasty at least 6 months after injury.
        - * Osteotomies likely required
    - Septal hematoma, if present, should be drained immediately.
      - ◊ Risk of infection, necrosis of underlying cartilage, and saddle nose deformity if septal hematoma is not drained expediently

- **Orbital fractures**
  - The frontal, zygomatic, maxillary, lacrimal, and ethmoid bones all contribute to the orbit's structure.
  - Optic canal transmits the optic nerve and ophthalmic artery.
  - The superior orbital fissure is lateral to the optic canal and houses CN III, IV, V, and VI.
    - Compression of these nerves results in superior orbital fissure syndrome—a surgical emergency.
  - The orbital apex is the posterior confluence of the orbit at the craniofacial junction, inclusive of all neurovasculature that passes intracranially via the optic canal, superior orbital fissure, and inferior orbital fissure. It is also the origin of the extraocular muscles.
    - Compression of the nerves passing through the superior orbital fissure with compression of the optic nerve results in orbital apex syndrome—a surgical emergency.
  - **Orbital roof fractures**
    - Rarely require repair, may require intracranial approach if operative intervention needed.
  - **Orbital medial wall, lateral wall, and floor fractures**
    - May result in diplopia, restricted eye movement, entrapment, enophthalmos, or exophthalmos.
      - ◊ Entrapment is a surgical emergency
        - * Entrapment requires release of any tissue trapped in the fracture and oftentimes placement of an implant, piece of fascia, cartilage, or gel film over the fracture.

        * Entrapment of the inferior rectus (as can be seen with orbital floor fractures) leads to limitation of extraocular movement (mainly up gaze, however can be both up and down and even all directions).
        * "White-eye fracture" in children (eye lacks chemosis and subconjunctival hemorrhage) is often associated with vagal reflex symptoms of nausea, vomiting, and bradycardia.
      ◊ Enophthalmos: enlargement of orbital volume which causes the globe to sink in.
        * Requires repair
    - "Orbital blowout fracture"—fracture of one or more orbital walls (often the floor) with orbital rims intact
      ◊ Usually occurs via blunt force to the globe
      ◊ Fractures of orbital floor can injure the infraorbital nerve (V2)
  ○ **Approaches**
    - Orbital floor
      ◊ Transconjunctival incision, with or without lateral canthotomy/cantholysis
      ◊ Subciliary incision
        * Either approach above can be combined with a gingivobuccal sulcus + endoscopic, transantral approach.
    - Lateral orbital rim
      ◊ Transconjunctival incision with lateral canthotomy/cantholysis
      ◊ Upper blepharoplasty incision
    - Medial orbital wall
      ◊ Pre-/transcaruncular incision
      ◊ Cutaneous external ethmoid incision
      ◊ Coronal incision
- **Naso-orbital ethmoidal (NOE) fractures**
  ○ Nasal bones and frontal processes of maxilla telescope posteriorly (due to the thin lamina papyracea of ethmoid bones), sparing orbits
  ○ Often present with telecanthus, pseudohypertelorism and loss of nasal dorsal height
    - Measure intercanthal distance
      ◊ Normal intercanthal distance: 30 to 35 mm.
    - Perform "bow-string test" (patient closes eyes, then lateral tension is applied to the upper and lower eyelids) to assess medial canthal stability.
    - An epicanthal fold may develop.
    - These findings may initially be subtle—important to recognize NOE fractures and repair in timely fashion.
      ◊ Delayed repair is significantly more challenging and often leads to unsatisfactory aesthetic outcomes.
  ○ Classified as Types I, II, or III depending on the status of the medial canthal ligament's attachment to bone.
    - Type I
      ◊ Medial canthal ligament is fixed to a moderately large bony fragment that can be fixated to surrounding bone with rigid fixation.
      ◊ Approaches (often used in combination): coronal incision, existing laceration, direct glabellar incision, transconjunctival incision, gingivobuccal sulcus incision
    - Type II
      ◊ Significant comminution: the ligament is attached to a small bony fragment—too small for rigid fixation
      ◊ Fixation via pre-/transcaruncular or transnasal wiring or permanent suture

- Type III
  - ◊ The medial canthal ligament is completely disrupted, detached. In these cases, the ligament must be directly repaired via transnasal wiring or permanent suture.
- Proper repair of Type II and III NOE fractures requires careful positioning of the ligament posteriorly, medially, and superiorly.
- A calvarial bone graft is required if there is a loss of nasal dorsal height.

- **Le Fort Fractures**
  - Repair centers on re-establishing occlusion and facial contour.
  - Repair typically requires maxillomandibular fixation (MMF) and the use of small plates (1.5-2.0mm) and screws to fixate bony fragments.
    - MMF is a means to fix occlusion.
      - ◊ Techniques used include:
        - * Erich arch bars: stainless steel bars with hooks for attaching wires or rubber bands, fixed to the teeth with wires.
        - * Modern arch bars: screwed to the bone of the maxilla and mandible with hooks for attaching wires or rubber bands.
        - * Teeth may be wired directly: Minne Ties, Ivy loops, Ernst ligatures.
        - * Screws with eyes or slots may be screwed directly into the bone of the maxilla and mandible, allowing wire to pass through the eyes/slots.
      - ◊ Ensure condyles are appropriately seated in temporomandibular joints prior to placement in MMF.
      - ◊ Take patient out of MMF once fractures have been reduced/fixated to ensure occlusion is maintained.
      - ◊ The surgeon may decide to remove the MMF device at the conclusion of the procedure.
  - **Le Fort I**
    - Horizontal maxillary fracture.
    - Fracture through maxilla, nasal septum, and pterygoid plates at a level just above the maxillary alveoli.
    - Repair involves establishing occlusion. If doing so reduces fracture (eg, minimally comminuted fracture), further repair may not be necessary. However, oftentimes, reduction and rigid fixation are applied.
    - Approach: gingivobuccal incision.
  - **Le Fort II**
    - Pyramidal fracture.
    - Fracture extends from the lateral maxillae above the alveoli, superiorly toward the orbit, crosses the inferior and medial orbit, crosses at or below the nasion, crosses the nasal septum and pterygoid plates.
    - Fixation performed at higher level compared to Le Fort I due to superior extension of the fractures.
      - ◊ Must determine if orbital exploration is indicated or not.
    - Risk of open-bite deformity
      - ◊ MMF with care to ensure maxillae are properly reduced prior to rigid fixation can help prevent this.
    - Rowe disimpaction forceps may be required if the maxilla is impacted.
    - Repair may require multiple surgical approaches:
      - ◊ Gingivobuccal sulcus incision
      - ◊ Transconjunctival incision

- **Le Fort III**
  - Complete craniofacial separation.
  - Fracture separates the zygomas from the temporal and frontal bones, crosses the lateral and medial orbits, nasion, nasal septum, pterygoid plates.
  - Pure Le Fort III fractures are extremely rare.
  - Repair may require multiple surgical approaches:
    - ◊ Coronal incision frequently used
      - ∗ Enables exposure of zygomatic arches, NOE region, orbital floors/medial orbits
    - ◊ Gingivobuccal sulcus incision may be required for lower maxillary fractures.

- **Zygomatic fractures**
  - The zygoma is an important aesthetic component of the face, providing the most lateral projection.
  - Functionally, it supports the vertical buttresses and serves as the attachment of the masseter muscle.
  - Two types of fractures associated with this region: zygomaticomaxillary complex (ZMC) fractures versus isolated zygomatic arch.
  - **ZMC fractures**
    - Occur at suture lines of the bones that articulate with the zygoma.
    - There are four suture lines:
      - ◊ Superior: zygomaticofrontal
      - ◊ Posterolateral: zygomaticotemporal
      - ◊ Medial: zygomaticomaxillary
      - ◊ Posterior: zygomaticosphenoid
    - ZMC fractures always include the orbital floor.
    - The ZMC is a complex three-dimensional structure and must be repositioned appropriately in all three dimensions.
  - **Approaches to ZMC fractures:**
    - Transconjunctival incision or subciliary incision:
      - ◊ Exposure to orbital floor.
    - Transconjunctival incision with lateral canthotomy/cantholysis:
      - ◊ Exposure to zygomaticosphenoid suture.
    - Upper blepharoplasty, infra- or suprabrow incision:
      - ◊ Exposure to zygomaticofrontal suture.
    - Gingivobuccal sulcus incision:
      - ◊ Exposure to zygomaticomaxillary suture.
      - ◊ This may also be used to access the inferior orbital rim but must take care to preserve the infraorbital nerve (V2).
    - Coronal incision:
      - ◊ For severe comminuted fractures requiring access to the zygomaticotemporal suture.
    - Following fracture reduction (may require Boies elevator, bone hook or Carroll-Girard screw) fixation is typically achieved with miniplates and screws.
  - **Zygomatic arch fracture**
    - Repair aimed at improving function (if arch is impacted on the underlying temporalis muscle causing trismus) and correcting cosmetic deformity.
    - **Approaches:**
      - ◊ Gingivobuccal sulcus (Keene) incision:
        - ∗ Boies elevator used to reduce arch laterally via this incision.

- ◊ Gilles incision:
  - * Incision in temporal region, down to temporalis muscle.
  - * Boies elevator placed deep to true temporalis fascia on the temporalis muscle and slides inferiorly, deep to the zygomatic arch to reduce it laterally.
- ◊ Severe comminution may require ORIF via coronal incision.

- **Lower third**
  - **Mandibular fractures**
    - Classified based on location(s) and severity.
      - ◊ Locations:
        - * Condylar
          - ▪ Fracture involves the intracapsular head of the condyle.
        - * Subcondylar
          - ▪ Fracture traverses the sigmoid notch and exits posteriorly, behind the angle of the mandible.
        - * Angle
          - ▪ Fracture occurs behind dentition, extending from posterior body to third molar.
        - * Ramus (less commonly fractured)
          - ▪ Fracture occurs between the superior border of the angle and the sigmoid notch.
        - * Coronoid process (less commonly fractured)
          - ▪ Fracture is anterior to the sigmoid notch.
        - * Body
          - ▪ Fracture between the mental foramen and the angle of the mandible.
        - * Symphysis
          - ▪ Fracture between the mental foramina (although some consider any fracture lateral to midline "parasymphyseal")
      - ◊ Fractures of the mandible may be simple, comminuted, non-displaced, displaced, and/or avulsive.
    - Dentition affects fracture location and management.
      - ◊ Determine if mandible is dentulous, edentulous, or atrophic edentulous.
        - * Age and tooth loss cause the alveolar bone to atrophy and can alter the way in which forces are distributed across mandible.
      - ◊ Alveolar fractures result from separation of the tooth-bearing segments from the mandible.
        - * Dental consultation often required.
    - **Principles of mandibular fracture repair:**
      - ◊ Re-establishing occlusion is critical. This may be achieved with MMF.
      - ◊ The goal of fixation is to stabilize the mandible, so forces of distraction become forces of compression in the area of the fracture.
        - * The mandible bears significant forces of mastication, and fixation must distribute these forces in a favorable way.
      - ◊ An arch bar can support the alveolar border; this can serve as a tension band.
      - ◊ Small plates (1.5-2.0mm) may also be used along the alveolar border; care must be taken to avoid tooth roots and the inferior alveolar nerve with monocortical screws only.
      - ◊ Mandibular reconstruction plates (MRPs) are strong, provide compression along the basal border of the mandible, and may be used for:

    * Areas of bone loss, as a bridge over the defect
    * Atrophic mandible, to stabilize weak bone
    * Comminuted fractures, to span the areas of comminution
      - Prior to application of a MRP, these bony fragments may first be fixed with wire or small plates.
  - Lag screws may also be used for compression.
  - Multiple surgical approaches are often required.
  - In pediatric patients:
    * Special care should be taken to avoid injury to tooth buds.
    * If titanium plates are used, they should be removed after approximately 6 to 8 weeks to prevent growth restriction or bony overgrowth.
    * Consider use of resorbable plates instead of titanium plates, this however is controversial.
- **Repair of mandibular fractures:**
  - Preoperative discussion with anesthesia regarding airway management is critical as patient will require placement in MMF.
    * Consider: nasotracheal intubation, submental intubation, or tracheotomy
  - Many non- or minimally displaced mandibular fractures that do not cause change in occlusion or excessive pain may be treated conservatively with watchful waiting and soft, no-chew diet for 6 weeks.
    * These cases, however, are in the minority.
  - **Condylar fracture:**
    * Typically treated with closed-reduction MMF
  - **Subcondylar fracture:**
    * Closed-reduction MMF
      - Minimally displaced, simple fracture.
    * ORIF if:
      - Condylar dislocation into middle fossa
      - Open fracture, grossly contaminated
      - Inability to achieve adequate occlusion
      - Concurrent comminuted maxillary fractures
    * Approaches to ORIF:
      - Endoscopic: requires specific expertise and instrumentation
      - Transoral, retromandibular, preauricular/facelift or submandibular incisions—increased risk of facial nerve injury
  - **Angle**
    * Closed reduction MMF
      - Nondisplaced, simple fracture
    * ORIF if:
      - At least minimally displaced, simple fracture.
      - All complex fractures.
      - Nondisplaced, simple fracture but patient preference to avoid MMF.
      - Champy (mini) plate may be used along the ideal line of osteosynthesis.
    * Approaches to ORIF:
      - Transoral, retromandibular, facelift or submandibular incisions
  - **Ramus**
    * Closed-reduction MMF
      - Minimally displaced, simple fracture

      - ORIF if:
        - Minimally displaced simple fracture and patient preference to avoid MMF.
        - At least moderately displaced simple fracture.
        - All complex fractures.
      - Approaches to ORIF:
        - Transoral, retromandibular, facelift or submandibular incisions
    - **Coronoid process**
      - Typically, no operative management required.
    - **Body**
      - Closed-reduction MMF.
        - Nondisplaced, simple fractures—however, not ideal as pull of the pterygomasseteric sling will often cause fracture displacement
      - ORIF
        - Preferred for nondisplaced, simple fracture.
        - All displaced, all complex fractures.
      - Approach to ORIF:
        - Transoral incision
    - **Symphysis**
      - ORIF
        - Preferred due to the torsional forces on the symphysis and parasymphysis during mastication
      - Approach:
        - Transoral, submental incision
- **Common complications**
  - Infection
    - May require drainage
    - The stability of the bone repair should be assessed
      - If stable:
        - Clean and culture wound, antibiotics
        - Consider hardware removal
      - If unstable or evidence of posttraumatic osteitis:
        - Clean and culture wound, antibiotics
        - Remove hardware and replace, with or without placement of cancellous bone graft
  - Malposition
    - May be significant or minimal, with or without a functional or cosmetic impact
      - Reoperation may be required if function compromised (ie, malocclusion)
      - Reoperation may be required if cosmetic deformity
  - Scars
    - Revise as needed
  - Eyelid malposition
    - Increased risk with repair of orbital floor fractures
    - May be prevented by performing lateral tarsal strip or canthopexy at the conclusion of the procedure or using a Frost stitch to stretch the lower lid during the immediate postoperative period
    - Mild may respond to massage
    - More significant may require surgical repair

- Lacrimal injuries
  - Best to identify preoperatively if present
- Nerve injuries
  - Best to identify preoperatively if present
    - ◊ Iatrogenic facial nerve injuries should be repaired if possible.
- Dental injuries
  - Tooth root injuries
    - ◊ Increased risk when using MMF screws and screw-in arch bars
- Missed fractures
  - NOE is most common.
- Sinus problems
- CSF leaks/meningitis

Questions

1. Which surgical approach to a ZMC fracture enables the best exposure of both the zygomaticofrontal suture and orbital floor?
   A. Transconjunctival incision with lateral canthotomy and cantholysis
   B. Gillies incision
   C. Intraoral gingivobuccal sulcus incision
   D. Upper blepharoplasty incision

2. Which of the following is unlikely to be appropriate management of an isolated anterior frontal sinus fracture?
   A. Observation with later injection of filler
   B. Open approach with graft overlay
   C. Frontal sinus cranialization
   D. Endoscopic approach with trephination

3. In a type II naso-orbital ethmoidal fracture, the medial canthal ligament is attached to
   A. The medial orbital wall
   B. Nothing; it is free-floating
   C. A fragment of bone too small to be fixated
   D. A small fragment of bone able to be fixated

4. The following are all indications for a mandibular reconstruction plate EXCEPT
   A. Atrophic edentulous mandible
   B. Comminuted fragments of mandibular bone in body of mandible
   C. Area of bone loss in ramus
   D. Condylar fracture

5. The following are all possible, reasonable approaches to a subcondylar fracture EXCEPT
   A. Transoral approach
   B. Submental approach
   C. Submandibular incision
   D. Retromandibular incision

Acknowledgements

We thank Robert M. Kellman, M.D. for his contribution to the Craniomaxillofacial Trauma chapter in the 12th edition of the K. J. Lee text, which served as a guide when developing this chapter for the 13th edition.

Bibliography

Guy MW, Brisett AE. Contemporary management of traumatic fractures of the frontal sinus. In: Boahene KDO, Brissett AE, eds. *Surgical Management of Facial Trauma*. 1st ed. Philadelphia, PA: Elsevier Inc; 2013.

Kellman R. Craniomaxillofacial trauma. In: Chan Y, Goddard JC, eds. *K. J. Lee's Essential Otolaryngology: Head and Neck Surgery*. 12th ed. New York, NY: McGraw Hill; 2019.

Kellman R. Maxillofacial trauma. In: Flint PW, Francis HW, Haughey BH, et al., eds. *Cummings Otolaryngology: Head and Neck Surgery*. 7th ed. Philadelphia, PA: Elsevier Inc; 2021.

Kochhar A, Byrne PJ. Surgical management of complex midfacial fractures. In: Boahene KDO, Brissett AE, eds. *Surgical Management of Facial Trauma*. 1st ed. Philadelphia, PA: Elsevier Inc; 2013.

Strong EB, Papel ID, Frodel JL, Holt GR, et al. Frontal sinus and naso-orbito-ethmoid fractures. In: Papel ID, Frodel JL, Holt GR, et al. Facial Plastic and Reconstructive Surgery, 4th ed. New York, NY: Thieme; 2016.

Part 8
Allergy

Chapter 58
Immunology and Allergy

The Immune System

A. Cells of the innate immune system
    i. Macrophages
        a. Cross capillaries and recruit other immune cells with cytokines
        b. Antigen-presenting cells allow communication from the innate to the adaptive immune system
        c. Polarize into M1 (proinflammatory) and M2 (anti-inflammatory) phenotypes, contributing to inflammation and tissue repair
    ii. Neutrophils
        a. Toxic to bacteria and fungi
        b. Can form neutrophil extracellular traps (NETs) to trap and kill pathogens
    iii. Mast cells
        a. Mast cell degranulation releases histamine and other cytokines triggering inflammatory cascade
            1. Vasodilation, increased blood flow, recruitment of neutrophils and macrophages
    iv. Eosinophils
        a. Toxic to bacteria and parasites
        b. Involved in allergic responses and asthma pathogenesis

- v. Basophils
    - a. Toxic to parasites and secrete histamines
    - b. Produce IL-4 and IL-13, contributing to Th2 responses in allergy
- vi. Natural killer (NK) cells
    - a. Signaled by infected host cells to destroy the infected cells
    - b. Account for 10% of circulating lymphocytes
    - c. Rarely found in lymph nodes
    - d. Positive for CD16 and express CD56 surface markers
    - e. Produce cytokines like interferon-gamma (IFN-γ), enhancing immune responses
- vii. Dendritic cells
    - a. Specialized macrophages found in the skin, mucosa, lymph nodes, spleen, and thymus
        1. Contact with external environment
    - b. Antigen-presenting cells
    - c. Include conventional dendritic cells (cDCs) and plasmacytoid dendritic cells (pDCs), each with specialized functions in immune activation and tolerance
- viii. Innate lymphoid cells (ILCs)
    - a. Recently identified group of innate immune cells lacking specific antigen receptors
    - b. Include ILC1, ILC2, and ILC3 subsets, analogous to T helper cell subsets (Th1, Th2, Th17)
    - c. Play roles in immunity, tissue remodeling, and maintaining homeostasis
    - d. ILCs contribute to immune defense, tissue remodeling, and maintenance of homeostasis, and are potential targets for novel therapies in allergic and inflammatory diseases

B. Adaptive immunity—coordinated, self-regulated response, with memory for prior antigen exposure and amplification in magnitude with successive antigen stimulation
- i. Nonreactivity to self
    - a. Recognize and eliminate foreign materials while avoiding harmful responses to host tissues
        1. Mediated by lymphocytes
            - B lymphocytes
                - (a) Produce antibodies and carry endogenously produced immunoglobulins (Ig) on surface
                    - Act as antigen receptors
                - (b) Maturation occurs in the bone marrow
                - (c) Naïve B cells differentiate into plasma cells or memory B cells upon encountering an antigen that matches their membrane-bound antibodies
                - (d) Memory B cells express identical membrane-bound receptors as its naïve parent cell
                - (e) Plasma cells secrete antibodies into circulation
                - (f) Act collaboratively with T cells and macrophages
                - (g) Account for 10% to 15% of circulating lymphocytes
                - (h) Positive for CD19, CD21
            - T lymphocytes
                - (a) Mature in the thymus
                - (b) Classification into subsets depends on the pattern of T-cell receptors (TCR)

(c) Can only recognize and bind to an antigen presented by an antigen-presenting cell on major histocompatibility complexes (MCH) class 1 or 2.
  - Class I: membrane-associated glycoproteins present on nearly all nucleated cells
  - Class II: normally expressed only on B lymphocytes, macrophages or dendritic cells, endothelial cells, and a few other cell lines

(d) Each MHC molecule contains an extracellular peptide-binding region and a pair of Ig-like domains that act as binding sites for CD4 and CD8 T cells

(e) CD2, CD3
  - Found on all T cells

(f) CD4 T cells/Helper T cells
  - 60% of peripheral T cells
  - Induce cytotoxic/suppressor T cells (CD8 cells)
  - TCR binds to MHC2

- Mature from naïve CD4 cells (TH0) into various subsets:

(a) Th1 cells
  - Participate in microbial immunity
  - Produce interleukin-2 (IL-2) and interferon gamma (IFN-γ) when activated
  - Activate macrophages and promote cell-mediated immune responses
  - Inhibit Th2 responses, balancing the immune system

(b) Th2 cells
  - Participate in the allergic response
  - Produce IL-4, 5, 6, and 10
  - Stimulate B cells
  - Involved in the recruitment and activation of eosinophils

(c) Th17 cells
  - Involved in immunity against extracellular bacteria and fungi
  - Produce IL-17, IL-21, and IL-22
  - Play a role in autoimmune diseases and inflammatory conditions

(d) Regulatory T cells (Tregs)
  - CD4 + CD25 cells/T regulatory cells
  - Regulate immune responses in vivo
  - Exert suppressor effects on effector T cells and APCs
  - Involved in prevention of autoimmunity
  - Involved in induction of immune tolerance
  - Play a central role in therapeutic effects noted with allergy immunotherapy
  - Express FOXP3 transcription factor, crucial for their development and function

- CD8 cells/cytotoxic T cells

(a) 20% to 30% of peripheral T cells

(b) Specifically kill target cells

(c) Lysis of virus-infected cells

(d) Lysis of tumor cells
  - Inhibit the response of B cells and other T cells
  - Important in immune tolerance

(e) Produce cytokines like IFN-γ and TNF-α

ii. Humoral immunity
   a. Mediated serum antibodies produced by plasma cells
   b. The primary function of humoral immunity is the defense against extracellular microbes and microbial toxins
   c. Antibodies are produced by plasma cells in the lymphoid organs and bone marrow, but antibodies perform their effector functions at sites distant from their production
   d. Antibodies may be derived from cells produced at the time of primary exposure and activated again through a secondary immune response mediated by memory B cells
   e. Features of an antibody
      1. Four polypeptide chains connected with disulfide bonds
      2. Two identical light polypeptide chains (25,000 MW)
         - The light chain determines light chain class—Kappa, Lambda
      3. Two identical heavy polypeptide chains (50,000-77,000 MW)
         - The heavy chain binds to host tissues and complement and determines Ig class
      4. Constant region (C-terminal end of the Ig molecule) or Fc fragment
      5. Variable region (N-terminal end) of Fab fragment
   a. Classes of immunoglobulins
      1. IgG
         - Major antibody involved in secondary immune responses
         - Important activity against viruses, bacteria, parasites, and some fungi
            (a) Only Ig class that crosses the placenta
               - Provides 3 to 6 months of immunity after birth
         - Fixes complement through the classic pathway
      2. IgM
         - Primary antibody associated with the early immune response
         - Pentamer associated with a J chain
         - Fixes complement through the classic pathway
      3. IgA
         - Predominant Ig in seromucinous secretions (saliva, tracheobronchial secretions)
         - Dimer associated with "secretory component" (prevents proteolysis by digestive enzymes) and J chain
      4. IgD
         - Found in large quantities on circulating B cells
         - May be involved in antigen-induced lymphocyte proliferation
      5. IgE
         - Involved in
            (a) Type I immediate hypersensitivity reactions
            (b) Anaphylaxis and atopy
         - Cell-associated IgE molecules of a particular antigenic specificity can be cross-linked by their appropriate antigen
         - Present in smallest amount of all of the five Ig classes
         - Hypersensitivity reactions (also known as the "Gell and Coombs" classes")
            (a) Type I: anaphylactic
               - Immediate hypersensitivity reaction
               - Symptoms apparent within minutes of exposure

- Upper respiratory symptoms
  - Sneezing, itching, rhinorrhea, congestion
- Lower respiratory symptoms
  - Cough, bronchospasm, wheezing
- Skin symptoms
  - Urticaria, angioedema, itching, wheeling
- Inciting agents
  - Inhalants, foods, drugs, insect stings
- Mechanism
  - Crosslinking of IgE molecules on mast cells
  - Degranulation of mast cells
  - Release of histamine

(b) Type II: cytotoxic

- Involved in various systemic hypersensitivities
  - Hemolytic anemia
  - Transfusion reactions
  - Hyperacute graft rejection
  - Goodpasture syndrome
  - Myasthenia gravis
- Inciting agents
  - Unknown
- Mechanism
  - IgG or IgM mediated
  - Antibodies react with antigens on cell surface
  - Activation of complement

(c) Type III: immune complex mediated

- Onset of symptoms may be delayed for up to days
- Involved in various system hypersensitivities.
  - Serum sickness
  - Poststreptococcal glomerulonephritis
  - Arthus reaction
  - Angioedema
  - GI intolerance
  - Systemic lupus erythematosus (SLE)
- Inciting agents:
  - Drugs
  - Bacterial products
  - Often unknown
- Mechanism:
  - Immune complexes are formed, usually with IgG antibodies
  - Complexes deposited in tissues
  - Activation of complement
  - Initiation of acute inflammatory response

(d) Type IV: delayed (cell-mediated) hypersensitivity

- Acute and chronic dermatitis
- Granulomatous diseases
  - Tuberculosis
  - Sarcoidosis
- Fungal diseases
  - Candidiasis

- Inciting agents
  - Poison ivy, sumac, oak
  - Cosmetics
  - Various metals and chemicals
  - Nickel
- Mechanism
  - Mediated by direct T-cell activation
  - Cell-mediated inflammation

iii. Cell-mediated immunity
   a. Mediated by T cells and their secreted cytokines and other related products.
   b. The adaptive immune response to antigens is mediated by T lymphocytes, which recognize specific antigens and produce cytokines that stimulate inflammation.
   c. Induction of cell-mediated immunity involves antigen recognition by T cells in peripheral lymphoid organs, proliferation of these T cells, and their differentiation into effector lymphocytes.
   d. The specificity of the immune response is due to T cells.
   e. Antigen-presenting cells (APCs)
      1. T cells respond to antigens presented by other cells in the context of MHC proteins
         - Proteins may be presented by macrophages, endothelial, or glial cells
         - Dendritic cells
         - APCs ingest and process the antigen
         - APCs present the antigen to T cells in association with Class II MHC molecules
         - In the spleen and thymus, these APCs may be important in the recognition of self-antigens
   f. T-cell activation
      1. Resting T cells are activated by cellular signaling
      2. When activated, these T cells
         - Proliferate
         - Differentiate
         - Produce cytokines and various effector functions
   g. Migration of activated T cells and other leukocytes
      1. Migration of leukocytes to sites of inflammation is stimulated by cytokines.
         - Cytokines induce the expression of adhesion molecules on endothelial cells and the chemotaxis of leukocytes.
      2. Previously activated effector and memory T cells migrate to the site of inflammation.
   h. Cytokines
      1. Proteins secreted by cells of the innate and adaptive immune system in response to stimulation with antigen and that mediate the function of these immune cells
      2. Produced in response to antigens and stimulate diverse cellular responses
      3. Stimulate growth and differentiation of lymphocytes
      4. Activate effector cells to eliminate microbial and other antigens
      5. Stimulate the development of hematopoietic cells
      6. Cytokines are often classified by their cellular sources or by their action on immune cells

- Lymphokines: cytokines produced by lymphocytes
- Interferons: potent antiviral agents
- Colony-stimulating factors: involved in maturation and systemic release of bone marrow precursor cells
- Tumor necrosis factors: principal mediators of acute inflammatory response to gram-negative bacteria
- Interleukins: cytokines produced by leukocytes that act on other leukocytes
  (a) Individual interleukins are assigned an IL number that is used to classify their function (eg, IL-1, IL-5)

7. Properties of cytokines:
   - Secretion is brief and self-limited.
   - Actions are often redundant.
   - Influence the synthesis and action of other cytokines.
   - Actions may be local and/or systemic.
   - Bind to specific membrane receptors on target cells to regulate gene expression.
8. Principal cytokines involved in the allergic response
   - IL-2
     (a) Derived from T cells
     (b) Growth factor for antigen-stimulated T cells and responsible for T-cell clonal expansion
     (c) Promotes the proliferation and differentiation of other immune cells
   - IL-3
     (a) Derived from CD4+ T cells
     (b) Promotes
       - Development and expansion of immature bone marrow elements
       - Mast cell proliferation
       - Eosinophil activation
   - IL-4
     (a) Derived from CD4+ T cells and mast cells
     (b) Principal cytokine that stimulates B-cell isotype switching to the IgE isotype
       - IgE is the primary immunoglobulin involved in the allergic response.
     (c) Stimulates the development of TH2 cells from naïve CD4+ cells
   - IL-5
     (a) Derived from CD4+ T cells
     (b) Activates eosinophils and links T-cell activation and eosinophilic inflammation
     (c) Stimulates the growth and differentiation of eosinophils and the activation of mature eosinophils
     (d) Involved in stimulating eosinophil chemotaxis to areas of inflammation
   - IL-9
     (a) Derived from Th2 cells
     (b) Contributes to mast cell expansion and mucus production
   - IL-10
     (a) Derived from activated macrophages and CD4+ T cells

(b) Inhibits
- Activated macrophages
- Cytokine synthesis in various cells

(c) Maintains homeostatic control of innate and cell-mediated immune reactions
(d) Suppresses antigen-presenting capacities of APCs
(e) Acts as an important regulator of the immune system

- IL-13
  (a) Functions are similar to IL-4
  (b) Induces adhesion molecules at sites of allergic inflammation contributing to increased populations of eosinophils and lymphocytes
- IL-17
  (a) Produced by Th17 cells
  (b) Promotes neutrophil recruitment and activation
  (c) Involved in autoimmune and inflammatory diseases
- IL-22
  (a) Produced by Th17 and other cells
  (b) Acts on epithelial cells to promote antimicrobial responses and tissue repair

Allergy for the Rhinologist

A. Allergy overview
  i. Allergic rhinitis is one of the most common diseases worldwide, affecting up to 40% of the global population, impacting both children and adults.
    a. Has a highly negative impact on quality of life
      1. Sleep disruptions and fatigue, irritability, decreased school and work performance, common reason for physician visits
  ii. Allergy is the most common disorder of immunity and affects 20% to 25% of all individuals in the United States.
  iii. Allergic reactions occur with exposure to normally harmless antigens among susceptible individuals.
  iv. The susceptibility to develop an allergic response is known as atopy, which implies a genetic predisposition toward the expression of allergic diseases.
    a. Atopic individuals demonstrate a skewing of T helper responses to the Th2 pattern.
    b. The overproduction of IgE antibodies in this setting creates a milieu in which allergic symptoms can be expressed.
    c. Recent studies have also highlighted the role of epithelial-derived cytokines like thymic stromal lymphopoietin (TSLP), IL-33, and IL-25 in initiating Th2 responses.
    d. IgE-mediated allergy/Th2-mediated inflammation are among the multiple etiologies for CRSwNP.
  v. In genetically predisposed individuals, an environmental protein antigen, commonly referred to as an allergen, stimulates CD4+ T cells to differentiate into TH2 effector cells.
  vi. A cascade of events occurs in which allergic symptoms occur through this immediate hypersensitivity response.

vii. Recent advances highlight the role of biologic therapies, such as anti IL-4 and lL-13, anti Il-5 and anti-IgE monoclonal antibodies, which have shown significant efficacy in treating in CRSwNP.

B. Sequence of events in immediate hypersensitivity responses
   i. Initial exposure to an antigen among susceptible individuals stimulates naïve T cells to differentiate into TH2 effector cells and activates innate lymphoid cells type 2 (ILC2s).
   ii. Activated Th2 cells and ILC2s secrete cytokines such as IL-4, IL-5, IL-9, and IL-13, and contact-mediated signals promote differentiation of B cells specific for that antigen into IgE-producing cells.
   iii. IgE produced by these cells circulates throughout the body and binds to high-affinity Fc receptors on the surfaces of circulating basophils and on tissue mast cells.
   iv. Subsequent reexposure to the antigen results in binding of the antigen to IgE molecules on the surface of mast cells and basophils.
   v. Crosslinking of adjacent IgE molecules initiates signal transduction in mast cells and basophils, resulting in the release of preformed mediators stored in cytoplasmic granules in these cells, as well as the rapid synthesis and release of other, newly formed mediators, including cytokines and chemokines that perpetuate the allergic response.
   vi. Clinical and pathological manifestations of the allergic response are due to the effects of these mediators on target cells.
      a. Early-phase reactions:
         1. Vascular leakage of plasma, vasodilation, smooth muscle stimulation, bronchoconstriction, acute inflammation
      b. Late-phase reactions:
         1. Recruitment of eosinophils, basophils, and other inflammatory cells
         2. Chronic inflammation and tissue remodeling

C. Specifics of the allergic response
   i. Production of IgE
      a. Type I immediate hypersensitivity reactions are primarily mediated by IgE antibodies
      b. Epithelial cells release cytokines such as thymic stromal lymphopoietin (TSLP), IL-33, and IL-25, which further promote Th2 differentiation and IgE production
   ii. Production of antigen-specific IgE antibodies
      a. Requires active collaboration between macrophages (APCs), T cells, and B cells
      b. Allergen exposure
         1. Introduced through the respiratory tract, GI tract, or skin
         2. Captured by dendritic cells that process the antigen
         3. Reacts with APCs that process the antigen
         4. Presented to appropriately sensitized T cells with interaction at the T-cell receptor
         5. B cells, in the presence of the APC, antigen, and sensitized T cells are stimulated to develop into plasma cells
         6. Plasma cells synthesize and secrete antigen-specific IgE
            - IgE-producing plasma cells are primarily located in the lamina propria of the skin, respiratory tract, and GI tract

iii. Binding of the IgE to mast cells
   a. IgE antibodies bind to mast cells
      1. Receptors on mast cells specific for the Fc region of the epsilon heavy chain
      2. IgE-laden mast cells are distributed throughout the body through passive transfer into the serum
   b. Mast cells:
      1. Located in perivascular connective tissue
      2. Basophils circulate in the blood and share similar functions with mast cells
      3. Contain up to 500,000 antigen-specific IgE antibodies on their surfaces
      4. Contain potent mediators of immediate hypersensitivity

iv. Reexposure to antigen
   a. The binding of IgE antibody to mediator cell receptors is directly related to serum IgE concentration.
      1. The higher the serum IgE level, the greater the binding of IgE to mast cells and basophils.
   b. The greater the patient sensitivity, the lesser antigen is required to initiate an allergic response.
   c. Antigen interaction with antigen-specific IgE bound to the surface of mast cells.
   d. Repeat allergen stimulation by the same specific allergen initiates the crosslinking of two or more mast cell-bound IgE molecules.
   e. Signal is transmitted to the cell interior that initiates a specific molecular response.
      1. Increased ratio of cyclic guanosine monophosphate (cGMP) to cyclic adenosine monophosphate (cAMP).
      2. Fc receptors are linked to a transmembrane coupling protein and adenylate cyclase.
      3. Coupling protein activates adenylate cyclase when cross-linking of antigen to two IgE antibodies occurs.
      4. Adenylate cyclase reduces adenosine triphosphate (ATP) to AMP.
      5. AMP decreased by kinase enhances mediator release.
   f. Preformed cytoplasmic granules.
      1. Migrate to the cell surface membrane
      2. Fuse with each other and with the cell membrane
      3. Extrude through the membrane and released into the external microenvironment
      4. Enhances the influx of Ca^2+ from the extracellular space
         - Release of mediators of type I anaphylaxis
         - Production of newly formed mediators, leukotrienes and prostaglandins, via the activation of arachidonic acid metabolism

v. Mast cell degranulation
   a. When triggered by an antigen, the mast cell membrane allows Ca^2+ influx, which triggers degranulation and the release of granule-associated preformed mediators
      1. Histamine
         - Main mediator of the allergic reaction
         - Tissue effects include
           (a) Vasodilation
           (b) Increased capillary permeability

(c) Bronchoconstriction
(d) Tissue edema
- Exerts effects through various receptor subtypes
  (a) H1 to H4 (H4 receptor is involved in immune modulation)
- Tryptase
  (a) Proteolytic enzymes
  (b) Serves as a marker for mast cell activation
- Heparin
  (a) Anticoagulant
  (b) Suppresses histamine production
  (c) Enhances phagocytosis
- Chemotactic factors
  (a) Involved in chemotaxis of both eosinophils and neutrophils
- Kininogenase
  (a) Promotes vasoactive mucosal edema

2. Newly generated inflammatory mediators are also released through metabolism of arachidonic acid
   - Leukotrienes (eg, LTC_4, LTD_4, LTE_4)
     (a) Formed through the lipoxygenase pathway
     (b) Potent mediators of inflammation
     (c) Vasoactive
     (d) Chemotactic
     (e) Involved in bronchoconstriction
   - Prostaglandins (eg, PGD_2)
     (a) Formed through the cyclooxygenase pathway
     (b) Involved in bronchoconstriction
     (c) Encourage platelet aggregation
     (d) Promote vasodilation
   - Platelet-activating factor (PAF)
     (a) Chemotactic for eosinophils
     (b) Stimulates other cells to release mediators
   - Cytokines (eg, IL-4, IL-5, IL-13, TNF-α)
     (a) Contribute to late-phase reactions and chronic inflammation

vi. Allergic signs and symptoms
  a. Eyes
    1. Allergic shiners: darkening under the eyes from chronic deposition of hemosiderin in tissues
    2. Long, silky eyelashes
    3. Periorbital edema and puffiness
    4. Dennie lines
       - Fine horizontal lines in the lower lids
       - Occur through spasms of Mueller muscles in the lids
    5. Conjunctival lymphoid aggregates
    6. Injection of the bulbar conjunctiva
    7. Itching and excessive tearing
  b. Nose
    1. Itching
    2. Supratip horizontal crease
       - Develops through chronic rubbing of the nose

3. Facial grimacing
4. "Allergic salute"
    - Characteristic rubbing of the nose with the heel of the hand
5. Nasal obstruction
    - Mucosal edema
    - Turbinate hypertrophy
    - Increased mucus secretion
6. Sneezing
7. Rhinorrhea
8. Pale, bluish mucosa

c. Mouth
1. Chronic mouth breathing (secondary to nasal obstruction)
2. Palatal itching
3. Nocturnal bruxism
4. High-arched palate in children

d. Pharynx
1. Dry, irritated, inflamed mucosa
    - Related to direct allergen exposure
    - Related to chronic mouth breathing
2. Repeated throat clearing
    - Also associated with laryngopharyngeal reflux
3. "Cobblestoning" of the posterior pharyngeal wall
    - Presence of lymphoid aggregates or patches on the posterior pharyngeal wall

e. Larynx
1. Intermittent dysphonia, increased tenacious mucus, throat clearing, cough

f. Lungs
1. Cough, wheezing, dyspnea, interference with sleep

vii. Phases of the allergic response

a. Early phase
1. Primarily histamine mediated
2. Occurs rapidly after exposure to a previously sensitized antigen
    - Usually occur within 5 to 10 minutes
    - Immediate symptoms can last for several hours
3. Symptoms primarily include itching, sneezing, tearing, wheezing, mild congestion, and rhinorrhea

b. Late phase (delayed)
1. Primarily mediated by newly generated mediators of inflammation and cellular infiltration
    - Leukotrienes, eosinophils
2. Occur after a delay
    - Generally begins in 4 to 8 hours after exposure
    - May occur after initial resolution of acute symptoms
    - Can last for 24 hours or more
3. Symptoms include increasing congestion, increased rhinorrhea, wheezing
4. Contributes to chronic inflammation and tissue remodeling

D. Four broad categories of allergic triggers

i. Inhalants: pollens, animal danders, molds
ii. Ingestants: foods, medications
iii. Injectables: medications, insect venom
iv. Contactants: nickel, poison ivy, medications

E. Inhalant allergy
   i. Seasonal allergy
      a. Occurs in relation to outdoor allergens
      b. Discrete identifiable seasons with onset, peak, and decline
         1. Spring, tree pollen
         2. Summer, grass pollen
         3. Fall, weed pollen
   ii. Perennial allergy
      a. Occurs primarily in relation to indoor allergens
         1. Dust mites, cockroach, indoor molds, animal danders
            - Present throughout the year with little or no seasonality
   iii. International (World Health Organization) classifies allergy according to the ARIA (Allergic Rhinitis and its Impact on Asthma) guidelines.
      a. Use categories based on persistence and severity of symptoms
         1. Intermittent allergic rhinitis
            - Less than 4 days a week or less than 4 weeks yearly
         2. Persistent allergic rhinitis
            - Greater than 4 days a week and greater than 4 weeks yearly
         3. Grades severity as mild or moderate/severe
            - Mild: no impact on quality of life or function
            - Moderate/severe: symptoms impact quality of life or function, for example, sleep, work, school performance
   iv. Seasonal (intermittent) allergic rhinitis
      a. Pollens from outdoor plants are released into the air at discrete times during the year
      b. Pollens need to be disbursed in the atmosphere in such a way as to come into contact with human populations and create symptoms
      c. Antigenicity of a pollen is determined by Thommen postulates:
         1. For a pollen to be an effective allergen, it must be
            - Windborne
            - Light enough to be carried large distances in the air
            - Produced in large quantities
            - Abundantly distributed in the environment
            - Able to be allergenic to sensitive individuals
      d. Distribution of allergens varies based on climate, elevation, and other local agricultural characteristics
      e. Effective management of seasonal allergy requires an awareness of the locally significant pollens in a specific geographic area
      f. Seasons for various classes of pollens can be broadly grouped as follows:
         1. Trees: winter and spring allergens, generally February to May
            - Birch, Oak, Maple, Sycamore, Cedar
         2. Grasses: later spring and summer allergens, generally April to August
            - Timothy, Johnson, Bermuda
         3. Weeds: later summer and fall allergens, generally July to first frost
            - Ragweed, Sage, Lamb quarter
   v. Perennial (persistent) allergic rhinitis
      a. Allergens are present in the environment year-round and are difficult to avoid
      b. Classes of perennial allergens include dust, dust mite, cockroach, animal dander, and indoor molds

c. Dust:
   1. Composite of various antigens rather than a discrete antigen
   2. Composed of dust mite and cockroach elements, human skin, fibers, paints, animal danders
   3. Dust is not generally tested or treated as a discrete antigen currently, but rather assessed and treated by its important component elements
d. Dust mites:
   1. Small arachnids present in large quantities around human habitation
   2. Two primary species important in US allergic disease
      - Dermatophagoides pteronyssinus
      - Dermatophagoides farina
   3. Primary antigenic proteins
      - DerP1 and DerF1
   4. Found primarily in humid environments at or near sea level
   5. Prefer 70° to 80°F and 35% to 70% relative humidity
   6. Most allergenic element of the dust mite is its feces
      - Highly allergenic and easily distributed
   7. Feed on human skin scales
   8. Found in large quantities in bedrooms
e. Animal sources
   1. Can be dander, urine, excrement
   2. Cat
      - Primary antigen is FelD1
      - Found in cat pelt, cat saliva, and cat urine
      - Highly allergenic and persistent in environment
   3. Dog
      - Primary antigen is CanD1
      - Often less allergenic than cat
      - Allergen is not well understood
   4. Mouse, rat, guinea pig, horse, etc.
      - Other animal danders may be significant in situations where individuals come into regular contact with these antigens
      - Rodent allergy appears to be increasing in frequency in the inner city
      - Lab workers may develop allergy to the lab animals in their care
f. Molds
   1. Molds that demonstrate significance in perennial allergy are generally found in or near the home
      - Indoor plants, moist areas indoors, basements, refrigerators, air-conditioning units
      - Associated with plants or decaying matter near the home outdoors
   2. Mold antigens vary widely in their size and their antigenicity
      - May promote both types I and IV responses
      - Leading offenders
        (a) Alternaria, Aspergillus, Curvularia, Hormodendrum, Cladosporium, Pullaria, Penicillium
   3. Recent studies have associated mold exposure with the development of asthma, especially in children
g. Cockroach
   1. Important allergen in inner-city environments that is difficult to avoid
   2. Very potent allergen, involved in both allergic rhinitis and asthma

3. Allergen appears to involve decaying whole-body antigens
   - May be secreted by the insect
4. Primary allergens include Bla g1 and Bla g2

Diagnosis of Allergic Disease

A. Diagnosis of allergy involves three elements
   i. History of the allergic patient
      a. Types of symptoms
         1. Nasal: sneezing, itching, rhinorrhea, congestion
         2. Ocular: tearing, itching, redness
         3. Lower respiratory: wheezing, cough, dyspnea
         4. Skin: itching, redness, swelling
         5. Gastrointestinal: abdominal pain, diarrhea, vomiting (in food allergies)
   ii. Magnitude of symptoms
   iii. Duration of symptoms
      a. Transient versus persistent
      b. Intermittent or persistent as per ARIA guidelines
   iv. Triggers to symptoms
      a. Inhalants, foods, contact irritants, medications
   v. Seasonality of symptoms
      a. Seasonal versus perennial
   vi. Family history of allergy
      a. First-degree relatives versus more distant
      b. History of allergic rhinitis, conjunctivitis, asthma
   vii. Present environments
      a. Home, school, work, time spent indoors versus outdoors
   viii. Past medical history
      a. Past and current treatment (medications, immunotherapy)
      b. History of comorbid conditions (eg, asthma, sinusitis, eczema)

B. Validated survey instruments
   i. Use is recommended to aid in diagnosis of allergic rhinitis and follow treatment response
   ii. Symptom severity surveys
      a. Total Nasal Symptom Score (TNSS)
         1. Rhinorrhea
         2. Nasal itching
         3. Sneezing
         4. Congestion
      b. Rhinoconjunctivitis Quality of Life Questionnaire (RQLQ)
      c. Nasal Obstruction Symptom Evaluation (NOSE)
      d. Sino-Nasal Outcome Test (SNOT-22)
         1. Includes assessment of nasal, sinus, and quality-of-life symptoms
   iii. Medication usage
      a. Daily medication score (DMS)
   iv. Disease prediction
      a. Respiratory allergy prediction
   v. Disease control
      a. Rhinitis control test

C. Physical examination of the allergy patient
    i. Overall appearance
        a. Presence of cough, sniffling, sneezing, allergic facies
    ii. Facial appearance
        a. Dennie lines, allergic shiners, periorbital edema, nasal crease
        b. Nasal rubbing, grimacing, or wiping
        c. Mouth breathing
        d. High-arched palate in children
    iii. Eyes
        a. Conjunctival redness or injection
        b. Conjunctival edema or tearing
        c. Periorbital dark circles (allergic shiners)
    iv. Nose
        a. Diagnostic nasal endoscopy is an option
            1. Can aid in exclusion of other causes of symptoms
        b. Size of inferior turbinates
        c. Color of nasal mucosa
            1. Pale, boggy mucosa in allergic rhinitis
        d. Presence of mucoid or mucopurulent secretion
        e. Position of nasal septum
        f. Nasal polyps
    v. Oral cavity/oropharynx
        a. Size of tonsils
        b. Presence of cobblestoning on posterior pharyngeal wall
        c. High-arched palate
    vi. Skin
        a. Eczema or atopic dermatitis lesions
        b. Urticaria (hives)
    vii. Lungs
        a. Presence of wheezing
        b. Use of accessory muscles of respiration
    viii. Cardiovascular
        a. Assess for signs of anaphylaxis in severe cases
D. Diagnostic testing of the allergic patient
    i. Specific allergen testing
        a. Designed to assess the presence of discrete allergens to which the patient shows hypersensitivity.
        b. Can be done through either in vivo (skin testing) or in vitro (serum testing) methods.
        c. Goal is to identify
            1. Whether the patient is allergic
            2. The antigens to which the patient is allergic
            3. The degree of sensitization
        d. Testing for inhalant allergens is safe and useful.
        e. A patient may have positive allergy tests without any allergic symptoms.
            1. Suggests that the patient is atopic, but may not have sufficient sensitization to be symptomatic
        f. Presence of symptoms is necessary to classify the patient as "allergic."
            1. Consideration of cross-reactivity between allergens (eg, pollen-food allergy syndrome)

g. In vivo allergy tests:
   1. Skin prick/puncture testing
      - Should be used in eligible patients when allergen immunotherapy is being considered
      - Recommended method of allergy testing
      - Provides rapid results (15-20 minutes)
      - Safe, with rare systemic reactions
   2. Skin intradermal testing
      - Often used to diagnose allergy
      - Can test sensitivity to other substances
        (a) Local anesthetics, neuromuscular blocking agents, antibiotics, contrast media
      - No longer recommended for food or chemical allergy
      - Can be used to
        (a) Determine starting point for allergen immunotherapy
        (b) Confirm skin prick testing
        (c) Higher risk of systemic reactions compared to skin prick testing
   3. Patch testing
      - Used for diagnosing contact dermatitis (Type IV hypersensitivity)
      - Involves applying allergens to the skin under occlusion for 48 hours
   4. Atopy patch testing
      - Combines features of skin prick testing and patch testing for diagnosing food allergies and atopic dermatitis
   5. Intradermal dilutional testing (IDT)
      - Less common in clinical practice than skin prick testing
      - Fivefold dilutions of each antigen are prepared and labeled from #1 through #6
      - IDT has been shown to have utility in the diagnosis of allergy and in guiding the preparation of sera for safe immunotherapy
      - Not standardized and generally not recommended for routine practice
   6. Component-resolved diagnostics
      - Uses purified allergen components to identify specific IgE sensitization patterns
      - Helps in risk assessment and management, especially in food allergies

h. In vitro allergy testing
   1. Immunoassays for specific IgE (eg, ImmunoCAP)
      - Measures the serum level of allergen-specific IgE
      - More sensitive and specific than older radioallergosorbent (RAST) tests
   2. Total serum IgE
      - Measurement of the total amount of nonspecific IgE.
      - High levels of total IgE ($\geq$ 100-150 IU/mL) suggest allergy or atopic disease.
      - Low levels of total IgE do not rule out the presence of allergy
        (a) Patients with low total IgE may still have one or more allergens that demonstrate significant levels of specific IgE.
      - Total IgE is nonspecific and can be useful as a screen, but low levels do not necessarily eliminate the presence of clinically significant allergy.
   3. Basophil activation test
      - Measures activation markers (eg, CD63, CD203c) on basophils in response to allergen exposure
      - Used in research and specialized settings

4. Molecular allergology
   - Assessment of specific IgE against individual allergen components
   - Improves diagnostic precision and management decisions
5. Indications for in vitro testing
   - Patients requiring allergy testing to determine the presence of allergy and to estimate degree of allergic sensitization
   - Patients not responding to environmental control and conservative medical management
   - Apprehensive children in whom allergy seems likely
   - Symptomatic patients with conditions in which in vivo skin testing is contraindicated (eg, dermatographism, eczema)
   - Patients on beta-blocking medications
   - Patients on antihistamines who are unwilling or unable to discontinue medications
   - Patients doing poorly on immunotherapy
   - Venom sensitivity
   - Diagnosis of IgE-mediated food sensitivity
   - Patients with extensive skin disease (eg, psoriasis, atopic dermatitis)
6. Contraindication for in vitro testing:
   - Cannot diagnose non–IgE-mediated disorders
   - Limited utility in conditions like eosinophilic esophagitis without IgE sensitization
7. Advantages of in vitro assays:
   - No risk of anaphylaxis
   - Eliminate variability of the skin response
   - Eliminates the need to avoid drugs that affect skin response
   - Safe for patients on beta-blockers
   - Allow testing for numerous antigens to be conducted on a single serum sample
   - Provide a quantitative assessment that can be used to estimate degree of allergic sensitization and for preparation of allergy sera for immunotherapy
   - Quantitative assessment may predict response to allergen immunotherapy
   - Demonstrate greater specificity than skin testing
   - Useful in patients with extensive skin disease or when skin testing is not feasible
8. Disadvantages of in vitro assays:
   - Generally more expensive than skin testing
   - Results may vary depending on the available assays
   - Results are not immediate like skin testing
   - Can be confounded by cross-reacting allergens and polysensitization
   - Lower sensitivity compared to skin prick testing in some allergens
   - May not correlate with clinical symptoms in all cases

ii. Nasal-specific IgE
   a. Local allergic rhinitis
      1. May affect up to 25% of the patients diagnosed with non-allergic rhinitis
      2. Production of local IgE and immune mediators in the nose itself, without systemic presence of IgE
      3. Diagnosis confirmed by
         - Nasal provocation test

- IgE in nasal secretions
  (a) Identify by nasal lavage, cellulose disks, mucosal biopsy, brushings
- There is no normative nasal IgE data
- Techniques have similar results.

4. Testing can be important for management
   - Allows for allergen avoidance
   - Allergen immunotherapy may be indicated

b. Not routinely performed due to practical limitations

iii. Nasal cytology
   a. Designed to evaluate for the presence of eosinophils versus neutrophils in the nasal mucus
   b. Rarely used, very nonspecific
   c. Three steps
      1. Sample nasal mucosa surface cells
      2. Stain with May-Grünwald-Giemsa method to identify inflammatory cells
         - Neutrophils, eosinophils, lymphocytes, mast cells
      3. Examine through optical microscopy to detect all cells
         - At least 50 microscopic fields
   d. Can detect
      1. Viruses, fungi, bacteria
   e. Allergic rhinitis
      1. Eosinophils > mast cells > basophils
   f. Nonallergic Rhinitis
      1. NARES (nonallergic rhinitis and eosinophilia syndrome)
         - Perennial rhinitis
         - Negative skin testing
         - Eosinophilia in nasal secretions
      2. NARMA (nonallergic rhinitis with mast cells)
      3. NARNE (nonallergic rhinitis with neutrophils)
      4. NARESMA (nonallergic rhinitis with eosinophils and mast cells
   g. Not widely used due to lack of standardization and limited clinical utility

Treatment of Allergy

A. All patients with allergies need to be actively involved in their treatment
   i. Education regarding allergic sensitivities and their management is essential for all allergy patients
   ii. Emphasizing patient-centered care and shared decision-making enhances treatment adherence and outcomes

B. The treatment of allergy generally relies on a three-pronged strategy, with the combination of these approaches individualized for each patient
   i. Environmental control/avoidance
   ii. Pharmacotherapy
   iii. Immunotherapy
      a. Biologic therapies are emerging as additional options for select patients

C. Environmental control:
   i. Involves decreasing the allergen load to which the patient is exposed by altering the environment of the patient

ii. While conceptually attractive, avoidance can be difficult to do and is of questionable efficacy in routine use
   a. However, environmental control measures are recommended as part of a comprehensive management plan, especially when targeted to specific allergens
   b. Pollens
      1. Difficult to avoid due to wide airborne distribution
      2. Avoidance of outdoor activities at times of greater pollen release
         - Pollen counts can be found on publicly available websites
      3. Avoidance should focus on residential management
         - Use of air-conditioners in the home
         - Keeping windows closed to prevent pollens from entering the indoor environment
         - Limit presence of offending plants in the immediate vicinity
         - Removing clothing and washing hair prior to entering bedrooms
      4. Avoidance has not been studied and clinical efficacy is unknown
      5. Studies suggest that these measures can reduce exposure and may alleviate symptoms, but complete avoidance is often impractical
      6. Physical barriers
         - Wrap-around eyeglasses
           (a) Significant improvement in ocular and nasal symptoms
         - Use of masks designed to filter pollen particles can reduce inhaled allergens during high pollen periods
         - Active nasal filter
           (b) Significant improvement in some nasal symptoms
   c. Molds
      1. Avoid damp environments
      2. Avoid dense landscaping with decaying organic material near the house
      3. Prevent moisture accumulation indoors around pipes, air conditioners, refrigerators, bathroom fixtures
      4. Regular cleaning and maintenance can reduce mold growth and spore dissemination
   d. Dust/dust mites
      1. Chemical techniques
         - The use of acaricides has limited efficacy; focus is on environmental modifications
      2. Use of synthetic carpets or elimination of carpets
      3. Regular and frequent vacuuming
         - HEPA vacuums distribute lesser levels of dust into the air and decrease symptoms in susceptible individuals.
      4. Regular changing of filters in the heating and air-conditioning systems
         - Using high-efficiency particulate air (HEPA) filters in HVAC systems can reduce airborne allergens.
      5. Use of impervious pillow and mattress covers on bedding
         - Significantly decreases antigen load
         - No difference in symptom severity
      6. Regular washing of bedding in hot (>140°F) water
      7. HEPA filters in the bedroom and other frequently occupied areas of the home
         - Filter must be of adequate capacity for size of room.

8. Combination of multiple environmental control measures may provide better symptom relief than single interventions.
9. While chemical agents like acaricides show limited efficacy, physical measures such as using allergen-impermeable mattress and pillow covers, reducing indoor humidity, and regular cleaning are recommended to minimize dust mite exposure

e. Animals
1. Removal or avoidance of the pet.
   - Studies site 4% of patients adhere to this recommendation.
2. Goal should be to decrease antigen exposure.
   - Pet washing at least twice a week to maintain significant antigen reduction.
     (a) Effectiveness is temporary and may not significantly reduce allergen levels.
   - Hypoallergenic animals have same levels of some allergenic antigens as nonhypoallergenic species.
   - Multimodality therapy is recommended.
   - Single modality has not been shown to improve symptoms.
3. Keeping pets out of the bedroom and using HEPA air purifiers may help reduce exposure.

f. Cockroach
1. Common in
   - Densely populated areas
     (a) Cities
   - Apartment/high occupant complexes
   - Homes in warm rural areas
2. Three key strategies
   - Education
     (a) House cleaning
     (b) Seal cracks in high infestation areas like the kitchen
   - Physical
     (a) Insecticides
     (b) Traps
   - Combination of education and physical methods
   - Either method has been shown to significantly decrease antigens and improve symptoms.
   - Pest control either professional or with insecticide traps is more effective at decreasing cockroach antigen load.
     (a) Traps are more cost-effective
   - Allergen reduction is difficult to maintain over time, especially in cities and densely populated complexes

D. Pharmacotherapy:
i. Primary treatment for majority of symptomatic allergic patients.
ii. Indicated in all patients with inhalant allergy.
iii. Treatment choice should be individualized based on symptom severity, patient preference, and response to therapy.
iv. Antihistamines
   a. Reduced nasal puritis, nasal obstruction, sneezing, and rhinorrhea
   b. Second-generation antihistamines are preferred due to better side-effect profiles

c. Have little effect on congestion
    1. Congestion driven significantly by late-phase mediators
    2. Exception: topically applied antihistamines have been shown to have clinically significant effects on reduction of nasal congestion
d. H2 blockers
    1. Ranitidine
        - Note that ranitidine has been withdrawn in many countries due to NDMA contamination concerns and is no longer recommended or available.
    2. Traditionally thought of as agents to decrease gastric acid secretion
    3. Not recommended for the treatment of allergic rhinitis
e. H1 blockers are classified by generation:
    1. First-generation oral antihistamines
        - Include agents such as diphenhydramine, chlorpheniramine, triprolidine, azatadine
        - Highly lipophilic
            (a) Cross the blood-brain barrier readily
            (b) Result in high incidence of sedation and central nervous system (CNS) suppressive effects
        - Highly anticholinergic
            (a) Drying of mucous membranes
            (b) Increase in mucus tenacity
            (c) Blurring of vision
            (d) Constipation
            (e) Urinary retention
        - May be accompanied with tachyphylaxis
            (a) Efficacy decreases with continued use
        - Inhibitors of CYP2D6
            (a) Involved in the metabolism of
                - TCAs
                - Some antipsychotics
                - Beta blockers
                - Anti-arrhythmics
                - Tramadol
        - Not recommended for the treatment of allergy
            (a) Have a significant negative impact on quality of life
    2. Second-generation oral antihistamines
        - Include medications such as loratadine, fexofenadine, cetirizine, desloratadine, levocetirizine
        - Lipophobic
            (a) Do not cross the blood-brain barrier as readily
            (b) Less likely to result in sedation or CNS effects
                - Can be dose related
            (c) Little or no anticholinergic activity
                - Safe to use in patients with asthma
            (d) Little if any tachyphylaxis
        - Recommended as first-line therapy for mild to moderate allergic rhinitis
        - Metabolized by CYP3A4
            (a) Be aware of the use of CYP3A4 inhibitors
        - Not cost prohibitive as many are available over-the-counter
        - Strongly recommended for the treatment of allergy

3. Topical antihistamines
   - Work directly through application at the target organ (eg, eye, nose)
   - Medications include azelastine, olopatadine
   - Rapid onset of action
   - Azelastine is as effective or superior to oral antihistamines for the treatment of nasal congestion
   - Intranasal antihistamines can be used alone or in combination with intranasal corticosteroids, depending on symptom severity and patient preference

v. Decongestants
  a. Administered either orally or topically to decrease nasal obstruction
  b. Have minimal effect on rhinorrhea, itching, or sneezing
  c. Work as alpha-1 agonists
  d. Bind to alpha-1 receptors on target organs
    1. Decrease vascular engorgement through vasoconstrictive mechanism
  e. Systemic decongestants
    1. Include pseudoephedrine and phenylephrine
       - Pseudoephedrine available only behind the pharmacy counter due to its ability to be converted chemically to methamphetamine
       - Phenylephrine has limited efficacy in symptom control
    2. Often combined with antihistamines to provide decongestant effect.
    3. Can be accompanied by significant alpha-adrenergic side effects.
       - Increased blood pressure in hypertensive patients
       - Loss of appetite
       - Insomnia
       - Increased cardiac symptoms
         (a) Tachycardia
         (b) Arrhythmia
  f. Topical decongestants
    1. Include oxymetazoline, phenylephrine, naphazoline, tetrahydrozoline.
    2. Work rapidly to decrease nasal congestion with excellent efficacy.
    3. Rapid rebound congestion can develop with use for as few as 3 days.
       - Leads to rhinitis medicamentosa, a severe representation of nasal congestion
    4. Option to use for short-term nasal decongestion (3 days or less).
    5. Have no effect on the other symptoms of allergic rhinitis (sneezing, rhinorrhea, nasal itching).

vi. Corticosteroids
  a. Can be used systemically or topically
  b. Block the generation and release of mediators and the influx of inflammatory cells
  c. Work on genetic transcription and protein synthesis in the nucleus of cells
  d. Wide range of effects is noted
    1. Cellular (mast cells, eosinophils, macrophages, lymphocytes, neutrophils)
    2. Humoral mediators (histamine, eicosanoids, leukotrienes, cytokines)
  e. Injectable corticosteroids:
    1. Rarely used in clinical practice
    2. Depot injections of corticosteroids are discouraged by current guidelines due to potentially significant prolonged adverse effects:

- Psychiatric (eg, psychosis, mood swings)
- Musculoskeletal (eg, joint and soft tissue abnormalities)
- Cataract formation
- Suppression of adrenal function

3. Not recommended for the routine treatment of allergic rhinitis

f. Oral corticosteroids:
1. Preferential to parenteral corticosteroids for the management of allergic rhinitis
2. Can be used for short courses in serious allergic inflammation
3. Often notice effects within 12 to 24 hours
4. Commonly used oral corticosteroids
    - Prednisone
    - Methylprednisolone
    - Dexamethasone
5. Because of their systemic adverse events the use of oral corticosteroids has been largely replaced by intranasal corticosteroids
6. Not recommended for routine use in allergic rhinitis

g. Topical corticosteroids
1. First-line therapy for moderate to severe allergic rhinitis
    - Strong recommendation for their use
    - Considered the most effective single-agent maintenance therapy
2. Can be used alone or in combination with other pharmacotherapies
    - Combination therapy with intranasal antihistamines may provide additional benefit
3. Increase local concentrations of effective agent with concurrent limitation of systemic absorption and adverse effects
4. Newer agents generally free of hypothalamic-pituitary-adrenal (HPA) axis suppression
5. Demonstrate broad local anti-inflammatory benefits and significant reduction in nasal and ocular symptoms
    - Secondary to reduced naso-ocular reflex
6. Variable onset
    - 3 to 5 hours up to 60 hours after first dose
    - Should start 2 weeks prior to pollen season
7. Daily dosing more efficacious than as-needed dosing
8. Agents
    - Fluticasone propionate
        (a) Widely available as a generic preparation
    - Fluticasone furoate
        (a) Indication for allergic rhinitis and labeled effectiveness for eye symptoms.
        (b) Approved for use down to age 2
    - Mometasone furoate
        (a) Indication for both allergic rhinitis and nasal polyps
        (b) Approved for use down to age 2
    - Budesonide
        (a) Only topical nasal corticosteroid with a pregnancy category B rating
    - Ciclesonide
        (a) Administered as a prodrug and activated by tissue esterases

9. Side effects
    - Epistaxis, dryness, local irritation. Aim spray away from septum
    - Rare septal perforation
    - No clinically relevant impact on ocular pressure, glaucoma, lens opacity, or cataract formation
    - Minimal impact on growth in children at recommended doses; monitoring may be considered

vii. Cromolyn sodium
  a. Mechanism of action
    1. Stabilizes mast cell membranes and inhibits degranulation and release of histamine
  b. Lipophobic without systemic absorption
    1. Free of systemic adverse effects
  c. Available in topical form for both ocular and nasal symptom
    1. Must be administered three to four times daily due to very short half-life
    2. Will not treat symptoms once exposure has occurred and mast cells have degranulated
    3. Best used prophylactically
  d. Inferior to intranasal corticosteroids
  e. Difficulty with compliance to frequent dosing regimen
  f. Can consider in patients who cannot take intranasal corticosteroids

viii. Leukotriene receptor antagonists
  a. Block the binding of leukotrienes to target cells
  b. Efficacy demonstrated in the treatment of allergic rhinitis
    1. Inferior to intranasal corticosteroids
  c. Systemic use also has therapeutic effect in lower airway disease
  d. Agent:
    1. Montelukast
      - Indicated for allergic rhinitis, asthma, and exercise-induced bronchospasm
      - Carries a boxed warning for serious neuropsychiatric events, including suicidal thoughts and actions; risks and benefits should be carefully considered
      - Indicated for use down to 6 months of age
      - Expensive compared to other therapies
      - Not recommended as first-line therapy or as monotherapy for allergic rhinitis
  e. Not recommended as first-line therapy or as monotherapy for allergic rhinitis
  f. Can be considered second-line therapy or when intranasal corticosteroids are contraindicated

ix. Intranasal anticholinergics
  a. Ipratropium bromide
    1. Decreases watery nasal secretions from seromucus glands
    2. Used to decrease rhinorrhea in rhinitis or colds
    3. Needs to be administered 2 to 3 times a day because of moderate half-life
    4. Use in combination with intranasal corticosteroids for rhinorrhea from allergic rhinitis is more effective than either agent alone
      - Can be used as adjuvant therapy in patients with persistent rhinorrhea despite intranasal corticosteroid use

x. Biologics
   a. Biologics are emerging therapies for severe allergic diseases; their role in allergic rhinitis is under investigation, indicated for eosinophilic asthma and CRswNP
   b. Omalizumab
      1. Inhibits binding of IgE to IgE receptors
         - Reduction of release of allergic mediators
      2. Approved for asthma and chronic idiopathic urticaria
      3. Not FDA-approved for allergic rhinitis but has shown efficacy in clinical trials; may be considered in select cases
   c. Mepolizumab
      1. Anti IL-5 monoclonal antibody
      2. Interrupts eosinophil chemotaxis, activation, and survival
      3. Induces eosinophil apoptosis
      4. Approved for severe eosinophilic asthma and CRSwNP
   d. Dupilumab
      1. Inhibits IL-4Rα required for IL-4 and IL-13 signaling
      2. Decreased Th2 inflammation/activation
      3. Decreased recruitment of eosinophils
      4. Approved for atopic dermatitis, asthma, and CRSwNP
   e. New biologics like tezepelumab are under investigation for potential use in allergic rhinitis and may represent future therapeutic options

xi. Nasal saline
   a. Studies have found improvements in symptomatic allergic rhinitis
   b. Isotonic vs hypertonic
      1. Isotonic saline use had improved mucociliary clearance
      2. In children, hypertonic saline irrigations showed significant improvement in nasal symptoms
   c. Combination with intranasal steroid use had increased symptom relief than either alone in both adults and children
      1. Also shows improved symptom control in combination with any first-line allergic rhinitis therapy
      2. Strongly recommended as adjunct therapy

E. Immunotherapy
   i. Process of administering allergen either subcutaneously or sublingually over time to induce allergic tolerance and reduction of allergic symptoms
      a. Both subcutaneous and sublingual administration of immunotherapy are both strongly recommended for the treatment of allergic symptoms.
      b. Treating for an adequate period of time:
         1. Immunotherapy generally is felt to require at least 3 to 5 years of regular administration to permit persistence of benefits after discontinuation.
   ii. Subcutaneous immunotherapy (SCIT)
      a. Treatment of IgE-mediated allergy
      b. Involves the injections of sequentially greater concentrations of allergens over time to induce hyposensitization and immune tolerance
      c. Begins with very dilute concentrations of allergenic sera, injected once or twice weekly, and advanced until maximal tolerability and delivery of adequate dosage of antigen is achieved

iii. Sublingual immunotherapy (SLIT)
   a. Involves the administration of allergens orally as aqueous/drops or tablets under the tongue to achieve hyposensitization and induce immune tolerance.
      1. Dosages may be given in fixed or escalating schedules
      2. FDA-approved SLIT tablets are available for certain allergens (eg, grass pollen, ragweed, house dust mite)

F. Surgical options
   i. To target symptoms refractory to medical therapies
   ii. Inferior turbinate reduction/outfracture
      a. Targets refractory nasal obstruction
   iii. Coblation and radiofrequency ablation
      a. Target the inferior turbinate, septal swell body, and nasal valve to address nasal obstruction
   iv. Cryoablation and radiofrequency ablation
      a. Significant improvement in total nasal symptom scores (TNSS) scores.
      b. Target the posterior nasal nerve.
      c. Emerging procedures such as endoscopic posterior nasal nerve ablation or ligation may be considered in select cases of allergic rhinitis.

G. Additional application of allergy in rhinology
   i. CRSwNP
      a. Th2 mediated inflammation associated with
         1. Allergy
         2. Nasal polyps
            - Elevated IL-5 and IL-13
            - Elevated eosinophils
      b. Inhalant allergy
         1. Specifically, dust mites, dust, cockroach
      c. Biologics such as dupilumab, mepolizumab, and omalizumab have been approved for the treatment of CRSwNP
   ii. Aspirin exacerbated respiratory disease (AERD)
      a. About 10% of patients with CRSwNP
      b. Type 2 inflammatory response
      c. Innate immune response
         1. Type 2 innate lymphoid cells → activation of mast cells
      d. Samter triad
         1. CRSwNP
         2. Respiratory reactions to aspirin and nonsteroidal anti-inflammatory drugs (NSAIDs)
            - Cyclooxygenase 1 (COX1) inhibitors
         3. Asthma
         4. Triad may develop over time
      e. Dysfunction in the arachidonic acid pathway
         1. NSAID COX1 inhibition + AERD (natural decrease in COX1) → excess proinflammatory activation of eosinophils, mast cells, and basophils
      f. AERD patients have high levels of tissue eosinophilia
      g. Aspirin desensitization is an established treatment option for AERD
      h. Biologics may also be effective in managing AERD symptoms

- iii. Central compartment atopic disease (CCAD)
  - a. Middle turbinate (MT) edema/polyposis
    - 1. Strong association between allergy/atopy
  - b. CCAD
    - 1. MT polypoid edema with progression to superior turbinate, posterior nasal septum (central nasal cavity structures)
    - 2. Sparing of lateral and superior sinus surfaces
  - c. May coexist with
    - 1. AERD
    - 2. Respiratory epithelioid hamartoma (REAH)
- iv. Allergic fungal rhinosinusitis (AFRS)
  - a. Eosinophilic subtype of CRSwNP
  - b. Bent and Kuhn Criteria
    - 1. Type I hypersensitivity
    - 2. Nasal polyposis
    - 3. CT findings
      - Expanded paranasal sinuses
      - Bony erosion
      - High-density materials within sinuses
    - 4. Eosinophilic mucin without fungal invasion
      - Necrotic eosinophils
      - Charcot-Leyden crystals
      - Fungal hyphae
    - 5. Positive fungal stain
      - Dematiaceous fungi
      - *Aspergillus*
  - c. Treatment includes surgery and corticosteroids; the role of antifungal therapy remains controversial
  - d. Upregulated pathways involved in T cell activation and the adaptive immune response
    - 1. Elevated serum total and fungal-specific IgE

Bibliography

Bachert C, Zhang N, Hellings PW, Bousquet J. Endotype-driven care pathways in patients with chronic rhinosinusitis. *J Allergy Clin Immunol*. 2018;5:1543-1551.

Brozek JL, Bousquet J, Agache I, et al. Allergic rhinitis and its impact on asthma (ARIA) guidelines – 2016 revision. *J Allergy Clin Immunol*. 2017;140:950-958.

Chan Y, Goddard JC. *K. J. Lee's Essential Otolaryngology Head and Neck Surgery*. 12th ed. New York, NY: McGraw-Hill.

Chang MT, Song S, Hwang PH. Cryosurgical ablation for treatment of rhinitis: a prospective multicenter study. *Laryngoscope*. 2020;130:1877-1884.

Ehmer D, McDuffie CM, Scurry WC, et al. Temperature-controlled radiofrequency neurolysis for the treatment of rhinitis. *Am J Rhinol Allergy*. 2022;36(1):149-156.

Khan Academy. Immune system. https://www.khanacademy.org/test-prep/mcat/organ-systems/the-immune-system.

Leatherman BD, Khalid A, Lee S, et al. Dosing of sublingual immunotherapy for allergic rhinitis: evidence-based review with recommendations. *Int Forum Allergy Rhinol*. 2015;5:773-783.

Orlandi RR, Kingdom TT, Smith TL, et al. International consensus statement on allergy and rhinology: rhinosinusitis 2021. *Int Forum Allergy Rhinol.* 2021;11(3):213-739.

Wise SK, Damask C, Roland L, et al. Internation consensus statement on allergy and rhinology: Allergic Rhinitis - 2023. *Int Forum Allergy Rhinol.* 2023 Apr;13(4):293-859.

Questions

1. Which is not thought to be involved in the allergy response?
   A. IL-4
   B. IL-5
   C. Th2 cells
   D. Th1 cells

2. A 56-year-old woman with hypertension and occasional shortness of breath is considering beginning SCIT. Which is an absolute contraindication to this course of treatment?
   A. Uncontrolled asthma
   B. Enalapril
   C. Trouble with transportation
   D. Concurrent food allergies

3. Which is considered first-line therapy for allergic rhinitis?
   A. Montelukast
   B. Omalizumab
   C. Azelastine
   D. Fluticasone

4. A patient who has been receiving SCIT for the last year came in for a shot an hour ago from a new vial, was observed for 30 minutes, and is now calling from home. The patient is complaining of nausea, diarrhea, and shortness of breath. What should you tell the patient to do immediately?
   A. Drive to the emergency room
   B. Take Benadryl
   C. Use epinephrine autoinjector
   D. Drink plenty of fluids

5. Which is false about using nasal saline for allergic rhinitis?
   A. Nasal saline used in conjunction with intranasal corticosteroids is superior to intranasal corticosteroids as monotherapy
   B. Hypertonic saline irrigations have been shown to be more beneficial for symptom control in children than isotonic saline
   C. Nasal saline is not recommended for use in the treatment of allergic rhinitis
   D. Isotonic saline may work by improving mucociliary clearance

Part 9
Review

Chapter 59
Highlights and Pearls

Embryology

A. Branchial (pharyngeal) apparatus
   i. (Arches: mesoderm
   ii. Pouches: endoderm
   iii. Clefts: between arches, ectoderm
B. Branchial arch derivatives: cranial nerve, muscle, cartilage, artery
   i. First arch (mandibular)
      a. Nerve: trigeminal (V)
      b. Muscle: muscles of mastication (masseter, temporalis, medial, and lateral pterygoid), floor of mouth muscles (mylohyoid, anterior belly of digastric), tensor tympani, tensor veli palatini
      c. Skeletal structure: Meckel cartilage (malleus, incus, mandible)
      d. Artery: maxillary
      e. Cleft derivatives: auricle, external auditory canal (EAC)
      f. Pouch derivatives: middle ear, eustachian tube
   ii. Second arch (hyoid)
      a. Nerve: facial (VII)
      b. Muscle: platysma, stapedius, posterior digastric, stylohyoid, muscles of facial expression

c. Skeletal structure: stapes superstructure, styloid process, stylohyoid ligament, lesser cornu/upper portion of hyoid
d. Artery: stapedial
e. Pouch and derivative: palatine tonsil

iii. Third arch
a. Nerve: glossopharyngeal (IX)
b. Muscle: stylopharyngeus
c. Skeletal structure: greater cornu/lower body of hyoid
d. Artery: common and internal carotid
e. Pouch and derivative: thymus, inferior parathyroid

iv. Fourth arch
a. Nerve: superior laryngeal (X)
b. Muscle: pharyngeal constrictors, cricothyroid, cricopharyngeus
c. Skeletal structure: laryngeal cartilages
d. Artery: right—subclavian, left—aortic arch
e. Pouch and derivative: superior parathyroid, parafollicular (c) cells of thyroid

v. Sixth arch
a. Nerve: recurrent laryngeal (X)
b. Muscle: intrinsic muscles of larynx
c. Skeletal structure: laryngeal cartilages
d. Artery: right—pulmonary artery, left—ductus arteriosus

C. Hillocks of His
i. Begins at fifth to sixth week of gestation from first and second branchial arches
ii. External ear develops from six small buds of mesenchyme
iii. Hillocks of His fuse during the 12th week
iv. First arch: 1) Tragus; 2) Helical crus; 3) Helix
v. Second arch: 4) Antihelix; 5) Antitragus; 6) Lobule (last to form)

D. Tongue
i. Anterior two-thirds of tongue form from:
a. Tuberculum impar in midline
b. Two lateral lingual prominences
ii. Posterior one-third of tongue forms from copula

E. Thyroid
i. At 3 to 4 weeks of gestation, starts as diverticulum of endoderm (first and second pharyngeal pouches) at the base of tongue (foramen cecum)
ii. Migrates inferiorly around fifth week of gestation, reaches final destination by seventh week of gestation
a. Connected to foregut by thyroglossal duct as it descends into neck; thyroglossal duct obliterates
b. Ultimobranchial body contributes to parafollicular C cells of thyroid

F. Nasal dermal sinus
i. *Foramen cecum*: anterior neuropore at anterior floor of cranial vault
ii. *Prenasal space*: potential space beneath nasal bone extending from anterior aspect of nasal bone to frontal bone/foramen cecum region
iii. *Fonticulus frontalis*: embryologic space between nasal and frontal bones
iv. Dura and nasal skin lie in close proximity and separate when foramen cecum closes
a. Persistent dural-dermal connection via foramen cecum and pre-nasal space (less frequently via fonticulus frontalis) produces gliomas, meningoceles, or nasal encephaloceles projecting from above. Projecting from below may be dermal sinuses or dermoids

G. Sinus
   i. *Ethmoturbinals:* series of ridges or folds on the lateral nasal wall that appear around eighth week of gestation
      a. First: Agger nasi (superior) and uncinate process (inferior)
      b. Second: Middle turbinate
      c. Third: Superior turbinate
      d. Fourth/fifth: Supreme turbinate
   ii. Maxillary sinus forms as furrows in lateral nasal wall at 8 to 10 weeks of gestation
   iii. Ethmoid sinuses form in second trimester
   iv. Sphenoid sinuses form in third month of gestation; pneumatize at 2 years of age
   v. Frontal sinuses form from anterior pneumatization into frontal bone; generally evident by 7 years of age

Anatomy

A. Skin
   i. *Epidermis*: stratum corneum, stratum granulosum, stratum lucidum, stratum spinosum, stratum basale
   ii. Dermis
   iii. Subcutis
B. Contents of skull base foramina B) (Figures 59-1 to 59-8)
   i. Cribriform plate—olfactory nerves (CN I)
   ii. Optic canal
      a. Optic nerve (CN II)
      b. Ophthalmic artery, first branch is the central retinal artery
      c. Central retinal vein

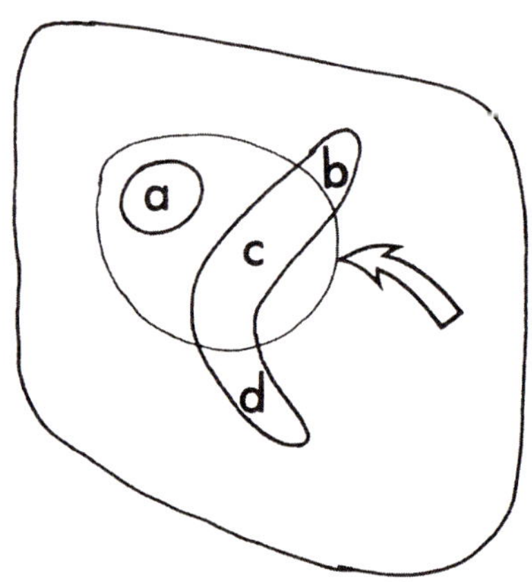

Figure 59-1 Left orbit. Arrow points to tendon of Zinn, which divides the orbital fissures into three compartments. Structures passing through (a) are the optic nerve and the ophthalmic artery. Structures passing through (b) are the trochlear nerve and the lacrimal and frontal divisions of V_1 as well as the supraorbital vein. Structures passing through (c) are the oculomotor and abducens nerves and the nasociliary division of V_1. Structures passing through (d) are the zygomaticofacial and zygomaticotemporal divisions of V_2 and the inferior ophthalmic vein.

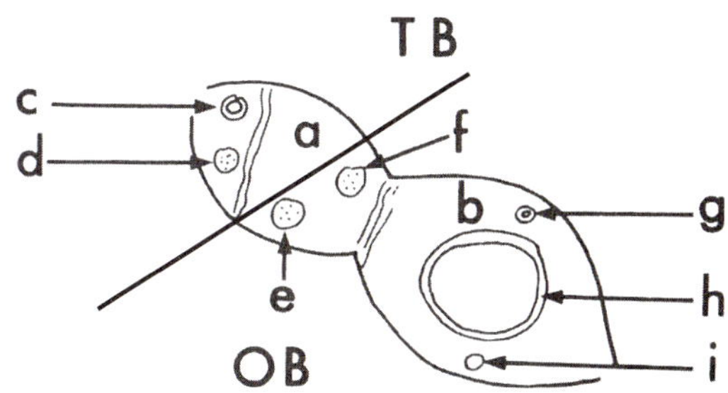

Figure 59-2 Right jugular foramen. (TB, temporal bone; OB, occipital bone; a, pars nervosa [contains c, inferior petrosal sinus; d, glossopharyngeal nerve]; b, pars vascularis [contains e, vagus nerve; f, accessory nerve; g, posterior meningeal artery; h, internal jugular vein; i, nodes of Krause.])

iii. Superior orbital fissure
   a. CN III (oculomotor), IV (trochlear), V1 (first branch of trigeminal), VI (abducens)
   b. Middle meningeal artery (orbital branch)
   c. Superior ophthalmic vein

iv. Inferior orbital fissure
   a. V2 branches (zygomatic nerves, sphenopalatine branch)
   b. Infraorbital artery and vein

v. Foramen rotundum—V2 branches

vi. Foramen ovale
   a. V3
   b. Accessory meningeal artery
   c. Emissary vein
   d. Lesser petrosal nerve

vii. Foramen spinosum—Middle meningeal artery

viii. Foramen lacerum
   a. Meningeal branch of ascending pharyngeal artery
   b. Emissary vein
   c. Internal carotid artery (partially traverses)
   d. Greater petrosal nerve

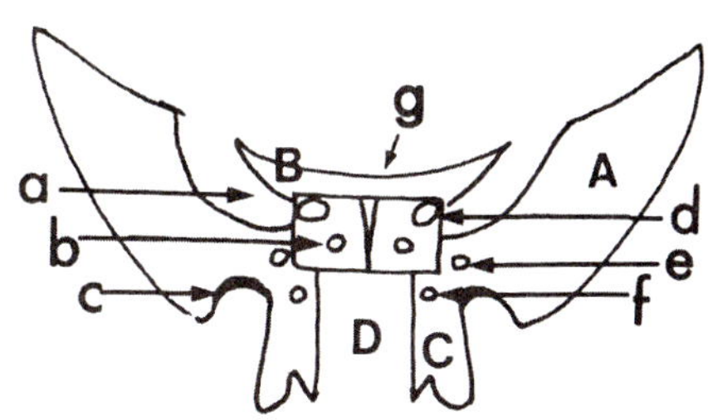

Figure 59-3 Sphenoid bone. (A, greater wing; B, lesser wing; C, pterygoid process; D, nasal cavity; a, foramen rotundum; b, pterygoid canal; c, jugum. Note: Pterygoid processes have medial and lateral plates [the lateral plate is the origin for both pterygoid muscles] and the hamulus [for tensor palati]).

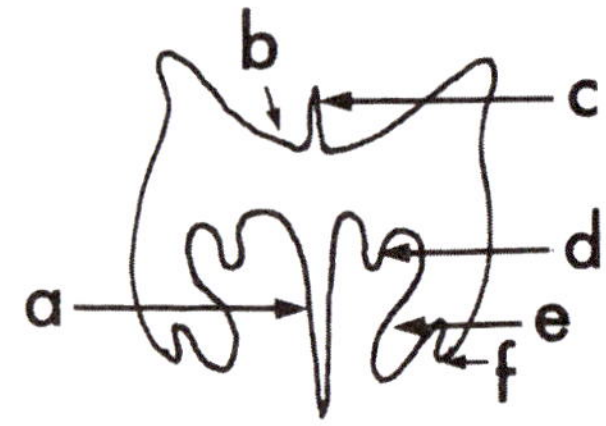

Figure 59-4 Ethmoid bone. (a, perpendicular plate; b, cribriform plate; c, crista galli, d, superior turbinate; e, middle turbinate; f, uncinate process.)

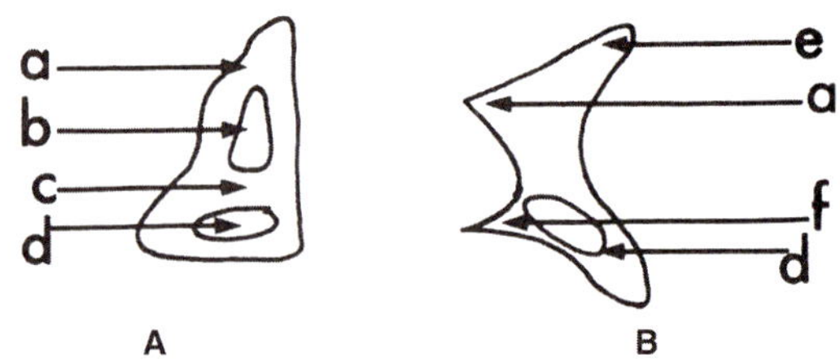

Figure 59-5 Right arytenoid. A. anterior view; B. lateral view. (a, colliculus; b, triangular pit; c, arcuate crest; d, oblong pit; e, corniculate; f, vocal process.)

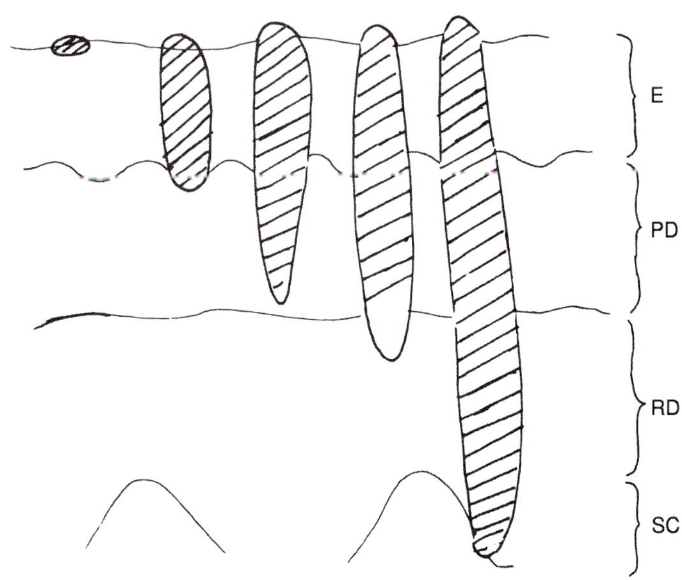

Figure 59-6 Clinicopathologic staging of melanoma. (E, epidermis; PD, papillary dermis; RD, reticular dermis; SC, subcutaneous tissue; BANS, back, upper arm, posterolateral neck, posterior scalp.)

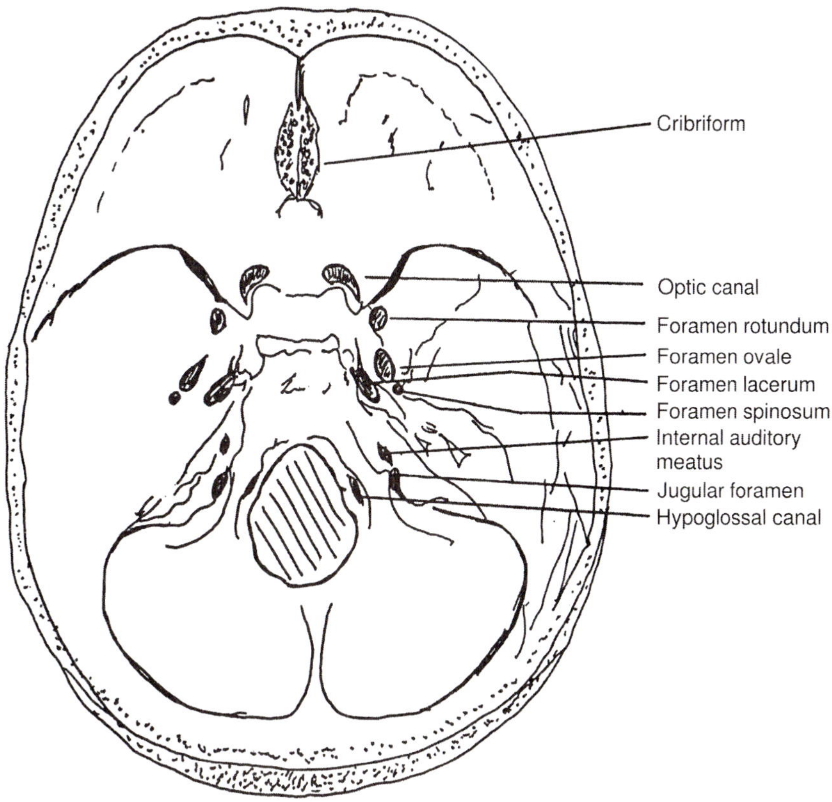

Figure 59-7 Base of skull, internal aspect.

ix. Internal auditory canal (IAC)
   a. CN VII (facial) including nervus intermedius, VIII (superior vestibular nerve, inferior vestibular nerve, cochlear nerve)
   b. Labyrinthine artery

x. Jugular foramen
   a. Pars nervosa (anterior)—Inferior petrosal sinus, CN IX (glossopharyngeal)
   b. Pars vascularis (posterior)—Jugular bulb, CN X (vagus) and XI (spinal accessory)

xi. Hypoglossal canal
   a. CN XII (hypoglossal)
   b. Emissary vein and lymphatics

xii. Foramen magnum
   a. CN XI (ascending spinal rootlets)
   b. Medulla oblongata
   c. Vertebral arteries
   d. Anterior and posterior spinal arteries

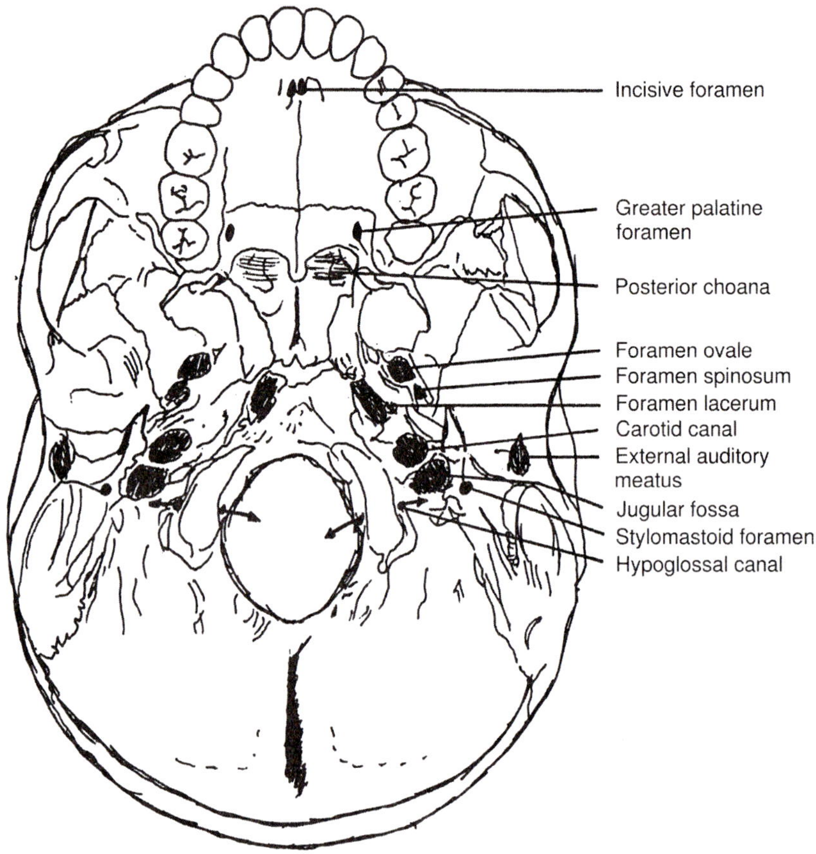

Figure 59-8 Base of skull, external aspect.

C. Bones of the skull
   i. Endochondral bones
      a. Petrous
      b. Occipital
      c. Ethmoid
      d. Mastoid
      e. Sphenoid
   ii. Membranous bones
      a. Frontal
      b. Lacrimal
      c. Nasal
      d. Maxillae
      e. Premaxilla
      f. Palate
      g. Mandible
      h. Vomer
      i. Sphenoid

j. Parietal
k. Zygoma
l. Tympanic ring
m. Squamosa
n. Bony modiolus

D. Cranial nerves
- i. Olfactory (I)
  - a. *Sensory* nerve only
  - b. Located in olfactory foramina in cribriform plate (anterior cranial fossa)
  - c. *Afferent pathway*: olfactory epithelium → olfactory nerve → olfactory bulb → primary olfactory cortex (prepyriform and entorhinal areas)
- ii. Optic (II)
  - a. *Sensory* nerve only
  - b. *Visual pathway*: optic nerve → optic chiasm → optic tract → lateral geniculate nucleus → optic radiation → primary visual cortex
- iii. Oculomotor (III)
  - a. *Mainly motor*: innervates levator palpebrae superioris, superior rectus, medial rectus, inferior rectus, and inferior oblique
  - b. *Autonomic*: lateral nucleus of Edinger-Westphal: preganglionic parasympathetic fibers to ciliary muscles and sphincter pupillae
- iv. Trochlear (IV)
  - a. *Motor* to superior oblique muscle
- v. Trigeminal (V)
  - a. *Somatic sensory*: sensory for pain, temperature, tactile sense from skin of face and forehead, mucous membranes of nose and mouth, teeth, and dura
    1. Proprioceptive inputs from teeth, periodontal ligaments, hard palate, and temporomandibular joint
    2. Stretch receptors for muscles of mastication
  - b. *Motor* to muscles of mastication (temporalis, masseter, and lateral and medial pterygoid), mylohyoid, anterior digastrics, tensor tympani, and tensor veli palatini muscles
  - c. Branches of mandibular nerve (V3)
    1. Trunk: Tensor tympani, Tensor veli palatini, Meningeal, Medial pterygoid
    2. Anterior divisions: Long buccal, Lateral pterygoid, Temporalis, Masseteric
    3. Posterior divisions: Auriculotemporal, Lingual, Inferior alveolar
- vi. Abducens (CN VI)
  - a. *Motor* to lateral rectus muscle
- vii. Facial (VII)
  - a. Nervus intermedius
    1. *Somatic sensory* for the EAC
    2. *Visceral afferent:* sensation from nose, palate, and pharynx, and taste from anterior two-thirds of tongue
    3. *Visceral efferent*: parasympathetic fibers traveling from the superior salivary nucleus via the nervus intermedius:
       - Chorda tympani to submandibular and sublingual glands
       - Greater superficial petrosal nerve (GSPN) to the pterygopalatine ganglion and then lacrimal gland and minor salivary glands to the palate and nasal cavity

b. *Motor* to stapedius, posterior belly of digastric, and muscles of facial expression
   1. Lower facial muscles receive only cross fibers, whereas upper facial muscles receive both crossed and uncrossed fibers.

viii. Vestibulocochlear (VIII)
   a. *Cochlear Nerve:*
      1. *Afferent*: spiral ganglion fibers ascend to dorsal and ventral cochlear nuclei → to ipsilateral superior olivary nucleus (or may cross via the reticular formation and the trapezoid body to opposite olivary nucleus) → ascend via lateral lemniscus → to inferior colliculus or the medial geniculate body → terminate in cortex of the superior temporal gyrus
      2. *Efferent:* innervate outer hair cells (OHC), auditory protection
   b. Superior vestibular nerve (*afferent)*: posterior and superior lateral semicircular canals and utricle—ascend to vestibular nuclei or descend via medial longitudinal fasciculus to vestibulospinal tract
   c. Inferior vestibular nerve (*afferent)*: saccule and horizontal semicircular canal

ix. Glossopharyngeal (CN IX)
   a. *Visceral afferent*: taste from posterior one-third of tongue to inferior (petrosal) ganglion and tractus solitarius to its nucleus
   b. *Somatic afferent*: sensation from oral cavity, oropharynx, and hypopharynx via the tractus solitarius
   c. *Visceral efferent*: inferior salivatory nucleus via Jacobson's nerve to the otic ganglion to the auriculotemporal nerve to the parotid gland
   d. *Motor* to stylopharyngeus muscle

x. Vagus (CN X)
   a. *Somatic sensory* via Arnold's nerve for EAC and posterior auricle
   b. *Motor* to striated muscles of the velum, pharynx, and larynx
   c. *Visceral afferent:* for receptors of respiration, cardiac activity, gastric secretions, and biliary function
   d. *Visceral efferent*: dorsal nucleus to smooth muscle of the esophagus, stomach, small intestine, upper colon, gallbladder, pancreas, lungs, and inhibitory fibers to the heart

xi Spinal accessory (CN XI)
   a. Cranially arises in nucleus ambiguous, special and general *visceral efferent* fibers that join the vagus and are distributed with it.
   b. Spinal portion arises from *motor* cells in the first five segments of cervical spinal cord, travels upward via the foramen magnum, across the occipital bone to the jugular fossa, where it pierces the dura and enters the neck via the jugular foramen to innervate the sternocleidomastoid and trapezius muscles.

xii. Hypoglossal (CN XII)—*motor* to the muscles of the tongue

E. Ganglia
   i. Ciliary ganglion (CN III): parasympathetic ganglion and receives
      a. Preganglionic, parasympathetic fibers from the Edinger-Westphal nucleus
      b. Postganglionic fibers to ciliary muscles and sphincter papillae muscles
   ii. Sphenopalatine ganglion (CN VII) receives
      a. Preganglionic, parasympathetic fibers via the GSPN from the superior salivary nucleus
      b. Postganglionic fibers innervate the lacrimal and minor salivary glands

  iii. Submandibular ganglion (CN VII) receives
    a. Preganglionic, parasympathetic fibers from the superior salivary nucleus via the chorda tympani
    b. Postganglionic fibers innervate the submandibular and sublingual glands
  iv. Otic ganglion (CN IX) receives
    a. Preganglionic, parasympathetic fibers from the inferior salivary nucleus via Jacobson's nerve
    b. Postganglionic fibers innervate the parotid gland.

F. Branches of the external carotid artery
  i. Superior thyroid artery: infrahyoid, superior laryngeal, sternomastoid, cricothyroid arteries
  ii. Ascending pharyngeal artery: prevertebral, pharyngeal, inferior tympanic branches
  iii. Lingual artery: suprahyoid, dorsalis linguae, sublingual arteries
  iv. Facial artery
    a. Inferior and superior labial, lateral nasal, and angular arteries
    b. Cervical branches: ascending palatine, tonsillar, submaxillary, submental arteries
  v. Occipital artery: sternomastoid and auricular arteries, meningeal branches
  vi. Posterior auricular artery: stylomastoid, stapedial, auricular, occipital branches
  vii. Superficial temporal artery: transverse facial and middle temporal arteries, anterior auricular branches
  viii. Internal maxillary artery
    a. Maxillary portion
    b. Anterior tympanic and deep auricular branches
    c. Middle and accessory meningeal arteries
    d. Inferior dental artery
    e. Pterygoid portion
      1. Deep temporal and pterygoid branches
      2. Masseteric and buccal arteries
    f. Sphenomaxillary portion
      1. (1) Posterior superior alveolar artery
      2. Infraorbital artery
      3. Descending palatine artery
      4. Vidian artery
      5. Pterygopalatine artery
      6. Sphenopalatine artery
      7. Posterior nasal artery

G. Segments of the internal carotid
  i. Cervical: no branches
  ii. Petrous (horizontal)
    a. Enters carotid canal and takes anterior turn toward cavernous sinus
    b. Caroticotympanic and vidian branches
  iii. Lacerum
  iv. Cavernous: abuts lateral sphenoid sinus
  v. Clinoid: enters dura
  vi. Ophthalmic
  vii. Communicating (terminal)

- H. Orbit
  - i. Composed of seven bones: maxilla, frontal, ethmoid, zygoma, sphenoid, palatal, and lacrimal
  - ii. Communicates with:
    - a. Infratemporal fossa via inferior orbital fissure
    - b. Pterygopalatine fossa via inferior orbital fissure
    - c. Middle cranial fossa via optic canal and superior orbital fissure
    - d. Nose via nasolacrimal duct
  - iii. Anterior ethmoid artery is approximately 24 mm posterior to the anterior lacrimal crest
  - iv. Posterior ethmoid artery is approximately 12 mm posterior to the anterior ethmoid artery
  - v. Optic nerve is approximately 6 mm posterior to the posterior ethmoid artery
- I. Upper eyelid
  - i. Skin
  - ii. Orbicularis oculi (CN VII)
  - iii. Orbital septum
  - iv. Prelevator fat (medial compartment with two fat pads and lateral compartment)
  - v. Levator palpebrae superioris (CN III)
  - vi. Superior tarsal muscle or Müller muscle (sympathetics)
  - vii. Conjunctiva
- J. Lower eyelid
  - i. Skin
  - ii. Orbicularis oculi
  - iii. Orbital septum
  - iv. Orbital fat (medial, central, and lateral compartments with inferior oblique muscle between the central and medial compartments)
  - v. Inferior tarsal muscle
  - vi. Conjunctiva
- K. HNS-related ophthalmology
  - i. *Pupillary reflex*: direct and consensual components
    - a. Optic nerve → optic tract → superior colliculus → pretectal area → visceral nuclei of oculomotor complex → preganglionic fibers via CN III to ciliary ganglion → postganglionic fibers from ciliary ganglion to sphincter of the iris
  - ii. Corneal reflex
    - a. Ophthalmic branch of the trigeminal nerve → motor nuclei of CN VII → orbicularis oculi
  - iii. *Argyle-Robertson pupil*: miotic pupils
    - a. Does not contract to light but does to accommodation (suggests syphilis)
  - iv. *Marcus-Gunn pupil*: pupil dilation in response to direct light (afferent pupillary defect)
    - a. Results from optic nerve injury with decreased afferent input to brain
  - v. Optic chiasm lesions may result in bitemporal hemianopsia, whereas optic tract lesions result in a contralateral hemianopsia
  - vi. Causes of unilateral proptosis in decreasing order of occurrence: infection → pseudotumor → dermoid → hemangioma/lymphangioma → rhabdomyosarcoma → leukemia → neurofibroma → optic nerve glioma → metastasis → paranasal tumor

L. Ear
  i. External auditory canal
    a. Lateral half is cartilage and medial half is bone
    b. *Fissures of Santorini*: small fenestrations within the anterior inferior cartilaginous EAC that can allow spread of infection to the parotid region and skull base
    c. *Foramen of Huschke*: embryologic remnant that may persist as a communication from the anterior inferior aspect of the medial EAC that can allow spread of tumors and infection to or from preauricular area/parotid
  ii. Tympanic membrane
    a. Pars tensa: three layers—squamous epithelium, fibrous layer, and cuboidal mucosal epithelium
    b. Pars flaccida (Shrapnell's membrane): squamous and cuboidal mucosal epithelium
    c. Blood supply
      1. *External*: deep auricular artery
      2. *Internal*: anterior tympanic artery
  iii. Middle ear
    a. Epitympanum: portion of middle ear superior to TM (first branchial arch structures)
      1. Contains head of malleus, body, and short process of incus, aditus ad antrum, epitympanic recess (adjacent to geniculate segment of facial canal)
      2. Bounded superiorly by tegmen tympani
    b. Mesotympanum: portion which can be visualized through TM (second branchial arch structures)
      1. Contains neck, anterior, and lateral (short) process of malleus, long and lenticular process of incus, stapes
    c. Hypotympanum: portion inferior to TM
      1. Contains eustachian tube orifice
      2. *Hyrtl's fissure*: an embryologic remnant that normally obliterates but may persist as a hypotympanic connection to the subarachnoid space
    d. Retrotympanum: contains facial recess and sinus tympani
    e. Protympanum: portion anterior to TM
    f. Ossicular chain
      1. Malleus: tensor tympani tendon originates from cochleariform process and connects to malleus neck
      2. Incus: lenticular process connects to stapes
      3. Stapes: stapedius tendon originates from pyramidal process
    g. *Prussak's space*: bounded by the scutum, lateral malleolar ligament, neck of malleus, anterior malleolar ligament, pars flaccida
    h. *Facial recess*: bounded by facial nerve (FN) posteriorly, chorda tympani anteriorly, and incudal buttress superiorly
    i. *Sinus tympani*: space medial to FN, bounded anteriorly by promontory, superiorly by facial canal, laterally by pyramidal eminence (subiculum beneath, ponticulus above)
    j. *Jacobson's nerve*: branch of CN IX that traverses the promontory and carries parasympathetics to the parotid gland
    k. *Arnold's nerve*: branch of CN X that supplies innervation to EAC

iv. Eustachian tube musculature:
   a. Levator and tensor veli palatini
   b. Salpingopharyngeus
   c. Dilator tubae
v. Facial nerve
   a. Course: facial motor nucleus → loops dorsomedially around abducens nucleus → exits at pontomedullary junction → joins nervus intermedius (nuclei are superior salivatory and nucleus solitarius) to become FN proper → intracranial (23-24 mm) → enters porus acousticus in anterior superior quadrant → intrameatal (8-10 mm) → angles 120 degrees anterior superior laterally → exits meatal foramen → labyrinthine (3-4 mm) → geniculate ganglion at processus cochleaformis → angles 75 to 90 degrees posteriorly → tympanic (10-11 mm) → gentle arc posterior laterally → at pyramidal eminence, it becomes the mastoid portion (13-15 mm) → dives toward stylomastoid foramen → extracranial segment → first major division at pes
   b. Blood supply:
      1. *Intracranial*: anterior inferior cerebellar artery (AICA)
      2. *Intrameatal*: labyrinthine artery
      3. *Labyrinthine*: not defined (watershed of labyrinthine and superior petrosal arteries)
      4. *Tympanic*: superior petrosal and stylomastoid arteries
      5. *Mastoid*: stylomastoid artery
vi. Internal auditory canal
   a. Facial nerve: motor plus nervus intermedius (anterosuperior)
   b. Cochlear nerve (anteroinferior)
   c. Superior (posterosuperior) and inferior (posteroinferior) vestibular nerve (posterosuperior)
   d. Labyrinthine artery and vein

M. Nose, paranasal sinuses, and nasopharynx
   i. *External nasal valve*: area in the vestibule, under the nasal ala, formed by the caudal septum, medial crura of the alar cartilages, alar rim, and nasal sill
   ii. *Internal nasal valve*: nasal septum, caudal margin of upper lateral cartilage, anterior end of inferior turbinate, floor of nose
   iii. *Septum*: quadrangular cartilage, perpendicular plate of the ethmoid, vomer
   iv. Ethmoid labyrinth is derived from four parallel bony lamellae
      a. Uncinate process
      b. Ethmoid bulla
      c. Ground lamella of middle and superior turbinates
   v. Three attachments of the middle turbinate:
      a. *Anterior*: parasagittal into cribriform plate
      b. *Middle*: coronal into lamina papyracea
      c. *Posterior*: axial into lamina papyracea
   vi. Blood supply to the nasal cavity
      a. Externally from dorsal nasal, angular, and superior labial arteries
      b. Superior septum supplied by anterior and posterior ethmoid, and sphenopalatine arteries
      c. Anterior septum supplied by *Kiesselbach plexus*
         1. Ethmoid arteries (branches of ophthalmic artery)
         2. Greater palatine artery

3. Sphenopalatine artery
4. Superior labial artery

vii. Blood supply to the adenoids
  a. Ascending palatine branch of facial artery
  b. Ascending pharyngeal artery
  c. Pharyngeal branch of internal maxillary artery
  d. Ascending cervical branch of thyrocervical trunk

N. Oral cavity
  i. Tongue
    a. Musculature: Genioglossus, styloglossus, hyoglossus, palatoglossus
    b. Innervation:
      1. *Motor*: CN XII (except palatoglossus—CN X)
      2. *Taste*: anterior two-thirds by CN VII (via chorda tympani), posterior one-third by CN IX
      3. *Sensation*: anterior two-thirds by CN V3, posterior one-third by CN IX
    c. Papillae
      1. *Fungiform*: most numerous
      2. *Circumvallate*: immediately anterior to foramen cecum and sulcus terminalis
      3. *Foliate*: laterally on the tongue
    d. Sulcus terminalis
      1. Inverted V-shape groove (posterior to circumvallate papillae) on tongue dividing anterior two-thirds and posterior one-third of tongue
      2. Foramen cecum lies at the posterior aspect of the sulcus terminalis

O. Pharynx
  i. Musculature: palatopharyngeus, stylopharyngeus, salpingopharyngeus, superior, middle, and inferior constrictors
    a. Innervation: CN X (except stylopharyngeus—CN IX)
    b. Inner musculature is longitudinal (palatopharyngeus, stylopharyngeus, salpingopharyngeus)
    c. Outer musculature is circular (constrictors)
    d. Passavant ridge is a constriction of the superior margin of the superior constrictor muscle
  ii. *Palatal musculature:* palatoglossus, palatopharyngeus, levator and tensor veli palatini, musculus uvulae
    a. Innervation: CNX (except tensor veli palatini—V3)
  iii. Pharyngeal constrictors
    a. *Superior*: spans from pharyngeal raphe and occipital bone to medial pterygoid, pterygomandibular ligament, and mandible
    b. *Middle*: spans from pharyngeal raphe to the hyoid bone
    c. *Inferior*: spans from pharyngeal raphe to the thyroid and cricoid cartilages
  iv. Killian triangle: site of least resistance between inferior constrictor and cricopharyngeus
    a. Zenker diverticulum tends to develop here—usually emanate from left posterior esophagus
  v. Blood supply to palatine tonsils
    a. Facial artery—tonsillar artery
    b. Ascending palatine artery → lingual artery → dorsal lingual branch
    c. Internal maxillary artery → descending and greater palatine arteries
    d. Ascending pharyngeal artery

P. Deep neck spaces
   i. Infratemporal fossa boundaries:
      a. *Superior*: greater wing of sphenoid, infratemporal crest
      b. *Anterior*: posterior curvature of maxillary bone
      c. *Medial*: lateral surface of lateral pterygoid plate
      d. *Lateral*: medial surface of mandibular ramus
      e. *Posterior*: spine of sphenoid, mandibular fossa
      f. *Inferior*: alveolar border of maxilla
   ii. Parapharyngeal space boundaries:
      a. *Superior*: skull base
      b. *Lateral*: mandible, medial pterygoid, parotid
      c. *Medial*: superior constrictor, buccopharyngeal fascia
      d. *Anterior*: pterygomandibular raphe, pterygoid fascia
      e. *Posterior*: carotid sheath, vertebral fascia
      f. *Interior*: lesser cornu of hyoid
      g. *Prestyloid*: internal maxillary artery, inferior alveolar nerve, lingual nerve, auriculotemporal nerve
      h. *Poststyloid*: carotid artery, internal jugular vein, CN IX to XII, cervical sympathetic chain
Q. Salivary glands
   i. Parotid gland:
      a. Duct: along a line from the tragus to the midportion of the upper lip
      b. *Parasympathetic*: inferior salivary nucleus → CN IX (Jacobson's nerve) enters middle ear via tympanic canaliculus → lesser superficial petrosal nerve (LSPN) via foramen ovale (otic ganglion → auriculotemporal branch of V3) → parotid gland
      c. *Sympathetic*: thoracic spinal cord → sympathetic trunk → superior cervical ganglion → external carotid artery → salivary glands
   ii. Submandibular and sublingual glands:
      a. *Parasympathetic:* Superior salivary nucleus → FN (nervus intermedius) → chorda tympani → leaves ear via petrotympanic fissure → lingual branch of V3 (in infratemporal fossa) → submandibular ganglion → submandibular and sublingual glands
      b. *Sympathetic*: see above
R. Neck triangles
   i. Anterior
      a. *Submental (1A)*: anterior digastrics, midline of neck, hyoid
      b. *Digastric (1B)*: mandible, anterior and posterior bellies of digastric
      c. *Carotid*: sternocleidomastoid muscle (SCM), posterior digastrics, anterior omohyoid
      d. *Muscular*: SCM, anterior omohyoid, midline of neck
   ii. Posterior
      a. *Occipital*: trapezius, SCM, posterior omohyoid
      b. *Supraclavicular*: clavicle, SCM, posterior omohyoid
   iii. Blood supply to the SCM
      a. Occipital artery
      b. Branches of superior thyroid artery
      c. Branches of thyrocervical trunk

S. Larynx
   i. Supraglottis
      a. From epiglottis to the level of the laryngeal ventricles
      b. Includes: epiglottis, aryepiglottic folds, arytenoids, false vocal folds, pre-epiglottic and paraglottic spaces
         1. *Pre-epiglottic space*: fat-filled space limited superiorly by the hyoid and posteriorly by the epiglottis
         2. *Paraglottic space*: fat-filled space lateral to false and true vocal folds
      c. *Quadrangular membrane*: poorly developed ligamentous membrane bounded by aryepiglottic fold, anterior surface of arytenoids, vestibular fold, and lateral epiglottis
   ii. *Glottis*: true vocal folds and anterior and posterior commissures
   iii. Subglottis
      a. From inferior aspect of the true vocal folds to the cricoid cartilage, lateral margin is conus elasticus
         1. *Conus elasticus*: arises from anterosuperior cricoids, sweeps up and medially to join anteriorly and attach to thyroid cartilage, and posteriorly to the vocal process of arytenoids, in between is the vocal ligament
   iv. Superior laryngeal nerve (SLN)
      a. Originate in the nodose ganglion of CN X, just inferiorly to the skull base
      b. External branch: *motor* to cricothyroid
      c. Internal branch: *sensory* to distal pharynx and larynx cephalad to true vocal cords
   v. Recurrent laryngeal nerve (RLN)
      a. *Motor* to laryngeal musculature except for cricothyroid and *sensory* for area below the level of true vocal cords.
      b. The most important laryngeal muscle of respiration and airway protection is posterior cricoarytenoid muscle (the only abductor).

Radiology

A. Computed tomography (CT)
   i. Uses tightly collimated x-ray beam that is absorbed by various body tissues differently.
   ii. Contrast is used to evaluate neck to highlight malignancy or infection.
   iii. Contrast is generally not needed for bony anatomy (sinus or temporal bone, for example).
B. Magnetic resonance imaging (MRI)
   i. Based on the varying response of body tissues to an applied and changing magnetic field
   ii. *T1-weighted images*
      a. Fat is high signal intensity (bright), muscles are intermediate, fluid is dark.
      b. Fat saturation is often applied to post-gadolinium T1-weighted images.
   iii. *T2-weighted images*: fluid is bright
   iv. Gadolinium contrast used to highlight pathology
C. Positron emission tomography (PET)
   i. Injection of positron-emitting radiopharmaceutical (^{18}F-florodeoxyglucose or FDG) highlights areas of increased metabolic activity

a. High negative predictive value
b. Asymmetric uptake can suggest malignancy
c. Used to assess for unknown primaries, posttreatment evaluation, and in searching for metastases

D. Ultrasound
i. Simple, quick, lack of radiation exposure
ii. Can be useful for evaluating multiple head and neck sites (eg, lateral and central neck, thyroid and parathyroid, larynx, salivary glands)
iii. US-guided fine-needle aspiration (FNA) a useful technique in the workup of neck, salivary, and thyroid lesions

E. Inner ear and temporal bone imaging
i. Cochlear malformations
a. *Mondini deformity triad*: bony and membranous cochlear dysplasia with 1.5 turns or less of cochlea, associated with enlarged vestibular aqueduct and minimal vestibular dilation
b. *Complete labyrinthine aplasia (Michel aplasia)*: complete aplasia of bony and membranous labyrinth, looks like solid bone

ii. Petrous apex
a. Arachnoid cyst
1. *CT*: fluid-filled mass without aggressive features
2. *MRI*: low on T1, bright on T2, no enhancement

b. Cholesteatoma
1. *CT*: soft tissue mass with bony erosion
2. *MRI*: intermediate on T1, bright on T2, no enhancement

c. Cholesterol granuloma
1. *CT*: expansile lesion
2. *MRI*: bright on T1 and T2, no enhancement

d. Chondrosarcoma
1. *CT*: bony erosion and soft tissue mass with calcifications
2. *MRI*: intermediate to low on T1, bright on T2, shows contrast enhancement

e. Mucocele
1. Like cholesterol granuloma

f. Petrous apicitis
1. *CT*: fluid-filled air cells +/– bony erosion
2. *MRI*: low on T1, bright on T2, may show contrast enhancement

g. Otosclerosis
1. CT: decreased density of bone anterior to oval window (fissula ante fenestram)
2. Ring of lucency around the cochlea (Halo sign)

iii. Cerebellopontine angle (CPA) lesions
a. Acoustic neuroma
1. *CT*: widening of IAC
2. *MRI*: intermediate on T1 and T2 (unless tumor is cystic), shows post-gadolinium enhancement; filling defect on high-resolution T2 images

b. Arachnoid cyst
1. *CT*: fluid-filled mass without aggressive features
2. *MRI*: low on T1, bright on T2, no enhancement

c. Epidermoid cyst
1. Like arachnoid cyst

d. Meningioma
   1. *CT*: intermediate intensity mass
   2. *MRI*: intermediate on T1 and T2 with increased post-gadolinium enhancement, "dural tail" seen on T1 postcontrast images

F. Nose and paranasal sinus imaging
   i. Esthesioneuroblastoma
      a. *CT*: homogeneous soft tissue mass with contrast enhancement and bony erosion and molding
      b. *MRI*: locally invasive soft tissue mass that is hypointense on T1, bright on T2, and enhances with gadolinium
   ii. Fungal sinusitis
      a. *Acute invasive*: aggressive soft tissue mass with bone and soft tissue destruction, contrast enhancement is often absent secondary to angioinvasion
      b. *Chronic invasive*: like allergic fungal sinusitis but with less fulminant course
      c. Allergic fungal sinusitis
         1. *CT*: soft tissue masses of multiple sinuses with mucosal thickening, sinus opacification, and bone remodeling
         2. Heterogeneous density is often seen because of inspissated secretions and increased iron content
   iii. *Mycetoma*: increased density and calcifications on CT
   iv. Inverting papilloma
      a. *CT*: mass extending from middle meatus into maxillary sinus and nasal cavity
      b. *MRI*: intermediate T1 and T2 signal intensity with postcontrast enhancement
   v. Juvenile nasal angiofibroma
      a. *CT*: contrast-enhancing mass with anterior displacement of the posterior maxillary sinus wall (*Holman-Miller sign*)
      b. *MRI*: prominent flow voids and post-gadolinium enhancement
   vi. Mucus retention cyst
      a. *CT*: low-intermediate density soft tissue mass
      b. *MRI*: intermediate on T1, bright on T2, variable contrast enhancement

G. Nasopharynx imaging
   i. Rhabdomyosarcoma
      a. *MRI*: aggressive process with isointense T1, intermediate T2, and post-gadolinium enhancement
   ii. Nasopharyngeal carcinoma
      a. *MRI*: soft tissue mass (often centered around fossa of Rosenmüller) with isointense T1, intermediate T2, and post-gadolinium enhancement
   iii. Tornwaldt cyst
      a. *CT*: hypodense
      b. *MRI*: bright on T1 and T2, with no enhancement

H. Neck imaging
   i. Salivary glands
      a. Contrast administration can help differentiate neoplastic from inflammatory conditions
   ii. Abscess
      a. *CT*: low-density mass with ring enhancement
   iii. Branchial cleft cyst
      a. *CT*: unilocular, cystic mass displacing the submandibular gland anteriorly and the SCM posteriorly

iv. Cystic hygroma
   a. *CT*: low density
   b. *MRI*: heterogeneous T1 and T2 without post-gadolinium enhancement

I. Paraganglioma (PGL) imaging
   i. *Duplex ultrasound:* hypervascular mass and its relationship to the carotid artery
   ii. *CT with contrast*
      a. Post-contrast enhancement
      b. If there is splaying of ICA and ECA (*Lyre sign*): likely a carotid body tumor
      c. If the mass pushes the carotid vessels laterally likely a sympathetic tumor
   iii. *MRI with gadolinium*
      a. Mild enhancement on T2, intense T1 postcontrast enhancement with "salt and pepper" appearance secondary to flow voids
   iv. Nuclear medicine: can be useful for screening in the setting of familial PGL syndromes

Pharmacology and Anesthesia

A. Local anesthetic
   i. Dosages: 1% solution equals 10 mg/mL
   ii. Amides (note "i's") lidocaine, bupivacaine, mepivacaine, prilocaine, ropivacaine, etc.
      a. Metabolized by liver dealkylation
      b. Higher incidence of allergy than esters
      c. Lidocaine: toxicity limit: 4.5 mg/kg without epinephrine (epi), 7 mg/kg with epi, max 300 mg
      d. Bupivacaine: toxicity limit: 2.5 mg/kg without epi, 3 mg/kg with epi
   iii. Esters: cocaine, procaine, chloroprocaine, tetracaine, benzocaine
      a. Metabolized by plasma and liver cholinesterase
      b. Cocaine
         1. Blocks uptake of epinephrine and norepinephrine
         2. Maximum dose: 200 to 300 mg
   iv. Toxicity
      a. Central nervous system (CNS) effects
         1. *Excitatory*: blurred vision, tingling, tinnitus, numbness, disorientation, sweating, seizures, sweating, vomiting
         2. *Inhibitory*: decreased level of consciousness, coma
      b. Cardiovascular system (CVS) effects
         1. Bradycardia, hypotension, cardiorespiratory arrest
      c. Management: airway, breathing, circulation, stop procedure/stop injection, oxygen, IV, fluids

B. Corticosteroids
   i. The body produces ~20 mg of cortisol/day, which is equivalent to 5 mg of prednisone, 4 mg of methylprednisolone, or 0.75 mg of Decadron
   ii. Tapers necessary after greater than 5 days of steroids
   iii. Side effects:
      a. Fluid imbalance
      b. Electrolyte disturbance
      c. Glycosuria

d. Susceptibility to infection
e. Hypertension
f. Hyperglycemia
g. Peptic ulcer disease
h. Osteoporosis
i. Cataracts
j. Behavioral disturbances
k. Cushingoid habitus
l. Central obesity
m. Acne
n. Hirsutism
o. Avascular necrosis

C. Antiemetics
   i. Emetic center in medulla—acetylcholine and histamine receptors
   ii. Chemoreceptor trigger zone in fourth ventricle—dopamine receptors
   iii. Phenothiazines—antidopaminergic and anticholinergic
   iv. Metoclopramide—antidopaminergic
   v. 5-HT3 receptor antagonist (*eg, ondansetron, granisetron, dolasetron*)
      a. Most common side effect: headache

D. Expectorants
   i. Stimulates secretions in respiratory tract via vagus nerve
   ii. Ammonium salts, iodide salts, guaifenesin

E. Malignant hyperthermia
   i. Associated with halogenated inhalational anesthetic agents and depolarizing muscle relaxants
   ii. Sudden increase in the calcium concentration in the muscle sarcoplasm due to either decreased uptake or excessive release of calcium from the sarcoplasmic reticulum—results in hyperkalemia
   iii. Treat with dantrolene, cooling, and supplemental oxygen, ICU admission

Antibiotic Classes

A. Aminoglycosides: gentamicin, tobramycin, amikacin, and neomycin
   i. Highly effective against *Pseudomonas*
   ii. Ototoxic (gentamicin primarily vestibulotoxic)

B. *Carbapenems*: meropenem, imipenem
   i. Broad-spectrum coverage
   ii. Used for serious hospital-acquired or mixed infections

C. Cephalosporins
   i. *First generation*: cephalexin, cefadroxil
      a. Primarily targeted toward gram-positive (*Streptococcus* and *Staphylococcus*) species (spp.)
      b. Includes some gram-negative spp. like *Escherichia coli*, *Proteus mirabilis*, and *Klebsiella*
   ii. *Second generation*: cefuroxime, cefaclor, cefprozil, cefpodoxime
      a. Good gram-positive coverage and increased coverage for *Haemophilus influenzae* and *Moraxella catarrhalis*

iii. *Third generation*: cefixime, ceftriaxone, ceftazidime, cefotaxime (no increased risk to PCN allergy cross reactivity)
    a. More active against gram-negatives: *H. influenzae, M. catarrhalis, Neisseria gonorrhoeae, Neisseria meningitides*
    b. Less active against gram positive and anaerobes
    c. Good CNS penetration
iv. *Fourth generation*: cefepime
    a. Provides the best cephalosporin coverage against *Pseudomonas aeruginosa*
v. *Fifth generation:* ceftaroline
    a. Coverage against methicillin-resistant *Staphylococcus aureus* (MRSA)

D. Clindamycin
  i. Highly effective against gram-positive and anaerobic organisms (ie, *Bacteroides fragilis*)
  ii. High concentrations in respiratory tissues, mucus, saliva, and bone
  iii. Increases risk for *Clostridium difficile*

E. Linezolid
  i. Alternative to vancomycin for MRSA
  ii. Can be given orally

F. Macrolides
  i. Concentrate in phagocytes
  ii. Poorly effective for mucosal biofilm-mediated infections such as otitis media (OM) and sinusitis
  iii. Erythromycin
    a. Primarily effective against streptococci, pneumococci, *M. catarrhalis* but also against *Mycoplasma, Chlamydia, Legionella,* diphtheria, and pertussis
    b. In combination with sulfa it is effective against *H. influenzae*
    c. Increases GI motility
  iv. Azithromycin and clarithromycin longer acting and effective for alveolar lung disease

G. Metronidazole
  i. Highly effective for obligate anaerobes, protozoa, and oral spirochetes
  i. First-line agent for pseudomembranous colitis

H. *Monobactam*: aztreonam
  i. Aerobic gram-negative coverage: *H. influenzae, N. gonorrhoeae, E. coli, Klebsiella, Serratia, Proteus, Pseudomonas*
  ii. Increases risk for gram-positive infection unless gram-positive coverage (ie, clindamycin) is added

I. Penicillins (β-lactam family)
  i. Penicillin (PCN) G and V
    a. *S. pyogenes, S. pneumoniae,* and actinomycosis
    b. Inactivated by penicillinase
  ii. Antistaphylococcal (penicillinase resistant): methicillin, oxacillin, cloxacillin, dicloxacillin, and nafcillin
    a. MRSA is resistant.
  iii. Aminopenicillins: ampicillin and amoxicillin
    a. More active against streptococci and pneumococci than PCN G and V
    b. Includes gram-negatives: *E. coli, Proteus,* and *H. influenzae*

- iv. Augmented PNC's: including β-lactamase inhibiting compounds—clavulanate, tazobactam
    - a. Restore aminopenicillin activity against *Staphylococcus, H. influenzae, M. catarrhalis*, and anaerobes
- v. Antipseudomonal: ticarcillin with clavulanate, piperacillin with tazobactam
    - a. *Pseudomonas, Proteus, E. coli, Klebsiella, Enterobacter, Serratia, B. fragilis*
    - b. Less effective than aminopenicillins against gram-positive upper respiratory bacteria

J. Quinolones: ciprofloxacin, levofloxacin, ofloxacin, moxifloxacin, gatifloxacin
- i. Active against *Pseudomonas*
- ii. Blackbox warning: tendinopathy, especially when combined with steroids
- iii. Respiratory quinolones (levofloxacin, gatifloxacin, and moxifloxacin) add coverage against *Streptococcus*, *Staphylococcus*, *H. influenzae*, and *M. catarrhalis*
- iv. Moxifloxacin adds anaerobic coverage

K. Tetracyclines
- i. Effective against *Mycoplasma*, *Chlamydia*, and *Legionella*
- ii. Used for acne, traveler's diarrhea, and nonspecific "flu" or atypical pneumonia
- iii. Stains tooth-forming enamel and should not be used under age 10 years or in pregnancy
- iv. Photosensitivity

L. TMP/SMX
- i. Effective adjuvant to immunosuppressive drugs for granulomatosis with polyangiitis (GPA—Wegener *granulomatosis*)
- ii. *Pneumocystis carinii*
- iii. Ineffective against *Strep*

M. Vancomycin
- i. Good gram-positive coverage including MRSA
- ii. Ototoxic intravenously (not ototoxic orally)
- iii. Oral formulation is second-line agent for pseudomembranous colitis

Infectious Diseases

A. Invasive fungal infections
- i. Acute invasive fungal sinusitis
    - a. Most commonly *Aspergillus fumigatus*
    - b. Clinical features
        1. Unilateral painless proptosis
        2. Sinusitis with pale, insensate mucosa
        3. Laryngeal involvement
        4. Bone erosion
    - c. Associated with immunosuppression or malignancy
        1. "Reversible" immunodeficiency (eg, DM): ~30% mortality
        2. "Irreversible" immunodeficiency: ~70% mortality
    - d. Workup
        1. Imaging
            - *CT:* unilateral edema, +/– bone erosion, +/– extension into surrounding soft tissue
            - *MRI:* loss of contrast enhancement, extra-sinus soft tissue involvement

2. Biopsy
   - *Aspergillus:* 45 degrees, branching, septate hyphae when grown on Sabouraud agar
   - Mucormycosis: 90 degrees, wide-angle branching septate hyphae
3. Treatment
   - Reversal of underlying immunosuppression if able
   - Surgical debridement—often requiring multiple debridements
   - Antifungal therapy

ii. Coccidiomycosis (San Joaquin Valley fever)
   a. *Coccidioides immitis*
   b. Involvement of skin, mucous membranes, thyroid, eyes, trachea, salivary glands, severe erosions of epiglottis
   c. Diagnosis
      1. Skin test
      2. Complement fixation
      3. CXR: "coin lesions"
      4. Treatment: amphotericin B

B. Cryptococcosis
   i. *Cryptococcus neoformans*
   ii. Predisposing factors: immunosuppression (incl HIV), lymphoma
   iii. Membranous nasopharyngitis, meningitis, hearing loss
   iv. Diagnosis: fluorescent antibody test
   v. Treatment: amphotericin B

C. Necrotizing fasciitis
   i. Progressive, rapidly spreading, inflammatory infection located in the deep fascia, with secondary necrosis of the subcutaneous tissues, subcutaneous emphysema
   ii. Seen in patients with trauma, recent surgery, or medical compromise (immunocompromised)
   iii. Pathogens: bacteria (polymicrobial)
      a. *S. pyogenes* (group A hemolytic streptococci) and *S. aureus:* most common
      b. Others: *Bacteroides, Clostridium perfringens* (classic gas-forming organism), *Peptostreptococcus, Enterobacteriaceae, Proteus, Pseudomonas, Klebsiella*
   iv. CT reveals necrosis, fascial thickening, and subcutaneous gas
   v. Treatment
      a. Strict glucose control
      b. Surgical debridement
      c. Broad-spectrum antibiotics (anaerobic and aerobic coverage)
      d. Consider hyperbaric oxygen

Head and Neck Manifestations of HIV

A. HIV-associated malignancies
   i. *Kaposi Sarcoma*
      a. An angioproliferative tumor caused by human herpes virus 8
      b. Incidence ~5%
      c. Presentation
         1. Occurs in head and neck up to 70% of cases
         2. Commonly presents in oral cavity (hard palate, gingiva, tongue), cutaneous areas

d. Workup: biopsy
e. Treatment: no curative therapy, role of surgery is palliative

ii. Lymphoma
a. Both non-Hodgkin and Hodgkin lymphoma occur at higher rate
b. Others include Burkitt, plasmablastic, CNS lymphoma
c. Commonly associated with Epstein-Barr virus (EBV)

iii. Nonmelanotic skin cancer
a. More common in immunosuppression and HIV
b. Basal cell carcinoma most common

B. HIV-associated inflammatory conditions
i. Salivary gland involvement
a. Benign lymphoepithelial cyst
1. Most common parotid lesion in HIV patients
2. Unilateral or bilateral
3. Associated cervical lymphadenopathy, sialadenitis, pain
b. Diffuse infiltrative lymphocytosis syndrome
1. Clinically similar to Sjögren syndrome
2. Diffuse parotid enlargement and sicca symptoms
ii. Facial lipoatrophy: fat atrophy in malar, buccal, melolabial, temporal regions
iii. Gingival and periodontal disease

C. HIV-associated infectious conditions
i. Oral candidiasis
ii. Oral histoplasmosis: *Histoplasma capsulatum*
a. Classically affects lungs and endemic to Ohio river valley in the United States
iii. Oral hairy leukoplakia: *EBV*

HNS-Related Rheumatology

A. Dermatomyositis and polymyositis
i. Idiopathic inflammatory myopathies characterized by symmetric proximal muscle weakness
ii. Difficulties phonating, dysphagia, aspiration, nasal regurgitation, and DM rashes
iii. Affects upper one-third of esophagus (striated)—associated dysphagia
iv. *Heliotrope rash*: reddish-violaceous eruption on the upper eyelids with accompanying eyelid swelling
v. Elevated plasma muscle enzymes

B. Relapsing polychondritis
i. Recurring inflammation of cartilaginous structures.
ii. Ninety percent of patients develop auricular chondritis and nonerosive inflammatory polyarthritis.
iii. Chondritis develops rapidly and resolves in 1 to 2 weeks.
iv. Recurrent episodes produce cartilaginous deformity.
a. Airway collapse may lead to death.
v. The erythrocyte sedimentation rate (ESR) is elevated.
vi. Steroids are used in severe cases.
vii. Up to 52% have cardiac abnormality → echo.

C. Rheumatoid arthritis
   i. Affects specific juvenile population and people in their 40s to 60s
   ii. Morning stiffness and subcutaneous rheumatoid nodules
   iii. Articular involvement
      a. Cricoarytenoid joints
         1. Best treatment for arytenoids involvement is steroids and NSAIDs
      b. Middle ear ossicles
      c. Temporomandibular joint
      d. Cervical spine
D. Scleroderma
   i. Heterogeneous group of disorders characterized by thickened, sclerotic/fibrotic lesions
   ii. Eighty percent of people have esophageal dysmotility
      a. Affects lower two-thirds (smooth muscle) of esophagus and dysphagia is usually the initial complaint
      b. Associated with decreased lower LES pressure
      c. Thirty-five percent develop facial tightness
      d. Twenty-five percent report sicca symptoms
   iii. Associated with CREST syndrome:
      a. *C*alcinosis
      b. *R*aynaud phenomenon
      c. *E*sophageal dysfunction
      d. *S*clerodactyly
      e. *T*elangiectasia
E. Sjögren disease
   i. Second most common connective tissue disease after RA
   ii. Peak incidence 40 to 60 years of age
   iii. Females to males (9:1)
   iv. Keratoconjunctivitis sicca and xerostomia
   v. Extraglandular symptoms may be seen in addition to primary exocrine gland pathology (ie, bronchiectasis)
   vi. Primary disease
      a. Not associated with connective tissue disorder
      b. Positive SS-A, SS-B, antinuclear antibodies (ANA), and ESR
   vii. Secondary disease
      a. Associated with connective tissue disorders (rheumatoid arthritis, systemic lupus erythematosus)
      b. Positive SS-A, ANA, and ESR
   viii. Patients with primary Sjögren disease have a risk for non-Hodgkin lymphoma
      a. Diagnosis: gold standard is abnormal minor salivary gland biopsy
   ix. Must be distinguished from sicca-like syndromes, which have xerostomia and/or xerophthalmia, negative tests, and normal biopsy
      a. Aging
      b. Medications (diuretics, anticholinergics, antihistamines, antidepressants)
      c. Other diseases (hepatitis, autoimmune disorders)
      d. Chronic dehydration
   x. Medications
      a. Pilocarpine (Salagen)—cholinergic agonist for post-XRT and Sjögren
      b. Cevimeline (Evoxac)—cholinergic agonist for Sjögren
      c. Dental rinses

F. Systemic lupus erythematosus (SLE)
  i. Malar and discoid rash, oral ulcerations, ulcers/perforation of nasal septum, inflammatory changes of larynx, dysphagia, sicca complex, and CN III, IV, V, VI, VII, and VIII neuropathy
  ii. ANA test—highly sensitive
  iii. Anti-dsDNA and anti-Sm antibodies—highly specific
G. Lupus anticoagulant
  i. A procoagulant
  ii. No special preoperative workup is required other than assuring the patient has sequential compression devices or subcutaneous heparin
H. Granulomatosis with polyangitis (*Wegener granulomatosis*)
  i. Classic triad of respiratory granulomas, vasculitis, and glomerulonephritis
  ii. Ninety percent have head and neck symptoms at presentation
    a. Nasal obstruction and discharge
    b. Mucosal ulcerations
    c. Epistaxis
    d. Saddle nose deformity
    e. Sinusitis
    f. Gingival hyperplasia
    g. Otologic disease (serous OM) occur 20% to 25%
    h. Laryngeal edema and ulceration
    i. Subglottic stenosis
  iii. Laboratory findings include elevated ESR, C-reactive protein, and cytoplasmic antineutrophil cytoplasmic antibody (C-ANCA)
    a. C-ANCA (65%-90% sensitive)—antibody against serine proteinase 3 antigen (PR3); other autoimmune vasculitides have perinuclear antibodies to cytoplasmic antigens within neutrophils (P-ANCA) against myeloperoxidase (MPO)
  iv. Biopsy confirms diagnosis
    a. Angiocentric, epithelial-type necrotizing granulomas with the presence of giant cells and histiocytes
  v. Treatment
    a. Steroids and cyclophosphamide
    b. Mild cases can be treated with trimethoprim/sulfamethoxazole and methotrexate instead of cyclophosphamide
    c. Plasma exchange has also been used for severe renal diseases
    d. Cartilaginous reconstruction for Saddle nose deformity
I. Eosinophilic granulomatosis with polyangiitis (*Churg-Strauss Vasculitis*)
  i. Asthma, eosinophilia (> 10%), sinusitis, pulmonary infiltrates, vasculitis with extravascular eosinophils, mono/polyneuritis
  ii. P-ANCA positive
J. Temporal arteritis (*giant cell arteritis*)
  i. Headaches, blindness
  ii. Biopsy: giant cells within the tunica media
  iii. Treatment: corticosteroids
K. Histiocytosis X (*Langerhans cell histiocytosis*)
  i. Family of granulomatous diseases of unknown etiology, proliferation of mature histiocytes
  ii. Histology: Birbeck granules (tennis racket-shaped structures) found in Langerhans cells

iii. Types
   a. Eosinophilic granuloma
      1. Children and adults
      2. Chronic course with osteolytic bone lesions (often frontal or temporal)
      3. Associated with proptosis, facial paralysis, acute mastoiditis, middle ear granulations, and TM perforations are common
      4. Surgical excision/debridement is the recommended treatment for single lesions
   b. Hand-Schüller-Christian disease
      1. Children and younger adults
      2. Subacute course with lytic skull lesions
      3. Associated with proptosis, diabetes insipidus, and pituitary insufficiency
      4. EAC polyps, mastoid and middle ear lesions causing ossicular erosion, acute mastoiditis, and facial paralysis
      5. Mandibular involvement with loss of teeth
      6. Chemotherapy and/or radiotherapy are recommended
   c. Letterer-Siwe disease
      1. Infants less than 2 years of age.
      2. Acute, rapidly progressive diseases characterized by fever, proptosis, splenomegaly, hepatomegaly, adenopathy, multiple bony lesions, anemia, thrombocytopenia, and exfoliative dermatitis.
      3. Chemotherapy is the treatment of choice, but the response is poor.
      4. Radiotherapy can be used for localized or unresponsive lesions.

L. Sarcoidosis
   i. Autoimmune disorder characterized by noncaseating granulomas involving many different organs.
   ii. Lungs and lymph nodes are most commonly involved.
      a. Cervical adenopathy is the most common head and neck manifestation.
   iii. Uveoparotid fever (*Heerfordt disease*)
      a. Uveitis, mild fever, nonsuppurative parotitis, and CN paralysis
   iv. Airway obstruction in sarcoidosis generally involves the supraglottis.
   v. Elevated angiotensin converting enzyme levels in ~70%.
   vi. *Histology:* Schaumann bodies, noncaseating granulomas.
   vii. Treatment
      a. Steroids ± methotrexate

HNS-related Neurology

A. Headache
   i. Intracranial pathology
      a. Traction headache: space-occupying lesion
         1. Papilledema, early morning headache, nausea, and vomiting
      b. Vascular
         1. Widespread vasodilation of cerebral vessels
         2. Aneurysm
         3. Subarachnoid hemorrhage
      c. Inflammatory
         1. Meningitis
         2. Cerebritis/encephalitis

ii. Tension headache
   a. Most common
   b. Bilateral, nonpulsating, mild-moderate severity, not associated with nausea and vomiting
iii. Vascular headache
   a. Distention of scalp arteries
   b. Triggered by menses, alcohol, stress
iv. Cluster headache
   a. Older age
   b. Affects men more than women (4:1)
   c. Occur in bouts
   d. Very severe unilateral headaches around eye and temporal region
   e. Pain accompanied by ipsilateral cranial autonomic features (hyperlacrimation, rhinorrhea)
   f. Treatment
      1. Abortive therapy: triptans (sumatriptan, zolmitriptan), ergotamine
      2. Preventive: beta blockers, calcium channel blockers
v. Trigeminal neuralgia (*tic douloureux*)
   a. Most often between 50s and 70s
   b. Women more than men (1.5:1)
   c. Sharp facial pain lasting seconds to minutes occurring multiple times daily
   d. Pain usually localized to V2/V3 distribution
vi. Migraine
   a. Family history
   b. Baseline hypersensitivity of brain, spreading cortical depression with activation of CN V
   c. One-third will have aura (sensory, motor, behavioral)
   d. Epiphenomena (photophobia, diarrhea)
   e. Headache may not be main complaint
      1. Vestibular, abdominal, ocular
   f. Treatment
      1. Abortive therapy: triptans (sumatriptan, zolmitriptan), ergotamine
      2. Preventive: Beta blockers, calcium channel blockers, antiepileptic drugs (AEDs), magnesium, riboflavin
vii. Inflammatory (sinusitis, dental, TMJ) headache

Otology

A. Audiology
   i. Range of human hearing is 20 to 20,000 Hz
   ii. Speech sounds are concentrated between 250 and 6000 Hz
   iii. *Decibel*: 10 log 10
   iv. Interaural attenuation is 0 dB for bone conduction (BC) and 40 to 60 dB for earphones
   v. When to mask
      a. Air conduction (AC) when test tone is 40 to 60 dB louder than bone thresholds of nontest ear.

b. BC when there is any difference between air conduction and bone conduction thresholds.
c. Masking dilemma occurs when there is bilateral 50 dB air–bone gap and requires special audiometric techniques.

vi. *Threshold*: lowest intensity level for a pure tone to be detected 50% of the time

vii. *Speech reception threshold (SRT)*: lowest intensity level required for patient to recognize 50% of bisyllabic words (spondee)
a. Should be within 10 dB of the pure tone average (PTA)

viii. Word recognition (WRS): patient's ability to recognize phonetically balanced monosyllabic words presented 30 to 40 dB above SRT

ix. Audiometry
a. Less than 6 months: ABR, DPOAE, *behavior observation audiometry* (warble tones)
b. 6 months to 3 years—ABR, distortion product otoacoustic emissions (DPOAE), *visual response audiometry* (child localizes to an object)
c. 3 to 6 years—conventional *play audiometry* (child performs an activity each time sound is heard)
d. Greater than 6 years—standard audiometry

x. Conductive hearing loss (CHL):
a. *10 to 30 dB*: TM perforation
b. *30 to 50 dB*: ossicular discontinuity and TM perforation
c. *Less than 50 dB*: otosclerosis
d. *50 to 60 dB*: ossicular discontinuity with intact TM

xi. Stenger test for pseudohypacusis, "functional" hearing loss, nonorganic loss, and malingering
a. Based on the principle that a listener will only hear the louder of two tones when identical tones of different intensity levels are presented to the two ears
b. Sound presented to both ears with "dead" ear louder than good ear
1. If true loss, patient will only hear in good ear
2. If malingering, will not acknowledge sound

xii. Special signs
a. *Carhart notch*: falsely depressed bone conduction scores at 2000 Hz suggestive of otosclerosis
b. *Recruitment*: increased signal intensity produces out-of-proportion perception of loudness, suggestive of cochlear hearing loss; lack of recruitment may indicate retrocochlear pathology
c. *Rollover*: paradoxical decrease in WRS with increasing loudness, classic finding of a retrocochlear pathology
d. *Tone decay/fatigue*: change of auditory threshold resulting from continued acoustic stimulation, suggestive of retrocochlear pathology

xiii. Tympanometry
a. *Type A*: normal
b. *Type As*: "S" hallow. Seen in otosclerosis, tympanosclerosis
c. *Type* Ad: "D"eep. Seen in ossicular discontinuity
d. *Type B*: flat. Seen in middle ear effusion or TM perforation
e. *Type C*: represents negative pressure as seen in eustachian tube dysfunction (ETD)

xiv. Acoustic reflex
a. Cochlea → CN VIII → cochlear nuclei and contralateral olivary complex via the trapezoid body → motor nucleus of CN VII → stapedius.
b. A unilateral stimulus results in bilateral contraction.

c. Abnormal result is decay to less than 50% of the original amplitude within 10 seconds—indicative of eighth nerve or brain stem lesion
d. Factors that can affect the acoustic reflex
    1. Conductive losses of 40 dB for the ear receiving the reflex-eliciting tone or as little as 10 dB for the probe ear
    2. Sensorineural hearing losses (SNHL) greater than 70 dB
    3. Eighth nerve lesions
    4. Seventh nerve lesion proximal to stapedius (ie, *Ramsay Hunt syndrome*)
    5. Multiple sclerosis
    6. Brain stem lesions
e. Eighth nerve or CNS lesions may have the following acoustic reflex responses:
    1. Normal reflexes
    2. Elevated reflex thresholds without decay
    3. Normal or elevated reflex thresholds with decay
    4. Absent reflexes

xv. Auditory brain stem response (ABR)
a. Brain stem function can be identified on ABR testing at approximately 28 weeks' gestational age with the appearance of waves I, III, and V. "Maturity" is not reached until approximately 18 months after birth.
b. Waves I-V represented by the mnemonic "EECOL"
    1. *Wave I*: distal *E*ighth nerve
    2. *Wave II*: proximal *E*ighth nerve
    3. *Wave III*: *C*ochlear nucleus
    4. *Wave IV*: Superior *o*livary complex
    5. *Wave V*: Lateral *l*emniscus
c. Normal waveform latencies
    1. I-III is 2.3 ms
    2. III-V is 2.1 ms
    3. I-V is 4.4 ms
d. Retrocochlear lesions should be suspected if ABR results show the following:
    1. Interpeak latency difference greater than 4.4 ms
    2. Interaural latency difference of wave V greater than 0.2 ms
    3. V_3-V_5 latency of greater than 2.1 ms

xvi. *Electrocochleography (ECOG)*: compares summating potential (SP) to compound action potential (AP)—AP similar to wave I in ABR
a. *High SP/AP ratio* (> 0.4) in Meniere's and superior semicircular canal dehiscence

xvii. Otoacoustic emissions
a. Produced by OHCs spontaneously or after acoustic stimulation
b. DPOAEs have the most clinical applications
c. Limitations: CHL, SNHL greater than 30 dB
d. Used to monitor newborn hearing, aminoglycoside-induced hearing loss, and to help differentiate between cochlear and retrocochlear causes of SNHL
e. Auditory neuropathy: normal OAEs, abnormal CN VIII

xviii. Occupational Safety and Health Administration limits for noise exposure:
a. 90 dB for 8 hours
b. 95 dB for 4 hours
c. 100 dB for 2 hours
d. 105 dB for 1 hour
e. 110 dB for 1/2 hour

B. Vestibular testing
   i. Components of vestibular testing
      a. Nystagmus evaluation
         1. Slow phase is driven by vestibulo-ocular reflex (VOR), and is measured in degree/second.
         2. Fast phase (saccade) is driven by the paramedian pontine reticular formation.
         3. Direction of nystagmus is determined by the direction of the fast phase.
         4. Frenzel goggles prohibit patient from being able to fixate, allow examiner to better visualize the eye movements.
         5. Peripheral nystagmus:
            - Usually horizontal ± torsional component
            - Decreases with visual fixation
         6. Central nystagmus
            - Vertical or purely torsional
            - Does not decrease with visual fixation
            - May change directions in different gaze positions
         7. Degrees
            - *First degree*: Nystagmus is present when looking laterally in the direction of the fast component.
            - *Second degree*: Nystagmus is present when looking laterally in the direction of the fast component and in neutral position.
            - *Third degree*: Nystagmus is present in three horizontal eye positions.
         8. Head-shaking nystagmus (HSN): Horizontal HSN can be seen in unilateral vestibular lesions.
         9. Positional: Dix-Hallpike maneuver
            - Vertical and torsional nystagmus toward downward ear (geotropic) indicates benign paroxysmal positional vertigo (BPPV).
         10. VOR/horizontal semicircular canal evaluation
            - Calorics: evaluates horizontal semicircular canal
              (a) Warm stimulus causes endolymph to rise and stimulate horizontal canal
              (b) COWS: Cold Opposite, Warm Same
            - Rotational chair for VOR
              (a) *Phase*: describes the *timing relationship* between head movement and the reflexive eye response.
              (b) If eyes and head move at the exact same velocity in opposite directions, they are *out of phase* (or 180 degrees).
              (c) *Phase lead*: Eye velocity is greater than head velocity.
              (d) Normal to have phase lead at low frequencies.
              (e) Abnormal phase leads at low frequencies—peripheral lesion.
              (f) Abnormal phase leads at all frequencies—central lesion.
              (g) *Phase lag*: Head velocity is greater than eye velocity.
              (h) Occurs in peripheral lesions or in presence of poor gains.
         11. Electronystagmography (ENG) incorporates nystagmus, VOR, horizontal semicircular canal, and oculomotor testing

C. External ear
   i. Aural atresia: absent ear canal and 40 to 65 dB air-bone gap
      a. Often sporadic
      b. Associated syndromes: *Treacher-Collins and Goldenhar*

c. Treatment options:
    1. Amplification (bone conduction aids)
    2. Bone anchored hearing aid (BAHA)
    3. Atresiaplasty
    4. Only 50% of aural atresia patients are surgical candidates
d. Surgical criteria evaluated by *Jahrsdoerfer criteria*

ii. Microtia
   a. RUM: *R*ight > left, *U*nilateral > bilateral (4:1), *M*ales > females (2.5:1)
   b. Classification:
      1. Type I—mild deformity (eg, lop ear, cup ear, etc.)
      2. Type II—all structures are present to some degree, but there is a tissue deficiency
      3. Type III—"Classic" microtia, significant deformity with few recognizable landmarks, lobule often present and anteriorly displaced, and canal atresia
      4. Best time to reconstruct is between 6 and 10 years
         - Ear reaches 85% of adult size by 5 years of age
         - Perform microtia surgery prior to atresia repair

iii. Frostbite
   a. Rapidly rewarm with gauze soaked in saline, that is, 38°C to 42°C/100.4°F to 107.6°F.
   b. Tissue should not be debrided upon rewarming as demarcation may take several weeks.
   c. Treat with topical antibiotic, ointment, and oral analgesics.

iv. Otitis externa
   a. Bacterial
      1. Often *S. aureus* and *P. aeruginosa*
      2. Treatment: topical antibiotics ± steroids
   b. Fungal
      1. Treatment: merthiolate (thimerosal), acetic acid, isopropyl alcohol, gentian violet, nystatin suspension, cream, ointment, or powder, topical azole

v. Malignant otitis externa
   a. Generally seen in diabetic, elderly, and immunocompromised patients
   b. Often *P. aeruginosa*
   c. Infection disseminates to skull base via fissures of Santorini
   d. Imaging
      1. Diagnosed with MRI or Technetium^{99} radioisotope scan and followed with gallium scan.
      2. CT: will only be clearly positive once 30% to 50% of the trabecular bone of the mastoid is destroyed.
   e. Treatment: antipseudomonal antibiotics for months and surgical debridement

vi. Exostoses
   a. Broad-based, bony lesions (multiple) of EAC secondary to cold water exposure
   b. Surgery required for CHL or cerumen impaction

vii. Osteoma
   a. Benign, pedunculated bony neoplasm (usually single) of the anterior EAC
   b. Surgery required for CHL or cerumen impaction

viii. Referred otalgia
   a. *CN V*: oral cavity, mandible, temporomandibular joint (TMJ), palate, preauricular region
   b. *CN VII*: EAC, postauricular region

c. *CN IX*: tonsil, tongue base, nasopharynx, eustachian tube, pharynx (via Jacobson's nerve)
d. *CN X*: hypopharynx, larynx, trachea (via Arnold's nerve)

D. Middle ear
   i. Cerebrospinal fluid (CSF) otorrhea
      a. Most common source in adults is tegmen mastoideum secondary to meningoencephalocele
      b. Associated with 6% of basilar skull fractures
      c. Ninety percent seal spontaneously
      d. Middle fossa leaks heal rapidly due to the extensive fibrosis promoted by the rich arachnoid mesh in this area
      e. Posterior fossa leaks close more slowly, as little arachnoid is present in this area
      f. Indications for repair
         1. Persistent leak for longer than 2 weeks despite bed rest with head elevation
         2. Recurrent meningitis
         3. Brain or meningeal herniation
         4. Penetration of brain by bony spicule
   ii. Cholesteatoma
      a. Congenital cholesteatoma
         1. Appears as a "pearl" in the middle ear space
         2. Usually develop from embryonic rest of epithelium in anterior-superior quadrant
         3. Often asymptomatic
         4. By definition, no previous ear infections
      b. Acquired cholesteatoma
         1. Usually develops from retraction of pars flaccida into Prussak's space (between pars flaccida and malleus neck).
         2. Epithelial migration or retraction pocket formation with internal desquamation, enzymatic erosion, and osteitis allows formation and progression of cholesteatoma.
         3. Most common location for cholesteatoma in middle ear is around the long process of the incus and stapes suprastructure.
         4. Common areas for residual disease following surgery include the sinus tympani, facial recess, and anterior epitympanum.
      c. Complications of cholesteatoma
         1. Erosion of horizontal semicircular canal
         2. Long process of the incus erosion
         3. Tympanic portion of FN is most commonly injured during surgery secondary to confusing anatomy and frequent nerve dehiscence
         4. Oval or round window fistulas should be patched with fascia and packed
      d. Treatment
         1. Canal-wall-up tympanomastoidectomy
            - Higher risk of persistent or recurrent cholesteatoma
            - Often requires second-look surgery within 1 year and possible delay of ossicular reconstruction
         2. Canal-wall-down tympanomastoidectomy
            - Highest rate of success on initial surgery
            - Requires meatoplasty
            - Indications: only hearing ear, contracted mastoid, labyrinthine fistula, EAC erosion

e. Reasons for a persistently draining mastoid cavity are:
   1. Inadequate meatoplasty
   2. Dependent tip cell
   3. High facial ridge
   4. Exposed eustachian tube

f. Reasons for subtotal cholesteatoma matrix resection:
   1. Adherence to the dura, semicircular canal, or FN
   2. Extends into the mesotympanum covering the footplate
   3. Performing canal-wall-down mastoid and will be using some residual matrix to line mastoid cavity

iii. Eustachian tube dysfunction
   a. The dilator tubae portion of the tensor veli palatini muscle is primarily responsible for eustachian tube opening.
   b. Tubal closure is passive.
   c. Chronic ETD can generate negative pressures to 600 cm H_2O with resultant retraction pocket formation and middle ear effusion.

iv. Otosclerosis
   a. Disease of abnormal bone remodeling
   b. Prevalence
      1. Onset usually between ages of 15 and 35
      2. Caucasian > Asian > African American
      3. Female > male (2:1)
      4. Multifactorial with genetic and environmental causes
         - Autosomal dominant with 40% penetrance
         - Hastened by pregnancy and menopause
      5. Eighty-five percent bilateral
      6. Usually begins in region anterior to oval window niche (fissula ante fenestram) resulting in stapes fixation and CHL
      7. Involvement of the cochlea may result in SNHL
      8. Increased osteoblastic and osteoclastic activity resulting in "spongiosis" and eventually resulting in bone with increased mineralization
      9. *Schwartze sign*: pinkish hue over promontory and oval window niche (represents region of thickened mucosa)
      10. Acoustic reflex testing:
          - Early in disease process—increased compliance
          - Late in disease process—decreased or absent reflex
      11. *Audiometry*: Air-bone gap (unusual to find air-bone gaps > 50 dB) with *Carhart notch*
      12. Differential diagnosis
          - Ossicular discontinuity
          - Ossicular fixation
          - Tympanosclerosis
          - Osteogenesis imperfecta
          - Third window conditions
      13. Treatment:
          - Amplification
          - Stapedectomy

v. Vascular anomalies
   a. Dehiscent carotid—pulsatile red mass in anteroinferior quadrant
   b. High-riding jugular bulb—bluish mass in posteroinferior quadrant

c. Persistent stapedial artery
   1. Branch of the petrous ICA
   2. Passes through obturator foramen of the stapes
   3. Gives off the middle meningeal artery (foramen spinosum is absent)
   4. Consider terminating surgery if encountered during stapedectomy
   5. CT may show absent foramen spinosum and widened fallopian canal

d. Glomus tympanicum

E. Ototoxicity: OHC death
   i. Ototoxic drugs preferentially affect OHCs at the basal turn of the cochlea
   ii. Salicylates, cis/carboplatin, aminoglycosides, loop diuretics, quinine, macrolides

F. Sudden SNHL (SSNHL)
   i. Decrease in hearing of 30 dB affecting at least three consecutive frequencies
   ii. Autoimmune pathologies:
      a. *Cogan syndrome*: interstitial keratitis and Meniere's like attacks of vertigo, ataxia, tinnitus, nausea, vomiting, and hearing loss
      b. Others: GPA, polyarteritis nodosa, temporal arteritis, Buerger disease (thromboangitis obliterans), and SLE
   iii. Idiopathic sudden SNHL
   iv. Traumatic
   v. Viral
      a. Increase in viral seroconversion in patients with idiopathic SSNHL compared with controls for cytomegalovirus, influenza B, mumps, rubeola, varicella zoster viruses
   vi. Treatment
      a. Oral steroids, salvage intratympanic steroid injections when patients have incomplete recovery from SSNHL 2 to 6 weeks after onset of symptoms
      b. No role for antivirals, thrombolytics, vasodilators to treat SSNHL
      c. Between 40% and 70% of patients recover some hearing without treatment
      d. Obtain MRI
   vii. Prognostic factors
      a. Good: minimal hearing loss, low-frequency loss, absence of vestibular symptoms, early treatment (within 3 days)
      b. Poor: older age, total deafness, vestibular symptoms, vascular risk factors, delayed treatment, systemic comorbidities (diabetes, hypertension, hyperlipidemia)

G. Auditory neuropathy:
   i. SNHL with poor word recognition scores
   ii. Normal OHC function but abnormal CN VIII function
   iii. Amplification and cochlear implants may be of little help

H. Vestibular disorders
   i. *BPPV*: seconds, no hearing loss, provoked by head movement
   ii. *Perilymphatic fistula (PLF)*: seconds, hearing loss, provoked by trauma, barotrauma, or stapes surgery
   iii. *Vestibular migraine*: minutes to hours, can precede headache, like Meniere's disease but without otologic symptoms
   iv. *Vertebrobasilar insufficiency*: minutes, accompany arterial hypotension (cardiac arrhythmia, orthostatic hypotension), patients with diabetes mellitus (DM), and atherosclerosis
   v. *Meniere disease*: hours, recurrent, hearing loss, tinnitus, aural fullness
   vi. *Delayed-onset vertigo (delayed endolymphatic hydrops)*: like Meniere disease but develops months or years after developing SNHL

vii. *Serous (toxic) labyrinthitis*: acute vertigo crisis in presence of OM, no hearing loss
viii. *Suppurative labyrinthitis*: acute vertigo crisis and hearing loss in presence of OM and fever
ix. *Labyrinthine fistula*: dizziness in patient with cholesteatoma
x. *Vestibular neuronitis*: acute crisis, hours to days, gradual improvement over days, present with no movement, no associated otologic symptoms
xi. *Viral labyrinthitis*: similar to vestibular neuronitis but with sudden hearing loss
xii. *Ototoxic*: vertigo and hearing loss following aminoglycoside use
xiii. *Acoustic neuroma*: hearing loss, tinnitus, and mild if any vestibular symptoms
xiv. *Multiple sclerosis*: vertigo frequently seen, common other findings: vertical nystagmus and internuclear ophthalmoplegia
xv. *Superior semicircular canal dehiscence syndrome (SSCD)*: vertigo, oscillopsia, symptoms generated by increased sound or pressure, CHL, diagnosed by CT temporal bone (VEMP also useful), treated avoidance measures or surgery
xvi. Special findings
    a. *Drop attacks*: crisis of Tumarkin (Meniere disease)
    b. *Vertigo with pressure changes (Hennebert sign) or noise (Tullio phenomenon)*: Meniere disease, PLF, SSCD, syphilis
xvii. Nonvestibular causes of vertigo
    a. CVA
    b. Multiple sclerosis
    c. Vertebrobasilar Insufficiency
    d. Normal pressure hydrocephalus
    e. Migraine-associated vestibulopathy
    f. Psychiatric: depression, anxiety, panic

I. Auditory aids
  i. Conventional hearing aids (HAs)—best for dynamic range of greater than 45db
  ii. Parameters for fitting HAs
    a. Most comfortable loudness (MCL): the level at which listening to words or speech is most comfortable (usually between 40 and 60 dB)
    b. Uncomfortable loudness (UCL): the level at which listening to words or speech is uncomfortably loud
    c. Loudness discomfort level (LDL): the level at which specific tones are painfully loud
    d. Dynamic range of HA: between UCL—SRT
  iii. *CROS*: Contralateral *R*outing *O*f *S*ound
    a. For patients with one good ear and one deaf ear
  iv. *BiCROS*: *B*ilateral *C*ontralateral *R*outing *O*f *S*ound
    a. For patients with one impaired ear and one deaf ear
  v. Bone conduction hearing aid: useful pre-BAHA/atresia/microtia surgery
  vi. *BAHA*
    a. For patients with unilateral conductive or mixed hearing loss who cannot otherwise wear traditional HAs (ie, chronic suppurative OM, atresia)
  vii. Cochlear implants
    a. Severe to profound SNHL with hearing in noise test (AZ Bio) scores of 50% in the implanted ear and 60% in the contralateral ear
    b. Pediatric pre- and post-lingual hearing loss
    c. Single-sided deafness
    d. *Transmission pathway*: microphone → external processor → receiver-stimulator → electrodes → spiral ganglion cells and eighth nerve → cochlear nucleus

e. Round window insertion or cochleostomy (placed anterior and inferior to the round window niche)
f. Electrode is ideally placed in scala tympani
g. Contraindications
   1. Cochlear or cochlear nerve aplasia

J. FN injury and disorders
   i. Sunderland classification
      a. First degree: *Neuropraxia*: pressure on nerve trunk. Blockage of axoplasm flow at site of injury
      b. Second degree: *Axonotmesis*: axonal and myelin injury. Axon degenerates distal to the site of injury and proximally to the next node of Ranvier. May develop Wallerian degeneration
      c. Third degree: *Neurotmesis*: injury to axon, myelin, and endoneurium. Poor prognosis
      d. Fourth degree: *Neurotmesis*: injury to axon, myelin, endoneurium, and perineurium. Poor prognosis
      e. Fifth degree: *Neurotmesis*: Injury to axon, myelin, endoneurium, perineurium, and epineurium (all layers of nerve sheath). Poor prognosis
   ii. *House-Brackmann* (HB) classification
      a. Grade I: normal
      b. Grade II: slight weakness/asymmetry with movement
      c. Grade III: obvious asymmetry with movement, possible synkinesis, complete eye closure
      d. Grade IV: incomplete eye closure, no forehead movement, asymmetry with movement
      e. Grade V: asymmetric at rest, minimal movement with effort
      f. Grade VI: no movement
   iii. Nerve testing
      a. Wallerian degeneration takes 48 to 72 hours to progress to extratemporal segments of FN. Electrophysiologic testing, nerve excitability test [NET], and electroneuronography [ENOG]) should not be done in first 3 days
      b. *NET*: 2.0 to 3.5 mA difference between sides suggests an unfavorable prognosis
      c. ENOG measures *compound muscle action potential* (CMAP)
         1. Greater than or equal to 90% degeneration of CMAP suggests poor recovery, indication for surgical exploration and decompression
         2. Should be performed daily until nadir is reached
      d. Electromyography (EMG) measures *motor unit potentials* (MUP)
         1. May be useful in first 3 days following injury
         2. Important for assessing reinnervation potential of the muscle *2 to 3 weeks after onset*
            - Fibrillation potentials suggest denervation
            - Polyphasic potentials seen in reinnervation
      e. *Indications for imaging*: progression of palsy over 3 weeks, recurrent palsy, facial hyperkinesis, development of associated cranial neuropathies. These symptoms may also suggest neoplastic involvement
   iv. Acute FN palsy
      a. Bell's (70%): diagnosis of exclusion
         1. Rapid onset (< 48 hours)
         2. May affect CN V to XII
         3. Believed to be viral (herpes simplex)

b. Herpes zoster (*Ramsay Hunt syndrome*) (15%)
   1. Cutaneous vesicles of EAC and conchal bowl
   2. Otalgia
   3. Higher incidence of cochlear and vestibular disturbances
c. Other symptoms related to FN paralysis
   1. Dysgeusia (chorda tympani)
   2. Hyperacusis (stapedius dysfunction)
   3. Decreased lacrimation (GSPN)
d. Treatment
   1. High-dose prednisone
   2. Acyclovir (option) if seen in first 3 days
   3. Valacyclovir may be more effective for Ramsay Hunt syndrome
e. Other notable causes of FN palsy
   1. Diabetes mellitus
   2. Infectious
      - Lyme disease—*Borrelia burgdorferi*
        (a) Unilateral greater than bilateral facial palsy (3:1)
        (b) "Bull's eye" rash
        (c) Tetracycline for adults, penicillin for children
      - Mononucleosis
      - Mumps
      - Otitis media (acute or malignant OM)
   3. Autoimmune
      - Sarcoidosis (uveoparotid fever: uveitis, fever, parotitis, CN paralysis)
      - GPA
      - Multiple sclerosis
      - Myasthenia gravis
   4. *Melkersson-Rosenthal syndrome*: unilateral facial palsy, facial edema, and fissured tongue (lingua plicata)
   5. *Guillain-Barré syndrome*: causes *bilateral* FN paralysis
   6. *Mobius syndrome*: bilateral facial and abducens nerve agenesis
   7. Hyperthyroidism
   8. Neoplasia
   9. Perinatal
      - FN at risk due to lack of mastoid tip
      - Compression by mother's sacrum or delivery forceps
      - Excellent spontaneous recovery
      - Elevated serum angiotensin-converting enzyme (ACE) usually confirms the diagnosis
   10. Trauma: penetrating wounds or temporal bone fracture

Immunology and Allergy

A. Antibodies
   i. IgA
      a. Found on mucus membranes
      b. Secreted as dimer and circulated as monomer
      c. Many bacteria contain IgA proteases

- ii. IgD: antigen receptor on B cells
- iii. IgE: Type I hypersensitivity, mediates TH-2 responses (allergic reactions)
- iv. IgG
  - a. Majority of antibody-based immunity
  - b. Placental transmission
  - c. Has function both extracellularly and intracellularly
  - d. Marker of previous infection
- v. IgM
  - a. First antibody seen in response to pathogen
  - b. On the surface of B cells
  - c. Pentamer—largest antibody
  - d. Marker of acute infection

B. Hypersensitivities (Gel and Coombs classification)
- i. Type I (atopic–classic allergic response)
  - a. Results from exposure to a particular antigen
  - b. Mediated by IgE
  - c. Results in mast cell degranulation and rapid inflammation
  - d. *Rhinitis, asthma, angioedema, anaphylaxis*
- ii. Type II (antibody dependent)
  - a. Mediated by IgG and IgM
  - b. Antibodies bind antigen and:
    1. Form complexes that activate classical pathway, the complement cascade, and membrane attack complex
    2. Function as markers for natural killer cells, which cause cell death
  - c. *Hashimoto thyroiditis, pemphigus*
- iii. Type III (immune complex)
  - a. Immune complexes of IgG and IgM form in the blood and are deposited in tissues
  - b. Activation of classical pathway, complement cascade, and membrane attack complex
  - c. *Rheumatoid arthritis, serum sickness,* and *lupus*
- iv. Type IV (cell-mediated/delayed type)
    1. T-cell mediated
    2. Takes 3 days to develop
    3. *Contact dermatitis, temporal arteritis, PPD-Mantoux test for tuberculosis*

C. Categories of allergic triggers:
- i. Inhalants (pollen, animal dander, molds)
  - a. Seasons for various classes or pollens:
    1. Trees—winter and spring, February to May
    2. Grasses—late spring and summer, April to August
    3. Weeds—late summer and fall allergens, July to frost
- ii. Ingestants (foods, medications)
  - a. Injectables (medications, insect venom)
  - b. Contactants (nickel, poison ivy, medications)

D. Types of specific allergen testing
- i. In vivo (serum testing)
  - a. Epicutaneous
    1. Introduction of the antigen into the epidermis only
    2. Include patch, scratch, prick, and puncture tests

3. Scratch testing has a highest false positive rate
4. Puncture and prick testing are excellent for screening for presence or absence of allergy to individual allergens

b. Percutaneous
1. Introduction of antigen into superficial dermis
2. Include various intradermal techniques
3. Single dilutional
 - Highly sensitive but less specific than prick or puncture testing
4. Intradermal dilutional testing (IDT)
 - Involves the sequential administration of fivefold diluted antigens, beginning with very dilute concentrations and progressively administrating more concentrated antigens until specific response obtained on the skin
 - Highly sensitive with very low level of systemic response

c. Not to be performed with patients on beta blockers (if need to use epinephrine, would lead to unopposed alpha-adrenergic stimulation)

ii. In vitro testing (RAST technique)
a. RAST measures the serum level of allergen-specific IgE.
b. Provides quantitative assessment of the degree of allergic sensitization.
c. It is more specific than skin testing.

E. Immunotherapy
i. Process of administrating allergen either subcutaneously or sublingually over time to induce allergic tolerance and reduction of allergic symptoms.
ii. The goal of immunotherapy is to shift the T cell response from a TH2 to TH1 phenotype.
iii. It increases specific IgG4 levels for the treated allergen.
iv. It requires at least 3 to 5 years of regular administration for continued benefits.

Rhinology

A. Chandler's classification of orbital cellulitis
i. Periorbital edema
ii. Periorbital cellulitis
iii. Subperiosteal abscess
iv. Orbital abscess
v. Cavernous sinus thrombosis

B. Chronic rhinosinusitis with (CRSwNP) or without nasal polyposis (CRSsNP)
i. CRSwNP phenotypes
a. Inflammatory polyps
b. Allergic fungal rhinosinusitis (AFRS)
1. Benign, noninvasive fungal disease
c. Diagnosis (Bent and Kuhn major criteria)
1. Type 1 hypersensitivity to fungi by history, skin tests, or serology
2. Nasal polyposis
3. Characteristic radiologic findings
 - CT: rim of hypointensity with hyperdense central material (allergic mucin) with ferromagnetic fungal elements

- MRI: peripheral hyperintensity with central hypointensity on both T1 and T2, central void on T2

4. Eosinophilic mucin (*Charcot-Leyden crystals*)
5. Noninvasive fungus in sinus contents

d. Aspirin-exacerbated respiratory disease (AERD)
   1. *Samter's triad*: aspirin sensitivity, asthma, nasal polyposis
e. Associated with medical conditions (eg, cystic fibrosis, Churg-Strauss)
f. Respiratory epithelial adenomatoid hamartoma
g. Rhinosporidiosis
   1. Endemic to Africa, Pakistan, India
   2. Red, friable nasal polyps, nasal obstruction, epistaxis

C. Differential diagnosis of nasal mass
   i. *Congenital*: glioma, encephalocele, dermoid, teratoma
   ii. *Infectious*: tuberculosis, rhinoscleroma, rhinosporidiosis
   iii. *Inflammatory/granulomatous*: allergic polyp, sarcoid
   iv. *Neoplasm (benign)*: squamous and Schneiderian papilloma, juvenile angiofibroma, paraganglioma, leiomyoma, schwannoma, adenoma
   v. *Neoplasm (malignant)*: squamous cell carcinoma (SCC), adenocarcinoma, adenoid cystic carcinoma, lymphoma, rhabdomyosarcoma, melanoma, Esthesioneuroblastoma, chordoma, plasmacytoma, histiocytosis X

D. Paranasal malignancy
   i. Maxillary > ethmoid > sphenoid > frontal sinuses.
   ii. Risk factors
      a. Wood dust
      b. Nickel
      c. Chromium
      d. Volatile hydrocarbons
      e. Organic fibers found in the wood, shoe, and textile industries
      f. Smoking
      g. Human papillomavirus (HPV) may be involved in the malignant transformation of inverting papilloma
   iii. Diagnosis
      a. Imaging
      b. Most patients have advanced disease at the time of diagnosis
         1. Exception: maxillary tumors inferior to Ohngren line

E. Anosmia
   i. Associated with
      a. Alzheimer disease
      b. Chronic rhinitis
      c. Chronic sinusitis
      d. Nasal polyps
      e. Nasal allergy
      f. Head trauma with/without cribriform fracture
      g. Postviral
      h. Malignancy of the nasal cavity/nasopharynx/ethmoid sinus/frontal sinus
      i. Psychiatric disorders
      j. Medications
      k. Nasal surgery
      l. Hypogonadism (Kallmann syndrome)

F. Nasal obstruction:
   i. Septal deviation, septal hematoma, turbinate hypertrophy, nasal narrowing, nasal valve collapse, tip ptosis, choanal atresia, nasopharyngeal obstruction/mass, trauma
   ii. Nasal tumor, foreign body
   iii. Inflammation due to nasal/sinus infection, allergy, granulomatous process, atrophic rhinitis (AR), septal abscess
   iv. Medication, hypothyroidism, pregnancy
   v. Psychogenic, hyperpatency (empty nose syndrome)
G. Septal perforation common differential diagnosis
   i. Iatrogenic
   ii. Cocaine use
   iii. Septal abscess
   iv. Nose picking
   v. Infections (eg, syphilis, tuberculosis, leprosy, rhinoscleroma)
   vi. Inflammatory (eg, GPA, sarcoidosis, lupus, other collagen vascular disease)
   vii. Neoplasms include nasal lymphoma and other malignancies
H. Craniopharyngioma
   i. Epithelial tumors derived from the Rathke cleft (embryonal precursor to the adenohypophysis)
   ii. Craniopharyngeal duct is the structure along which the eventual adenohypophysis and infundibulum migrate—tumors can occur anywhere along the course of this duct (pharynx, sella turcica, third ventricle)
   iii. Clinical presentation
      a. Headaches
      b. Visual loss (possible bitemporal hemianopsia)
      c. Optic atrophy
      d. Hypopituitarism
      e. Enlargement of sella turcica
      f. Parasellar calcifications
   iv. Differential diagnosis
      a. Optic glioma
      b. Primary pituitary tumors
      c. Parasellar metastases
I. Nasopharyngeal carcinoma
   i. Presenting symptoms
      a. Cervical lymphadenopathy
      b. Epistaxis
      c. Serous effusion
      d. CN VI paralysis
      e. Commonly arises at the fossa of Rosenmüller
      f. Male > female (2.5:1)
      g. Increased incidence in population from southern China
      h. Associated with EBV infection—can follow EBV as a marker
   ii. Treatment: radiation therapy
      a. No neck dissection unless for persistent disease
J. Tornwaldt cyst
   i. Most common congenital nasopharyngeal lesion
   ii. Develops in the midline as the notochord ascends through the clivus to create the neural plate

Laryngology

A. True vocal fold (TVC)
   i. Superior edge of cricothyroid ligament
   ii. 1.7 mm in thickness
   iii. Layers
      a. Stratified squamous epithelium
      b. Superficial layer of lamina propria (corresponds to Reinke's space)
      c. Vocal ligament
         1. Intermediate layer of lamina propria
         2. Deep layer of lamina propria
      d. Vocalis muscle
B. Phonation
   i. Air from the lungs causes Bernoulli effect and vocal fold vibration.
   ii. Mucosal wave produces a fundamental tone accompanied by several nonharmonic overtones.
   iii. Sound is modified by the volume of airflow, movements of the vocal tract, and the degree of vocal cord tension.
   iv. Voice fundamental frequency increases in aging men but decreases in aging women.
C. Benign lesions
   i. Amyloidosis
      a. Extracellular deposits of insoluble fibrillar proteins.
      b. Glottis most common site of airway involvement.
         1. Deposition in true and false vocal folds and the ventricles
      c. Biopsy is the mainstay of diagnosis.
         1. Classic Congo red staining: apple green birefringence
      d. Surgical excision is mainstay of treatment.
   ii. Chondroma
      a. Firm, smooth lesion usually involving posterior cricoid cartilage
      b. Treatment is surgical excision
   iii. Cysts
      a. Mixed group of benign lesions that may involve any laryngeal structure except for the free edge of TVCs
      b. Lined with ciliated pseudostratified columnar (respiratory) epithelium, columnar epithelium, squamous epithelium, or a combination of all three
      c. *Ductal cysts (75%)*: Develop from an obstructed mucous duct, which subsequently leads to cystic dilation of the mucous gland
      d. *Saccular cysts* (24%)
         1. Disorders of the saccule represent a spectrum from enlarged saccule to laryngocele to saccular cyst
         2. Mucous-filled dilations of the laryngeal saccule
         3. Anterior saccular cysts protrude anteromedially between the true and false vocal folds
         4. Lateral saccular cysts extend superolaterally to involve the false vocal cord, aryepiglottic fold, and vallecula and may extend to the extralaryngeal tissues via the thyrohyoid membrane
   iv. Laryngopharyngeal reflux
      a. Erythema and edema
      b. Pachydermia
      c. Pseudosulcus

v. Granuloma
   a. Develop from extrinsic trauma (ie, intubation, GERD)
   b. Arise posteriorly in the region of the vocal process of the arytenoids
   c. Treat: speech therapy, anti-reflux pharmacotherapy, and removal of source of trauma

vi. Granular cell tumor
   a. Yellow lesion on posterior one-third of vocal fold
   b. Also found on the tongue, skin, breast, subcutaneous tissues, and respiratory tract
   c. Histology shows pseudoepitheliomatous hyperplasia
   d. ~3% become malignant
   e. Treatment: conservative excision

vii. Nodules
   a. Develop from vocal trauma
   b. Bilateral white lesions often found at the junction of the anterior one-third and posterior two-thirds of the vocal fold
   c. Treatment: speech therapy

viii. Polyps
   a. Associated with vocal trauma and smoking
   b. Unilateral, pedunculated lesion commonly found between anterior one-third and posterior two-thirds of the vocal fold
   c. Treatment: excision (microflap)

ix. Recurrent respiratory papillomatosis
   a. Juvenile onset
      1. Usually between 2 and 4 years
      2. Manifests as hoarseness and stridor
   b. Adult onset
      1. Occasionally solitary or more localized than juvenile-onset
   c. Self-limited disease
   d. Associated with HPV 6 and 11
   e. Papilloma virus resides in the superficial epithelial layer
   f. Occult sites: nasopharynx and undersurface of the true vocal folds
   g. Treatment
      1. Microlaryngoscopy with stripping and/or CO_2 laser/microdebridement
      2. Intralesional injections
         - Avastin: inhibits vascular endothelial growth factor A
         - Cidofovir: inhibits viral DNA polymerase
      3. HPV vaccination
      4. Indol-3-carbinol: natural derivative of cruciferous vegetables

x. Reinke edema
   a. Associated with smoking
   b. Accumulation of fluid in superficial layer of lamina propria
   c. Bilateral, edematous changes of vocal fold
   d. Treatment: smoking cessation, surgery in severe cases

xi. Sarcoidosis
   a. Epiglottis is the most common site of involvement
   b. Pale pink, turban-like epiglottis

xii. Tuberculosis
   a. Most seen in the interarytenoid area and the laryngeal surface of the epiglottis

D. Malignant lesions
   i. Risk factors:
      a. Tobacco and alcohol use
      b. HPV 16 and 18
      c. GERD
      d. Radiation exposure
   ii. Dysplasia risk of malignant transformation
      a. Mild to moderate: 10%
      b. Severe: 20% to 30%
   iii. Types
      a. SCC (> 90%)
      b. Minor salivary gland malignancies
         1. Adenoid cystic carcinoma
         2. Mucoepidermoid carcinoma
         3. Chondrosarcoma—posterior cricoid cartilage
   iv. Fixed cords are usually the result of involvement of the thyroarytenoid muscle
   v. Staging—different schemas for supraglottis, glottis, and subglottis
   vi. Treatment
      a. Glottic CIS—serial microlaryngoscopy, stripping, laser excision
      b. Chondrosarcoma—narrowly excised without postoperative radiation
      c. Stage I and II SCC: surgery or XRT (comparable oncologic outcome)
      d. Stage III and IV SCC: chemoradiation (organ preservation) or surgery ± radiation
      e. Surgical approaches
         1. Cordectomy
            - For T1 vocal fold malignancies, dysplastic vocal fold lesions
            - Contraindications: impaired vocal fold mobility, extension to thyroid cartilage, supra/subglottic extension
         2. Transoral laser microsurgery (TLM)
            - For T1/2 malignancies
            - Contraindications: extralaryngeal spread, unable to preserve cricoid and arytenoid cartilages, inability to gain endoscopic access
         3. Transoral robotic surgery
            - Most used for supraglottic laryngeal cancer
            - Particularly good outcomes (80-100% locoregional control rates)
         4. Supraglottic laryngectomy
            - For T1/2 supraglottic tumors, T3 supraglottic tumors with pre-epiglottic space invasion, tumor extending to base of tongue
            - Contraindications: glottic involvement, invasion of cricoid or thyroid cartilage, bilateral involvement of the arytenoids, poor pulmonary function
         5. Hemilaryngectomy
            - For bulky T1/2 glottic cancer (can involve anterior commissure), less than 1 cm subglottic involvement
            - Contraindications: large T3 or any T4 tumor, arytenoid fixation, thyroid cartilage invasion, pre-epiglottic space invasion, poor pulmonary function
         6. Supracricoid laryngectomy
            - For T3 glottic lesions with TVC fixation and impaired arytenoid mobility or T4 glottic lesions with minimal thyroid cartilage invasion

- Contraindications: arytenoid fixation, significant pre-epiglottis spread, invasion of cricoid or thyroid cartilage, poor pulmonary function
- Removes entire thyroid cartilage, bilateral true and false vocal folds, paraglottic space but spares the cricoid, hyoid, and at least one arytenoid

7. Total laryngectomy
   - For T3 and T4 tumors with cartilaginous invasion and extralaryngeal/neck involvement, salvage treatment or nonfunctional larynx

E. Vocal cord paralysis
   i. Vocal cord position
      a. RLN—*Paramedian*
      b. Vagal—*Lateral/intermediate* and patient will have *hypernasal* speech
   ii. Vocal cord medialization
      a. Injection laryngoplasty:
         1. Temporary: carboxymethylcellulose, gel foam, hyaluronic acid, calcium hydroxyapatite, collagen
         2. Permanent: Teflon, fat
      b. Medialization laryngoplasty +/− arytenoid adduction
   iii. Gutman sign SLN paralysis. In the normal individual, lateral pressure over the thyroid cartilage causes an increased voice pitch, whereas anterior pressure causes a decrease. In SLN paralysis, the reverse is true.

F. Tracheal resection/reconstruction:
   i. Airway lengthening techniques
      a. Mobilization after blunt dissection of the larynx and trachea (3 cm)
      b. Incision of the annular ligaments on one side of the trachea proximal to the anastomosis and on the opposite side distally (1.5 cm)
      c. Laryngeal release
         1. Suprahyoid (5 cm)
         2. Infrahyoid (often results in dysphagia)
      d. Neck flexion (1-2 cm)

G. Neurolaryngology
   i. Hyperfunctional disorders
      a. Paradoxical vocal fold motion (spasmodic dysphonia)
         1. A focal dystonia of the larynx, that is, laryngeal hyperresponsiveness
         2. Can be triggered by irritants, allergens, exercise induced
         3. Types
            - Adductor: strained and strangled voice with glottic breaks, difficulty with vowels (80-89)
            - Abductor: breathy voice breaks or whispering voice, unvoiced consonants (60-69)
         4. Treatment: voice therapy, Botulinum toxin injection
      b. Tremor: rhythmic oscillations of a body part or segment
      c. Myoclonus: sudden brief muscle contractions
   ii. Hypofunctional disorders
      a. Amyotrophic lateral sclerosis
         1. Flaccid-spastic mixed dysarthria, progressive weakness affects voice and swallowing
      b. Myasthenia gravis: vocal fatigue, which improves with rest
         1. Evaluate with edrophonium (tensilon test)

iii. Mixed disorders
   a. Parkinsonism
      1. Voice symptoms: poor breath support, monotone voice
      2. Treatment: Lee-Silverman voice therapy, injection laryngoplasty, laryngeal framework surgery
   b. Multiple sclerosis
      1. Voice symptoms: spastic, slurred speech

H. Venturi jet ventilation
   i. Used in endoscopic procedures (pediatric and adult), endolaryngeal laser procedures
   ii. Complications: hypoventilation, pneumothorax, pneumomediastinum, subcutaneous emphysema, abdominal distention, mucosal dehydration, distal seeding of malignant cells or papillomavirus particles

I. Trachea
   i. Differential diagnosis of hemoptysis
      a. Acute: pneumonia, neoplasm, foreign body, aspiration, pulmonary infarct, acute bronchitis, infection (bronchitis, abscess, tuberculosis), iatrogenic (tracheotomy, intubation, bronchoscopy, needle biopsy)
      b. Chronic: tuberculosis, bronchial carcinoma
      c. Recurrent: chronic bronchitis, neoplasm, bronchiectasis, cystic fibrosis, pulmonary hypertension, Osler-Weber-Rendu syndrome, arteriovenous fistula, cardiovascular disease
      d. Investigations: chest x-ray, endoscopy, cytology, culture, bronchogram, lung scan
   ii. Stenosis
      a. Congenital, extrinsic, idiopathic, or posttraumatic
      b. Commonly seen in patients requiring ventilatory support
      c. Overinflated balloon cuffs (> 25 mm Hg) result in mucosal ischemia and loss, inflammation, scarring, granulation tissue
      d. Treatment: antireflux measures, incision (laser or cold) and dilation, ± mitomycin C application, tracheal resection

J. Esophagus
   i. Upper one-third: skeletal muscle
   ii. Lower two-thirds: smooth muscle
   iii. Physiology of swallowing
      a. Oral phase: bolus preparation with tongue against hard palate
      b. Pharyngeal phase
         1. Nasopharyngeal closure: constriction of superior constrictor (Passavant's ridge) and tensor and levator veli palatini
         2. Breathing cessation and glottic closure
         3. Bolus propulsion: base of tongue elevation and contraction of pharyngeal constrictors
         4. Laryngeal elevation: stylopharyngeus, stylohyoid, and salpingopharyngeus
         5. Epiglottic rotation
         6. Dilation of cricopharyngeus
      c. Esophageal phase: bolus propelled by muscular wave
   iv. Benign disease
      a. Achalasia
         1. Lack of peristalsis
         2. Failure of esophageal sphincter (LES) relaxation
         3. Caused by degeneration of Auerbach plexus

4. "Birds beak" esophagus on esophagram
5. Treatment
   - Medical
     (a) Calcium channel blockers
     (a) Botox of the LES
   - Surgical
     (a) Dilation
     (b) Heller myotomy: gold standard
     (c) LES myotomy and partial fundoplication

b. Gastroesophageal reflux disease/laryngopharyngeal reflux
   1. Results from LES relaxation and abnormalities in esophageal peristalsis
   2. May lead to Barrett esophagitis
   3. Symptoms
      - Classic: heartburn, regurgitation
      - Atypical: laryngospasm, cough, hoarseness, globus sensation, wheezing
   4. Diagnosis:
      - History
      - Response to over-the-counter antacids or trial PPI
      - Esophageal manometry
      - pH-impendence monitoring
      - Esophagoscopy
   5. Treatment
      - Behavioral: weight loss, smoking cessation, dietary modification, elevate head of bed
      - Medications: OTC meds, H2 blockers, PPI, promotility agents (metoclopramide), sodium alginates
      - Surgery: Nissen fundoplication

c. Zenker's diverticulum
   1. Occurs in posterior wall of Killian triangle
      - Symptoms
        (a) Dysphagia
        (b) Regurgitation of undigested food
        (c) Halitosis
      - Diagnosis: esophagram
      - Treatment: endoscopic versus transcervical approaches

d. Esophageal webs
   1. Slowly progressive dysphagia
   2. Commonly develop on anterior wall
   3. Associated with Plummer-Vinson syndrome
      - Esophageal web
      - Iron deficiency anemia
      - Hypothyroidism
      - Gastritis
      - Cheilitis
      - Glossitis

v. Malignant lesions
   a. Barrett esophagitis
      1. Metaplasia of esophageal mucosal epithelium from squamous to columnar
      2. May progress to carcinoma in 10% to 15% of cases
      3. Treatment: PPI ± fundoplication

b. Esophageal carcinoma
   1. Male more than female (5:1)
   2. Associations
      - Barrett esophagitis
      - Alcohol
      - Tobacco
      - Achalasia
      - Oculopharyngeal syndrome
      - Caustic burns
      - Plummer-Vinson syndrome
      - Pernicious anemia
   3. Symptoms
      - Dysphagia is the most common symptom
      - Odynophagia
      - Weight loss
      - Hoarseness
   4. Cancers arising in upper third are SCC, lower usually adenocarcinoma
   5. Treatment: surgery

Benign Head and Neck

A. Angioedema
   i. Causes
      a. Allergy
      b. ACE inhibitor use
      c. Familial—C1 esterase deficiency
   ii. Treatment
      a. ABC's: Airway protection
      b. Meds: Steroids, H_1 and H_2 blockers, epinephrine (if allergy)

B. Benign cutaneous neoplasms
   i. *Actinic keratosis*: small lesions of epidermal proliferation. May evolve (1%) into squamous cell carcinoma (SCC)
   ii. *Chondrodermatitis nodularis helicis/antihelices*: ulcerative lesion of helix or antihelix. Results from pressure and may be treated with surgical excision
   iii. *Keratoacanthoma*: fast-growing tumors that are difficult to distinguish from SCC. Distinguished from malignancy by absence of epithelial membrane antigen
   iv. *Nevi*
      a. *Intraepithelial*: benign
      b. *Junctional*: premalignant
      c. *Intradermal*: benign
      d. *Blue (Spitz)*: benign
   v. *Seborrheic keratosis*: originate in keratinocytes and increase with age. May have various colors (tan, brown, black), "pasted on" appearance. Easily treated with curettage

C. Dental pathology
   i. Amalgam tattoo—tattoo of gingiva from dental amalgam
   ii. Enamel discoloration—antibiotic (tetracycline) exposure prior to eruption

- iii. Odontogenic cysts and tumors
  - a. Dentigerous (follicular) cyst—defect in enamel formation. Results in unerupted tooth crown. Ameloblastoma formation occurs in cyst wall
  - b. Lateral periodontal cyst—small lucent cysts (usually at mandibular premolars)
  - c. Primordial cyst—rare cyst that develops instead of a tooth
  - d. Periapical/radicular cyst—most common. Burned-out tooth infection
  - e. Odontogenic keratocyst—can arise from any cyst. Distinguished by keratinizing lining. Aggressive and difficult to remove. Need larger resection. Part of basal cell nevus syndrome (*Gorlin syndrome*)
  - f. Nonodontogenic cysts—bone cysts, aneurysmal bone cyst, gingival cysts
  - g. Ameloblastoma—most common odontogenic tumor. Benign but locally aggressive. Wide excision (eg, segmental mandibulectomy)

D. TMJ disorder
- i. Associated with
  - a. Bruxism
  - b. Dental trauma or dental surgery
  - c. Mandibular trauma/abnormalities/asymmetry
  - d. Myofascial or cervical tension
- ii. Treatment begins with soft diet, warm compresses, and nonsteroidal anti-inflammatory drugs. A thorough dental/maxillofacial evaluation is advised

E. Granular cell tumor
- i. Nonulcerated, painless nodules with insidious onset and slow growth
- ii. Involves tongue in 25% of cases
- iii. Histology shows pseudoepitheliomatous hyperplasia
- iv. ~3% malignant transformation
- v. Treatment: conservative excision

F. Immunosuppression (acquired/iatrogenic) results in an increase in lymphoproliferative disorders and should be kept in mind when evaluating lesions of Waldeyer ring, salivary glands, or cervical nodes

G. Infections
- i. Candidiasis
  - a. Predisposing factors
    1. Antibiotics, steroids
    2. Infants, elderly
    3. Diabetes, malnutrition, immunosuppression
  - b. Clinical features
    1. Patches of creamy white pseudomembrane
    2. Odynophagia
    3. Dysphagia
    4. Angular cheilitis
    5. Laryngitis
  - c. Diagnosis—culture on Sabouraud medium
  - d. Treatment—topical or oral antifungals
- ii. Herpangina—Coxsackie A virus (hand, foot, and mouth disease)
  - a. Minute vesicles on the anterior tonsillar pillars and soft palate
- iii. Histoplasmosis
  - a. Endemic in Missouri and Ohio River valleys
  - b. Clinical features
    1. Lung involvement
    2. Rhinitis, pharyngitis, epiglottitis

3. Nodular lesions of tongue, lip, and oral mucosa (oral lesions much more common than in *Blastomyces* and *Coccidioides*)
4. Dirty white mucosa or true cords

c. Pathology—epithelioid granulomas
d. Diagnosis
1. Skin test
2. Complement fixation
3. Latex agglutination
4. Laryngeal lesions require direct laryngoscopy (DL) and biopsy with fungal stains

e. Treatment—antifungals

iv. Pharyngitis
a. Symptoms: throat pain, fever, pharyngeal erythema/exudates, cervical lymphadenopathy in the absence of coryza, cough, and hoarseness
b. Pathogens
1. *Streptococcus pyogenes* (most important pathogen)
2. *Staphylococcus aureus*
3. *Streptococcus pneumoniae*
4. *Moraxella catarrhalis*
5. *Haemophilus influenzae*
6. *Mycoplasma pneumoniae* (may account for ~30% of adult pharyngitis)
7. *Corynebacterium diphtheriae*
8. Gonococcal

c. Treatment—antimicrobial therapy

H. Paragangliomas (PGL)
i. Rule of 10's: 10% bilateral, 10% familial, 10% malignant
ii. Arise from extra-adrenal paraganglionic cells derived from the neural crest
iii. Correct terminology based on location (ie, carotid, jugulotympanic, vagal, etc.)
iv. Incidence in head and neck: carotid (50-60%) > jugulotympanic > vagal
v. Hereditary PGL syndromes: von-Hippel Lindau, neurofibromatosis, MEN2a/b
vi. Familial PG syndromes: are familial 10% of the time, mutations in succinate dehydrogenase subunits, autosomal dominant
vii. Risk of malignant transformation by site of origin: Orbit and laryngeal (25%), vagal (10-15%), jugulotympanic (5%), carotid (2-5%)
viii. Capable of producing vasoactive substances
a. Catecholamines, norepinephrine, dopamine, somatostatin, vasoactive intestinal polypeptide, calcitonin
b. If patient has headache, palpitations, flushing, diarrhea, or HTN
1. Obtain 24-hour urine vanillylmandelic acid and serum catecholamine levels
2. Consider abdominal CT to rule out concomitant adrenal pheochromocytoma

ix. Radiology
a. Arteriography is the gold standard.
b. CT shows postcontrast enhancement and MRI shows mild enhancement on T2 image, intense postcontrast enhancement, and "salt and pepper" appearance secondary to flow voids.

x. Histology shows
a. Chief cells (amine precursor and uptake decarboxylase cells)
b. Sustentacular cells (modified Schwann cells) organized in clusters known as Zellballen

xi. Carotid PGL (carotid body tumor)
  a. Located in the adventitia of the posteromedial aspect of the bifurcation of the common carotid artery
  b. Slow-growing, painless neck mass, often pulsatile and mobile in a horizontal axis, not vertical
  c. May have hoarseness, vocal cord paralysis, or dysphagia
  d. Arteriography reveals characteristic splaying of the internal and external carotid arteries (*Lyre sign*)
  e. Treatment:
    1. Surgery ± preoperative embolization
    2. Radiation may be used as primary therapy

xii. Jugular and tympanic PGL (glomus tympanicum and jugulare)
  a. Most common tumor of the middle ear
  b. Female more than male (4:1)
  c. May present with *pulsatile tinnitus*, aural fullness, hearing loss, and cranial neuropathies
  d. Examination may show vascular middle ear mass, which exhibits blanching of mass with positive pneumatic otoscopy (*Browns sign)*
  e. Gold standard of diagnosis is arteriography
  f. Treatment: Surgery ± preoperative embolization versus Radiation therapy

xiii. Vagal PGL (glomus vagale)
  a. Located within the perineurium of the vagus nerve, commonly arise from the nodose ganglion (inferior ganglion of vagus nerve)
  b. More common in females
  c. Often present with a painless neck mass with tongue weakness, hoarseness, dysphagia, and Horner syndrome
  d. Radiography reveals vascular lesion that displaces the internal carotid artery anteromedially
  e. Treatment
    1. Surgery ± preoperative embolization
    2. In certain situations (recurrent tumor, incomplete resection, and elderly patients) stereotactic radiation may be used as primary therapy

I. Peripheral nerve sheath tumors
  i. Schwannomas
    a. Encapsulated, round tumor derived from Schwann cells
    b. Adherent or partially displacing involved nerve
    c. Histology shows Antoni A and Antoni B tissue
    d. Treatment—surgery (can often preserve nerve function)
  ii. Neurofibroma
    a. More common than schwannomas
    b. Nonencapsulated, fusiform tumor
    c. Intertwined with involved nerve
    d. Associated with von Recklinghausen disease (neurofibromatosis type 1 [NF-1])
    e. Treatment—surgery (often lose nerve function)

J. Fibro-osseous lesions
  i. Unrelated group of lesions sharing the same histologic features as their common denominator (benign cellular fibrous tissue containing variable amounts of mineralized material)
  ii. Diagnosis is often impossible by microscopy alone and requires clinical and radiographic information

a. Osseous dysplasia cementoma
   1. Asymptomatic, reactive lesion
   2. Occurs predominantly in African American women over age 20
   3. Most common location is anterior mandibular periapical alveolar bone
   4. X-ray findings: early lesion show periapical lucency or multiple lucencies resembling periapical granuloma or cyst, but tooth is always vital
b. Fibrous dysplasia
   1. Develops in first to second decade of life
   2. Diffuse, painless bony swelling with facial deformity
   3. Does not cross midline
   4. Types:
      - Monostotic (most common)
      - Polyostotic
      - Disseminated (*McCune-Albright*)
      - Juvenile aggressive: rapidly growing, markedly deforming lesion of maxilla that destroys tooth buds and is refractory to treatment
   5. Radiologic findings
      - *Ground glass*, multilocular, radiolucent, or irregularly mottled opaque and lucent
      - Fusiform tapered expansion
      - Diffuse margins
      - Involves and incorporates lamina dura and cortical bone
c. Ossifying fibroma
   1. Benign, locally aggressive neoplasm
   2. The most common site in adults is the mandible
   3. Causes painless bulge in cortical bone
   4. Radiologic findings
      - Well-demarcated lucency
      - Causes divergence of tooth roots
   5. Treatment: conservative curettage

K. Osteomas
   i. Benign, slow growing, osteogenic
   ii. Usually affect the bones of the face and skull
   iii. Usually painless, but may cause pain, headache, or facial pressure
   iv. Sites of predilection
      a. Mandible, temporal bone, paranasal sinuses (frontal (80%) > ethmoid > maxillary > sphenoid)
   v. Treat with surgical excision
   vi. Associated with Gardner syndrome
      b. Autosomal dominant
      c. Colon polyps, osteomas, soft tissue tumors
         1. Polyps have 40% rate of malignant degeneration—recommend colonoscopy

L. Nutritional deficiencies
   i. Vitamin B_2 (riboflavin)—atrophic glossitis, angular cheilitis, gingivostomatitis
   ii. Vitamin B_6 (pyridoxine)—angular cheilitis
   iii. Vitamin B_{12}—pernicious anemia, tongue with lobulations and possible shiny, smooth, and red appearance
   iv. Vitamin C—scurvy, gingivitis, and bleeding gums
   v. Iron deficiency—oral mucosa is gray and tongue is smooth and devoid of papillae
   vi. Nicotinic acid—angular cheilitis

M. Pemphigus
    i. Types
        a. Vulgaris—rapid acute form
        b. Vegetans—indolent chronic form
    ii. Affects the oral cavity in approximately two-thirds of cases
    iii. In those with oral cavity involvement, about half subsequently develop skin lesions
        a. Suprabasal *intraepidermal* bullae
    iv. Autoantibodies are present in the epithelial intercellular substance
    v. Biopsy: acantholysis, and there is a positive *Nikolsky sign*
    vi. All areas of the gastrointestinal tract can become involved
    vii. Treatment: steroids

N. Pemphigoid
    i. Types
        a. Bullous—oral lesions are seen in one-third of patients
        b. Benign mucous membrane—usually limited to the oral cavity and conjunctiva
    ii. *Subepidermal* bullae are present and tend to be smaller than pemphigus and more tense
    iii. No acantholysis is present and Nikolsky sign is negative
    iv. Autoantibodies are present to the basement membrane
    v. Treatment: steroids, penicillamine may allow healing in resistant cases

O. Premalignant lesions
    i. Leukoplakia
        a. Hyperkeratotic lesion
        b. Five percent to 10% will progress to SCC
    ii. Erythroplakia
        a. Granular, erythematous region
        b. Often seen in association with leukoplakia
        c. Fifty percent will show dysplasia or carcinoma in situ (CIS) on biopsy

P. Eagle syndrome
    i. Dysphagia associated with a calcified stylohyoid ligament or an elongated styloid process
    ii. Calcified stylohyoid ligament is an incidental finding in about 4% of the normal population
    iii. Treatment: surgery through transoral or transcervical approach

Salivary Gland

A. Salivary duct—acinus (surrounded by myoepithelial cells) → intercalated duct → striated duct → excretory duct

B. Saliva
    i. Made in the acinus and modified in the duct
    ii. High in potassium and low in sodium
    iii. Parotid secretions are watery (due to increased serous cells), low in mucin, and high in enzymes
    iv. Submandibular and sublingual secretions are thicker due to increased levels of mucin
    v. Important in dental hygiene and antibacterial activity (IgA)

- C. Nonneoplastic disease
  - i. Infectious
    - a. Mumps (viral parotitis)
    - b. Paramyxovirus
      1. Affects children 4 to 6 years of age
      2. Bilateral parotid swelling
      3. Other symptoms: encephalitis, meningitis, nephritis, pancreatitis, orchitis
      4. Self-limited disease
    - c. HIV
  - ii. Sialadenitis
    - a. Acute
      1. Seen in debilitated and dehydrated patients
      2. *Staphylococcus aureus* (50-90%), *S. pyogenes/pneumoniae, H. influenzae*
      3. Treatment:
         - Anti-*Staphylococcus* antibiotics
         - Warm compresses
         - Massage
         - Hydration
         - Sialagogues
    - b. Chronic
      1. Recurrent, painful enlargement of gland
      2. Caused by decreased salivary flow (sialolith, stasis)
      3. Recurrent inflammatory reactions → progressive acinar destruction with fibrous replacement and sialectasis
      4. Treatment
         - Hydration, sialagogues, massage
         - Salivary duct dilation
         - Salivary endoscopy, occasional sialoadenectomy
    - c. Granulomatous
      1. Chronic unilateral or bilateral swelling with minimal pain
      2. Actinomycosis
         - Acute illness inflammation and trismus
         - Chronic illness—firm, progressively enlarging, painless facial mass with increasing trismus, often confused with a parotid tumor
         - Draining sinus tracts are common
         - *Actinomyces israelii*
           - (a) Culture: branching, anaerobic, or microaerophilic gram-positive rods (must be grown on blood agar in anaerobic conditions), sulfur granules
         - Associations: Mucous membrane trauma, poor oral hygiene, dental abscess, diabetes, immunosuppression
         - Treatment
           - (a) Penicillin (4-6 weeks)
           - (b) Incision and drainage required in some cases
      3. Cat scratch disease
      4. Sarcoid—uveoparotid (*Heerfordt disease*) consists of uveitis, mild fever, nonsuppurative parotitis, and CN paralysis
      5. Tuberculosis
      6. GPA (*Wegener granulomatosis*)

iii. Noninfectious
  a. Sialolithiasis
    1. Most commonly affects the submandibular glands (80%)
    2. Sixty-five percent of parotid sialoliths are radiolucent and 65% of submandibular sialoliths are radiopaque
    3. Pain and swelling of affected gland
    4. Treatment
      - Sialolithotripsy (ultrasonic, pulsed dye laser)
      - Endoscopic removal
      - Sialodochoplasty (open removal)
  b. Sjögren disease
  c. Xerostomia
    1. Commonly seen with aging, radiation therapy, Sjögren disease, dehydration, diabetes, and medications
    2. Medications
      - Chemoprotectants such as amifostine can help prevent radiation-induced xerostomia
      - Pilocarpine—cholinergic agonist
      - Cevimeline—cholinergic agonist, approved for Sjögren disease but sometimes used as second-line therapy for postradiation xerostomia
  d. Necrotizing sialometaplasia
    1. Benign, self-healing, inflammatory process of salivary gland tissue
    2. Most seen in nasal cavity, parotid gland, sublingual gland, palate, retromolar trigone, lip, and tongue
    3. Histology shows lobular necrosis and pseudoepitheliomatous hyperplasia
    4. *Treatment*: observation with expectant recovery in 6 to 12 weeks

D. Neoplastic disease
  i. One percent of all head and neck tumors
  ii. Eighty percent of tumors occur in parotid and 75% to 80% of these are benign
  iii. Fifteen percent of tumors occur in submandibular gland and 50% to 60% of these are malignant
  iv. Five percent of tumors in minor salivary gland and 80% of these are malignant
  v. Benign tumors
    a. Pleomorphic adenoma (benign mixed tumor)
      1. Most common salivary gland neoplasm
      2. Most common location is the parotid; 90% occur in the tail of the superficial lobe
      3. Slow-growing, painless, and firm mass
      4. Histology shows epithelial, myoepithelial, and stromal elements
      5. Treatment: excision with a cuff of normal tissue
      6. Risk of conversion to carcinoma ex-pleomorphic adenoma
        - Risk is 1.5% within first 5 years, increases to 10% if observed for more than 15 years
    b. Warthin tumor (papillary cystadenoma lymphomatosum)
      1. Second most common benign parotid neoplasm
      2. Rarely seen outside of parotid gland
      3. Seen in older white males
      4. Associated with smoking
      5. Slow-growing, painless, and firm mass

6. Histology—papillary projections, cystic spaces, lymphoid stroma
7. Treatment: excision

c. Oncocytoma
1. Less than 1% of all salivary gland tumors
2. Seen in older individuals
3. Slow-growing, painless, and firm mass
4. Histology shows sheets, nests, or cords of oncocytes (granular-appearing cells)
5. Treatment: excision with a cuff of normal tissue

d. Malignant tumors
1. Most seen in fifth to sixth decade
2. Asymptomatic mass 60% to 85%
3. CN VII paralysis ~10%
4. Mucoepidermoid carcinoma
   - Most common salivary gland malignancy (parotid 45%-70%)
   - Derived from excretory duct cells
   - Histology: mixed cystic and solid components, hallmark is presence of three cell types—mucous, squamous, intermediate
   - Low grade
     (a) Slow growing, painless mass
     (b) Prominent cystic component, higher ratio of mucous to epidermoid cells
     (c) Smaller, partially encapsulated, with a long history
     (d) Treatment: surgery without adjuvant treatment
   - High grade
     (a) Rapidly enlarging, +/− pain
     (b) More solid component, higher ratio of epidermoid to mucous cells
     (c) At times mistaken for SCC on pathology
     (d) Fifty percent metastasis rate
     (e) Twenty-five percent present with facial paralysis
     (f) Treatment: surgery with postop radiation
5. Adenoid cystic
   - Second most common parotid malignancy
   - Most common submandibular and minor salivary gland malignancy
   - Notorious for infiltrative growth with recurrences and spread
     (a) Tendency for *perineural invasion* and skip lesions
     (b) Lung is most common site of metastasis
   - Three histologic subtypes: cribriform, tubular, and solid
   - Prognosis depends on cell type: tubular (best) > cribriform > solid (worst)
   - Treatment: surgery with postoperative radiation
   - Lung is most common site of metastasis (often late, fatal)
6. Polymorphous low-grade adenocarcinoma
   - Almost exclusively of minor salivary glands
   - Most common site is palate (junction or hard and soft palate)
   - Treatment: complete excision
7. Malignant mixed tumor
   - *Carcinosarcoma* (true malignant mixed tumor)
     (a) Rare, two-third parotid, 15% submandibular gland, 15% palate
     (b) Contains sarcomatous and carcinomatous histologic components
     (c) Average survival less than 2.5 years

- *Carcinoma ex-pleomorphic adenoma*
  - (a) Malignant transformation within pre-existing pleomorphic adenoma
  - (b) Slow-growing mass which suddenly increases in size
  - (c) Only contains epithelial cells

8. Acinic cell carcinoma
   - Greater than 90% occur in parotid
   - Derived from acinar and intercalated duct cells
   - Low to intermediate-grade malignancy
   - Histology: serous acinar cells and cells with clear cytoplasm
   - Calcification may be prominent
   - Treatment: wide surgical excision
   - Radiation is ineffective
   - Metastases are rare, but tend to be hematogenous to bone and lungs
9. Squamous cell carcinoma
   - Rare
   - Derived from excretory duct cells
   - Must exclude
     - (a) Metastatic SCCA
     - (b) Invasive SCCA
     - (c) High-grade mucoepidermoid carcinoma
   - Treatment: wide excision and postop radiation

E. Frey syndrome
   i. Preauricular gustatory sweating
   ii. Parasympathetic salivary nerves from the auriculotemporal nerve innervate the sweat glands of the skin flap
   iii. Diagnosed by Minor's starch-iodine test
   iv. Treatment: topical antiperspirant, topical glycopyrrolate, or topical atropine
   v. Prevention: make thick skin flap during exposure for parotidectomy

Endocrine

A. Thyroid
   i. Follicle
      a. Spheroidal, cyst-like compartment with follicular epithelium, colloid center, parafollicular cells, capillaries, connective tissue, and lymphatics
      b. Principal component of colloid is large, iodinated glycoprotein called thyroglobulin
   ii. Hormones
      a. Thyroid hormone
         1. Thyroid peroxidase is responsible for iodination of thyroglobulin molecules
         2. Iodinated thyroglobulin molecules are coupled to form T3 and T4
         3. T3 and T4 are mostly bound to carrier proteins (> 99%)
         4. T3 is most biologically active
         5. T4 (90%) > T3 (10%) eventually released into bloodstream
      b. Thyroid-stimulating hormone (TSH)
         1. Elevated reflects hypothyroidism
         2. Decreased levels should be studied in conjunction with T4 levels
         3. Low TSH and high T4—*hyperthyroidism*

4. Low TSH and low T4—*secondary hypothyroidism* (possible nonthyroidal illness)
5. Low TSH and normal T4—*early or mild hypothyroidism*
6. Normal T3—*subclinical hyperthyroidism*
7. High T3—*T3 toxicosis*

c. Calcitonin
1. Produced in thyroid C cells
2. Reduces blood calcium levels
3. Used as a marker in medullary thyroid cancer

d. Thyroglobulin
1. Useful marker in thyroid cancer: values above 10 mg/dL indicate persistent disease

e. Antithyroid peroxidase antibodies—elevated in Hashimoto thyroiditis
f. Thyroid-stimulating antibody—elevated in Graves' disease

iii. Thyroid nodules
a. Clinically apparent in 4% to 7% of the population (W > M 5:1)
b. Most are benign with carcinoma being detected in 5% of all lesions
c. Findings of concern
1. Age less than 20, men greater than 40, women greater than 50
2. Male
3. Size greater than 4 cm
4. History of radiation exposure
5. Family history
6. Rapid growth

d. Fine-needle aspiration (FNA)
1. Nodules greater than or equal to 1 cm
2. Most accurate tool for selecting patients requiring surgery, has increased the percentage of malignant nodules excised by 60% to 100% and reduced percentage of benign nodules excised by 34% to 70%
3. Overall accuracy exceeds 95%
4. Bethesda criteria (and predicted risk of malignancy):
   - Nondiagnostic (1-4%)
   - Benign (0-3%)
   - Atypia of undetermined significance (AUS) or follicular lesion of underdetermined significant (FLUS) (5-15%)
   - Follicular neoplasm or suspicious for follicular neoplasm (15-30%)
   - Suspicious for malignancy (60-75%)
   - Malignant (97-99%)

e. Thyroid scintigraphy—utilizes radioisotopes of iodine or Technetium^{99}
1. Less cost-effective and more controversial than FNA
2. Considered primary test in two scenarios
3. Low TSH (autonomous nodule)
4. Suspicion for Hashimoto thyroiditis
5. Sometimes used after FNA reveals microfollicular pattern to further distinguish between autonomous adenomas and cold lesions, which may represent follicular carcinoma

f. Ultrasound
1. More detail than scintigraphy
2. Most cost-effective way of screening for thyroid adenoma
3. Reveals additional nodules in 20% to 48% of patients referred for solitary nodule

g. Adenomas
   1. Monoclonal neoplasms arising from follicular epithelium or Hürthle cells
   2. May be autonomous
   3. May be macrofollicular or microfollicular on FNA
      - Macrofollicular adenomas are benign.
      - Microfollicular adenomas that do not exhibit vascular or capsular invasion are considered benign.
   4. Treatment
      - Nontoxic
        (a) Macrofollicular: may be watched; less than or equal to 20% will decrease in nodule size with T4 therapy
        (b) Microfollicular: surgical excision to evaluate for capsular or vascular invasion
   5. Toxic adenomas
      - Beta blockers
      - Thionamide therapy (methimazole and propylthiouracil)
        (a) Inhibits thyroperoxidase, blocks T3 and T4 synthesis
        (b) Propylthiouracil blocks the peripheral conversion of T4 to T3
            i. Black box warning: liver failure
      - I^{131} ameliorates hyperthyroidism and reduces total thyroid volume by 45% in 2 years
      - Surgery

h. Colloid nodules
   1. Develop within multinodular goiters
   2. Focus of hyperplasia within the thyroid architecture
   3. Macrofollicular on FNA and benign
   4. Treatment
      - I^{131} (hyperthyroidism)
      - Surgery (hyperthyroidism or aerodigestive compromise)
      - T4 has been shown to interfere with goitrogenesis and prevent new nodule formation but does not reduce the size of solitary thyroid nodules

i. Cysts
   1. Primarily develop from degenerating adenomas
   2. Suddenly appearing or painful neck mass may represent a hemorrhagic cyst
   3. 0% to 3% contain malignant cells (often papillary)
   4. Treatment
      - FNA for benign cysts—25% to 50% disappear after aspiration
      - Surgery

iv. Thyroiditis
   a. Hashimoto thyroiditis
      1. Lymphocytic infiltration, germinal center formation, Hürthle cells, and follicular atrophy
      2. Elevated antithyroid peroxidase antibodies
      3. Thyroid lymphoma usually arises from Hashimoto thyroiditis
      4. Treat resultant hypothyroidism with T4
   b. Lymphocytic thyroiditis
      1. Painless, postpartum thyroiditis
      2. Hyperthyroidism followed by hypothyroidism
      3. Self-limited

- c. Riedel's struma
  1. Inflammatory process of unknown etiology
  2. Woody goiter fixed to surrounding structures and progressive aerodigestive symptoms
- d. Subacute granulomatous thyroiditis (SGT)
  1. Most common cause of *painful* thyroid
  2. Viral etiology
  3. Hyperthyroidism followed by hypothyroidism
  4. Self-limited
- e. Top causes of hyperthyroidism
  1. Graves' disease
     - Females 20 to 40
     - Immunoglobulins that bind with the TSH receptor
     - Accumulation of glycosaminoglycans in tissues leading to
       - (a) Exophthalmos
       - (b) Dermopathy (pretibial myxedema)
       - (c) Osteopathy
     - Treatment
       - (a) Beta blockers
       - (b) Thionamides
       - (c) Radioactive iodine
       - (d) Subtotal thyroidectomy
  1. Toxic multinodular goiter
  2. Autogenous adenoma
  3. SGT
  4. Hashimoto thyroiditis
  5. Iatrogenic
  6. Excessive iodine intake

v. Well-differentiated thyroid carcinoma
- a. AMES staging better than Hay's AGES
  1. *A*ge, *M*etastases, *E*xtent of primary tumor, *S*ize
  2. Low risk:
     - Men < 40 and women < 50 without distant metastases
     - Men > 41 and women greater than 51, with no metastases, tumor confined to the thyroid gland and less than 5 cm in diameter
  3. High risk:
     - Patients with distant metastases
     - Men greater than 41 and women greater than 51 with extrathyroidal tumor (or major capsular involvement for follicular) and greater than or equal to 5 cm in diameter
- b. Papillary thyroid carcinoma (PTC)
  1. 60% to 70% of thyroid malignancies
  2. Spontaneous
  3. Cystic
  4. Associated with familial colonic polyposis (*Gardner syndrome*) and familial goiter and skin hamartomata (*Cowden disease*)
  5. Hashimoto's increases risk for lymphoma but protective against PTC
  6. Lymphotropic with high rate of nodal metastasis
  7. Histology: papillae, lack of follicles, *psammoma bodies*, large nuclei, and prominent nucleoli (*Orphan Annie eye*)

c. Follicular thyroid carcinoma
   1. Ten percent of thyroid malignancies
   2. Unifocal
   3. Occur more frequently in iodine-deficient areas
   4. Hematogenous spread with higher rate of distant metastasis
   5. Hürthle cell carcinoma is a more aggressive subtype of follicular carcinoma
   6. Differentiated from follicular adenoma by pericapsular vascular invasion

d. Treatment
   1. Surgery is primary therapy
   2. Ten-year survivals of 98% (papillary) and 92% (follicular)
   3. I^{131} imaging (and ablation with 30 to 50 mCi for subtotal thyroidectomy patients) should be performed 4 to 6 weeks after surgery. Postoperative I^{131} ablation reduces local and regional recurrence and disease-specific mortality in high-risk patients
   4. Indications for postoperative I^{131}
      - Primary tumor greater than 4 cm
      - Gross extrathyroidal extension
      - Known or suspected distant metastasis
      - Extensive vascular invasion
      - Greater than 5+ lymph nodes
      - Presence of postoperative thyroglobulin greater than 5 to 10 ng/mL
   5. Following treatment, patients should receive T4 to minimize potential TSH stimulation of tumor growth
   6. Repeat thyroid scintigraphy when thyroglobulin is greater than 5 mg/mL

e. Medullary thyroid carcinoma
   1. Five percent of thyroid malignancies
   2. Seventy percent sporadic, 30% familial
   3. Multiple endocrine neoplasia (MEN) 2a—medullary thyroid carcinoma, pheochromocytoma, hyperparathyroidism
   4. MEN 2b—medullary thyroid carcinoma, pheochromocytoma, mucosal neuromas
   5. Familial non-MEN medullary thyroid carcinoma (FMTC)
   6. *RET* proto-oncogene is associated with MEN 2a and 2b
      - *RE*arranged during *T*ransfection
      - *RET* is a tyrosine kinase
      - Arises from parafollicular C cells and secretes calcitonin
      - Tendency for paratracheal and lateral node involvement
      - Histology shows sheets of amyloid-rich cells
   7. Treatment:
      - Total thyroidectomy with neck dissection for cervical disease
        (a) Recommend thyroidectomy at age 6 years in MEN 2a and at 2 years in MEN 2b
      - Follow with serum calcitonin

f. Anaplastic thyroid carcinoma
   1. Less than 5% of thyroid malignancies
   2. Extremely aggressive and uniformly fatal
   3. Twenty percent history of DTC
   4. Ninety percent have regional or distant spread at presentation
   5. Treatment: palliative with chemoradiation

g. Lymphoma
    1. Primary thyroid lymphoma is rare
    2. Non-Hodgkin lymphoma most common
    3. Association with Hashimoto thyroiditis

B. Parathyroid disease
  i. Differential for hypercalcemia: CHIMPANZEES
    a. Calcium supplements
    b. Hyperparathyroidism
    c. Iatrogenic
    d. Multiple myeloma, milk-alkali, meds (lithium)
    e. Parathyroid hyperplasia, adenoma
    f. Alcohol
    g. Neoplasm
    h. Zollinger-Ellison Syndrome
    i. Excessive Vit D
    j. Excessive Vit A
    k. Sarcoid
  ii. Hyperparathyroidism
    a. Primary
      1. Frequently seen in 30- to 50-year-old postmenopausal women
      2. Usually caused by isolated parathyroid adenoma (85%)
      3. Associated with MEN 1 (Werner) and MEN 2a
      4. Symptoms: painful bones (arthralgia), kidney stones (nephrolithiasis), abdominal groans (constipation, nausea/vomiting, pancreatitis), psychic moans (depression), and fatigue overtones. Cardiovascular: HTN and arrhythmias
      5. Localization
        - Ultrasound—60% to 90% sensitivity for localizing a single adenoma
        - Sestamibi scan—uses Technetium^{99}, initially taken up in thyroid and parathyroids. Over time, Sestamibi washes out of thyroid and remains in parathyroids
          (a) Scan has 70% to 100% sensitivity.
          (b) Limited in adenomas less than 5 mm, multigland disease (ie, four-gland hyperplasia), coexisting thyroid pathology, and previous surgery
        - 4D CT: time-lapsed imaging of the neck
      6. Treatment:
        - Parathyroidectomy
          (a) Intraoperative parathyroid hormone (PTH) monitoring may be helpful. Half-life of PTH is 3 to 5 minutes. Decrease in PTH of 50% at 10 minutes indicates likely success
    b. Secondary: results from hypocalcemia secondary to renal disease
    c. Tertiary: autonomous secretion of PTH following prolonged period of secondary hyperparathyroidism
    d. Reimplantation may be used in setting of four-gland hyperplasia
    e. Hypocalcemia after uneventful removal of solitary parathyroid adenoma may indicate "hungry bone syndrome," caused by adenoma's prior suppression of other parathyroids

iii. Parathyroid carcinoma
   a. Rare
   b. From the parenchymal cells of parathyroid glands
   c. Slow growth, tends to be indolent tumor
   d. ~80% are symptomatic or have metabolic abnormality
      1. ~40% have palpable neck mass
   e. Associated with local infiltration and invasion into surrounding structures
   f. Pulmonary metastasis most common distant metastasis
   g. Treatment: surgical excision

Head and Neck Oncology Considerations

A. Cutaneous malignancy
   i. Basal cell carcinoma
      a. Most common cutaneous malignancy in adults
      b. Risk factors
         1. High association with ultraviolet (UV) exposure
         2. Ionizing radiation
         3. Immunosuppression
         4. Nevoid basal-cell carcinoma syndrome (*Gorlin syndrome*)
         5. Xeroderma pigmentosum
      c. Low risk for metastases but may become locally aggressive
      d. Subtypes
         1. Superficial
            - Slow-growing, nonaggressive, scaly, erythematous plaques
            - Treatment: 5-FU, cryotherapy, photodynamic therapy, curettage, or Mohs
         2. Nodular
            - Histology with cells of decreased cytoplasm and "palisading" nuclei
            - Pearly papules with telangiectatic borders
            - Local excision (5 mm margins) or Mohs excision
         3. Sclerosing/morpheaform
            - Small stands of tumor extend out from central lesion (skip lesions) resulting in high recurrence rates and large surgical defects
         4. Basosquamous
            - Characterized by squamous differentiation and keratinization
            - Can be mistaken for SCC
            - Mohs or wide local excision
   ii. SCC
      a. Second most common cutaneous malignancy in adults
      b. Risk factors
         1. Precursor lesions: actinic keratosis (1-2/5% transformation to SCC)
         2. Cumulative UV exposure
         3. Fair skin
         4. Age greater than 50
         5. Smoking
         6. Scarring skin lesions
            - *Marjolin ulcer*: aggressive, ulcerating SCC in area of previous trauma, inflammation, or scar

c. May result in nodal disease and distant metastases
d. *Bowen disease*: SCC in situ (5% progress to invasive SCC). Cryotherapy and photodynamic therapy
e. Well differentiated
    1. Squamous cells in cords with "intercellular bridges" and "keratin pearls"
    2. Stain for cytokeratins
    3. Mohs or wide local excision
f. Poorly differentiated
    1. Few intercellular bridges and keratin pearls
    2. Mohs or wide local excision with 1 cm margins

iii. Melanoma
a. Third most common cutaneous malignancy in adults
b. Twenty-five percent of cutaneous melanomas are in head and neck sites
c. Risk factors
    1. Frequent, intermittent exposure to intense sunlight
    2. Tanning beds
    3. Fair skin
    4. Family history
    5. Congenital nevi
d. *Histological markers*: S-100 (highly sensitive), Melan A, HMB-45 ("*H*uman *M*elanoma *B*lack"—antibody against melanoma antigen) (highly specific)
e. Premalignant lesions
    1. Congenital nevi: characteristics of benign nevus but present at birth
    2. Dysplastic nevus: irregular/indistinct borders
    3. Lentigo maligna: melanoma in situ
    4. Atypical junctional melanocytic hyperplasia: lesion between nevus and lentigo maligna
f. Melanoma subtypes
    1. Superficial spreading: most common (70%)
        - Usually develop from preexisting nevi
        - Radial growth
    2. Nodular (15-30%)
        - Early invasion and vertical growth
    3. Lentigo maligna melanoma: when lentigo maligna violates the papillary dermis
    4. Desmoplastic (2%)
        - Neurotropic
g. *ABCDEs*: *A*symmetry, irregular *B*orders, *C*olor variation, *D*iameter (> 6 mm), *E*volving lesion
h. *Prognostic factors*: thickness, ulceration, satellite lesions, and lymph node involvement
i. *Subsite prognosis* (worst to best): scalp > ear > cheek > neck
j. Biopsy: Do not do shave biopsy. Need to assess depth, so perform excisional biopsy with 1- to 2-mm margins
k. Treatment
    1. *Lentigo maligna*: square technique, Mohs, Woods light with 5 mm margins
    2. Wide surgical excision with sentinel lymph node biopsy if lesion is greater than 1.0 mm Breslow depth

3. Sentinel node dissection: offered to all patients with a clinically negative nodal basin and a primary melanoma greater than 1 mm in depth. It may be considered in melanoma 0.76 to 1 mm in thickness with adverse features including lymphovascular invasion, age less than 40, significant vertical growth phase, increased mitotic rate.
4. *Lesions under 2 mm Breslow depth*: 1-cm margins
5. *Lesions over 2 mm Breslow depth*: 2-cm margins
6. Radiation
7. Interferon

B. Genetics:
   i. C-myc: most commonly mutated proto-oncogene in head and neck cancer
   ii. p53: most commonly mutated tumor suppressor gene in head and neck cancer
   iii. HPVs 16 and 18
      a. Implicated in oropharyngeal SCC
      b. E6 gene inhibits p53 (p53 is a tumor suppressor)
      c. E7 gene inhibits Rb (Rb is a tumor suppressor)

C. Cervical metastases from occult primary tumors (unknown primary)
   i. Five percent present with adenopathy
   ii. Squamous is predominant histologic type
   iii. Ninety percent of primaries eventually found with repeated examination, biopsies, and scanning
   iv. Most commonly from Waldeyer's ring, pyriform sinus
   v. Perform HPV testing on FNA if SCC
   vi. Workup:
      a. Exam and laryngoscopy
      b. FNA any suspicious node—test for HPV (EBV if HPV negative)
      c. Panendoscopy—biopsy suspicious lesions
      d. If direct laryngoscopy is not fruitful, consider ipsilateral palatine and lingual tonsillectomy
      e. Trans-Oral Robotic Surgery lingual tonsillectomy

D. Chyle fistula
   i. Can result from dissection in the supraclavicular fossa
   ii. Low output: less than 500 to 700 mL/24 h:
      a. Pressure and a low-fat diet
      b. If using hyperalimentation, medium-chain triglycerides can be used as a caloric source
      c. Octreotide has been shown to help resolve chyle fistulas
   iii. High output: greater than 500 to 700 mL/24 h
      a. Exploration and ligation

E. Flaps
   i. Regional skin and fascial
      a. Deltopectoral—first to fourth perforators from internal mammary artery
      b. Paramedian forehead—supratrochlear artery
      c. Pericranial—supraorbital and supratrochlear
      d. Temporoparietal—superficial temporal
   ii. Myocutaneous
      a. Latissimus dorsi—thoracodorsal artery
      b. Pectoralis major—thoracoacromial artery and internal mammary artery perforators
      c. Platysma—occipital, postauricular, facial, superior thyroid, and transverse cervical

- d. Sternocleidomastoid—occipital artery (loops around 12th CN) superior thyroid artery, transverse cervical artery
- e. Trapezius—occipital, dorsal scapular, and transverse cervical arteries

iii. Osteomyocutaneous
- a. Pectoralis major with rib (see above)
- b. Sternocleidomastoid with clavicle (see above)
- c. Trapezius with scapular spine (see above)

iv. Free flaps
- a. Fibula—peroneal artery
  1. Evaluate preop blood supply with imaging
- b. Iliac crest—deep circumflex iliac artery
- c. Jejunum—superior mesenteric arterial arcade
- d. Lateral arm—posterior radial collateral artery
- e. Lateral thigh—profunda femoris artery
- f. Latissimus dorsi—thoracodorsal artery
- g. Radial forearm—radial artery
- h. Rectus—deep inferior epigastric artery
- i. Scapula—body from circumflex scapular artery, tip—angular artery

F. Indications for postoperative radiation therapy
- i. Advanced stage
- ii. Close or positive margins
- iii. Lymph node involvement
- iv. Extracapsular spread
- v. Perineural invasion
- vi. PORT should be started ideally by 6 weeks after resection

Facial Plastics and Reconstruction

A. Fitzpatrick scale
- i. Type I: very white—always burns, never tans
- ii. Type II: white—burns easily, tans minimally
- iii. Type III: white to olive—sometimes burns, slowly tans to light brown
- iv. Type IV: brown—burns minimally, always tans to dark brown
- v. Type V: dark brown—rarely burns, tans well
- vi. Type VI: black—never burns, deeply pigmented

B. Aging
- i. Decrease in overall collagen and decrease in the ratio of Type I to Type III
- ii. Analysis: examine upper, mid, and lower face, neck for
  - a. Ptosis
  - b. Loss of Volume
  - c. Environmental/Sun Damage
    1. Sun exposure is the most significant factor in premature aging

C. Injectables
- i. Botulinum toxin
  - a. Binds to cholinergic nerve terminals—irreversibly binds and cleaves SNARE proteins at *presynaptic* junction
    1. Prevents acetylcholine vesicle docking/ultimate release

b. New neuromuscular junctions develop in 3 to 4 months
c. Complications: ptosis, "frozen" appearance
1. Treat ptosis with iopidine drops PRN, ~1 to 2 weeks

ii. Hyaluronic acids
a. Highly hydrophilic—attracts water
b. Dissolved by hyaluronidase—natural as well as injectable forms
c. Complications: vascular compromise, embolism, blindness

iii. Collagen
a. Animal derivatives
b. Early complication: allergy, requires skin testing prior
c. Late complication: granulomatous/precipitation reactions

D. Skin resurfacing

i. General
a. Endpoint is determined by punctate bleeding and shammy cloth appearance of the papillary dermis.
b. Accutane causes sebaceous gland atrophy and must be discontinued 6 months prior to dermabrasion or laser resurfacing.
c. Treat resurfacing patients with antiviral prophylaxis.

ii. Chemical peels
a. Indications: fine rhytids and solar damage
b. Agents
1. Glycolic acid
  - Penetration is time dependent
  - Mildest results, but least complications
2. Trichloroacetic acid
  - Intermediate-to-deep peel
  - 10-25%—intraepidermal
  - 30-40%—papillary dermis
  - 45-50%—reticular dermis
3. Phenol (with croton oil)—keratolysis and keratocoagulation

c. Complications
1. Hypopigmentation
  - Pigmented areas may lose pigmentation temporarily or permanently
  - Peels for pigmentation must be superficial
2. Irregular hyperpigmentation
3. Perioral scarring
4. Prominent skin pores
5. Phenol toxicity—headache, nausea, hypertension, hyperreflexia, central nervous system depression, and cardiotoxicity (arrhythmias); treated with aggressive hydration

iii. Dermabrasion
1. Surgical procedure requires dermabrader and carries infectious transmission risk
2. Complications
  - Transient post inflammatory hyperpigmentation
  - Hypopigmentation
  - Milia

- iv. Laser
    - a. Types
        1. CO_2 (10,600 nm)
        2. Erbium:YAG (2940 nm)
    - b. Following laser resurfacing, bio-occlusive dressings provide a pathway of proper moisture and humidity, decreasing epithelial closure time by up to 50%
    - c. Complications
        1. Transient post inflammatory hyperpigmentation
        2. Long term hypopigmentation
        3. Infection (bacterial, viral, fungal)
    - d. Healing timetable
        1. 5 days—epidermis regenerates
        2. 7 days—epidermis loosely attached to dermis
        3. 2 weeks—new collagen deposited, fills out dermis, giving youthful appearance
        4. 1 month—pigmentation returns, milia possible, and requires opening
        5. 6 months—epidermis normal thickness
        6. 10 months—dermis normalizes

E. Rhytidectomy
- i. Goals: reduce jowling, decrease laxity of skin and platysma, submental lipectomy
- ii. Ideal candidate
    - a. Nonsmoker
    - b. Normotensive
    - c. Good skin tone
    - d. Strong facial bones and chin
    - e. Sharp cervicomental angle (high and posterior hyoid bone)
- iii. Anatomy
    - a. Superficial musculoaponeurotic system (SMAS)
        1. Continuous with temporoparietal fascia, lower orbicularis oculi, zygomaticus muscle, dermis of upper lip, and platysma
        2. Overlies parotid fascia posteriorly and masseteric fascia anteriorly
    - b. Facial nerve
        1. Temporal branch
            - Within temporoparietal fascia
            - Can be found between 0.8 and 3.5 cm anterior to the EAC (*Pitanguy's line*)
        2. Zygomatic and buccal
            - Lay deep to the SMAS
            - Buccal branch may be injured during rhytidectomy but often not appreciated on examination
        3. Greater auricular nerve: most injured nerve during rhytidectomy
- iv. Types
    - a. Subcutaneous
    - b. Composite
    - c. SMAS imbrication versus plication
    - d. Sub-SMAS
    - e. Deep plane
        1. More invasive technique, bigger lift, longer lasting, higher risk to FN

v. Complications
  a. Most common area for skin loss is in postauricular region
  b. Most common complication is hematoma (1-8%)
    1. Major risk factor: systolic blood pressure greater than140
  c. Facial nerve injury 1%, 90% recover

F. Brow lift
  i. Anatomical relationships
    a. Consider brow position *before* performing blepharoplasty.
    b. Ideal brow position
      1. Woman—arc above the orbital rim with its apex above the lateral limbus
      2. Male—rest on superior orbital rim
    c. Temporal branch of FN is lateral to plane of dissection. The sentinel vein indicates its location.
    d. Corrugator and procerus muscles are often partially resected at the time of surgery.
      1. Procerus muscle: horizontal glabellar wrinkles
      2. Corrugator supercilia: vertical glabellar wrinkles
  ii. Approaches
    a. Coronal
      1. For total forehead and brow elevation, excellent longevity
      2. Disadvantages: elevates hairline, less fine-tuning of brow
    b. Pretrichial
      1. For high hairline and elongated forehead
      2. Disadvantages: exposed scar, scalp hyposthesia
    c. Midforehead
      1. For those with prominent forehead wrinkles, receding hairline, very thin hair
      2. Disadvantages: exposed scar, not good for lateral elevation
    d. Direct
      1. For accurate brow elevation, preserves forehead sensation, corrects brow asymmetry
      2. Disadvantages: treats brow only, does not address lateral rhytids
    e. Browpexy
      1. For mild brow ptosis
      2. Disadvantages: prolonged eyelid edema, possible brow asymmetry
    f. Endoscopic
      1. For high hairline (preserves hairline), least invasive, no vertical forehead lengthening
      2. Disadvantages: less fine-tuning of brow position

G. Blepharoplasty
  i. Definitions
    a. Dermatochalasis: excess eyelid skin laxity
    b. Blepharoptosis: abnormal low-lying upper lid margin
    c. Blepharochalasis: uncommon condition involving recurrent episodes of marked eyelid edema
    d. Hering's law of equal innervation
      1. Can lead to overactivity of normal side as it is trying to compensate for weak ptosis side
      2. Cover ptotic eye for 30 minutes and retracted eye will settle into normal position
    e. Festoons: prolapsed orbicularis oculi

- ii. Anatomy
  - a. The thickness of the eyelid skin is on average 1/100 in.
  - b. Levator aponeurosis inserts into the orbicularis and dermis to form the upper eyelid crease
    1. This is usually 10 mm from the lid margin in Caucasians and absent in the Asian eyelid
- iii. Preoperative assessment
  - a. Ophthalmologic history
  - b. Basic eye exam: visual acuity, extraocular movements
  - c. Schirmer test (> 10 mm in 5 minutes is normal)
  - d. Snap test of lower lid. If abnormal (> 1 second), consider lower lid pexy to prevent ectropion
  - e. Evaluate for negative vector. If present, consider fat repositioning of lower lid fat to prevent hollowed-out appearance
- iv. Medical contraindications
  - a. Hypothyroid myxedema
  - b. Allergic dermatitis
  - c. Dry eye syndrome
- v. Complications
  - a. Upper lid
    1. Lagophthalmos (over-resection of soft tissue)
    2. Ptosis (injury to levator muscle)
  - b. Lower lid
    1. Ectropion
    2. Inferior oblique injury
    3. Epiphora (punctal eversion due to wound contraction, edema)
  - c. Pain, proptosis, and ecchymosis suggest hematoma
    1. Orbital decompression with cantholysis/canthopexy

H. Rhinoplasty

- i. Anatomy
  - a. Nasion—nasofrontal suture
  - b. Rhinion—junction of nasal bones and upper lateral cartilage (ULC)
  - c. Supratip break—transition between cartilaginous dorsum and apex of lower lateral cartilage (LLC)—ideal is 6 mm
  - d. Tip—apex of LLC
  - e. Infratip break (double break)—junction between medial lower lateral crura and intermediate lower lateral crura
  - f. Subnasale—nasal base
  - g. Pogonion—most anterior portion of chin
  - h. Menton—most inferior point of chin
  - i. External valve—opening of the nostrils
  - j. Internal valve—nasal septum, caudal margin of ULC, inferior turbinate, and floor of nose
  - k. Frankfort horizontal plane—high point of external auditory canal to orbital rim is parallel to floor
  - l. Major tip support
    1. Shape, size, strength of LLC
    2. Attachment of LLC's to ULC's
    3. Attachment of medial crura of LLC to caudal septum

- ii. Considerations
  - a. Chin position
    1. Perpendicular dropped from Frankfurt horizontal at nasion
       - Male chin—2 mm anterior to line
       - Female chin—2 mm posterior to line
    2. Retrognathic chin may make nose appear overprojected
    3. Dorsal hump may make chin appear underprojected
  - b. Nasal length should be two-thirds of the midfacial height (glabella to subnasale)
  - c. Nasal projection should be 50% to 60% of nasal length (3 cm-4 cm-5 cm right triangle) or the same as the width of the alar base
  - d. 50% to 60% of nasal projection should be anterior to upper lip
  - e. Base of nose should equal intercanthal distance
  - f. Nasofrontal angle—115° to 130°
  - g. Nasolabial angle—90° to 115°
  - h. 2 to 4 mm of columella should be visible on profile
- iii. Systematic nasal analysis
  - a. Skin thickness
  - b. Frontal view
    1. Upper, middle, lower third
    2. Straightness
    3. Width
    4. Brow-tip aesthetic line
    5. Collapse of sidewall
  - c. Profile view
    1. Dorsum
    2. Projection
    3. Rotation
  - d. Base view
    1. Symmetry
    2. Columella-lobule relationship
    3. Caudal septum
    4. External valve collapse
  - e. Internal exam
    1. Septum, turbinates, internal valve collapse
- iv. Approaches
  - a. Endonasal—marginal and intercartilaginous incisions to deliver lateral crura
    1. Technically difficult
    2. Faster healing
    3. Ideal for minimal tip work (ie, cephalic trim)
  - b. Open—marginal and transcolumellar incisions
    1. Ideal approach for tip work, complex deformity
    2. May result in decreased tip projection (requires placement of caudal strut)
    3. Longer healing times
- v. Techniques
  - a. The tip
    1. Increasing tip projection
       - Transdomal suturing, lateral crural steal, cartilage tip grafts, columellar strut grafts

2. Decreasing tip projection
   - Positioning medial crura more posteriorly relative to caudal septum, shortening medial or lateral crura
3. Increasing tip rotation
   - Shortening lateral crura while keeping medial crura length constant
4. Decreasing tip rotation
   - Lengthening lateral crura while keeping medial crura length constant, changing medial crura relative to caudal septum

b. Nasal valves
1. External valve
   - Sutures: lateral crural spanning suture, lateral crural flaring suture
   - Grafts: alar rim graft, batten graft resting on top of lateral crura, lateral crural strut graft, alar spreader graft
2. Internal valve
   - Sutures: flaring suture, suspension suture
   - Grafts: batten graft, spreader graft, butterfly graft,

c. Dorsal hump
1. Address tip-supratip first
2. Resection of cartilaginous and bony dorsum
3. Osteotomies often required to address open-roof deformity (lateral osteotomies last)

d. Complications
1. Alar notching may result from over-resection of LLC's
2. Inverted V: collapse of upper lateral cartilages.
3. Open-roof deformity: inadequate osteotomies (usually lateral osteotomies) following resection of dorsal hump
4. Pollybeak deformity: excessive bony dorsum resection with under resection of cartilaginous septum, loss of tip projection, or scar formation at supratip
5. Saddle nose deformity: over-resection of dorsum
6. Rocker deformity: due to osteotomy placed superior to medial canthus

I. Facial nerve

i. General principles of FN rehabilitation
a. Spontaneous regeneration (observation)
b. Facial nerve neurorrhaphy
   1. Epineural suturing
   2. Perineural suturing
c. Facial nerve cable graft
d. Nerve or muscle transposition
e. Microneurovascular transfer
f. Static procedures

ii. Approach to FN paralysis
a. Flaccid versus spasmodic paralysis
b. New (< 2 years) versus old (> 2 years) injury

iii. General algorithm
a. Injury less than 2 years
   1. Short-segment resection: primary neurorrhaphy
   2. Long-segment resection: cable grafting (sural or great auricular nerve)
   3. Proximal stump sacrifice: crossover grafts (CNXII-VII jump, facial-facial, masseteric-VII jump)

b. Injury more than 2 years
    1. Muscle transposition: temporalis rotation, masseter rotation
    2. Free tissue transfer: gracilis or latissimus dorsi free flap

J. Otoplasty
  i. Auriculomastoid angle—30 degrees
  ii. Distance from helical rim to skull is 1 to 2 cm
  iii. Most common abnormality is conchal protrusion. Treat with conchal setback with sutures (Furnas procedure)
  iv. Lack of antihelical fold. Treat with creation of antihelical fold (Mustardé technique)
  v. Perform around 6 years of age
  vi. Telephone ear can result from over resection of conchal cartilage

K. Skin grafting
  i. Steps of healing
    a. Imbibition: derives nutrients from underlying recipient bed (first 24 hours)
    b. Inosculation: small vessel growth into graft (2-3 days)
    c. Angiogenesis: new and permanent vessels grow into graft (4-7 days)

L. Local flaps
  i. Classification
    a. By blood supply
      1. Random: no named blood supply
      2. Axial: named blood supply
    b. By configuration: rhombic, bilobed, etc.
    c. By method of transferring flap
      1. Advancement
        - Unipedicle
        - Bipedicle
        - V-Y
        - Hinged flaps
      2. Pivotal
        - Rotation
        - Transposition: bilobe, rhombic
        - Interpolated: paramedian forehead, melolabial cheek

M. Lip reconstruction
  i. Wedge excision with primary closure, defects up to 30% of lip length
  ii. Abbe-Estlander
    a. Defects between 30% and 60% of lip length
    b. Flap has a width of 50% of the defect
  iii. Karapandzic
    a. Total lip reconstruction
    b. Preserves neurovascular bundles
    c. Results in microstomia
  iv. Bernard-Burrow
    a. Lower lip reconstruction—brings cheek skin medially

N. Scar management
  i. Appropriate time for revision is 1 year
  ii. Skin elasticity is greatest during infancy (children are more likely to form hypertrophic scars)

- iii. Keloids are more common in patients with Fitzpatrick Type III skin and above
  - a. High recurrence rate (45-100%) following excision
- iv. Scar is Type I collagen
- v. Wound Strength
  - a. Three percent at 1 week
  - b. Thirty percent at 4 weeks
  - c. Eighty percent at final maturation
- vi. Collagen production: peak at 1 week, lasts for 2 to 3 weeks
- vii. Treatments:
  - a. Massage
  - b. Topical silicone (gels, sheets, cream)
  - c. Steroids—can be used at any time, decrease metabolism in scar
  - d. Dermabrasion
  - e. Surgery
    1. Simple excision
       - Used for shorts scars (< 2 cm) and those that fall in Relaxed Skin Tension Lines
       - Maintain 3:1 ratio to avoid standing cutaneous deformity
    2. W-plasty and geometric broken line—helps camouflage long scars opposed to RSTLs
    3. Z-plasty—lengthens and reorients scar
       - 30 degrees → lengthens 25% → rotates 45 degrees
       - 45 degrees → lengthens 50% → rotates 60 degrees
       - 60 degrees →lengthens 75% → rotates 90 degrees

O. Hair restoration
- i. Androgenic Alopecia: male-pattern baldness (men>>women)
  - a. Hair loss is mediated by dihydrotestosterone
  - b. Medications
    1. Minoxidil: vasodilator, increases hair follicle width
    2. Finasteride: inhibits 5α reductase
- ii. Surgery
  - a. Grafts.
    1. Micrografts: one to two hairs
    2. Minigrafts: three to six hairs
    3. Follicular grafts: hair in its natural grouping of one to four hairs surrounded by adventitial sheath
    4. Takes 10 to 16 weeks for hair to start growing
       - Consider pattern of hair loss and expected future loss when implanting
  - b. Flaps:
    1. Juri flap—based on superficial temporal artery
       - Most robust, immediate effect
  - c. Advancement: Hairline advancement—“reverse browlift”

P. Lasers
- i. Work by selective thermolysis
- ii. Hair removal
  - a. Ruby (694 nm)
  - b. Alexandrite (755 nm)
  - c. Diode laser (800 nm)
  - d. Nd:YAG laser (1064 nm)

iii. Tattoo—Ruby (694 nm)
   a. Black easiest to remove, yellow/greens difficult
iv. Skin resurfacing
   a. Erbium:YAG (2940 nm)
   b. CO_2 (10,600 nm)
v. Vascular lesions
   a. Potassium titanyl phosphate (KTP) (532 nm)
   b. Pulsed dye laser (585 nm)
vi. Cutting bone
   a. Ho:YAG (2070 nm)
   b. Erbium:YAG (2940 nm)

Pediatrics

A. Adenotonsillar disease
   i. Tonsillitis
      a. Common pathogens
         1. *Streptococcus pyogenes* (most important treatable pathogen)
         2. *Streptococcus viridans*
         3. *Staphylococcus aureus*
         4. *Haemophilus influenzae*
      b. Adult tonsils show mixed infections, and three-fourths of patients have β-lactamase-producing organisms
      c. Classic finding in *S. pyogenes* infection is a tonsillar exudate
      d. EBV (mononucleosis) causes abundant exudates
      e. Complications
         1. Peritonsillar abscess with potential spread to the deep neck spaces
   ii. Indications for tonsillectomy and/or adenoidectomy (paradise criteria)
      a. Seven episodes of acute tonsillitis in 1 year, 5 episodes per year for 2 years, 3 episodes per year for 3 years (tonsillectomy)
      b. Peritonsillar abscess (tonsillectomy)
      c. Chronic tonsillitis (tonsillectomy)
      d. Obstructive sleep apnea (adenotonsillectomy)
      e. Adenotonsillar hypertrophy with dysphagia, speech abnormalities, and occlusive abnormalities (adenotonsillectomy)
      f. Studies suggest that adenoidectomy, regardless of adenoidal size, is helpful in children with chronic OM with effusion requiring multiple sets of tubes
B. Ciliary dysmotility
   i. Numerous forms
   ii. Clinical tests of ciliary function using methylene blue and saccharin
   iii. Electron microscope study of cilia biopsy in glutaraldehyde
   iv. Kartagener syndrome
         1. Lacks dynein side arms on A-tubules
         2. Triad of recurrent sinusitis, bronchiectasis, and situs inversus
C. Cleft lip (CL) and cleft palate (CP)
   i. 2:1 girls to boys have isolated CP.
   ii. 2:1 boys to girls have isolated CL.
   iii. CPs are associated with syndromes, lip not so much.

iv. Genetic associations
   a. Nonsyndromic
      1. Seventy percent of cleft lips +/− palates
      2. Thirty percent of isolated cleft palates
   b. Syndromes associated with cleft lip +/− palate
      1. Van der Woude (lower lip pits, hypodontia)
      2. CHARGE
         - *C*oloboma
         - *H*eart defects
         - Choanal *A*tresia
         - *R*etarded growth
         - *G*enital hypoplasia
         - *E*ar abnormality
      3. Velocardiofacial (22q deletion/DiGeorge)
      4. Down
   c. Syndromes associated with isolated cleft palate
      1. Stickler (myopia and Pierre-robin sequence)
      2. Velocardiofacial
      3. Kabuki
      4. Down

v. Risk factors for CL/CP
   a. Single gene transmission
      1. Highest risk when one child and one parent have a cleft (18%)
   b. Chromosome aberrations
   c. Teratogens: alcohol, thalidomide, vitamin A
   d. Environmental: amniotic band syndrome, maternal diabetes

vi. Classification
   a. Lip
      1. Microform cleft: dehiscence of orbicularis oris without overt clefting of epidermis
      2. Incomplete cleft: dehiscence of epidermis, orbicularis oris, and mucosa. Nasal sill and floor intact
      3. Complete cleft: dehiscence of epidermis, orbicularis oris, mucosa extending into nasal floor
   b. Palate
      1. Bifid uvula
      2. Submucous cleft
         - Classic findings: bifid cleft, zona pellucida, posterior palate notch at midline
      3. Incomplete cleft: dehiscence of mucosa and palatal muscles but does not extend fully through entire secondary palate
      4. Complete cleft: dehiscence extending through entire secondary cleft
      5. Tessier cleft: facial clefting

vii. CL anatomical relationships
   a. Ipsilateral maxillary hypoplasia
   b. Ala on cleft side displaced *inferiorly, laterally, posteriorly*
   c. *Shortened medial crus, elongated lateral crus*
   d. Caudal septum, columella, nasal tip is deviated to the non-cleft side

viii. CP anatomical relationships
   a. Levator veli palatini, which normally forms a sling across the palate, is oriented parallel to the cleft.
   b. Tensor veli palatini runs in a more anterior-posterior direction resulting in ETD and the need for tympanostomy tubes.

ix. When to repair:
   a. CL: (rule of 10s):10 weeks, 10 lb, hemoglobin of 10
   b. CP: 10 to 18 months (when deciduous molars arrive). Cleft palate flaps are designed to reconstruct muscular sling and are based on the descending palatine, which is in the greater palatine foramen
      1. Lengthening—V to Y and Furlow Z-plasty
      2. Posterior flaps—pharyngeal flap and sphincter pharyngoplasty

D. Cystic fibrosis
   i. AR disease (*CFTR* gene) of children and young adults
   ii. Generalized dysfunction of exocrine glands
   iii. Features
      a. Pancreatic insufficiency
      b. Chronic obstructive pulmonary disease/bronchiectasis/pneumonia
      c. Malabsorption
      d. Cirrhosis of the liver
      e. Nasal polyps/chronic sinusitis
      f. High sweat chloride/salt wasting
      g. Dehydration
   iv. Diagnosis—sweat chloride values greater than 60 meq/L
   v. Aggressive management of polyps and sinusitis with steroids, regular sinus irrigations with tobramycin, and endoscopic sinus surgery
   vi. Children who undergo polypectomy alone will experience a 90% recurrence

E. Down syndrome considerations
   i. Frequent upper respiratory infections
   ii. Frequent OM secondary to ETD
   iii. Abnormal nasopharynx shape
   iv. Poor tone of tensor veli palatini

F. Esophageal atresia and tracheoesophageal fistula (TEF)
   i. Associated with VACTERL
      a. *V*ertebral
      b. *A*nal
      c. Cardiac
      d. *T*racheo*E*sophageal
      e. *R*enal
      f. *L*imb abnormalities
   ii. Also associated with VATER syndrome
   iii. Types
      a. Esophageal atresia with distal TEF—most common (85%)
      b. Esophageal atresia without TEF—second most common (7%)

G. Caustic ingestion
   i. Bases (alkali) cause most esophageal injuries (60-80%)
      a. Sodium, potassium, and ammonium hydroxide
      b. *Liquefactive necrosis* with full-thickness burns

ii. Acids are less harmful than bases
   a. Bleach, lysol
   b. *Coagulative necrosis*
   c. Coagulum limits penetration of acid and prevents full-thickness burns
iii. Diagnosis
   a. Evaluate chin, lips, tongue, and palate for evidence of burns
      1. Severity of oral cavity burns does not correlate with esophageal symptoms but can help in diagnosis
   b. CXR to rule out free air
   c. Esophagoscopy 24 to 48 hours after injury
      1. Do not advance esophagoscope past ulcers or circumferential burns
      2. Children presenting after 48 hours should have esophagram
iv. Treatment
   a. Steroids
   b. Antibiotics
   c. Varying opinions exist regarding the placement of a nasogastric tube at the time of esophagoscopy
   d. Strictures are often treated with esophageal dilation

H. Foreign bodies
   i. Children less than 6 years of age do not possess molars to grind nuts and raw vegetables
   ii. A foreign body should be ruled out if a child has unilateral wheezing
   iii. Tracheal/bronchial
      a. Stridor/wheezing
      b. Cough without associated illness
      c. Recurrent or migratory pneumonia
      d. Acute aphonia
   iv. Esophageal
      a. Odynophagia
      b. Drooling
      c. Vomiting/spitting
      d. Airway compromise due to impingement of posterior trachea
   v. Radiograph
      a. CXR
         1. Visualize foreign body
         2. Evaluate for atelectasis on the side affected
         3. Overinflation due to air trapping
      b. Lateral decubitus
         1. Evaluates for mediastinal shift
         2. Uninvolved side down results in shift of mediastinum down secondary to gravity
         3. Involved side down results in no shift due to air trapping
   vi. Anesthesia
      a. Deep inhalational
      b. Allows patient to spontaneously ventilate
      c. Topical lidocaine on vocal cords vs neuromuscular paralysis
   vii. Five levels at which a foreign body is likely to lodge in the esophagus
      a. Cricopharyngeus muscle
      b. Thoracic inlet

- c. Level of aortic arch
- d. Tracheal bifurcation
- e. Gastroesophageal junction

viii. Ingestion of disc battery
- a. Contains lithium, NaOH, KOH, mercury
- b. 1 hour—mucosal damage
- c. 2 to 4 hours—damage to muscular layer
- d. 8 to 12 hours—potential perforation
- e. If battery passed into stomach, demonstrated by x-ray
  1. Send home and monitor stool for battery
  2. Repeat x-ray if not passed in 4 to 7 days
  3. With larger batteries (23 mm), repeat x-ray in 48 hours following observation of battery in stomach
  4. If still in stomach, remove endoscopically

I. Hereditary hearing loss

i. 1/1000 children born with hearing loss. 50/50 nongenetic versus genetic

ii. Nongenetic or acquired
- a. Most commonly CMV
- b. Other etiologies: idiopathic, hypoxia, hyperbilirubinemia, nongenetic conditions (Goldenhar, Fabry)
- c. TORCH infections
  1. *T*oxoplasmosis
  2. *O*ther (ie, syphilis)
  3. *R*ubella: "Cookie bite" audiogram, cataracts, cardiac malformations
  4. *C*ytomegalovirus
  5. *H*erpes
  6. *H*IV

iii. Genetic (50%)
- a. Nonsyndromic (2/3)
  1. Autosomal recessive-DNFB (75%)
     - Most commonly connexin 26 (the protein) on gene GJB2/6
  2. Autosomal dominant—DNFA
  3. X-linked fixation of stapes with perilymphatic gusher
- b. Syndromic (1/3)
  1. Autosomal dominant (*WANT BCS*)
     - *W*aardenburg: SNHL, vestibular abnormalities, dystopia canthorum, pigmentary changes of the eyes, skin, and hair (ie, white forelock)
     - *A*pert: flat CHL due to stapes fixation, syndactyly, craniosynostosis
     - *N*eurofibromatosis 2: Bilateral acoustic neuromas. Candidates for auditory brain stem implants
     - *T*reacher-Collins (mandibulofacial dysostosis): CHL, SNHL, or mixed, midface hypoplasia, micrognathia, malformed ears, lower lid coloboma, downward slanting eyes
     - *B*ranchio-oto-renal: branchial apparatus abnormalities (clefts, cysts, or fistulas), preauricular pits, hearing loss (SNHL, CHL, or mixed), and renal malformations
     - *C*rouzon: CHL, craniosynostosis, maxillary hypoplasia, ocular hypertelorism with exophthalmos, mandibular prognathism
     - *S*ticklers: SNHL or mixed, flattened facial appearance with Pierre Robin sequence, myopia

2. Autosomal recessive (*PUJ*)
    - *P*endred: SNHL, euthyroid goiter. Patients have abnormal perchlorate uptake test (reduced thyroid radioactivity over time). Associated with Mondini malformation and EVA
    - *U*sher: SNHL, retinitis pigmentosa ± vestibular symptoms. Most common syndrome to affect the eyes and ears. Diagnosed with electroretinogram
    - *J*ervell/Lange-Nilsen: SNHL, prolonged QT with syncopal events and sudden death
3. X-linked
    - Alport: SNHL, renal failure with hematuria, and ocular abnormalities

iv. Enlarged vestibular aqueduct syndrome
a. Most common inner ear abnormality in children with congenital hearing loss
b. Associated with Mondini malformation, Pendred syndrome, and branchio-otorenal syndrome
c. Upper limit of normal is less than or equal to 1.5 mm at the midpoint of the aqueduct
d. Progressive SNHL (or mixed hearing loss) that may worsen in a stepwise fashion
e. Hearing loss may worsen after minor trauma: avoid contact sports.
f. Treatment
1. Hearing aids
2. Cochlear implantation

J. Nasal anomalies
i. Midline nasal masses
a. Dermoid
1. Ectodermal and mesodermal tissues (hair follicles, sweat glands, sebaceous glands, etc.)
2. Commonly on the lower third of nasal bridge ± overlying tuft of hair
3. CT scan may reveal skull base defect and intracranial involvement via foramen cecum
4. External surgical excision

b. Glioma
1. Males > females (3:1)
2. Glial cells in a connective tissue matrix with or without a fibrous connection to the dura via fonticulus frontalis
3. No fluid-filled space connected to the subarachnoid space
4. Firm and noncompressible
5. Intranasal gliomas most often arise from the lateral wall and are more often associated with dural attachment (35%)
6. External excision unless dural connection

c. Encephalocele
1. Herniation of meninges ± brain through fonticulus frontalis
2. Connected to subarachnoid space (contains CSF)
3. Nasofrontal, nasoethmoid, naso-orbital, or skull base
4. Soft, compressible intranasal lesions (may be confused for polyps)
5. Positive *Furstenberg sign*: mass expands with crying
6. CT and MRI to evaluate for skull base defect and neural tissue
7. Intracranial then extracranial excision

d. Choanal atresia
    1. Neonates are obligate nasal breathers until approximately 6 weeks of age
    2. Failure to pass a 5 or 6 Fr catheter at least 3 cm into the nasal cavity
    3. "FURB"
        - *F*emale predominance.
        - *U*nilateral atresia is more common (2/3) and presents later in childhood. Initial approaches are usually transnasally, although transpalatal approaches have less recurrence
        - *R*ight side is more common
        - Ninety percent have a *B*ony and/or cartilaginous component, 10% mucosal only
    4. Fifty percent are associated with congenital anomaly
    5. CHARGE association
    6. Bilateral atresia presents at birth with cyclical apnea and crying, and urgently requires an oral airway and surgical correction before hospital discharge

K. Teratomas
  i. Tumors of pluripotent embryonal cells
  ii. Majority recognized by 1 year
  iii. Ten percent occur in the head and neck
    a. Orbital
    b. Nasal
    c. Nasopharynx
    d. Oral cavity
    e. Neck
  iv. Dermoid cyst
    a. Most common
    b. Contains epidermal and mesodermal remnants
    c. Polypoid masses covered with skin and epidermal appendages
    d. In neck, occur in submental region deep to or superficial to mylohyoid membrane
        1. Superficial lesions may be confused with ranula
        2. May cause obstruction of breathing or deglutition
        3. Excision is the treatment of choice
  v. Teratoid cyst
    a. Composed of all three germ layers
    b. Cystic with an epithelial lining
    c. Differentiation of tissues is minimal
  vi. Teratoma
    a. Composed of all three germ layers
    b. Usually solid
    c. Cellular differentiation allows recognition of organ structure
    d. Often fatal
  vii. Epignathi—oropharyngeal origin
    a. Composed of all three germ layers
    b. Most differentiated of all forms. Complete organs and body parts identifiable
    c. Often arise from midline or lateral basisphenoid and protrude through mouth
    d. Often fatal

L. Neck masses
   i. Congenital
      a. Branchial cleft abnormalities
         1. May exist as either cysts, sinuses, or fistulae
         2. Often present after URI
         3. In general, these anomalies form within its branchial arch derivatives, and form superficial to the next branchial arch structure
         4. First branchial cleft cyst
            - Type I (rare): EAC duplication
            - Type II: passes through parotid gland, below the angle of the mandible, and open in the anterior neck above the level of the hyoid bone. Relation to FN is variable (may pass medial to or bifurcate around nerve)
         5. Second branchial cleft cyst
            - *Most common* type (70-90%)
            - *Pathway*: anterior border of SCM → deep to platysma, stylohyoid, and posterior digastric → superficial to CN IX and XII → between external and internal carotid artery → tonsillar fossa
         6. Third branchial cyst
            - Predominantly left sided (~90%)
            - *Pathway*: anterior border of SCM → deep to CN IX → deep to internal carotid artery → penetrates thyrohyoid membrane (superior to SLN) → pyriform sinus
      b. Dermoid cyst
         1. Midline mass composed of mesoderm and ectoderm (hair follicles, sebaceous glands, and sweat glands)
         2. Frequently misdiagnosed as thyroglossal duct cysts
         3. Does not elevate with tongue protrusion
      c. Laryngocele
         1. Enlargement of the laryngeal saccule
         2. Internal causes distention of false vocal cord and aryepiglottic fold
         3. External presents as compressible, lateral neck masses that penetrate the thyrohyoid membrane
      d. Plunging ranula
         1. May pierce the mylohyoid and present as a paramedian or lateral neck mass
         2. Fluid with elevated levels of protein and salivary amylase
         3. Excision in continuity with the sublingual gland of origin
      e. Sternocleidomastoid tumor of infancy
         1. Similar presentation as torticollis (chin pointed toward opposite side)
         2. May result from hematoma during delivery
         3. Physical therapy
      f. Thyroglossal duct cyst
         1. Most common midline mass
         2. Results from failure of involution of thyroglossal duct
         3. Asymptomatic midline mass at or below the hyoid bone that elevates with tongue protrusion
         4. Confirm normal thyroid tissue with US prior to surgical excision with Sistrunk procedure

ii. Inflammatory/infectious
   a. Viral—most common cause of pediatric lymphadenitis
      1. Rhinovirus, adenovirus, and enterovirus
      2. EBV—patients may develop pink, measles-like rash if given amoxicillin
   b. Bacterial
      1. Most common bacterial cause of cervical adenitis is *S. aureus* and group A streptococci.
      2. Parapharyngeal and retropharyngeal spaces are the most common neck spaces to be involved in pediatric neck abscesses.
      3. *Lemierre syndrome*—septic thrombophlebitis of the internal jugular vein resulting in spiking fevers and neck fullness.
   c. FNA if mass persists past 4 to 6 weeks
   d. Cat scratch disease
      1. Most common cause of chronic cervical adenopathy in children
      2. History of contact with cats
      3. *Bartonella henselae*
      4. Warthin-Starry stain shows small pleomorphic gram-negative rods
   e. Tuberculosis
      1. "Scrofula"
      2. Single large cervical lymph node
      3. Skin may turn violaceous color
      4. Purified protein derivative (PPD) is usually reactive
      5. Isoniazid, ethambutol, streptomycin, and rifampin
   f. Atypical mycobacteria
      1. Rarely exhibit fever or systemic symptoms
      2. CXR is usually normal, and PPD reactions are normal or only intermediate in reactivity
      3. Notoriously resistant to traditional antituberculous agents
      4. Chronic draining sinuses often develop

iii. Noninfectious
   a. Rosai-Dorfman disease: self-limited, nontender cervical lymphadenopathy
   b. Kawasaki disease
      1. Cervical lymphadenopathy
      2. Erythema of lips and tongue ("strawberry tongue")
      3. Erythema and peeling of hands and feet
      4. Rash
      5. Treat with aspirin and gamma-globulin to prevent coronary artery aneurysms

iv. Neoplasms
   a. Juvenile nasopharyngeal angiofibroma (JNA)
      1. Occurs in young boys
      2. Originates near sphenopalatine foramen
      3. Highly vascular tumor that results in nasal obstruction and epistaxis
      4. CT classically shows *Holman-Miller sign* (anterior bowing of posterior maxillary sinus wall)
      5. Treatment
         - Preoperative angioembolization
         - Surgical resection ± radiation

b. Lymphoma
   1. Most common pediatric malignancy
   2. FNA (under sedation if necessary) with appropriate staining techniques to determine the cell of origin
   3. Chest x-ray
   4. Intravenous pyelogram
   5. Bone marrow aspirate, and scans as indicated
   6. Overall mortality 30%
   7. Stages
      - 1—localized
      - 2—limited above diaphragm with systemic symptoms
      - 3—diffuse disease

c. Rhabdomyosarcoma
   1. Most common soft tissue malignancy of the head and neck in children
   2. Sites of involvement
      - Orbit
      - Neck
      - Face
      - Temporal bone
      - Tongue
      - Palate
      - Larynx
   3. Often presents before age 10
   4. Rapid growth
   5. Usually embryonal subtype
   6. Orbital tumors are unique in that they tend toward locally aggressive behavior, but metastasize rarely (the converse is true of other sites)
   7. Chemotherapy and radiation are the main modalities of treatment after biopsy-proven diagnosis
   8. Increased survival (81% vs 51%) in patients with nonorbital, parameningeal disease who were treated with chemoradiation/radiation
      - Surgery is reserved for unresponsive lesions and residual disease following chemoradiation.

M. Stridor
   i. Inspiratory: supraglottis and glottis
   ii. Biphasic: subglottis
   iii. Expiratory: trachea
   iv. Timing
      a. Most common cause of stridor at *two days* is vocal cord paralysis
      b. At *two weeks*: laryngomalacia
      c. At *two months:* hemangioma
      d. At *two years:* papilloma
   v. By subsite
      a. Laryngeal (60%)
         1. Laryngomalacia (60%)
         2. Subglottic stenosis (20%)
         3. Vocal cord palsy (13%)
         4. Others (7%)

b. Tracheal (15%)
  1. Tracheomalacia (45%)
  2. Vascular compression (most commonly aberrant subclavian artery) (45%)
  3. Stenosis (5%)
  4. Bronchial (5%)

c. Infection (5%)
  1. Croup
     - Parainfluenzae virus
     - "Barking" cough
  2. Epiglottitis
     - Historically with *H. influenzae*
     - HIB vaccine has significantly decreased incidence
  3. Bacterial tracheitis
     - *Staphylococcus aureus*
     - Obstructive tracheal casts
     - Intubation, pulmonary toilet, suctioning, and possible bronchoscopy

d. Other (15%)

vi. Laryngomalacia
  a. Most common cause of stridor in children (generally biphasic)
  b. Most common congenital laryngeal abnormality
  c. Often seen in association with other findings resulting from delay in development of neuromuscular control (ie, gastroesophageal reflux, central or obstructive apnea, hypotonia, failure to thrive, and pneumonia)
  d. Endoscopic findings
     1. Anterior collapse of arytenoid mucosa (hooding)
     2. Short aryepiglottic folds
     3. Posterior collapse of epiglottis
     4. Omega-shaped epiglottis
  e. Typically self-limited, supraglottoplasty necessary in ~10%

vii. Subglottic stenosis
  a. Newborn infants have a subglottic lumen that averages 6 mm in diameter; 5 mm is regarded as borderline normal, and 4 mm is stenotic
  b. Formula for pediatric endotracheal (ET) tube selection: (age in years + 16)/4
  c. In an emergency, choose the ET tube closest to the size of the patient's pinky finger
  d. High association of subglottic stenosis in Down syndrome patients
  e. Myer-Cotton grading
     1. Grade I—0% to 50% obstruction
     2. Grade II—51% to 70% obstruction
     3. Grade III—71% to 99% obstruction
     4. Grade IV—complete obstruction
  f. Treatment
     1. Grade I and mild Grade II may be observed or treated with incision/dilation
     2. Grade III and IV will require trach and open repair with
        - Anterior cricoid split (neonates)
        - Laryngotracheal reconstruction (LTR)
        - Cricotracheal resection

viii. Complete tracheal rings are associated with pulmonary slings in 30% of cases.
ix. Vocal cord paralysis
   a. Second most common congenital laryngeal abnormality
   b. Most commonly idiopathic
   c. Most common congenital CNS abnormality—*Arnold-Chiari malformation*
   d. Best treatment for unilateral pediatric vocal cord paralysis is speech therapy

N. Vascular lesions
i. Hemangiomas
   a. Lesion is small at birth and has a 6- to 12-month proliferative phase
   b. Strawberry or bruised appearance
   c. Suspect visceral involvement in patients with three or more cutaneous lesions
   d. Suspect glottic or subglottic involvement in neonates with progressive stridor and cutaneous hemangiomas of the face
   e. Occurs more commonly in the left posterolateral quadrant
   f. PHACE syndrome
      1. *P*osterior fossa malformations
      2. *H*emangiomas (usually of the face)
      3. *A*rterial abnormalities
      4. Coarctation of the aorta
      5. *E*ye abnormalities
   g. Spontaneous involution occurs over 2- to 10-year period at a rate of 10% per year (ie, 50% by 5 years, 70% by 7 years, etc.)
   h. Treatment
      1. Observation
      2. Medical/surgical therapy
         - Often reserved for symptomatic infants
         - Steroids
           (a) Oral or intralesional injection for periorbital, nasal, or lip lesions
               ○ Periorbital injections can result in blindness
         - Laser
           (a) CO_2 laser (10,600 nm) and pulsed dye laser (585 nm) are currently favored for debulking symptomatic mucosal lesions (ie, subglottic)
         - Excision
           (a) Early lesions—to avoid systemic medical therapy and social trauma
           (b) Stable lesions following involution

ii. Vascular malformations
   a. Arteriovenous malformations (AVMs)
      1. Usually present at birth and grows with patient
      2. Eventually develop pulsations secondary to arterial blood flow
      3. Differentiated from hemangioma or capillary malformation by MRI/A or US
      4. Eventually may lead to heart failure
      5. Surgical excision is the gold standard, but selective arterial embolization may be used as an adjunct or for palliation
   b. Capillary malformations
      1. "Port wine stain"
      2. Present at birth and distribution remains constant (grows with patient)

3. Syndromes
    - *Sturge-Weber*
        (a) Capillary malformation of V_1 distribution with calcification and loss of meninges and cortex
        (b) Results in glaucoma and seizures
    - *Osler-Weber-Rendu*
    - Hereditary hemorrhagic telangiectasia (HHT)
        (a) Capillary malformations of skin, mucous membranes, brain, liver, and lungs
        (b) Commonly have severe and recurrent epistaxis

c. Venous malformations
1. Usually not detected at birth
2. Lesion enlarges in dependent position and has a blue hue
3. Treatment
    - Compression
    - Sclerotherapy—alcohol-based agents frequently used for craniofacial lesions
    - Surgery—usually performed after sclerotherapy

d. Lymphatic malformations (cystic hygroma)
1. Usually present at birth and primarily involve the head and neck.
2. Lesions are progressive
3. MRI is gold standard for radiologic evaluation
4. Macrocystic and microcystic lesions
5. Treatment
    - Surgical excision—gold standard but has high recurrence rate
    - Sclerotherapy—*OK-432* (*Streptococcus* that has treated with penicillin), doxycycline
    - CO_2 laser used for glottic involvement.
        (a) Diffuse disease may require tracheostomy and gastrostomy tube

O. Velopharyngeal dysfunction
i. Intelligibility of speech is affected more by articulation rather than resonance
ii. "M," "n," and "ng" are normal nasal consonants, and their production is associated with an open velopharyngeal port
iii. The hypernasal child nasalizes nonnasal phonemes /d/, /b/, /t/
iv. Diagnosis
    a. Endoscopic evaluation of Passavant ridge
    b. Videofluoroscopy
v. Treatment
    a. Speech therapy directed toward articulation and increasing resonance
    b. Prosthetics
        1. Indicated in children whose gap is large because of little to no motion of the velopharyngeal sphincter
    c. Palatal lift: not indicated in a child with a short palate
    d. Surgery
        1. Pharyngeal flap
            - Success depends on lateral wall motion
            - Caution must be taken to create ports less than 20 mm^2 to prevent continued nasal escape; ports that are of insufficient size may result in chronic nasopharyngitis, anterior rhinorrhea, and otitis

2. Posterior wall augmentation
   - Increase anteroposterior (AP) projection of the posterior pharyngeal wall to contact velum
   - Injectables (ie, gelfoam, teflon, collagen)
3. Sphincter pharyngoplasty
   - Designed to create a dynamic pharyngeal sphincter using posterior tonsillar pillar flaps

P. Facial paralysis
   i. Approximately 90% of congenital facial paralysis resolves spontaneously.
   ii. Frequently caused by traumatic delivery (cephalopelvic disproportion, dystocia, high forceps delivery, intrauterine trauma).
   iii. If no resolution after a period of observation, ENOG can be used to determine excitability.
   iv. CT and MRI may be required for adequate evaluation.

Sleep

A. Obstructive sleep apnea (OSA)—1/5 American adults has at least mild OSA
   i. Apnea: complete cessation of airflow for at least 10 seconds
   ii. Hypopnea: reduction in airflow greater than 30% for at least 10 seconds with greater than 4% oxyhemoglobin desaturation or reduction of airflow greater than 50% for at least 10 seconds with greater than 3% oxyhemoglobin desaturation
   iii. Respiratory effort-related arousal: sequence of breaths for at least 10 seconds with increasing respiratory effort that terminates with an arousal
   iv. Apnea-hypopnea index (AHI): number of apneas and hypopneas per hour of total sleep time—grades severity of OSA
   v. AHI grading system
      a. Children: less than 1 = normal, 1 to 5 = mild; 5 to 10 = moderate greater than 10 = severe
      b. Adults: less than 5 = normal, 5 to 15 = mild; 15 to 30 = moderate; greater than 30 = severe
   vi. Symptoms
      a. Loud snoring
      b. Restless sleep
      c. Daytime hypersomnolence
      d. Morning headaches
      e. Decreased productivity
      f. Lethargy
      g. Depression
   vii. Long-term sequelae:
      a. Intellectual deterioration
      b. Impotence
      c. Cardiac arrhythmias
      d. Pulmonary hypertension
   viii. Diagnosis
      a. Physical exam
         1. BMI: obesity is a common finding
         2. Neck circumference

3. Occlusion/retrognathia
4. Nasal cavity
5. Tongue and tonsil size
6. Laryngoscopy
   - Müller maneuver: endoscopic evaluation in awake patient with forced inspiratory effort against closed mouth and nose

b. Polysomnogram: in lab, portable (at home)

ix. Medical treatment
   a. Positive airway pressure (CPAP, BiPAP)
   b. Oral appliances: tongue retaining device, mandibular repositioning device
   c. Adjunctive therapy
      1. Treatment of allergies and sinusitis
      2. Weight loss

x. Surgical treatment
   a. Basics
      1. For those with low adherence to PAP therapy
      2. Must address site of obstruction
   b. Nasal: septoplasty, adenoidectomy, inferior turbinate reduction, nasal valve reconstruction
   c. Palate: palatal radiofrequency ablation, uvulopalatopharyngoplasty, expansion pharyngoplasty
   d. Oropharynx: tonsillectomy, lateral pharyngoplasty, hypoglossal nerve stimulation
   e. Hypopharynx: lingual tonsillectomy, partial midline glossectomy, mandibular osteotomy and genioglossal advancement, hyoid myotomy and suspension, tongue-suspension suture, axillo-mandibular osteotomy and advancement
   f. Hypoglossal nerve stimulation
      1. Electrical stimulation of CN XII improves neuromuscular tone of pharynx during sleep. Particularly the genioglossus and transverse/vertical intrinsic musculature. Want to exclude retractors (hyoglossus, styloglossus)
      2. FDA indications
         - Age greater than 18 years
         - AHI 15 to 65/h with less than 25% central/mixed events
         - PAP failure/noncompliance
         - No complete concentric collapse at the velum on drug-induced sleep endoscopy
         - BMI less than 32 to 35
      3. Predictors of success
         - Females
         - Older individuals
         - Lower BMI
         - Higher preop AHI
         - Lower pre-implant CPAP pressures
      4. Predictors of poor outcomes
         - High BMI
         - Mouth breathing predicts worse outcomes with upper airway stimulation

B. Non-OSA sleep disorders
   i. Insomnia
   ii. Central sleep apnea: apnea without respiratory effort. May be sign of brain stem issue/compression

- iii. Narcolepsy
  - a. Diagnosis
    - 1. Multiple latency sleep test
    - 2. Low *CSF hypocretin* levels
  - b. Treated with modafinil
- iv. Restless leg syndrome
  - a. Eighty-five percent associated with periodic limb movements of sleep
  - b. May be a sign of iron deficiency
  - c. Treatment: dopaminergic agents, benzos, opioids, antiepileptics, iron

Trauma

A. Temporal bone fractures
- i. Management
  - a. Priority is airway/head injury/c-spine management.
  - b. Symptoms include FN injury, hearing loss, vertigo, CSF otorrhea, TM perforation, hemotympanum, canal laceration.
- ii. Fracture patterns
  - a. More accurately classified as otic-capsule sparing or otic-capsule involving
- iii. Most common cause of a persistent CHL associated with temporal bone fractures is incudostapedial joint dislocation.
- iv. The most common cause of posttraumatic vertigo is concussive injury to the membranous labyrinth.
- v. CSF leaks have 20% association with temporal bone fractures (usually temporary and resolve without surgery).

B. Orbital floor fractures
- i. Indication for surgical repair of orbital floor blowout fractures
  - a. Rapid onset of intraorbital bleeding and decreased visual acuity
  - b. Occulobradycardic reflex: more common in pediatric floor fractures
  - c. Diplopia lasting more than 7 days
  - d. Entrapment
  - e. Enophthalmos greater than 2 mm or involvement of one-third to one-half of the orbital floor
- ii. The most common error in orbital floor reconstruction is failure to repair the posterior orbital floor.
- iii. Ideal time for surgical repair is 10 to 14 days (only urgent is entrapment with oculocardiac reflex activation)
  - a. After repair is complete, forced duction test is performed.
- iv. Inappropriate repair may result in enophthalmos and hypo-ophthalmos

C. Nasal bone fractures
- i. 40% to 45% of all facial fractures
- ii. Evaluate for external defects, septal deviation, septal hematoma, epistaxis, and CSF rhinorrhea
  - a. Untreated septal hematoma may progress to septal abscess or result in saddle nose deformity
- iii. Closed reduction should be ideally performed within hours of the accident or maybe delayed from 5 to 10 days

D. Naso-orbital-ethmoid (NOE) fractures
   i. Orbital swelling and telecanthus
   ii. Often results in skull base fracture with CSF leak
   iii. Types
      a. Type I: single, noncomminuted fragment of bone without medial canthal tendon disruption
      b. Type II: comminution of bone, but medial canthal tendon is still attached to segment of bone
      c. Type III: comminution of bone with disruption of medial canthal tendon
   iv. Goal of surgery is to accurately reconstruct the nasal root, into which the medial canthal tendon inserts.
      a. Normal intercanthal distance is 3 to 3.5 cm.
      b. Medial canthal tendons may need to be reapproximated with wire.
E. Maxillary fractures
   i. LeFort fractures (midface separation with mobile palate, may have different types for each half of the face. All require pterygoid fractures)
      a. Type I: palate separated from midface. Involves the pterygoid plates
      b. Type II: involves pterygoid plates, frontonasal maxillary buttress, and skull base. Often results in CSF leak
      c. Type III: involves pterygoid plates, frontonasal maxillary buttress, and frontozygomatic buttress. Results in craniofacial separation
F. Mandibular fractures
   i. Second most fractured bone in facial trauma
   ii. Occlusion
      a. Postoperative result should be patient's preop occlusion
      b. Class I: normal. First maxillary molar has four cusps (mesiobuccal, mesiolingual, distobuccal, and distolingual). *Mesiobuccal cusp of the first maxillary molar fits in mesiobuccal groove of first mandibular molar*
      c. Class II: retrognathic (mesiobuccal cusp of first maxillary molar is between first mandibular molar and the second premolar)
      d. Class III: prognathic
   iii. Condyle, angle, and body are most common fracture locations.
   iv. Bilateral fractures occur greater than 50% of the time (ie, parasymphysial and contralateral subcondylar).
   v. Compressive forces occur along the inferior rim, and areas of tension develop along the superior rim.
   vi. Favorable vs unfavorable fractures
      a. Favorable: reduced by musculature
      b. Unfavorable: displaced/distracted by musculature
   vii. Open fractures require prophylactic antibiotics
      a. Mandibular osteomyelitis after fracture is associated with a fracture through a tooth root.
   viii. Treatment
      a. Maxillomandibular fixation (MMF)
         1. Reestablishes preinjury occlusion
         2. Classically used for uncomplicated subcondylar fractures and fractures with gross comminution or soft tissue loss
         3. Contraindications for closed reduction with MMF include
            - Multiple comminuted fractures
            - Elderly patients

- Severe pulmonary disease
- Children
- Mentally handicapped/seizures
- Alcoholic
- Pregnant

b. Open reduction internal fixation
  1. Rapid and dependable bony union with limited morbidity and complication rates
  2. Placement of plates to overcome distracting forces and take advantage of compressive forces
  3. Properly positioned miniplates can take advantage of dynamic compressive forces
  4. Champy defined areas for fixation of miniplates along the ideal osteosynthesis lines

G. Laryngeal fractures
  i. Primary objective is securing airway
  ii. Evaluate with fiberoptic examination and CT
  iii. Classification
    a. Group 1: minor hematoma, small laceration, no fracture
    b. Group 2: airway compromise: edema/hematoma, no cartilage exposure, nondisplaced fracture
    c. Group 3: airway compromise: massive edema, mucosal tears, exposed cartilage, VC immobility, displaced fracture
    d. Group 4: cricotracheal separation

H. Cervical injuries
  i. Zones of the neck
    a. 1: sternal notch to cricoid cartilage
    b. 2: cricoid cartilage to angle of mandible
    c. 3: angle of mandible to skull base
    d. General trend away from mandatory exploration of all penetrating neck wounds; immediate surgery always prudent for immediately life-threatening injuries
      1. Angiography and esophagram are often used to obtain further information in nonimmediately emergent cases.
      2. Angiography is usually the first-line treatment for Zones 1 and 3.
    e. For Zone 2, surgical exploration (angiography is generally not needed) is frequently the first-line treatment, especially with any of the following symptoms:
      1. Subcutaneous emphysema
      2. Hemoptysis
      3. Hematemesis
      4. Hematoma
      5. Significant bleeding
      6. Dysphagia
      7. Dysphonia
      8. Neurologic injury
    f. Air embolism
      1. Associated with head and neck trauma or venous perforation during routine head and neck procedures.
      2. "To-and-fro" murmur and decreased cardiac output can be seen with ultrasound.

3. Place patient in Trendelenburg (head down) and left lateral decubitus position (this traps air in the right ventricle and prevents ejection into pulmonary system).
4. Cardiac puncture may be required for aspiration of air.

Selected Histologic Findings

A. Actinomycosis: sulfur granules
B. Adenoid cystic carcinoma
   i. Cribriform—"Swiss cheese"
   ii. Tubular
   iii. Solid
C. Allergic fungal sinusitis: Charcot-Leyden crystals
D. Amyloidosis: apple-green birefringence after staining with Congo red dye
E. Aspergillus: 45-degree branching, septate hyphae when grown on Sabouraud agar
F. Basal cell carcinoma: basaloid cells, palisading of cells
G. Blastomycosis: pseudoepitheliomatous hyperplasia, broad-based budding hyphae
H. Cat scratch disease: Warthin-Starry stain showing pleomorphic gram-negative rods
I. Chordoma: physaliferous cells
J. Esthesioneuroblastoma
   i. Homer-Wright rosette
   ii. Flexner-Wintersteiner rosette
K. Fungal sinusitis: stain with methenamine silver
L. Granular cell tumor-pseudoepitheliomatous hyperplasia: can be confused with malignancy
M. Hashimoto thyroiditis: lymphocytic infiltrate, germinal centers, Hürthle cells, follicular atrophy
N. Hemangiopericytoma: Zimmerman cells
O. Histiocytosis X: Birbeck granules (tennis racket-shaped structures) found in Langerhans cells
P. Histoplasmosis: epithelioid granulomas, pseudoepitheliomatous hyperplasia
Q. Hodgkin disease: Reed-Sternberg cells—"Owl eyes"
R. Melanoma: S100, Melan A, HMB 45
S. Meningioma: psammoma bodies
T. Mucor: aseptate, wide branching
U. Necrotizing sialometaplasia: pseudoepitheliomatous hyperplasia
V. Paraganglioma: Type 1 chief cells and Type 2 Sustenacular cells, Zellballen = balls of cells
W. Pemphigus: acantholysis and positive Nikolsky sign
X. Pleomorphic adenoma: epithelial, myoepithelial, and stromal elements (benign mixed tumor)
Y. *Pneumocystis carinii*: cysts and trophozoites
Z. Rhinoscleroma: granulation, pseudoepitheliomatous hyperplasia, Russell bodies, and Mikulicz cells
AA. Sarcoidosis: Schaumann bodies and asteroids within giant cells
AB. Schwannoma: Antoni A and B cells
AC. Squamous Cell Carcinoma

i. Well differentiated: squamous cells in cords with intercellular bridges (desmosomes at the electron microscopic level) and keratin pearls
ii. Verrucous carcinoma: church-spire keratosis and broad rete pegs with pushing margins

AD. Smooth muscle tumors: vimentin positive on pathology
AE. Syphilis: endolymphatic hydrops (bowing of Reissner membrane) with mononuclear leukocyte infiltration and osteolytic lesions of the otic capsule
AF. Thyroid cancer
i. Papillary: papillae, lack of follicles, large nuclei with prominent nucleoli (Orphan Annie eye), psammoma bodies
ii. Follicular: need to see invasion of tissue outside capsule of follicle to diagnose cancer
iii. Medullary: sheets of amyloid-rich cells
iv. Anaplastic: undifferentiated cells

AG. Warthin tumor: papillary cystadenoma lymphomatosum
AH. Wegener granulomatosis: angiocentric, epithelial-type necrotizing granulomas with giant cells and histiocytes

Selected Syndromes

A. *Albright syndrome*: polyostotic fibrous dysplasia, precocious puberty, and café au lait spots
B. *Alport*: SNHL, renal failure with hematuria, and ocular abnormalities
C. *Arnold-Chiari syndrome*: cerebellar crowding at foramen magnum with cranial neuropathies and hydrocephalus
D. *Basal cell nevus syndrome*: BCC, cysts of maxilla and mandible, ocular abnormalities
E. *Behcet syndrome*: Symptom complex of oral and genital ulcers, iritis. Cause unknown but may be viral or autoimmune related
F. *Branchio-otorenal syndrome*: branchial apparatus abnormalities (clefts, cysts, or fistulas), hearing loss (SNHL, CHL, or mixed) and renal malformations
G. *Churg Strauss Syndrome:* Eosinophilic granulomatosis with polyangiitis, results in vasculitis and allergic airway hypersensitivity
H. *Cogan syndrome*: interstitial keratitis and Meniere's-like attacks of vertigo, ataxia, tinnitus, nausea, vomiting, and hearing loss
I. *Cowden disease*: familial goiter, skin hamartomata, and well-differentiated thyroid carcinoma
J. *Dandy syndrome*: oscillopsia caused by bilateral loss of vestibular function
K. *Gardner syndrome*: familial colonic polyposis, osteomata, soft tissue tumors, and well-differentiated thyroid carcinoma
L. *Gradenigo syndrome*: otorrhea, retro-orbital pain, and lateral rectus palsy
M. *Heerfordt disease* (uveoparotid fever): seen in sarcoid patients with uveitis, mild fever, nonsuppurative parotitis, and CN paralysis
N. *Jerville-Lange-Nielsen*: SNHL, prolonged QT with syncopal events, and sudden death
O. *Kawasaki disease*: cervical lymphadenopathy, erythema of lips and tongue ("strawberry tongue"), erythema and peeling of hands and feet, rash. Treat with aspirin and gamma-globulin to prevent cardiac complications
P. *Lemierre syndrome*: septic thrombophlebitis of the internal jugular vein because of infection resulting in spiking fevers and neck fullness

Q. *McCune-Albright Syndrome:* triad of polyostotic fibrous dysplasia, precocious puberty, and café-au-lait spots
R. *NF-2*: bilateral acoustic neuromas
S. *Osler-Weber-Rendu syndrome* (hereditary hemorrhagic telangiectasia): capillary malformations of skin, mucous membranes, brain, liver, and lungs. Commonly have severe and recurrent epistaxis. Check lung and brain MRI for arteriovenous malformations
T. *Pendred*: SNHL, euthyroid goiter. Patients have abnormal perchlorate uptake test
U. *Pierre Robin sequence*: retrognathia, retrodisplacement of the tongue, and respiratory compromise. Patients also often have CP
V. *Plummer-Vinson syndrome*: iron deficiency anemia, dysphagia secondary to esophageal webs, hypothyroidism, gastritis, cheilitis, glossitis
W. *Rosai-Dorfman disease*: self-limited, nontender cervical lymphadenopathy
X. *Stickler*: SNHL, flattened facial appearance with Pierre Robin sequence, myopia
Y. *Sturge-Weber*: capillary malformation of V_1 distribution with calcification and loss of meninges and cortex. Results in glaucoma and seizures
Z. *Treacher-Collins syndrome* (mandibulofacial dysostosis): CHL, midface hypoplasia, micrognathia, malformed ears, lower lid coloboma, down-slanting eyes
AA. *Usher*: SNHL, retinitis pigmentosa ± vestibular symptoms. Most common syndrome to affect the eyes and ears
AB. *Von-Hippel-Lindau disease*: bilateral endolymphatic sac tumors, cavernous hemangiomas (cerebellum, brain stem, retina), renal cell carcinoma
AC. *Von Recklinghausen disease* (NF-1): Café au lait spots and neurofibromas
AD. *Waardenburg syndrome*: SNHL, vestibular abnormalities, dystopia canthorum, pigmentary changes of the eyes, skin, and hair (ie, white forelock)

Selected Eponyms

A. Argyle-Robertson pupil: miotic pupils. Does not contract to light but does to accommodation (suggests syphilis)
B. Battle sign: ecchymosis over the mastoid process indicative of a temporal bone or posterior fossa fracture
C. Bezold abscess: abscess in digastric groove of SCM, result of mastoiditis
D. Brown sign: blanching of glomus tympanicum with positive pneumatoscopic pressure
E. Chvostek sign: facial twitch by tapping the distribution of the facial nerve, hypocalcemia
F. Crisis of Tumarkin: drop attacks
G. Eagle syndrome: dysphagia associated with a calcified stylohyoid ligament or an elongated styloid process
H. Furstenberg sign: encephaloceles expand with crying, jugular vein compression, due to increased intracranial pressure
I. Gradenigo syndrome: otorrhea, retro-orbital pain, and lateral rectus palsy secondary to irritation of CN VI within Dorello's canal
J. Griesinger sign: edema and tenderness over the mastoid cortex associated with thrombosis of the mastoid emissary vein because of lateral sinus thrombosis
K. Gutman sign: In the normal individual, lateral pressure over the thyroid cartilage causes an increased voice pitch, whereas anterior pressure causes a decrease. In SLN paralysis, the reverse is true

L. Hennebert sign: vertigo with pressure changes
M. Hitzelberger sign: numbness of ear canal in response to CN VII injury from acoustic neuroma
N. Holman Miller sign: anterior bowing of posterior wall of maxillary sinus, indicative of JNA
O. Lyre Sign: splaying of ICA and ECA with carotid body tumor in the middle
P. Marcus-Gunn pupil: pupil dilation in response to direct light (afferent pupillary defect). Results from optic nerve injury with decreased afferent input to brain
Q. Marjolin ulcer: a skin ulceration at the site of an old scar, often from burns, with propensity for malignant degeneration
R. Meleney ulcer: associated with *S. aureus* and nonhemolytic streptococci
S. Schwartze sign: pinkish hue over promontory and oval window niche (represents region of thickened mucosa) in otosclerosis
T. Tullio phenomenon: noise-induced vertigo, usually a sign of superior semicircular canal dehiscence

Bibliograhpy

1. Chan Y, Goddard JC. *K. J. Lee's Essential Otolaryngology*. 12th ed. 2019.
2. Anderson BW, Kortz MW, Black AC, et al. *Anatomy, Head and Neck, Skull.* [Updated 2023 Nov 9]. StatPears Publishing; 2024.
3. Mehta RP. Surgical treatment of facial paralysis. *Clin Exp Otorhinolaryngol*. 2009:2(1)1-5.
4. Holty JE, Guilleminault C. Surgical options for the treatment of obstructive sleep apnea. *Med Clin North Am*. 2010 May;94(3):479-515.

Questions

1. What paraganglioma site of origin is associated with the highest risk of malignant transformation?
   A. Vagal
   B. Jugulotympanic
   C. Carotid
   D. Larynx

2. What midline nasal mass is related to failure of involution of the foramen cecum?
   A. Encephalocele
   B. Nasal dermoid
   C. Rathke cleft cyst
   D. Glioma

3. What fibro-osseous lesion is associated with McCune-Albright syndrome?
   A. Fibrous dysplasia
   B. Ossifying fibroma
   C. Osteoma
   D. Osseous dysplasia

4. Which patient with well-differentiated thyroid carcinoma is considered to have low risk factors?
   A. A 40-year-old woman with a 3.5 cm thyroid tumor
   B. A 42-year-old man with a small tumor without extrathyroidal extension
   C. A 54-year-old woman with a 5 cm thyroid tumor
   D. A 25-year-old woman with a 1.5 cm tumor with capsular involvement

5. The pathogenesis of HPV-related oropharyngeal squamous cell carcinoma is associated with all the following aberrations in molecular biology **except**
   A. p53 inactivation
   B. C-myc mutation
   C. TP53 mutation
   D. Rb inhibition

Answers to Chapter Questions

CHAPTER 1
1. C
2. B
3. D
4. C
5. B

CHAPTER 2
1. B
2. D
3. D
4. B
5. A

CHAPTER 3
1. B
2. E
3. A
4. C
5. E

CHAPTER 4
1. C
2. D
3. B
4. B
5. D

CHAPTER 5
1. E
2. C
3. B
4. C
5. B

CHAPTER 6
1. D
2. B
3. D
4. C
5. A

CHAPTER 7
1. C
2. D
3. A
4. A
5. A

CHAPTER 8
1. A
2. B
3. B
4. A
5. B

CHAPTER 9
1. D
2. D
3. C
4. C
5. D

CHAPTER 10
1. D
2. C
3. C
4. B
5. C

CHAPTER 11
1. D
2. D
3. C
4. D
5. C

CHAPTER 12
1. B
2. D
3. C
4. B
5. E

CHAPTER 13
1. B
2. D
3. E
4. B
5. A

CHAPTER 14
1. A
2. C
3. C
4. B
5. C

CHAPTER 15
1. A-II; B-III; C-I
2. A
3. B
4. D
5. D

CHAPTER 16
1. E
2. A
3. C
4. B
5. C

CHAPTER 17
1. B
2. D
3. G
4. C
5. B

CHAPTER 18
1. A
2. B
3. E
4. B
5. E

CHAPTER 19
1. B
2. D
3. C
4. C
5. D

CHAPTER 20
1. C
2. A
3. D
4. B
5. C

CHAPTER 21
1. A
2. A
3. C
4. True
5. C

CHAPTER 22
1. C
2. E
3. B
4. E
5. A

CHAPTER 23
1. C
2. A
3. D
4. C
5. D

CHAPTER 24
1. B
2. B
3. C
4. D
5. A

CHAPTER 25
1. B
2. C
3. A
4. B
5. D

CHAPTER 26
1. B
2. A
3. B
4. C
5. D

CHAPTER 27
1. D
2. D
3. C
4. B
5. A

CHAPTER 28
1. A
2. B
3. C
4. D
5. D

CHAPTER 29
1. C
2. A
3. A
4. D
5. B

CHAPTER 30
1. B
2. A
3. A
4. C
5. D

CHAPTER 31
1. C
2. B
3. C
4. B
5. B

CHAPTER 32
1. B
2. C
3. C
4. B
5. D

CHAPTER 33
1. B
2. C
3. A
4. E
5. E

CHAPTER 35
1. B
2. C
3. C
4. D
5. A

CHAPTER 36
1. C
2. D
3. D
4. D
5. E

CHAPTER 37
1. C
2. C
3. B
4. A
5. B

CHAPTER 38
1. C
2. A
3. A
4. E
5. E

CHAPTER 39
1. A
2. C
3. C
4. D
5. C

CHAPTER 40
1. A
2. C
3. B
4. C
5. C

CHAPTER 41
1. A
2. D
3. C
4. C
5. D

CHAPTER 42
1. C
2. D
3. C
4. C
5. B

CHAPTER 43
1. E
2. B
3. A
4. C
5. B

CHAPTER 44
1. B
2. D
3. C
4. C
5. D

CHAPTER 45
1. E
2. E
3. A
4. B
5. B

CHAPTER 46
1. D
2. A
3. A
4. A, B, C
5. A

CHAPTER 47
1. D
2. C
3. C
4. D
5. B

CHAPTER 48
1. D
2. B
3. C
4. C
5. C

CHAPTER 49
1. F
2. D
3. B
4. A
5. B

CHAPTER 50
1. C
2. C
3. D
4. A
5. A

CHAPTER 51
1. C
2. B
3. C
4. D
5. D

CHAPTER 52
1. C
2. C
3. B
4. D
5. C

CHAPTER 53
1. C
2. B
3. A
4. A
5. A
6. E

CHAPTER 54
1. D
2. D
3. C
4. C
5. B

CHAPTER 55
1. C
2. D
3. A
4. B
5. C

CHAPTER 56
1. A
2. D
3. E
4. B
5. A

CHAPTER 57
1. A
2. C
3. D
4. D
5. B

CHAPTER 58
1. D
2. A
3. D
4. C
5. C

CHAPTER 59
1. D
2. B
3. A
4. A
5. B

Index

Note: Page numbers followed by f indicate figures; those followed by t indicate tables.

J